Essentials of Paramedic Care

VOLUME 1

Canadian Edition

BRYAN E. BLEDSOE

D.O., F.A.C.E.P., EMT-P

Emergency Department Staff Physician
Baylor Medical Center—Ellis County
Waxahachie, Texas
and
Clinical Associate Professor of Emergency Medicine
University of North Texas Health Sciences Center
Fort Worth, Texas

ROBERT S. PORTER

M.A., NREMT-P

Senior Advanced Life Support Educator
Madison County Emergency Medical Services
Canastota, New York
and
Flight Paramedic
AirOne, Onondaga County Sheriff's Department
Syracuse, New York

RICHARD A. CHERRY

M.S., NREMT-P

Clinical Assistant Professor of Emergency Medicine
Assistant Residency Director
SUNY Upstate Medical University
Syracuse, New York

DWAYNE E. CLAYDEN

M.E.M., Paramedic

Assistant to the Medical Director
The City of Calgary Emergency Medical Services
Calgary, Alberta

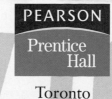

PEARSON

Prentice
Hall

Toronto

Library and Archives Canada Cataloguing in Publication

Essentials of paramedic care/Bryan E. Bledsoe ... [et al.]. — Canadian ed.

Includes index.
ISBN 0-13-120305-3 (vol. 1)
ISBN 0-13-120306-1 (vol. 2)

1. Emergency medicine—textbooks. 2. Emergency medical technicians—handbooks, manuals, etc.
I. Bledsoe, Bryan E., 1955–

RC86.7.E88 2006   616.02'5   C2004-906406-1

0-13-120305-3

Vice President, Editorial Director: Michael J. Young
Executive Editor: Samantha Scully
Executive Marketing Manager: Cas Shields
Developmental Editor: Pamela Voves
Production Editor: Marisa D'Andrea
Copy Editor: Dawn Hunter
Proofreader: Rohini Herbert
Production Coordinator: Patricia Ciardullo
Manufacturing Coordinator: Susan Johnson
Literary Permissions and Photo Researcher: Amanda McCormick
Indexer: Belle Wong
Page Layout: Jansom
Art Director: Julia Hall
Interior and Cover Design: Anthony Leung
Cover Image: Mike Powell, Getty Images

8   12

Printed and bound in the United States.

Notices

It is the intent of the authors and publisher that this textbook be used as part of a formal paramedic education program taught by a qualified instructor. The care procedures presented here represent accepted competencies and practices in Canada. They are not offered as a standard of care.

Paramedic-level prehospital care in Canada is to be performed under the specific paramedic competencies available in each province and territory. These competencies are specific for Primary Care Paramedics (PCP), Advanced Care Paramedics (ACP), and Critical Care Paramedics (CCP). Medically delegated acts can only be performed by a paramedic certified by a licensed medical physician or base hospital physician. It is the reader's responsibility to know and follow local protocols and follow their scope of practice associated to the system to which they belong. Also, it is the reader's responsibility to remain current of emergency care procedures and changes to their scope of practice.

NOTICE ON DRUGS AND DRUG DOSAGES

Every effort has been made to ensure that the drug dosages presented in this textbook are in accordance with nationally accepted standards. When applicable, the dosages and routes have been taken from the American Heart Association's Advanced Cardiac Life Support Guidelines. It is the responsibility of the reader to be familiar with the drugs used in his or her system, as well as the dosages specified by medical direction. The drugs presented in this book should only be administered by direct order of a licensed physician, whether verbally or through accepted orders.

NOTICE ON GENDER USE

The authors have made a great effort to treat the use of the two genders equally. The chapters alternate in their use of gender by applying male pronouns in one chapter and female pronouns in the next. (Exceptions exist in situations that are specifically related to only one gender.)

NOTICE ON PHOTOGRAPHS

Please note that many of the photographs contained in this book are of actual emergency situations. As such, it is possible that they may not accurately depict current, appropriate, or advisable practices of emergency medical care. They have been included for the sole purpose of giving general insight into real-life emergency settings.

DEDICATION

This book is respectfully dedicated to the paramedics who toil each day in an environment that is unpredictable, often dangerous, and constantly changing. They risk their lives to aid the sick and the injured, driven only by their love of humanity and their devotion to this profession we call emergency medical services.

We remember the EMS, fire, and law enforcement personnel who have made the ultimate sacrifice for their communities and our nation. May they never be forgotten.

Brief Contents

Detailed Contents

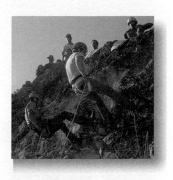
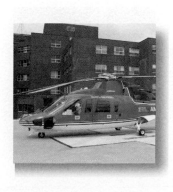

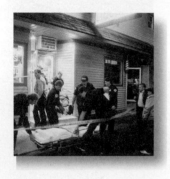

DIVISION 2 PATIENT ASSESSMENT 217

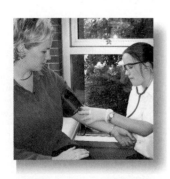

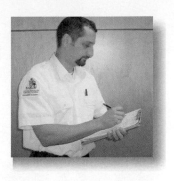

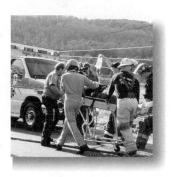

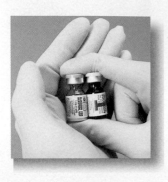

CHAPTER 14   GENERAL PRINCIPLES OF PHARMACOLOGY   688

CHAPTER 15   MEDICATION ADMINISTRATION   761

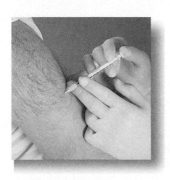

Preface

Congratulations on your decision to further your EMS career by undertaking the course of education required for certification as a paramedic! The world of paramedic emergency care is one that you will find both challenging and rewarding. Whether you will be working as a volunteer or paid paramedic, you will find the field of advanced prehospital care very interesting.

This two-volume textbook program is derived from Brady's best-selling *Paramedic Care: Principles & Practice* (Volumes 1–5). Ideal for paramedic refresher and abbreviated paramedic programs, this book is based on the Canadian National Paramedic Competencies and is organized into five divisions.

The first division, entitled Introduction to Prehospital Care, addresses the medical-legal aspects of all levels of paramedic care in Canada as well as general ambulance operational systems. Included in this division are incident commands through mass casualty incidents, rescue awareness and operations, and hazardous material and crime scene incidents. The second division, Patient Assessment, builds on the patient assessment skills of a paramedic with special emphasis on advanced patient assessment at the scene. It also introduces the reader to basic anatomy and physiology, as well as pathophysiology, principles of pharamacology, and drug administration. Trauma Emergencies, the third division of the text, discusses advanced prehospital care from the mechanism of injury analysis to shock/trauma resuscitation. The fourth division of the text, Medical Emergencies, is the most extensive and addresses multiple levels of paramedic care involving medical emergencies. The last division addresses Special Considerations including neonatology, pediatrics, geriatric emergencies, chronic patients, the challenged patient, and assaulted or abused patients. An appendix that cross-references the text with the National Occupational Competency Profiles developed by the Paramedic Association of Canada concludes both volumes.

SKILLS

The psychomotor skills of fluid and medication administration, advanced airway care, electrocardiography (ECG) monitoring and defibrillation, and advanced medical and trauma patient care are best learned in the classroom, skills laboratory, and clinical and field settings. Common advanced prehospital skills are discussed in the text as well as outlined in the accompanying procedure sheets. Review these before and while practising the skill. It is important to point out that this or any other text cannot teach skills. Care skills are only learned under the watchful eye of a paramedic instructor and perfected during your clinical and field internship.

HOW TO USE THIS TEXTBOOK

Essentials of Paramedic Care, Canadian Edition, is designed to accompany a paramedic education program that includes ample classroom, practical laboratory, in-hospital clinical, and prehospital field experiences. These educational experiences must be guided by instructors and preceptors with special training and expertise in their areas of participation in your program.

It is intended that your program coordinator will assign reading from the text in preparation for each classroom lecture and discussion section. The knowledge gained from reading this text will form the foundation of the information you will need in order to function effectively as a paramedic in your EMS system. Your instructors will build on this information to strengthen your knowledge and understanding of advanced prehospital care so that you may apply it in your practice. The in-hospital clinical and prehospital field experiences will further refine your knowledge and skills under the watchful eyes of your preceptors.

The workbook that accompanies this text can also assist in improving classroom performance. It contains information, sample test questions, and exercises designed to assist learning, and can be very helpful in identifying the important elements of paramedic education, in exercising the knowledge of prehospital care, and in helping you self-test your knowledge.

Essentials of Paramedic Care presents the knowledge of emergency care in as accurate, standardized, and clear a manner as is possible. However, each EMS system is uniquely different, and it is beyond the scope of this text to address all differences. You must count heavily on your instructors, the program coordinator, and ultimately the program medical director to identify how specific emergency care procedures are applied in your system.

CHAPTER CONTRIBUTORS

We wish to acknowledge the remarkable talents and efforts of the following people who contributed to *Essentials of Paramedic Care.* Individually, they worked with extraordinary commitment on this new program. Together, they form a team of highly dedicated professionals who have upheld the highest standards of EMS instruction.

CANADIAN CONTRIBUTORS

Ronald Bowles, B.Ed., M.Ed. Technology, EMA II. Manager, Instructional Design, Paramedic Academy, Justice Institute of British Columbia, New Westminster, British Columbia. *All chapters, Volumes 1 and 2.*

Kevin Branch, BHSc., PHC, ACP Coordinator, Paramedic Programs, Cambrian College, Sudbury, Ontario. *All chapters, Volumes 1 and 2.*

Heather MacKenzie-Carey, B.Sc., EMT-P, M.Sc. (Disaster Management), Bridgewater, Nova Scotia. *Chapters 37 and 41*

U.S. CONTRIBUTORS

Beth Lothrop Adams, M.A., R.N., NREMT-P; ALS Coordinator, EHS Programs; Adjunct Assistant Professor, Emergency Medicine, The George Washington University. *Chapters 30, 39, 40*

J. Nile Barnes, B.S., NREMT-P; Associate Professor of EMS Professions, Austin Community College, Austin, Texas; Paramedic, Williamson County (Texas) EMS Department. *Chapter 1*

Brenda Beasley, R.N., B.S., EMT-P; EMS Program Director, Calhoun College, Decatur, Alabama. *Chapter 42*

Sandra Bradley, Pleasant Hill, California. *Chapter 45*

Lawrence C. Brilliant, M.D., F.A.C.E.P.; Clinical Assistant Professor, Department of Primary Care Education and Community Services, Hahnemann University; Emergency Physician, Doylestown Hospital, Doylestown, Pennsylvania. *Chapters 23, 28*

Eric C. Chaney, M.S. NREMT-P; Administrator, Office of the State EMS Medical Director, Maryland Institute for Emergency Medical Services Systems, Baltimore, Maryland. *Chapter 1*

Elizabeth Coolidge-Stolz, M.D., Medical Writer, Health Educator, North Reading, Massachusetts. *Chapters 30, 32, 33*

Robert A. De Lorenzo, M.D., F.A.C.E.P.; Lieut. Colonel, Medical Corps, US Army; Brooke Army Medical Center. *Chapters 20, 21*

Kate Dernocoeur, B.S. EMT-P, Lowell, Michigan. *Chapters 1, 5*

Clyde Deschamp, M.Ed., NREMT-P; Chairman and Assistant Professor, Department of Emergency Medical Technology; Director, Helicopter Transport, University of Mississippi Medical Center. *Chapter 37*

James W. Drake, B.S., NREMT-P; Instructor, Department of Emergency Medical Technology, School of Health Related Professions, University of Mississippi Medical Center, Jackson, Mississippi. *Chapter 15*

Robert Elling, M.P.A., NREMT-P; Professor, American College of Prehospital Medicine; Faculty Member, Institute of Prehospital Emergency Medicine, Hudson Valley Community College, Troy, New York. *Chapter 3*

Robert Feinberg, EMT-P, PA-C, Emergency Medicine, Wayne, Pennsylvania. *Chapter 24*

Joseph P. Funk, M.D., F.A.C.E.P.; Peachtree Emergency Associates, Piedmont Hospital, Atlanta, Georgia. *Chapter 28*

Kathleen G. Funk, M.D., F.A.C.E.P.; Emergency Medicine Physician, Atlanta, Georgia. *Chapter 28*

Eric W. Heckerson, R.N., M.A., NREMT-P; EMS Coordinator, Mesa Fire Department, Mesa, Arizona. *Chapters 1, 22, 29, 37, 38*

Chris Hendricks, NREMT-P, Field Instructor; Paramedic, Pridemark Paramedics, Boulder, Colorado. *Chapter 46*

Sandra Hultz, B.S., NREMT-P; EMS Instructor, University of Mississippi Medical Center, Jackson, Mississippi. *Chapter 1*

Jeffrey L. Jarvis, M.S., EMT-P; Medical Student, University of Texas Medical Branch, Galveston, Texas. *Chapter 14*

Deborah Kufs, R.N., B.S., C.C.R.N., C.E.N., NREMT-P; Clinical Instructor, Hudson Valley Community College, Institute for Prehospital Emergency Medicine, Troy, New York. *Chapters 35, 43*

Daniel Limmer, EMT-P, Frederick, Maryland. *Chapters 3, 38*

William Marx, D.O.; Associate Professor of Surgery and Critical Care; Director, Surgical Critical Care SUNY Upstate Medical University, Syracuse, New York. *Chapter 26*

Michael O'Keefe, NREMT-P; EMS Training Coordinator, Vermont Department of Health. *Chapter 1*

John M. Saad, M.D.; Medical Director of Emergency Services, Navarro Regional Hospital, Corsicana, Texas; Medical Director of Emergency Services, Medical Center at Terrell, Terrell, Texas. *Chapters 34, 36*

John S. Saito, M.P.H., EMT-P; Director, EMS/Paramedic Education; Assistant Professor, Oregon Health Sciences University, School of Medicine, Department of Emergency Medicine, Portland, Oregon. *Chapters 13, 37*

Jo Anne Schultz, B.A., NREMT-P; Paramedic, Lifestar Ambulance Inc., Salisbury, Maryland; Level II Emergency Medical Services Instructor, Maryland Fire and Rescue Institute, University of Maryland; Paramedic Instructor, Maryland Institute of Emergency Medical Services Systems, University of Maryland; ACLS, BTLS, and PALS instructor. *Chapters 11, 36, 41*

Craig A. Soltis, M.D., F.A.C.E.P.; Assistant Professor of Clinical Emergency Medicine, Northeastern Ohio Universities College of Medicine; Chairman, Department of Emergency Medicine, Forum Health, Youngstown, Ohio. *Chapters 25, 35*

Marian D. Streger, R.N., B.S.N., C.E.N., Cleveland, Ohio. *Chapters 11, 45*

Matthew R. Streger, M.P.A., NREMT-P; Deputy Commissioner, Cleveland Emergency Medical Services, Cleveland, Ohio. *Chapters 3, 44, 46*

Emily Vacher, Esq., M.P.A., EMT-CC; Associate Director of Judicial Affairs, Syracuse University, Syracuse, New York. *Chapter 2*

Kevin Waddington, EMT-P, MedStar, Fort Worth, Texas. *Chapter 28*

Gail Weinstein, M.A., EMT-P; Director of Paramedic Training, State University of New York Upstate Medical University, Syracuse, New York. *Chapter 43*

Howard A. Werman, M.D., F.A.C.E.P.; Associate Professor of Clinical Emergency Medicine, The Ohio State University College of Medicine and Public Health, Columbus, Ohio; Medical Director, Med-Flight of Ohio. *Chapter 27*

Matthew S. Zavarella, B.S.A.S., NREMT-P, CCTEMT-P; Director Prehospital Education, Medical College of Ohio, Toledo, Ohio. *Chapters 13, 32*

DEVELOPMENT AND PRODUCTION

The tasks of writing, editing, reviewing, and producing a textbook the size of *Essentials of Paramedic Care (Volumes 1 and 2)* are complex. Many talented people have been involved in developing and producing this new program.

First, the authors would like to acknowledge the support of Samantha Scully and Leslie Carson. We also thank Pamela Voves, Development Editor, for this project. Special thanks go to Patricia Ciardullo, Production Coordinator, and Marisa D'Andrea, Production Editor, who skillfully supervised all production stages to create the final product you now hold. We are grateful to Rohini Herbert and Dawn Hunter, Copyeditors, for their hard work on these volumes. In developing our art and photo program, we were fortunate to work with yet additional talent—leaders within their professions.

We also wish to thank John Fader, B.Sc., ACP (Professor and Coordinator, Fleming College Paramedic Program, Peterborough, Ontario) and Sean C. Fisher of the Manitoba Emergency Services College for their technical review of the volumes.

MEDICAL REVIEW BOARD

Our special thanks to the following physicians for their review of material in our paramedic program. Their reviews were carefully prepared, and we appreciate the thoughtful advice and keen insight each shared with us.

Dr. Robert De Lorenzo, Lieutenant Colonel, Medical Corps, U.S. Army; Associate Clinical Professor of Military and Emergency Medicine, Uniformed Services University of Health Sciences.

Dr. Edward T. Dickinson, Assistant Professor and Director of EMS Field Operations in the Department of Emergency Medicine, University of Pennsylvania School of Medicine in Philadephia.

Dr. Howard A. Werman, Associate Professor, Department of Emergency Medicine, The Ohio State University College of Medicine and Public Health, Columbus, Ohio.

INSTRUCTOR REVIEWERS

The reviewers of *Essentials of Paramedic Care* have provided many excellent suggestions and ideas for improving the text. The quality of the reviews has been outstanding, and the reviews have been a major aid in the preparation and revision of the manuscript. The assistance provided by these EMS experts is deeply appreciated.

Ron Bowles, Justice Institute of British Columbia
Kevin Branch, Cambrian College
Ian Dailly, Justice Institute of British Columbia
Carl Damour, The Michener Institute for Applied Health Sciences

John Fader, Fleming College
Sean C. Fisher, Manitoba Emergency Services College
Ralph Hofmann, Durham College of Applied Arts and Technology
Steve Pilkington, Southern Alberta Institute of Technology
Jim Whittle, Algonquin College

Prehospital emergency personnel, like all health-care workers, are at risk for exposure to bloodborne pathogens and infectious diseases. In emergency situations, it is often difficult to take or enforce proper infection control measures. However, as a paramedic, you must recognize your high-risk status.

Infection control is designed to protect emergency personnel, their families, and their patients from unnecessary exposure to communicable diseases.

Laws, regulations, and standards regarding infection control include:

* *Canadian Centre for Disease Guidelines.* The CCDC has published extensive guidelines regarding infection control. Proper equipment and techniques that should be used by emergency response personnel to prevent or minimize risk of exposure are defined.

* *The Canadian Occupational Safety and Health Administration Act.* This Act mandates that all employees within a workplace be protected from harm through lack of safety or lack of safety equipment. Each province and territory has variations to this Act and specifics associated with professions and trade occupations.

* *National Fire Protection Association Guidelines.* The NFPA is a national organization that has established specific guidelines and requirements regarding infection control for emergency response agencies, particularly fire departments in Canada.

BODY SUBSTANCE ISOLATION PRECAUTIONS AND PERSONAL PROTECTIVE EQUIPMENT

Emergency response personnel should practise body substance isolation (BSI), a strategy that considers all body substances potentially infectious. To achieve this, all emergency personnel should utilize personal protective equipment (PPE). Appropriate PPE should be available on every emergency vehicle. The minimum recommended PPE includes the following:

* *Gloves.* Disposable gloves should be donned by all emergency response personnel *before* initiating any emergency care. When an emergency incident involves more than one patient, you should change gloves between patients. When gloves have been contaminated, they should be removed as soon as possi-

ble. To remove gloves, first hook the gloved fingers of one hand under the cuff of the other glove. Then pull that glove off without letting your gloved fingers come in contact with bare skin. Then, slide the fingers of the ungloved hand under the remaining glove's cuff. Push that glove off, being careful not to touch the glove's exterior with your bare hand. Always wash your hands after gloves are removed, even when the gloves appear intact. Paramedics on the scene should utilize alcohol-based cleansers to wash their hands until a facility is readily available.

* *Masks and Protective Eyewear.* Masks and protective equipment should be present on all emergency vehicles and used in accordance with the level of exposure encountered. Proper eyewear and masks prevent a patient's blood and body fluids from spraying into your eyes, nose, and mouth. Masks and protective eyewear should be worn together whenever blood spatter is likely to occur, such as in arterial bleeding, childbirth, endotracheal intubation, invasive procedures, oral suctioning, and cleanup of equipment that requires heavy scrubbing or brushing. Both you and the patient should wear masks whenever the potential for airborne transmission of disease exists.

* *HEPA Respirators.* Due to the resurgence of tuberculosis (TB), prehospital personnel should protect themselves from TB infection through use of a high-efficiency particulate air (HEPA) respirator, a design approved by the National Institute of Occupational Safety and Health (NIOSH). It should fit snugly and be capable of filtering out the tuberculosis bacillus. The HEPA respirator should be worn when caring for patients with confirmed or suspected TB. This is especially important when performing "high-hazard" procedures, such as administration of nebulized medications, endotracheal intubation, or suctioning.

* *Gowns.* Gowns protect clothing from blood splashes. If large splashes of blood are expected, such as during childbirth, wear impervious gowns.

* *Resuscitation Equipment.* Disposable resuscitation equipment should be the primary means of artificial ventilation in emergency care. Such items should be used once and then disposed of.

Remember, the proper use of personal protective equipment ensures effective infection control and minimizes risk. Use *all* protective equipment recommended for any particular situation to ensure maximum protection.

Consider *all* body substances potentially infectious and *always* practise body substance isolation.

HANDLING CONTAMINATED MATERIAL

Many of the materials associated with emergency response become contaminated with possibly infectious body fluids and substances. These include soiled linen, patient clothing, dressings, and used care equipment, including intravenous needles. It is important that you collect these materials at the scene and dispose of them appropriately to ensure your safety as well as that of your patients, their family members, bystanders, and fellow caregivers. Properly dispose of any contaminated materials according to the recommendations outlined below.

* Handle contaminated materials only while wearing the appropriate personal protective equipment.
* Place all blood- or body-fluid-contaminated clothing, linen, dressings, patient-care equipment, and supplies in properly marked bio-hazard bags and ensure they are disposed of properly.
* Ensure that all used needles, scalpels, and other contaminated objects that have the potential to puncture the skin are properly secured in a puncture-resistant and clearly marked sharps container.
* Do not recap a needle after use, stick it into a seat cushion or other object, or leave it lying on the ground. This increases the risk of a needle-stick injury.
* Always scan the scene before leaving to ensure that all equipment has been retrieved and all potentially infectious material has been bagged and removed.
* Should you be exposed to an infectious disease, have contact with body substances with a route for system entry (such as an open wound on your hand when a glove tears while moving a soiled patient), or receive a needle-stick injury from a used needle, alert the receiving hospital and contact your service's infection control officer immediately.

Following these recommendations will help protect you and the people you care for from the dangers of disease transmission.

A Great Way to Learn and Instruct Online

The Pearson Education Canada Companion Website is easy to navigate and is organized to correspond to the chapters in this textbook. Whether you are a student in the classroom or a distance learner you will discover helpful resources for in-depth study and research that empower you in your quest for greater knowledge and maximize your potential for success in the course.

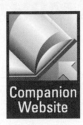
Companion
Website

[www.pearsoned.ca/bledsoe]

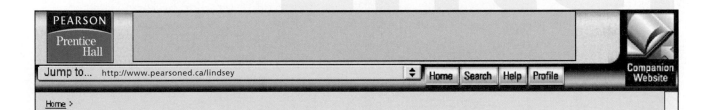

PEARSON
Prentice
Hall

Jump to...   http://www.pearsoned.ca/lindsey   ⬧   Home Search Help Profile

Companion
Website

Home >

PH Companion Website

Essentials of Paramedic Care, Canadian Edition, Volumes 1 and 2, by Bledsoe/Porter/Cherry/Clayden

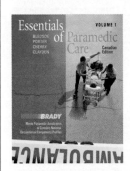

Student Resources

The modules in this section provide students with tools for learning course material. These modules include:

- Chapter Objectives
- Destinations
- Quizzes
- PowerPoint Presentations
- Glossary
- Flashcards

In the quiz modules, students can send answers to the grader and receive instant feedback on their progress through the Results Reporter. Coaching comments and references to the textbook may be available to ensure that students take advantage of all available resources to enhance their learning experience.

Instructor Resources

The modules in this section provide instructors with additional teaching tools. Downloadable PowerPoint Presentations and an Instructor's Manual are just some of the materials that may be available in this section. Where appropriate, this section will be password protected. To get a password, simply contact your Pearson Education Canada Representative or call Faculty Sales and Services at 1-800-850-5813.

EMPHASIZING PRINCIPLES

CHAPTER 9

Documentation

Objectives

After reading this chapter, you should be able to:

1. Identify the general principles regarding the importance of EMS documentation and ways in which documents are used. (pp. 412–414)
2. Identify and properly use medical terminology, medical abbreviations, and acronyms. (pp. 415, 417–420)
3. Explain the role of documentation in agency reimbursement. (p. 413)
4. Identify and eliminate extraneous or nonprofessional information. (p. 425)
5. Describe the differences between subjective and objective elements of documentation. (pp. 425–427)
6. Evaluate a finished document for errors and omissions and proper use and spelling of abbreviations and acronyms. (pp. 422, 424–425)
7. Evaluate the confidential nature of an EMS report. (p. 435)
8. Describe the potential consequences of illegible, incomplete, or inaccurate documentation. (pp. 422, 424–425)

Continued

Chapter Objectives with Page References

Each chapter begins with clearly stated **Objectives** that follow the N.O.C.P. curriculum. Students can refer to these objectives while studying to make sure they fully understand the material. Page references after each objective indicate where relevant content is covered in the chapter.

Key Terms

Reinforcement of **Key Terms** helps students master new terminology.

Key Points

Key Points in the margins help students identify and learn the fundamental principles of paramedic practice.

Content Review

Content Review summarizes important content and gives students a format for quick review.

THINKING UNDER PRESSURE

✳ **autonomic nervous system** part of the nervous system that controls involuntary actions.

When you must make a critical decision, physical influences may help or hinder your ability to think clearly. Your **autonomic nervous system**, which controls your involuntary actions, may respond by secreting "fight or flight" hormones. These hormones will enhance your visual and auditory acuity and will improve your reflexes and muscle strength. However, they may also impair your ability to think critically and diminish your ability to assess and concentrate. In these instances, you will revert to your most basic instincts. Many an inexperienced paramedic has been "mentally paralyzed" by a complicated, critical call. With experience, you will learn to manage your nervousness and maintain a steadfast, controlled demeanour.

✳ **pseudo-instinctive** learned actions that are practised until they can be done without thinking.

One way to enhance your ability to remain in control is to raise your technical skills to a **pseudo-instinctive** level. This means that you do not have to concentrate on them to perform them. For example, you do not think about tying your shoelaces, you just tie them. Such "muscle memory" is essential when performing emergency medical skills. When you set up an salbutamol nebulizer treatment, for instance, you automatically fit together the pieces of the device and administer the treatment without hesitation. This way you can concentrate on your patient's condition, controlling the scene, and managing the multitude of items that usually complicate any emergency call. Concentrating on more than one thing simultaneously is difficult, if not impossible.

Maintaining your composure, especially during a chaotic, complicated call, is key to developing a management plan for the best patient outcome.

MENTAL CHECKLIST

Thinking under pressure is not easy. Maintaining your composure, especially during a chaotic, complicated call is key to developing a management plan for the best patient outcome. Developing a routine mental checklist is a good way to stay focused and systematic. Pilots work through their preflight checklists routinely before ever turning over their engines. Medical clinicians develop acronyms and mnemonics to remember critical elements during stressful incidents. For example, when conducting a primary assessment, use the acronym MS-ABC. Use OPQRST to elicit your patient's present history, or use SAMPLE when time is critical. You can adopt the following checklist any time you must make a critical decision.

Content Review

MENTAL CHECKLIST
- Scan the situation.
- Stop and think.
- Decide and act.
- Maintain control.
- Reevaluate.

Scan the Situation Stand back, and scan the situation. Sometimes, you can miss subtle signs if you focus too narrowly on one aspect of your patient's problem. Look for environmental factors and other not-so-obvious clues. For example, your patient lies unconscious and cyanotic on the floor. You rule out any airway, breathing, or circulation problems. No medical history is available and no medication bottles are present. When you detect a fruity odour on your patient's breath, you suspect diabetic ketoacidosis.

Stop and Think Do not do anything without stopping and weighing your actions. Consider all of your options before you act. Remember that for every action, there is a reaction. Know what reactions to expect, and anticipate their possible harmful effects. For example, after administering lidocaine, monitor your patient closely for the expected benefits (eradication of ventricular tachycardia) and early signs of toxicity (numbness and tingling to the lips, drowsiness, nausea).

Decide and Act Once you have assessed the situation, make your decision, and act confidently. Announce your management plan to your crew with a combination of authority, confidence, and respect. Convey the feeling that you

Tables and Illustrations

Tables and **illustrations** offer visual support to enhance students' understanding of paramedic principles and practice.

Table 9-1 | STANDARD CHARTING ABBREVIATIONS

Patient Information/Categories

Asian	A	Medications	Med
Black	B	Newborn	NB
Chief complaint	CC	Occupational history	OH
Complains of	c/o	Past history	PH
Current health status	CHS	Patient	Pt
Date of birth	DOB	Physical exam	PE
Differential diagnosis	DD	Private medical doctor	PMD
Estimated date of confinement	EDC	Review of systems	ROS
Family history	FH	Signs and symptoms	S/S
Female	♀	Social history	SH
Hispanic	H	Visual acuity	VA
History	Hx	Vital signs	VS
History and physical	H&P	Weight	Wt
History of present illness	HPI	White	W
Impression	IMP	Year-old	y/o
Male	♂		

Body Systems

Abdomen	Abd	Gynecological	GYN
Cardiovascular	CV	Head, eyes, ears, nose, and throat	HEENT
Central nervous system	CNS	Musculoskeletal	M/S
Ear, nose, and throat	ENT	Obstetrical	OB
GastroIntestinal	GI	Peripheral nervous system	PNS
Genitourinary	GU	Respiratory	Resp

Common Complaints

Abdominal pain	abd pn	Lower back pain	LBP
Chest pain	CP	Nausea/vomiting	n/v
Dyspnea on exertion	DOE	No apparent distress	NAD

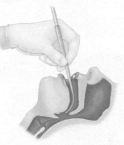

FIGURE 7-20   Suction fluids from your patient's airway.

Stridor signals a potentially life-threatening airway obstruction.

The high-pitched inspiratory screech of stridor is caused by a life-threatening upper airway obstruction that may be due to a foreign body, severe swelling, allergic reaction, or infection. If you suspect a foreign body obstruction and your patient exhibits poor air movement, a weak cough, or a diminishing mental status, immediately deliver abdominal thrusts (Heimlich manoeuvre) to dislodge the object. If your patient is less than one year old, use back blows and chest thrusts instead of abdominal thrusts. If these manoeuvres are ineffective, remove the object under direct laryngoscopy with Magill forceps.

Other causes of stridor require vastly differently approaches. Upper respiratory infections, such as croup or epiglottitis, call for blow-by oxygen and a quiet ride to the hospital; respiratory burns demand rapid endotracheal intubation; and anaphylaxis necessitates vasoconstrictor medications. Since these vastly different management techniques are potentially life threatening when applied inappropriately, your correct field diagnosis is critical. If your patient presents with stridor, take time to evaluate the history and clinical signs and symptoms for foreign body obstruction (sudden onset while eating), epiglottitis (fever, illness, drooling, inability to swallow), respiratory burns (history of facial burns, hoarseness), and anaphylaxis (hives, history of allergies).

The softer, expiratory whistle of wheezing is caused by constricted bronchioles, the smaller, lower airways. You will hear it in such cases as asthma, bronchitis, emphysema, or other causes of bronchospasm. Bronchiolitis, a lower respiratory infection, often causes these sounds in infants and young children. Wheezing patients require a bronchodilator medication to dilate the bronchioles and reduce airway resistance.

If your patient is not moving air, he is in respiratory arrest. Immediately provide ventilation with a bag-valve mask. Ventilate adult patients at a minimum of 12 breaths per minute and all children at a minimum of 20 breaths per minute. If you cannot ventilate the lungs, reposition the head and neck and try again. If there is still no air movement, assume a complete obstruction and begin measures to correct it.

Once you have cleared the airway, keeping it open may require constant attention.

Once you have cleared the airway, keeping it open may require constant attention. In these cases, insert a basic airway adjunct to help keep the tongue from blocking the upper airway. If your patient is unconscious and lacks a gag reflex, insert an oropharyngeal airway. If he has a gag reflex or significant orofacial trauma,

---

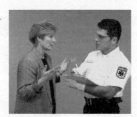

FIGURE 5-2   If the patient cannot provide useful information, gather it from family members or bystanders.

BLINDNESS

Blind patients present special problems. They need you to identify yourself immediately, since they cannot see your uniform. Always announce yourself, and explain who you are and why you are there. If possible, take your patient's hand to establish a personal contact and to show him where you are. Remember that nonverbal communications, such as hand gestures, facial expressions, and body language, are useless in these cases. Your voice is your only tool for effective communication.

TALKING WITH FAMILIES OR FRIENDS

You will often encounter patients who cannot give you any useful information. In these cases, find a third party who can augment the patient history and offer a useful adjunct to the patient's answers (Figure 5-2). The typical case is the postictal patient who cannot describe his seizure activity to you. Another example is learning from a friend that your patient's spouse died in an automobile accident just three weeks ago. Now you better understand why your patient appears depressed and suicidal. Make sure that patient confidentiality is a priority when you accept personal information from a family member, friend, or bystander. Patient assessment is a process of comprehensive history and secondary assessement.

SUMMARY

This chapter dealt with taking a good history. Although it presented the patient history in its entirety, common sense will determine which parts are appropriate for a given situation. Most of a paramedic's work is patient contact. It is making a connection with people in crisis. Patients most often comment on the attitudes of their paramedics. How well did they relate to them? Did they make them feel at ease? Did they care for them? Patients rarely comment on a paramedic's technical skills. Top-notch paramedics are technically skillful and treat all their patients with dignity and compassion. This begins with the history taking.

End-of-Chapter Summary

Each end-of-chapter **Summary** reviews the main topics covered.

EMPHASIZING PRACTICE

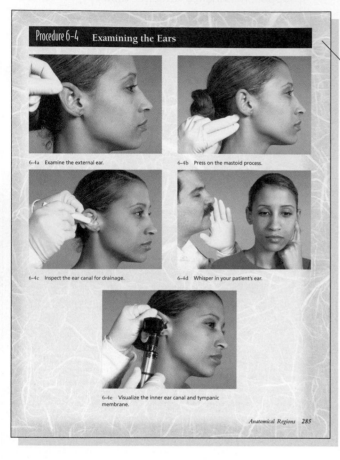

Procedure 6-4 Examining the Ears

6-4a Examine the external ear.

6-4b Press on the mastoid process.

6-4c Inspect the ear canal for drainage.

6-4d Whisper in your patient's ear.

6-4e Visualize the inner ear canal and tympanic membrane.

Anatomical Regions **285**

Procedure Scans

Newly photographed **Procedure Scans** provide step-by-step visual support on how to perform skills included in the DOT curriculum.

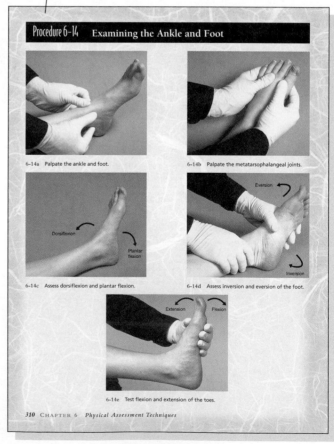

Procedure 6-14 Examining the Ankle and Foot

6-14a Palpate the ankle and foot.

6-14b Palpate the metatarsophalangeal joints.

6-14c Assess dorsiflexion and plantar flexion.

6-14d Assess inversion and eversion of the foot.

6-14e Test flexion and extension of the toes.

310 CHAPTER 6 *Physical Assessment Techniques*

Documentation

Covered thoroughly throughout the text, **proper documentation techniques** are critical to ensuring provider protection on the job as well as patient safety during the transition of care.

Prehospital Care Report
FOR BLS FR USE ONLY

FIGURE 9-4   Complete both the narrative and check-box sections of every PCR.

Medical Calculations

Mathematical examples are provided to give students practice in medical calculations, a critical skill in prehospital care.

CALCULATING DOSAGES FOR ORAL MEDICATIONS

The following example illustrates how to calculate the volume of a specific drug dosage:

Example 1. A physician orders you to administer 90 mg of acetaminophen to a pediatric patient. The liquid acetaminophen is packaged as a concentration of 500 mg in 8 mL of solution. How much of the medication will you administer?

Because you cannot see the 90 mg of acetaminophen, you must convert this weight to a volume. To do so you need these facts:

$$\text{desired dose} = 90 \text{ mg}$$
$$\text{dosage on hand} = 500 \text{ mg}$$
$$\text{volume on hand} = 8 \text{ mL}$$

Use the formula to calculate the dosage's volume:

$$\text{volume to be administered} = \frac{\text{volume on hand (8 mL)} \times \text{desired dose (90 mg)}}{\text{dosage on hand (500 mg)}}$$

$$\text{volume to be administered} = (8 \times 90)/500$$
$$\text{volume to be administered} = 720/500$$
$$\text{volume to be administered} = 1.44 \text{ mL}$$

Administer 1.44 mL of solution to deliver 90 mg of acetaminophen.

Another way to calculate drug dosages is the ratio (fraction) and proportion method. A ratio (fraction) illustrates a relationship between two numbers. A proportion is the comparison of two numerically equivalent ratios. Using the variable x, the above problem can be stated this way:

$$8 \text{ mL}/500 \text{ mg} = x \text{ mL}/90 \text{ mg}$$

To solve the problem, cross-multiply the numerals:

$$\frac{8}{500} = \frac{x}{90}$$
$$720 = 500x$$
$$\frac{720}{500} = x$$
$$1.44 = x$$
$$x = 1.44 \text{ mL}$$

Math Summary 1

$$x \text{ mL} = \frac{8 \text{ mL} \times 90 \text{ mg}}{500 \text{ mg}}$$
$$x \text{ mL} = \frac{720}{500}$$
$$x \text{ mL} = 1.44$$

Math Summary 2

$$\frac{8 \text{ mL}}{500 \text{ mg}} = \frac{x \text{ mL}}{90 \text{ mg}}$$
$$x \text{ mL} = \frac{720}{500}$$
$$x = 1.44 \text{ mL}$$

CONVERTING PREFIXES

The following example shows how to calculate the volume to be administered when the desired dose, the dosage on hand, and the volume on hand are not all expressed in metric units with the same prefix.

Example 2. A physician orders you to give 250 mg of a drug via IV bolus. The multidose vial contains 2 grams of the drug in 10 mL of solution. How much of the medication should you administer?

Because the desired dose is expressed as *milli*grams, the dosage on hand must be converted from grams to milligrams. In the metric system, 2 grams equal 2000 milligrams. You now know:

$$\text{desired dose} = 250 \text{ mg}$$
$$\text{dosage on hand} = 2000 \text{ mg}$$
$$\text{volume on hand} = 10 \text{ mL}$$

TEACHING AND LEARNING PACKAGE

FOR THE INSTRUCTOR

The following resources are available to aid instructors:

Instructor's Resource CD-ROM for Volume 1 and Volume 2 with Instructor's Resource Manual, TestGen, and PowerPoint Slides (ISBN 0-13-197285-5)

The Instructor's Resource CD-ROM contains all print and technology supplements on a single CD-ROM. Enjoy the freedom to transport the entire package to the office, home, or classroom. This enables you to customize any of the ancillaries, print only the chapters or materials that you wish to use, or access any item from the package within the classroom. This CD-ROM provides the following resources:

Instructor's Resource Manual The Instructor's Resource Manual contains everything needed to teach curriculum that is based on the Canadian National Paramedic Competencies. The manual provides a variety of teaching strategies for each chapter that are intended to help convey information to the broadest range of students. Included are:

- lecture outlines
- innovative teaching strategies
- suggestions for additional resources
- student activities handouts for reinforcement and evaluation

Pearson TestGen This special computerized test item file enables instructors to view and edit existing questions, add questions, generate tests, and print the tests in a variety of formats. Powerful search and sort functions make it easy to locate questions and arrange them in any order desired. TestGen also enables instructors to administer tests on a local area network, have the tests graded electronically, and have the results prepared in electronic or printed reports. The Pearson TestGen is compatible with IBM or Macintosh systems.

PowerPoint Slides PowerPoint Slides, which provide key points covered in each chapter, are included to aid instructors in the presentation of text material.

Downloadable Instructor Supplements The Instructor's Resource Manual and PowerPoint Slides are available for downloading at www.pearsoned.ca, Pearson's online catalogue. Search for this text within the catalogue and then click on "Instructor" to access the supplements in a protected area for instructors.

FOR THE STUDENT

Student Workbook (Volume 1: ISBN 0-13-120307-X; Volume 2: ISBN 0-13-120308-8)

A student workbook with review and practice activities accompanies *Essentials of Paramedic Care*. The workbook includes multiple-choice questions, fill-in-the-blank questions, labelling exercises, case studies, and special projects, along with an answer key with text page references.

ONLINE RESOURCES

Companion Website This free site, located at **www.pearsoned.ca/bledsoe**, is tied chapter by chapter to the text. It reinforces student learning through interactive online study guides, quizzes based on the new curriculum, and links to important EMS-related internet resources.

DIVISION 1
INTRODUCTION TO PREHOSPITAL CARE

CHAPTER 1

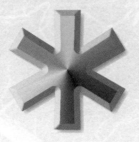

Introduction to Prehospital Care

Objectives

Part 1: Introduction to Advanced Prehospital Care (begins on p. 6)

After reading Part 1 of this chapter, you should be able to:

1. Describe the relationship between the paramedic and other members of the health professions. (p. 6)
2. Identify the attributes and characteristics of the paramedic. (p. 7)
3. Explain the elements of paramedic

education and practice that support its stature as a profession. (p. 7)
4. Define and give examples of the expanded scope of practice for the paramedic. (p. 8)

Part 2: EMS Systems (begins on p. 8)

After reading Part 2 of this chapter, you should be able to:

1. Describe key historical events that influenced the national development of emergency medical services (EMS) systems. (pp. 10–12)
2. Define the following terms: EMS systems (p. 12), licensure (p. 18), certification (p. 18), profession (p. 18), professionalism (p. 24), ethics (p. 25),

Continued

peer review (p. 25), medical direction (p. 14), protocols (p. 15).

3. Identify national groups that are important to the development, education, and implementation of EMS, as well as the role of provincial or territorial associations, the Paramedic Association of Canada (PAC), and the roles of various EMS standard-setting agencies. (p. 20)

4. Identify the standards (components) of an EMS system. (p. 12)

5. Differentiate among EMS provider levels: emergency medical responder, primary care paramedic, advanced care paramedic, and critical care paramedic. (p. 18)

6. Describe what is meant by "citizen involvement in the EMS system." (pp. 15–16)

7. Discuss the role of the EMS physician in providing medical direction and prehospital care as an extension of the physician, the benefits of online and offline medical direction, and the process for the development of local policies and protocols. (pp. 14–15)

8. Describe the relationship among the physician on the scene, the paramedic on the scene, and the EMS physician providing online medical direction. (pp. 14–15)

9. Describe the components of continuous quality improvement, and analyze its contribution to system improvement, continuing medical education, and research. (pp. 23–25)

10. Describe the importance, basic principles, process of evaluating and interpreting, and benefits of research. (pp. 25–26)

Part 3: Roles and Responsibilities of the Paramedic (begins on p. 26)

After reading Part 3 of this chapter, you should be able to:

1. Describe the attributes of a paramedic as a health-care professional. (pp. 30–34)

2. Describe the benefits of continuing education for paramedics and the importance of maintaining the paramedic licence or certification. (p. 35)

3. List the primary and additional responsibilities of paramedics. (pp. 27–30)

4. Define the role of the paramedic relative to the safety of the crew, the patient, and bystanders. (pp. 27–28)

5. Describe the role of the paramedic in health-education activities related to illness and injury prevention. (pp. 29–30)

6. Describe examples of professional behaviours in the following areas: integrity, empathy, self-motivation, appearance and personal hygiene, self-confidence, communication, time management, teamwork and diplomacy, respect, patient advocacy, and careful delivery of service. (pp. 32–34)

7. Identify the benefits of paramedics teaching in their communities. (pp. 29–30)

8. Analyze how the paramedic can benefit the health-care system by supporting primary care for patients in the prehospital setting. (pp. 28–29)

9. Describe how professionalism applies to the paramedic while on and off duty. (p. 31)

Continued

Part 4: The Well-Being of the Paramedic (begins on p. 35)

After reading Part 4 of this chapter, you should be able to:

1. Discuss the concept of wellness and its benefits, the components of wellness, and the role of the paramedic in promoting wellness. (p. 35)

2. Discuss how cardiovascular endurance, weight control, muscle strength, and flexibility contribute to physical fitness. (pp. 35–40)

3. Describe the impact of shift work on circadian rhythms. (p. 49)

4. Discuss the contributions that periodic risk assessments and warning sign recognition make to cancer and cardiovascular disease prevention. (p. 37)

5. Differentiate proper from improper body mechanics for lifting and moving patients in emergency and nonemergency situations. (pp. 38–40)

6. Describe the problems that a paramedic might encounter in a hostile situation and the techniques used to manage the situation. (p. 53)

7. Describe the considerations that should be given to using escorts, dealing with adverse environmental conditions, using lights and siren, proceeding through intersections, and parking at an emergency scene. (pp. 53–54)

8. Discuss the concept of "due regard for the safety of all others" while operating an emergency vehicle. (p. 54)

9. Describe the equipment available for self-protection in a variety of adverse situations, including body substance isolation steps for protection from airborne and bloodborne pathogens. (pp. 40–42, 53, 54–56)

10. Given a scenario in which equipment and supplies have been exposed to body substances, plan for the proper cleaning, disinfection, or disposal of the items. (pp. 42–43)

11. Describe the benefits and methods of smoking cessation. (p. 38)

12. Identify and describe the three phases of the stress response, factors that trigger the stress response, and causes of stress in EMS. (pp. 47–50)

13. Differentiate between normal or healthy and detrimental physiological and psychological reactions to anxiety and stress. (pp. 50–51)

14. Describe behaviour that is a manifestation of stress in patients and those close to them and describe how that behaviour relates to paramedic stress. (pp. 50–51)

15. Identify and describe the defence mechanisms and management techniques commonly used to deal with stress, and the components of critical incident stress management (CISM) and provide examples of situations in which CISM would be beneficial to paramedics. (pp. 50, 51–52)

16. Given a scenario involving a stressful situation, formulate a strategy to help adapt to the stress. (pp. 47–52)

17. Describe the stages of the grieving process (Kübler-Ross) and the unique challenges for paramedics in dealing with themselves, adults, children, and special populations concerning their understanding or experience of death and dying. (pp. 44–47)

18. Given photos of various motor-vehicle collisions, assess scene safety and propose ways to make the scene safer. (pp. 53–54)

Continued

Part 5: Illness and Injury Prevention (begins on p. 54)

After reading Part 5 of this chapter, you should be able to:

1. Describe the incidence, morbidity, and mortality, and the human, environmental, and socioeconomic impact of unintentional and alleged unintentional injuries. (pp. 54–56)
2. Identify health hazards and potential crime areas within the community. (pp. 59–60)
3. Identify local, municipal, and community resources available for physical and socioeconomic crises. (pp. 56–57, 61)
4. List the general and specific environmental parameters that should be inspected to assess a patient's need for preventive information and direction. (pp. 59–60)
5. Identify the role of EMS in local, municipal, and community prevention programs. (pp. 55, 56–61)
6. Identify the injury and illness prevention programs that promote safety for all age populations. (pp. 59–62)
7. Identify patient situations in which the paramedic can intervene in a preventive manner. (pp. 59–62)
8. Document primary and secondary injury prevention data. (pp. 61–62)

Part 6: Ethics in Advanced Prehospital Care (begins on p. 63)

After reading Part 6 of this chapter, you should be able to:

1. Define ethics and morals and distinguish between ethical and moral decisions in emergency medical service. (pp. 63–66)
2. Identify the premise that should underlie the paramedic's ethical decisions in prehospital care. (p. 65)
3. Analyze the relationship between the law and ethics in EMS. (p. 63)
4. Compare and contrast the criteria used in allocating scarce EMS resources. (pp. 71–72)
5. Identify issues surrounding advance directives in making a prehospital resuscitation decision and describe the criteria necessary to honour an advance directive in your province or territory. (pp. 67–68)

Part 7: Lifting and Moving Patients (begins on p. 74)

After reading Part 7 of this chapter, you should be able to:

1. Define body mechanics. (p. 74)
2. Discuss the guidelines and safety precautions that need to be followed when lifting a patient. (pp. 74–75)
3. Describe the power lift and the power grip. (pp. 75–76)
4. Explain how good posture and physical fitness can contribute to your well-being as an EMS provider. (pp. 77–78)
5. Describe the indications for an emergency move. (p. 79)
6. Describe the indications for assisting in nonemergency moves. (pp. 82–84)
7. Describe additional types of emergency moves, such as the piggyback carry, one-rescuer crutch, one-rescuer cradle carry, and firefighter's drag. (pp. 81–82)
8. Discuss the various devices associated with moving a patient in the out-of-hospital arena. (pp. 85–87)
9. Discuss the principles of loading and securing the stretcher into, and unloading the stretcher from, an ambulance. (pp. 87–88)
10. Explain the rationale behind properly lifting and moving patients. (pp. 74–75)
11. Explain the rationale behind an emergency move. (p. 79)

INTRODUCTION

Congratulations on your decision to become a paramedic. Before you begin this rewarding endeavour, it is important to understand what the job of a paramedic entails.

Emergency medical services (EMS) has made significant advances over the past 30 years. Not that long ago, the ambulance was simply a vehicle that provided rapid, horizontal transportation to the hospital. Today, equipped with the latest in equipment and technology, the ambulance is truly a mobile emergency room. Today, the paramedic is a highly trained health-care professional.

Part 1: Introduction to Advanced Prehospital Care

DESCRIPTION OF THE PROFESSION

The primary task of the paramedic is to provide emergency medical care in a prehospital environment, extending the care of the emergency physician to the patient in the field. To function as a paramedic, you must have fulfilled the prescribed requirements of the appropriate licensing or credentialling body. Paramedics may only function under the direction and licence of an EMS system's medical director. Because of this, the paramedic must also be approved by the system's medical director before being permitted to practise.

There are many different types of EMS system designs and operations. As a paramedic, you may work for a municipal city service, hospital, fire department, private ambulance service, police department, or other operation. Regardless of the type of service you work for, as a paramedic, you are an essential component in the continuum of care. Furthermore, paramedics often serve as a link between various health resources. Although paramedics continue to fill the well-defined and traditional role of 911 response, they also find themselves taking on a wide variety of additional responsibilities. The emerging roles and responsibilities of the paramedic include public education, health promotion, and participation in injury and illness prevention programs. Because of the need to cut costs, you may be charged with ensuring that your patient gets to the appropriate health-care facility, which may be a facility other than the hospital emergency department. Thus, the paramedic may begin to function as a facilitator of access to care as well as an individual treatment provider.

Paramedics must always strive toward maintaining high-quality health care. You must always be an advocate for your patient and ensure that the patient receives the best possible care—without regard to age, gender, type of complaint, socioeconomic status, religion, or nationality.

Paramedics are responsible and accountable to the system medical director, their employer, the public, and their peers. Although this may seem like a difficult standard to meet, if you always act in the best interests of the patient, you will seldom have problems.

PARAMEDIC CHARACTERISTICS

As a paramedic, you must be a confident leader who can accept the challenge and responsibility of the position. You must have excellent judgment and be able to prioritize decisions and act quickly in the best interests of the patient. You must be able to develop a rapport with a wide variety of patients so that, for example, you can safely interview hostile patients and communicate with members of diverse cultural groups and the various ages within those groups. Overall, you must be able to function independently at an optimum level in a nonstructured, constantly changing environment. The job is never easy and is always challenging.

> *You must be a confident leader, able to function independently at an optimum level in a nonstructured, constantly changing environment. The job is never easy and is always challenging.*

THE PARAMEDIC: A TRUE HEALTH PROFESSIONAL

Despite its relative youth as a profession, the field of emergency medical services is now recognized as an important part of the health-care system. As a paramedic, you must never take this status for granted. Instead, you must always strive to earn your acceptance as a **health-care professional**. Consider the completion of your initial paramedic course to be the start of your professional education, not the end. Participate in continuing education programs. Frequently review and practise skills, especially those less frequently used. Participate in routine peer-evaluation, and assume an active role in professional and community organizations.

> ***** **health-care professional**
> a properly trained and licensed or certified provider of health care.

> *You must always strive to earn your status as a health-care professional.*

A major step toward the recognition of EMS as a true health-care profession was the increase in the standards of education for prehospital personnel. In Canada, health care, including prehospital care, is a provincial or territorial responsibility. Each province and territory has developed its own operational models and supporting educational structures. A significant advance for paramedic education in Canada was the development of a National Occupational Competency Profile (NOCP) by the Paramedic Association of Canada in conjunction with Human Resources and Development Canada. The NOCP, introduced in March 2000, established a comprehensive framework for standardizing the fragmented paramedic educational programs across Canada. The NOCP serves as a reference point for provincial or territorial bodies seeking to facilitate the mobility of paramedics between provinces and territories. The NOCP may become the blueprint for a national registry exam.

> *The National Occupational Competency Profile is the key to defining a national scope of practice for EMS in Canada.*

As a paramedic, you must actively participate in the design, development, evaluation, and publication of research on topics relevant to your profession. For years, paramedic practice was based on anecdotal data and tradition. EMS adapted hospital-based procedures and equipment for use in the field. Only during the 1990s did we truly begin applying the scientific method to various aspects of prehospital practice. Surprisingly, we found little or no scientific data to support many of our prehospital practices. As a result of research, many traditional EMS treatments have been abandoned or refined. Equipment is now designed specifically for the uncontrolled conditions and unique demands of the paramedic. Many questions about paramedic practice are still unanswered, and these can only be answered by sound, ongoing scientific research. Results of this research are published in journals and form part of operational quality assurance and improvement programs.

> *Participation in research projects relevant to EMS is an important part of your profession as a paramedic.*

Another essential aspect of a health professional is acceptance and adherence to a code of professional ethics and etiquette. The public must feel confident that for the paramedic, the patient's and public's interests are always placed above personal, corporate, or financial interests. You must never forget that the patient is your primary concern.

> *An essential aspect of a health professional is acceptance and adherence to a code of professional ethics and etiquette. The patient is always your primary concern.*

EXPANDED SCOPE OF PRACTICE

Paramedics have a very bright future. New technologies and therapies bring the emergency department to the patient. Paramedics must be willing to step into these expanding roles, or persons from other health-care disciplines will fill them. Many aspects of prehospital care can give you the opportunity to work in an environment other than the typical 911-response vehicle:

- *Critical care transport.* Paramedics manage complicated inter-hospital transports—typically from one intensive care unit to another—in specially equipped ambulances or aircraft designed to provide a higher level of care.
- *Primary health care.* An emerging trend in health care is to keep patients with nonemergency problems out of the hospital emergency department. As a result, the EMS system is becoming involved in triaging and directing patients to the proper nonhospital facilities. In some cases, paramedics with additional skills can provide cost-effective, convenient medical care in the field or home.
- *Tactical EMS.* Paramedics accompany specially trained law enforcement officers on such tactical operations as hostage rescue, drug raids, and similar high-risk emergencies. The tactical paramedic is a member of the operations team but is also trained to provide sophisticated, prolonged, definitive patient care.
- *Industrial medicine.* Paramedics specially trained in occupational health are used to staff construction sites, oil rigs, and other facilities in which unique skills are required. These personnel may also serve as safety officers and inspectors.
- *Sports medicine.* Many sports teams hire paramedics to complement their trainers. In this role, paramedics participate in pregame preparation and assume responsibility for injury prevention. They are also trained to deal with injuries specific to the sport, such as orthopedic injuries, with the goal of returning players to action as quickly and safely as possible.
- *Heavy urban search and rescue (HUSAR).* Paramedics are an integral part of these multidisciplinary groups. HUSAR teams are groups of search, rescue, medical, and technical specialists that can rapidly assemble and deploy to disaster areas.
- *Other specialty teams.* Other multidisciplinary teams are formed to deal with specific public safety issues. Paramedics are increasingly participating in specialized HAZMAT (hazardous materials), rescue, and emergency response groups.

Paramedics are now stepping into such nontraditional roles because of their unique education and ability to think and work independently.

Paramedics are now stepping into new, nontraditional roles because of their unique education and ability to think and work independently.

Part 2: EMS Systems

✱ **emergency medical services (EMS) system** a comprehensive network of personnel, equipment, and resources established for delivering aid and emergency medical care to the community.

An **emergency medical services (EMS) system** is a comprehensive network of personnel, equipment, and resources established to deliver aid and emergency medical care to the community. An EMS system comprises both prehospital and in-hospital components. The prehospital component includes:

- Members of the community who are trained in first aid and cardiopulmonary resuscitation (CPR)

- A communications system that allows public access to emergency services dispatch and allows EMS providers to communicate with one another
- EMS providers, including paramedics
- Fire/rescue and hazardous-materials services
- Public utilities, such as power and gas companies
- Resource centres, such as regional poison control centres
- Medical control

The in-hospital component includes:

- Emergency nurses
- Emergency physicians
- Ancillary services, such as radiology and respiratory therapy
- Specialty physicians, such as trauma surgeons and cardiologists
- Rehabilitation services

A typical request for EMS begins with citizen activation when someone contacts a 911 dispatch centre. EMS dispatch collects essential information and sends out the closest appropriately staffed and equipped unit. In many EMS systems, the dispatcher also provides prearrival instructions to the caller.

The first EMS provider at the scene may be a police officer, firefighter, lifeguard, teacher, or other community member who has been trained as an **emergency medical responder (EMR)**. The EMR's role is to stabilize the patient until more advanced personnel arrive. The next EMS provider likely to arrive depends on the type of EMS system. In most areas, the dispatcher will send either a **basic life support (BLS)** or an **advanced life support (ALS)** ambulance. Other EMS systems use a tiered response, sending multiple levels of emergency care personnel to the same incident. In still other areas, ALS personnel respond to every incident, regardless of the level of care needed.

Once care has been initiated, EMS providers must quickly decide on the medical facility to which the patient should be transported, based on the type of care needed, transport time, and local protocols. Where specialty centres have been designated (such as pediatric, trauma, and burn centres), it may be necessary to transport the patient to a facility other than the closest hospital. At the receiving medical facility, an emergency nurse or physician assumes responsibility, and the patient is assigned a priority of care. If needed, a surgeon or other specialist will be summoned.

✱ **emergency medical responders (EMR)** are responders who provide first-aid skills until more advanced personnel arrive.

✱ **basic life support (BLS)** refers to such basic life-saving procedures as artificial ventilation and cardiopulmonary resuscitation (CPR, automated defibrillation) generally provided by EMS personnel trained at the primary care paramedic (PCP) level.

✱ **advanced life support (ALS)** refers to such advanced life-saving procedures as intravenous therapy, drug therapy, intubation, and manual defibrillation, cardioversion/pacing provided by advanced care paramedics (ACP) or critical care paramedics (CCP).

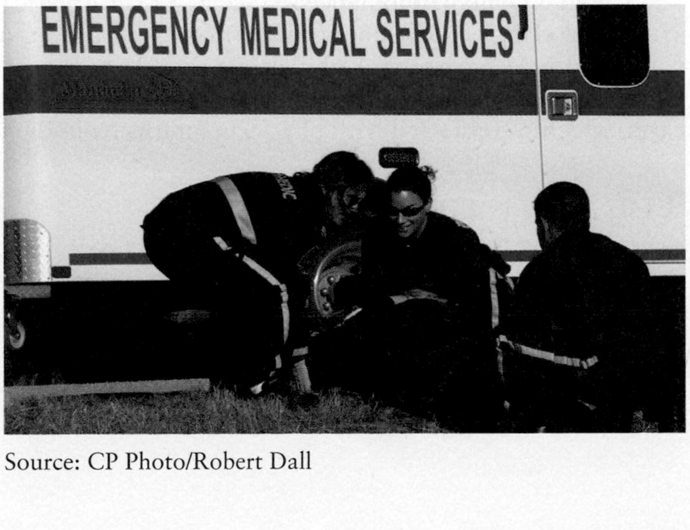

Source: CP Photo/Robert Dall

FIGURE 1-1   The advanced care paramedic (ACP) is generally the highest level of prehospital care provider for ground ambulances and the leader of the prehospital care team.

HISTORY OF EMS

ANCIENT TIMES

Emergency medicine has a very long history. Emergency medicine may be traced back to biblical times, when it was recorded that a "good Samaritan" provided care to a wounded traveller by the side of a road. In fact, about 4000 to 5000 years ago, Sumerians inscribed clay tablets with some of the earliest medical records. Similar to EMS protocols today, the tablets provided step-by-step instructions for care based on the patient's description of symptoms, as well as instructions on how to create and administer medications. The most striking difference between these first "protocols" and EMS today is the absence of a secondary assessment (physical exam).

In 1862, the Egyptologist Edwin Smith purchased a papyrus scroll dating to about 1500 B.C.E. It contained 48 medical case histories with data arranged in head-to-toe order and in order of severity, an arrangement very similar to today's patient assessment. One section, the "Book of Wounds," explains the treatment of such injuries as fractures and dislocations.

At about the same time, King Hammurabi of Babylon created a code of laws known today as the "Code of Hammurabi." A section of the code regulated medical fees and penalties based on the social class of the patient. For example, if a surgeon operated successfully on a commoner, he would be paid only half of what his fee would be if he had operated on a rich man. If a surgeon caused the death of a rich man, the surgeon's hand would be cut off, but if a slave died under his care, he only had to replace the slave.

THE NINETEENTH CENTURY

During the Napoleonic Wars of the early nineteenth century, one of Napoleon's chief surgeons, Jean Larrey, formed the ambulance volante, or "flying ambulance," which focused efforts on providing emergency surgery as close to the battlefield as possible. Though the ambulance volante was little more than a covered horse-drawn cart, Larrey is credited with the development of the first prehospital system that used **triage** and transport.

* **triage** a method of sorting patients by the severity of their injuries.

Between 1861 and 1865, during the American Civil War, a nurse named Clara Barton coordinated care for the sick and injured. Defying army leaders, she persisted in going to the front, where wounded men suffered and often died from lack of the simplest medical attention. She organized the triage and transport of injured soldiers to improvised hospitals in nearby houses, barns, and churches away from the battlefield.

The first civilian ambulance service in North America was formed about the same time (1865) in Cincinnati, Ohio. Four years later, in 1869, the New York City Health Department Ambulance Service began operating out of Bellevue Hospital. The ambulances of both services were specially designed horse-drawn carts, which were staffed with physician interns from the various hospital wards.

THE TWENTIETH CENTURY

The high mortality rate of soldiers during World War I was associated with an average evacuation time of 18 hours. As a result, in World War II, a system was created in which battlefield ambulance corps transported wounded soldiers from the front lines to the echelons (levels) of care. However, many of the echelons were so far from the battlefield and each other that there were huge delays in patient care. In many cases, it was often days from the injury itself to definitive surgery.

During the Korean and Vietnam conflicts, great advances in the patient care delivery system were made. The wounded soldier was treated on the battlefield when the injury occurred and evacuated by helicopter to a field hospital to receive definitive surgery. In Vietnam, in many cases, this occurred within 10 to 20 minutes. Once stabilized and able to be moved (generally within 24 to 48 hours), the patient would be flown by jet to Clark Air Force Base in the Philippines for further treatment. The decreased time before definitive care and the advances in medical procedures significantly reduced mortality rates.

Throughout history, significant advances in **trauma** care occurred during wartime. However, until the late 1960s, few areas in North America provided adequate civilian prehospital emergency care. Medical care began in the hospital emergency department. Rescue techniques were crude, ambulance attendants poorly educated, and equipment minimal. Police, fire, and EMS personnel had no radio communication. Proper medical direction was not available, and the only interaction between physicians and EMS personnel was at the receiving facility.

✻ trauma a physical injury or wound caused by external force or violence.

EARLY EMS

In the late 1960s, ambulance services were provided by a wide variety of municipal services, fire- and police-based services, hospitals, private operators, funeral homes, and volunteers. As demands for additional services and increased training grew, early EMS systems with formal training, communications, and medical direction began to develop across Canada. In many areas, fragmented operations were amalgamated into municipal, regional, or even provincial or territorial services. In the late 1960s, many provinces and territories were creating basic emergency medical technician (EMT) programs, often following the American models and curriculum. By the 1970s, Calgary and some communities in Ontario had early advanced life support (ALS) programs. ALS was soon available in parts of Quebec, Toronto, and in British Columbia through the newly formed B.C. Ambulance Service. However, many of these initiatives continued to exist only at municipal, regional, or provincial or territorial levels, and there was little coordination of these emerging prehospital systems at a national level.

In the United States, EMS was pushed by several federal initiatives. In 1966, the National Academy of Sciences, National Resource Council published "Accidental Death and Disability: The Neglected Disease of Modern Society." This White Paper spelled out deficiencies in prehospital emergency care. It suggested guidelines for the development of EMS systems, the training of prehospital emergency medical providers, and the upgrading of ambulances and their equipment. This publication set off a series of federal and private initiatives including the National Highways Safety Act, the establishment of the U.S. Department of Transportation (DOT), and funding for a variety of EMS projects and systems. In 1969, the Emergency Medical Technician-Ambulance program was made public. The first American paramedic curriculum followed in 1977.

Canadian EMS has remained a provincial or territorial responsibility. Each province and territory developed its own systems and educational programs built on its unique historical and operational needs. Most have a mix of basic, intermediate, and ALS programs, often based on the American DOT curriculum. However, in adapting to local operations, these programs have become difficult to compare. Through the 1980s and 1990s, some provinces and territories retained EMT and EMT-paramedic designations, while others developed their own models. British Columbia trained three levels of emergency medical assistants (EMA), while Ontario created the emergency medical care assistant (EMCA) designation.

In 1988, in the United States, the National Highway Traffic Safety Administration (NHTSA) established the Statewide EMS Technical Assessment Program.

It defines elements necessary to all EMS systems. Although these elements have not been formally adopted by Canadian EMS, they are often referred to by Canadian EMS systems. Briefly, the essential elements are:

- *Regulation and policy.* Each state (province or territory) must have laws, regulations, policies, and procedures that govern its EMS system. It also is required to provide leadership to local jurisdictions.
- *Resources management.* Each state (province or territory) must have central control of EMS resources so that all patients have equal access to acceptable emergency care.
- *Human resources and training.* A standardized EMS curriculum should be taught by qualified instructors, and all personnel who transport patients in the prehospital setting should be adequately trained.
- *Transport.* Patients must be safely and reliably transported by ground or air ambulance.
- *Facilities.* Every seriously ill or injured patient must be delivered in a timely manner to an appropriate medical facility.
- *Communications.* A system for public access to the EMS system must be in place. Communication among dispatchers, the ambulance crew, and medical control and hospital personnel must also be possible.
- *Trauma systems.* Each state (province or territory) should develop a system of specialized care for trauma patients, including one or more **trauma centres** and rehabilitation programs. It also must develop systems for assigning and transporting patients to those facilities.
- *Public information and education.* EMS personnel should participate in programs designed to educate the public. The programs are to focus on the prevention of injuries and how to properly access the EMS system.
- *Medical direction.* Each EMS system must have a physician as its medical director. This physician delegates medical practice to nonphysician caregivers and oversees all aspects of patient care.
- *Evaluation.* Each state (province or territory) must have a **quality improvement (QI)** system in place for continuing evaluation and upgrading of its EMS system.

Many EMS providers fail to realize that each component of the EMS system has gone through many stages of development. In spite of the advances of more than 40 years, startling differences in the quality of prehospital care exist across Canada.

TODAY'S EMS SYSTEMS

Though EMS systems across the country and the world vary, certain elements are essential to ensure the best possible patient care. *In Canada, there is no one method of provision of prehospital care. EMS systems in Canada vary across provinces and territories and even across cities and towns.*

TYPES OF EMS SERVICES

The provision of EMS is a provincial or territorial responsibility. The following list describes some of the models that have developed in Canada. Note that the following services are given only as examples and that EMS systems

---

✱ **trauma centre** medical facility that has the capability of caring for the acutely injured patient. Trauma centres must meet strict criteria to use this designation.

✱ **quality improvement (QI)** an evaluation program that emphasizes service and uses customer satisfaction as an indicator of system performance.

change over time. Canadian EMS services may be provided by the following types of agencies:

- Provincial or territorial service
- Municipal service
- Fire-based service
- Hospital-based service
- Private operator
- Volunteer service

Provincial or Territorial Service
EMS is often regulated through provincial or territorial agencies but delivered through a variety of agencies. In British Columbia, B.C. Ambulance Service was created in 1974 to serve as the sole provider of EMS in B.C.

Municipal, Upper Tier, and Regional Municipality Services
In many provinces and territories, provision of EMS is delegated to the municipality. Cities, such as Calgary and Winnipeg, maintain EMS departments separate from other emergency services (fire and police) within the municipal structure. In Ontario, the province sets EMS standards, but service may be delivered through municipal or provincial organizations.

Fire-Based Service
EMS is provided within a fire department structure in municipalities, such as Fort McMurray and Lethbridge in Alberta, or Riverview in New Brunswick. Fire-based EMS may operate independently but under the administrative structure of the department. In a dual-trained model, members may rotate between firefighting and EMS duties.

Hospital-Based Service
Hospital-based EMS services can be found in Fredericton and Saint John in New Brunswick or St. John's in Newfoundland and Labrador. This type of service allows paramedics to maintain close relationships with nurses and physicians. In some models, paramedics may also assume duties within the hospital.

Private Operator
Some systems contract EMS services to a private operator. Performance clauses establish expectations for such things as levels of service, response times, and so on.

Volunteer Services
Some small towns, rural areas, and isolated communities maintain EMS services through a volunteer network. These members often take training on their own time and at their own expense and receive little compensation for their service to the community.

EMS SYSTEMS

In essence, EMS is made up of a series of systems within a system. The integration of these systems and the cooperation of all participants help ensure the best quality of emergency care. These systems include the following:

- Medical direction
- Public information and education
- Communications
- Education and certification
- Patient transport
- Receiving facilities

- Mutual aid and mass-casualty preparation
- Quality improvement and quality assurance
- Research
- System financing
- Certification and licensing of personnel

MEDICAL DIRECTION

An EMS system must retain a **medical director**—a physician who is legally responsible for all clinical and patient-care aspects of the system. Prehospital medical care provided by nonphysicians is considered an extension of the medical director's licence; that is, prehospital care providers are the medical director's designated agents, regardless of who their employers may be.

The medical director's role in an EMS system is to:

- Educate and train personnel
- Participate in personnel and equipment selection
- Develop clinical protocols in cooperation with expert EMS personnel
- Participate in quality improvement and problem resolution
- Provide direct input into patient care
- Interface between the EMS system and other health-care agencies
- Advocate within the medical community
- Serve as the "medical conscience" of the EMS system, including advocating for quality patient care

In addition to the responsibilities listed above, the medical director is the ultimate authority for all online (direct) and offline (indirect) **medical direction**.

Online Medical Direction

Online medical direction occurs when a qualified physician gives direct orders to a prehospital care provider by either radio or telephone, or RIM devices (these are similar to pagers but have tiny keyboards for writing text). Toronto critical care paramedics use RIM devices and the internet to send patient information and receive orders (see Figure 1-2). In some jurisdictions, medical direction may be delegated to a registered nurse (RN) or to a paramedic. In all circumstances, ultimate online responsibility remains with the medical director.

Online medical direction offers several benefits to the patient, including immediate medical consultation and use of telemetry to provide instant diagnostic information to the medical director. In most systems, online consultations can be recorded for review and quality improvement.

At the emergency scene, the provider with the highest level of training in the delivery of prehospital emergency care should be in charge. When a nonaffiliated physician, or **intervener physician,** is on scene and online medical direction does not exist, the paramedic may relinquish responsibility to the physician. However, the intervener physician must first identify himself, demonstrate a willingness to accept responsibility, and document the intervention as required by the local EMS system. If treatment differs from established protocol, the intervener physician must accompany the patient in the ambulance to the hospital. If an intervener physician is on scene and online medical direction does exist, the online physician is ultimately responsible. In case of a disagreement, the paramedic must take orders from the online physician.

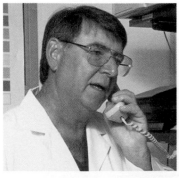

FIGURE 1-2 The medical director can provide online guidance to EMS personnel in the field.

Offline Medical Direction

Offline medical direction refers to medical policies, procedures, and practices that a medical director has set up in advance of a call. It includes prospective medical direction, such as guidelines on the selection of personnel and supplies, training and education, and protocol development. It also includes retrospective medical direction, such as auditing, peer review, and other quality assurance processes.

Protocols are the policies and procedures of an EMS system. They provide a standardized approach to common patient problems, a consistent level of medical care, and a standard for accountability. Based on such protocols, the online physician can assist prehospital personnel in interpreting the patient's complaint, understanding assessment findings, and providing the appropriate treatment. Protocols are designed around the four Ts of emergency care:

- *Triage.* Guidelines that address patient flow through an EMS system, including how system resources are allocated to meet the needs of patients
- *Treatment.* Guidelines that identify procedures to be performed on direct order from medical direction and procedures that are preauthorized protocols called **standing orders**
- *Transport.* Guidelines that address the mode of travel (air versus ground) based on the nature of the patient's injury or illness, the condition of the patient, the level of care required, and estimated transport time
- *Transfer.* Guidelines that address receiving facilities to ensure that the patient is admitted to the one most appropriate for definitive care

Protocols also are established for special circumstances, such as do not resuscitate (DNR) orders, sexual abuse, abuse of children or elderly people, patients who refuse treatment, termination of CPR, and intervener physicians. Although protocols standardize field procedures, they should allow the paramedic the flexibility to improvise and adapt to special circumstances.

PUBLIC INFORMATION AND EDUCATION

The public is an essential, yet often overlooked, component of an EMS system. EMS should have a plan to educate the public on recognizing an emergency, accessing the system, and initiating basic life support procedures.

Recognizing an emergency can save lives. The Heart and Stroke Foundation of Canada reports that cardiovascular disease accounted for 78 942 Canadian deaths in 1999. Many patients delay calling for help when symptoms occur. If the patient and bystanders are taught to recognize the emergency and call for help in time, many deaths can be prevented.

The second aspect of public education is system access. Citizens must know how to activate EMS in an emergency to avoid life-threatening delays. Whether access is by way of 911 or a local emergency phone number, the number should be well publicized, and citizens should be taught how to give the necessary information to the emergency medical dispatcher.

Finally, after recognizing an emergency and activating EMS, citizens must know how to provide basic life support assistance (BLS), such as cardiopulmonary resuscitation (CPR) and bleeding control after major trauma. Abundant research indicates that a relationship exists between EMS response times and mortality (death) rates of patients. Communities have proven that when many citizens are trained in BLS—and a rapid advanced life support (ALS) response occurs—a larger number of patients can be successfully resuscitated.

* **offline medical direction** refers to medical policies, procedures, and practices that medical direction has set up in advance of a call.

* **protocols** the policies and procedures for all components of an EMS system.

* **standing orders** preauthorized treatment procedures; a type of treatment protocol.

Content Review

FOUR Ts OF EMERGENCY CARE
- Triage
- Treatment
- Transport
- Transfer

Public involvement now includes bystander defibrillation, including the Public Access Defibrillation (PAD) initiative. With the development of automated external defibrillator (AED) technology, it is now possible to place affordable, portable AEDs in the homes of cardiac patients and in public places.

COMMUNICATIONS

The communications network is the heart of a regional EMS system. A communications plan should include the following:

- *Citizen access.* A well-publicized universal number, such as 911, provides direct citizen access to emergency services. Multiple community numbers add life-threatening minutes to emergency response times. Enhanced 911, or E-911, automatically gives the location of the caller, instantly routes the call to the appropriate emergency service (fire, police, or EMS), and has instant callback capability.
- *Single control centre* (Figure 1-3). One control centre that can communicate with and direct all emergency vehicles within a large geographical area is best. Ideally, all public service agencies should be dispatched from the same communications centre.
- *Operational communications capabilities.* With these capabilities, EMS dispatch can manage all aspects of system response and assess the system's readiness for the next response. Emergency units can communicate with each other and with other agencies during mutual aid and disaster operations. Hospitals also can communicate with other hospitals in the region to assess specialty capabilities.
- *Medical communications capabilities.* EMS providers can communicate with the receiving facility and medical control and, in many areas, transmit electrocardiographic (ECG) telemetry signals to the online physician. Hospitals also can communicate with each other to facilitate patient transfer.
- *Communications hardware.* Radios, consoles, pagers, cell phone transmission towers, repeaters, telephone landlines, and other telecommunications equipment are required.
- *Communications software.* Software includes radio frequencies and, in many systems, satellite and high-tech computer programs that track ambulances. Procedures, policies consistent with Canadian Radio-television and Telecommunications Commission (CRTC) standards and local protocols, and backup communications plans for disaster operations are essential.

Emergency Medical Dispatcher (EMD)

* emergency medical dispatcher (EMD) EMS person medically and technically trained to assign emergency medical resources to a medical emergency.

The **emergency medical dispatcher (EMD)** is crucial to the operation of EMS. EMDs not only send ambulances to the scene, but they also make sure that system resources are in constant readiness to respond. EMDs must be both medically and technically trained. The course should be standardized and include certification by a government agency.

EMS Dispatch

Emergency medical dispatching is the nerve centre of an EMS system. It should be under the full control of the medical director and the EMS agency. In general, EMS system status management relies on projected call volumes and locations to

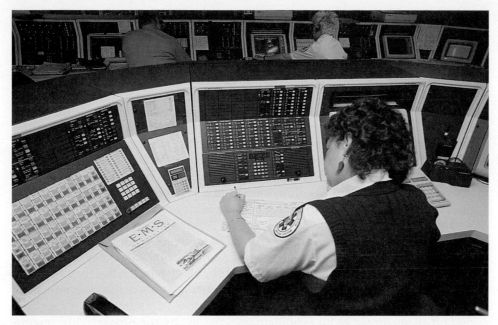

FIGURE 1-3   The ideal communications centre can communicate with and control the movement of all emergency units within an EMS system.

strategically place ambulances and crews. This method helps reduce response times. Another management method, "priority dispatching," was first used by the Salt Lake City Fire Department. Using a set of medically approved protocols, EMDs are trained to medically interrogate a distressed caller, prioritize symptoms, select an appropriate response, and give life-saving prearrival instructions.

In 1974, the Phoenix Fire Department introduced a prearrival instruction program developed by medically trained dispatchers. In that program, callers initiate life-saving first aid with the dispatcher's help while they wait for emergency units to arrive on scene. In 1985, the Seattle EMS system initiated a successful program of instructing callers in CPR. Prearrival instruction may result in increased liability, but the liability risk of *not* providing it may far outweigh the risk of providing it.

An effective EMS dispatching system places the first responding units on scene within four minutes of the onset of the emergency. Brain resuscitation will not be successful unless there is proper BLS intervention (CPR) within four minutes. Studies also suggest that defibrillation within eight minutes can reverse sudden-death mortality. So, the goal of emergency response is BLS care in less than four minutes and ALS care in less than eight minutes after the event. High-performance systems meet this standard more than 90 percent of the time.

An effective EMS dispatching system places BLS care on scene within four minutes of onset and ALS care in less than eight minutes.

EDUCATION AND CERTIFICATION

EMS education includes both initial and continuing programs. *Initial education* programs are the original training courses for prehospital providers. *Continuing education* programs include refresher courses for recertification and periodic inservice training.

Initial Education

A paramedic's initial education usually consists of a course of study in prehospital care. Standards for the programs are usually set at the provincial or territorial level. With the release of the Paramedic Association of Canada's National Occupational Competency Profile (NOCP), many training programs have chosen to participate in a national accrediting process administered by the Canadian Medical Association. The NOCP specifies competencies for emergency medical responders, primary care paramedics, advanced care paramedics, and critical care paramedics.

Once initial education is completed, the paramedic may become either certified, licensed, or registered, depending on the province or territory. **Certification** is the process by which an agency or association grants recognition to an individual who has met its qualifications.

Licensure is a process of occupational regulation. Through licensure, a regulatory agency grants permission to engage in a given trade or **profession** to an applicant who has attained the degree of competency required to ensure the public's protection.

Many provinces and territories require paramedics to be *registered* before working as a paramedic in that jurisdiction. *Registration* is accomplished at the emergency medical responder level or one of the three paramedic levels by meeting several requirements. First, the registrant must have successfully completed a course of education for the level of registration for which they are applying. The registrant then completes an examination provided by the provincial or territorial regulating agency or its delegate, and successful registrants receive a registration number that allows them to work in that province or territory.

For example, provincial associations register EMS personnel in Alberta and Saskatchewan. The Ministry of Health registers personnel in Ontario but before being able to practise, a paramedic must be certified by the local base hospital medical director. In Manitoba, EMS personnel are licensed through the government. Graduates of the Justice Institute of British Columbia (JIBC) are certified at their education level but receive the licensure required to operate as paramedics in B.C. from the Ministry of Health EMA Licensing Branch.

Reciprocity is the process by which an agency grants automatic certification or licensure to an individual who has comparable certification, licensure, or registration from another agency. For example, some provinces and territories grant reciprocity to paramedics who are certified in another province or territory. The individual must complete a registration process as outlined by the individual province or territory.

Levels of Prehospital Care

A number of certification levels for prehospital care providers are available in Canada. At a national level, the Paramedic Association of Canada has identified four levels:

1. Emergency medical responder (EMR)
2. Primary care paramedic (PCP)
3. Advanced care paramedic (ACP)
4. Critical care paramedic (CCP)

Practitioner Levels
The following descriptions are based on the NOCP established by the Paramedic Association of Canada (PAC). Note that paramedics may only perform those procedures that they are licensed for. The NOCP may contain procedures that are not used operationally in some provinces or territories. For example, a PCP training program may contain symptom relief protocols that are not licensed

✱ certification the process by which an agency or association grants recognition and the ability to practise to an individual who has met its qualifications.

✱ licensure the process by which a regulatory agency grants permission to engage in a given occupation to an applicant who has attained the degree of competency required to ensure the public's protection.

✱ profession refers to the existence of a specialized body of knowledge or skills.

✱ reciprocity the process by which an agency grants automatic certification or licensure to an individual who has comparable certification or licensure from another agency.

within a specific jurisdiction. It is your responsibility as a professional to know the limits of your licence. Each level builds on the competencies of the previous level. Thus, an ACP is expected to meet all of the competencies of the PCP, in addition to the competencies specified at the ACP level.

Emergency Medical Responder (EMR)
An emergency medical responder may act as a first responder or take an entry-level position in some EMS systems. EMRs are responsible for primary assessment, BLS treatments and interventions, and the provision of safe and prudent care. In some agencies, EMRs may provide transport. The EMR competency profile does not include controlled or delegated medical acts.

Primary Care Paramedic (PCP)
The PCP is the largest group of paramedic practitioners in Canada. PCPs may be volunteer or career paramedics and may operate in any EMS setting. PCPs perform patient assessment, treat medical conditions and injuries, and perform delegated medical acts, such as the administration of specific medications, semiautomated defibrillation, and IV maintenance. PCPs are expected to build a sound knowledge of anatomy, physiology, and pathophysiology and to demonstrate excellent problem-solving and decision-making skills.

Advanced Care Paramedic (ACP)
Advanced care paramedics provide enhanced levels of care, using ALS procedures and protocols. ACPs most often operate in suburban, urban, air ambulance, and military settings. ACP may also be available in some rural areas. In many systems, PCP is a prerequisite to ACP training. ACPs build on their PCP foundation to provide additional levels of assessment and treatment. ACP competencies include advanced techniques, invasive procedures, pharmacological interventions, and delegated medical acts for managing life-threatening conditions involving airway, breathing, and circulation.

Critical Care Paramedic (CCP)
The critical care paramedic is the highest level described by the NOCP. CCPs extend ACP competencies to function in large urban and air ambulance services. CCPs are expected to perform thorough patient assessment, interpret laboratory and radiological data, demonstrate advanced decision-making and differential discrimination skills, and manage patients autonomously and with consultation of medical authorities. The CCP profile includes a wide range of controlled and delegated medical acts, including the use of invasive hemodynamic monitoring devices.

Paramedic Association of Canada
In 1988, the PAC replaced the Canadian Society of Ambulance Personnel (CSAP). The PAC is Canada's only national EMS organization representing prehospital practitioners. The PAC currently has more than 14 000 members located in divisional chapters in British Columbia, Alberta, Saskatchewan, Manitoba, Ontario, Quebec, New Brunswick, Nova Scotia, Yukon, and the Canadian Armed Forces.

Regulation of Paramedic Practice and Approval of Training Programs

The delivery of health care is a provincial or territorial responsibility. Although federal laws affect such areas as controlled drugs and medical devices, communications, and transport, the regulation and delivery of EMS services are governed by provincial and territorial bodies. Some jurisdictions, such as the Canadian Armed Forces, remain within the federal jurisdiction.

Content Review

LEVELS OF
PREHOSPITAL CARE

- Emergency medical responder
- Primary care paramedic
- Advanced care paramedic
- Critical care paramedic

Each province or territory sets its own scope of practice and practitioner classification system. Training programs must meet appropriate standards. Graduates of a recognized training program may apply for certification or licensure, based on current jurisdictional standards.

The NOCP gives licensing and professional bodies a way to compare programs from different jurisdictions and creates a mechanism for allowing mobility between EMS systems. In the future, the NOCP may become a blueprint for a national registry.

Training agencies may choose to participate in a voluntary accreditation process established by the Canadian Medical Association (CMA). The CMA's *Requirements for Accreditation* uses the NOCP to establish levels for accreditation at the PCP, ACP, and CCP levels. Many provinces and territories have begun adapting their curriculum to meet or exceed the NOCP levels.

Professional Organizations

Belonging to a professional organization is a good way to keep informed and share ideas. Canadian EMS organizations include the following:

- Ambulance Paramedics of British Columbia
- Alberta College of Paramedics
- Saskatchewan Paramedic Association
- Paramedic Association of Manitoba, Inc.
- Ontario Paramedic Association
- Paramedic Professional Association of Quebec/Association Professionnelle des Paramédics du Québec
- Nova Scotia College of Paramedics
- Paramedic Association of New Brunswick
- Paramedic Association of Prince Edward Island
- Paramedic Association of Yukon

Many EMS organizations in the United States accept members from other countries:

- National Association of Emergency Medical Technicians (NAEMT)
- National Association of Search and Rescue (NASAR)
- National Association of State EMS Directors (NASEMSD)
- National Association of EMS Physicians (NAEMSP)
- National Flight Paramedics Association (NFPA)
- National Council of State EMS Training Coordinators (NCSEMSTC)

These are just some examples of organizations through which EMS providers can enrich themselves and pursue their particular interests. Such organizations assist in the development of educational programs, operational policies and procedures, and the implementation of EMS.

Professional Journals

The following is just a partial list of the many journals available to keep the paramedic aware of the latest changes in this ever-changing industry. They also offer an opportunity for EMS professionals to write and publish articles:

- *Annals of Emergency Medicine*
- *EAU FAU Magazine*
- *Emergency Medical Services*
- *Canadian Emergency News*
- *Emergency*
- *Journal of Emergency Medical Services*
- *Journal of Emergency Medicine*
- *Journal of Pediatric Emergency Medicine*
- *Journal of Trauma*
- *Prehospital Emergency Care*

PATIENT TRANSPORT

Patients who are transported under the direction of an EMS system should be taken to the nearest appropriate medical facility whenever possible. Medical direction should designate that facility, based on the needs of the patient and the availability of services. In some cases, the patient's need for special services (such as care for burns) means designating a facility that is not always nearby. At other times, the closest facility will be designated for stabilization of the patient while transfer is arranged. The ultimate authority for this decision remains with medical direction.

Patients may be transported by ground or air. Today, trauma care systems use law enforcement, municipal, hospital-based, private, and military helicopter transport services to transfer patients. Fixed-wing aircraft also are used when patients must be transported long distances, usually more than 320 km.

All transport vehicles must be licensed and meet local and provincial or territorial requirements. For example, in Alberta, all ambulances must meet the requirements of Alberta Health before entering into service. Each ambulance must also meet those requirements during a yearly inspection.

Currently, no federal regulations specify ambulance design and manufacturing requirements. Generally, ambulance services in Canada follow specifications from the United States known as DOT KKK 1822 specs. Over the years, the "KKK" specifications have had a significant influence on ambulance manufacturing, in both the United States and Canada.

In 1974, in response to a request from the DOT, the General Services Administration developed the "KKK-A-1822 Federal Specifications for Ambulances." This was the first attempt at standardizing ambulance design. The act defined the following basic types of ambulances:

- *Type I.* A conventional cab and chassis on which a module ambulance body is mounted, with no passageway between the driver's compartment and the patient's compartment
- *Type II.* A standard van, body, and cab form an integral unit; most have a raised roof
- *Type III.* A specialty van with forward cab, integral body, and a passageway from driver's compartment to patient's compartment

In 1980, the revision "KKK-A-1822A" aimed at improving ambulance electrical systems by designing a low-amperage lighting system to replace antiquated light bars and beacons. In 1985, another revision, "KKK-A-1822B," specified changes based on National Institute for Occupational Safety and Health (NIOSH) standards. These include reduced internal siren noise, engine temperatures, and exhaust emissions; safer cot-retention systems; wider axles; handheld spotlights; battery conditioners for longer life; and venting systems for oxygen compartments.

RECEIVING FACILITIES

Not all hospitals are equal in emergency and support service capabilities. So, how do you get the right patient to the right facility in an appropriate amount of time? EMS systems categorize hospitals according to their ability to receive and treat emergency patients. EMS coordinators use these categories to quickly identify the most appropriate facility for definitive treatment or life-saving stabilization. Regionalizing available services also helps give all patients reasonable access to the appropriate facility. Burn, trauma, pediatric, psychiatric, perinatal, cardiac, spinal, and poison centres are examples of specialty service facilities that offer high-level care for specific groups of patients in a wide region. Large EMS systems should designate a resource hospital that will coordinate specialty resources and ensure appropriate patient distribution.

To select the appropriate receiving facility for your patient, it is important to know which facilities in your area offer the following services:

- Fully staffed and equipped emergency department
- Trauma care capabilities
- Operating suites available 24 hours a day, seven days a week
- Critical care units, such as postanesthesia recovery rooms and surgical intensive care units
- Cardiac facilities with on-staff cardiologists
- Neurology department that provides a stroke team
- Acute hemodialysis capability
- Pediatric capabilities, including pediatric and neonatal intensive care units
- Obstetric capabilities, including facilities for high-risk delivery
- Radiological specialty capabilities, such as computerized tomography (CT) and magnetic resonance imaging (MRI)
- Burn specialization for infants, children, and adults
- Acute spinal-cord and head-injury management capability
- Rehabilitation staff and facilities
- Clinical laboratory services
- Toxicology, including hazmat decontamination facilities
- Hyperbaric oxygen therapy capability
- Microvascular surgical capabilities for replants
- Psychiatric facilities

In Canada, the Trauma Association of Canada accredits hospitals based on the guidelines of the American College of Surgeons and incorporating their own guidelines. The Trauma Association of Canada recommends three levels of trauma centre designation:

1. Tertiary centre (TTC)
2. District trauma centre (DTC)
3. Primary trauma centre (PTC)

Tertiary Trauma Centre (TTC)

A tertiary trauma centre (TTC) is a pediatric or adult centre that has been designated and funded by a provincial or territorial Ministry of Health. A TTC is the regional referral. It is often a teaching hospital affiliated with a university and involved in trauma research. It is the regional referral centre for seriously injured patients. The TTC is accredited by and follows the Trauma Association of Canada guidelines. One of the most important guidelines is the availability of a 24-hour trauma response team to provide prompt resuscitation and treatment to seriously injured patients.

District Trauma Centre (DTC)

A district trauma centre (DTC) is designated by a health authority and may function as a trauma centre in smaller communities or support a tertiary centre. A DTC may be a teaching hospital and affiliated with a university or community facility. The DTC provides 24-hour trauma team response to provide prompt resuscitation and treatment of injured patients. It must comply with quality improvement programs and participate in a comprehensive data collection program.

Primary Trauma Centre (PTC)

A primary trauma centre (PTC) is designated by the health authority and is accredited by its regional accredited trauma program. A PTC is usually a smaller rural medical centre or nursing station that provides initial triage for all trauma situations. This centre refers all but minor trauma patients to its district trauma centre.

A fourth designation may be given to specialty referral centres, which offer unique services. They include burn, pediatric, psychiatric, perinatal, cardiac, spinal, and poison centres.

Ideally, all receiving facilities should have the following capabilities: an emergency department with an emergency physician on duty at all times, surgical facilities, a lab and blood bank, x-ray capabilities available around the clock, and critical and intensive care units. They should have a documented commitment to participate in the EMS system, a willingness to receive all emergency patients in transport, and medical audit procedures to ensure quality care and medical accountability. Finally, receiving facilities should exhibit a desire to participate in multiple-casualty preparedness plans.

MUTUAL AID AND MASS-CASUALTY PREPARATION

Since the resources of any one EMS system can be overwhelmed, a mutual-aid agreement ensures that help is available when needed. Such agreements may be between neighbouring departments, municipalities, systems, or provinces or territories. Cooperation must transcend geographical, political, and historical boundaries.

Each EMS system should have a disaster plan for catastrophes that can overwhelm available resources. There should be a coordinated central management agency, integration of all EMS system components, and a flexible communications system. Frequent drills should test the plan's effectiveness and practicality.

Each EMS system should have a disaster plan that is practised frequently.

QUALITY ASSURANCE AND IMPROVEMENT

The only acceptable quality of an EMS system is excellence. Many EMS systems in Canada have adopted a manual released by the United States National Highway Traffic Safety Administration (NHTSA) in 1997 as a template for quality

The only acceptable quality of an EMS system is excellence.

improvement. The manual, "A Leadership Guide to Quality Improvement for Emergency Medical Services Systems" recommends the following components:

- Leadership
- Information and analysis
- Strategic quality planning
- Human resources development and management
- EMS process management
- EMS system results
- Satisfaction of patients and other stakeholders

* **quality assurance (QA)** a program designed to maintain continuous monitoring and measurement of the quality of clinical care delivered to patients.

A **quality assurance (QA)** program monitors and measures the quality of clinical care delivered to patients through the evaluation of such objective data as response times, adherence to protocols, patient survival, and other key indicators. QA programs document the effectiveness of the care provided. They also help identify problems and areas that need improvement. A common complaint about QA programs is that they tend to identify only the problems and therefore focus only on punitive corrective action. Thus, prehospital personnel often view QA programs negatively.

* **continuous quality improvement (CQI)** a program designed to refine and improve an EMS system, emphasizing customer satisfaction.

As a result, many EMS systems have taken QA a step further with a **continuous quality improvement (CQI)** program. A CQI program emphasizes customer satisfaction and includes evaluations of such aspects as billing and maintenance. In contrast to QA programs, CQI focuses on recognizing, rewarding, and reinforcing good performance. The dynamic process of CQI includes six basic steps:

1. Researching and identifying system-wide problems
2. Elaborating on the probable causes
3. Listing possible solutions
4. Outlining a plan of corrective action
5. Providing the resources and support needed to ensure the plan's success
6. Reevaluating results continually

Content Review

GUIDELINES FOR QUALITY IMPROVEMENT
- Leadership
- Information and analysis
- Strategic quality planning
- Human resources development and management
- EMS process management
- EMS system results
- Satisfaction of patients and other stakeholders

In general, EMS quality can be divided into two categories: "take-it-for-granted" quality and service quality.

"Take-It-for-Granted" Quality

People must be able to take it for granted that EMS will respond quickly to a 911 call and act at the highest level of **professionalism,** providing care that is safe, appropriate, and the best that is available.

* **professionalism** refers to the conduct or qualities that characterize a practitioner in a particular field or occupation.

When considering a new medication, process, or procedure, we must follow rules before permitting its use in EMS. These rules, often called **rules of evidence,** were developed by Joseph P. Ornato (M.D., Ph.D.). They include the following guidelines:

* **rules of evidence** guidelines for permitting a new medication, process, or procedure to be used in EMS.

- *There must be a theoretical basis for the change.* That is, the change must make sense based on relevant medical science.
- *There must be ample research.* Any device or medication for patient care must be justified by adequate scientific human research.
- *It must be clinically important.* The device, medication, or procedure must make a significant clinical difference to the patient. For example, a defibrillator may mean the difference between living

and dying for some patients, while colour-coordinated stretcher linen has little clinical significance.

- *It must be practical, affordable, and teachable.* Some medical devices remain too expensive and too impractical for use in routine prehospital emergency care.

Another way to accomplish "take-it-for-granted" quality improvement is through the ongoing education of personnel. Paramedics can improve their skills by reading, taking classes, soliciting feedback on clinical performance from receiving hospitals, and following up on patients. **Peer review**—the process of EMS personnel reviewing each other's patient reports, emergency care, and interactions with patients and families—is another way for paramedics to improve their knowledge and skills.

Ethics are the standards that govern the conduct of a group or profession. Prehospital providers at all levels have an ethical responsibility to their patients and to the public. The public expects excellence from the EMS system, and we should accept no less than excellence from ourselves.

Service Quality

In the business world, service quality is called "customer satisfaction." This is the kind of quality that individual customers get excited about, feel good about, and tell stories about. These are the little extras that exceed a customer's expectations and elicit thank-you letters. Prime examples of customer satisfaction include such patient statements as: "You fed my cat before we left." "You remembered my name and introduced me to the nurse." "You held my hand." "You seemed like a friend when I needed one."

Customer satisfaction can be created or destroyed with a simple word or deed. A significant part of the way we communicate with one another is through body language and tone of voice. Paramedics who genuinely care about their patients communicate it in many subtle ways. From the patient's perspective, this is much more important than IVs, backboards, and ECGs.

RESEARCH

The future enhancement of EMS is strongly dependent on the availability of quality research. The current trend of introducing "new and improved" ideas or new high-tech equipment to existing procedures must be evaluated scientifically. Unfortunately, many EMS protocols and procedures in use today have evolved without clinical evidence of usefulness, safety, or benefit to the patient.

One area that will rely heavily on research is funding. EMS systems need to be accountable for their actions and are being required to validate their effectiveness. The Ontario Prehospital Advanced Life Support (OPALS) study is an initiative that is looking at the outcomes of advanced life support (ALS) in Canada. Restrictions on reimbursement will drive the push for quality EMS research. Outcome studies will also be required to justify funding and ensure the future of EMS.

Future EMS research must address the following:

- Which prehospital interventions actually reduce morbidity and mortality?
- Are the benefits of certain field procedures worth the potential risks?
- What is the cost-benefit ratio of sophisticated prehospital equipment and procedures?
- Is field stabilization possible, or should paramedics begin immediate transport in every case?

peer review an evaluation of the quality of emergency care administered by an individual, which is conducted by that individual's peers (others of equal rank). Also, an evaluation of articles submitted for publication.

ethics the rules or standards that govern the conduct of members of a particular group or profession.

Customer satisfaction can be created or destroyed with a simple word or deed.

The future enhancement of EMS is strongly dependent on the availability of quality research.

- Identify a problem, explain the reason for the proposed study, and state the hypothesis or a precise question.
- Identify the body of published knowledge on the subject.
- Select the best design for the study, clearly outline all logistics, examine all patient-consent issues, and get them approved through the appropriate investigational review process.
- Begin the study, and collect raw data.
- Analyze and correlate your data in a statistical application.
- Assess and evaluate the results against the original hypothesis or question.
- Write a concise, comprehensive description of the study for publication in a medical journal.

Current EMS practice must be justified by hard clinical data derived from an objective, valid program of ongoing research. EMS providers at all levels share the responsibility for identifying research opportunities, conducting peer review programs, and publishing the results of their projects. As leaders in the prehospital care environment, paramedics should set an example in the development of and for participation in research projects.

Prehospital research is covered in detail in Appendix B of this volume.

SYSTEM FINANCING

In Canada, a wide variety of EMS system designs are used. As previously discussed, EMS can be provincial or territorial, hospital-based, fire- or police-department based, a municipal service, a private commercial business, a volunteer service, or some combination. Major differences exist in methods of EMS system financing, ranging from fully tax-subsidized municipal or provincial or territorial systems to all-volunteer squads supported solely by contributions.

EMS funding can come from many sources. The most common is fee-for-service revenue, which may be generated from provincial or territorial health insurance plans, private insurance companies, specialty service contracts, or private paying patients. In some cases, funding comes from EMS response fees and funding from either a municipality or a province or territory. Most of these revenue sources are called "third-party payers" because payment comes from someone other than the patient. Reimbursement may also be based on the level of care the patient receives during transport.

Part 3: Roles and Responsibilities of the Paramedic

The roles and responsibilities of the paramedic are dramatically different from the way they were 10 years ago. Today, paramedic emergency care is an enormous responsibility for which you must be mentally, physically, and emotionally prepared. You will be required to have a strong knowledge of **pathophysiology** and of the most current medical technology. You will have to be capable of maintaining a professional attitude while making medical and ethical decisions about severely injured and critically ill patients (Figure 1-4). You will be required to provide not only competent emergency care but also emotional support to your patients and their families.

* **pathophysiology** the study of how disease affects normal body processes.

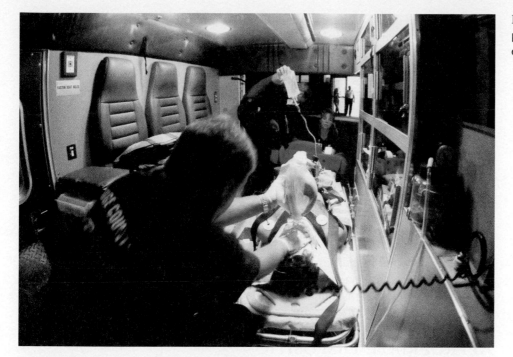

FIGURE 1-4 A paramedic provides emergency medical care to ill and injured patients.

PRIMARY RESPONSIBILITIES

A paramedic's responsibilities include emergency medical care for the patient and a variety of other responsibilities before, during, and after a call.

PREPARATION

Preparation includes making sure that inspection and routine maintenance have been completed on your emergency vehicle and on all equipment. It means re-stocking medications and intravenous solutions and checking their expiration dates. In addition, you must be very familiar with:

- All local EMS protocols, policies, and procedures
- Communications system hardware (radios) and software (frequency utilization and communication protocols)
- Local geography, including populations during peak usage times, and alternative routes during rush hours
- Support agencies, including services available from neighbouring EMS systems and the methods by which efforts and resources are coordinated

RESPONSE

During an emergency response, remember that personal safety is your number-one priority. If your ambulance crashes en route to an incident because of speeding or running red traffic lights, you will be of no benefit to the patient. Always follow basic safety precautions en route to an incident. Wear a seatbelt, obey posted speed limits, and monitor the road for potential hazards.

You must also get to the scene in a timely manner. Make certain you know the correct location of the incident and, en route, request any additional personnel or services that you think may be needed. Don't wait to ask for such assis-

> **Content Review**
>
> **PRIMARY RESPONSIBILITIES**
> - Preparation
> - Response
> - Scene assessment
> - Patient assessment
> - Patient management
> - Disposition and transfer
> - Documentation
> - Cleanup, maintenance, and review

tance after you get to a chaotic scene. Learn to anticipate potential high-risk situations based on dispatch information and experience. For example, if any of the following is reported to be on scene, you may need to call for assistance:

- Multiple patients
- Motor-vehicle collisions
- Hazardous materials
- Rescue situations
- Violent individuals (patients or bystanders)
- Reported use of a weapon
- Knowledge of previous violence

PATIENT ASSESSMENT AND MANAGEMENT

Your primary responsibilities as a paramedic involve scene assessment and primary assessment and management of the patient (Figure 1-5). These topics will be discussed fully in subsequent chapters. Keep in mind that your primary concern is the safety of yourself, your crew, the patient, and bystanders.

APPROPRIATE DISPOSITION

As noted earlier, the mode of transport and the selection of the receiving facility are critical decisions to be made for your patient. For example, you might opt for ground or air transport. You might choose the nearest medical facility or a facility with special treatment capabilities, such as burn care or hyperbaric oxygen therapy.

Most patients request transport to the nearest medical facility. Other patients may ask you to transport them to a facility outside your call area. Even though the requested facility may be appropriate for the patient, there may be an equally appropriate hospital that is closer. Remember, you are responsible for patient care and, therefore, also ultimately responsible for selecting the transport destination. When in doubt, contact online medical direction for advice and support.

In some areas, paramedics have well-defined protocols that allow them to treat patients at the scene and transfer them to facilities other than a hospital. For example, a child cuts his arm on a shard of glass. He has a simple five-centimetre laceration. Instead of transporting the patient to the hospital, using resources that are not needed for this patient, and incurring a costly emergency department fee, the paramedics contact medical direction and request permission to transport the child to a local outpatient centre.

Another type of disposition is "treat and release," in which paramedics assess the patient and provide emergency care. If they determine there is no need for further medical attention, they contact medical direction and request orders not to transport.

One example is treat and release criteria used by Calgary EMS for hypoglycemic and narrow complex tachycardia patients. After treatment, patients are evaluated following specific criteria to determine their suitability for release.

PATIENT TRANSFER

You may be required to provide patient transfer from one facility to another. Often, these transfers are routine. Other times, the transfer may involve unstable patients or patients with special needs. When you are assigned to transport a patient, you share the responsibility—with the receiving and accepting physician—for the treatment and care of the patient. Ensure that you are able to continue or initiate care that the patient requires during transport. If necessary,

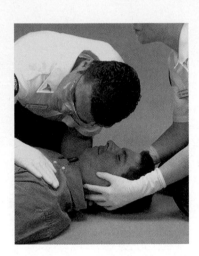

FIGURE 1-5 During the primary assessment of your patient, you will look for and immediately treat any life-threatening conditions.

arrange for a medical escort to manage procedures or equipment that you are not licensed or trained to use. When you are in doubt about the patient's stability for the duration of transport, or about the capabilities of the receiving facility, contact medical direction.

Before removing the patient from a hospital, request a verbal report from the primary care provider (usually a registered nurse or a physician). Request a copy of essential parts of the patient's chart, including a summary of the patient's past and present medical history. However, if the results of diagnostic tests taken at the facility are not ready when you are prepared to leave, do not delay patient transport. The data can be faxed, emailed, or telephoned to the receiving facility.

Your first priority during transport is the patient. If necessary, while en route, contact the receiving facility, and provide them with an estimated time of arrival (ETA) and an update on the patient's condition. On arrival, seek out the contact person (usually a registered nurse or physician). Provide that person with an updated patient report, including any treatment or changes in status while en route. All documents provided by the sending facility should be turned over to the receiving care provider along with a copy of your call report. If required by your service, obtain appropriate billing or insurance information at this time.

DOCUMENTATION

Maintaining a complete and accurate written patient care report is essential to the flow of patient information, to research efforts, and to the quality improvement of your EMS system. Documentation will be discussed in detail in Chapter 9.

RETURNING TO SERVICE

Once you have completed patient care, turned the patient over to the hospital staff, and completed all documentation, immediately prepare to return to service (Figure 1-6). Clean and decontaminate the unit, properly discard disposable materials, restock supplies, and replace and stow away equipment. If necessary, refuel the unit on the way back to your station or post. Review the call with crewmembers, including any problems that may have occurred. Such a dialogue can lead to solutions that enhance the delivery of quality patient care. Finally, the paramedic team leader should check crewmembers for signs of critical incident stress and assist anyone who needs help.

ADDITIONAL RESPONSIBILITIES

The role of the paramedic involves duties in addition to those associated with emergency response. They may include training civilians in CPR, EMS demonstrations and seminars, teaching first-aid classes, organizing prevention programs, and engaging in professional development activities. All involve taking an active role in promoting positive health practices in your community.

COMMUNITY INVOLVEMENT

Prehospital providers should take the lead in helping the public learn how to recognize an emergency, how to provide basic life support (BLS), and how to properly access the EMS system. A successful effort can save lives. Providing educational programs can also encourage positive health practices in the community. The SMARTRISK program founded in 1992 by pediatrician Dr. Robert Conn has become one of the leading injury-prevention groups in Canada, and it enjoys international recognition and support. SMARTRISK is a national non-

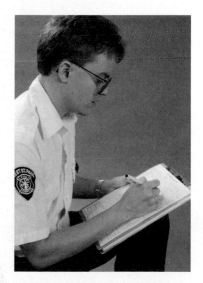

FIGURE 1-6 A paramedic's responsibility does not end with delivering the patient to the emergency department. Documentation, restocking, and a call critique are as important as the call itself.

profit organization dedicated to preventing injuries and saving lives. The five key messages of SMARTRISK are Buckle Up, Drive Sober, Look First, Wear the Gear, and Get Trained. This program provides an opportunity for paramedics to provide injury-prevention training within the community.

To decide what injury-prevention projects need to be developed in a community, EMS systems often conduct illness- and injury-risk surveys. For example, an EMS service reviews call reports for a six-month period and finds they responded to 10 vehicle collisions at railroad crossings. A public safety campaign directed at the safe crossing of railroad tracks may be appropriate. Once an EMS service has identified a problem and target audience, they should seek community agencies—including the local political structure—to assist in the development, promotion, and delivery of the campaign.

Additional benefits of community involvement are the following: It enhances the visibility of EMS, promotes a positive image, and puts forth EMS personnel as positive role models. It also creates opportunities to improve the integration of EMS with other health-care and public safety agencies through cooperative programs.

COST CONTAINMENT

Promoting wellness and preventing illness and injury will be important components of EMS in the future. Some systems have already begun to direct resources toward the development of prevention and wellness programs that decrease the need for emergency services. The theory is that the cost of the services provided to the community will decrease if the burden on the system is decreased.

One strategy is to establish protocols that specify the mode of transportation for nonemergency patients. Some systems already operate vans rather than ambulances to transport such patients to and from nursing facilities or from their residences to a doctor's office. Though an additional expense to the system, this service reduces emergency equipment costs and the demand for emergency personnel. The result is a decrease in the overall operating expense.

Another strategy being used in many areas of the country is having EMS and hospitals team up to provide an alternative to the emergency department. They transport patients to freestanding outpatient centres or clinics, which ultimately reduces the cost of care to the patient and the system. The development of such alliances will undoubtedly continue. However, caution should be taken to ensure that the patient always receives the appropriate emergency care based on need, not cost.

CITIZEN INVOLVEMENT IN EMS

Citizen involvement in EMS helps give "insiders" an outside, objective view of quality improvement and problem resolution. Whenever possible, members of the community should be used in the development, evaluation, and regulation of the EMS system. When considering the addition of a new service or the enhancement of an existing one, community members should help establish what is needed. After all, they are your "customers," and their needs are your priority.

PROFESSIONALISM

The word profession *refers to a specialized body of knowledge or skills.*

⚷

A paramedic is a member of the health-care professions. The word *profession* refers to a specialized body of knowledge or skills. Generally self-regulating, a profession will have recognized standards, including requirements for initial and ongoing education. When you have satisfied the initial education requirements as a paramedic, you may then be either certified or licensed. The EMS profession has regulations that ensure that members maintain standards. For the paramedic, these regulations come in the form of periodic recertification with a specified amount of continuing education time.

The term *professionalism* refers to the conduct or qualities that characterize a practitioner in a particular field. Health-care professionals promote quality patient care and pride in their profession, setting and striving for the highest standards and earning the respect of team members and the public. Attaining professionalism requires an understanding of what distinguishes the professional from the nonprofessional.

PROFESSIONAL ATTITUDES

A commitment to excellence is a daily activity. While on duty, health-care professionals place their patients first; nonprofessionals place their egos first. True professionals establish excellence as their goal and never allow themselves to become complacent about their performance. They practise their skills to the point of mastery and then keep practising them to stay sharp and to improve. They also take refresher courses seriously because they know they have forgotten some things and because they are eager for new information. Nonprofessionals believe their skills will never fade.

Professionals set high standards for themselves, their crew, their agency, and their system. Nonprofessionals aim for the minimum standard and can be counted on to take the path of least resistance. Professionals critically review their performance, always seeking ways to improve. Nonprofessionals look to protect themselves, hide their inadequacies, and place blame on others. Professionals check out all equipment before the emergency response. Nonprofessionals hope that everything will work, supplies will be in place, batteries will be charged, and oxygen levels will be adequate.

A professional paramedic is responsible for acting in a professional manner both on and off duty. Remember, the community you serve will judge other EMS providers, the service you work for, and the EMS profession as a whole by your actions.

Professionalism is an attitude, not a matter of pay. It cannot be bought, rented, or faked. Although it is a young profession, EMS has achieved recognition as a bona fide **allied health profession**. This gain in professional stature is the result of many hard-working, caring individuals who refused to compromise their standards. Always strive to maintain that level of performance and commitment.

PROFESSIONAL ATTRIBUTES

Leadership

Leadership is an important but often forgotten aspect of paramedic training. Paramedics are the prehospital team leaders (Figure 1-7). They must develop a leadership style that suits their personalities and gets the job done. Although there are many successful styles of leadership, certain characteristics are common to all great leaders:

- Self-confidence
- Established credibility
- Inner strength
- Ability to remain in control
- Ability to communicate
- Willingness to make a decision
- Willingness to accept responsibility for the consequences of the team's actions

A commitment to excellence is a daily activity.

A professional paramedic is responsible for acting in a professional manner both on and off duty.

✱ **allied health professions** ancillary health-care professions, apart from physicians and nurses.

Content Review

PROFESSIONAL ATTRIBUTES
- Leadership
- Integrity
- Empathy
- Self-motivation
- Professional appearance and hygiene
- Self-confidence
- Communication skills
- Time management skills
- Diplomacy and teamwork
- Respect
- Patient advocacy
- Careful delivery of service

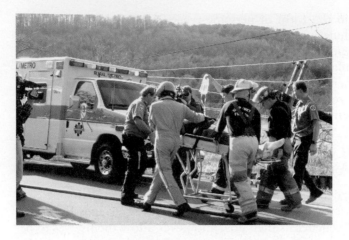

FIGURE 1-7 As the leader of the EMS team, the paramedic must interact with patients, bystanders, and other rescue personnel in a professional and efficient manner.

The successful team leader knows the members of the crew, including each one's capabilities and limitations. Ask crewmembers to do something beyond their capabilities and they will question your ability to lead, not their ability to perform.

Integrity

The patient and other members of the health-care team assume that you, as a paramedic, have integrity. The single most important behaviour that you will be judged by is honesty. Your work will often put you in the patient's home or in charge of the patient's wallet and other personal possessions, such as jewellery and items left in a vehicle. You must be trustworthy. The easiest way to lose respect is to be dishonest. Additionally, in acting as an agent of the medical director, you are entrusted with carefully following protocols, providing the best possible care, and accurately documenting it.

Empathy

One of the most important components of successful interaction with a patient and family is empathy. To have empathy is to identify with and understand the circumstances, feelings, and motives of others. As a professional, you will often have to place your own feelings aside to deal with others, even when you are having a bad day. Paramedics who act in a professional manner can show empathy by:

- Being supportive and reassuring
- Demonstrating an understanding of the patient's feelings and the feelings of the family
- Demonstrating respect for others
- Having a calm, compassionate, and helpful demeanour

Self-Motivation

You will often work without direct supervision, and so it is up to you to be able to motivate yourself and establish a positive work ethic. Ways to create a positive work ethic are the following:

- Completing assigned duties without being asked or told to do so
- Completing all duties and assignments without the need for direct supervision

- Correctly completing all paperwork in a timely manner
- Demonstrating a commitment to continuous quality improvement
- Accepting constructive feedback in a positive manner
- Taking advantage of learning opportunities

Appearance and Personal Hygiene

From the moment you arrive at the scene of an emergency, you are judged by the way you present yourself. Good appearance and personal hygiene are critical. If you have a sloppy appearance, your patient may suspect that your medical care will be sloppy, too. Slangy, foul, abusive, or off-colour language is not acceptable and will alienate you from your patients. Your appearance, as well as your behaviour, is vital to establishing credibility and instilling confidence.

From the moment you arrive at the scene of an emergency, you are judged by the way you present yourself.

Always wear a clean, pressed uniform. Multiple pagers, holsters with tape hanging from them, or rubber gloves pulled through a belt loop simply do not give you a professional appearance. Also, avoid wearing an abundance of patches and pins on your uniform. Remember that it is the care you provide, not the patches and pins you wear, that will impress the patient. Keep hair off the collar. If facial hair is allowed, keep it neat and trimmed. A light-coloured T-shirt that closely matches the uniform shirt colour may be worn under your uniform shirt, which should be buttoned up, with only the top collar button open. Wearing jewellery, other than a wedding ring, a watch, or small plain earrings for a female, is unprofessional. Long fingernails that have the potential to puncture protective gloves also should be avoided.

Your appearance, as well as your behaviour, is vital to establishing credibility and instilling confidence.

Self-Confidence

The patient and family will not trust you if they sense you do not trust yourself. A lack of self-confidence shows and is the basis of many lawsuits. The easiest way to gain self-confidence is to accurately assess your strengths and limitations, and then seek every opportunity to improve any weaknesses. Also, keep in mind that self-confidence does not equal cockiness. When a self-confident paramedic is presented with a complex situation, he will ask for assistance.

The easiest way to gain self-confidence is to accurately assess your strengths and limitations, and then seek every opportunity to improve any weaknesses.

Communication

Communication is a skill often underestimated in EMS. Providing emergency care in the prehospital environment requires constant communication with the patient, the family, and bystanders, as well as with other EMS providers, dispatch, medical control, and rescuers from other public agencies. Communication skills are discussed in detail in later chapters.

Time Management

The experienced paramedic who plans, prioritizes tasks, and organizes them to make maximum use of time will generally be more effective in the field. A paramedic with good time-management skills is punctual for shifts and meetings and completes such tasks as paperwork and maintenance duties on or ahead of schedule.

The experienced paramedic who plans, prioritizes tasks, and organizes them to make maximum use of time will generally be more effective in the field.

Some simple time-management techniques that you can use are making lists, prioritizing tasks, arriving at meetings or appointments early, and keeping a personal calendar. By implementing just one or two of these techniques, you may find your schedule is more manageable and less stressful.

Teamwork and Diplomacy

The paramedic is a leader. Leadership implies the ability to work with other people—to foster teamwork. Teamwork requires diplomacy, or tact and skill in dealing with people, even when you are under siege from the patient or family. Diplomacy requires paramedics to place the interests of the patient or team ahead of their own interests. It means listening to others, respecting their opinions, and being open-minded and flexible when it comes to change. A strong leader of any team realizes that success requires the support of all team members. A confident leader will:

- Place the success of the team ahead of personal self-interests
- Never undermine the role or opinion of another team member
- Provide support for members of the team, both on and off duty
- Remain open to suggestions from team members and be willing to change for the benefit of the patient
- Openly communicate with everyone
- Above all, respect the patient, other care providers, and the community he serves

Respect

To respect others is to show—and feel—deferential regard, consideration, and appreciation for them. A paramedic respects all patients and provides the best possible care to all of them, no matter what their race, religion, sex, age, or economic condition. Showing that you care for a patient's or family member's feelings, being polite, and avoiding the use of demeaning or derogatory language toward even the most difficult patients are simple ways to demonstrate respect.

Patient Advocacy

A paramedic is an advocate for patients, defending them, protecting them, and acting in their best interests. As a health-care professional, you are expected to look beyond the immediate presentation of your patient. Often, paramedics are the only ones in the health-care chain who see patients in their home settings. You play a role in identifying situations in which patients require assistance, such as possible child abuse, elder abuse, inability to cope, or assault. Know what community resources are available and what policies are in place for identifying and intervening in these types of situations. Except in cases in which your safety is threatened, you should always place the needs of your patient above your own.

Careful Delivery of Service

Professionalism requires the paramedic to deliver the highest quality of patient care with very close attention to detail. Examples of behaviours that demonstrate a careful delivery of service include:
- Mastering and refreshing skills
- Performing complete equipment checks
- Operating the ambulance carefully and safely
- Following policies, procedures, and protocols

CONTINUING EDUCATION AND PROFESSIONAL DEVELOPMENT

Only through continuing education and recertification can the public be assured that quality patient care is being delivered consistently. After you are certified or licensed, you have an important responsibility to continue your personal and professional development. Remember, everyone is subject to the erosion of knowledge and skills over time. Use this as a rule of thumb: As the volume of calls decreases, training should correspondingly increase. Refresher requirements and courses vary across Canada, but the goal is the same: to review previously learned materials and to receive new information.

Since EMS is a relatively young profession, new technology and data emerge rapidly. Make a conscious effort to keep up. A variety of journals, seminars, computer newsgroups, and learning experiences are available to help. So are professional EMS organizations at the local, provincial or territorial, and national levels. Additionally, by participating in activities designed to address work-related issues—such as case reviews and other quality improvement activities, mentoring programs, research projects, multiple-casualty incident drills, in-hospital rotations, equipment in-services, refresher courses, and self-study exercises—you can expect substantial career growth.

> *The paramedic must continually strive to stay abreast of changes in EMS.*

Part 4: The Well-Being of the Paramedic

Well-being, or wellness, is a fundamental aspect of top-notch performance in EMS. It includes your physical well-being as well as your mental and emotional well-being.

This section discusses the many elements of well-being. If you listen now and enhance your knowledge later, you stand a good chance of enjoying a long and rewarding career of helping others—all because you helped yourself.

> *Well-being is a fundamental aspect of top-notch performance.*

BASIC PHYSICAL FITNESS

The benefits of achieving acceptable physical fitness are well known. They include a decreased resting heart rate and blood pressure, increased oxygen-carrying capacity, increased muscle mass and metabolism, and increased resistance to illness and injury. Quality of life is enhanced, as is self-image. Other benefits are improved mental outlook, reduced anxiety levels, and enhanced ability to maintain sound motor skills throughout life.

CORE ELEMENTS

Core elements of physical fitness are cardiovascular endurance (aerobic capacity), muscular strength, and flexibility. Like a three-legged stool, if any one of the three is deficient, the whole becomes unstable. Each is equally important.

Be careful about plunging into a well-intentioned effort to get in shape. For example, before starting an exercise or stretching regimen, it can be helpful to measure your current state of fitness. There are various methods of assessing the three core elements of fitness. Many EMS agencies have access to facilities where precise assessment methods—with trained personnel—are available. Take advantage of any information available to you.

Content Review

BASICS OF PHYSICAL FITNESS

- Cardiovascular endurance
- Strength and flexibility
- Nutrition and weight control
- Disease prevention
- Freedom from harmful habits and addictions
- Back safety

Muscular strength is achieved with regular exercise that may be isometric or isotonic. **Isometric exercise** is active exercise performed against stable resistance, in which muscles are exercised in a motionless manner. **Isotonic exercise** is active exercise during which muscles are worked through their range of motion. Weight lifting is an obvious way to achieve muscular strength, and it is excellent all-around training for the body. Rotate among training the muscles of your upper body and shoulders, chest and back, and lower body. Do abdominal exercises daily. Take time to get in-depth information about the best approach from a trainer or other knowledgeable person.

Cardiovascular endurance results from exercising at least three days a week vigorously enough to raise your pulse to its target heart rate (Table 1-1). There is no need to become a marathon runner to gain aerobic capacity. Try a brisk walk, or ride a stationary bike while watching TV. Make it a daily habit. Even modest exercise helps. Walking briskly from the outer reaches of the employee parking lot, using stairs whenever possible, and playing actively with your children can all count toward physical fitness.

Flexibility seems to be the forgotten element of fitness. Without an adequate range of motion, your joints and muscles cannot be used efficiently or safely. A body builder with tight hamstrings may be as much at risk for a back injury as anyone else. To achieve (or regain) flexibility, stretch the main muscle groups regularly. Try to stretch daily. Never bounce when stretching; this causes microtears in muscle and connective tissues. Hold a stretch for at least 60 seconds. A side benefit of good flexibility is prevention or reduction of back pain. Stretching is an excellent TV-time activity. If you are interested, consider studying yoga.

NUTRITION

Good nutrition is fundamental to your well-being because your food is your fuel. So, in addition to eating balanced meals, you must also eat in moderation and limit fat consumption. *Canada's Food Guide to Healthy Eating* includes the dietary guidelines from the Nutrition Recommendations (1990). One key to eating well is to learn the major food groups and eat a variety of foods from them daily:

- *Grain products*. 5 to 12 servings per day, for complex carbohydrates, B vitamins, and fibre. Choose whole grain and enriched products more often.
- *Vegetables and fruit*. 5 to 10 servings per day, for iron, vitamins A and C, and folate, potassium, and fibre. Chose dark green and orange vegetables and orange fruit more often.

Table 1-1	FINDING YOUR TARGET HEART RATE

1. Measure your resting heart rate. (You will use this number later.)
2. Subtract your age from 220. This total is your estimated maximum heart rate.
3. Subtract your resting heart rate from your maximum heart rate, and multiply that figure by 0.7.
4. Add the figure you just calculated to your resting heart rate.

EXAMPLE: In a 44-year-old woman whose resting heart rate is 52, maximum heart rate would be 176 (220 – 44). Maximum heart rate minus resting heart rate is 124 (176 – 52). Multiply 124 by 0.7 for a value of 86.8. Resting heart rate plus the calculated figure is 138.8 (52 + 86.8). Rounded up, this person's target heart rate is 140 beats per minute.

- *Milk products.* Adults, 3 to 4 servings per day, for calcium, protein, and vitamins A and D. Choose lower-fat milk products more often.
- *Meat and alternatives.* 2 to 3 servings per day, for protein, zinc, iron, and B vitamins. Choose leaner meats, poultry, and fish, as well as dried peas, beans, and lentils more often.

Avoid or minimize intake of fat, salt, sugar, cholesterol, and caffeine. For example, you can avoid a dose of fat by eating lean instead of marbled meat. An apple is far more nutritious than a slice of apple pie. In general, aim for a diet that is approximately 40 percent carbohydrates, 40 percent protein, and 20 percent fat. Food portions also have a significant impact on body weight. Even a well-planned, healthy diet can result in weight gain if the portions are too large. Note that snacking is a weight-gain trap. Plan to eat low-calorie snacks, and buy them *before* you get hungry. Food labels (Figure 1-8) contain abundant information about nutritional content. Learn to read them. Standardization of food labels has made this easier. Be sure to check the serving size to avoid misinterpreting the food's overall nutritional value.

The servings noted above are guidelines and may vary depending on your age, body size, and activity level, and whether you are male or female. For those who are younger and very active, the higher recommended serving numbers may be appropriate. If you are older and less active, the lower serving numbers may be appropriate for you.

Eating on the call, as EMS providers must often do, can be less detrimental if you plan ahead and carry a small cooler filled with whole-grain sandwiches, cut vegetables, fruit, and other wholesome foods. If you must buy food, stop at a local market instead of the fast-food place next door. Buy fresh fruit, yogurt, and sensible deli selections. They are more nutritious and much cheaper than fast foods. Monitor your fluid intake. Your body needs plenty of fluids to flush food through your system and eliminate toxins. Fill a "go-cup" with fresh ice water when you stop by the emergency department instead of spending your money on soft drinks.

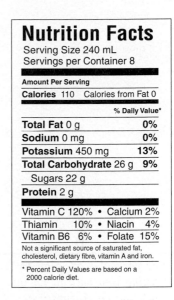

FIGURE 1-8 Example of a standardized food label.

PREVENTING CANCER AND CARDIOVASCULAR DISEASE

Exercising and eating well can help prevent both cancer and cardiovascular disease. Although for the typically youthful EMS provider, the likelihood of being hit by either of these diseases seems remote, it happens. You can do a lot to prevent it. Minimizing stress through healthy stress management practices, for example, can work wonders. In addition, assess yourself and your family history.

Exercise will improve cardiovascular endurance, help lower blood pressure, and tip the balance of your body composition favourably—all good measures against cardiovascular disease. Know your cholesterol and triglyceride levels, and keep them in check. For women who are menopausal, be informed about the risks and benefits of using hormone replacement therapy (particularly estrogen). Diet can also do much to minimize the chances of getting certain cancers. Certain foods, such as broccoli and high-fibre foods, can help reduce the incidence of cancer; others, such as charcoal-cooked foods, can increase it. The connection between sun exposure and skin cancer is well known. Use sunblock and wear sunglasses and a hat when you can. Watch out for the warning signs of cancer, such as blood in the stools (even in young people, especially men), a changing mole, unexplained weight loss, unexplained chronic fatigue, and lumps. Be sure to include appropriate periodic risk-assessment screening and self-examination habits in your personal well-being program. That includes tests like mammograms or prostate exams as you age.

HABITS AND ADDICTIONS

Many people who work in high-stress jobs overuse and abuse such substances as caffeine and nicotine. These bad habits are rampant in EMS. Each can contribute to such long-term diseases as cancer and cardiovascular disease. Choose a healthier lifestyle, and avoid overindulging in these and other harmful substances, such as alcohol. For example, smoking cessation programs are usually easily found locally or on the internet. Whatever it takes, the message is clear: get free of addictions, particularly those that threaten your well-being. Substance abuse programs, nicotine patches, 12-step groups—all exist to help you help yourself. But the first step has to be yours.

BACK SAFETY

EMS is physically demanding. Of the host of movements needed (scrambling down embankments, climbing ladders or trees, squeezing into narrow spaces, and so on), none will be more frequent than lifting and carrying equipment and patients. To avoid back injury, you must keep your back fit for the work you do. You also must use proper lifting techniques each time you pick up a load, whether the load is heavy or light.

Back fitness begins with conditioning the muscles that support the spinal column. These are the guy wires that stabilize the spine, much the way cables help keep telephone poles upright. Note that the muscles of the abdomen are also crucial to overall spinal-column strength and safe lifting. Never perform old-fashioned situps. They can seriously strain your lumbar spine. Instead, use abdominal crunches, which target only the stomach muscles. Consult an exercise coach or trainer for specifics.

Pay particular attention to keeping your back fit for the work you do. Always use the proper techniques for lifting and moving patients and equipment.

Correct posture will minimize the risk of back injury (Figures 1-9A and 1-9B). Good nutrition helps maintain healthy connective tissue and intervertebral discs. Excess weight contributes to disc deterioration. So does smoking. Thus, proper weight management and smoking cessation are relevant to back health. Finally, adequate rest gives the spine non-weight-bearing time to nourish discs and repair itself.

Proper lifting techniques should ideally be taught by and practised with a trainer who understands the variety of challenges faced by EMS providers. Important principles of lifting are as follows:

- Move a load only if you can safely handle it.
- Ask for help when you need it—for *any* reason.
- Position the load as close to your body and centre of gravity as possible.
- Keep your palms up whenever possible.
- Do not hurry. Take the time you need to establish good footing and balance. Keep a wide base of support with one foot ahead of the other.
- Bend your knees, lower your buttocks, and keep your chin up. If your knees are bad, do not bend them more than 90 degrees.
- "Lock in" the spine with a slight extension curve, and tighten the abdominal muscles to support spinal positioning.
- Always avoid twisting and turning.
- Let the large leg muscles do the work of lifting, not your back.
- Exhale during the lift. Do not hold your breath.
- Given a choice, push. Do not pull.

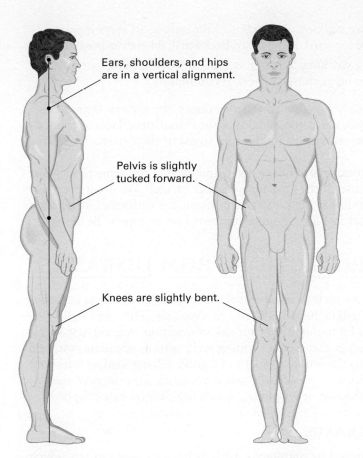

Ears, shoulders, and hips are in a vertical alignment.

Pelvis is slightly tucked forward.

Knees are slightly bent.

FIGURE 1-9A Correct standing posture.

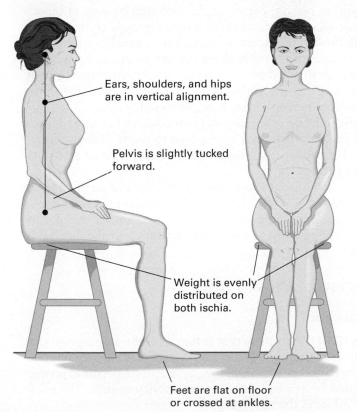

Ears, shoulders, and hips are in vertical alignment.

Pelvis is slightly tucked forward.

Weight is evenly distributed on both ischia.

Feet are flat on floor or crossed at ankles.

FIGURE 1-9B Correct sitting posture. Note the straight line from ear through shoulder and hip and from knee to arch of foot.

- Look where you are walking or crawling. Take only short steps if you are walking. Move forward, rather than backward, whenever possible.
- When rescuers are working together as a team to lift a load, only one person should be in charge of verbal commands.

Heed your own body's signals. You are stronger some days than others. Know when you are physically depleted because of exhaustion, lack of food, or minor illness. Use volunteers wisely, and be sure to ask if their backs are strong enough for the job.

Never reach for an item, or attempt to lift it, and twist at the same time. Most back injuries occur because of the cumulative effect of such low-level everyday stresses. Everything you do for back safety can mean the difference between a long and rewarding career in EMS and one shortened by an injury. Be careful!

PERSONAL PROTECTION FROM DISEASE

Treat all blood and other body fluids as if they are infectious, and take appropriate body substance isolation (BSI) precautions whenever you treat a patient.

In recent years the emphasis on infection control has focused on the most devastating diseases, such as HIV/AIDS, hepatitis B, and tuberculosis (TB)—and rightly so. Fortunately, you can do a lot to minimize your risk of infection. A good first step is to do the things promoted in this chapter. Eating well, getting adequate rest, and managing stress are among the building blocks of a good defence against infection. In addition, it is a good idea to periodically assess your risk for infection, such as noticing when you are rundown or when your hands are dangerously chapped.

INFECTIOUS DISEASES

✱ **infectious disease** any disease caused by the growth of pathogenic microorganisms, which may be spread from person to person.

Infectious diseases are caused by **pathogens,** such as bacteria and viruses, which may be spread from person to person. For example, infection by way of bloodborne pathogens can occur when the blood of an infected person comes in contact with another person's broken skin (cuts, sores, chapped hands) or by way of parenteral contact (stick by a needle or other sharp object). Infection by airborne pathogens can occur when an infected person sneezes or coughs, causing body fluids in the form of tiny droplets to be inhaled or to come in contact with the mucous membranes of another person's eyes, nose, or mouth.

✱ **pathogens** microorganisms capable of producing disease, such as bacteria and viruses.

HIV/AIDS, hepatitis B, and TB are diseases of great concern because they are life threatening. However, a paramedic can be exposed to many different infectious diseases. See Table 1-2 for some common ones, their modes of transmission, and their **incubation periods.**

✱ **incubation period** the time between contact with a disease organism and the appearance of the first symptoms.

Even when someone is carrying pathogens for disease, signs of an illness may not be apparent. For this reason, *you must consider the blood and body fluids of every patient you treat as infectious.* Safeguards against infection are mandatory for all medical personnel. They involve a form of infection control called body substance isolation (BSI).

✱ **body substance isolation (BSI)** a strict form of infection control that is based on the assumption that all blood and other body fluids are infectious.

INFECTION-CONTROL PRACTICES

Body Substance Isolation

✱ **personal protective equipment (PPE)** equipment used by EMS personnel to protect against injury and the spread of infectious disease.

Body substance isolation (BSI) is a strategy that is based on the assumption that all blood and body fluids are infectious. It dictates that all EMS personnel take BSI precautions with every patient. To achieve this, appropriate **personal protective equipment (PPE)** should be available in every emergency vehicle. The minimum recommended PPE includes the following:

- *Protective gloves.* Wear disposable protective gloves before initiating any emergency care. When an emergency involves more than one

Table 1-2 COMMON INFECTIOUS DISEASES

Disease	Mode of Transmission	Incubation Period
AIDS (acquired immune deficiency syndrome)	AIDS- or HIV-infected blood via intravenous drug use, semen and vaginal fluids, blood transfusions, or (rarely) needle sticks; mothers also may pass HIV to their unborn children	Several months or years
Hepatitis B, C	Blood, stool, or other body fluids, or contaminated objects.	Weeks or months
Tuberculosis	Respiratory secretions, airborne or on contaminated objects	2 to 6 weeks
Meningitis, bacterial	Oral and nasal secretions	2 to 10 days
Pneumonia, bacterial and viral	Oral and nasal droplets and secretions	Several days
Influenza	Airborne droplets or direct contact with body fluids	1 to 3 days
Staphylococcal skin infections	Contact with open wounds or sores or contaminated objects	Several days
Chicken pox (varicella)	Airborne droplets, or contact with open sores	11 to 21 days
German measles (rubella)	Airborne droplets; mothers may pass it to unborn children	10 to 12 days
Whooping cough (pertussis)	Respiratory secretions or airborne droplets	6 to 20 days
SARS (severe acute respiratory syndrome)	Body fluids and droplets	3 to 7 days

patient, change gloves between patients. When gloves have been contaminated, remove and dispose of them properly as soon as possible (Figures 1-10A and 1-10B).

- *Masks and protective eyewear.* These should be worn together whenever blood or body fluid spatter is likely to occur, such as with arterial bleeding, childbirth, endotracheal intubation and other invasive procedures, oral suctioning, and cleanup of equipment that requires heavy scrubbing or brushing. Both you and your patient should wear masks whenever the potential for airborne transmission of disease exists.

- *HEPA and N-95 respirators.* Due to the resurgence of TB and the emergence of SARS, you must protect yourself from infection by using a high-efficiency particulate air (HEPA) or N-95 respirator. Wear one whenever you care for a patient with confirmed or suspected TB or SARS, especially during procedures that involve the airway, such as the administration of nebulized medications, endotracheal intubation, or suctioning.

- *Gowns.* Disposable gowns protect your clothing from splashes. If large splashes of blood are expected, such as with childbirth, wear an impervious gown.

- *Resuscitation equipment.* Use disposable resuscitation equipment as your primary means of artificial ventilation in emergency care.

These garments and equipment will assist you in achieving, to the extent possible, the universal precautions recommended by the Health Canada and the Laboratory Centre for Disease Control (LCDC). BSI precautions also include handwashing and the proper cleaning, disinfection, or sterilization of equipment.

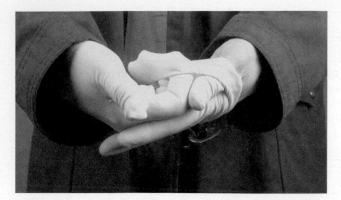

FIGURE 1-10A   To remove gloves, first hook the gloved fingers of one hand under the cuff of the other glove. Then pull that glove off without letting your gloved fingers come in contact with bare skin.

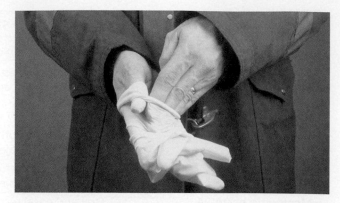

FIGURE 1-10B   Then slide the fingers of the ungloved hand under the remaining glove's cuff. Push that glove off, being careful not to touch the glove's exterior with your bare hand.

Content Review

HANDWASHING
- Lather with soap and water.
- Scrub for at least 15 seconds.
- Rinse under running water.
- Dry on a clean towel.

The transfer of infectious disease is also minimized through the use of appropriate work practices and equipment especially engineered to minimize risk. For example, use disposable invasive equipment once, and then dispose of it properly. Launder reusable clothing with infection control in mind.

Probably the most important infection-control practice is handwashing as soon as possible after every patient contact and decontamination procedure. First, remove any rings or jewellery from your hands and arms. Lather your hands vigorously front and back, for at least 15 seconds up to 5 to 8 cm above the wrist. Lather and rub between your fingers and in the creases and cracks of your knuckles. Scrub under and around the fingernails with a brush. Rinse well under running water, holding your hands downward so that the water drains off your fingertips. (Surgeons hold hands upward so water drains toward the elbow. This is to protect the patient; however, it is not required in handwashing after patient contact.) Dry your hands on a clean towel. Plain soap works perfectly well for handwashing. When soap is not available, use an antimicrobial handwashing solution or an alcohol-based foam or towelette.

Vaccinations and Screening Tests

Immunizations against many illnesses are available. Get them. Your EMS system may make many immunizations mandatory. Even nuisance illnesses can be avoided if you get vaccinated. Immunizations are available for rubella (German measles), measles, mumps, chicken pox, and other childhood diseases, as well as for tetanus/diphtheria, poliomyelitis, influenza, hepatitis B, and Lyme disease. Some, such as tetanus, may require booster shots periodically, so monitor your personal medical history well. Also, arrange for regular TB screenings.

Decontamination of Equipment

Any personal protective equipment (PPE) designed for a single use should be properly disposed of after use. The same is true of medical devices designed for a single use. Such materials should be discarded in a red bag marked with a biohazard seal (Figure 1-11). Needles and other sharp objects should be discarded in properly labelled, puncture-proof containers. Containers should be disposed of according to local guidelines.

Nondisposable equipment that has been contaminated must be cleaned, disinfected, or sterilized:

- **Cleaning** refers to washing an object with soap and water. After caring for a patient, wash down your work areas with approved soaps. Throw away single-use cleaning supplies in a proper biohazard container.
- **Disinfecting** includes cleaning with a disinfecting agent, which should kill many microorganisms on the surface of an object. Disinfect equipment that had direct contact with the intact skin of a patient, such as backboards and splints. Use a commercial disinfectant or bleach diluted in water (1 part bleach to 100 parts water, or follow local guidelines).
- **Sterilizing** is the use of a chemical, or a physical method—such as pressurized steam—to kill all microorganisms on an object. Items that were inserted into the patient's body (a laryngoscope blade, for example) should be sterilized by heat, steam, or radiation. There are also approved solutions for sterilization.

If your equipment needs more extensive cleaning, bag it, and remove it to an area designated for this purpose. Disposable work gloves worn during cleaning and decontamination should be properly discarded. If your clothing has become contaminated, bag the items, and wash them in accordance with local guidelines. After removing contaminated clothing, take a shower before dressing again.

Postexposure Procedures

By definition, an **exposure** is any occurrence of blood or body fluids coming in contact with nonintact skin, the eyes, or other mucous membranes, or parenteral contact (needle stick). In most areas, an EMS provider who has had an exposure should (Figure 1-12) do the following:

- Immediately wash the affected area with soap and water.
- Get a medical evaluation.
- Take the proper immunization boosters.
- Notify the agency's infection-control liaison.
- Document the circumstances surrounding the exposure, including the actions taken to reduce chances of infection.

In general, the EMS provider should cooperate with the incident investigation and comply with all required reporting responsibilities and time frames.

✱ **cleaning** washing an object with such cleaners as soap and water.

✱ **disinfecting** cleaning with an agent that can kill some microorganisms on the surface of an object.

✱ **sterilizing** use of a chemical or physical method, such as pressurized steam, to kill all microorganisms on an object.

✱ **exposure** any occurrence of blood or body fluids coming in contact with nonintact skin, mucous membranes, or parenteral contact (needle stick).

Follow your EMS system guidelines on all management and documentation of any exposure to a patient's blood or body fluids.

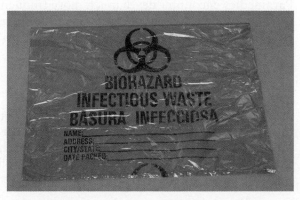

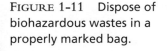

FIGURE 1-11 Dispose of biohazardous wastes in a properly marked bag.

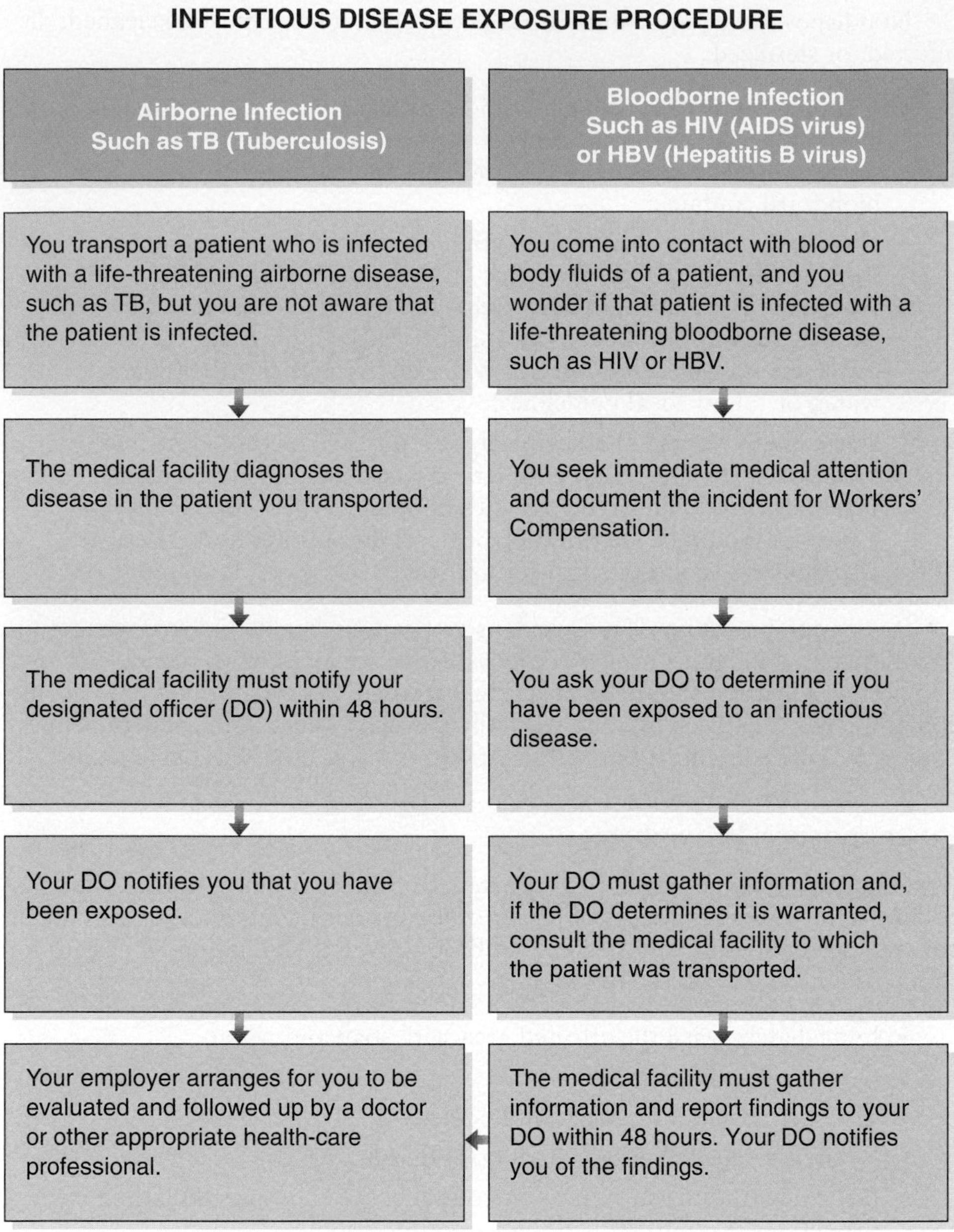

Figure 1-12 An American federal regulation, called the Ryan White Comprehensive AIDS Resources Emergency (CARE) Act, outlines procedures to follow after an occupational exposure to HIV, hepatitis B, diphtheria, meningitis, plague, hemorrhagic fever, rabies, or TB. In Canada, a similar law is being considered but has not yet been enacted.

INFECTIOUS DISEASE EXPOSURE PROCEDURE

Airborne Infection Such as TB (Tuberculosis)	Bloodborne Infection Such as HIV (AIDS virus) or HBV (Hepatitis B virus)
You transport a patient who is infected with a life-threatening airborne disease, such as TB, but you are not aware that the patient is infected.	You come into contact with blood or body fluids of a patient, and you wonder if that patient is infected with a life-threatening bloodborne disease, such as HIV or HBV.
The medical facility diagnoses the disease in the patient you transported.	You seek immediate medical attention and document the incident for Workers' Compensation.
The medical facility must notify your designated officer (DO) within 48 hours.	You ask your DO to determine if you have been exposed to an infectious disease.
Your DO notifies you that you have been exposed.	Your DO must gather information and, if the DO determines it is warranted, consult the medical facility to which the patient was transported.
Your employer arranges for you to be evaluated and followed up by a doctor or other appropriate health-care professional.	The medical facility must gather information and report findings to your DO within 48 hours. Your DO notifies you of the findings.

DEATH AND DYING

Paramedics encounter death much more frequently than most other people do. They often see it as it happens. These encounters can lead to a sense of cumulative overload, which the paramedic needs to recognize and deal with in a healthy manner.

LOSS, GRIEF, AND MOURNING

A longstanding taboo against discussing death and dying changed when grief pioneer Elisabeth Kübler-Ross braved the backlash to meet with terminally ill hospital patients to discuss their feelings about death and dying. Before then, it was assumed that dying people did not want to talk about the experience. What Kübler-Ross learned is that there are five predictable stages of loss:

- *Denial, or "not me."* This is the inability or refusal to believe the reality of the event. It is a defence mechanism, during which the patient puts off dealing with the inevitable end of life.
- *Anger, or "why me?"* The patient's anger is really frustration related to his inability to control the situation. That anger can focus on anyone or anything.
- *Bargaining, or "okay, but first let me..."* In the patient's mind, he tries to make a deal to buy additional time to put off or change the expected outcome.
- *Depression, or "okay, but I haven't..."* The patient is sad and despairing, often mourning things not accomplished and dreams that will not come true. The patient withdraws, or retreats, into a private world, unwilling to communicate with others.
- *Acceptance, or "okay, I'm not afraid."* The patient may come to realize his fate and achieve a reasonable level of comfort with the anticipated outcome. At this stage, the family may need more support than the patient does.

Because paramedics encounter death and dying often, there is a mistaken belief that they can handle it better. However, paramedics are human, too. Let yourself deal with death and dying when they occur. Do not refuse the support of friends and family. Do not try to "tough it out." Use every opportunity to process a specific incident in a healthy manner, through appropriately grieving the losses that have an impact on you.

Grief is a feeling. Mourning is a process. A grieving person feels mostly sadness or distress. A person in mourning is immersed in the process of displaying and ultimately dissipating the feelings of grief. The sense of loss is predictably most intense immediately after the news is received. Although numerous models for the mourning process exist, a good rule of thumb is that after the loss of a close friend or relative, a period of one year of mourning is normal.

On initially hearing the news of a death, a person experiences incapacitating grief that is so acute it blocks out everything else in the environment. Typically, the feeling lasts for 5 to 15 minutes. When you deliver the news of a death, remember that a survivor cannot function during this grief spike. After delivering the news, wait until it has passed and the survivor is ready and able to receive information and make decisions.

A period of intense feelings continues for around four to six weeks following the grief spike. Feelings may include loss, anger, resentment, sadness, and even guilt, depending on the relationship and the circumstances surrounding the death. Gradually, the intensity and immediacy of the loss fades into a phase dominated by a sense of loneliness, which lasts about six months. Finally, a period of recovery ensues. The survivor begins to view the loss more objectively and rediscovers an interest in living. Key to the process of mourning is the passage of significant dates and anniversaries, such as birthdays, holidays, and the monthly (then annual) date when the loss occurred.

How different people cope with difficult experiences, such as death, varies. If you are dealing with a child, understand that children's perceptions are different from adults' (see Table 1-3 for a summary). This is true of all the special populations you will encounter, such as the elderly and people with mental disabilities. The elderly, for example, may be particularly concerned about the effects of the loss on other family members, about further loss of their own independence, and about the costs of a funeral and burial. There are many responses to death among different peoples and cultures as well. Be flexible, and be ready for anything.

Given enough time, a person experiencing a significant loss usually works through the five predictable stages: denial, anger, bargaining, depression, and acceptance.

Table 1-3	NEEDS AND EXPECTATIONS OF CHILDREN REGARDING DEATH	
Age Range	**Characteristics**	**Suggestions**
Newborn to age 3	Senses that something has happened in family, and notices that there is much activity in the household. Realizes that people are crying and sad. Watch for irritability and changes in eating, sleeping, or other behavioural patterns.	Be sensitive to the child's needs. Try to maintain consistency in routines. Maintain consistency with significant people in child's life.
Ages 3 to 6	Believes death is a temporary state and may ask continually when the person will return. Believes in magical thinking and may feel responsible for the death or feel that it is punishment for their own behaviour. May be fearful of catching the same illness and dying, or may believe that everyone else he loves will die also. Watch for changes in behaviour patterns with friends and at school, difficulty sleeping, and changes in eating habits.	Emphasize that the child was not responsible for the death. Reinforce that when people are sad, they cry and that crying is normal and natural. Encourage the child to talk about or draw pictures of his feelings or to cry.
Ages 6 to 9	May prefer to hide or disguise feelings to avoid looking babyish. Is afraid significant others will die. Seeks out detailed explanations for death and differences between fatal illness and "just being sick." Has an understanding that death is real but may believe that those who die are too slow, weak, or stupid. Fantasizes in an effort to make everything the way it was. Denial is most common coping skill.	Talk about the normal feelings of anger, sadness, and guilt. Share your own feelings about death. Do not be afraid to cry in front of the child. This and other expressions of loss help give the child permission to express his feelings.
Ages 9 to 12	Begins to understand the irreversibility of death. May seek details and specifics of the situation and may need repeated, explicit explanations. Hard-won sense of independence becomes fragile and may show concern about the practical matters of his lifestyle. May try to act "adult" but then regress to earlier stage of emotional response. When threatened, expresses anger toward the ill or deceased person, himself or herself, or other survivors.	Set aside time to talk about feelings. Encourage sharing of memories to facilitate grief response.
Ages 12 to 18	Demanding developmental processes are an awkward fit with need to take on different family roles. Retreats to safety of childhood. Feels pressure to act as an adult while still coping with skills of a child. Suppresses feelings in order to "fit in," leaving teen isolated and vulnerable.	Encourage talking but respect need for privacy. See if a trusted, reliable friend or adult can provide appropriate support. Locate support group for teens.

WHAT TO SAY

As do not resuscitate (DNR) orders and other prehospital death situations increase, EMS personnel are more often placed in the position of telling people that someone has died. It would be nice to have a script for those difficult moments, but the reality is that you have to assess the scene and the people in each situation to determine the safest and most compassionate way to deliver the sad news.

In terms of safety, you never know how people will respond, even if you know them. Most people accept the news quietly. However, some allow their grief to flood out of them in very physical ways, such as throwing things, kicking walls, or screaming and running in circles. Before speaking, consciously position yourself between them and the door or other escape route. Remember, initially the grief spike has its grip on the survivors. You can do little except give them a safe, private place to get through it. Also, for safety, do not deliver the news to a large group. Ask the primary people (no more than four or five) to step aside with you to a private place. Let them tell the others in their own way.

Find out who is who among the survivors. Do not make assumptions. Then, address the closest survivor, preferably in a way that shows compassion. That is, avoid standing above the survivor. Instead, sit or squat so that your eyes are at the same level. If the survivor is alone, call for a friend, neighbour, clergy member, or relative. When possible, wait to tell the survivor the news until that person has arrived.

Introduce yourself by name and function ("My name is Kate. I'm a paramedic with the Ambulance Service."). A careful choice of words is helpful. Although it may seem blunt, use the words "dead" and "died," rather than euphemisms that may be misinterpreted or misunderstood. Use eye contact gently and, if appropriate, touch an arm or hold a hand. Basic elements of your message should include the following:

- The loved one has died.
- There is nothing more anyone could have done.
- Your EMS service is available to assist the survivors if needed. (Sometimes, medical emergencies occur in survivors in the wake of such stressful news.)
- Information about local procedures for out-of-hospital death, such as the inspection of the scene by the medical examiner or coroner, and so on.

Do not include statements about God's will or relief from pain or any subjective assumption. You do not know the people well enough to know the details about their relationship or their religious preferences.

WHEN IT IS SOMEONE YOU KNOW

Many paramedics are called to serve in small communities, in which calls often involve people you know. Elements of this are both rewarding and heart-rending. People may be greatly relieved to see a familiar, trusted face among the EMS team. There also is a lot of support for paramedics in small communities because you are there to help others during their most fearful moments. However, being involved when the life of someone you know is threatened—or lost—can have a powerful impact on your own emotions. If it is too much, you must find a way to manage the stress. Often, you must grieve as well. Your well-being demands it.

STRESS AND STRESS MANAGEMENT

Many aspects of EMS are stressful. Stress, according to researcher Hans Selye, is "the nonspecific response of the body to any demand." The word **stress** also refers to a hardship or strain, or a physical or emotional response to a stimulus. A person's reactions to stress are individual. They are affected by previous exposure to the stressor, perception of the event, general life experience, and personal coping skills.

✱ **stress** a hardship or strain; a physical or emotional response to a stimulus.

* **stressor** a stimulus that causes stress.

A stimulus that causes stress is known as a **stressor.** Stress is usually understood to generate a negative affect, or *distress,* in an individual. There is also "good" stress, which is called *eustress* (for example, seeing a lost loved one for the first time in years). However, even eustress generates physiological and psychological signs and symptoms.

Adapting to stress is a dynamic, evolving process. As a person adapts, he develops the following:

- *Defensive strategies.* Although sometimes helpful for the short term, these strategies deny and distort the reality of a stressful situation.
- *Coping.* This is an active process during which a person confronts the stressful situation and changes or adjusts as necessary. Coping may not serve as the best strategy for the long term.
- *Problem-solving skills.* These skills are regarded as the healthiest approach to everyday concerns. Reflected in the ability to analyze a problem and recognize multiple options and potential solutions, mastery generally comes only as a result of extensive experience with similar situations.

EMS has abundant stressors, which provide many opportunities for the development of problem-solving skills. There are administrative stressors, such as the wait for calls, shift work, loud pagers, and inadequate pay. There are scene-related stressors, such as violent and abusive people, flying debris, vomit, loud noises, and chaos. There are emotional and physical stressors, such as fear, demanding bystanders, abusive patients, frustration, exhaustion, hunger or thirst, and the lifting of heavy objects.

Environmental stress may take the form of siren noise, inclement weather, confined work spaces, infectious diseases, and the frequent urgency of rapid scene responses and life-or-death decisions. In addition, the often difficult world of EMS can strain a paramedic's family relationships and possibly lead to conflicts with supervisors and coworkers. Add this to the common personality traits of paramedics, which include a strong need to be liked and often unrealistically high self-expectations, and the combination can lead to disturbing feelings of guilt or anxiety. All these stressors take a toll on the paramedic.

Your job in managing stress is to learn these things:

- *Your personal stressors.* Each person has an individual list. What is stressful to you may be enjoyable to someone else. What was stressful to you last year may be replaced by new stressors this year.
- *Amount of stress you can take before it becomes a problem.* Stress occurs in a tornado-like continuum. It starts with a few breezes, but it can increase in force until it is whirling out of control. Stopping the "storm" early is key to your well-being. You need to know which stress responses are early indicators for you so that you can deal with them at that point.
- *Stress management strategies that work for you.* Again, this is totally individual. Those who seek personal well-being must become well-versed about personally appropriate options.

If a person piles on stressor after stressor without regard for the consequences, the results are likely to be bad. Stress-related disease is avoidable if you make a habit of doing what is necessary to preserve your personal well-being.

To manage stress, identify your own personal stressors, the amount of stress you can take before it becomes a problem, and what specific stress-management techniques work for you.

There are three phases of a stress response: alarm, resistance, and exhaustion. At the end comes a period of rest and recovery.

Content Review

PHASES OF A STRESS RESPONSE
- Alarm
- Resistance
- Exhaustion

- *Stage I: Alarm.* The alarm phase is the "fight-or-flight" phenomenon. It occurs when the body physically and rapidly prepares to defend itself against a perceived threat. The pituitary gland begins by releasing adrenocorticotropic (stress) hormones. Hormones continue to flood the body via the autonomic nervous system, coordinated by the hypothalamus. Epinephrine and norepinephrine from the adrenal glands increase heart rate and blood pressure, dilate pupils, increase blood sugar, slow digestion, and relax the bronchial tree. This reaction ends when the event is recognized as not dangerous.

- *Stage II: Resistance.* This stage starts when the individual begins to cope with the stress. Over time, an individual may become desensitized or adapted to stressors. Physiological parameters, such as pulse and blood pressure, may return to normal.

- *Stage III: Exhaustion.* Prolonged exposure to the same stressors leads to exhaustion of an individual's ability to resist and adapt. Resistance to all stressors declines. Susceptibility to physical and psychological ailments increase. A period of rest and recovery is necessary for a healthy outcome.

It would be great if we could manage each stressor to the point of recovery before the next one hits, but that is not how it works. Typically, people are still dealing with one stress (or the same ongoing one, such as the chronic stress of shift work) when additional stressors pile on, resulting in cumulative stress. If stress accumulates without intervention, the consequences can be serious.

SHIFT WORK

There will always be shift work in EMS. Because EMS is a 24-hour, 7-days-a-week endeavour, someone has to be functional at all times. This is inherently stressful because of disruptions in the biorhythms of the body, known as **circadian rhythms,** and sleep deprivation.

Circadian rhythms are biological cycles that occur approximately every 24 hours. These include hormonal and body temperature fluctuations, appetite and sleepiness cycles, and other bodily processes. When life patterns disrupt the circadian rhythms, biological effects can be stressful. For example, sleep deprivation is common among people who work at night. The inherent dangers to paramedics are clear. If you have to sleep in the daytime, there are some tips to minimize the stress:

✳ **circadian rhythms** physiological phenomena that occur at approximately 24-hour intervals.

- Sleep in a cool, dark place that mimics the nighttime environment.
- Stick to sleeping at your **anchor time** (times you can rest without interruption), even on days off. Do not try to revert to a daytime lifestyle on days off. For example, if you work 9 p.m. to 5 a.m. and your anchor time is 8 a.m. to 12 noon, then go to bed "early" on days off, and sleep from 8 a.m. to 3 p.m on workdays.
- Unwind appropriately after a shift in order to rest well. Do not eat a heavy meal or exercise right before bedtime.
- Post a "day sleeper" sign on your front door, turn off the phone's ringer, and lower the volume of the answering machine.

✳ **anchor time** set of hours when a night-shift worker can reliably expect to rest without interruption.

SIGNS OF STRESS

A variety of factors can trigger a stress response. They include the loss of something valuable, injury or the threat of injury, poor health or nutrition, general frustration, and ineffective coping mechanisms. Remember, each individual is susceptible to different stressors and therefore has a different constellation of signs and symptoms.

These signs and symptoms (Table 1-4) are a blessing because they are the body's way of warning that corrective stress management is needed. The warnings typically are mild at first, but left uncorrected, they will build in intensity until you are forced to rest. If it means having a heart attack or collapsing, that is what the body will do. So, pay attention. If you catch a warning sign of excessive stress early and manage it, there is no need to reach the extreme end-point commonly referred to as **burnout**.

✳ **burnout** occurs when coping mechanisms no longer buffer stressors, which can compromise personal health and well-being.

COMMON TECHNIQUES FOR MANAGING STRESS

There are two main groups of defence mechanisms and techniques for managing stress: beneficial and detrimental. Detrimental techniques may provide a temporary sense of relief, but they will not cure the problem. They only make things worse. They include substance abuse (alcohol, nicotine, illegal and prescription drugs), overeating or other compulsive behaviours, chronic complaining, freezing out or cutting off others and the support they could give you, avoidance behaviours, and dishonesty about your actual state of well-being ("I'm just fine!").

It is far better for you to spend your energy on beneficial, or healthy, techniques that serve to dissipate the accumulation of stress and promote actual recovery. In situations in which your stress response threatens your ability to handle the moment, you can:

- *Use controlled breathing.* Focus attention on your breathing. Take in a deep breath through your nose. Then, exhale forcefully but steadily through your mouth so that you can hear the air rush out. Press all the air out of your lungs with your abdomen. Do this two or more times, until you feel steadier. This technique helps reduce your adrenaline levels and slow your heart rate so that you can do your job appropriately.

- *Reframe.* Mentally reframe interfering thoughts, such as "I can't do this" or "I'm scared." Be sure to deal with the thoughts later, or they will continue to interfere with the performance of your duties.

- *Attend to the medical needs of the patient.* Even if you know the people involved, do not let those relationships interfere with your responsibilities as an EMS provider. Later, when it is appropriate to do so, address your stress about the call.

For long-term well-being, the best stress-management technique is to take care of yourself—that is, eat properly, exercise regularly, and take time off!

For long-term well-being, one of the best stress management techniques is to take care of yourself—physically, emotionally, and mentally. Remember that regular exercise does not have to be extreme. Do something that you enjoy and find relaxing. At stressful times, pay especially close attention to your diet. If you smoke, make it a goal to quit.

Create a non-EMS circle of friends, and renew old friendships or activities. Take a vacation or a few days off. Say "no!" to the next offer of an overtime shift. Listen to music, meditate, and learn positive thinking. Try the soothing techniques of guided imagery and progressive relaxation. Some paramedics have even quit EMS for a while. You can make many choices. The key principle is to generate positive options for yourself, and keep choosing them until you have recovered.

Table 1-4 WARNING SIGNS OF EXCESSIVE STRESS

Physical	Cognitive
Nausea/vomiting	Confusion
Upset stomach	Shortened attention span
Tremors (lips, hands)	Calculation difficulties
Feeling uncoordinated	Memory problems
Diaphoresis (profuse sweating), flushed skin	Poor concentration
	Difficulty making decisions
Chills	Disruption in logical thinking
Diarrhea	Disorientation, decreased level
Aching muscles and joints	of awareness
Sleep disturbances	Seeing an event repeatedly
Fatigue	Distressing dreams
Dry mouth	Blaming someone
Shakes	
Headache	
Vision problems	
Difficult, rapid breathing	
Chest tightness or pain, heart palpitations, cardiac rhythm disturbances	

Emotional	Behavioural
Anticipatory anxiety	
Denial	Change in activity
Fearfulness	Hyperactivity, hypoactivity
Panic	Withdrawal
Survivor guilt	Suspiciousness
Uncertainty of feelings	Change in communications
Depression	Change in interactions with others
Grief	Crying spells
Hopelessness	Change in eating habits
Feeling overwhelmed	Increased or decreased food intake
Feeling lost	Increased smoking
Feeling abandoned	Increased alcohol intake
Feeling worried	Increased intake of other drugs
Wishing to hide	Being overly vigilant to environment
Wishing to die	Excessive humour
Anger	Excessive silence
Feeling numb	Unusual behaviour
Identifying with victim	

CRITICAL INCIDENT STRESS MANAGEMENT (CISM)

Uniquely stressful situations that arise in EMS are known as **critical incidents,** or events that have a powerful emotional impact that can cause acute stress reactions. Such events are not common, even by EMS standards. They include:

* Injury or death of an infant or child

* **critical incident** an event that has a powerful emotional impact on a rescuer that can cause an acute stress reaction.

- Injury or death of someone known to EMS personnel
- Injury, death, or suicide of an EMS worker
- Extreme threat to an EMS worker
- Disasters or multiple-casualty incidents (especially when most of the victims are dead)
- Injury or death of a civilian caused by EMS operations
- Incidents that draw unusual media attention
- Prolonged incidents
- Other significant events

Critical incidents will affect you, so take advantage of your EMS system's critical incident stress management (CISM) services.

A critical incident can affect a single crew or an entire agency. It also tends to generate intense, rapid-onset stress responses. Critical incident stress is managed by a system of related interventions called **critical incident stress management (CISM)**. These interventions are best performed by regional, nonpartisan, multidisciplinary teams comprising EMS peers (fire, police, paramedics, dispatchers, and so on) in combination with specifically trained mental health workers. The components of CISM are the following:

✻ critical incident stress management (CISM) a system of related interventions usually performed by regional, nonpartisan, multidisciplinary teams comprising EMS peers and specifically trained mental health workers.

- *Preincident stress training.* For all EMS personnel in the service area (fire, police, EMS, dispatchers, and so on), preincident education occurs during initial education and in subsequent training sessions.
- *On-scene support.* Techniques for reducing crisis-induced stress on scene include regular rest intervals, replacement of food and fluids, limited exposure to the incident, and a change in assignments.
- *Advice to command staff* during a large-scale incident.
- *Initial discussion.* This is a spontaneous, postcall, initial airing of crew responses. It is a process of simply talking about the incident. It is not intended as a critique. A trained member of a CISM team is present and can provide excellent emotional support during discussions.
- *Defusing.* Held two to four hours, but not more than 12 hours, postevent, a **defusing** is a short, informal meeting that provides a chance for crews to vent their feelings about the incident. A CISM-trained peer usually conducts it.
- *Demobilization.* **Demobilization** is an on-scene CISM service in which a site is established and staffed as a transition point between a large-scale situation and going off duty or back to regular duty. What goes on is not a critique but, rather, a chance to give crews time to regroup before reentering everyday life.
- *Critical incident stress debriefing.* The **critical incident stress debriefing (CISD)** is a formal, structured, carefully planned intervention. It is done 24 to 72 hours post event by a trained CISM team, including mental health providers and peer supporters.
- *Follow-up services.* Sometimes, the CISM team follows up with additional meetings to allow a safe environment for crews to grapple with ongoing reactions to the situation.
- *Special debriefings to nonemergency community groups.*
- *Spouse and family education and support.*
- *Individual consultations.*

✻ defusing a short, informal type of debriefing held within hours of a critical incident.

✻ demobilization establishment and staffing of a transition point to provide crews time to regroup between a large-scale critical stress situation and going off duty or back to regular duty.

✻ critical incident stress debriefing (CISD) a process used to help rescuers work through their responses to a critical incident within 24 to 72 hours after the event.

GENERAL SAFETY CONSIDERATIONS

The topic of scene safety is vast and requires career-long attention. Considering the many problems that can occur, it is impressive how few injuries there are. Your risks include violent people, environmental hazards, structural collapse, motor vehicles, and infectious disease. Many of these hazards can be minimized with protective equipment, such as helmets, body armour, reflective tape for night visibility, footwear with ankle support, and BSI precautions against infectious diseases. Whatever protective equipment you have should be used.

INTERPERSONAL RELATIONS

Safety issues that arise in prehospital care often stem from poor interpersonal relations. Paramedics are public ambassadors of health care. Interpersonal safety begins with effective communication. If you can build a rapport with the strangers you have been sent to serve, you will gain their trust. Suspicious, angry, upset people are far more likely to be defensive and inflict harm than those who see a reason to trust what you are doing.

Building rapport depends on the ability to put your personal prejudices aside. Everyone has prejudices. But as a representative of an institution far greater than yourself, you must never allow them to interfere with appropriate patient and bystander management. In fact, go beyond curbing prejudice, and challenge yourself to treat every person you meet with dignity and respect.

You can begin by paying attention to the rich array of cultural diversity in Canada and learning to see those differences as valuable and positive. In particular, learn about the different cultural backgrounds of people in your area and how to work with them effectively. For example, although you may like a lot of eye contact, understand that it is regarded as more polite in several cultures to avoid eye contact. Therefore, someone showing you esteem might avoid eye contact with you. This is not wrong; it is just different. Listen well to the stories of other people, and see what you can learn. When a person can accept differences easily, it becomes easier to work toward win-win situations on the streets.

Treat every person you meet with dignity and respect, no matter what their race, sex, age, religion, economic background, or present condition.

ROADWAY SAFETY

Roadways are unsafe places. There are good books, classes, and mentors to help you become aware of the various roadway hazards. Learn the principles of the following:

- Safely following an emergency escort vehicle
- Managing intersections when traffic is moving in several directions
- Noting hazardous conditions, such as spilled hazardous materials (gasoline, industrial chemicals, and so on), downed power lines, and proximity to moving traffic; and also noting adverse environmental conditions
- Evaluating the safest parking place when arriving at a roadway incident
- Safely approaching a vehicle in which someone is slumped over the wheel
- Practising patient compartment safety—in particular, bracing yourself against sudden deceleration or swerving to avoid roadway hazards; and making a habit of hanging on consistently, especially when changing positions
- Safely using emergency lights and siren

One of the greatest hazards in EMS is the motor vehicle. Be sure to obey roadway laws and follow all driving safety guidelines.

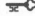

An ambulance escort can create additional hazards. Inexperienced ambulance operators often follow the escort vehicle too closely and are unable to stop when the escort does. Inexperienced operators also may assume that other drivers know that an ambulance is following an escort. In fact, other drivers do not know and often pull out in front of the ambulance just after the escort vehicle passes.

Multiple-vehicle responses can be just as dangerous, especially when responding vehicles travel in the same direction close together. When two vehicles approach the same intersection at the same time, not only may they fail to yield to each other, but other drivers may also yield for the first vehicle only and not to the second one. Extreme caution must be taken when approaching intersections.

Certain equipment is intended to promote your safety on roadways. For example, to be visible to oncoming drivers, who may have dirty, smeared, pitted windshields and may not be sober, wear reflective tape and orange or lime-green safety vests. In fact, you also may be issued other protective gear, especially if you are in the fire service. Using respiratory protection, gloves, boots, turnout coat and pants (or coveralls), and other specialty safety equipment is the mark of an aware, professional paramedic. Ask nonmedical personnel to set out cones or other safety markers if needed. Leave some emergency lights flashing, but be careful not to blind oncoming drivers.

To park safely at a roadway incident, make it a habit to scan each individual setting. Notice curves and hilltops and the volume and speed of surrounding traffic. Ideally, park in the front of a crash site on the same side of the street. This facilitates access to the patient compartment and equipment, and it protects you from traffic coming from behind. However, when responding to such an incident as "person slumped behind wheel," maintain the defensive advantage by staying behind the vehicle, and use spotlights to "blind" the person until you know there are no hostile intentions. Walk to the vehicle with cautious alertness until you are sure it is not a trap.

The use of seatbelts in the front of an ambulance should be an obvious habit, both for safety and for role modelling. Less obvious is the use of safety restraints in the patient compartment. An improper assumption is that the paramedic is too busy attending the patient and passengers to wear a seatbelt. However, buckling into a seatbelt for a safer ride is, in fact, possible during much or most of ambulance transport times. Death and major disability are common among personnel in the patient compartment during a crash. For your well-being, wear a seatbelt whenever possible, even in the back of the ambulance.

Because ambulances represent help and hope, it is doubly tragic when a paramedic crewmember is involved in a motor-vehicle crash caused by the misuse of lights and siren. Lights and siren are tools, not toys. They are the paramedic's means for gaining quick access to people in dire need. Those who misuse the mandate to operate them chip away at the public's trust in EMS. Whether using lights and siren or not, in most jurisdictions, the paramedic has a legal responsibility to drive with "due regard for the safety of all others." As a professional, you are obligated to study and use safe driving practices at all times.

Part 5: Illness and Injury Prevention

Injury is one of our nation's most important health problems.

How often do EMS crews respond to incidents that could easily have been prevented? How often have you thought to yourself "I wish there was something I could have done" in the wake of senseless circumstances surrounding an accidental injury or illness? But what if EMS personnel asked questions before an incident occurred? How many injuries could be prevented? How many lives could be saved? This section focuses on these questions and discusses illness and injury prevention as a paramedic's crucial duty and responsibility.

EPIDEMIOLOGY

The numbers surrounding Canada's urgent health problems are staggering. The Alberta Centre for Injury Control and Research reports that injury is the number-one killer of Canadians under the age of 45 years. The following information is a small portion of the information collected by the Alberta Centre for Injury Control and Research.

- Injury is one of our nation's most important health problems.
- Each year in Canada 34 000 people are admitted to hospital with brain injuries—that's more than 90 people injured per day.
- Twice as many males as females experience head injuries.
- Wearing a helmet reduces the risk of head injury by 85 percent and brain injury by 88 percent.
- Every day in Alberta at least one person is killed in motor-vehicle collisions.
- Motor-vehicle collisions are the leading cause of unintentional injury for Albertan's under age 30.
- Firearms result in more than 1300 deaths in Canada each year.
- Ninety-five percent of farm-related deaths are of males.
- Most pedestrian injuries involving children occur within one block of their home.
- One in 25 Canadians will attempt suicide at some point in their lives.
- Falls are the second-leading cause of injury-related deaths among seniors aged 65 and older.
- Suicide is the fifth-leading cause of death in Canada.

As well, the following facts are provided by the U.S. Department of Transportation:

- Injury surpassed stroke as the third-leading cause of death in the United States, and it is the leading cause of death in people ages 1 to 44.
- Unintentional injuries result in nearly 70 000 deaths and millions of nonfatal injuries each year. The leading causes of death from unintentional injuries are motor-vehicle collisions, fires, burns, falls, drownings, and poisonings.
- For every one death caused by injury, there are an estimated 19 hospitalizations and 254 emergency department visits.

Injuries result from interaction with potential hazards in the environment, which means that they may be predictable and preventable.

Though many people believe that injuries "just happen," evidence shows that injuries result from interaction with potential hazards in the environment.

Thus, it has been suggested that MVAs (motor-vehicle accidents) should be called MVCs (motor-vehicle collisions), since driving drunk or at 120 km/hr and crashing is no accident. In other words, many injuries may be predictable and preventable. The study of the factors that influence the frequency, distribution, and causes of injury, disease, and other health-related events in a population is called **epidemiology.**

Concepts related to epidemiology that you should know include **years of productive life,** a calculation made by subtracting the age at death from 65. (For example, in a liability suit concerning the death of a 45-year-old, a jury might assess damages based on the deceased's loss of 20 years as a wage earner.) Another con-

✱ epidemiology the study of factors that influence the frequency, distribution, and causes of injury, disease, and other health-related events in a population.

✱ years of productive life age at death subtracted from 65.

✱ injury intentional or unintentional damage to a person resulting from exposure to mechanical or any other form of energy or from absence of essentials, such as heat or oxygen.

✱ injury risk a situation that puts people in danger of injury.

✱ injury-surveillance program ongoing systematic collection, analysis, and interpretation of injury data important to public health practice.

✱ teachable moment the time shortly after an injury when patients and observers may be more receptive to teaching about how similar injuries may be prevented in the future.

✱ primary prevention keeping an injury or illness from ever occurring.

✱ secondary prevention medical care after an injury or illness that helps prevent further problems from occurring.

✱ tertiary prevention rehabilitation after an injury or illness that helps prevent further problems from occurring.

The more than 14 000 EMS registered with the Paramedic Association of Canada compose a great arsenal in the war to prevent injury and disease.

EMS organizational commitment is vital to the development of prevention activities.

cept is **injury,** which refers to the intentional or unintentional damage to a person resulting from acute exposure to thermal, mechanical, electrical, or chemical energy or from the absence of such essentials as heat and oxygen. An accident is an *unintentional injury,* but an injury that is purposefully inflicted either on the self (e.g., suicide) or on another person (e.g., homicide) is an *intentional injury.* Intentional injuries make up about one-third of all injury deaths. Other categories of intentional injury include rape, assault, and domestic, elder, and child abuse.

Other concepts related to epidemiology include **injury risk,** which is a real or potentially hazardous situation that puts people in danger of sustaining injury. As medical professionals, EMS providers should assess every scene and situation for injury risk and help provide statistics as part of an **injury-surveillance program**— the ongoing systematic collection, analysis, and interpretation of injury data essential to the planning, implementation, and evaluation of public health practice.

An injury-surveillance program must also include a component for the timely dissemination of data to those who need to know. The final link in the injury-surveillance chain is the application of these data to prevention and control. **Teachable moments** occur shortly after an injury when the patient and observers remain acutely aware of what has happened and may be more receptive to teaching about how similar injury or illness could be prevented in the future.

By becoming involved in injury prevention, EMS providers can focus on **primary prevention,** or keeping an injury from ever occurring. Medical care and rehabilitation activities that help prevent further problems from occurring are referred to, respectively, as **secondary prevention** and **tertiary prevention.**

PREVENTION WITHIN EMS

Even armed with the best equipment and technology, EMS providers cannot save every life. However, by working as partners in public health and safety, members of the EMS community can go beyond their normal daily routine and work with the public to prevent avoidable illness and injury.

EMS providers are widely distributed in the population, often reflecting the composition of their communities. They are often considered champions of the health-care consumer and are welcome in schools and other community institutions. Medical personnel are high-profile role models and, as such, can have a significant impact on the reduction of injury rates. In rural areas, EMS providers are sometimes the most medically educated individuals, often looked to for advice and direction. Essentially, the more than 14 000 EMS providers registered with the Paramedic Association of Canada compose a great arsenal in the war to prevent injury and disease.

ORGANIZATIONAL COMMITMENT

EMS organizational commitment is vital to the development of prevention activities in the following areas:

- *Protection of EMS providers.* The leadership of EMS agencies must ensure that policies are in place to promote response, scene, and transport safety. The appropriate body substance isolation (BSI) equipment and personal protective equipment (PPE) should be issued to protect against exposure to bloodborne and airborne pathogens as well as environmental hazards. An overall commitment to safety and wellness should be emphasized and supported.
- *Education of EMS providers.* A buy-in from employees at every level is key to the success of any prevention program. EMS managers

have the responsibility of instructing employees in the fundamentals of primary prevention. Public and private sector specialty groups may be called on for specific training (Figure 1-13). EMS providers should also have the skills and training necessary to defend against violent patients or other hostile attackers. Classes in on-scene survival techniques should be commonplace in every EMS agency.

- *Data collection.* Monitoring and maintaining records of patient illnesses and injuries is essential in determining trends and in developing and measuring the success of prevention programs. Each agency should contribute data to local, regional, provincial or territorial, and national systems that track such information.

- *Financial support.* An agency's internal budget should show support for prevention strategies as a priority. If necessary, support must be sought from outside the organization. Large corporations are often willing to donate funds in exchange for stand-by coverage at an event or company function. Provincial or territorial highway ministries may offer funding for traffic-related projects, such as those involving child safety seats, seatbelts, and drunk driving. Advertising agencies may contribute billboards for safety messages and public service announcements. Partnerships with local hospitals can result in advertising safety messages in newsletters and flyers. Such community groups as Mothers Against Drunk Driving (MADD) also are great resources for initiating community and school programs.

- *Empowerment of EMS providers.* Frontline personnel are the ultimate factor in achieving success in a prevention program. Managers should identify, encourage, foster, and reward employee interest, support, and involvement. In addition, managers should rotate assignment to prevention programs and provide salary for off-duty injury prevention activities.

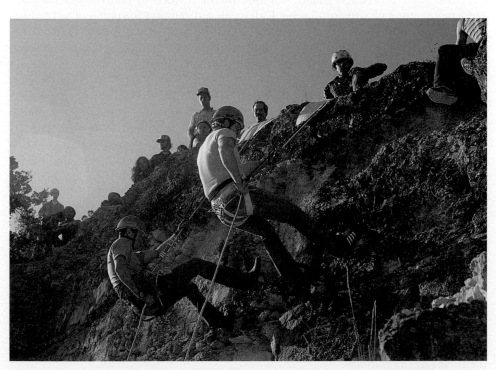

FIGURE 1-13   Training in specialized safety procedures should be available to you.

Content Review

ORGANIZATIONAL COMMITMENT

- Protect EMS providers.
- Provide initial and continuing education.
- Collect and distribute illness and injury data.
- Empower EMS personnel.

Content Review

EMS ILLNESS AND INJURY PREVENTION

- Take BSI precautions.
- Maintain physical fitness, and use proper lifting and moving techniques.
- Manage stress.
- Seek professional care when needed.
- Drive safely.

Safety is always your first priority.

EMS has a responsibility to prevent injury and illness not only among EMS workers but also among members of the public.

EMS PROVIDER COMMITMENT

Illness and injury prevention should begin at home and be carried over into the workplace. The priority for EMS providers is to protect themselves from harm. Employers have an obligation to provide a safe environment. Written guidelines and policies should promote wellness and safety among employees, emphasizing the following areas (Part 4 of this chapter provided more information on the points listed):

- Body substance isolation precautions
- Physical fitness
- Stress management
- Professional care and counselling
- Safe driving
- Proper lifting techniques

SCENE SAFETY

Safety is always your first priority. Once your unit is dispatched to a call, evaluate the dispatch information before arrival. Focus your attention on response and equipment needed. On arrival, park the unit in the safest and most convenient place to load the patient as well as to leave the scene. Consider traffic, road conditions, and all other possible hazards. Directing traffic is primarily the responsibility of local law enforcement agencies. The safest method for traffic control at serious vehicle collisions is to stop all traffic and reroute it to different roads. This is for the safety of patients, bystanders, and rescue personnel.

Note that if you are called to an area with potential health hazards, such as an industrial park or a chemical plant or an area with high crime rates, approach the scene with caution. Be sure to protect yourself appropriately. If you do not have adequate protection or are not specifically trained to control specific hazards, never enter a hazardous scene. Call in specialized teams, such as a hazardous materials crew, if necessary. Law enforcement agencies should be contacted for any violent, potentially violent, or dangerous scene, including those involving domestic abuse or other crimes. Do not enter the scene until you are cleared by the appropriate agency.

If the scene is safe to enter, be sure to wear reflective clothing to provide added protection on the scene. With BSI precautions in place, approach patients with your safety in mind. Determine the mechanisms of injury (forces that caused injury) or the nature of illness. Treat the patient according to protocol.

After patient care is addressed and a transport decision is made, make sure your unit is secure before departure. Have your partner check the outside of the unit to make certain that all doors are secured. The patient should be secured on an ambulance stretcher with at least three straps and shoulder straps if available. If a family member is allowed to accompany the patient, that person should be placed in the passenger seat in the front compartment with vehicle restraints in place.

PREVENTION IN THE COMMUNITY

As a component of health care, EMS has a responsibility to not only prevent injury and illness among EMS workers but also to promote prevention among the members of the public.

AREAS OF NEED

Infants and Children

According to Statistics Canada, more than 20 000 babies born to Canadian mothers in 1996–1997 were considered to have low birth weights (less than 2500 g). Low birth weight is a key indicator of poor health at the time of birth. Babies born too small or too soon are far more likely to die in the first year of life. Low birth weight and prematurity contribute to serious disabilities, such as mental retardation, cerebral palsy, seizure disorders, and blindness.

Health Canada reports that in 1995, 2321 infants died before their first birthday. Of concern is the fact that 1584 (68 percent) of these deaths occurred in the neonatal period (less than 28 days of age). In 60 percent of these cases, respiratory distress syndrome, short gestation period, and low birth weight were contributing factors. Congenital anomalies accounted for 33 percent of neonatal deaths. The good news is that the Canadian infant mortality rate has fallen steadily since the early 1960s. In fact, next only to Japan, Canada has experienced the most dramatic decline in infant mortality in the past 35 years. In spite of the decline, the mortality rate is considered high (6.1/1000) when compared with Finland (3.9), Sweden (4.2), and Japan (4.3).

Despite our efforts in injury prevention, injury is still the number-one killer of children, causing approximately 480 deaths per year. However, for every child who dies due to injury, another 63 require hospitalization. According to the Canada Safety Council, motor-vehicle collisions account for 41 percent of the deaths. Drowning is the second-leading cause of death in children at 15 percent, followed by intentional harm at 14 percent. In contrast, one in six fatalities to children in the United States involves a firearm.

In the case of deaths due to motor-vehicle collisions, most children killed are pedestrians or cyclists. One concern is that children today walk or cycle far less than children of previous generations. Their lack of familiarity and exposure to the risks in traffic situations may be a contributing factor. For children between the ages of 10 and 14, bicycle injuries are the third-leading cause of injury.

Of special concern is the potential for head injuries. The effects of a head injury can leave a child with a permanent brain injury. The injury may impair speech, cause learning disabilities, and affect everything from memory to mood. Safe Kids Canada reports that about 500 children under 15 years of age are hospitalized each year for head injuries caused by cycling accidents.

In motor-vehicle collisions, young children are easily thrown on impact. Because a young child's head is large in proportion to the body, unrestrained children tend to fly head first into the windshield or out of the car when a collision occurs. The back seat is the best seat for children 12 years old or younger. In this location, the properly restrained child is least likely to sustain injuries in a crash. Car safety seats and seat belts can prevent most severe injuries to passengers of all ages if they are used correctly. Air bags are designed to save people's lives when used with seatbelts, and they can protect drivers and passengers who are correctly buckled in.

Infants and toddlers are commonly injured by cars backing up in driveways or parking lots. Children between the ages of five and nine typically dart out into traffic and are struck by cars. Children riding bicycles can be injured when they collide with cars or other fixed objects or when they are thrown from bicycles. The most serious bicycle-related injuries are head injuries, which can cause death or permanent brain damage.

Falls are the most frequent cause of injury to children younger than six years old. In the United States, about 200 children die from falls each year. Fire and burn injuries occur in the highest numbers in the very young. Most are caused by scalding from a hot liquid, such as when children grab the handles of pots on the stove and spill the contents.

Content Review

AREAS IN NEED OF PREVENTION ACTIVITIES

- Low birth weight
- Unrestrained children in motor vehicles
- Bicycle-related injuries
- Household fire and burn injuries
- Unintentional firearm-related deaths
- Alcohol-related motor-vehicle collisions
- Fall injuries in the elderly
- Workplace injuries
- Sports and recreation injuries
- Misuse or mishandling of medications
- Early discharge of patients

In this modern age of mass media and the internet, children and young adults are bombarded with an incredible amount of information and are often faced with some of the same stressors as adults. Sometimes, those stressors become overwhelming. One of the most troubling recent trends is the number of violent acts among young people, occurring in the form of self-destructive behaviour, gang violence, and assaults. In addition, firearm injury is becoming more common because of the accessibility of handguns to children. Injuries and deaths often occur when children and adolescents take guns to school. The number of firearm deaths has doubled since 1953. About 15 percent of all firearm-related deaths are unintentional, often resulting from improper handling and lack of safety mechanisms.

Geriatric Patients

Falls account for the largest number of preventable injuries for persons over 75 years of age. The elderly are at increased risk of injury from falls as a result of slower reflexes, failing eyesight and hearing, and arthritis. Falls frequently result in fractures, since the bones become weaker and more brittle with age.

The aging process also places the elderly at greater risk for serious head injury as well as other injuries. Although many geriatric patients are completely coherent, many others suffer from some degree of dementia. Alzheimer's disease is merely one of the mental conditions that can affect the elderly. The associated confusion can contribute to dangerous behaviours, such as wandering away from home or into a roadway.

Motor-Vehicle Collisions

As noted earlier, EMS and law enforcement have long referred to vehicular collisions as motor-vehicle accidents (MVAs). However, the term motor-vehicle collision (MVC) more accurately reflects the fact that no collision is an accident: something caused the crash to occur. Such crashes are responsible for more than half of all deaths from unintentional injuries. Alcohol use is a factor in about half of all motor-vehicle fatalities.

Work and Recreation Hazards

In the workplace, back injuries account for 22 percent of all disabling injuries. Injuries to the eyes, hands, and fingers are responsible for another 22 percent. Even the quietest office setting can be hazardous. Never underestimate the potential dangers in an area that appears to be safe. Copy machines, electrical cords, faulty wiring, and shoddy building construction can be hazardous.

Sports injuries are commonly seen in persons of all ages due to the increased popularity of and participation in outdoor recreational activities. Football, soccer, baseball, as well as running, hiking, and biking are among popular sports that can result in fractures, dislocations, sprains, and strains.

Medications

When an illness or injury occurs and treatment is sought, medications are often part of the treatment regimen. These medications are occasionally taken improperly (too much or not enough), or they are taken by others, sometimes causing serious medical problems. Medications of any kind should be taken only by those for whom they are prescribed. They should be stored according to label directions. They should also be continued until the prescription is completed. Following the physician's, the pharmacist's, and the label directions is imperative.

Early Discharge

Many health regions have mandated shorter hospital stays and early discharges from the hospital, urgent care centres, and other outpatient facilities. Such policies often result in more patients who are home sooner with illnesses that are less completely treated. These patients may call on 911 for supportive care and intervention.

IMPLEMENTATION OF PREVENTION STRATEGIES

The following is a list of prevention strategies that you should be able to implement:

- *Preserve the safety of the response team.* Always remember that your first priority is your safety and the safety of your fellow crewmembers. The next priorities are the patient and, finally, bystanders. Do what you can and what is within your training to maintain a safe and secure working area. Do not hesitate to contact backup units and law enforcement personnel if necessary.

- *Recognize scene hazards.* Assess the scene for potential risks or dangers before entering. Be aware of your surroundings. Is there anyone or anything that could cause harm to you, your crew, or the patient? Does the mechanism that injured the patient still pose a threat to the rescuers? Are there any hazardous materials in the area? Has any crime been committed? Are there structural risks? Are there temperature extremes for which you are unprepared? Are there suspicious conditions, such as unsafe ice or water hazards? Call for the appropriate assistance. Do not enter or approach until it is safe to do so.

- *Document findings.* Document your patient-care findings at the end of every call. Note that EMS patient forms often can be designed to include specific data on injury prevention in order to benefit researchers and implement future prevention programs. Such a form should include space to describe scene conditions at the time of EMS arrival, the mechanism of injury, and any risks that were overcome. If protective devices were used (or not used) during the emergency, these should be documented, too. (See Figure 1-14 for an example.)

- *Engage in on-scene education.* Take advantage of a teachable moment to decrease future emergency responses. Remain objective, nonjudgmental, and nonthreatening. Inform your listeners of how they can prevent the recurrence of a similar emergency and, if needed, instruct them on the use of protective devices.

- *Know your community resources.* Determine what your patient's needs are and how you may assist him. Your patient may require a referral to an outside agency, such as a prenatal clinic, a social service organization that offers food, shelter, clothing, mental health resources, or counselling, or other agency. Your system may also allow for referral or transport to a clinic, urgent care facility, or alternative health-care centre. Be aware of the presence of both licensed and unlicensed daycare centres in your area. Encourage parents to provide preexisting consent for treatment and transport in case of illness or injury at a daycare facility. Follow local protocol to report suspected abuse situations. Consider developing a social service resource guide for your organization to provide solutions and ideas for these and other situations.

> ### Content Review
>
> #### PREVENTION STRATEGIES
> - Preserve the safety of the response team.
> - Recognize scene hazards.
> - Document findings.
> - Engage in on-scene education.
> - Know community resources.
> - Conduct a community needs assessment.

- *Conduct a community needs assessment.* Conducting a needs assessment will assist in identifying community priorities. Consider the following:

  – Childhood and flu immunizations
  – Prenatal and well-baby clinics
  – Eldercare clinics
  – Defensive driving classes
  – Workplace safety courses
  – Health clinics (co-sponsored by local hospitals or health-care organizations)
  – Prevention information on your agency's website

The population you serve and its ethnic, cultural, and religious makeup may affect the needs and approaches that are most appropriate. Also, consider community members who have a learning disability or a physical disability. These are just a few of the ideas that may be appropriate for your organization.

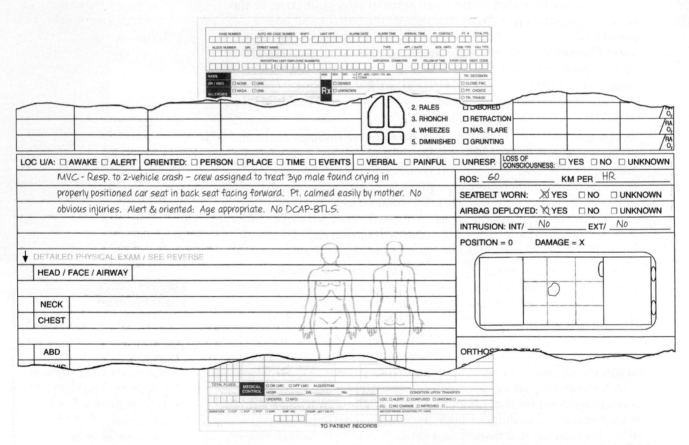

FIGURE 1-14 Documentation of primary and secondary injury prevention data.

Part 6: Ethics in Advanced Prehospital Care

When asked what the most difficult part of the job is, most paramedics do not say "ethics." Nonetheless, a significant percentage of calls do pose possible ethical conflicts, for example, regarding refusal of care, choice of hospital destination, and advance directives. So, whether or not you are consciously thinking about ethics, you are almost certain to be called on periodically in your work to decide what the ethical thing to do is.

OVERVIEW OF ETHICS

Ethics and morals are closely related concepts. **Morals** are generally considered social, religious, or personal standards of right and wrong. **Ethics** more often refers to the rules or standards that govern the conduct of members of a particular group or profession. Both ethics and morals address a question Socrates asked: "How should one live?"

✱ **morals** social, religious, or personal standards of right and wrong.

✱ **ethics** the rules or standards that govern the conduct of members of a particular group or profession.

RELATIONSHIP OF ETHICS TO LAW AND RELIGION

Ethics and the law have a great deal in common, but they are distinct. In general, laws have a much narrower focus. Laws frequently describe what is wrong in the eyes of society. Ethics goes beyond what is wrong and examines what is right, or good. As a result, the law frequently has little or nothing to say about ethical problems. In fact, laws themselves can be unethical, for example, laws that once perpetuated racial segregation. Even though ethics and the law are different, ethical discussions can sometimes benefit from techniques developed in the law. In particular, the law emphasizes impartiality, consistency, and methods to identify and balance conflicting interests.

Just as ethics differs from the law, it also differs from religion. In a pluralistic society, such as ours, ethics must be understood by and apply to people who hold a broad range of religious beliefs or no religious beliefs at all. Thus, ethics cannot derive from a single religion. It is true, however, that religion can enhance and enrich a person's ethical principles and values.

MAKING ETHICAL DECISIONS

Many approaches exist for determining how a medical professional should behave. One is to say that each person must decide how to behave and that whatever decision the person makes is acceptable. This is known as *ethical relativism*. However, people typically do not find ethical relativism satisfactory. For example, no reasonable person would say that it was acceptable for the Nazis to behave as they did. A similar approach is to say, "Just do what is right." This sounds fine, but different people have different beliefs about what is "right." Even the Golden Rule—"Do unto others as you would have them do unto you"—is not a sufficient guideline. What happens when the care provider's desires and values differ from the patient's? It becomes clear that reason and logic must be used and emotion must be excluded as much as possible from the decision-making process.

Reason must be used and emotion must be excluded as much as possible from the decision-making process.

CODES OF ETHICS

Over the years, a number of organizations have drafted codes of ethics for the members of their organizations. The Canadian Medical Association has a code of ethics for physicians. The Canadian Association of Emergency Physicians has a code of ethics specifically for emergency physicians. The Canadian Nurses Association and the National Emergency Nurses Affiliation both have codes for practitioners in their fields. In 1948, the World Medical Association adopted the Oath of Geneva. The Paramedic Association of Canada (PAC) has a code of ethics that can be found on its website, www.paramedic.ca.

Most codes of ethics address broad humanitarian concerns and professional etiquette. Few provide solid guidance on the kind of ethical problems commonly faced by practitioners. For example, a paramedic is expected to work in an uncontrolled environment that is sometimes dangerous. A person who is unwilling to enter a scene until every risk has been eliminated is not acting in accordance with the expectations of the profession. Conversely, a paramedic is expected to refrain from entering a hazardous area until the risks have been made manageable. Common sense should help in resolving such conflicts as these.

National Code of Ethics

The PAC developed a National Code of Ethics that describes the values and standards for the profession of prehospital medical care in Canada. The purpose of the National Code of Ethics is to:

1. Define and clarify ethical principles
2. Identify the basic moral commitments of prehospital emergency medical practitioners
3. Serve as a source for education and reflection
4. Serve as a tool for self-evaluation and peer review

The values are broad ideals of prehospital care and the standards are moral obligations that have their basis in the emergency prehospital values. Standards tend to be more specific than values.

In the National Code of Ethics, PAC lists three ethical problems faced by prehospital care:

1. Ethical violations occur when practitioners neglect or fail to meet their moral obligations to their patients.
2. Ethical dilemmas arise when ethical reasons both for and against a particular course of action are present and one option must be selected. There is usually a conflict between two ethical principles.
3. Ethical distress occurs when practitioners experience the imposition of practice that provokes feelings of guilt, concern, or distaste.

The function of the Code of Ethics is to educate the public about the profession's aspirations, ethical values, standards, and disciplinary governance of the professions' behaviour.

THE FUNDAMENTAL QUESTIONS

The single most important question a paramedic has to answer when faced with an ethical challenge is, "What is in the patient's best interests?"

The single most important question a paramedic has to answer when faced with an ethical challenge is, "What is in the patient's best interests?" Usually, the answer is obvious, but not always. For example, what is in the best interests of a terminally ill patient who goes into cardiac arrest—to resuscitate or not to start resuscitation in order to prevent further suffering?

A paramedic must be very cautious in accepting a family's description of what a patient desires. The family members are often under a great deal of stress when the paramedic encounters them. The paramedic must also realize that the family may not agree with the patient's desires. They may be led to substitute their own desires for the patient's.

Under ideal circumstances, a written statement describing the patient's desires will be available. In many jurisdictions, such a statement (which meets other specified provincial or territorial and local requirements) is required by law before a paramedic may elect not to start resuscitation efforts. In less extreme circumstances, the patient may state verbally what he wants you to do and not do. It may sometimes be difficult for a paramedic to agree to or to comply with a patient's wishes, but as long as the patient is competent and the desires are consistent with good practice, the paramedic is obligated to respect the patient's wishes. For example, the paramedic would need to respect the wishes of a patient who clearly requires hospitalization but refuses to go. The paramedic should use good judgment and persuasion skills to convince the patient to seek medical attention.

FUNDAMENTAL PRINCIPLES

A common approach to resolving problems in **bioethics** today is to employ four fundamental principles or values: beneficence, nonmalfeasance, autonomy, and justice.

- **Beneficence** is related to a more familiar term, *benevolence*. Both come from Latin and concern doing good. However, *benevolence* means the desire to do good (usually the main reason people become paramedics), whereas *beneficence* means actually doing good (the paramedic's obligation to the patient).

- **Nonmalfeasance** means *not* doing harm. (*Malfeasance* means doing harm, the opposite of *beneficence*.) Few medical interventions are without risk of harm. Under the principle of nonmalfeasance, however, the paramedic is obligated to minimize that risk as much as possible. This includes, for example, making the scene safe and protecting the patient from impaired or unqualified health-care providers. The Latin phrase, *primum non nocere*, which means "first, do no harm," sums up nonmalfeasance very well.

- **Autonomy** refers to a competent adult patient's right to determine what happens to his own body, including treatment for medical illnesses and injuries. Under ordinary conditions, a patient must give consent before the paramedic can begin treatment. There are, of course, exceptions to this (see the discussion of consent later in this chapter and in Chapter 2), but the implication is that the paramedic must be truthful in describing to the patient his condition and the risks and benefits of treatment. It also implies respect for the patient's privacy.

- **Justice** refers to the paramedic's obligation to treat all patients fairly, without regard to sex, race, ability to pay, or cultural background, among other conditions.

RESOLVING ETHICAL CONFLICTS

The paramedic needs to have a system for resolving ethical conflicts. One such method of resolving ethical issues is illustrated in the following scenario:

You represent your service at the regional EMS coordinating agency. The head nurse for the emergency department of a large hospital mentions how recent cutbacks in support staff have led to difficulty retrieving patients' medical records in a timely manner. This problem has led to a number of difficulties in treating patients. As a result, the emergency

* bioethics ethics as applied to the human body.

* beneficence the principle of doing good for the patient.

* nonmalfeasance the obligation not to harm the patient.

* autonomy a competent adult patient's right to determine what happens to his own body.

First, do no harm (primum non nocere).

---

* justice the obligation to treat all patients fairly.

department (ED) was considering asking incoming ambulances to give patients' names and dates of birth on the radio. This would give the ED staff additional time to search for the patient's medical records.

You consider the issue's ethical aspects. First, you identify the problem: Is it justifiable to breach patient confidentiality in order to expedite the retrieval of medical records? Second, you list the possible actions that might be taken in this situation:

- Provide all patients' names and dates of birth on the radio.
- Continue, as now, to identify patients only by age and sex.
- Provide selected patients' names and dates of birth on the radio.

To reason out an ethical problem, first state the action in a universal form. Then, list the implications or consequences of the action. Finally, compare them with relevant values, as follows:

1. *State the action in a universal form. Describe what should be done, who should do it, and under what conditions.* For example, EMS (who) will volunteer names and dates of birth for all patients (what) on the radio (condition).

2. *List the implications, or consequences, of the action.* Positive consequences: The ED will be able to get records sooner for patients who have records at that hospital. There will be no change for most patients because hospital records are often irrelevant to emergency care. The ED admitting staff may be able to admit patients more quickly. Negative consequences: Patients' names and dates of birth will be broadcast to thousands of people listening with scanners. In the long term, people with scanners will learn more about patients who go to the hospital via EMS. Because private information may be broadcast, patients may become reluctant to call EMS. Conceivably, more burglaries may occur at homes of patients who use EMS.

3. *Compare the consequences with relevant values.* A list of values that pertain to this case might include beneficence, nonmalfeasance, autonomy, and confidentiality. That is, if EMS provided names and dates of birth for all patients on the radio, what would be the benefit to the patient (beneficence)? A few patients might be cared for sooner because their records arrived sooner. Most patients will see no benefit because they have no records at that hospital or time is not a significant issue (such as for a laceration that requires sutures). Autonomy suffers under this arrangement because the patient is not given the opportunity to consent (or decline). The patient's name and date of birth go out over the air without permission. And, in this case, malfeasance and confidentiality are intertwined. There is potential for harm to the patient and to future patients who lose faith in the EMS system's ability to maintain privacy.

Since the possible consequences of providing all patients' names and dates of birth on the radio are not compatible with the values we consider important and relevant, you must go back and test another action using this same method.

What about the second option, simply to continue the current policy of identifying all patients over the radio only by age and sex? The consequences might be that people listening to scanners can learn about the patients that EMS is transporting but not their identities, and a few patients may get delayed care because their records do not arrive quickly enough. A comparison with relevant values reveals that patient confidentiality and patient confidence in EMS are unchanged, but the patients who might benefit from earlier arrival of their records may be suffering.

What about the third option, to provide names and dates of birth of selected patients, for example, those in serious condition whose treatment must not be delayed? A comparison with relevant values shows that there is potential benefit for selected patients, a breach of confidentiality for those patients, but no breach of confidentiality for any other patients. So, the scenario may conclude as follows:

The third option sounds closer to being acceptable, but you wonder if there is a way to further limit loss of confidentiality. You suggest revising the request: "EMS broadcasts the names and dates of birth of selected patients (1) *who meet predetermined criteria,* and (2) *when there is no other private means of communication available.*" This strictly limits the loss of confidentiality to patients who may benefit from it and encourages both EMS and the ED to find other, less public means of identifying patients. For example, having someone at the scene telephone the ED to relay the patient's name and date of birth privately.

The method described above is useful when you encounter a new ethical problem and time is not an issue. In situations in which time is limited, an abbreviated method can sometimes be used. First, ask yourself whether the current problem is similar to other problems for which you have already formulated a rule. If the answer is yes, follow that rule. If the answer is no, analyze the potential action against three tests suggested by K.V. Iserson in *Ethical Issues in Clinical Emergency Medicine*: the impartiality test, the universalizability test, and the interpersonal justifiability test.

- *Impartiality test*—asks whether you would be willing to undergo this procedure or action if you were in the patient's place. This is really a version of the Golden Rule (Do unto others as you would have them do unto you), which helps reduce the possibility of bias.

- *Universalizability test*—asks whether you would want this action performed in all relevantly similar circumstances, which helps the paramedic to avoid short-sightedness.

- *Interpersonal justifiability test*—asks whether you can defend or justify your actions to others. It helps ensure that an action is appropriate by asking the paramedic to consider whether other people would think the action reasonable.

When there is little time to consider a new ethical problem, these three questions can help a paramedic navigate murky waters, allowing him to find an acceptable solution in a short time.

ETHICAL ISSUES IN CONTEMPORARY PARAMEDIC PRACTICE

The preceding discussion described principles and methods for dealing with ethical issues. The following discussion is meant to help you apply those principles to several commonly encountered situations as well as some less common situations you may face.

RESUSCITATION ATTEMPTS

Consider the following scenario:

You are leaving the emergency department in your ambulance when a man jumps out of a window of the hospital and lands on the road in front of you. Your partner stops the vehicle, and you grab your kit. As

Content Review

SOLVING AN ETHICAL PROBLEM
1. State the action in a universal form.
2. List the implications or consequences of the action.
3. Compare them with relevant values.

you reach the patient, a breathless aide runs out the door and says, "Don't do anything! He's got a DNR order!" How does this affect the care you administer? Your instincts say treat him now and let the hospital sort things out later if he survives.

In this case, your instincts are probably steering you in the right direction for a number of reasons. First, provincial and territorial law requires that you see the order and verify its legitimacy in some manner. In this case, the order is not available for you to see, and so you are under no legal obligation to withhold care.

Second, if the patient is alive (as he appears to be), even a valid DNR order would not prevent you from assessing the patient and administering basic care, including comfort care.

Third, the principle of nonmalfeasance says you should do no harm. Refraining from helping him might cause irreversible harm, perhaps death. The principle of beneficence also urges you to help the patient. The potential conflict arises when you consider autonomy. The competent patient of legal age has a right to determine what happens to his body, but you are unable to verify his wishes regarding resuscitation.

The conclusion of the scenario is as follows:

You and your partner go ahead and assess the patient. He responds to verbal stimuli by moaning, his airway is open, ventilations are adequate, and he has several lacerations and apparent fractures. Since you are literally in front of the hospital, you limit your interventions to quick immobilization on a spine board with bleeding control and oxygen by mask. You rapidly move him to the ED and turn him over to the team there.

Later, you discover that he had originally been admitted for evaluation of new-onset seizures. When the doctors told him that he might have a brain tumour, he signed a DNR form. Fortunately, no tumour was found and his prognosis is actually quite good. The trauma team finds no life-threatening injuries from his fall and expects him to be able to begin psychiatric treatment before he leaves the hospital. This additional information makes you very glad you decided to go ahead with treatment.

Provinces and territories are increasingly passing laws or regulations allowing prehospital personnel to withhold certain treatment when the patient has a DNR order. A valid order consists of a written statement describing interventions a particular patient does not want to have that is recognized by the authorities of that province or territory. (See Chapter 2 for the legal aspects of DNR orders.)

Paramedics spend a great deal of time and energy learning how to assess and treat patients with life-threatening problems. It becomes difficult, then, for a paramedic to watch someone die without doing something to try to stop it. You must nonetheless respect the patient's wishes when a competent patient has clearly communicated what he really wants. DNR orders make this easier because they typically must be signed or approved by a physician, increasing the likelihood that the decision was carefully made.

When no such order exists, however, it becomes more difficult for the paramedic to determine what the patient's wishes truly are. Family members may be able to describe the patient's desires, but they can have conflicts of interest that make their statements less credible. For example, the patient may have accepted his impending death before his family has. They may want you to attempt resuscitation when that was clearly against the patient's expressed wishes. A less common situation is one in which the patient wants all resuscitation efforts but the family does not because they do not want to prolong their own suffering or they have other less noble motivations.

The general principle for paramedics to follow in such cases as these is: "When in doubt, resuscitate." This usually satisfies the principles of beneficence and nonmalfeasance, admittedly perhaps at the expense of autonomy, but one of the biggest advantages to this approach is that, unlike the alternative, it is reversible. If you refrain from attempting resuscitation, it is certain that the patient will die. If you attempt resuscitation, there is no guarantee the patient will survive, but the patient can be removed from life-sustaining equipment later if that is deemed appropriate. Another advantage is that there will be more time later to sort out competing interests.

What about not attempting resuscitation when the situation appears futile? This option may appear attractive at first glance. After a little investigation, though, the issue becomes much more complex. How would a reasonable person or society define "futile"? Except at the extreme ends of the spectrum, no consensus exists on what constitutes a futile attempt at resuscitation. In addition, there is the issue of who would actually make the decision that a resuscitation attempt is futile in a particular case. Is it the experienced paramedic who has seen very few lives saved under similar circumstances or the new paramedic who is still excited about the prospect of saving lives every day? How can it be fair to have such wide disparities in such an important decision? Clearly, the concept of futility does not provide a useful guide for whether or not to attempt resuscitation.

Another related topic is what to do when an advance directive is presented to you after you have begun resuscitation. Once you have verified the validity of the order and the identity of the patient, you are obligated ethically (and perhaps legally, depending on your jurisdiction) to cease resuscitation efforts. This can be a very difficult situation for you emotionally, but you have an obligation to respect the patient's autonomy and stop doing something he did not want. Follow your local protocols regarding procedures for cessation of resuscitation efforts.

> *The general principle for paramedics to follow is, "When in doubt, resuscitate."*

CONFIDENTIALITY

Consider this scenario:

> You are called at one o'clock in the morning to a local hotel for a man reported to be unresponsive (but breathing) at the front desk. When you arrive, one of the guests at the hotel meets you and tells you he found the clerk slumped over in his chair, apparently unconscious, with what smelled like alcohol on his breath.
>
> You approach the patient. His skin appears normal, and he is moving air well. He does not respond when you call him by the name on his name tag, Howard. He has a strong, regular radial pulse that is within normal limits. You do not smell anything except for a faint minty odour. When you shake his shoulder and call his name again, he opens his eyes, looks around, and asks, "Who are you?"
>
> You explain to Howard that you were called by a concerned guest who could not wake him up. Howard says he is fine now and does not want to go to a hospital. He is alert and oriented to person, place, and time. He denies any complaints, takes no medications, and has no past medical history. His vital signs are within normal limits. He denies any alcohol intake or use of any other drugs. The secondary assessment is unremarkable.
>
> By your protocols and standard operating procedures, you have no reason to attempt to force the patient to go to a hospital. You complete the appropriate documentation for a refusal of transport and are leaving the lobby when the guest who called 911 stops you. "Aren't

you going to take him to the hospital?" he asks. No, you reply, he does not want to go. "But what if there's a fire in the hotel and he's passed out and unable to help guests evacuate?"

This makes you stop and think, and you begin to weigh the rights of the hotel guests against the rights of your patient.

Your obligation to the patient is to maintain as confidential the information you obtained as a result of your participation in this medical situation. If you reported his condition to hotel management, what would you report? You have found no objective evidence that he was under the influence of alcohol or drugs. Depending on the jurisdiction you are in, you may actually have a legal obligation to maintain confidentiality under such circumstances as these. However, what if there is an emergency in which the desk clerk's assistance is needed and he is unable to provide it? That is a conceivable but unlikely possibility. There is no clear and present danger that would require you to report.

There are many reasons to respect confidentiality in general. In an emergency, a patient assumes that he can be honest with these strangers who have come to help because they will protect his privacy. If that trust were violated without sufficient cause, patients might very well be embarrassed or humiliated. This would undermine the public's trust in EMS. If word got around that private information was being made public, patients might not be forthcoming in giving their medical histories, potentially leading to disastrous consequences. For example, a man who had recently taken sildenafil (Viagra) for erectile dysfunction might deny taking it before you give him nitroglycerine. The drug interaction in this case is potentially serious, possibly even fatal.

There are nonetheless times when it is appropriate and necessary to breach confidentiality. Every province and territory has laws requiring the reporting of certain health facts, such as births, deaths, particular infectious diseases, child neglect and abuse, and elder neglect and abuse. These last requirements have the most applicability to EMS. They are considered justifiable reasons to breach confidentiality because, in the eyes of society, the benefit to someone who is defenceless (protection from harm and perhaps even death) and to the public (a safer environment for children and the elderly) outweighs the right to privacy of a particular person. A valid court order is also considered a reasonable justification for breaching confidentiality. So is a clear threat by a patient to a specific person, as is having to inform other health-care professionals who will care for the patient.

Clearly, patient confidentiality is an important principle but not an inviolable one. When determining whether it is appropriate to breach confidentiality, take into account the probability of harm, the magnitude of the expected harm, and alternative methods of avoiding harm that do not require encroaching on confidentiality.

In the scenario above, factors do not justify breaching confidentiality. The person who called 911 for emergency assistance, however, is under no such obligation. The scenario ends as follows:

You inform the hotel guest that you are unable to discuss the case with anyone because of confidentiality. However, you point out, the guest is not under the same obligation. He replies, "OK, you may not be able to do anything about it, but I'm calling the manager!"

CONSENT

Consider this scenario:

Bob, a 58-year-old male, has been having crushing substernal pain radiating to his left arm for several hours. He also is pale, sweaty, and nauseated. He denies shortness of breath. His condition remains unchanged after you give him oxygen and nitroglycerine. When you ask Bob which hospital he wants to go to, he tells you, "I'm not going to any hospital." Surprised, you find it difficult to understand why someone in this much pain would not want to go to a hospital.

You try to enlist the help of relatives over the telephone (Bob lives alone), but they are unable to persuade the patient. He has no regular physician, and so that option is not available to you. Finally, you decide to try online medical direction. While you are waiting for the physician to come to the phone, you wonder: If the patient continues to refuse, can you force him to go? How can you act in the best interests of a patient who refuses to accept what you feel certain is best for him?

A competent patient of legal age has the fundamental right to decide what health care he will receive and will not receive. This is at the core of patient autonomy. To exercise this right, a patient must have the information necessary to make an informed decision, the mental faculties to weigh the risks and benefits of various treatment options, and the freedom from restraints that might hamper the ability to exercise his options (such as threats).

It is sometimes appropriate to use the doctrine of implied consent to force the patient to go to the hospital. For the paramedic to use this approach, the patient must be unable to give consent. Typically, the doctrine is invoked when the patient is unable to communicate, but it also can be employed when the patient is incapacitated because of drugs, illness, or injury. In the scenario above, however, the patient shows no signs of being incapacitated. He is alert and oriented, making judgments and answering questions in a manner completely compatible with competence. The fact that the patient refuses something you recommend does not, in itself, indicate that he is incompetent.

Before you leave the patient, you must not only do the things you need to do to protect yourself legally, but you must also assure yourself that the patient truly understands the issues at hand and is able to make an informed decision. As difficult as it may be for you, if the patient is able to do these things, you may have to accept the patient's desires and leave him.

ALLOCATION OF RESOURCES

Paramedics do not usually think of themselves as guardians of finite resources, but occasionally they are. The most obvious example of this occurs when more patients are present than the paramedic is able to manage, such as in a multiple-casualty incident (MCI). While learning how to provide emergency medical care for multiple patients at the same scene, you might ask: What are the ethics of triage?

Several possible approaches are used in parcelling out scarce resources. Patients could all receive the same amount of attention and resources (true parity). They could receive resources based on need. Or they could receive what someone has determined they have earned.

The civilian method of triage, in which the most seriously injured patients receive the most care, is based on need. This method is intended to produce the most good for the most people. However, other methods of triage are in use. Military triage, for example, has traditionally concentrated on helping the least seriously injured because this approach produces the greatest number of soldiers who can return to duty. When international events are staged in a city, typically one or more ambulances are dedicated for the use of the prime minister and other visiting dignitaries. These ambulances are not to be used for anyone else. Because these officials are considered extremely important and because many others need them, the typical order of care is changed.

A controversy exists in emergency medicine as to whether or not celebrities should be treated ahead of others. The argument for doing so typically emphasizes the disorder brought to the ED by the presence of a celebrity and the need to get the person out of the ED as quickly as possible to restore normal operation. The argument against takes the position that giving preferential treatment to a celebrity is an affront to justice and fairness.

All of these methods have their proponents for different situations. The key to resolving the issue of allocation of scarce resources is to examine the competing theories in light of the circumstances at hand.

OBLIGATION TO PROVIDE CARE

Those who provide emergency care have a special obligation to help all those in need. Many other health-care professionals are free to pick and choose their patients, accepting only those who have health insurance or who can themselves pay for the services delivered by the health-care professional. This is not the case in emergency medicine. Paramedics, like other emergency professionals, are obligated to provide medical care for those in need without regard to ability to pay.

Another situation is offering assistance when off duty. In Canada, paramedics are not required by law to stop and render help when they encounter someone in need of emergency care. However, they have a strong ethical obligation to do so. This does not extend to situations in which the paramedic would put himself in danger (such as getting into a car teetering on the edge of a cliff), if assisting would interfere with important duties owed to others (such as leaving young children unattended in a car), or when someone else is already providing assistance. In return, society offers limited liability in the form of Good Samaritan statutes (as discussed in Chapter 2).

TEACHING

When patients call for EMS, they generally expect to receive care from qualified, credentialled individuals. EMS systems with students working in them should make sure students are clearly identified by the uniform they wear. The paramedic acting as preceptor should also, when appropriate, inform patients of the presence of a student and request the patient's consent before the student performs a procedure. This sounds more cumbersome than it actually is. Patients who are unable to consent obviously do not fall into this category. Implied consent is invoked in this case. Patients who are able to consent are frequently very understanding of the student's need for experience. As long as the preceptor stresses that he is overseeing the student, the vast majority of patients consent.

Another issue related to students is how many attempts they should be allowed in order to perform such procedures as intravenous placement and endotracheal intubation before the preceptor steps in. Factors to consider include the student's skill level, the anticipated difficulty of the procedure, and the relative importance of the procedure. It is important to have a limit, at least initially, for the number of times a student will be allowed to attempt a procedure. Such a number will need to be decided by each system in consultation with the medical director.

PROFESSIONAL RELATIONS

As a health-care professional, the paramedic answers to the patient. As a physician extender, the paramedic answers to a physician medical director. As an employee (or volunteer), the paramedic answers to the EMS system. These competing interests can sometimes make life difficult. Each can lead to ethical challenges.

In general, three potential sources of conflict exist between paramedics and physicians. One possibility is a case in which a physician orders something the paramedic believes is contraindicated. For example, suppose a physician ordered a paramedic to transport a critical blunt-trauma patient without attempting any intravenous access, either at the scene or en route during the anticipated 45-minute transport. This order would run counter to standard medical practice.

A different situation arises when the physician orders something the paramedic believes is medically acceptable but not in the patient's best interests. For example, imagine you are transporting a patient with stable vital signs who is complaining of abdominal pain. In accordance with your protocols, you and your partner have each tried twice to start an IV line without success. The patient's veins are some of the worst you have ever seen, and you have no expectation that you will be successful on further attempts. The patient experienced considerable pain with each attempt and is now crying, asking you not to try any more. The physician, however, insists you continue attempts to gain access.

A third potential source of conflict is the situation in which the physician orders something the paramedic believes is medically acceptable but morally wrong. For example, you are ordered to stop CPR on a young male found in cardiac arrest after blunt trauma. His initial rhythm of asystole has remained unchanged, and you know it is usually associated with death. Nonetheless, although there is a very slim chance of recovery for the patient if you continue your resuscitation efforts, you would not be able to live with yourself if you did not at least try.

In each of the three cases, it is certainly appropriate for the paramedic to start by confirming the order and asking the physician to repeat it. If the order is confirmed, the medic would be prudent to ask the physician for an explanation, given the controversial nature of the orders. The next steps will depend on the physician's explanation, the patient's condition, the need for the intervention in the judgment of the paramedic, the feasibility of performing the intervention (like gaining IV access), and the amount of time available to discuss the issue.

Ultimately, the paramedic must determine how the patient's interests are best served. This typically does not lead to conflict, but on occasion the paramedic may run into situations like the ones described above. In these cases, the paramedic must consider the competing interests of beneficence, nonmalfeasance, autonomy, and justice; the roles of the physician and the paramedic; the relative confidence (or lack thereof) the paramedic has in his own medical and ethical judgments; how far the paramedic is willing to go as an advocate for his patient; and the degree of risk acceptable to the paramedic in contravening physician orders.

It is important for the paramedic to understand that no matter what decision he makes, he will have to defend it. The explanation that he was just following the doctor's orders (or, conversely, just doing what he felt was right) will not be sufficient in and of itself. A paramedic is expected to be more than a robot. He is expected to simultaneously be a physician extender, working under a physician's licence, and a clinician with the ability and independence to recognize and question inappropriate orders. The paramedic should also understand that he is not expected to act in ways he feels are immoral. However, if the individual's morals are significantly out of step with the expectations of the profession, he needs to consider changing his profession.

Disagreements with physician orders happen rarely. Usually, they are the result of poor communication (such as saying one thing while meaning another or static interfering with the radio transmission) or lack of sufficient information. Conflicts with physicians that reach the level in the examples above are fortunately rare. When they happen, the paramedic must be willing to be an advocate for the patient and act in the patient's best interests.

RESEARCH

EMS research is only in its infancy, but it will clearly become more important and more common as the field establishes the foundation necessary to introduce, modify, and justify field interventions. As this occurs, paramedics will become instrumental in implementing research protocols and gathering data.

The goal of patient care is to improve the patient's condition. The goal of research is to help the future. The two goals are not the same, and so patients must be protected from untoward outcomes as much as possible.

One very important way of protecting the patient is by gaining the patient's expressed consent. Consent presents several difficulties. One is the concern that a patient experiencing an emergency may not be able to truly consent because of the emotional pressures he is feeling. This pressure may occur in spite of the paramedic's best efforts to explain matters calmly and impartially.

Another concern is with the patient who is unable to consent. An excellent example of this occurs in cardiac arrest research. By the very nature of the problem being studied, the investigators will be unable to gather consent from the patient. In this case, an ethics committee or review board would approve or deny the study on the basis of the ethical implications of consent. The goal of patient care is to improve the patient's condition, and any study in which the patient would be compromised would not be approved. A paramedic participating in such a study needs to be familiar with these rules and their implications.

Although many interventions have been tested and found to be life saving, there are, unfortunately, documented instances of patients denied treatment for life-threatening conditions in the name of research in the United States (e.g., the Tuskegee syphilis research project in which treatment for the disease was withheld). The paramedic has an obligation to prevent such things from happening in EMS research.

Part 7: Lifting and Moving Patients

After receiving emergency care, a patient may need to be handled or transported. If this is done improperly, the patient may be injured further. It is your responsibility to see that the patient is not subjected to unnecessary pain or discomfort.

SECTION 1: BODY MECHANICS

BASIC PRINCIPLES

As a paramedic, you may be asked to lift and carry both patients and heavy equipment. If you do it incorrectly, you could cause yourself injury, strain, and life-long pain. With planning, good health, and skill, you can do your job with minimum risk to yourself.

Apply the principles of proper lifting and moving every day. Practise enough so that they become automatic. Make them a habit that increases your safety and performance, even in the most stressful emergencies.

Body mechanics refers to the safest and most efficient methods of using your body to gain a mechanical advantage. It includes the following:

- *Use your legs, not your back, to lift.* To move a heavy object, use the muscles of your legs, hips, and buttocks, plus the contracted muscles of your abdomen. These muscles let you safely generate a lot of power. Never use the muscles in your back to help you move or lift a heavy object.

FIGURE 1-15 Keep weight close to the body as it is lifted.

- *Keep the weight of the object as close to your body as possible.* Reach across a short distance to lift a heavy object (Figure 1-15). Back injury is much more likely to occur when you reach across a long distance to lift an object.

- *Stack your posture.* Visualize your shoulders stacked on top of your hips and your hips on top of your feet. Then, move as a unit. If your shoulders, hips, and feet are not aligned, you could create twisting forces that can harm your lower back.

- *Reduce the height or distance you need to move the object.* Get closer to the object, or reposition it before you try to lift. Lift in stages, if you need to.

Lifting and moving patients is an important responsibility. Many lifts and moves are routine, while others require quick thinking and skill.

Apply the principles of body mechanics to lifting, carrying, moving, reaching, pushing, and pulling. The key to preventing injury during all these tasks is correct alignment of the spine. Keep a normal inward curve in the lower back. Keep the wrists and knees in normal alignment. Whenever possible, let the equipment to do the lifting for you.

In an emergency, teamwork is essential. Just as a football coach positions players according to ability, rescuers should, too. It can help capitalize on their abilities to ensure the best outcome in any emergency.

All members on a team should be trained in the proper techniques. Problems can occur when team members are greatly mismatched. The stronger partner can be injured if the weaker one fails to lift. The weaker one can be injured if he tries to do too much. Ideally, partners in lifting and moving should have adequate and equal strength and height. Know your physical abilities and limitations. Respect them. Consider the weight of the patient, and recognize the need for help.

Team members also need to communicate during a task, clearly and frequently. Use commands that are easy for team members to understand. Verbally coordinate each lift from beginning to end.

THE POWER LIFT

The power lift is a technique that offers you the best defence against injury. It also protects the patient on a stretcher with a safe and stable move. It is especially useful for rescuers who have weak knees or thighs. Remember, when performing the power lift, keep your back locked, and avoid bending at the waist (Figures 1-16A to 1-16C). Follow these steps:

1. Place your feet a comfortable distance apart. For the average-size person, this is usually about shoulder width. Taller rescuers might prefer a little wider stance.

2. Turn your feet slightly outward. Most people find that this helps them feel more comfortable and more stable.

3. Bend your knees to bring your centre of gravity closer to the object. As you bend your knees, you should feel as though you are sitting down, not falling forward.

4. Tighten the muscles of your back and abdomen to splint the vulnerable lower back. Your back should remain as straight as you can comfortably manage, with your head facing forward in a neutral position.

5. Keep your feet flat, with your weight evenly distributed and just in front of the heels.

6. Place your hands a comfortable distance from each other to provide balance to the object as it is lifted. This is usually at least 25 cm apart.

7. Always use a power grip to get maximum force from your hands. Your palms and fingers should come in complete contact with the object, and all fingers should be bent at the same angle (Figure 1-17).

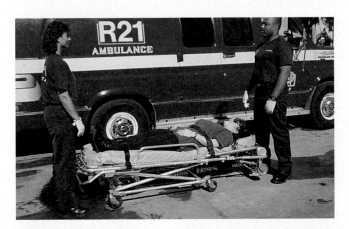

FIGURE 1-16A   Get in position.

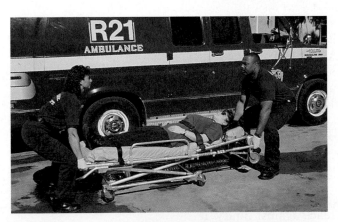

FIGURE 1-16B   Lift in unison, keeping your back locked, knees bent, and feet flat.

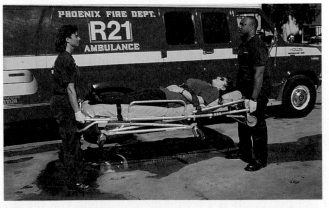

FIGURE 1-16C   Stand straight, making sure your back remains locked.

8. As the lifting begins, your back should remain locked as the force is driven through the heels and arches of your feet. Your upper body should come up before the hips do.

9. Reverse these steps to lower the object.

POSTURE AND FITNESS

Posture is a much overlooked part of body mechanics. When people spend a great deal of time sitting or standing, poor posture can easily tire the back and stomach muscles. This can only make back injury more likely.

One extreme of poor posture is the swayback (Figure 1-18). In this example, the stomach is too far forward and the buttocks too far back, causing extreme stress on the lower back. Another extreme is the slouch, the shoulders are rolled forward, putting increased pressure on every region of the spine.

Be aware of your posture. While standing, your ears, shoulders, and hips should be in vertical alignment. Your knees should be slightly bent and your pelvis slightly tucked forward (Figure 1-19).

When sitting, your weight should be evenly distributed on both ischia (the lower portion of your pelvic bones; Figure 1-20). Your ears, shoulders, and hips should be in vertical alignment. Your feet should be flat on the floor or crossed at the ankles. If possible, your lower back should be in contact with the support of the chair.

Finally, proper body mechanics will not protect you if you are not physically fit. A proactive, well-balanced physical fitness program should include flexibility training, cardiovascular conditioning, strength training, and nutrition.

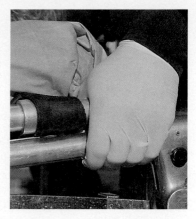

FIGURE 1-17   The power grip.

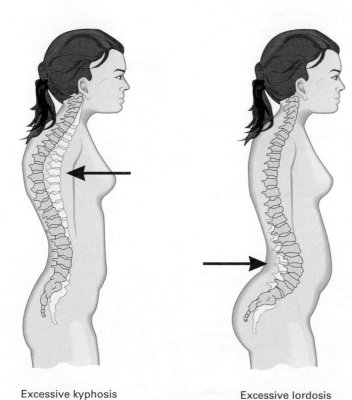

Excessive kyphosis
(slouch)

Excessive lordosis
(swayback)

FIGURE 1-18   Slouch and swayback are extremes of poor posture.

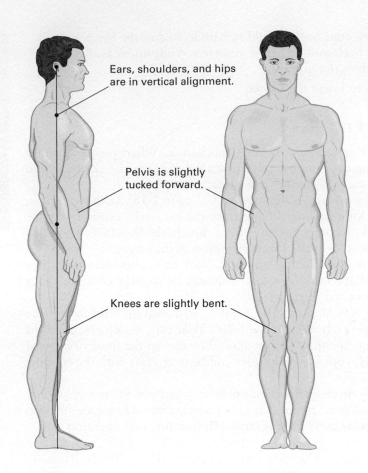

FIGURE 1-19 Proper standing position.

Ears, shoulders, and hips are in vertical alignment.

Pelvis is slightly tucked forward.

Knees are slightly bent.

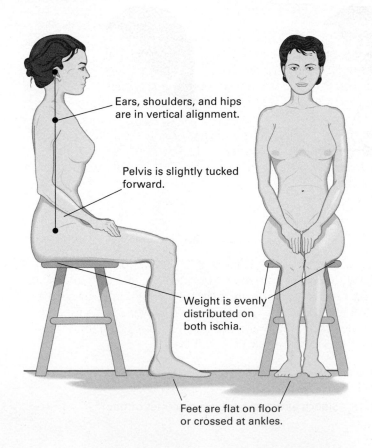

FIGURE 1-20 Proper sitting position.

Ears, shoulders, and hips are in vertical alignment.

Pelvis is slightly tucked forward.

Weight is evenly distributed on both ischia.

Feet are flat on floor or crossed at ankles.

SECTION 2: PRINCIPLES OF MOVING PATIENTS

EMERGENCY MOVES

The top priority in emergency care is to maintain a patient's airway, breathing, and circulation (ABCs). However, if the scene is unstable or poses an immediate threat, you may have to move the patient first. Follow local protocols.

In general, when there is no threat to life, provide emergency medical care. Make an emergency move only when there is an immediate danger to the patient. The following are examples of situations in which you may make an emergency move:

- *Fire or threat of fire.* Fire should always be considered a grave threat, not only to patients but also to rescuers.
- *Explosion or the threat of explosion.*
- *Inability to protect the patient from other hazards at the scene.* Examples of hazards include an unstable building, a rolled-over car, spilled gasoline and other hazardous materials, an unruly or hostile crowd, and extreme weather conditions.
- *Inability to gain access to other patients who need life-saving care.* For example, this may occur at the scene of a car crash involving two or more patients.
- *When life-saving care cannot be given because of the patient's location or position.* For example, a patient in cardiac arrest must be supine on a flat, hard surface for you to perform CPR properly. If that patient is sitting on a chair, an emergency move must be made in order for you to provide life-saving care.

The greatest danger in an emergency move is the possibility of worsening a spine injury. To provide as much protection to the spine as possible, pull the patient in the direction of the long axis of the body.

It is impossible to move a patient from a vehicle quickly and, at the same time, protect the spine. So, move the patient from the vehicle immediately only if one of the five conditions described above exists.

If the patient is on the floor or the ground, use one of the following emergency moves. Be sure never to pull the patient's head away from the neck and shoulders. If there is time, you may want to bind the patient's wrists together with a cravat or gauze. This will make the patient easier to move, and it will help protect his hands and arms from injury.

Shirt Drag

To perform a shirt drag, do the following (Figure 1-21). First, fasten the patient's hands or wrists loosely with a cravat or gauze to protect them during the move. Then, grasp the shoulders of the patient's shirt (not a T-shirt). Pull the shirt under the patient's head to form a support. Then, using the shirt as a "handle," pull the patient toward you. Be careful not to strangle the patient. The pulling should engage the patient's armpits, not the neck.

Blanket Drag

To perform a blanket drag, do the following (Figure 1-22). First, spread a blanket alongside the patient. Gather half of it into lengthwise pleats. Roll the patient away from you onto his side, and tuck the pleated part of the blanket as far under as you can. Then, roll the patient back onto the centre of the blanket, preferably onto his back. Wrap the blanket securely around the patient. Grabbing the part of the blanket that is under the patient's head, drag the patient toward you.

If you do not have a blanket, you can use a coat in the same way.

Shoulder or Forearm Drag

To perform a shoulder drag, do the following (Figure 1-23). First, stand at the patient's head. Then, slip your hands under the patient's armpits from the back. If you must drag the patient a long distance and need a better grip, then perform a forearm drag. Position yourself as you would in a shoulder drag. After you slip your hands under the patient's armpits, grasp the patient's forearms and drag the patient toward you. Use your own forearms as a support to keep the patient's head, neck, and spine in alignment.

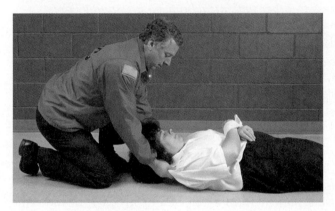

FIGURE 1-21   Shirt drag.

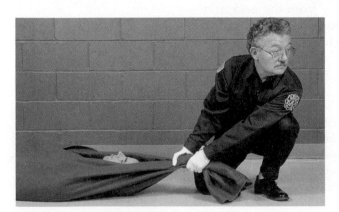

FIGURE 1-22   Blanket drag.

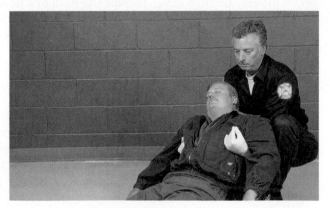

FIGURE 1-23   Shoulder drag.

Other Emergency Moves

Other emergency moves include the piggyback carry, one-rescuer crutch, one-rescuer cradle carry, firefighter's drag, and others (Figures 1-24A to 1-24E and 1-25A to 1-25D).

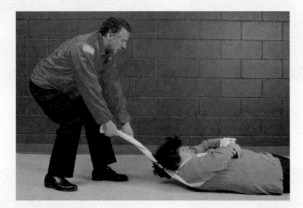

FIGURE 1-24A   Sheet drag.

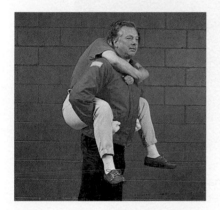

FIGURE 1-24B   Piggyback carry.

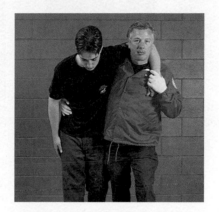

FIGURE 1-24C   One-rescuer crutch.

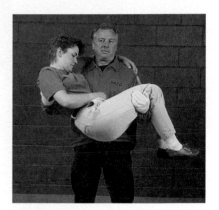

FIGURE 1-24D   Cradle carry.

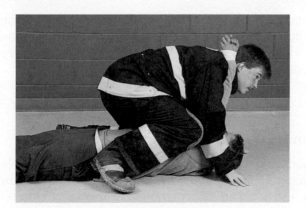

FIGURE 1-24E   Firefighter's drag.

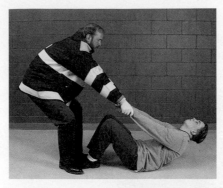

FIGURE 1-25A Grasp the patient's wrists.

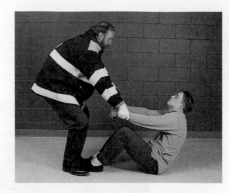

FIGURE 1-25B Stand on the patient's toes, and pull.

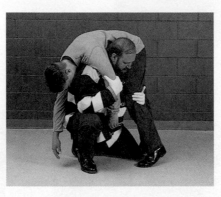

FIGURE 1-25C Pull the patient over your shoulder.

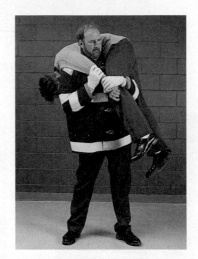

FIGURE 1-25D Pass an arm between the patient's legs, and grasp the arm nearest you.

NONEMERGENCY MOVES

Nonemergency moves, or nonurgent moves, are generally performed with other rescuers. They require no equipment and may take less time than such moves as a blanket drag. However, do not use them with possible spine-injured patients, since they offer no spinal protection.

Nonemergency, or nonurgent, moves include the direct ground lift and extremity lift.

Direct Ground Lift

The direct ground lift requires two or three rescuers. It is valuable when the patient is unable to sit in a chair and when a stretcher cannot be brought close to the patient. It is difficult if the patient weighs more than 75 kg, is on the ground or some other low surface, or is uncooperative.

Position the stretcher as close to the patient as possible. Undo the stretcher straps, lower the railings, and clear any equipment off the mattress. Tell the patient what you are going to do. Then, warn the patient to remain still in order to maintain your balance. If possible, place the patient's arms on his chest.

To perform a direct ground lift, follow these steps (Figures 1-26A to 1-26D):

1. Line up on one side of the patient. If possible, line up on the least injured side.

2. Kneel on one knee, preferably the same side for all rescuers.

3. Have the first rescuer cradle the patient's head by placing one arm under the neck and shoulder. The rescuer must place his other arm under the patient's lower back.

4. Have the second rescuer place one arm under the patient's knees and the other arm above the buttocks.

5. If a third rescuer is available, have him place both arms under the patient's waist. The other two rescuers should slide their arms up to the middle of the back and down to the buttocks as appropriate.

6. On signal, all rescuers, as a unit, should lift the patient to the level of their knees. Then, with a gentle rocking motion, as a unit, roll the patient toward your chests until he is cradled in the bends of your elbows. Tuck the patient's head in toward your chest.

7. On signal, the rescuers should stand up and carry the patient to the stretcher.

8. To lower the patient onto the stretcher, reverse the steps.

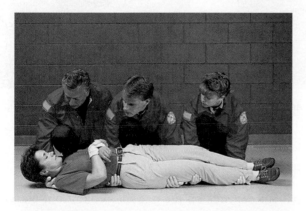

FIGURE 1-26A   Kneel on one knee on the least injured side.

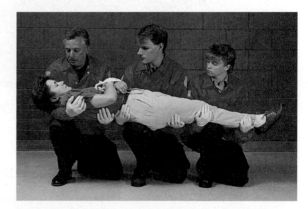

FIGURE 1-26B   In unison, lift the patient to knee level.

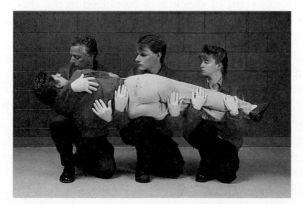

FIGURE 1-26C   Slowly turn the patient toward you.

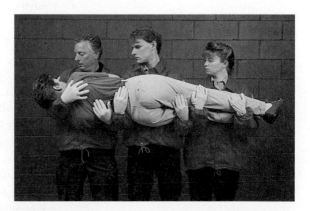

FIGURE 1-26D   In unison, rise to the standing position.

Extremity Lift

Do not use the extremity lift if the patient has injuries to his arms or legs. Use this lift to move a patient from a chair or the floor to the stretcher. Two rescuers are needed to perform the lift (Figures 1-27A and 1-27B).

1. Take a position at the patient's head. The other rescuer should kneel at the patient's side by the patient's knees.
2. Place one hand under each of the patient's shoulders, reaching through to grab the patient's wrists.
3. The second rescuer should slip his hands under the patient's knees.
4. On signal, both of you can then move the patient to the desired location.

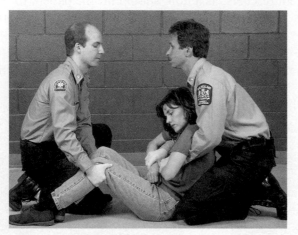

FIGURE 1-27A   Move up to a crouch and then to the standing position.

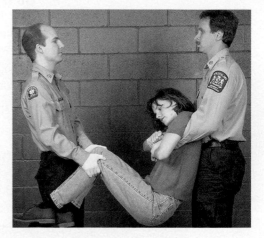

FIGURE 1-27B   Get in position at the head and feet of the patient.

POSITIONING THE PATIENT

How you position a patient depends on the patient's condition. General guidelines include the following:

- Unless there is a life-threatening emergency, a patient who has been injured should not be moved until a primary assessment is completed.
- A patient who shows signs of shock may be placed in the shock position. If it will not aggravate injuries to the legs or spine, this is done by elevating the supine patient's legs by 20 to 30 cm.
- A patient who has pain or breathing problems may get in any position that makes him more comfortable, unless the injuries prevent it. Generally, a patient who has breathing difficulties will want to sit up. A patient with abdominal pain will want to lie on his side with the knees drawn up.
- A conscious patient who is nauseated or vomiting should be allowed to remain in a position of comfort. However, you should always be positioned so you can manage the patient's airway if needed.
- An unconscious patient who is not injured should be placed in the recovery position. Many ambulances are configured with the stretcher against the driver-side wall. Rolling the unconscious patient onto his left side allows you to better monitor him during transport.

SECTION 3: EQUIPMENT

Become completely familiar with the equipment used to move patients in your EMS system. To decide which to use, base your decision on the patient's condition, the environment in which he is found, and the resources available. Generally, the best way to move a patient is the easiest way that will not cause injury or pain.

Let your equipment do the work, whenever possible. Drag or slide the patient (not lift) whenever you can. If you must lift a patient, do it with a device designed for that purpose. As a rule, carry a patient only as far as absolutely necessary. Make sure you have adequate help. If you do not have it, get it. Never risk injuring yourself.

Typical equipment used in EMS includes various types of stretchers, the stair chair, and backboards.

STRETCHERS

A standard stretcher, or cot, has wheeled legs. It also has a collapsible undercarriage that makes it possible to load it into an ambulance (Figure 1-28).

A portable stretcher is lightweight, folds compactly, and is easy to clean. It does not have an undercarriage and wheels. It is comfortable to rest on, especially if the head is padded. It is valuable when there is not enough space for a standard stretcher or when there are many patients. It comes in a variety of styles. The most common has an aluminum frame with canvas fabric (Figures 1-29 and 1-30).

A scoop, or orthopedic, stretcher splits into two or four sections (Figure 1-31). Each section can be fitted around a patient who is lying on a relatively flat surface. It is used in confined areas where larger stretchers will not fit. Once secure in a scoop stretcher, the patient can be lifted and moved to a standard one. To operate a scoop stretcher, split it apart lengthwise. Carefully slide it under the patient from both sides. Then, lock the brackets at each end, and lift the patient.

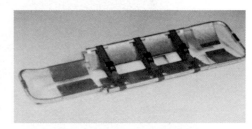

FIGURE 1-28   Standard stretcher.

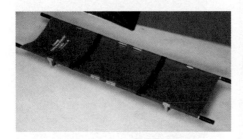

FIGURE 1-29   Pole stretcher.

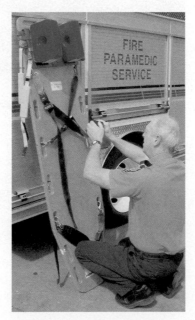

FIGURE 1-30   Portable ambulance stretcher.

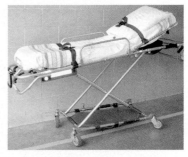

FIGURE 1-31   Scoop or orthopedic stretcher.

STAIR CHAIRS

Moving patients up or down stairs dramatically increases the potential for rescuers to be injured. The safest way to do it is with a stair chair. A stair chair is a lightweight folding device. It has straps to confine the patient, wheeled legs, a grab bar below the patient's feet, and handles that extend behind the patient's shoulders.

When you use a stair chair (Figures 1-32A to 1-32C), make sure that as many people as necessary are helping. A spotter is needed to help manoeuvre the stair chair down stairs. The spotter should continually tell how many stairs are left and what conditions are ahead. A spotter also can place his hand on the back of the rescuer who is moving backward to help steady the rescuer.

Rescuers carrying a patient in a stair chair should keep their backs in a locked position. They should flex at the hips instead of at the waist, bend at the knees, and keep the arms (and the weight of the chair) as close to their bodies as possible. Once off the stairs, the patient can be transferred to a more conventional stretcher.

Stair chairs work well for patients in respiratory distress who need to be moved up or down stairs. The sitting position does not worsen the patient's breathing problems.

BACKBOARDS

There are both long and short backboards (Figures 1-33A to 1-33E). A long backboard is approximately 2 m long, which means it can stabilize the patient's entire body. It is used for patients with suspected spine injury who are lying down.

A short backboard is 1 to 1.25 m long and can stabilize the patient down to the hips. It is used to stabilize a patient with suspected spine injuries who is in a sitting position.

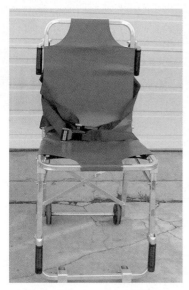

FIGURE 1-32A   Stair chair.

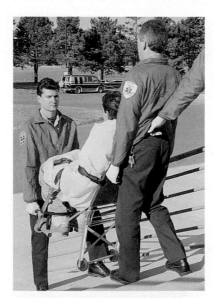

FIGURE 1-32B   Moving a patient up steps with a third rescuer as spotter.

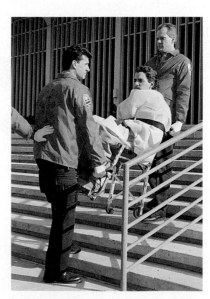

FIGURE 1-32C   Moving a patient down steps with a third rescuer as spotter.

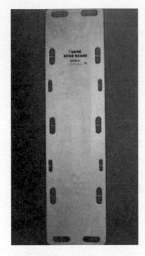

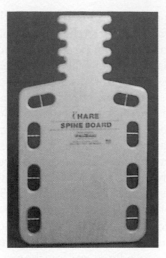

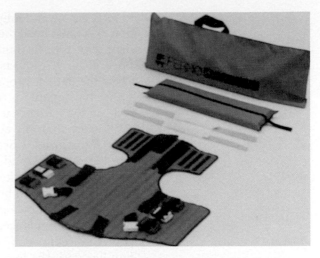

FIGURE 1-33A
Traditional wooden
long backboard.

FIGURE 1-33B Short
backboard.

FIGURE 1-33C Vest-type immobilization device.

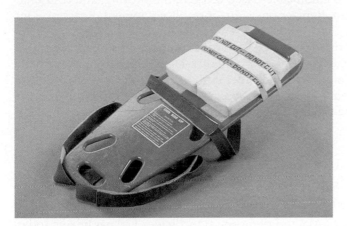

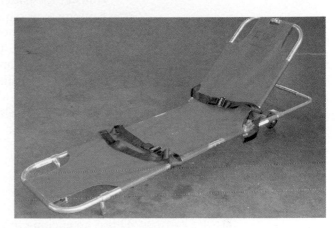

FIGURE 1-33D Short backboard.

FIGURE 1-33E Long backboard.

Both the long and short backboards feature handholds and straps. Most are made of synthetic material that will not absorb blood and are easy to clean. Regardless of whether you use a long or short backboard, always maintain manual support of the patient's head and neck in the normal anatomical position. Maintain that support until the patient is *fully* secured to the backboard.

You will learn more about managing and packaging spinal patients in Chapter 24, Spinal Trauma.

LOADING AND UNLOADING STRETCHERS

You may encounter a variety of stretcher styles and ambulance designs. Ensure that you review the mechanics of your stretcher and stretcher securing system.

Most stretchers have handles for releasing the undercarriage at the end of the stretcher and along one side.

Use an appropriate lift or transferring device to place the patient on the stretcher. Ensure that your patient is positioned and covered properly. Most stretchers allow you to position a patient supine, to raise the head of the stretcher to semi-sitting and fully upright positions, or to raise the feet of the stretcher. Note that you must keep the head of the stretcher flat if you want to position your patient semi-prone. Many stretchers can be shortened to allow travel through confined areas. Use sheets, blankets, and other covers as per policy in your system. Once the patient is positioned, raise the side bars and use the stretcher straps to secure the patient for transport. Some stretchers include shoulder straps that help restrain the patient's torso when the ambulance accelerates or brakes.

Ensure that any equipment required for ongoing treatment and monitoring is safely secured. Check all equipment before moving the patient. Ensure that bandages, splints, and immobilization devices are secure and that tubes, airways, ECG leads, and IV sites are intact and in place. Do not place equipment, such as monitors or oxygen bottles, directly on the patient. Some EMS systems use specially designed brackets or clips to secure equipment to the stretcher.

At the ambulance, prepare the patient and stretcher for loading. Lower IV poles and remove any equipment that is attached to the sides of the stretcher. Be familiar with the loading procedures and mechanics of your system's stretcher and securing systems. Communicate with your partner and any other emergency medical responders who are assisting you to ensure smooth loading. Double-check that the stretcher is secure before entering the ambulance.

Transfer the patient to ambulance-based oxygen, monitoring, and resuscitation equipment as required. Replace or secure portable equipment. Reassess your patient before transport.

When you arrive at your destination, you must prepare the patient for transfer out of the ambulance. Change from ambulance-based equipment to portable systems. Move IV bags, monitors, and other equipment to the stretcher. Ensure that the patient and all equipment are secure. Communicate with your partner and patient as you release the stretcher from its docking mechanisms and take it from the ambulance.

SUMMARY

This is an exciting time for EMS and prehospital medicine. The paramedic today is a true health-care professional who can have a significant impact on health care.

EMS has evolved over many years. Today, a comprehensive EMS system provides a continuum of care by professionals, from the emergency medical dispatcher, emergency medical responder, and the paramedic to hospital and rehabilitative staff, from the mechanic who maintains the ambulance fleet to the medical control physician. It is a total team effort. The paramedic is the leader of the prehospital emergency medical team. You must undertake the responsibility of preparing yourself to do the job and of continually updating your knowledge and skills. The best paramedics are those who make a commitment to excellence.

As a paramedic, you must attend first to your own well-being and maintain your health and fitness in order to help others and to be a positive role model. Additionally, each member of EMS shares the responsibility of promoting wellness and preventing illness and injury among coworkers and in the community.

As a paramedic, you also have the responsibility to act ethically by acquiring a foundation in ethical values and having a system for making ethical decisions.

The best paramedics are those who make a commitment to excellence.

CHAPTER 2

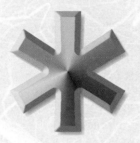

Medical-Legal Aspects of Prehospital Care

Objectives

After reading this chapter, you should be able to:

1. Differentiate among legal, ethical, and moral responsibilities. (pp. 90–91)
2. Describe the basic structure of the Canadian legal system and differentiate between civil law and criminal law. (pp. 91–93)
3. Differentiate between licensure and certification. (p. 96)
4. List reportable problems or conditions and to whom the reports are to be made. (pp. 96–97)
5. Define: Abandonment (pp. 108–109); Advance directives (pp. 110–111); Assault (p. 109); Battery (p. 109); Breach of duty (p. 98); Confidentiality (p. 103); Consent (expressed, implied, informed, involuntary) (pp. 104–106); Do Not Resuscitate orders (p. 111); Duty to act (p. 98); Emancipated minor (p. 106); False imprisonment (p. 109); Immunity (pp. 97, 100); Liability (pp. 91, 98–102); Libel (p. 104); Minor (p. 106); Negligence (pp. 98–101); Proximate cause (p. 100); Scope of practice (pp. 95–96); Slander (p. 104); Standard of care (pp. 98–99); Tort (p. 93)
6. Discuss the legal implications of medical direction. (pp. 95, 101–102)
7. Describe the four elements necessary to prove negligence. (pp. 98–100)

Continued

INTRODUCTION

To practise competent prehospital care today, paramedics must become familiar with the legal issues they are likely to encounter in the field. As a paramedic, you must be prepared to make the best medical decisions and the most appropriate legal decisions. This chapter addresses general legal principals in addition to specific laws and legal concepts that affect the paramedic's daily practice.

Because laws vary among provinces and territories in Canada and protocols can vary regionally within each province or territory, the information contained in this chapter is not a substitute for competent legal advice. Just like the practice of medicine, the practice of law involves some art and some science, and it is always heavily dependent on the unique facts of each situation. If you are faced with a specific legal issue, you must rely on the advice of an attorney.

LEGAL DUTIES AND ETHICAL RESPONSIBILITIES

As a paramedic, you have specific legal duties. Failure to perform your job appropriately can result in civil, professional, or criminal sanction. If, for example, you sexually abuse a patient, you can face a criminal charge. At the same time, the patient can sue you in civil court. Your professional association can also come after you—all because of the one action.

Your best protection from **liability** (legal responsibility) and possible sanction is to perform a systematic patient assessment, provide the appropriate medical care, and maintain accurate and complete documentation of all incidents, in accordance with what a reasonable and prudent paramedic would do in similar circumstances.

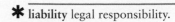
* **liability** legal responsibility.

A paramedic is responsible for meeting ethical standards. Ethical standards are not laws; they are principles that identify desirable conduct by members of a particular group. Although the phrasing of ethical guidelines varies, they all share common goals. Your ethical responsibilities generally include:

- Promptly responding to the needs of every patient
- Treating all patients and their families with courtesy and respect
- Maintaining mastery of your skills and medical knowledge
- Participating in continuing education and refresher training
- Critically reviewing your performance and seeking improvement
- Reporting honestly and with respect for patient confidentiality
- Working cooperatively and respectfully with other emergency professionals

Your best protection from liability is to perform systematic assessments, provide appropriate medical care, and maintain accurate and complete documentation.

In addition, you will encounter moral issues. Morality concerns right and wrong as governed by individual conscience. In your career, always strive to meet the highest legal, ethical, and moral standards when providing patient care.

In Canada, various governments have placed what are ethical parameters into statutes. For example, in Alberta, Section 13 of the EMT Regulation, "Duties of Registered Members," states:

A registered member shall

(a) execute duties in a safe and competent manner being guided at all times by the welfare and best interests of the patient;
(b) work within the scope of practice and the registered member's ability and within the limitations or conditions placed on the provision of service by the medical director;
(c) conduct affairs with respect to the discipline so as not to bring discredit to the discipline;
(d) maintain current knowledge and skill in the practice of emergency care and upgrade knowledge and skill with the development of new procedures and equipment;
(e) work to promote high standards of research, training, and performance for registered members;
(f) work in cooperation with colleagues and other health-care personnel;
(g) refer any incompetent, illegal, or unethical conduct by colleagues or other health-care personnel to the appropriate authorities;
(h) hold in confidence all information learned in the health-care setting respecting the patient unless failure to disclose would endanger the patient or a third party or the disclosure is required by law.

THE LEGAL SYSTEM

The legal system in Canada has two regimes. Quebec operates under a system based on the French Code Napoleon and has a civil law–common law fused system. The other provinces and territories, and the federal government, use a system based on English common law, and all federal laws must be written in both French and English.

The Criminal Code of Canada is the only criminal legislation in Canada, and it is under federal jurisdiction. The Code is enacted and amended by the federal government, but the provinces and territories have jurisdiction to deal with minor noncriminal offences, such as environment offences.

Quebec's Civil Code (le droit civil) was first enacted in 1866. It was replaced in 1991 with a consolidated code incorporating the many amendments that had been made since 1866. The Civil Code is a collection of general rules and ideals that guide the conduct of the courts and the citizenry and that outline the laws. The Civil Code deals with property rights, wills, contracts, and noncriminal interaction between parties. In addition to the Civil Code, other legislation addresses the areas dealt with in common law by the other provinces and territories.

The historical laws of Canada's Aboriginal people also affect the courts. Aboriginal sentencing practices tend to focus less on pure punishment and more on healing.

Canada's political structure is that of a federation; that is, the provinces and territories are united and have a central (federal) government based in Ottawa. The British North America Act, 1867, divided the areas that the federal government is responsible for (e.g., waterways) from those of the provinces and territories (e.g., regulation of professionals). This split gives both Parliament and the provincial and territorial legislatures the power to make laws, albeit in different areas. Health care is a provincial and territorial domain, and each jurisdiction has developed its own EMS models, certification levels, and practices.

Unlike the United States, which has most of its constitutional law in its Constitution, Canada was created by a law made not in North America, but in Great Britain. The British North America Act, 1867, created the Dominion of Canada by uniting Upper Canada, Lower Canada, Nova Scotia, and New Brunswick. A second constitutional document, the Constitution Act, 1982, cut Canada's final legal ties to Great Britain. Although the Queen remains the head of state for Canada, she is represented in Ottawa by the governor general and in each province and territory by a lieutenant governor.

Sources of Law

As a general concept, the Canadian Constitution is the supreme law (subject to the right of each province and territory to override laws that are found to be unconstitutional). When federal laws conflict with provincial or territorial laws, the federal laws govern. Regulations that conflict with their governing statute fall in the face of that statute. Codes of conduct from professional associations likely take precedence over the policies of any organization.

Canada has four primary sources of law: constitutional law, common law, legislative (or statutory) law, and administrative (or regulatory) law.

Constitutional Law

✳ **constitutional law** law based on the Canadian Constitution.

Constitutional law entrenches certain fundamental principles within the supreme law of Canada. The Canadian Constitution comprises two sections: the Constitutional Acts, 1867 to 1975, and the Constitution Act, 1982. Entrenched as Part I of the Canadian Constitution is the Canadian Charter of Rights and Freedoms, which provides certain guarantees for citizens. For example, Section 2(a) of the Charter provides for freedom of conscience and religion.

Common Law

✳ **common law** law derived from society's acceptance over time of customs and norms. Also called *case law* or *judge-made law.*

Common law, also called *case law* or *judge-made law,* originated in the English legal system and is derived from society's acceptance over time of customs and norms. Common law changes and grows over the years. As a part of common law, precedents set by the courts are binding on lower courts and generally followed by other courts of the same level.

Legislative Law

Legislative law (or statutory law) does not come from court decisions. It is created by law-making or legislative bodies. Statutes are enacted at the federal, provincial/territorial, and local levels by the legislative branches of government. Examples of legislative bodies include the federal House of Commons, provincial and territorial legislatures, city councils, and district boards. Legislative law generally takes precedence over common-law decisions; however, the courts can use the Constitution to strike down legislative laws that conflict with constitutional rights.

Administrative Law

Administrative law (or regulatory law) is enacted by an administrative or government agency at either the federal or the provincial/territorial level. Administrative agencies, such as the Occupational Safety and Health Administration (OSHA) or any of the Colleges of Paramedics, will take a statute enacted by a legislative body and produce the rules and regulations necessary to implement that statute. These agencies are given the authority to make regulations based on that statute; to enforce the rules, regulations, and statutes under its authority; and to hold administrative hearings to assign penalties for any violations of its rules. The right to regulate professions is granted as part of administrative law.

Categories of Law

Canada has two general categories of law: civil law and criminal law. **Criminal law** deals with crime and punishment. It is an area of law in which the federal, provincial/territorial, or local government will prosecute an individual on behalf of society for violating laws meant to protect society. Homicide, rape, and burglary are examples of criminal offences. Violations of criminal laws are punished by imprisonment, fines, or a combination of the two.

Civil law deals with noncriminal issues, such as personal injury, contract disputes, and matrimonial matters. In civil litigation, which involves conflicts between two or more parties, the *plaintiff* (person initiating the litigation) will seek to recover damages from the *defendant* (person against whom the complaint is made). **Tort** (Latin for "wrong") law is a branch of civil law that deals with civil wrongs committed by one individual against another (rather than against society). Tort law claims include negligence, medical malpractice, assault, battery, and defamation. Defamation includes written defamation, or libel, and spoken defamation, or slander.

Canada's federal court has its own Court of Appeal. All courts in Canada eventually appeal to the Supreme Court of Canada, which is the last level of appeal. Canada differs from the United States in that Canada has a national Criminal Code, a statute that provides for some offences to be heard in the superior court of each province or territory, and others to be heard in the lower courts. Criminal laws in the United States change from state to state.

The provincial or territorial court system is the location for most cases in which a paramedic may become involved. In *trial courts,* a judge or jury determines the outcome of individual cases. Each province and territory has superior courts, with judges appointed by the federal government, and provincial or territorial courts, with judges appointed by the premier. *Appellate courts* hear appeals of decisions by trial courts or other appeals courts. The decisions of appellate courts may set precedents for later cases and are binding on lower courts.

ANATOMY OF A CIVIL LAWSUIT

Being sued or even being called to testify at a trial can be very unsettling. A basic understanding of the legal system can help, as it will explain what to expect. Remember, just because someone sues you does not mean that you have done anything wrong. The following is a brief description of the components of a civil lawsuit.

- *Incident.* For example, a person is driving on a road and fails to see a stop sign. When the car passes through the intersection, it hits another car and that driver sustains several injuries.

- *Investigation.* The injured driver's attorney makes a preliminary inquiry into the facts and circumstances surrounding the incident to determine whether the case has merit.

- *Statement of Claim.* The injured driver (now called the "plaintiff") commences the lawsuit by filing a complaint with the court. The complaint contains such information as the names of the parties, the legal basis for the claim, and the damages sought by the plaintiff. A copy of the complaint is served on the defendant. In Canada, this document is called a Statement of Claim.

- *Statement of Defence.* The defendant's attorney then prepares an answer, which addresses each allegation made in the complaint. The answer is then filed with the court, and a copy is given to the plaintiff's attorney. In Canada, this document is called a Statement of Defence.

- *Discovery.* Before any lawsuit appears in front of a judge or jury, both parties to an action participate in pretrial discovery. At this stage of the lawsuit, all relevant information about the incident is shared so that the parties can prepare trial strategies. Discovery often results in settlement of cases once the evidence is tested and reviewed by all the parties. Discovery may include:

  - *An examination before trial,* also called an examination for discovery, which allows a witness to answer questions under oath with a court stenographer present.

  - *An interrogatory.* Used by either side, this is a set of written questions that require written responses.

  - *Requests for document production,* which entitle each side to request relevant documents that are not protected by solicitor-client privilege, including the patient care report, records of the receiving hospital, any subsequent medical records, police records, and other records necessary to help prove or defend the lawsuit. This request is usually made before the deposition, and you may be cross-examined on those documents and your answers recorded. There are complex rules with regard to what documents you must produce. Courts in Canada have recently held that tape recordings and electronic records (i.e., email) are documents for the purposes of document production.

- *Trial.* A trial will commence at the lowest-level provincial or territorial court that has the jurisdiction to hear the matter. In many provinces and territories, these courts are called "superior" courts. The amount of money being sought for damages may also dictate which court the matter is heard in. At the trial, each side will be given the opportunity to present all relevant evidence and testimony from witnesses.

- *Decision.* After deliberations, the judge or jury determines the guilt or liability of the defendant and then decides the amount of damages to award the plaintiff.

- *Appeal.* After the jury's decision is entered by the court, either party may be entitled to an appeal. Generally, grounds for an appeal are limited to errors of law made by the court. Appeals will not be heard at the lower-level court but by the higher-level appellate court.
- *Settlement.* Settlement can occur at any stage of the lawsuit. Generally, the defendant will offer the plaintiff an amount of money that is less than the amount for which she is being sued, without any admission of liability on the part of the defendant. The plaintiff may then agree to accept the reduced amount on the condition, for example, that she will no longer pursue the case and will acknowledge that notwithstanding payment by the defendant of money, there is no admission of error on the part of the defendant.

LAWS AFFECTING EMS AND THE PARAMEDIC

Most laws that affect EMS and paramedics are provincial or territorial laws. Although these laws vary across provinces and territories, they share common principles.

Scope of Practice

The range of duties and skills paramedics are allowed and expected to perform is called the **scope of practice.** Usually, the scope of practice is set by provincial or territorial law or regulation and in some locales by local medical direction. Often, a province or territory has a general "medical practice act" that governs the practice of medicine and other statutes for individual health-care professions. For example, in Nova Scotia, registered nurses are subject to the Registered Nurses Act, and in Alberta, paramedics are regulated by the Alberta College of Paramedics in accordance with the Health Disciplines Act. In Canada, most EMS professionals act in accordance with their own provincial or territorial regulations.

Physicians are very involved in the practice of paramedics, as all provinces and territories require some form of medical direction. As you learned in Chapter 1, paramedics may function only under the direct supervision of a licensed physician through a delegation of authority. Generally, paramedics should follow orders given by online and offline medical direction. However, they should not blindly follow orders that they know are medically inappropriate. In fact, damages have been awarded against individuals who followed the direction of a physician, when they knew, or ought to have known, that the directions were inappropriate and the course of action resulted in injury to the patient.

The circumstances under which an order from medical direction may be legitimately refused include being ordered to provide a treatment that is beyond the scope of your training and that is inconsistent with established protocols or procedures and being ordered to administer a treatment that you reasonably believe will be harmful to the patient. For example, imagine that a paramedic is en route to the hospital with a 100-kg patient who is having 15 multifocal premature ventricular contractions (PVCs) per minute. The treatment protocol for such a condition is to administer 1–1.5 mg/kg of lidocaine, or 100–150 mg to a 100-kg patient. The online physician orders the paramedic to administer 1 g (1000 mg) of lidocaine. The paramedic knows this amount of medication will seriously harm the patient. What should she do? The paramedic should first raise the concern with the physician. If the physician still insists, the paramedic should refuse to follow the order and should document the incident thoroughly on the patient care report. Such an incident should be reported to the management team as soon as appropriate, as many problems can be resolved successfully if attended to early in the process.

Content Review

COMPONENTS OF A CIVIL LAWSUIT
- Incident
- Investigation
- Statement of Claim
- Statement of Defence
- Discovery
- Trial
- Decision
- Appeal
- Settlement

✱ **scope of practice** range of duties and skills paramedics are allowed and expected to perform.

You may function as a paramedic only under the direct supervision of a licensed physician through a delegation of authority.

Every EMS system should have a policy in place to guide paramedics in dealing with intervener physicians (on-scene licensed physicians who are professionally unrelated to the patient and who are attempting to assist with patient care). Generally, such a policy requires that certain conditions be met before the paramedic allows the intervener physician to assume control of patient care. That is, the physician must be properly identified to the paramedic, licensed to practise medicine in the province or territory, willing to accept the responsibility of continuing medical care until the patient reaches the hospital, and willing to document the intervention as required by the local EMS system. Some systems have successfully used cards printed with their policy on intervener physicians that are handed to the person offering to assist. No physician should be upset with a request for verification of her licence. Refusal or a histrionic reaction should raise red flags for the paramedic. Every EMS system has its horror stories of citizens pretending to be physicians attending at calls.

Licensure and Certification

Other laws that directly affect the paramedic's ability to practise relate to certification and licensure requirements. *Certification* is the recognition granted to an individual who has met the qualifications to participate in a certain activity. It is usually given by a certifying agency (not necessarily a government agency) or professional college or association. In Alberta, after successfully completing an approved paramedic program and passing the required exams, a person will become a registered emergency medical technologist-paramedic and by statute may use the initials "EMT-P" after her name.

Licensure is a process used to regulate occupations. Generally, a governmental agency, such as a provincial or territorial medical board, grants permission to an individual who meets established qualifications to engage in a particular profession or occupation. Certification or licensure, or perhaps both, may be required by your provincial, territorial, or local authorities for you to practise as a paramedic. In British Columbia, paramedics receive certification from their training agency and then must apply for and maintain a licence from a provincial licensing body to practise in the field.

Most provinces and territories have laws that govern paramedic practice and set out the requirements for certification, licensure, recertification, and relicensure. It is your responsibility to fully understand the EMS laws and regulations in your province or territory.

Motor-Vehicle Laws

As with other EMS-related laws, motor-vehicle laws vary across jurisdictions. Generally, special motor-vehicle laws govern the operation of emergency vehicles and the equipment they carry. These laws apply to such areas as vehicle maintenance and use of the siren and emergency lights. It is important that you become familiar with the laws of your province or territory. Keep up to date with local regulations, too. Generally, the laws allow EMS vehicles to exceed posted speed limits and to breach other vehicle traffic laws in an emergency, when it is safe and reasonable to do so.

Mandatory Reporting Requirements

Each province and territory enacts different laws designed to protect the public. For example, most provinces and territories have laws that require health-care workers to report to local authorities any suspected spousal abuse, child abuse and neglect, and elder abuse. In many jurisdictions, violent crimes, such as sexual assault, gunshot wounds, and stab wounds, must be reported to law enforcement. Emergencies that threaten public health, such as animal bites and communicable diseases, also must be reported to the proper authorities. The content of such reports and to whom they must be made is set by law, regulation, or policy. Become familiar with the circumstances under which you are required to make a report. If you fail to make a required report, you may be criminally, professionally, and civilly liable for your inaction.

Legal Protection for the Paramedic

In addition to the laws that protect patients, legislative bodies have enacted laws to protect paramedics. For example, some jurisdictions have enacted laws that criminally punish a person who commits assault or battery against a paramedic while she is providing medical care. Others have laws prohibiting the obstruction of paramedic activity.

Immunity, or exemption from legal liability, is another form of protection. Governmental immunity is a judicial doctrine that prohibits a person from bringing a lawsuit against a government without its consent. However, most jurisdictions today have waived their immunity rights, and courts are becoming increasingly likely to strike down the ones that still exist. This type of liability protection, even if allowed under law, generally serves to protect only the government agency, not the individual paramedic. Therefore, you should not rely on governmental immunity to protect you from claims of negligence.

Almost every province and territory has **Good Samaritan laws,** which provide immunity to people who assist at the scene of a medical emergency. Although these laws vary, generally, they protect a person from liability if that person acts in good faith, is not negligent (most jurisdictions will cover acts of simple negligence but not ones of gross negligence), acts within her scope of practice, and does not accept payment for services. The Good Samaritan laws of many jurisdictions have been expanded to protect both paid and volunteer prehospital personnel. In Canada, there is no positive duty to assist; therefore, a paramedic is not *legally* required to stop and assist. However, once you start to assist, you must continue, stopping only in accordance with acceptable standards.

As a paramedic, you should also become familiar with local laws and regulations governing the use of physical restraints for dangerous or violent patients. There also may be regulations governing entry into restricted areas, such as military installations, prisons, nuclear power plants, and sites with hazardous materials. Since the laws affecting paramedic practice vary across jurisdictions, your agency should obtain the advice of an attorney to minimize potential exposure to liability.

Other laws are designed to protect the paramedic in the event of exposure to bloodborne or airborne pathogens. For example, in the United States, the Ryan White Comprehensive AIDS Resources Emergency Act (Ryan White CARE Act) requires hospitals and EMS agencies to create a notification system to provide information and assist the paramedic when an exposure occurs. This law allows the paramedic who has potentially been exposed to certain diseases (such as hepatitis B, AIDS, and tuberculosis) access to medical records to determine whether the patient has tested positive for, or is exhibiting signs and symptoms of, an infectious disease. The Ryan White CARE Act is a federal law, but many states have enacted similar or even more comprehensive laws to protect paramedics. It is important for each agency to appoint an infection control officer and for this individual to implement protocols and an appropriate infection control plan. In Canada, although a proposed law is being considered, it has not yet been enacted.

COMMONLY MANDATED REPORTS
- Spouse abuse
- Child abuse and neglect
- Elder abuse
- Sexual assault
- Gunshot and stab wounds
- Animal bites
- Communicable diseases

✳ **immunity** exemption from legal liability.

✳ **Good Samaritan laws** laws that provide immunity to certain people who assist at the scene of a medical emergency.

LEGAL ACCOUNTABILITY OF THE PARAMEDIC

As a paramedic, you are required to provide a level of care to your patients that is consistent with your education and training and equal to that of any other competent paramedic with equivalent training. You also are expected to perform your duties in a reasonable and prudent manner, as would any other paramedic in a similar situation. Any deviation from this standard might open you to allegations of negligence and liability for any resulting damages.

NEGLIGENCE AND MEDICAL LIABILITY

* **negligence** deviation from accepted standards of care recognized by law for the protection of others against the unreasonable risk of harm.

Negligence is defined as a deviation from accepted standards of care recognized by law for the protection of others against the unreasonable risk of harm. It can result in legal accountability and liability. In the health-care professions, negligence is synonymous with malpractice.

Components of a Negligence Claim

In a negligence claim against a paramedic, the plaintiff must establish and prove four particular elements in order to prevail: a duty to act, a breach of that duty, actual damages to the patient or other individual, and proximate cause (causation of damages).

* **duty to act** a formal contractual or informal legal obligation to provide care.

First, the plaintiff must establish that the paramedic had a **duty to act.** That is, she must prove that the paramedic had a formal contractual or informal legal obligation to provide care. Note that the act of voluntarily assuming care of a patient may imply that there was a duty to act, which creates a continuing duty to act. For example, in some jurisdictions if an off-duty paramedic witnesses a person choking, the paramedic may be under no legal duty to act. However, if that paramedic initiates care, then she has a duty to continue care. The rationale behind this rule is if bystanders see that a victim is being helped, they may walk away. If the paramedic rendering assistance walks away after initiating treatment but not completing it, the patient may actually be left in a worse condition than if the paramedic had never tried to help.

Duties that are expected of the paramedic include the following:

- The duty to respond to the scene and render care to ill or injured patients
- The duty to know and obey federal, provincial/territorial, and local laws and regulations
- The duty to operate the emergency vehicle reasonably and prudently, consistent with the road conditions
- The duty to provide care and transport to the expected standard of care
- The duty to provide care and transport consistent with the paramedic's scope of practice and local medical protocols
- The duty to continue care and transport through to appropriate conclusions

> ## Content Review
> ### ELEMENTS OF NEGLIGENCE
> - Duty to act
> - Breach of that duty
> - Actual damages
> - Proximate cause

* **breach of duty** an action or inaction that violates the standard of care expected from a paramedic.

* **standard of care** the degree of care, skill, and judgment expected under like or similar circumstances from a similarly trained, reasonable paramedic in the same community.

Second, the plaintiff must prove there was a **breach of duty** by the paramedic. A paramedic always must exercise the degree of care, skill, and judgment that would be expected under like circumstances from a similarly trained, reasonable paramedic in the same community. The **standard of care** specific to the paramedic's practice is generally established by court testimony from expert witnesses (often other paramedics) and reference to published codes, standards, criteria, and guidelines applicable to the situation. A breach of duty may occur by **malfeasance, misfeasance,** or **nonfeasance:**

- *Malfeasance* is the performance of a wrongful or unlawful act by the paramedic. For example, a paramedic commits malfeasance if she assaults a patient.
- *Misfeasance* is the performance of a legal act in a manner that is harmful or injurious. For example, a paramedic commits misfeasance when she inadvertently intubates a patient's esophagus, fails to confirm tube placement, and leaves the tube in place.
- *Nonfeasance* is the failure to perform a required act or duty. For example, it would be an act of nonfeasance to fail to fully immobilize a collision victim who is complaining of neck and back pain.

Unlike criminal cases, which require proof "beyond a reasonable doubt," civil cases require only a proof of guilt by a "preponderance of evidence." In most cases, the burden of proving negligence rests on the plaintiff. In Canada, in the past, when it is difficult to prove negligence, a plaintiff could invoke the doctrine of **res ipsa loquitur,** which is Latin for "the thing speaks for itself."

To support a claim of res ipsa loquitur, the complainant had to prove that the damages would not have occurred in the absence of somebody's negligence, the instruments causing the damages were under the defendant's control at all times, and the patient did nothing to contribute to her own injury. After the doctrine of res ipsa loquitur was invoked in court, the burden of proof shifted from the plaintiff to the defendant. Many cases in which res ipsa loquitur would have been successful were settled out of court.

Res ipsa loquitur is no longer applicable in Canada. Justice Major, speaking for the Supreme Court of Canada, stated that, even in respect of negligence,

> Whatever value *res ipsa loquitur* may have once provided is gone. Various attempts to apply the so-called doctrine have been more confusing than helpful. Its use has been restricted to cases where the facts permitted an inference of negligence and there was no other reasonable explanation for the accident. Given its limited use, it is somewhat meaningless to refer to that use as a doctrine of law.
>
> It would appear that the law would be better served if the maxim was treated as expired and no longer used as a separate component in negligence actions. After all, it was nothing more than an attempt to deal with circumstantial evidence. [*Fontaine v. British Columbia* (1997), 41 C.C.L.T. (2d) 36, at 48 (S.C.C.)]

One situation in which little proof is required occurs when the paramedic violates a statute and injury to a plaintiff results. Some laws state that if a statute is violated and an injury results, a person will be guilty of *negligence per se,* or automatic negligence. For example, if a paramedic, who is driving in nonemergency mode, fails to stop at a red light and hits a pedestrian, the paramedic's negligence is obvious. She violated vehicular and traffic statutes that prohibit a vehicle from running a red light and is therefore guilty of negligence per se.

After a duty to act and a breach of that duty have been proven, **actual damages** is the third required element of proof in a negligence claim. That is, the plaintiff must prove that she was actually harmed in a way that can be compensated by the award of monetary damages. This is an essential component. A lawsuit cannot be won if the paramedic's action caused no ill effects. The plaintiff must prove that she suffered compensatable physical, psychological, or financial damage, such as

✱ malfeasance a breach of duty by performance of a wrongful or unlawful act.

✱ misfeasance a breach of duty by performance of a legal act in a manner that is harmful or injurious.

✱ nonfeasance a breach of duty by failure to perform a required act or duty.

Always exercise the degree of care, skill, and judgment expected under like circumstances from a similarly trained, reasonable paramedic in the same community.

✱ res ipsa loquitur a legal doctrine invoked by plaintiffs to support a claim of negligence, it is a Latin term that means "the thing speaks for itself."

✱ actual damages refers to compensatable physical, psychological, or financial harm.

medical expenses, lost wages, lost future earnings, conscious pain and suffering, or, when the suit claim is brought by someone else, wrongful death.

In addition, the plaintiff may seek punitive (punishing) damages. These are infrequent and awarded only when a defendant commits an act of gross negligence or willful and wanton misconduct. An act of ordinary negligence, such as accidentally allowing an IV to infiltrate, will not support an award of punitive damages. If punitive damages are awarded to the plaintiff, most insurance policies will not cover them. Therefore, the paramedic may become personally liable for any punitive damages awarded to the plaintiff.

Finally, to prove negligence, the plaintiff must show that the paramedic's action or inaction was the **proximate cause** of the damages; that is, the action or inaction of the paramedic immediately caused or worsened the damage suffered by the plaintiff. For example, a cardiac patient who breaks his arm during an ambulance collision en route to the hospital will likely be able to prove that the injuries resulted from the incident; that is, the collision was the proximate cause of the injuries. However, a patient with a sprained wrist who happens to suffer a stroke while in the ambulance would have difficulty proving the ambulance ride was the proximate cause of the stroke.

Proximate cause is also thought of in terms of whether the damage was foreseeable. To show the existence of proximate cause, the plaintiff needs to prove that the damage to the patient was reasonably foreseeable by the paramedic. This is usually established by expert testimony. For example, imagine that a paramedic negligently crashes the ambulance into a telephone pole. As a result, two people are injured—the patient who was in the back of the ambulance and, two blocks away, a baby who was dropped by his mother when the loud crash startled her. It should be easy for the patient to prove proximate cause because it was reasonably foreseeable that an ambulance crash could hurt passengers. However, if the woman who dropped her baby sued the paramedic, she probably would not be able to establish proximate cause. Although the crash was the reason her baby was injured, it was not a foreseeable injury resulting from the ambulance crash.

Defences to Charges of Negligence

The following is a list of potential defences to negligence:

- *Good Samaritan laws.* If the paramedic can establish that her actions, albeit negligent, were protected by a Good Samaritan law, liability may be avoided. Good Samaritan laws are a shield against a lawsuit for simple negligence. Note that such laws generally do not protect providers from acts of gross negligence, reckless disregard, or willful or wanton conduct, and they do not prohibit the filing of lawsuits.

- *Governmental immunity.* These laws do not offer much protection for the individual paramedic accused of negligence. Though governmental immunity laws vary across provinces and territories, the current legal trend is toward limiting this type of protection.

- *Statute of limitations.* This law sets the maximum period during which certain actions can be brought in court. After the time limit is reached, no legal action can be brought, whether or not a negligent act occurred. Statutes of limitations vary across the country, and so carefully review the laws in your jurisdiction. The limitation period could range from 2 to 10 years, based on when the negligence was discovered. Note that the statutes may vary for different negligent acts and for cases involving children.

* **proximate cause** action or inaction of the paramedic that immediately caused or worsened the damage suffered by the patient.

- *Contributory or comparative negligence.* Some provincial or territorial laws will reduce or eliminate a plaintiff's award of damages if the plaintiff is found to have caused or worsened her own injury. For example, imagine that a patient involved in a car crash complains of neck pain but refuses to let the paramedics properly immobilize her spine. The paramedics explain the risks of refusing treatment, but the patient signs a "release-from-liability" form. Later, the patient learns that she has permanent spinal-cord damage and sues the paramedics for negligence. Many courts will find that the paramedics were not negligent, because by refusing necessary treatment, the patient exacerbated her own injury.

If you are accused of negligence, you may be able to avoid liability if you can establish a defence to the plaintiff's claim.

The test that a court of law or professional college would use in reviewing the actions of any paramedic issues that come before them would be to structure the issue as a question. For example, in any case involving alleged negligence by paramedics, the question would be, "Did the paramedics in this case meet the required standard of care required, and if not, were they the cause of any resulting damages?"

As for what the "legal standard of care" is, the legal test, or question, a court or professional college will use will always be, "What would a reasonable and prudent, or cautious, paramedic with equal training do in the same situation in light of the state of medical science at the time of the event?" If the paramedics did what reasonable and prudent paramedics would do, or perhaps even more, then they met the standard required. If they did less than what reasonable and prudent paramedics would have done, then they were negligent.

These are very complex questions; therefore, every case is multifactorial, and the opinion as to whether or not a paramedic would likely be found liable is dependent on the facts of the case.

To protect yourself against claims of negligence, you should receive appropriate education, training, and continuing education; receive appropriate medical direction, both online and offline; always prepare accurate, thorough documentation; have a professional attitude and demeanour at all times; always act in good faith; and use your own common sense. In addition, it is essential for all paramedics to be covered by liability insurance. Although many employers and agencies carry coverage, in Canada, some are required by statute to carry only a minimal amount of insurance. It is a good idea to consider obtaining your own insurance because your agency's coverage may be inadequate.

It is essential for all paramedics to be covered by liability insurance.

SPECIAL LIABILITY CONCERNS

Medical Direction

If a paramedic makes a mistake in the field and is sued by the injured patient, it is possible that the patient will also sue the paramedic's medical director and the online physician. The online physician may be liable to a patient for giving the paramedic medically incorrect orders or advice, for refusing to authorize the administration of a medically necessary medication, or for directing an ambulance to take a patient to an inappropriate medical facility.

A paramedic's medical director may be liable to the patient for the negligent supervision of the paramedic. For the patient to be successful in this type of claim, she would have to prove that the physician breached a duty to supervise the paramedic and that breach was the proximate cause of the patient's injuries. Examples include the medical director failing to establish medication protocols or standing orders consistent with the current standards of medical practice for the paramedic to use in the field; the medical director observing and then failing to correct a paramedic's poor intubation technique; or the medical director receiving complaints of inappropriate care by a paramedic and then failing to effectively investigate and resolve the problem. A common defence from medical directors is that they responded in accordance with acceptable standards, relying on what proved to be incorrect information from the paramedic. Hence, any damage is a result only of the paramedic's negligence.

Borrowed Servant Doctrine

As a paramedic, you may find yourself in the position of supervising other emergency care providers, such as emergency medical responders or primary care paramedics. You may have a student on practicum for whom you are responsible. It is your responsibility to make sure these people perform their duties in a professional and medically appropriate manner. Depending on the degree of supervision and the amount of control you have, you may be liable for any negligent act they commit. This is called the "borrowed servant" doctrine. For it to apply, the paramedic accused of negligence must have taken the employees of another employer under her control and exercised supervisory powers over them.

Ride-Alongs

A growing number of EMS systems have civilians who ride along for educational or media purposes. Even if the individual signs a waiver, the paramedic is still responsible for the person's safety; after all, the paramedic is the expert in this environment—she knows the risks and dangers. A prompt and full briefing for ride-alongs is of great assistance if the paramedic needs to defend an action for alleged negligence by a person injured while on a ride-along.

Civil Rights

In addition to suing you for negligence, a patient may be able to sue you under certain circumstances for violating her civil rights if you fail to render care for a discriminatory reason. As a paramedic, you may not withhold medical care for such reasons as race, creed, colour, gender, national origin, or in some cases, ability to pay. Also, all patients should be provided with appropriate care, regardless of their status, condition, or disease (including AIDS/HIV, tuberculosis, and other communicable diseases).

Off-Duty Paramedics

Liability also may arise in a situation in which an off-duty paramedic renders assistance at the scene of an illness or injury. As noted earlier, generally, any person who provides basic emergency first aid to another person is protected from liability under a Good Samaritan law. However, when the off-duty paramedic provides advanced life support, a problem may arise. In most jurisdictions, paramedics cannot practise advanced skills unless they are practising within an EMS system. To employ, while off duty, paramedic skills and procedures that require delegation from a physician may constitute the crime of practising medicine without a licence. Learn the law in your jurisdiction.

PARAMEDIC-PATIENT RELATIONSHIPS

The relationship you establish with your patient is a very important one. Not only must you provide the best medical care, but you also have legal and ethical duties to protect the patient's privacy and treat her with honesty, respect, and compassion.

Confidentiality

All records related to the emergency care rendered to a patient must be kept strictly confidential. Keeping patient **confidentiality** means that any medical or personal information about a patient—including medical history, assessment findings, and treatment—will not be released to a third party without the express permission of the patient or legal guardian. The right to confidentiality belongs to the patient; however, under specific circumstances, a patient's confidential information may be released:

* *Patient consents to the release of the records.* A patient may request a copy of her own medical records for any reason. If the patient is a child, consent for release of medical records must be obtained from the child's parent or other legal guardian. The request should be accepted only if it is in writing, specifically authorizes the agency to release the records, and contains the patient's signature (or other authorized signature). If the request so directs, it is permissible to forward the records to the patient's physician, insurance company, lawyer, or any other party the patient specifies. Be sure your agency retains a copy of the consent document.

* *Other medical care providers have a need to know.* For example, it is not a breach of patient confidentiality to discuss the patient's condition with online medical direction or to give a patient report to an emergency department nurse on arrival at the hospital. This is permitted because it allows medical care appropriate for the patient to be continued. It is not acceptable, however, to discuss confidential patient information with medical providers who have no responsibility for the patient's care.

* *EMS is required by law to release a patient's medical records.* Records may be requested by a court order that is signed by a judge, or they may be requested by *subpoena* (a command to appear at a certain time and place to give testimony). When an agency receives a court order or subpoena, it is good practice to consult with a lawyer to make sure the order is valid and for assistance with compliance. Failure to comply with a court order or subpoena may result in severe penalties.

* *There are third-party billing requirements.* For EMS agencies that bill patients for services, it is generally necessary to release certain confidential information to receive reimbursement from private insurance companies. If possible, the agency should obtain patient authorization for this purpose.

The law penalizes breach of confidentiality. The improper release of information may result in a lawsuit against the paramedic for defamation (libel or slander), breach of confidentiality, breach of contract, or invasion of privacy. If found guilty, the paramedic may be responsible for paying money damages to the patient.

Defamation

Defamation occurs when a person makes an intentional false communication that injures another person's reputation or good name. A patient may sue a paramedic for defamation if the paramedic communicates an untrue statement about a patient's character or reputation without legal privilege or consent. Defamation can occur in written form or through verbal statements.

---

* confidentiality the principle of law that prohibits the release of medical or other personal information about a patient without the patient's consent.

* defamation an intentional false communication that injures another person's reputation or good name.

✱ libel the act of injuring a person's character, name, or reputation by false statements *made in writing* or through the mass media with malicious intent or reckless disregard for the falsity of those statements.

✱ slander act of injuring a person's character, name, or reputation by false or malicious statements *spoken* with malicious intent or reckless disregard for the falsity of those statements.

Libel is the act of injuring a person's character, name, or reputation by false statements *made in writing* or through the mass media with malicious intent or reckless disregard for the falsity of those statements. Allegations of libel can be avoided by completing an accurate, professional, and confidential patient care report. Do not use slang and value-loaded words or phrases in your report (for example, do not refer to a patient as "stupid" or use any derogatory race-based terms). Since many jurisdictions consider the patient care report part of the public record, never write anything on it that could be considered libellous.

Slander is the act of injuring a person's character, name, or reputation by false or malicious statements *spoken* with malicious intent or reckless disregard for the falsity of those statements. An allegation of slander can be avoided by limiting oral reporting of a patient's condition to appropriate personnel only. Note that many EMS systems record ambulance-hospital radio transmissions, and scanners, which give the public access to EMS transmissions, are common. Therefore, information transmitted over the radio should be limited to essential matters of patient care. In most cases, the patient's name and address should not be transmitted over the radio.

Many of the cases dealing with defamation and EMS arise from statements and notations that are written as expressions of humour. Be careful when making statements or notations that at the time seem amusing but can be misconstrued by third-party readers.

Invasion of Privacy

A paramedic may be accused of invasion of privacy for the release of confidential information, without legal justification, regarding a patient's private life, which might reasonably expose the patient to ridicule, notoriety, or embarrassment. That includes, for example, the release of information regarding HIV status or other sensitive medical information. The fact that released information is true, while a pure defence in a defamation action, is not a defence to an action for invasion of privacy.

CONSENT

✱ consent the patient's granting of permission for treatment.

By law, you must get a patient's consent before you can provide medical care or transport. **Consent** is the granting of permission to treat and need not be in writing, but it must be valid. More accurately, consent is the granting of permission to touch. It is based on the concept that every adult of sound mind has the right to determine what should be done with her own body. Touching a patient without appropriate consent may subject you to charges of assault and battery, and a civil lawsuit for battery. The same test of consent is required for a patient to refuse treatment.

✱ competent able to make an informed decision about medical care.

A patient must be **competent**, or have capacity, in order to give or withhold consent. A competent adult is one who is lucid and able to make an informed decision about medical care. She understands your questions and recommendations and understands the implications of her decisions about medical care. Although there is no absolute test for determining competency, keep the following factors in mind when making a determination: the patient's mental status, the patient's ability to respond to questions, statements regarding the patient's competency from family or friends, evidence of impairment from drugs or alcohol, or indications of shock. You must be in a position to prove that given what you observed and were told, a reasonable and prudent paramedic with equal training in the same situation would also have concluded that the patient understood the nature and purpose of treatment and the consequences of giving consent to treat or not to treat.

By law, you must get a patient's consent before you can provide medical care or transport.

If in doubt, treat. It is much easier to defend against a patient claiming you were in error for treating than it is to defend against the estate of a deceased patient.

Informed Consent

Conscious, competent patients have the right to decide what medical care to accept. However, for consent to be legally valid, it must be **informed consent,** or consent given based on full disclosure of information. That is, a patient must understand the nature, material risks, and benefits of any procedures to be performed. Before providing medical care, you must explain the following to the patient in a manner she can understand:

* The nature of the illness or injury
* The nature of the recommended treatments
* The risks, dangers, and benefits of those treatments
* The alternative treatment possibilities, if any, and the related risks, dangers, and benefits of accepting each one
* The dangers of refusing treatment, including transport

Informed consent must be obtained from every competent adult before treatment may be initiated. As consent is a process and not merely a one-time event, any conscious, competent patients may revoke consent at any time during care and transport. In most jurisdictions, a patient must be 18 years of age or older to give or withhold consent. Generally, a child's parent or legal guardian must give informed consent before treatment of the child can begin treatment.

Expressed, Implied, and Involuntary Consent

There are three more types of consent: expressed, implied, and involuntary. **Expressed consent** is the most common. It occurs when a person directly grants permission to treat—verbally, nonverbally, or in writing. Often, the act of a patient requesting an ambulance is considered an expression of a desire to be treated. However, just because the patient consents to a ride to the hospital does not mean she has consented to all types of treatment (such as the initiation of an IV or the administration of medications). You must obtain consent for each treatment you plan to provide. Consent from the patient does not always need to be granted verbally. It may be expressed by allowing care to be rendered.

Unconscious patients cannot grant consent. When treating them or any patient who requires emergency intervention but is mentally, physically, or emotionally unable to grant consent, treatment depends on **implied consent** (sometimes called "emergency doctrine"). That is, it is assumed that the patient would want life-saving treatment if she were able to give informed consent. Implied consent is effective only until the patient no longer requires emergency care or until the patient regains competence. The law does not allow for waiting until a patient who initially refused treatment becomes unconscious to say you have implied consent.

Occasionally, a court will order patients to undergo treatment, even though they may not want it. This is called **involuntary consent.** It is most commonly encountered with patients who must be held for mental-health evaluation or as directed by law enforcement personnel who have the patient under arrest. It also is used on occasion to force patients to undergo treatment for a disease that threatens the community at large (tuberculosis, for example). Law-enforcement personnel often will accompany patients who are undergoing court-ordered treatment.

* **informed consent** consent for treatment that is given based on full disclosure of information.

* **expressed consent** verbal, nonverbal, or written communication by a patient that she wants to receive medical care.

* **implied consent** consent for treatment that is presumed for a patient who is mentally, physically, or emotionally unable to grant consent. Also called *emergency doctrine*.

* **involuntary consent** consent to treatment granted by the authority of a court order.

Consent issues also can arise when a paramedic is called by law-enforcement officials to treat a sick or injured prisoner or arrestee. The officers may tell you that they have the legal authority to give consent to treatment for the patient simply because the patient is in police custody. However, a competent adult in police custody does not necessarily lose the right to make medical decisions for herself. In fact, many prisoners have successfully sued health-care providers for rendering treatment without consent. Generally, forced treatment is limited to emergency treatment necessary to save life or limb or treatment ordered by the court. Be sure that you are familiar with your local protocols and laws on this issue. This situation can lead to legal liability for EMS.

Special Consent Situations

In the case of a **minor** (depending on provincial or territorial law, this is usually a person under the age of 18), consent should be obtained from a parent, legal guardian, or court-appointed custodian. The same is true of a mentally incompetent adult. If a responsible person cannot be located and the child or mentally incompetent adult is suffering from an apparent life-threatening injury or illness, treatment may be rendered under the doctrine of implied consent. Again, if in doubt, treat.

Generally, an **emancipated minor** is considered an adult. This is a person under 18 years of age who is married, pregnant, a parent, a member of the armed forces, or financially independent and living away from home. Each case is fact dependent, and the courts look at several factors. As an adult, an emancipated minor may legally give informed consent, notwithstanding the general rule that anyone else under the age of 18 may not grant informed consent.

Withdrawal of Consent

A competent adult may withdraw consent for any treatment at any time. However, refusal must be informed. That is, the patient must fully understand the risks of not continuing treatment or transport to the hospital. A common example of a patient withdrawing consent occurs after a hypoglycemic patient regains full consciousness with the administration of dextrose. The patient should be encouraged—*but cannot be forced*—to go to the emergency department. If she is competent, the patient may refuse transport. In such cases, advanced life support measures, such as IV fluids, which were initiated when the patient was unconscious, should be discontinued. The patient also should complete a release-from-liability form (Figure 2-1).

Refusal of care by a patient must be informed and properly documented.
⚷

Sometimes, patients choose to accept one recommended treatment but refuse others. For example, a patient involved in a motor-vehicle crash may refuse to be fully immobilized but ask to be transported to the hospital. It is very important for you to do everything in your power to be sure she understands why spinal precautions are necessary and what may happen if they are not taken. If a competent adult continues to refuse care, be sure to thoroughly document the reason for refusal and your attempts to convince the patient to change her mind. Have the patient and a witness sign a release-from-liability form.

Refusal of Service

Not every EMS run results in the transport of a patient to a hospital. Emergency care should always be offered to a patient, no matter how minor the injury or illness may be. However, often, the patient will refuse. If this occurs, you must:

- Be sure that the patient is legally permitted to refuse care; that is, the patient must be a competent adult.

```
REFUSAL OF TREATMENT AND TRANSPORT

I, THE UNDERSIGNED, HAVE BEEN ADVISED THAT MEDICAL ASSISTANCE ON MY BEHALF IS
NECESSARY AND THAT REFUSAL OF SAID ASSISTANCE AND TRANSPORT MAY RESULT IN
DEATH, OR IMPERIL MY HEALTH. NEVERTHELESS, I REFUSE TO ACCEPT TREATMENT OR
TRANSPORT AND ASSUME ALL RISKS AND CONSEQUENCES OF MY DECISION AND RELEASE
THE AMBULANCE SERVICE AND ITS EMPLOYEES FROM ANY LIABILITY ARISING FROM
MY REFUSAL.

                                              _____
                                                  SIGNATURE OF PATIENT

_____
         WITNESSED BY
                                              _____
                                                    DATE SIGNED
```

FIGURE 2-1   Example of a "release-from-liability" form.

- Make multiple and sincere attempts to convince the patient to accept care.
- Enlist the help of others, such as the patient's family or friends, to convince the patient to accept care.
- Make certain that the patient is fully informed about the implications of the decision and the potential risks of refusing care.
- Consult with online medical direction.
- Have the patient and a disinterested witness, such as a police officer, sign a release-from-liability form. If the police officer or other such person is hesitant to witness the signature, assure the witness that, in fact, they are only verifying that they saw the patient sign the refusal.
- Advise the patient to call you again for help if necessary.
- Attempt to get the patient's family or friends to stay with the patient.
- Document the entire situation thoroughly and accurately on your patient care report.

Remember, the refusal of care must be informed. That is, the patient must be told of and understand all possible risks of refusal. Decisions not to transport should involve medical direction. It is a good idea to put the patient directly on the phone with the online physician. If all efforts fail, be sure to thoroughly document the reasons for refusal and your efforts to change the patient's mind. If an online physician was involved, it is a good idea to obtain her signature on your patient care report if possible. Refer to Chapter 9, Documentation, for examples of documentation of refusal of service. Be very careful and thorough with refusal of care situations; they can be extremely risky for EMS.

Problem Patients

As a paramedic, you will occasionally encounter a "problem patient," one who is violent, a victim of a drug overdose, an intoxicated adult or minor, or an ill or injured minor with no adult available to provide consent for medical treatment. Such a patient can present you with a medical-legal dilemma. For example, consider the patient who has allegedly taken an overdose of medication. Concerned family members may panic and activate the EMS system. However, on your arrival at the scene, you find the patient alert, oriented, denying that she has taken any medication, and refusing to give consent for treatment or transport.

In such a case as this, attempt to develop trust and some rapport with the patient. If she continues to refuse and remains alert and oriented, a refusal form should be completed and witnessed by a police officer. If the patient will not sign the form, have a police officer or family member sign it, indicating that the patient verbally refused care. If, however, the situation becomes dangerous, or you have reason to suspect the patient has tried to injure herself, police officers or family members should consider legal measures to force the patient to receive treatment.

The intoxicated person who refuses treatment and transport also poses a problem for the paramedic. Every effort should be made to encourage the patient, keeping in mind that just because a person is intoxicated does not mean she is not competent. You should encourage your patient to accept care and transport to the hospital. If the patient refuses, explain in a calm and detailed manner the implications of refusal. However, if you determine that the patient cannot understand the nature of her illness or the consequences of refusal, then the patient may not refuse treatment because she is not competent to do so. Involve law enforcement at this point. If the patient is competent to make such a decision, then have her sign a refusal form. Your conversation with the patient and the refusal should be witnessed by a disinterested third party, such as a police officer.

Regardless of the type of problem patient, always document the encounter in detail. Your records should include a description of the patient, the results of any secondary assessment (or reasons for the lack of one), important statements made by the patient and other persons at the scene, and the names and addresses of any witnesses. If you are going to include an important statement from the patient or witnesses in your patient care report, write the exact statement in quotation marks (this includes profanity). Courts generally take a very dim view of EMS persons being subjected to verbal abuse by citizens.

Ideally, a police officer should respond to the scene in the case of all problem patients and should either sign the patient care report as a witness or, if the paramedic's safety is at risk, accompany the patient and paramedic to the emergency department. Unless you are in a dual role, be very clear where the need for law enforcement begins and your job as EMS provider ends.

LEGAL COMPLICATIONS RELATED TO CONSENT

Consent to treatment has many legal complications. If the paramedic does not obtain the proper consent to treat or fails to continue appropriate treatment, she may be liable for damages based on a tort cause of action, such as abandonment, assault, battery, or false imprisonment.

Abandonment

Abandonment is the termination of the paramedic–patient relationship without providing for the appropriate continuation of care still needed and desired by the patient. You cannot initiate patient care and then discontinue it without sufficient reason. You cannot turn the care of a patient over to personnel who have less training than you without creating potential liability for an abandonment action. For example, a paramedic who has initiated advanced life support should not turn the patient over to an emergency medical responder or primary care paramedic for transport.

> Involve the police, and document in detail any encounter with a "problem patient."

* abandonment termination of the paramedic–patient relationship without assurance that an equal or greater level of care will continue.

Abandonment can occur at any point during patient contact, including in the field or in the hospital emergency department. Physically leaving a patient unattended, even for a short time, may also be grounds for a charge of abandonment. If, for example, you leave a patient at a hospital without properly turning over care to a physician or nurse, you may be liable for abandonment. It is always a good idea to have the nurse or physician to whom you have passed responsibility for patient care sign your patient care report.

Assault and Battery

Failure to obtain appropriate consent before treatment could leave the paramedic open to allegations of assault and battery. **Assault** is defined as unlawfully placing a person in apprehension of immediate bodily harm without consent. For example, your patient states that she is scared of needles and refuses to let you start an IV. If you then show her an IV catheter and bring it toward her arm as if to start an IV, you may be liable for assault.

    Battery is the unlawful touching of another individual without consent. It would be battery to actually start an IV on a patient who does not consent to such treatment. A paramedic can be sued for assault and battery in both criminal and civil contexts and additionally be subject to professional sanction.

✱ **assault** an act that unlawfully places a person in apprehension of immediate bodily harm without consent.

✱ **battery** the unlawful touching of another individual without consent.

False Imprisonment

False imprisonment may be charged by a patient who is transported without consent or who is restrained without proper justification or authority. False imprisonment is defined as intentional and unjustifiable detention of a person without consent or other legal authority, and it may result in civil or criminal liability. Like assault and battery, a charge of false imprisonment can be avoided by obtaining and documenting appropriate consent.

    This problem is a particular dilemma when trying to treat psychiatric patients. In most cases, you can avoid allegations of false imprisonment by having a law enforcement officer apprehend the patient and accompany you to the hospital. If no officer is available, you should attempt to consult with medical direction and carefully judge the risks of false imprisonment charges against the benefits of detaining and treating the patient. You should determine whether medical treatment is immediately necessary and whether the patient poses a threat to herself or to the public when you are making your decision to treat or transport.

✱ **false imprisonment** intentional and unjustifiable detention of a person without consent or other legal authority.

REASONABLE FORCE

If it is safe to do so, you may use a reasonable amount of force to control an unruly or violent patient. The definition of **reasonable force** depends on the amount of force necessary to ensure that the patient does not cause injury to herself, to you, or to others. Excessive force can result in liability for the paramedic. Force used as punishment will be considered assault and battery for which the patient may be able to recover damages and the paramedic may face criminal charges. When you believe it is necessary to use force, involve law enforcement if possible.

    The use of restraints may be indicated for a combative patient. Restraints must conform to your local protocols. Restraining devices typically used by EMS providers include straps, jackets, and restraining blankets. In this circumstance, an EMS team's goal is to use the least amount of force necessary to safely control the patient causing the least amount of discomfort. If the use of restraints is indicated, involve law enforcement officials.

✱ **reasonable force** the minimal amount of force necessary to ensure that an unruly or violent person does not cause injury to herself or to others.

PATIENT TRANSPORT

The transport of patients to a health-care facility is an integral part of the patient-care continuum. During transport to a health-care facility, be sure to maintain the same level of care as was initiated at the scene. This means that if you, as a paramedic, initiate advanced emergency care procedures, you must either ride with the patient to the hospital or ensure that another paramedic will accompany the patient. If you fail to do so and the patient is harmed as a result, you may be liable for abandonment.

One area of great potential liability for paramedics is emergency vehicle operation. It is essential that you become familiar with your provincial/territorial and local laws. The laws that provide exemptions from driving rules and regulations may allow you, for example, to drive at a rate of speed in excess of a posted speed limit, but if you are negligent at any time during the operation of your vehicle, you will not be protected from liability.

Another issue that will arise is patient choice of destination. If you work in a small area with only one hospital, you are not likely to encounter difficulties. However, many paramedics work in areas that have many hospitals and medical centres to choose from. Lawsuits involving facility selection have increasingly been brought by patients. Some have sued the paramedics, claiming negligence based on the failure to transport to the nearest or most appropriate hospital.

In general, facility selection should be based on patient request, patient need, and facility capability. Local written protocols, the paramedic, online medical direction, and the patient should all play a role in facility selection. The patient's preference, however, should be honoured unless the situation or the patient's condition dictates otherwise.

> During transport of a patient to a health-care facility, be sure to maintain the same level of care as was initiated at the scene.

RESUSCITATION ISSUES

Advances in medical technology have saved and prolonged thousands of lives. However, in some instances, the use of sophisticated medical technology may only prolong pain and suffering. When a person is seriously injured or gravely ill, family members must make difficult decisions regarding the medical care to be provided, including the use or withdrawal of life-support systems.

Generally, you are under obligation to begin resuscitative efforts when summoned to the scene of a patient who is unresponsive, pulseless, and not breathing. Sometimes, however, you will determine that resuscitation is not indicated. This occurs with patients who have a valid do not resuscitate (DNR) order, with patients who are obviously dead (decapitated, for example), with patients who have obvious tissue decomposition or extreme dependent lividity (gravitational pooling of blood in dependent areas of the body), with patients who are at a scene that is too hazardous to enter, or in mass-casualty situations.

Always follow your provincial or territorial laws, local protocols, and medical direction. The role of medical direction should be clearly delineated and included in your agency's protocols. If you are authorized to determine that resuscitative efforts are not indicated, be sure to thoroughly document your decision and the criteria on which it was based.

ADVANCE DIRECTIVES

In Canada, each province and territory has some form of legislation dealing with this issue. This legislation requires hospitals and physicians to provide patients and their families with sufficient information to make informed decisions about medical treatment and the use of life-support measures, including cardiopulmonary resuscitation (CPR), artificial ventilation, nutrition, hydration, and blood transfusions.

Patients and their families are therefore more likely than ever to have prepared a written statement of the patient's own preference for future medical care, or an **advance directive**. An advance directive is a document created to ensure that certain treatment choices are honoured when a patient is unconscious or otherwise unable to express her choice of treatments. Advance directives come in a variety of forms. The most common encountered in the field are living wills, durable powers of attorney for health care, and DNR orders.

The types of advance directives recognized in each jurisdiction are governed by provincial and territorial law and local protocols. Medical direction must establish and implement policies for dealing with advance directives in the field. Those policies should clearly define the obligations of a paramedic who is caring for a patient with an advance directive. They should also provide for reasonable measures of comfort to the patient and emotional support to the patient's family and loved ones. Some jurisdictions do not allow paramedics to honour living wills in the field, but do allow them to honour valid DNR orders. Be sure you are familiar with your provincial or territorial law and local policies.

Living Will

A **living will** is a legal document that allows a person to specify the kinds of medical treatment she wants to receive should the need arise. For example, many jurisdictions allow patients to include in living wills their wishes concerning dying in a hospital or at home, receiving CPR, and donating their organs and tissues. In addition, patients with prolonged illnesses sometimes invoke the right to choose a person who may make health-care decisions for them in the event that their mental functions become impaired. They might formalize this decision by way of a special notation in a living will. They may also do this through execution of a document called a "durable power of attorney for health care" or "health-care proxy." Living wills, once signed and witnessed, are effective until they are revoked, usually in writing, by the patient.

Be sure you know your local protocols concerning living wills. If any question arises on scene, contact medical direction for instructions.

Do Not Resuscitate Orders

A **do not resuscitate (DNR) order** is a common type of advance directive. Usually signed by the patient and her physician, the DNR order is a legal document that indicates to medical personnel which, if any, life-sustaining measures should be taken when the patient's heart and respiratory functions have ceased. DNR orders generally direct EMS personnel to withhold CPR in the event of a cardiac arrest. When you honour a DNR order, do not simply pack up your equipment and leave the scene. You still may have the patient's family and loved ones to attend to. Provide emotional support as appropriate.

DNR orders pose a particular problem in the field. Paramedics are often called to nursing homes or residences where they find a patient in cardiac arrest and in need of resuscitation. As a rule, you are legally obligated to attempt resuscitation. If a physician has written a specific order to avoid it, the paramedics should not have been summoned. Even so, people tend to panic and will call for help. Valid DNR orders should be honoured as your protocols allow. Note, however, that if there is any doubt as to the patient's wishes, resuscitation should be initiated.

You may be requested to treat a patient as a "slow code" or "chemical code only." This treatment is not legally permitted. Cardiac resuscitation is an all-or-nothing proposition. Treating a cardiac arrest with only medications would mean abandoning airway management and defibrillation. To do so, even at the request of the family, amounts to negligence and must be avoided.

* **advance directive** a document created to ensure that certain treatment choices are honoured when a patient is unconscious or otherwise unable to express her choice of treatment.

* **living will** a legal document that allows a person to specify the kinds of medical treatment she wants to receive should the need arise.

Content Review

ADVANCE DIRECTIVES
- Living wills
- Durable powers of attorney for health care
- DNR orders
- Organ donor cards (such as found on a driver's licence)

* **do not resuscitate (DNR) order** a legal document, usually signed by the patient and her physician, that indicates to medical personnel which, if any, life-sustaining measures should be taken when the patient's heart and respiratory functions have ceased.

Suppose that paramedics arrive at a home and are met by the anxious parents of a 17-year-old patient who has cancer. The paramedics are told that the patient has written an advance directive stating that attempts at resuscitation are not to be made. What do the paramedics do? If the patient is awake and has the basic requirements necessary to allow her to grant consent (voluntary, patient with capacity, referable, and informed), then the paramedics need only ask the patient. In any event, the best rule for paramedics as to whether to treat or not is, for obvious reasons, if in doubt, treat.

What paramedics should do in the scenario suggested depends on the province or territory that the paramedics are working in. One problem with giving consideration to an advance directive is that some provinces and territories have legislation that deals with the issue of consent, and some do not.

If the situation above occurred in Ontario and it became an issue whether or not the paramedics had valid consent to treat, the court would likely look at several sources, decide which sources had precedence, and (after taking into consideration the totality of all the sources), make a decision.

In Ontario, consent to health care is governed, in part, by the Health Care Consent Act, 1996, which replaced the previous Consent to Treatment Act, 1992, and also the Substitute Decisions Act, 1992. The current Health Care Consent Act, 1996, lists several types of health practitioners to whom that Act applies. Although such professionals as members of the colleges of audiologists, dental hygienists, dietitians, dentists, and massage therapists are listed, paramedics are not. So, although that law does not apply to paramedics, a court of law may consider what that act states, especially with regard to capacity to make decisions.

In Ontario, advance directives are made pursuant to the Substitute Decisions Act, 1992, S.O. 1992, c. 30. Under that statute, when dealing with "contracts," the Act states that a person who is 18 years of age or more is "presumed to be capable of entering into a contract." Yet, with regard to "personal care," which includes health-care decisions, a person who is 16 years of age is "presumed to be capable of giving or refusing consent in connection with her own personal care." So, in Ontario, 16 years of age is legislated as the age of consent for health care. This is different in other provinces and territories, such as Alberta.

In Alberta, advance directives are governed by the Personal Directives Act RSA 2000, c. P-6, which denotes at section 3 that only people who are at least 18 years of age may make a personal directive. The Act also notes that persons who are at least 18 years of age are presumed to understand the nature and effect of a personal directive. However, in many cases, people 16 years of age have been allowed to make decisions regarding their own health care, and people 17 years of age have been denied the right to make their own decisions.

As noted by Justice Moen, of the Alberta Court of Queen's Bench in 2001, Canadian law is clear:

> Regardless of age, a child is capable of consenting (or refusing consent) if she is able to appreciate the nature and purpose of the treatment and the consequences of giving or refusing consent. If the child has this capacity, the child's consent is both necessary and sufficient; the parents' consent is not required, nor can they override the child's decision. (E.I. Picard and G.B. Robertson, *Legal Liability of Doctors and Hospitals in Canada* [3d ed.], Toronto: Carswell, 1996, at 72-3.)

In the same case, looking at the issue of a mature minor, the court analyzes whether the patient appreciates the nature and purpose of the treatment and the consequences of refusing the treatment. Factors indicative of a minor's ability to consent may include the age of the minor, the maturity of the minor, the nature and extent of the minor's dependence on the parent(s), and the complexity of the treatment. The nature and extent of the minor's dependence goes to the ability of the minor to make an independent decision without coercion and influence of a parent or a guardian.

If legislation that sets out an age for consent has been enacted, then the common law principle (judge-made law) is replaced. That does not mean it is ignored; it means that the decision of the minor is not necessarily the ruling one. This legislation of the age of consent has occurred in Ontario and Alberta, with different ages of 16 and 18, respectively. So, notwithstanding that the patient may well be a mature minor, the courts have held that where legislative parameters exist, the court and all persons exercising authority should take into consideration the opinions of the child. But the courts have determined that "take into consideration" is not equivalent to "follow," and the court must always do what is in the best interests of the child. In Alberta and Ontario, although a mature minor's opinions are considered, they cannot automatically be followed.

Under legislation with an age set out, the court and other people exercising authority over the minor do the analysis, balance all factors, and make a conclusion. It is not a clear case of a higher level of law winning over a lesser law.

In the above scenario, in Ontario, the child may well have been able to provide an advance directive, and if that directive meets all the requirements of the Substitute Decisions Act, 1992 of Ontario, the paramedics could follow the advance directive and not be bound by the opinion of the family. However, in Alberta, the paramedics could not because only a person 18 years of age could make a personal directive. If the person were conscious, and assuming they had capacity, then the court would look at what the patient wanted.

Potential Organ Donation

Advances in medicine have led to an increased number of organ transplantations. As organs and tissues are in very high demand and short supply, many EMS systems are now becoming a vital link in the organ procurement and transplantation process. Some have developed protocols that specifically address organ viability after a patient's death. These include providing circulatory support through IV fluids and CPR and ventilatory support via endotracheal tube. Whether or not your EMS has protocols in place for potential organ donation, it is important for you to consult with online medical direction when you have identified a patient as a potential donor.

Death in the Field

Whether you arrive at the scene of a patient who has died before your arrival or you make an authorized decision to terminate resuscitative efforts, a death in the field must be appropriately dealt with and thoroughly documented. Follow provincial/territorial and local protocols, and contact medical direction for guidance.

CRIME AND ACCIDENT SCENES

You may be called to treat a patient at a crime scene. You must not sacrifice patient care to preserve evidence or to become involved in detective work. You can best assist investigating officers by properly treating the patient and by doing your best to avoid destroying any potential evidence. As a paramedic, your responsibilities at a crime scene include the following:

- If you believe a crime may have been committed on the scene, immediately contact law enforcement if they are not already involved.
- Protect yourself and the safety of other EMS personnel. Your safety should always be your primary consideration. You will not be held liable for failing to act if a scene is not safe to enter.

- Once a crime scene has been deemed safe, initiate patient contact and medical care.
- Do not move or touch anything at a crime scene unless it is necessary to do so for patient care. Observe and document the original placement of any items moved by your crew. If the patient's clothing has holes made by bullets or a knife, leave the clothing intact if possible. If the patient has an obvious mortal wound, such as decapitation, try not to touch the body at all. Do your best to protect any potential evidence.
- If you need to remove items from the scene, such as an impaled weapon or bottle of medication, be sure to document your actions and notify investigating officers.

Preserve evidence at a crime scene whenever possible.

Treat the scene of an accident in the same way. Ensure your own safety and the safety of your crew, and treat your patients as medically indicated.

DOCUMENTATION

The treatment of your patient does not end until you have properly documented the entire incident. A complete patient care report is your best protection in a negligence action. In fact, a well-written report may actually discourage a plaintiff from filing a claim in the first place. In general, a plaintiff's attorney will request copies of all medical records, including the paramedic's report, before filing a lawsuit. If the paramedic's report is sloppy, incomplete, or otherwise not well written, this may encourage the plaintiff to sue.

A well-documented patient care report has the following characteristics:

- *It is completed promptly after patient contact.* It should be made in the course of business, not long after the event. Any delay could cause you to forget important observations or treatments. If possible, a copy of the completed report should be left with the emergency department staff before you leave the hospital. This copy will become part of the patient's permanent medical records. Never delay patient care to attend to a patient care report.
- *It is thorough.* The main purpose is not simply to record patient data; it is also meant to support the diagnosis and treatment that you provided to the patient. All actions, procedures, and administered medications should be documented. Remember: If you did not write it down, you did not do it.
- *It is objective.* Avoid the use of emotional and value-loaded words. They are irrelevant, have the potential to make your report look unprofessional, and may be the cause of a libel suit.
- *It is accurate.* Be precise, and avoid abbreviations and jargon that are not commonly understood. Try to limit your report to information that you have personally seen or heard. If you document something that you do not have personal knowledge of, indicate the source of your information. Document your observations, not your assumptions, and do not draw a medical conclusion that you are not competent to make. For example, you cannot conclusively diagnose a patient as having pneumonia. You can, however, report your suspicion of pneumonia and document consistent findings.
- *It maintains patient confidentiality.* Follow your agency's policies regarding the release of patient information. Whenever possible, patient consent should be obtained before release of information.

Intentional alteration of a medical record amounts to an admission of guilt by the paramedic. If a patient care report is found to be incomplete or inaccurate, a written amendment should be attached with the date and time the amendment was written, not the date of the original report. Send a copy of the addendum to the receiving hospital to become a part of the patient's medical records. Medical records need to be maintained for a period prescribed by federal and provincial/territorial laws; the time varies up to 10 years after the call. Become familiar with the record-retention requirements in your jurisdiction.

> *A patient care report should never be altered after it is filed.*

SUMMARY

It is in your best interests to learn and follow all provincial/territorial laws and local protocols related to your practice as a paramedic. Be sure to receive good training, and keep current by pursuing continuing education, reading professional journals, and obtaining recertification or relicensure as required by local law. Always act in good faith, and use your common sense. High-quality patient care and high-quality documentation are always your best protection against liability.

CHAPTER 3

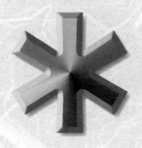

Operations

Objectives

Part 1: Ambulance Operations (begins on p. 120)

After reading Part 1 of this chapter, you should be able to:

1. Identify current local and provincial standards that influence ambulance design, equipment requirements, and staffing of ambulances. (pp. 120–125)
2. Discuss the importance of completing ambulance vehicle, equipment, and supply checklists. (pp. 122–123)

3. Discuss factors used to determine ambulance stationing and staffing within a community. (pp. 124–125)
4. Describe the advantages and disadvantages of air medical transport and identify conditions and situations in which air medical transport should be considered. (pp. 130–133)

Part 2: Medical Incident Command (begins on p. 133)

After reading Part 2 of this chapter, you should be able to:

1. Explain the need for the incident management system (IMS) or incident command system (ICS) in managing emergency medical services incidents. (p. 134)

2. Define the terms multiple-casualty incident (MCI), disaster management, open or uncontained incident, and closed or contained incident. (pp. 133, 137, 150)

Continued

3. Describe the essential elements of scene assessment when arriving at a potential MCI. (pp. 136–137)
4. Describe the role of paramedics and the EMS system in planning for MCIs and disasters. (pp. 135–136, 151, 152)
5. Describe the functional components (command, finance, logistics, operations, and planning) of the incident management system. (pp. 135–141)
6. Differentiate between singular and unified commands and identify when each is most applicable. (pp. 135–136)
7. Describe the role of command, the need for command transfer, and procedures for transferring it. (pp. 135, 136, 138)
8. Differentiate among incident command structures used at small-, medium-, and large-scale incidents. (pp. 135–136)
9. Explain the local or regional threshold for establishing command and implementation of the incident management system, including MCI declaration. (pp. 135–136)
10. List and describe the functions of the following groups and leaders in ICS as it pertains to EMS incidents: safety, logistics, rehabilitation, staging, treatment, triage, transport, extrication and rescue, disposition of deceased and morgue, and communications. (pp. 137–138, 140–141, 142–150)
11. Describe the methods and rationale for identifying specific functions and leaders for the functions in ICS. (pp. 135–136, 138)
12. Describe the role of both command posts and emergency operations centres in MCI and disaster management. (pp. 136, 138–139, 140–141)

13. Describe the role of the on-scene physician at multiple-casualty incidents. (p. 147)
14. Define triage and describe the principles of triage. (pp. 142, 145–146)
15. Describe the START (simple triage and rapid transport) method of initial triage. (pp. 143–145)
16. Given colour-coded tags and numerical priorities, assign the following terms to each: immediate, delayed, hold, deceased. (pp. 143, 145–146)
17. Define primary and secondary triage and describe when primary and secondary triage techniques should be implemented. (p. 143)
18. Describe the need for and techniques used in tracking patients during multiple-casualty incidents. (pp. 138, 143–145, 148)
19. Describe the techniques used to allocate patients to hospitals and track them. (pp. 148)
20. Describe the modifications of telecommunications procedures during multiple-casualty incidents. (pp. 137–138, 149, 156)
21. List and describe the essential equipment to provide logistical support to MCI operations, including airway, respiratory, and hemorrhage control; burn management; and patient packaging or immobilization. (p. 146)
22. List the physical and psychological signs of critical incident stress and describe the role of critical incident stress management sessions in MCIs. (pp. 140, 148–149, 152)
23. Describe the role of table top exercises and small and large MCI drills in preparation for MCIs. (pp. 151–152)

Part 3: Rescue Awareness and Operations (begins on p. 152)

After reading Part 3 of this chapter, you should be able to:

1. Define the term rescue and explain the medical and mechanical aspects of rescue operations. (p. 153)
2. Describe the phases of a rescue operation and the role of the paramedic at each phase. (pp. 157–161)
3. List and describe the personal protective equipment needed to safely operate in the rescue environment,

highway encounters, violent street incidents, residences, and "dark houses." (pp. 202–204, 204–208)

3. Describe the warning signs of potentially violent situations. (pp. 202–204, 204–208)
4. Explain the emergency evasive techniques for potentially violent situations, including threats of physical violence, firearms encounters, and edged weapons encounters. (pp. 201–213)
5. Explain the EMS considerations for the following types of violent or potentially violent situations: gangs and gang violence, hostages or sniper situations, clandestine drug labs, domestic violence, and people with emotional disturbances. (pp. 204–208)

6. Explain the following techniques: field "contact and cover" procedures during assessment and care, evasive tactics, and concealment techniques. (pp. 208–213)
7. Describe the police evidence considerations and techniques to assist in evidence preservation. (pp. 213–215)
8. Given several crime scene scenarios, identify potential hazards, determine whether the scene is safe to enter, and provide care, preserving the crime scene as appropriate. (pp. 201–215)

INTRODUCTION

Although patient care is your core responsibility as a paramedic, operations are also a critical part of your job. You are already familiar with many aspects of EMS operations through your prior basic training and your experience. However, because the safety of so many people—the EMS team, patients, and bystanders—depends on effective and efficient operations, it is important to review and practise operational procedures regularly so that they become second nature and can be performed smoothly, especially during a high-stress emergency.

This chapter discusses the paramedic responsibilities involved in five aspects of EMS operations: Part 1, Ambulance Operations; Part 2, Medical Incident Command; Part 3, Rescue Awareness and Operations; Part 4, Hazardous Materials Incidents; and Part 5, Crime Scene Awareness.

Part 1: Ambulance Operations

Good ambulance operations depend on effective ambulance maintenance as well as operations. In addition to the communication and dispatch skills described in Chapter 8, you should be proficient in these five areas: ambulance standards, maintenance of ambulance equipment and supplies, ambulance stationing, safe ambulance operations, and the use of air medical transport.

AMBULANCE STANDARDS

EMS operations and standards are set at the provincial and territorial level in Canada. Each province and territory is responsible for establishing its own requirements for vehicles and equipment. Transport Canada sets overall vehicle safety standards through the Canadian Motor Vehicle Safety Standards. Modification and equipping of ambulances may then be set through provincial or territorial government agencies. Specific regulations and guidelines may be set by regulatory agencies or at the operational level, depending on how EMS is structured. These standards, regulations, and guidelines are influenced by national and international trends and practices.

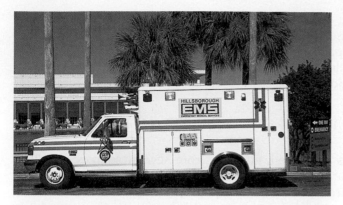

FIGURE 3-1A   Type-I ambulance.

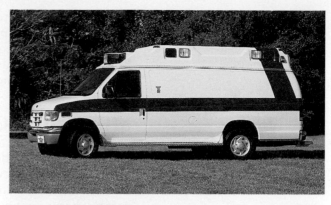

FIGURE 3-1B   Type-II ambulance.

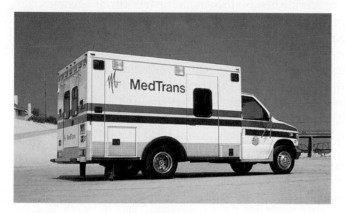

FIGURE 3-1C   Type-III ambulance.

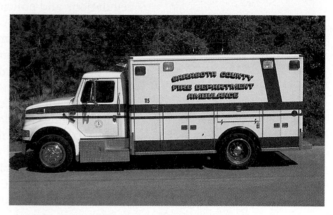

FIGURE 3-1D   Medium-duty ambulance.

These standards tend to be generic, affordable, and politically feasible. Regulatory agencies usually set **minimum standards,** rather than a **gold standard,** for operations. In other words, they establish the lowest acceptable level at which units will be allowed to operate. The regulations and guidelines set by local or regional EMS systems and operators tend to be much more detailed and often approach a gold standard.

✱ **minimum standards** lowest or least allowable standards.

✱ **gold standard** ultimate standard of excellence.

AMBULANCE DESIGN

The changing nature of EMS has led to the development of a number of styles and designs for ambulances. There are no federal or provincial or territorial standards in Canada for ambulance design. However, ambulance manufacturers use a set of specifications—the DOT KKK 1822D specs—developed by the U.S. General Services Administration Automotive Commodity Center. These specifications identify three basic ambulance designs:

- Type I—conventional truck cab-chassis with modular body
- Type II—standard van, forward control integral cab-body
- Type III—specialty van, forward control integral cab-body

In addition to these designs (Figure 3-1), there is also a medium-duty ambulance rescue vehicle, designed to handle heavier loads. As well, many EMS systems have developed specialty vehicles for specific operational roles. For example, B.C. Ambulance Service has deployed a number of vehicles stocked for handling multiple-patient and mass-casualty situations. Toronto EMS uses a series of emergency response units, smaller vehicles that cannot transport patients but are staffed and equipped with primary care or advanced care paramedics. EMS operators have developed buses and other vehicles as mobile command centres and for communications, supplies, mass-casualty incidents, and disasters.

MEDICAL EQUIPMENT STANDARDS

Equipment specifications and standards arise from several sources. Workers' Compensation or occupational health and safety regulations in most provinces and territories set standards for ambulance equipment that includes disinfecting agents, sharps containers, biohazardous material bags, HEPA masks, and personal protective equipment (PPE). In some jurisdictions, equipment standards, regulations and policies are established by provincial or territorial agencies.

These standards often list minimum types and amounts of equipment that must be carried in ambulances. Individual EMS services and operators usually specify actual stock amounts and suppliers. EMS medical direction committees sometimes list the medications and equipment that paramedics should carry. For example, where advanced care paramedics are trained to obtain a 12-lead ECG, the medical advisory committee or service operator may specify the brand of equipment in order to standardize care. These standards may be influenced by guidelines established by national and international medical and EMS associations.

Regional or local operators may add to these standards to meet the particular demands of their operating context. Thus, crews in isolated or rural areas may carry extra kits and supplies for dealing with multiple patients. EMS operators in coastal or northern communities may stock specialized hypothermia equipment.

CHECKING AMBULANCES

Check your ambulance, equipment, and supplies at the start of each shift. On each shift, an essential duty is completion of the ambulance equipment and supply checklist. A typical checklist includes the following:

The shift checklist makes the work environment safer by ensuring mechanical maintenance and the availability of personal protection equipment.

- Patient infection control, comfort, and protection supplies
- Primary and secondary assessment equipment
- Equipment for the transfer of the patient
- Equipment for airway maintenance, ventilation, and resuscitation
- Oxygen therapy and suction equipment
- Equipment for assisting with cardiac resuscitation
- Supplies and equipment for immobilization of suspected fractures
- Supplies for wound care and treatment of shock
- Supplies for childbirth
- Supplies, equipment, and medications for the treatment of acute poisoning, snakebite, chemical burns, and diabetic emergencies
- Basic and advanced life support equipment, medications, and supplies
- Safety and miscellaneous equipment
- Information on the operation and inspection of the ambulance itself

Routine, detailed shift checks of the ambulance can minimize risks. Many services, for example, hold a "stretcher day" once a week. Routine preventive maintenance makes it less likely that a faulty stretcher will cause an injury to a patient or paramedic. Medication expiration dates should be checked each shift, and older, unexpired drugs marked so they will be used first. In services that use prescription medications, such as narcotics, paramedics should sign for these medications at the beginning and end of each shift.

Ensure that all electronic equipment (such as monitors, defibrillators, and radios) is functioning and has fresh batteries. Go through your kits, and replace any dated or depleted stocks. Restock equipment and supplies in the ambulance as well. Although ambulances often have similar configurations, they are often stocked differently in each station. Make sure that you know the location of key items, such as resuscitation equipment and medications. Finally, ensure that all equipment is properly and safely secured.

Perform a vehicle check at the start of each shift. Most services have established standard operating procedures (SOPs) and checklists for start-of-shift vehicle checks, ongoing maintenance schedules, and criteria for removing a vehicle from service. Although it is not your responsibility to service the ambulance, you must be aware of the vehicle check and maintenance requirements in your system. Review fleet bulletins, station postings, and your vehicle's log for any items that may affect your vehicle. Check with the off-going crew to ensure that the vehicle is in good operating condition.

Your vehicle check should include inspecting the exterior (including all lights and sirens), the cab, under the hood, and all operating equipment. Individual ambulances have different configurations and equipment packages. Become familiar with the layout and controls in your ambulance. Many ambulance operators have a checklist or policy that specifies what items you should inspect. Report any deficiencies and arrange for their correction. If scheduled maintenance is due, check with your administrative officer. Follow your SOP for removing a vehicle from service. You should "tag out" a vehicle if you note conditions that you reasonably believe may cause an accident, injury to the crew or patients, or damage to other property.

Clean and disinfect the vehicle as required by your service. Most services routinely clean the ambulance at the start of each shift and after each call, and schedule more thorough "deep cleans" on a regular basis. Some agencies document the procedure. Wash the exterior and clean all interior surfaces following your service's SOPs. Ensure that you use appropriate cleaning and disinfecting supplies and procedures. Note that occupational health and safety regulations in many jurisdictions require EMS operators to have an exposure control plan that specifies cleaning requirements and the methods of cleaning up blood and other body fluid spills. If there is no specific SOP in your service, document cleaning and disinfecting on the shift checklist.

Finally, you should do all scheduled tests, maintenance, and calibrations on specific medical equipment. Items that should be regularly checked include the following:

- Automated external defibrillator (AED)
- Glucometer
- Cardiac monitor
- Oxygen systems
- Automated transport ventilator (ATV)
- Pulse oximeter
- Suction units
- Laryngoscope blades
- Lighted stylets
- Penlights
- Capnography
- Automatic BP cuffs
- Any other battery-operated equipment

Expiration dates on medications should be checked each shift, and the older, unexpired drugs marked appropriately so that they will be used first.

It is your responsibility to report ambulance and equipment problems or failures to your supervisor in a manner prescribed by the SOPs for your service.

✱ **deployment** strategy used by
an EMS agency to manoeuvre
its ambulances and crews in an
effort to reduce response times.

✱ **demographic** pertaining to
population makeup or changes.

✱ **peak load** the highest volume
of calls at a given time.

✱ **primary area of responsibility
(PAR)** stationing of ambulances at specific high-volume
locations.

✱ **system status management
(SSM)** a computerized personnel and ambulance deploy-
ment system.

✱ **tiered response system** system
that allows multiple vehicles
to arrive at an EMS call at different times, often providing
different levels of care or
transport.

The manoeuvring of ambulances and crews to minimize response times is known
as **deployment**. Deployment is based on a number of factors: location of the facilities to house ambulances, location of hospitals, anticipated call volume, and
geographic and traffic considerations. Ideally, deployment decisions take into account both past community responses and projected **demographic** changes. The
highest volume of calls, or **peak load**, should be described in terms of both day
of the week and time of day.

In communities that do not have multiple strategically located stations, services
often deploy ambulances to wait for calls at specific high-volume locations. Such
stationing locations are known as **primary areas of responsibility (PAR)**. These same
ambulances may be relocated throughout the day as the population moves—to
work or to school—and as other ambulances in the community respond to calls.
The size of a PAR may differ from a few city blocks to a larger location, such as
"northeast sector of town." Size depends on the number of ambulances available
and the expected call volume. One sophisticated deployment strategy that has become popular is **system status management (SSM)**. SSM is a computerized personnel and ambulance deployment system designed to meet service demands with fewer
resources and to ensure appropriate response time and vehicle location.

TRAFFIC CONGESTION

In deployment, traffic congestion must be taken into account as well as special
situations, such as a grade-level railroad. Some communities, for example, station ambulances on both sides of the tracks. Other special considerations include
daily activities, such as commuter traffic and school bus schedules. Other considerations include sporting events, VIP appearances, and public gatherings.

National guidelines help communities set the standards. For example, a cardiac arrest victim should receive defibrillation within the first four minutes and
ALS within eight minutes. A system's standards for reliability must take into account the time frames for such calls. An example of such a standard might be response within four minutes to 90 percent of the priority-one calls (cardiac
arrests, respiratory complaints, and motor vehicle collisions).

To meet reliability standards, many communities use a **tiered response system**.
Tiered systems may include police, fire, or other public safety personnel who are
trained as emergency responders. These emergency medical responders have
training in basic life support and automatic external defibrillator (AED) and can
generally be at the patient's side within four minutes. In some communities, a second tier of primary care paramedics (PCP) are the next level of response, followed
by advanced care paramedics (ACP) ideally within eight minutes. Other systems,
such as in Toronto, place paramedics in emergency response units with the goal
of quick response, followed by ambulance backup. The ideal system for your area
will depend on such considerations as available personnel, available training, and
many other factors.

OPERATION STAFFING

How many paramedics should be assigned to a unit? This is a complex decision.
Some services see units staffed by two ACPs as the gold standard. Several systems
strive for this model, such as the City of Calgary EMS. Other systems, such as
Toronto EMS and the B.C. Ambulance Service, used a tiered response model in
which basic life support units staffed by PCPs are supported by advanced life
support ACP units. However, even in these systems, advanced life support units
are sometimes staffed with mixed ACP/PCP crews. Other systems increase the
availability of ACP units by specifically staffing with mixed ACP/PCP crews. In

this model, the supporting PCP member may have additional training and may perform specific advanced procedures under the direct supervision of the ACP member. Because community needs and resources vary so widely, unit staffing will in all likelihood continue to be settled locally.

In general, ambulance staffing should take peak load into account. Some services vary shift times to ensure ample coverage for the busiest days and times of day. Services should also take into account the need for **reserve capacity**—the ability to muster additional crews when all ambulances are on call or when resources are taxed by a multiple-casualty incident. Some services fulfill this need by asking off-duty personnel to carry pagers or to volunteer for backup.

Finally, standards for ambulance operators (drivers) and for driving the vehicle itself are usually determined at the local service level.

* **reserve capacity** the ability of an EMS agency to respond to calls beyond those handled by the on-duty crews.

SAFE AMBULANCE OPERATIONS

Patients, family members, motorists, and other EMS providers are injured—sometimes fatally—in ambulance collisions. In addition to personal injuries, ambulance collisions exact a high toll: vehicle repair or replacement, lawsuits, downtime from work, increased insurance premiums, and damage to your agency's reputation in the community.

Most safety-minded ambulance operators agree that the days of "blowing through" an intersection at high speeds with lights blazing and siren blasting have come and gone.

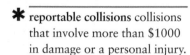

EDUCATING PROVIDERS

The first part of any education program is recognizing and defining the problem. No national Canadian statistics on ambulance collisions exist. However, several studies on ambulance accidents have been completed, and their experience can be a starting point. The following statistics come from an analysis of 22 years of **reportable collisions**—accidents involving more than $1000 in vehicle damage or a personal injury—in New York State. During 1974–1996, New York recorded 7756 reportable ambulance collisions involving 64 fatalities and 10 636 injuries. The first rule in medical practice is "do no harm," and yet these collisions by emergency vehicles harmed a considerable number of people.

* **reportable collisions** collisions that involve more than $1000 in damage or a personal injury.

The data collected by New York provide a profile of the typical ambulance collision. Inclement weather accounted for a relatively small number of the accidents. About 18 percent occurred on rainy days, 16 percent on cloudy days, and 6 percent on days with snow, sleet, hail, or freezing rain. The majority (55 percent) took place on clear days. Some 67 percent took place during daylight hours. Head-on collisions accounted for only 1 percent of the collisions. The largest number (41 percent) occurred when the ambulance struck another vehicle or was itself struck laterally or at a right angle. Approximately 21 percent resulted from side-swiping or overtaking another vehicle. Another 12 percent occurred during a right or left turn.

Probably the most important observation from the data is that nearly three-quarters (72 percent) of all collisions took place at intersections. Most safety-minded ambulance operators agree that the days of "blowing through" an intersection at high speeds with lights blazing and siren blasting have come and gone. Yet, nearly half of all collisions took place at locations with a traffic control device. Another third took place at locations with no traffic device or sign at all.

Based on the New York statistics, the profile of a typical ambulance collision might be: *a lateral collision that takes place on a dry road during daylight hours on a clear day in an intersection with a traffic light.* Typically, when ambulance operators respond in poor weather conditions, they try to drive with a bubble of safety around the vehicle. Maybe the bubble should be there all the time!

In British Columbia, most ambulance accidents involve backing up. Use of a spotter whenever possible is a simple way to eliminate this type of preventable accident.

REDUCING AMBULANCE COLLISIONS

If you have the opportunity to develop programs to reduce ambulance collisions in your community, consider implementing the following actions or standards:

- Routine use of driver qualification checklists and driver's licence checks, either through the local police or the Ministry of Transportation
- Demonstrated driver understanding of preventive mechanical maintenance, including a vehicle operator checklist and a procedure for reporting any problems found during the check or while driving the vehicle
- Provision of plenty of hands-on driver training, using experienced and qualified field officers. A 4500–10 900 kg ambulance requires a much longer stopping distance than the 1100 kg pickup truck that an operator drove to work. The goal is to prevent an inexperienced driver from being stopped by a light pole—or another car—after sliding through an intersection
- Implementation of a slow-speed course to ensure that operators know how to use mirrors, back up, park, and handle ambulance-sized vehicles—including accurate estimation of braking distance and turn radius
- Training that ensures that operators know how to react to emergency situations, such as the loss of brakes, the loss of power steering, a stuck accelerator, a blownout tire, or vehicle breakdown
- Demonstrated driver knowledge of both the primary and backup routes to all hospitals in your service response area
- Demonstrated driver understanding of the rules, regulations, and laws that your Department of Motor Vehicles has established, for drivers in general and for ambulance operators in particular

STANDARD OPERATING PROCEDURES

Each EMS agency should have standard operating procedures (SOPs) pertaining to the operation of its vehicles. At a minimum, they should spell out the following:

- Procedure for qualifying as an ambulance operator
- Procedure for handling and reporting an ambulance collision
- Process for investigating and reviewing each collision
- Process for implementing quality assurance in the aftermath of a collision
- Method for using a **spotter** when backing up a vehicle (Figure 3-2)
- Use of seat belts in the ambulance, and the procedure for transporting a child passenger under 18 kg
- Guidelines on what constitutes an emergency response and the exemptions that may be taken under provincial or territorial laws
- Guidelines on prudent speed; proper travel in and the circumstances for using oncoming lanes; and safe negotiation of intersections
- Circumstances and procedures for use of escorts
- A policy of zero tolerance for driving the vehicle under the influence of alcohol or any drugs

✱ spotter the person behind the left rear side of the ambulance who assists the operator in backing up the vehicle.

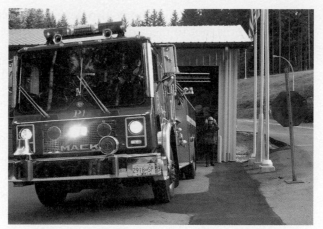

FIGURE 3-2 Use of a spotter.

THE DUE REGARD STANDARD

Provincial and territorial laws pertaining to ambulance operation tend to be similar and to include the legal concept of **due regard.** Essentially, due regard exempts ambulance drivers from certain laws but at the same time holds them to a higher standard.

Provincial and territorial laws typically exempt ambulance drivers who are operating in an emergency from posted speed limits, posted directions of travel, parking regulations, and requirements to wait at red lights. However, ambulances are rarely or never exempt from prohibitions against passing over a railroad crossing with the gates down and passing a school bus with flashing red lights.

Although the laws are often liberal in their exemptions, they place the responsibility for use of these exemptions squarely on the shoulders of the drivers. The laws often say, for example, "the foregoing exemptions do not relieve the operator of an emergency vehicle from acting with due regard for the safety of all persons." Such language sets a higher standard for ambulance operators than for almost any other driver. Nowhere else in the motor vehicle laws are drivers held accountable for the safety of all other motorists!

The moral is this: As an ambulance operator, you will always be held to a higher standard than other drivers. You must be attentive and prepared to shoulder the responsibilities that come with the profession that you have chosen.

LIGHTS AND SIREN: A FALSE SENSE OF SECURITY

As a general rule, do not rely solely on lights and siren to alert other motorists of your approach. Studies have shown that most motorists do not see or hear your ambulance until it is within 30 metres of their vehicles. Even so, the siren is the most commonly used—and abused—audible warning device. Before you decide to turn on the siren, consider the following points:

- Motorists are less inclined to yield to an ambulance when the siren is continually sounded.
- Many motorists feel that the right-of-way privileges given to ambulances are abused when sirens are sounded.
- Inexperienced motorists tend to increase their driving speeds by 6 to 10 km per hour when a siren is sounded.
- The continuous sound of a siren can possibly make sick or injured patients feel worse by increasing their anxiety.

* due regard legal terminology found in the motor vehicle laws of most provinces and territories that sets a higher standard for the operators of emergency vehicles.

Ambulances are rarely or never exempt from prohibitions against passing over a railroad crossing with the gates down or passing a school bus with flashing lights.

As a general rule, do not rely solely on lights and siren to alert other motorists of your approach.

The role of lights and siren in the modern emergency response situation has diminished. Recent data have shown that lights and siren shave only a few seconds off response time but significantly increase the possibility of injury to the responding crew.

- Ambulance operators may also develop anxiety from sirens used on long runs, not to mention the possibility of hearing problems.

Some provinces, territories, and services have specific laws and SOPs that address the use of sirens. Some useful guidelines include:

- Vary the pitch and mode of the siren to increase other drivers' awareness of the siren.
- Never assume all motorists will hear your siren.
- Assume that some motorists will hear your siren but choose to ignore it.
- Be prepared for panic and erratic manoeuvres when drivers do hear your siren.
- Never use the siren to scare someone.

Some provinces, territories, and services have specific laws or SOPs that address the use of lights and sirens. For example, in B.C., ambulances are granted exemptions from specific motor vehicle regulations provided they are showing lights and sirens. Note that these privileges are only in effect if both lights and siren are on. Some SOPs limit the privileges granted by the Motor Vehicle Act in their jurisdictions. Although ambulances in B.C. and Alberta may exceed the speed limit and proceed through traffic control signals (e.g., red lights or stop signs), both B.C. Ambulance Service and Calgary EMS have policies restricting ambulance speed and requiring units to come to a complete stop before proceeding through red lights or stop signs. Calgary policy further requires ambulances on emergency runs to stop at uncontrolled railway or C-Train tracks or stopped school buses with lights flashing.

Whenever the ambulance is on the road, day or night, turn on the headlights to increase its visibility. Alternating headlamps should only be used at night if they are installed in a secondary lamp. Probably the most useful light is the one in the centre of the cowling on the front hood. This light can usually be easily seen in the rearview mirror of the car in front of you.

Each corner of the ambulance should have large flashers that blink in tandem or unison to help oncoming vehicles identify the location and size of the ambulance. Consider the latest research when designing or picking the lighting on your ambulance. At present, recommendations lean toward the use of single-beam bulbs and strobes instead of relying on one type of lighting system. The most important point is visibility. The vehicle must be clearly visible from 360 degrees to all other motorists and pedestrians.

ESCORTS AND MULTIVEHICLE RESPONSES

Use of a police escort for ambulances is rarely recommended—except when the ambulance needs guidance in an unfamiliar district.

Use of a police escort for ambulances is rarely recommended—except when the ambulance needs guidance in an unfamiliar district. Ambulances and police cars have different braking distances. If an ambulance follows a police car too closely, it can easily rear end the car. Also, the vehicles have different acceleration speeds. An ambulance may have trouble keeping up with a police car. A gap often develops, allowing other vehicles to pull in between. Finally, other motorists may not realize that the two vehicles are travelling together. After the police car speeds by, a vehicle may pull in front of an ambulance.

Multivehicle responses pose similar dangers. Additional danger occurs when two emergency vehicles approach an intersection at the same time. Besides confusing motorists and pedestrians, the potential for an intersection collision increases dramatically. Often, motorists fail to yield the right of way to the first emergency vehicle, the second, or both.

Even if you pay attention to other calls in your district, do not assume you are aware of them all. To avoid warning perpetrators, for example, the police often respond to incidents without announcing their approach. Always negotiate an intersection assuming that you may meet another emergency vehicle.

PARKING AND LOADING THE AMBULANCE

Whenever you arrive first at the site of a motor-vehicle collision, assess the scene for potential hazards. Establish a danger zone, parking at least 30 m from the wreckage upwind and uphill (if possible) to avoid fire or any escaping hazardous liquids or fumes. If there is no fire or escaping liquids or fumes, park at least 15 m from the wreckage. If possible, assign a crew member to handle traffic until the police arrive to take control of the task.

If your ambulance is the first emergency vehicle on the scene, park before the wreckage so your warning lights can alert approaching motorists. Then, set up flares or nonincendiary warning devices as quickly as possible. If the scene has already been secured, park beyond the wreckage to avoid being exposed to traffic. If command has already been established by an on-scene EMS unit, you may receive prearrival instructions.

Always be aware of potential traffic hazards. Many EMS providers have been seriously injured or killed when struck by passing motorists. As much as possible, try not to expose your crew or your patient to traffic. Keep in mind that rear ambulance doors often obstruct warning lights when they are opened to load the patient. Also, studies have shown that red revolving lights attract drunk or tired drivers. Consider pulling off the road, turning off your headlights, and using just the amber rear sealed blinkers that flash in tandem or in unison to help oncoming motorists identify the size and location of your vehicle.

THE DEADLY INTERSECTION

Recall that New York statistics reveal 72 percent of all ambulance collisions occur in intersections. Exercise extreme caution whenever you approach an intersection. Keep in mind the braking distance of your ambulance, the effectiveness of lights and siren, the rules of the road, the SOPs of your service, the acceleration needed to get through the intersection safely, and more. Helpful tips include the following:

- Stop at all red lights and stop signs, and then proceed with caution.
- Always proceed through an intersection slowly.
- Make eye contact with other motorists to ensure they understand your intentions.
- If you are using any of the exemptions offered to you as an emergency vehicle, such as passing through a red light or a stop sign, make sure you warn motorists by appropriately flashing your lights and sounding the siren.
- Remember that lights and siren only "ask" the public to yield the right of way. If the public does not yield, it may be because they misunderstand your intentions, cannot hear the siren due to noise in their own vehicles, or cannot see your lights. Never assume that other motorists know what you plan to do at the intersection.
- Always go around cars stopped at the intersection on their left (driver's) side. In some instances, this may involve passing into the oncoming lane, which should be done slowly and very cautiously. You invite trouble when you use a clear right lane to sneak past a group of cars at an intersection. If motorists are doing what they

should do under motor vehicle laws, they may pull into the right lane just as you attempt to pass.

- Know how long it takes for your ambulance to cross an intersection. This will help you judge whether you have enough time to pass through safely.
- Watch pedestrians at an intersection carefully. If they all seem to be staring in another direction, rather than at your ambulance, they may well be looking at the fire truck headed your way.
- Remember that an ambulance may weigh more than 4500 kg, a medium duty vehicle 10 900 kg. Even at speeds as slow as 50 km per hour, these vehicles will not stop quickly. When negotiating an intersection, consider "covering the brake" to shorten stopping distance.

UTILIZING AIR MEDICAL TRANSPORT

✱ aeromedical evacuations transport by helicopter or fixed-wing aircraft.

Air medical transport involves fixed-wing aircraft and rotorcraft. Air rescues are commonly referred to as **aeromedical evacuations,** or medevac.

FIXED-WING AIRCRAFT

Fixed-wing aircraft generally are employed when patients require transport over distances of more than 150 km. They may also be used to bring patients injured far from their homes to hospitals nearer to where they live. EMS units may also respond to medical emergencies aboard commercial aircraft that have been forced to land. Most major airlines now carry AEDs as part of their first-aid equipment, so you can expect to find almost anything when called to a landing strip.

ROTORCRAFT

The type of air transport that you will most likely encounter as a paramedic will involve rotorcraft, or helicopters. The use of helicopters for medical rescue grew out of their proven benefit during the Korean War and the conflict in Vietnam. Today, air medical transport programs are becoming more common in Canada (Figure 3-3). Many agencies now have the ability to order medically equipped helicopters to traumatic incidents requiring rapid response. They also use helicopters to transport patients from the field, especially in rural areas, to specialized hospitals. Finally, helicopters can provide quick inter-hospital transport of critically ill or injured patients.

ADVANTAGES AND DISADVANTAGES OF AIR TRANSPORT

Aeromedical transport offers a number of advantages and disadvantages. Advantages include more rapid transport in many situations, access to remote areas, access to specialty units (e.g., neonatal intensive care units, replantation units, transplant centres, burn centres), access to personnel with specialized skills (e.g., surgical airway, thoracotomy, rapid sequence intubation, critical care), and access to specialty supplies (e.g., aortic balloon pumps).

Disadvantages of aeromedical evacuation include weather and environmental restrictions to flying, altitude limitations, and airspeed limitations. Depending on the specific aircraft, cabin size can also restrict the number of crew members, the amount of equipment carried on board, and the configuration of

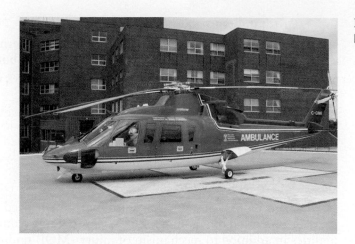

FIGURE 3-3 A hospital-based helicopter.

the stretcher. In smaller aircraft, such as the commonly used Bell LongRanger®, size limits the crew to the pilot and one flight medic or flight nurse. It also restricts the procedures that can be done on the patient during flight.

In the case of helicopter transport, in-flight climate control systems may not meet normal expectations. The thin walls of the fuselage do not allow much space for thermal insulation. Expect the "ship" to be hot in summer and cool in winter. Inside lighting is limited, otherwise the glare might enter the pilot's compartment, severely affecting his vision. Even though there is a curtain between the patient's compartment and the pilot, the lights still must be kept low, making ongoing patient assessment a challenge for the flight crew.

Finally, helicopter transport costs a lot of money. Some communities simply cannot afford to have a program.

ACTIVATION

Local and provincial or territorial guidelines may exist for the use of air medical transport in your area. Just as the public should access EMS by a single point (i.e., 911), ideally there should be a single access point for air medical transport in your region. To be effective, the need for medevac should be considered as early as possible. The decision should take into consideration the pilot's input, particularly regarding the safety of weather conditions, potential landing sites, and terrain.

Consider the need for medevac as early as possible.

INDICATIONS FOR USE

The indications for patient transport by helicopter include medical emergencies, trauma emergencies, and search and rescue missions. Factors that may warrant the need for air medical transport include the following:

Stable patients who are accessible to ground vehicles are best transported by ground vehicles.

Clinical Criteria

- Trauma score < 12
- Glasgow Coma Scale < 10
- Penetrating trauma to abdomen, pelvis, chest, neck, or head
- Spinal cord or spinal column injury or any injury producing paralysis or lateralizing signs
- Partial or total amputation of an extremity (excluding digits)
- Two or more long bone fractures or pelvis fracture

- Crush injury to abdomen, chest, or head
- Major burns or burns to face, hands, feet, or perineum; burns with respiratory involvement; electrical or chemical burns
- Patients in serious traumatic event < 12 or > 55 years of age
- Patients with near-drowning injuries
- Adult patients with
  —Systolic BP < 90 mmHg
  —Respiratory rate < 10 or > 35 per minute
  —Heart rate < 60 or > 120 per minute
  —No response to verbal stimuli

The mechanism of injury may also indicate the need for air transport. However, keep in mind that a number of local programs require physiological abnormalities in addition to mechanism of injury (MOI) findings:

Mechanism of Injury

- Vehicle rollover with unbelted passengers
- Vehicle striking pedestrian > 30 km/hr
- Falls > 3 m
- Motorcycle victim ejected at > 30 km/hr
- Multiple victims

Difficult Access

- Wilderness rescue
- Ambulance egress or access impeded by road conditions, weather, or traffic

Time or Distance Factors

- Transport to trauma centre > 15 minutes by ground ambulance
- Transport time to local hospital by ground ambulance greater than transport time to trauma centre by helicopter
- Patient extrication time > 20 minutes
- Utilization of local ground ambulance results in absence of ground ambulance coverage for local community

EMS operators do not generally perform rescue missions involving special means of access, such as rappelling out of helicopters. Rescue operations are usually undertaken by specially trained and equipped teams from such agencies as Department of National Defence Search and Rescue, local fire or rescue departments, or search and rescue groups.

> *It is important to weigh the risks versus benefits before using a helicopter for EMS patient transport.*
>
>

PATIENT PREPARATION AND TRANSFER

Be familiar with any special considerations that must be taken into account prior to loading the patient. For example, you may need to immobilize the patient on a specific type of backboard. Smaller helicopters might accept only a certain size backboard, while larger helicopters might accommodate an entire stretcher. Also, some helicopter services limit the length of the patient when supine, which could alter your method of immobilizing a fractured femur. In this instance, a standard traction splint may extend the leg too far to fit inside the aircraft.

Some agencies specify procedures to limit the spread of bloodborne pathogens in the helicopter. You might, for instance, be required to wrap the packaged patient in a disposable blanket or to place the patient in a body bag. It will also be necessary to convert IV bags to pressure infuser bags. The patient may need to be intubated prior to flight due to the limited area around the airway once the patient is on board. Depending on altitude, you may find it useful to put fluid in the air cuffs of tubes, such as Foley catheters or endotracheal (ET) tubes, since the fluid will not expand or contract as gases do at varying altitudes.

Since it is difficult to assess a patient's pulmonary sounds in a helicopter, ensure tube placement by visualization, observation of symmetrical chest expansion and condensation in the ET tube, positive colour changes, or a reading with an end-tidal carbon dioxide detector. Pulse oximeter readings will also be useful.

Remember that air pressure is changed by altitude, which affects IV bags, air cuffs of tubes, and the use of a PASG.

SCENE SAFETY AND THE LANDING ZONE

The medical helicopter industry has suffered a number of very serious crashes, especially in the mid-1980s. Recently, great strides have been made in improving the safety of helicopter transport. An important factor in bringing about these changes has been the focus on safety among flight personnel.

Flight crews should familiarize all EMS personnel in their region with their procedures and expectations. This will go a long way toward maintaining a safe scene and defining a safe landing zone (LZ) for the incoming helicopter. All paramedics should be able to select an appropriate LZ. As a rule, a helicopter requires an LZ of approximately 30 by 30 m (about 30 large steps on each side) on ground with less than an eight-degree slope. Paramedics should also be able to describe the terrain, major landmarks, estimated distance to the nearest town, and other pertinent information to the pilot on a designated frequency.

The LZ, as well as the approach and departure path, should be clear of wires, towers, vehicles, people, and loose objects. Most flight crews suggest that EMS crews mark the LZ with a single flare in an upwind position. During night operations, never shine a light into the pilot's eyes. This could cause temporary blindness or interfere with depth perception.

Once the aircraft has landed, approach it with extreme caution and only on approval of the flight crew. Make sure all loose objects, such as pillows and linens, are secured on the stretcher. Allow the flight crew to direct loading of the patient. Stay clear of the tail rotor at all times. Approach in a crouch. A sudden gust of wind can cause the main rotor to dip to a point as close as four feet from the ground. If the helicopter has landed on an incline, approach from the downhill side. Keep all vehicles at least 30 m away from the helicopter. Do not allow anyone to smoke within 60 m of the aircraft.

Part 2: Medical Incident Command

Occasionally, paramedics are called on to treat more than one patient at a time. The multipatient incident may result from a motor-vehicle collision (MVC), an apartment fire, a gang fight, or any number of other scenarios. During your career, you can also expect to respond to a much larger **multiple-casualty incident (MCI)**, also known as a mass-casualty incident (Figure 3-4). The MCI can involve "everyday" incidents, such as a bus and tractor-trailer collision; disasters

✳ **multiple-casualty incident (MCI)** incident that generates large numbers of patients and that often makes traditional EMS response ineffective because of special circumstances surrounding the event; also known as a mass-casualty incident.

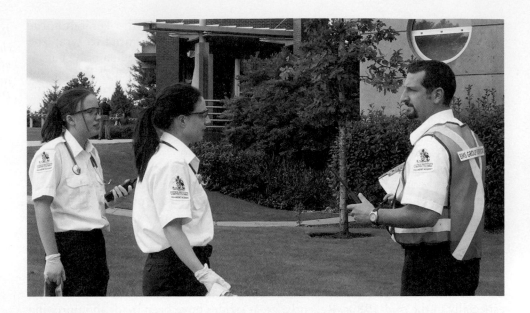

The same techniques and tools used to respond to a multiple-patient MVC will be used to manage a major MCI.

such as tornadoes, train wrecks, airline crashes; or even a terrorist event. Some districts define an MCI as any incident involving three or more patients. Others set the level for an MCI at five, seven, or more patients. In a disaster, the number of patients can reach the hundreds or thousands.

ORIGINS OF THE INCIDENT MANAGEMENT SYSTEM

Based on the confusion surrounding several major fires in the 1970s, the fire service took the lead in organizing responses to large-scale emergencies. The result was several versions of the incident command system (ICS)—a management program designed to control, direct, and coordinate emergency response resources. In recent years, the various ICS systems have been merged into the comprehensive, standardized **incident management system (IMS)**. It is a national system used for the management of multiple casualty incidents, involving assumption of responsibility for command and designation and coordination of such elements as triage, treatment, transport, and staging. Although the incident command system was originally developed for use at major fires, the standardized IMS has been adopted by law enforcement, EMS, hospitals, and industry.

 incident management system (IMS) national system used for the management of multiple casualty incidents, involving assumption of responsibility for command and designation and coordination of such elements as triage, treatment, transport, and staging; sometimes called the incident command system.

REGULATIONS AND STANDARDS

There are no federal Canadian regulations or standards regarding use of Incident Command or Incident Management Systems. Provincial, territorial, and regional standards vary, and you should be familiar with the system in use in your jurisdiction. For example, B.C. government organizations, including the B.C. Ambulance Service, are mandated to use the incident command system as outlined by the B.C. Emergency Response Management System (BCERMS).

A UNIFORM, FLEXIBLE SYSTEM

With its uniform terminology and approach, the incident management system has a number of advantages. First, an IMS can supersede jurisdictional and geographical boundaries to provide a well-organized response to routine and large-scale emergencies. Second, an IMS has the flexibility to respond to emergencies in both the public and the private sectors.

The following sections focus on the major functional areas of IMS. Use the mnemonic **C-FLOP** to keep these areas in mind:

C   command
F   finance and administration
L   logistics
O   operations
P   planning

COMMAND AT MASS-CASUALTY INCIDENTS

The most important functional area in the incident management system is **command**. The incident commander (IC)—also known as the officer in command (OIC) or the incident manager (IM)—is the individual who runs the incident (Figure 3-5). Establishing command at a multiagency, multijurisdictional incident can be complicated. If provincial, territorial, or local law does not decide the issue, the decision should be part of a preexisting MCI plan.

The ultimate authority for decision making rests with the incident commander. Because it would be too confusing or impossible for all on-scene personnel to report directly to the IC, the IC delegates certain functions and responsibilities to others. In this way, the IC maintains a reasonable **span of control,** or number of people or tasks that a single individual can monitor. Depending on the scope of the incident, the span of control may range from three to seven people with an average of five.

SINGULAR VERSUS UNIFIED COMMAND

At small incidents with limited jurisdictions, **singular command** usually works best. For example, a traffic accident may involve the local fire department, EMS, and police. The three agencies might agree that the fire department should assume overall command, thus creating a singular command situation. In incidents with

✱ **C-FLOP** mnemonic for the main functional areas with the IMS—command, finance and administration, logistics, operations, and planning.

✱ **command** the individual or group responsible for coordinating all activities and who makes final decisions on the emergency scene; often referred to as the incident commander (IC) or officer in charge (OIC).

The ultimate authority for decision making rests with the incident commander.

✱ **span of control** number of people or tasks that a single individual can monitor.

✱ **singular command** process in which a single individual is responsible for coordinating an incident; most useful in single-jurisdictional incidents.

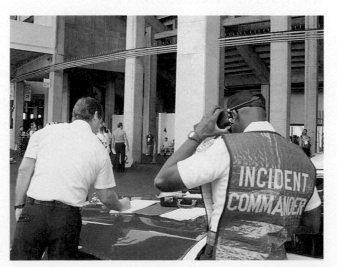

FIGURE 3-5   The incident commander takes overall charge of the incident.

unified command process in which managers from different jurisdictions—law enforcement, fire, EMS—coordinate their activities and share responsibility for command.

command post (CP) place where command officers from various agencies can meet with each other and select a management staff.

Generally, when two or more units respond to an emergency or when casualties include two or more patients, you should implement the incident management system.

Never forget the importance of assigning command early in an incident.

Successful handling of any MCI involves coordination of all key personnel—whether it be two people, twenty, or more.

If you arrive first on the scene, you must observe and protect all rescuers, including yourself, from hazards.

overlapping responsibilities or jurisdictions—such as terrorist attacks, explosions, sniper or hostage situations, and large-scale disasters—a **unified command** will be established. In these cases, law enforcement, fire, and EMS from several jurisdictions will coordinate their activities.

In establishing a unified command, the co-managers try to achieve balanced decision making. Together, they identify and access the agencies or organizations that might be needed at the scene, such as local Red Cross, emergency social services, health department, public works, and so on. They select sector leaders and establish reasonable and unified spans of control. Finally, the commanders determine the need for public information officers and liaison with the media.

When the incident management system is expanded or the scene is large, co-managers set up a **command post (CP)**, where command officers from various agencies can meet and confer. Because a command post may operate for weeks, the site should be selected carefully. Access to telephones, restrooms, and shelters should be taken into account. Also, the command post should be close enough to the scene so that officers can monitor operations but far enough away so that they are outside the direct operational area. Persons operating on the scene, members of the media, and bystanders should not have routine access to the CP.

ESTABLISHING COMMAND

An MCI may be declared when an incident produces multiple patients, has circumstances that make scene management challenging, or significantly taxes the available resources of a system. Generally, when two or more units respond to an emergency or when casualties include two or more patients, you should implement the incident management system.

As a rule, the first arriving unit establishes command. If you are the first to arrive, depending on the scope of the incident and local protocols, you and your partner will most likely fill the roles of incident commander and triage officer—at least until other units arrive. Never forget the importance of assigning command early in an incident. Most MCIs are won or lost in the first 10 minutes. Without incident command, emergency personnel may freelance. They may fail to prioritize patients, underestimate the severity of the incident, or delay requesting additional resources. Successful handing of any MCI involves coordination of all key personnel—whether it be two people, twenty, or more.

INCIDENT ASSESSMENT

Scene assessment is an integral part of establishing command. Survey the scene through the windshield of your vehicle as you arrive on the scene. Do not exit the vehicle until you have identified all the elements of the incident and noted any potential hazards. At an MVC, for example, do not miss the vehicle partially hidden in the woods or the pool of gasoline near your vehicle. Once you have determined the visible scope of an incident and any obvious hazards, relay this information to dispatch.

In managing an MCI, you must keep in mind three main priorities: life safety, incident stabilization, and property conservation.

Life Safety

Life safety is always your top priority. If you arrive first on the scene, you must observe and protect all rescuers, including yourself, from hazards. Then, and only then, will you attend to patients with immediate life threats. Keep in mind, however, that the needs of the many usually outweigh the needs of the few. If you commit to caring for the first patient that you encounter, you may neglect 10 other critical patients lying nearby. If you are the incident commander, remember that responsibility for triage belongs to the triage officer. At a small-scale incident, the IC may end up triaging some patients. Even so, the triage officer assumes the main responsibility for sorting patients into categories based on the severity of their injuries.

Incident Stabilization

Your second priority is incident stabilization. To achieve this goal, quickly identify whether the situation is an **open incident** or a **closed incident.** An open incident, also known as an uncontained incident, has the potential to generate more patients at any time. A fire that traps people inside an office building is an example. You may find several patients when you arrive on the scene. However, additional patients—including firefighters—may soon appear. As a result, the IC must anticipate the need for additional resources. Whenever you command an open incident, remember this point: It is better to call too many resources than too few.

In the case of a closed or contained incident, such as a multivehicle collision, the injuries have usually already occurred by the time you arrive. Yet, even a so-called closed incident carries the potential for additional hazards, such as an undetected gas leak or further injury to patients wandering about the scene. Stabilizing the incident to prevent further injuries helps ensure a smoother and more successful management of an MCI.

Property Conservation

The third priority is conservation of property. Rescue personnel must never damage property unless it is absolutely necessary for achieving the first two priorities, life safety and incident stabilization. Property conservation includes protection of the environment where operations are staged.

IDENTIFYING A STAGING AREA

Identification of a staging area is part of scene assessment. At MCIs involving hazardous materials or structural fires, for example, you must note wind speed and direction. The staging area and command post must lie well beyond the reach of any fumes, smoke, water, chemicals, or other hazardous materials.

Once you establish command of an MCI, choose both a primary and a secondary staging area. Keep in mind the main purpose of a staging area—organization of resources in one place for quick and easy deployment. Position the primary staging area as close to the scene as possible without compromising safety. Make sure the site has good access and exit points to ensure the flow of emergency vehicles. The secondary staging area should ideally lie in a different direction. This will provide you with a contingency plan in case the primary staging area becomes unusable. Conditions that may force a change in staging areas include altered traffic patterns, shifts in wind direction, or restricted access due to the deployment of fire hoses or other special equipment.

INCIDENT COMMUNICATIONS

Communications are the cornerstone of the incident management system. Once command is established, the incident commander has a responsibility to relay this information to dispatch. Then, as soon as possible, the IC should transmit a preliminary report that includes the following data: type of incident, approximate

✴ open incident an incident that has the potential to generate additional patients; also known as an uncontained incident or an unstable incident.

✴ closed incident an incident that is not likely to generate any further patients; also known as a contained incident or a stable incident.

Whenever you command an open incident, remember this point: It is better to call too many resources than too few.

Communications are the cornerstone of the incident management system.

number of patients by priority, request for additional resources, staging instructions, and a plan of action. If a fixed command post is required, the IC should communicate the location of this site as well.

Once an MCI has been declared, further communications should be moved to a secondary, or tactical, channel. The IC must be able to supply the information necessary to coordinate resources. That is the whole purpose of the IMS. Use of a secondary channel will also prevent an IC from interfering with the communications by other jurisdictions or from overwhelming the primary EMS channel.

Remember that communications will involve units from different jurisdictions and perhaps different districts. One of the foundations of incident management is the use of common terminology. Eliminate all radio codes, which may have different meanings in different places, and use only plain English. In fact, it may be preferable to avoid radio codes even in routine operations. Then there will be no need to even think about switching to plain English when you assume command of an MCI.

RESOURCE UTILIZATION

Most EMS units will require additional ambulances, personnel, equipment, and medical supplies. In many cases, they will also require specialized equipment and perhaps the help of public or private agencies.

The primary role of an incident commander is the strategic deployment of all necessary resources at an incident, which means setting goals and determining the tactics needed to accomplish these goals. The IC must continually assess the effectiveness of a given strategy or plan.

To ensure flexibility, an IC should radio a brief progress report approximately every 10 minutes until the incident has been stabilized. The report should state established goals, tactics, and resources and any progress or lack of progress. This forces an IC to monitor an operation, adapt to changing circumstances or to eliminate ineffective tactics entirely. Subordinates should deliver similar reports to the IC so that he can properly evaluate the overall operation.

COMMAND PROCEDURES

Several procedures help an incident commander to manage an MCI. First and foremost, all personnel must be able to recognize the IC. The incident management system calls for the IC and other officers to wear special reflective vests. The vests can be colour coded to functional areas and may have the officer's title on the front and back. Such vests should be worn whenever the IMS is utilized, even at smaller incidents. By making a basic set of vests available on every response unit, especially for command and triage, personnel will get in the habit of wearing and recognizing the vests prior to a major incident.

An IC can also benefit from the use of a worksheet or clipboard. An IMS worksheet should include basic information on the incident, a small area to sketch the scene, and a checklist of important items to remember. It might also include a section to record on-scene units and personnel, their assignments, and relevant patient information, particularly transport data. Many commercial paper and computer products are available for this purpose.

You will find a worksheet especially useful when transferring command, as often happens when higher ranking officers arrive on the scene. Command is only transferred face to face, with the current IC conducting a short but complete briefing on the incident status. A higher ranking officer does not become IC simply by his arriving—a briefing must take place. The worksheet serves as an outline for the briefing.

The primary role of an incident commander is the strategic deployment of all necessary resources at an incident.

Command is only transferred face to face, with the current incident commander conducting a short but complete briefing on the incident status.

TERMINATION OF COMMAND

As the incident progresses, resources will be reassigned or released. For example, an IC who transfers command to a higher ranking officer may become an aide to the new IC or be assigned to a totally new IMS role. Eventually, resources will be **demobilized,** or released for use elsewhere in the EMS system. Once the incident has progressed to the point at which the IMS is no longer needed, command should be terminated. A final progress report should be delivered to the communications centre. All units will then return to routine rules of operation.

The point at which command terminates depends on the incident. Some high-impact incidents, such as natural disasters or terrorist events, may last for weeks. However, not all agencies will have a significant presence for the long term. EMS may have a strong initial response, for example, but may simply have a single ambulance stand by for the long term. Other agencies may be released entirely from the incident if their services are no longer needed.

SUPPORT OF INCIDENT COMMAND

Incident command is supported by four sections or functional areas: finance/administration, logistics, operations, and planning. Each section has a place within the IMS and is headed by a **section chief.** However, all four areas may not be established at every incident. At small- or medium-sized incidents, for example, operations may be the only section implemented. At large-scale or long-term incidents, finance and administration, logistics, and planning may be activated. These sections may not be staffed with EMS personnel. However, they may help coordinate some EMS activities.

In addition, officers handling public information, safety, outside liaisons, and critical stress debriefing may report to the IC. Together, they are known as the **management staff,** or command staff. Management staff and section chiefs compose and carry out **staff functions.**

As a paramedic, it is more important for you to know how the incident management system works than to be an expert in specific job functions. Figure 3-6

✳ **demobilized** resources—personnel, vehicles, and equipment—released for use outside the incident when they are no longer needed at the scene.

✳ **section chief** officer who supervises major functional areas or sections; reports to the incident commander.

✳ **management staff** officers that handle public information, safety, outside liaisons, and critical stress debriefing; also known as the command staff.

✳ **staff functions** officers who perform supervisory roles in the IMS, rather than actually performing a task.

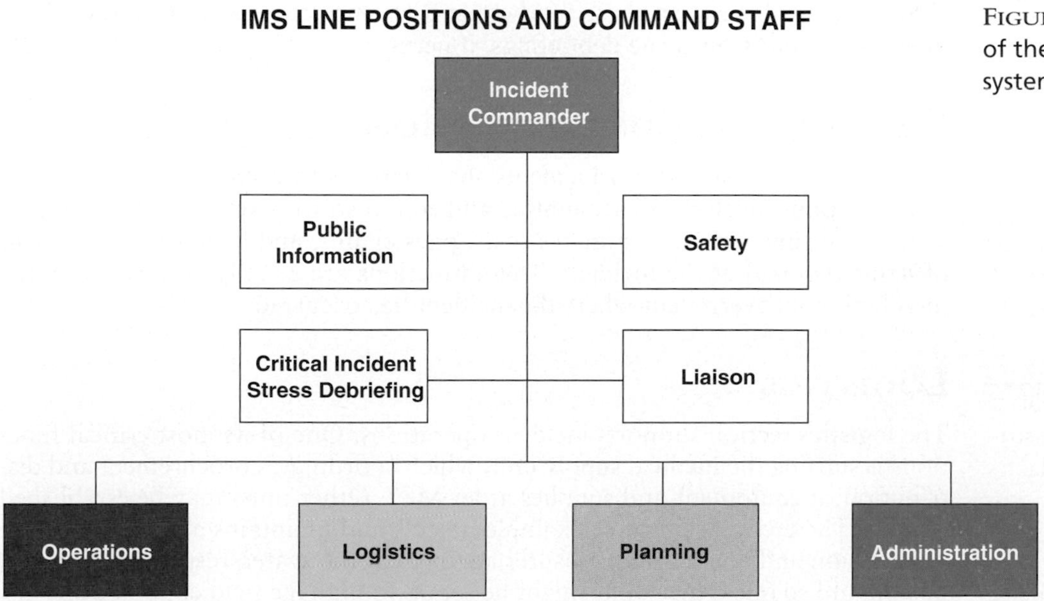

IMS LINE POSITIONS AND COMMAND STAFF

FIGURE 3-6   Basic elements of the incident management system.

and the following sections give you a quick overview of the basic elements of the incident command system.

MANAGEMENT STAFF

The management staff can play an important role in supporting the incident commander, particularly at major incidents or disasters.

Safety Officer

safety officer monitors all on-scene actions and ensures that they do not create any potentially harmful conditions.

The **safety officer** may hold the most important role at an MCI. This person—or, in some cases, team of people—monitors all on-scene actions and ensures that they do not create any potentially harmful conditions. Some of the areas that must be monitored include infection control, use of personal protective equipment, crowd control, lifting of patients and equipment, and quality of scene lighting. Under the IMS, the safety officer has the authority to stop any action that is deemed an immediate life threat.

Liaison Officer

liaison officer coordinates all incident operations that involve outside agencies.

The **liaison officer** coordinates all incident operations that involve outside agencies, such as other emergency services, disaster support networks, private industry representatives, government agencies, and more. The liaison officer makes sure these outside resources are connected with the appropriate functional areas and are deployed effectively.

Public Information Officer (PIO)

public information officer (PIO) collects data about the incident and releases it to the press.

Although you may not have a preexisting relation with the media in your community, a major incident will put your unit in the public spotlight. The **public information officer** collects data about the incident and releases them to the press.

Critical Incident Stress Management (CISM) Team

critical incident stress management (CISM) team monitors the emotional status of all on-scene personnel and provides the necessary support.

The **CISM team** monitors the emotional status of all on-scene personnel. The CISM team will support these workers and attempt to reduce the stress. They may also conduct on-scene debriefings, if necessary.

FINANCE AND ADMINISTRATION

finance and administration is responsible for maintaining records for personnel, time, and costs of resources or procurement; reports directly to the IC.

On large-scale or long-term incidents the **finance and administration** staff assumes responsibility for all accounting and administrative activities. It keeps personnel and time records, estimates costs, pays claims, and handles procurement of items required at the incident. These functions are usually performed by the jurisdictional government where the incident has occurred.

LOGISTICS

logistics supports incident operations, coordinating procurement and distribution of all medical resources.

medical supply unit coordinates procurement and distribution of equipment and supplies at an MCI.

facilities unit selects and maintains areas used for rehabilitation and command.

The **logistics** section supports incident operations. One of its most critical functions is staffing the **medical supply unit,** which coordinates procurement and distribution of equipment and supplies at an MCI. Other units may be established as well. The **facilities unit,** for example, selects and maintains areas used for rehabilitation and command. It ensures adequate food, water, restrooms, lighting, power, and so on. Other units might be set up to manage field communications, on-scene medical care for workers, and so on.

OPERATIONS

Whatever work needs to be performed at an incident takes place under **operations.** This section carries out tactical objectives, directs front-end activities, participates in planning, modifies the action plan, maintains discipline, and accounts for personnel. In short, operations gets the job done.

As will be explained later, operations may have many **branches**—functional levels based on primary roles or geography. Branches organized by role might include sections within EMS, rescue, fire, law enforcement, and so on. Branches based on geography might include the operations at various locations.

PLANNING

Planning helps formulate the overall action plan and oversees changes in that plan. It collects such information as weather reports, documents incident actions, and develops contingency plans. It ensures that written SOPs for **mutual aid**—agreements for sharing departmental resources—are activated or fulfilled. The planning section operates according to the principle of "anything that can go wrong will go wrong," using past incidents to anticipate troubles that might arise at the current incident. When command and operations must switch tactics, planning provides the necessary strategic support.

DIVISION OF FUNCTIONS

There are several ways to divide functions at an incident. The choice depends on the scope of an MCI, the structure of your department, the implementation of singular or unified command, and so on. If you are an IC, one of your jobs will be to organize line functions—that is, operations—in the most effective manner. Figure 3-7, for example, shows the functional levels within a typical EMS branch.

BRANCHES

Command may establish any number of branches organized by primary role or geography. Branches are supervised by branch directors, who report to the section chief for their functional area. The EMS branch director supervises all patient care and transport operations. Rescue may be an independent branch or may report to the director of EMS or fire.

GROUPS AND DIVISIONS

Branches may be further organized into groups or divisions. Groups are based on function, while divisions are based on geography. As an example, think of triage as a group and the responders working on the third floor of a multi-floor incident as a division. The supervisors of groups and divisions, in turn, report to the branch director.

UNITS

Groups and divisions can be broken into task-specific groups called units, supervised by unit leaders, who report to the group or division supervisor.

SECTORS

Depending on the type of IMS in your area, you may hear the term *sectors.* **Sector** is an interchangeable name for a branch, group, or division. However, it does not

* **Operations** carries out directions from command and does the actual work at an incident.

* **branches** functional levels within the IMS based upon primary roles and geographic locations.

* **Planning** provides past, present, and future information about an incident.

* **mutual aid** agreements or plans for sharing departmental resources.

* **Sector** interchangeable name for a branch, group, or division; does not, however, designate a functional or geographical area.

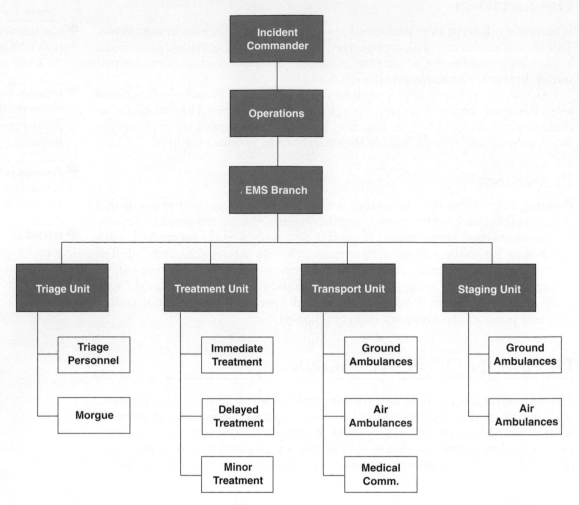

IMS EMS BRANCH

FIGURE 3-7   Example of branches that may operate in a major incident.

designate a functional or geographical area. Individuals who supervise a sector are often called sector officers.

FUNCTIONAL GROUPS WITHIN AN EMS BRANCH

The flexibility of the incident management system is founded on the ability to implement only the areas that are needed at an incident.

The incident management system operates under the "tool box" theory. Do not remove a tool from the toolbox unless you actually need it. The flexibility of IMS is founded on the ability to implement only the areas needed at an incident. This holds for all areas of IMS, including branches, groups, sectors, divisions, and specific areas where EMS operates. At many EMS incidents, the basic IMS organization in Figure 3-8 will provide all the "tools" you need.

TRIAGE

＊ triage act of sorting patients based on the severity of their injuries.

Triage is the act of sorting patients based on the severity of their injuries. In order to do the most good for the most people, you need to determine which patients need immediate care to live, which will live despite delays in care, and which will die despite receiving medical care. Because triage will direct subsequent operations, it is one of the first functions performed at an MCI. Therefore, all personnel should be trained in triage techniques and all response units should carry triage equipment. The triage group supervisor may act independently or may supervise the triage group/sector.

Primary and Secondary Triage

Triage occurs in phases. **Primary triage** takes place early, when you first contact patients, and provides a basic categorization of sustained injuries. It must be done quickly and efficiently so that command can determine on-site treatment needs and resources. Universally recognized triage categories include:

* **primary triage** triage that takes place early in the incident, usually on first arrival.

Category	Colour	Priority
Immediate	Red	Priority-1 (P-1)
Delayed	Yellow	Priority-2 (P-2)
Hold	Green	Priority-3 (P-3)
Deceased	Black	Priority-0 (P-0)

Secondary triage takes place throughout the incident as patients are collected, moved to treatment areas, and receive care. A patient's condition may change, requiring you to upgrade or downgrade the triage category.

* **secondary triage** triage that takes place after patients are moved to a treatment area to determine any change in status.

The START System

The most widely used triage system is **START,** an acronym for simple triage and rapid transport, a system developed at Hoag Memorial Hospital in Newport Beach, California. START's easy procedures allow for rapid sorting of patients into the preceding categories. START does not require a specific diagnosis. Instead, it focuses on these signs or symptoms (Figure 3-9):

* **START** acronym for the most widely used disaster triage system; stands for simple triage and rapid transport.

* Ability to walk
* Respiratory effort
* Pulses/perfusions
* Neurological status

Ability to Walk You initiate the START system by asking patients who can walk to get up and come to you. Any patients who can comply, despite their injuries, are categorized "green" and the appropriate tags are placed on the patients. Because patients who can walk will walk, you should make every effort to confine them to one site. There is enough confusion at an MCI without having the "walking wounded" wandering around the scene.

Content Review

SIGNS AND SYMPTOMS IN START

Can get up and walk
Has an open airway
Has respirations of more than 30/min
Follows commands

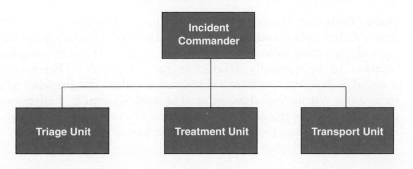

BASIC IMS ORGANIZATION
EMS OPERATIONS

FIGURE 3–8 Organization for a small- to medium-sized incident.

START TRIAGE SYSTEM

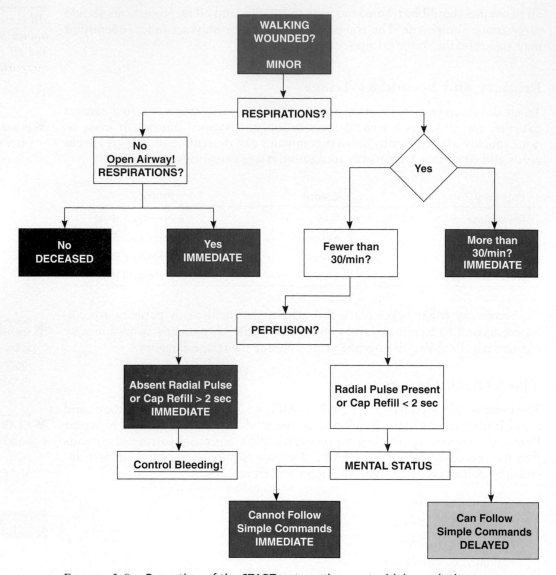

FIGURE 3-9   Operation of the START system, the most widely used triage system.

Respiratory Effort Next, you begin to triage the nonwalking patients. Remember to keep the focus on tagging patients. Your only treatment effort should be directed toward correction of airway problems and severe bleeding. Begin by assessing breathing. If patients are not breathing, open their airways manually. Tag patients who start to breathe spontaneously "red," those who fail to respond "black." For those who are breathing, quickly assess respiratory rate. Patients with respirations above 30/min should be tagged "red." If respirations are fewer than 30/min, go to the next assessment step.

Pulse/Perfusion Assessment of circulatory status can be accomplished in two ways: radial pulses and capillary refill. Delayed capillary refill (more than two seconds) is a poor indicator of perfusion in adults. It can be compromised by cold weather or be normally delayed in certain people. Therefore, the preferred method of assessing perfusion is the radial pulse. The presence of a radial pulse indicates a systolic blood pressure of at least 90 mmHg. Patients with absent radial pulses will be triaged "red." If patients have respirations fewer than 30/min and a present radial pulse, go to the next assessment step.

Neurological Status You now quickly assess mental status. Use this quick test: Ask patients to grip both your hands. If they can perform this simple task, categorize them Priority-2 or "yellow." If they cannot follow such simple commands, categorize them Priority-1 or "red."

Triage Tagging or Labelling

As already mentioned, you should attach a colour-coded tag to each patient whom you have triaged. Tagging offers these advantages:

- Alerts care providers to patient priorities—that is, provides organization of treatment
- Prevents retriage of the same patient
- Serves as a tracking system during transport and treatment

Commercial tags are available, such as the METTAG (Figure 3-10). However, you can also use coloured surveyor's tape. Each has its advantages and disadvantages. Tags provide tear-off strips that help you count patients in each

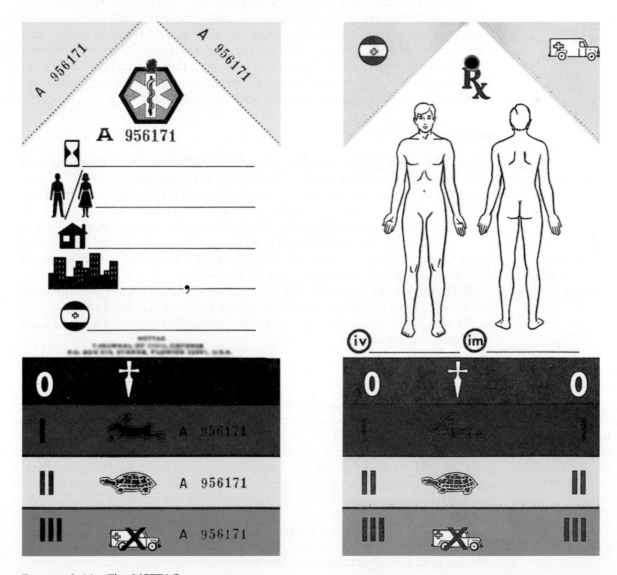

FIGURE 3-10   The METTAG.

triage category. Tags also make it easier to track patients, record treatment information, and indicate a patient's location in a transport accident. But tags can be damaged in wet weather, and tear-off strips can make it difficult to change patient categories. Surveyor's tape is less expensive but does not allow you to count patients during triage. Also, black tape cannot be easily seen at night.

Some systems combine use of both tags and tape. Others use tags only when immediate transport is unavailable or when patients need to be sorted into separate treatment areas. Whatever tagging method you use, it must be easy to use and provide rapid visual identification of priorities.

The Need for Speed

Although you must not become committed to single-patient care during triage, that does not mean you do nothing. Simple care—opening airways and direct pressure on profuse bleeding—can save lives early in an incident. The triage officer should carry infection control supplies, oral airways, and trauma dressings as well as tags or tape, a portable radio to communicate with the incident commander, a command vest, and a flashlight (at night).

Ideally, it will take less than 30 seconds to triage each patient. However, that means it will take five minutes to triage 10 patients, more than 20 minutes to triage 40 patients, and so on. The simple decision to add triage personnel can dramatically reduce triage time and speed up treatment and transport. They can act individually or be assigned to units. Either way, they report to the triage officer, who, in turn, relays information to the IC. After completing triage, personnel can be reassigned to other units, such as treatment.

The simple decision to add personnel can dramatically reduce triage time and speed treatment and transport.

MORGUE

You should collect patients who are triaged "black," or deceased (Priority-0), in an area away from treatment. This area, known as the **morgue,** should be access-controlled so that bystanders or the media cannot enter it. In determining the disposition of the deceased, you will need to work closely with the medical examiner, coroner, law enforcement, and other appropriate agencies. Once a morgue is established, it will be supervised by a **morgue officer.** This person may report to the TO or the treatment officer. In many cases, these supervisors will assist in selecting and securing an area for the morgue.

Keep in mind the importance of having a preexisting plan for managing situations with large numbers of fatalities. Special facilities may be required to care for the victims. In addition, responders may require the support of a CISM team or members of the clergy.

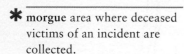 **morgue** area where deceased victims of an incident are collected.

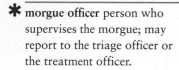 **morgue officer** person who supervises the morgue; may report to the triage officer or the treatment officer.

TREATMENT

When the number of patients exceeds the number of ambulances available for transportation, you will need to collect patients into treatment areas. The **treatment group supervisor** controls all actions in the treatment group/sector. Those who carry patients to the treatment area should work in teams of four to prevent lifting injuries. As patients arrive in the treatment area, conduct secondary triage to determine whether their status has changed. Patients should then be separated into functional treatment areas based on their category: red (immediate, P-1), yellow (delayed, P-2), or green (hold, P-3).

Essential equipment for a treatment area includes airway maintenance supplies, oxygen and delivery devices, bleeding control supplies, and burn management supplies as well as immobilization and transport devices, such as stretchers, spine boards, or other equipment to move patients.

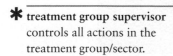 **treatment group supervisor** controls all actions in the treatment group/sector.

Red Treatment Unit

This area provides care for all critical patients. As a result, command or logistics will assign the bulk of medical resources to this unit. Providers with ALS skills usually report to the red treatment area so that they can stabilize patients and prepare them for transport. Because medical resources can be quickly used up, a supply system is necessary to support this operation. Finally, this is the place where any on-scene physicians or nurses should be utilized.

Yellow Treatment Unit

Teams of responders carry all noncritical patients to this unit for stabilization. Although these patients are not as critical as those in the red area, ALS procedures may still be necessary. A patient with an isolated femur fracture, for example, will probably be categorized yellow. Although this patient does not require immediate intervention or transport, he may still require an intravenous line and eventual surgical intervention.

Green Treatment Unit

Ambulatory patients report to the green area, where they are prepared for transport. Very little care is necessary in this area, but these patients still require monitoring in case their conditions deteriorate. In such instances, they will be triaged and moved to the appropriate treatment area.

Supervision of Treatment Units

Each of the preceding units is supervised by a **treatment unit leader,** who reports to the treatment group supervisor. The leader's job requires extreme flexibility to ensure that patients receive adequate care. Patient conditions can change and responders, equipment, or supplies may not be available in the subarea. As a result, communications must be carefully coordinated. The treatment group supervisor must be apprised of activities in each subarea. He must also help coordinate operations with other functional areas, particularly command, triage, and transport.

* **treatment unit leaders** EMS personnel who manage the various treatment units and who report to the treatment group supervisor.

ON-SCENE PHYSICIANS

At some high-impact or long-term incidents, physicians may support EMS. For example, they may be better able to make difficult triage decisions, perform advanced triage and treatment, or perform emergency surgery to extricate a patient as a last resort. Physicians also provide direct supervision and medical direction over paramedics in the treatment area, removing the need to operate under standing orders or radio contact. A contingency plan should outline when and how physicians respond to and operate at an MCI.

STAGING

Ambulances may be the most precious resource at a mass-casualty incident. As a result, ambulances must be staged as they arrive to allow proper access to the scene and, more importantly, egress with the patients. If ambulances arrive before they are needed to treat patients, they should be kept in a **staging** area under a **staging officer.** This area may be a roadway, a parking lot, or some other site where the units can wait until they are deployed by command.

* **staging** locations where ambulances, personnel, and equipment are kept in reserve for use at an incident.

* **staging officer** supervises the staging area and guards against premature commitment of resources and freelancing by personnel; reports to the branch director.

Depending on local protocols, drivers or crew members will be required to wait with the vehicles until they are needed for transport. A staging pool keeps personnel from "freelancing" and ensures their availability for quick deployment. It also prevents premature commitment of resources. If ambulances are required for immediate transport, the staging area can serve as a loading area for patients.

TRANSPORT

The **transport supervisor** coordinates operations with the staging officer and the treatment supervisor. His job is to get patients into the ambulances and routed to hospitals. If you are assigned to this role, you will need to be flexible in determining the order in which patients are packaged and loaded. You may, for example, elect to place two critical patients in one ambulance for transport to a trauma centre. If you decide that the ambulance provider cannot adequately care for two critical patients, you may instead decide to transport one critical and one noncritical patient. You may also take into account the facilities at a given hospital and avoid overwhelming its resources with critical patients.

The routing of patients to hospitals is as important as getting them into the ambulances. Early in the incident, your communications centre should contact local hospitals and determine how many patients in each triage category they can handle. You must also consider any specialties that a hospital may have—trauma centres, burn units, neurological teams, and so on. Keep in mind, too, that many patients may have left the scene before the arrival of EMS and transported themselves to the closest hospital.

A transport supervisor needs to implement some type of tracking system or destination log, which ideally will include each patient's triage tag number; triage priority; age, gender, and major injuries; transporting unit; hospital destination; departure time; and patient's name if possible. The tracking sheet not only helps organize activities at an MCI, but it also proves invaluable in reconstructing the incident later. In addition, this record will help document on-scene patient care.

EXTRICATION OR RESCUE

Extrication, or rescue, may be a branch or a group. If it is considered an EMS function, it will be a group (sector) under the EMS branch. If it is a fire department function, it may be under the fire branch. If the rescue is extensive or long term, the operation may be its own branch. The extrication or rescue group removes patients from entanglements and arranges for them to be carried to treatment areas. The operation has many facets and may require specialized personnel and equipment. During extended operations, treatment personnel will need to work in this area and begin patient care prior to removal.

Depending on the circumstances, personnel operating in this area will need personal protective equipment, including helmets, eye protection, gloves, breathing apparatus, and protective clothing. Some of the rescue tools may also require specific support materials, such as gasoline, electricity, or compressed air. Extrication or rescue is a very dangerous area, and all efforts should be taken to ensure that operations are well supervised and safe.

REHABILITATION

At extended operations, a special rehabilitation area should be established to support on-scene responders. Arrangements should be made with logistics to ensure the necessary food, water, and medical monitoring supplies.

Ideally, rescuers should regularly rotate through a dedicated rehabilitation area away from the incident. The site should provide thermal control and shelter from fumes, crowds, or the media. In this environment, rescuers can rest and hydrate themselves. Medical personnel operating in this area will take the vital signs of rescuers and watch for signs of fatigue or incident stress. A predetermined threshold should be established so that rescuers with abnormal vitals are removed from the operation. This is especially important during extremely hot or cold conditions.

Provision should also be made for a **rapid intervention team.** If possible, an ambulance and crew should be dedicated to stand by outside the staging area in case a rescuer becomes ill or injured. Unfortunately, the demands of a large-scale MCI sometimes prevent implementation of this aspect of the IMS.

COMMUNICATIONS

It cannot be said too often that communications form the cornerstone of the incident management system. Therefore, it helps to review some basic rules.

First, think about what you are going to say before you say it. Does the message really need to be transmitted over the radio? Remember that the frequencies at an MCI will already be congested with messages. As a result, you should try to prevent as much unnecessary radio traffic as possible.

Second, key up your radio before transmitting. Wait one second after pressing the button to speak. This allows your radio to begin transmitting effectively—and all other radios to begin listening—before you begin your message. Keep in mind that missed messages mean missed chances at increased coordination and efficiency.

Third, acknowledge each message with feedback to ensure that you understood it. For example, the message "Staging from Transport, send two ambulances" should not be acknowledged with "Staging received." It should be answered with "Staging received, send two ambulances."

Other rules include points already covered: the use of plain English instead of radio codes; the need for a common radio channel among command, groups (sectors), divisions, and units; face-to-face communications when appropriate; and respect for the lines of communication established by the IMS. In other words, report to the person you are supposed to report to.

EMS Communications Officer

At large-scale incidents, the incident management system provides for an **EMS communications officer,** also known as the EMS COM or the MED COM. This person works closely with the transport supervisor to notify hospitals of incoming patients. A dedicated radio channel works best for this purpose. The EMS COM will not deliver complete patient reports, which would increase the communications traffic. Instead, he will transmit the basic information collected by the transport supervisor, such as the number of Priority 1 patients en route to a hospital, the expected arrival time, and so on.

Alternative Means of Communication

Remember that your primary radio system may not always work at an MCI. Disasters can knock out radio towers and power. Frequencies can be overwhelmed. Telephone lines can be down. Radio batteries can fail. As a result, alternative means of communication should be included in every MCI preplan and should be practised regularly. You might use cellular phones, mobile data terminals, alphanumeric pagers, fax machines, or other technology to overcome the failure of your primary radio system. When all else fails, runners can be used to hand-deliver

A predetermined threshold should be established so that rescuers with abnormal vitals are removed from the operation.

✱ **rapid intervention team** ambulance and crew dedicated to stand by in case a rescuer becomes ill or injured.

✱ **EMS communications officer** notifies hospitals of incoming patients from an MCI; reports to the transport officer and may also be called the EMS COM or MED COM.

messages around the incident scene. Although there are obvious limitations to this method, it may be your last resort. Know how to use it.

DISASTER MANAGEMENT

Disasters can alter the routine operating procedures used at high-impact events. For example, disasters can damage a region's infrastructure, preventing the operation of railroads, hospitals, radio systems, and so on. If a disaster occurs in your jurisdiction, you will be a victim as much as a responder, which is why outside assistance is often required. As a rule, **disaster management** occurs in the following four stages: mitigation, planning, response, and recovery.

✽ **disaster management** management of incidents that generate large numbers of patients, often overwhelming resources and damaging parts of the infrastructure.

MITIGATION

Mitigation involves the prevention or limiting of disasters in the first place. For example, the public safety community tries to prevent people from building houses on flood plains or from putting up structures unable to withstand the impact of natural phenomena or terrorist attacks. In addition, most communities today have early warning systems to alert people to such emergencies as hurricanes, tornadoes, volcanic eruptions, or earthquakes.

PLANNING

As already indicated, planning is integral to the successful management of all high-impact emergencies. Every community should take part in a hazard analysis, rate these hazards according to their likelihood, and then devise relocation plans or evacuation procedures as needed. When possible, every effort should be made to keep people in their natural social groupings. That is, provide home-based relocation instead of removing people to hospitals and clinics when they are not injured. If you must evacuate people, use whatever means you have to spread the message frequently and with urgency. Alert people to the nature of the disaster, estimated time of impact, and expected severity. Advise people of safe routes out of the area and appropriate destinations.

Critical to any successful disaster plan will be provision for an efficient communication system in case the primary system fails. Decide, for example, where a central communications centre might be established for people needing help. Set up guidelines on the use of radios by all EMS personnel. Make arrangements for portable radios and recorders as necessary.

RESPONSE

In a disaster, there is a great disparity between casualties and resources. The event overwhelms the natural order and causes a great loss of property or life. A disaster almost always requires outside assistance and alternative operating plans. In general, you will follow incident management system guidelines.

RECOVERY

Recovery involves the return of your department, your jurisdiction, and your community to normal as soon as possible. Actions taken will vary with the nature of the disaster and the disaster plan. You may be involved with the reunion of families, follow-up care, and support of the personnel charged with handling potential hazards, such as collapsed buildings, highways, and so on.

MEETING THE CHALLENGE
OF MASS-CASUALTY INCIDENTS

As implied by the preceding sections, you will never be more challenged in your EMS career than when you respond to an MCI. The routine actions that you perform every day will suddenly become more difficult or, in some cases, impossible because of the stress of the incident. For this reason, you should anticipate various problems and work to overcome them.

COMMON PROBLEMS

Things can—and do—go wrong at MCIs and disasters. One way to avert or minimize complications is to anticipate them. As the saying goes, "Forewarned is forearmed." Studies of past incidents have revealed the following common problems, any of which can hinder the success of the operation:

- Lack of recognizable EMS command in the field
- Failure to provide adequate widespread notification of an event
- Failure to provide proper triage
- Lack of rapid "initial" stabilization of patients
- Failure to move, collect, and organize patients rapidly into a treatment area
- Lack of appropriate equipment and supplies
- Overly time-consuming patient care
- Premature transport of patients
- Improper or inefficient use of in-field personnel
- Improper distribution of patients to medical facilities
- Failure to establish an accurate patient-tracking system
- Inability to communicate with on-scene units, regional EMS agencies, or other personnel
- Lack of command vests for all IMS officers or supervisors
- Lack of adequate training or practice of rescuers at an MCI
- Lack of drills among regional agencies involved in the IMS
- Lack of proper community assessment, preplanning, and contingency plans

PREPLANNING, DRILLS, AND CRITIQUES

Anticipate any problems that may occur and work toward removing them. Anything that can be planned in advance should be planned in advance.

The first step is a complete assessment of the potential hazards—both natural and human—that could occur in your area. If you live in Saskatchewan, for example, you might not worry about hurricanes, but tornadoes are a very real possibility. Sites of potential incidents in almost any community include chemical or nuclear plants, factories or mines, schools, jails, sporting arenas, entertainment centres, railroads, airports, and so on.

Then, develop a plan that outlines the SOPs and protocols for potential incidents. You will not, of course, be able to plan for every possible scenario. If you develop 100 preplans, for example, you can expect to be summoned to scenario 101 or 102—that is, the unscripted event. For this reason, you must develop contingency plans for worst-case scenarios. For example, how would you communicate with ambulances if something or someone knocked out the dispatch centre? What would you do if the local hospital suddenly became unusable because of chemical contamination?

Then, test the preplan. Start small. Tabletop drills, for example, are a good place to begin. Once you have worked out the wrinkles, distribute the plan to everyone in your department, surrounding departments, local police, fire departments, hospitals—in short, to anyone who could be involved. Ensure that the necessary mutual aid agreements are in place and that the appropriate personnel know about these agreements.

Then, make sure that all personnel who could show up at an MCI have received proper training in the use of the IMS. As you have learned, the emergency responders on the scene will often determine the course of an event. Run or take part in drills so that you can gain practice in MCI operations and large-scale use of the incident management system. Again, start small. Use local drills within your department to help familiarize personnel with the system. Then, aim for large-scale drills that involve outside agencies.

Finally, never say, "It will never happen here." Experience has proven time and again that mass-casualty incidents and disasters can occur almost anywhere and at any time. Make it part of your professional training to be ready to act as an incident commander—the person charged with running the IMS.

Never say, "It will never happen here."

CRITICAL INCIDENT STRESS MANAGEMENT

As you already know, every EMS professional faces the possibility of critical incident stress (CIS)—the powerful emotional response to a catastrophic event. The response can begin during the event or immediately after. There can also be a delayed response, such as a flashback during a later call. Reactions can be physical, emotional, behavioural, or a combination of all three.

For this reason, you or your agency should make provisions for use of specially trained critical incident stress management (CISM) teams of local **trauma intervention programs (TIP)**. Such resources will provide access to mental health workers or other specially trained personnel who are familiar with emergency operations. CISM team members should circulate around the scene of a high-impact incident to spot anyone exhibiting a stress reaction. Others should be available for debriefing after an event.

At smaller incidents, a CISM team will probably not be activated. For this reason, you and other members of your crew should be aware of the signs or symptoms of a stress reaction. Be ready to help each other. For more on the management of stress within an EMS agency or unit, see Chapter 1.

✱ **trauma intervention programs (TIP)** mental health workers and citizen volunteers specially trained to provide assistance to anyone emotionally traumatized by a crisis event.

Part 3: Rescue Awareness and Operations

What do you do when your patient is pinned beneath a vehicle, trapped in a collapsed building, or injured climbing a rock face or crawling into a cave? When people get injured or stranded in such situations, often somebody must first rescue the patient before emergency medical care can even begin.

ROLE OF THE PARAMEDIC

It is not practical to train every paramedic in every rescue specialty (Figure 3-11). It is possible, though, to train all paramedics to an "awareness level." Awareness training teaches recognition of hazards and understanding of the need for additional expertise at the scene. Failing to train paramedics in rescue awareness will end in the injury or death of EMS personnel, patients, or both.

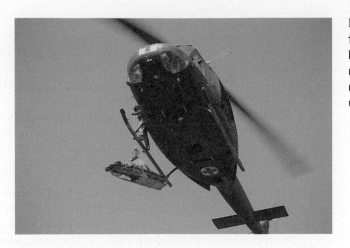

FIGURE 3-11 It is impossible for an individual paramedic to be highly trained in all types of rescue. Instead, specialized rescue teams should be utilized.

Rescue involves a combination of medical and mechanical skills. If a rescue unit does not have medical training, your unit provides the balance. In any rescue situation, treatment begins at the site of the incident. If the patient can be accessed in any way, treatment may start before the patient is actually released from entrapment. Once medical care begins, it continues throughout the incident. The trick is to balance the medical and mechanical rescue skills. Teams must coordinate efforts to meet both the medical and physical needs of the patient.

The role of EMS in a rescue operation varies from area to area. Some localities, for example, may require additional training beyond the awareness level. In general, however, all paramedics should have the proper training and personal protective equipment (PPE) to allow them to access the patient, provide assessment, and establish incident command.

As the first on scene, paramedics should understand the hazards associated with various environments—extreme heat or cold, potentially toxic atmospheres, unstable structures, and so on. They should also be able to recognize when it is safe or unsafe to access the patient or attempt a rescue. If you deem an environment safe and if you have the training to effect a rescue, you should at least participate in the rescue under the guidance of individuals with additional expertise. You should also understand the rescue process so that you can decide when various treatments are indicated or contraindicated.

The following pages focus on considerations that apply to most rescue situations—rescuer PPE and safety, the seven general phases of a rescue operation, and a "rescue awareness level" for the following environments:

- Surface water—for example, "low head" dams, flat water, moving water
- Hazardous atmospheres—for example, confined spaces, trenches, hazmat incidents
- Highway operations—for example, unstable vehicles, hazardous cargoes, volatile fuels
- Hazardous terrains—for example, high-angle cliffs, off-road wilderness areas

PROTECTIVE EQUIPMENT

Personal and patient safety equipment are paramount in any rescue. Some of the equipment discussed here have application in many rescue situations. Other pieces of gear are appropriate to specific environments or conditions.

The application of safety equipment—both to the rescuers and to the patient—is paramount in any rescue situation.

RESCUER PROTECTION

In all rescues, EMS personnel should wear highly visible clothing. Ideally, PPE should fit the situation, but gear can be adapted. In fact, most PPE has not been specifically designed for EMS use. Instead, it has been borrowed from other fields, such as firefighting, mountaineering, caving, occupational safety, and more. The use of adapted gear has resulted from the lack of a national uniform reporting system to identify risk-related exposures for EMS personnel. Future risk management and PPE design should be driven by such data. At a minimum, the following equipment should be available:

- *Helmets.* The best helmets have a four-point, non-elastic suspension system, most of which are designed to withstand a greater impact than the two-point system in construction hard hats. Avoid helmets with nonremovable "duck bills" in the back, which often cannot be worn in tight spaces. A compact firefighting helmet that meets CSA standards is adequate for most vehicle and structural applications, climbing helmets for confined space and technical rescues, and padded rafting or kayaking helmets for water rescues.

- *Eye protection.* Two essential pieces of eye gear are goggles, vented to prevent fogging, and industrial safety glasses. These should be CSA approved. Do not rely on the face shields found in fire helmets. They usually provide inadequate eye protection.

- *Hearing protection.* High-quality earmuff styles provide the best hearing protection. However, you must also think about practicality, convenience, availability, and environmental considerations. In high-noise areas, for example, you might use the multibaffled rubber earplugs used by the military or the sponge-like disposable earplugs.

- *Respiratory protection.* Surgical masks or commercial dust masks prove adequate for most occasions. These should be routinely carried on all EMS units.

- *Gloves.* Leather gloves usually protect against cuts and punctures. They allow free movement of the fingers and ample dexterity. Heavy, gauntlet-style gloves are too awkward for most rescue work.

- *Foot protection.* The best general boots for EMS work are high-top, steel-toed, shank boots with a coarse lug sole to provide traction and prevent slipping. For rescue operations, lace-up boots offer greater stability and better ankle support and don't come off as easily as pull-on boots when walking through deep mud. Insulation may be useful in colder working environments.

- *Flame or flash protection.* Every service should have an SOP calling for the use of flame or flash protection whenever the potential for fire exists. Turnout gear, coveralls, or jump suits all offer some arm and leg protection, help prevent damage to your uniform (Figure 3-12), and are quick and easy to apply. For protection against the sharp, jagged metal or glass at motor vehicle collisions or structural collapses, turnout gear generally works best. For limited flash protection, choose gear made from Nomex®, PBI®, or flame-retardant cotton. For high visibility, pick bright colours, such as orange or lime, and reflective trim or symbols. Some services use highly visible gear or orange safety vests at all highway operations—day and night. Insulated gear or jumpsuits are helpful in cold environments, but they can also increase heat stress during heavy work or in high ambient temperatures.

For protection against the sharp, jagged metal or glass at motor vehicle collisions or structural collapses, turnout gear generally works best.

- *Personal flotation devices (PFDs).* If your service includes areas where water emergencies can result, your unit should carry PFDs that meet the Fisheries and Oceans Canada and Transport Canada standards for flotation. They should be worn whenever operating on or around water. Attach an easily accessible knife, strobe light, and whistle to the PFD.
- *Lighting.* Many rescuers carry at least a flashlight or, better yet, a headlamp that can be attached to a helmet for hands-free operation. Consider the long-burning headlamps commonly worn by mountaineers and found through catalogues, the internet, or climbing and camping stores.
- *Hazmat suits or SCBA (self-contained breathing apparatus).* These should only be made available to the personnel trained to use them. Most services or regions have special hazmat units to provide the highly specialized support for rescues involving toxic substances.
- *Extended, remote, or wilderness protection.* If your unit provides service to a remote or wilderness area, have a backcountry survival pack preloaded with PPE for inclement weather (cold, rain, snow, wind), provisions for personal drinking water (iodine tablets/water filter), snacks for a few hours (energy gels or bars), temporary shelter (tent/tarp/bivouac ["bivy"] sack), butane lighter, and some redundancy in lighting in case of light source failure.

PATIENT PROTECTION

Many of the considerations for rescuer safety also apply to patients, with several significant differences. A patient protective equipment cache should include the following:

- *Helmets.* Patients usually do not require the same heavy-duty helmets as rescuers. Less expensive, construction-style hard hats provide adequate protection against minor hazards. However, if you anticipate greater danger, as in climbing or caving rescues, outfit patients with the same high-grade helmets as rescuers would use.
- *Eye protection.* Vented goggles, held in place by elastic bands, are ideal. They are not as easily dislodged as safety glasses. You might also use workshop face shields.
- *Hearing and respiratory protection.* Apply the same considerations as for yourself. Earplugs are usually adequate for hearing protection.
- *Protective blankets.* You should have a variety of protective blankets. Inexpensive vinyl tarps do a good job of protecting patients from water, weather, and most debris. Aluminized rescue blankets protect from fire, heat, or glass dust. Commercially available wool blankets provide excellent insulation from the cold. Plastic shielding (the kind used by landscapers) and plastic trash bags of many sizes and weights are also very useful. One 200-L drum liner is large enough to cover a single patient. It can serve as a disposable blanket, poncho, vapour barrier, or, in a wilderness situation, bivy sack.
- *Protective shielding.* Circumstances may call for more substantial protective equipment. All rescue teams should be trained to use backboards and other commonly found equipment as shields to protect patients from fire, weather, falling rock or debris, glass, or other sharp-edged objects. Shields specifically designed for a Stokes

Personal flotation devices should be worn whenever operating on or around water.

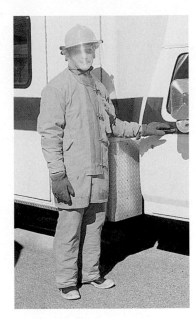

FIGURE 3-12 Full protective gear, including turnout gear, eye protection, helmet, and gloves.

Content Review

CHECKLIST FOR BACKCOUNTRY SURVIVAL PACK

PPE for inclement weather
Provisions for drinking water
Snacks for a few hours
Temporary shelter
Butane lighter
Redundant light sources

Always be sure to avoid covering the patient's mouth and nose during rescue operations.

basket should be available. Keep in mind, however, that a device that shields a patient from debris or the elements may also limit rescuers' access to the patient.

SAFETY PROCEDURES

As you already know, safety—your own and that of your crew—is your first priority. Yet, in rescue situations, a number of factors prod you to take action—your own desire to access the patient for treatment, the urging of people to "do something," the patient's cries for help, the presence of media, frustration at rescuers' lack of medical experience, and more. However, one mistake can spell disaster for you, your crew, or the entrapped victim. One way to curb "heroics" is by establishing rescue SOPs, determining crew assignments, and, above all else, preplanning scenarios well in advance of actual rescues.

RESCUE SOPs

Standard operating procedures (SOPs) are the nuts and bolts of effective EMS practice. At rescue situations, all teams should have written safety procedures familiar to everyone. Contents should include sections on all types of anticipated rescues. Each section should specify required safety equipment, required or prohibited actions, and any rescue-specific modifications in assignments. SOPs should include a statement requiring a safety officer and an explanation of that person's relationship to incident command. Ideally, the safety officer should be someone with the knowledge and authority to intervene in unsafe situations. This person makes the "go or no go" decision in the operation.

CREW ASSIGNMENTS

EMS units must anticipate crew assignments and special needs before the rescue operation takes place.

Search-and-rescue planners often use personnel screening to determine the participants. Programs exist to identify the physical capabilities of crew members. In addition, psychological testing is recommended. It may even be desirable to screen for specific traits, such as phobias. For example, a rescuer's inordinate fear of heights or small spaces should be taken into account when assigning duties. There must be regular practice of any dangerous rescue techniques that members of a unit may be trained to perform (Figure 3-13).

PLANNING

Planning starts with identification of potential rescue locations, structures, or activities within your area and then evaluates the training and equipment needed to manage each event. The plan considers efficient use of existing resources and anticipates the need for additional equipment, rescuers, and expertise.

Practice exercises with specialized rescue teams will give you and your unit ample opportunity to utilize the IMS as it applies to rescue situations.

Due to the intensity and length of many rescue operations, provisions must be made for the maintenance and rotation of rescue personnel, as discussed earlier for multiple-casualty events. On-scene diets should be high in complex carbohydrates and low in sugars and fats. Fluid replacement should consist of diluted (at least 50 percent) electrolyte solutions, such as those found in sports drinks. The classic coffee-and-donuts regimen should be avoided altogether.

Planning should be part of a broader regional emergency rescue plan, to be tested and modified in practice exercises. When possible, specialized groups, such as high-angle teams, should take part. These "test-runs" will provide ample opportunity to practise the IMS as it applies to rescue situations.

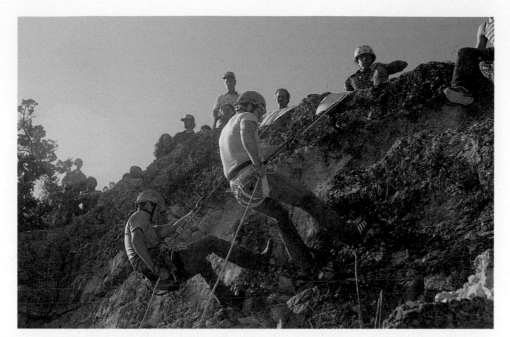

RESCUE OPERATIONS

As already mentioned, many types of rescue operations include technically difficult procedures, very specialized equipment, or both. *They should be attempted only by personnel with special training and experience in these areas.* Some of these special rescue operations will be examined later. But first, you need to be aware of the general approach to most rescue situations. Although procedures vary from area to area and rescue to rescue, most calls go through seven general phases: arrival and scene assessment, hazard control, patient access, medical treatment, disentanglement, patient packaging, and removal and transport.

PHASE 1: ARRIVAL AND SCENE ASSESSMENT

Scene assessment begins with the dispatcher's call. Although the dispatcher's message may indicate a rescue situation, you must still evaluate the environment and potential risks. On arrival, you or another paramedic must quickly establish medical command and appoint a triage officer. You must also conduct a rapid scene assessment, determine the number of patients, and notify dispatch of the magnitude of the event. Now is the time to implement the IMS, any mutual-aid agreements, and the procedures for contacting off-duty personnel or backup ALS units.

Prompt recognition of a rescue situation and identification of the specific type are essential. You may be summoned to a structural collapse, vehicle rollover, or climbing accident. Each holds the potential for entrapment and the need for specialized crews and equipment. Be careful not to overestimate your capability to handle a rescue. Individual acts of courage may be called for, but safety comes first. If in doubt, err on the side of safety.

In calling for backup, *don't undersell overkill.* Remember that it is always easier to send back a rescue crew than to rectify a tragedy caused by too few rescuers or hasty heroics. Realistically, evaluate the time needed to access and evacuate a patient. Use the IMS to shave off valuable response minutes.

Rescue operations should only be attempted by personnel with special training and experience in these areas.

Content Review

PHASES OF A RESCUE OPERATION

Arrival and scene assessment
Hazard control
Patient access
Medical treatment
Disentanglement
Patient packaging
Removal/transport

Be careful not to overestimate your capability to handle a rescue situation. In calling for backup, follow this precaution: "Don't undersell overkill."

PHASE 2: HAZARD CONTROL

Identify on-scene hazards quickly and clearly. You must often deal with these hazards before even attempting to reach the patient to avoid risk to yourself and other crewmembers. Control as many of hazards as possible, but don't attempt to go beyond your training or skills. Some situations, for example, involve chemical spills, radiation, gas leaks, explosives, or other dangerous substances. You will need to employ a hazmat team and confine your actions to a safe area. Electric wires hold a "double threat" for fire and shock.

The very environment in which you stand can be risk filled. Look around to determine the possibility of lightning, avalanches, rock slides, cave-ins, and so on. Ensure that all personnel wear appropriate PPE, and never forget traffic hazards. The following list is just a sampling of other potential hazards:

- Poisonous or caustic substances
- Biological agents or germ-infected materials
- Swift moving currents, floating debris, or contaminated water
- Confined spaces, such as vessels, trenches, mines, or caves
- Extreme heights or icy rock faces, especially in mountainous areas
- Possible psychological instability, as often experienced in hostage crises, urban violence, mass hysteria, or individual emotional trauma on the part of either the patient or the crew

PHASE 3: PATIENT ACCESS

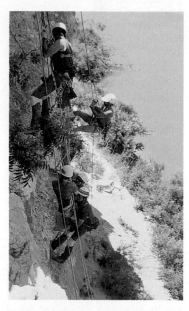

Access triggers the technical beginning of the rescue.

After controlling hazards, you will then attempt to gain access to the patient or patients. First, formulate a plan. Determine the best method to gain access and deploy personnel. Take steps to stabilize the patient's location. For example, look for threats of structural collapse, cave-ins, or vehicle rollover.

Access is the technical beginning of the rescue. This is the point at which you or the command and safety officers must honestly evaluate the training and skills needed to access the patient. Untrained, poorly equipped, or inexperienced rescue personnel must not put their safety—and the safety of others—at risk by attempting foolhardy, heroic rescues.

Key medical, technical, and command personnel must confer with the safety officer on strategy. To ensure that everyone understands and supports the plan, a formal briefing should be held for rescuers before the operation begins. Even with well-trained personnel and adequate equipment, rescue efforts can be poorly executed because team members do not understand the "big picture" or do not know what is expected of each member of the team.

PHASE 4: MEDICAL TREATMENT

After devising a plan, medical personnel can begin to make patient contact (Figure 3-14). A paramedic has three general responsibilities during this phase:

- Initiation or patient assessment and care as soon as possible
- Maintenance of patient care procedures during disentanglement
- Accompaniment of the patient during removal and transport

FIGURE 3-14 Assessment and care may need to be modified, depending on the on-scene environment and any special hazards.

If you are treating the patient, as conditions allow, quickly conduct a primary assessment. The next critical steps include rapid trauma assessment for the patient with a significant MOI and medically oriented recommendations to the evacuation team.

A patient's condition may change dramatically during disentanglement and removal. Therefore, first, identify and care for existing problems. Second, anticipate changing patient conditions and the assistance and equipment needed to cope with them. Continually evaluate risks to both rescuers and patient. In many situations, the best overall patient care requires rapid stabilization and immediate removal. Final positive patient outcome may depend on initial sacrifice of definitive patient care so that the patient and rescuers can be removed from imminent danger. Examples of such situations include the following:

- Injured, stranded high-rise window cleaners; workers on water, radio, or TV towers; high-rise construction workers
- Workers or bystanders involved in a trench cave-in
- Persons stranded in swift-running, rising water
- Patients entrapped in vehicles with an associated fire
- Patients overcome by life-threatening atmospheres
- Victims entrapped with unstable or volatile hazardous materials

In such cases, rapid transport of a nonstabilized patient to a safer location may be justified by the risk of injury to the rescuers and exposure of the patient to even greater complications. Rapid movement might be required even though the transport will aggravate existing patient injuries. Generally, management for the entrapped patient has the same foundation as all emergency care:

- Primary assessment of the MS-ABCs (mental status; airway, breathing, circulation)
- Management of life-threatening airway, breathing, and circulation problems
- Immobilization of the cervical spine (C-spine)
- Splinting of major fractures
- Packaging with consideration to patient injuries, **extrication** requirements, and environmental conditions
- Ongoing reassessment during the transport phase

Patient management during a rescue often follows the same protocols used "on the street." However, some specifics may be, or should be, significantly different. Differences result mainly from the lengthy time periods often required to access, disentangle, or evacuate the patient. EMS personnel are trained in rapid stabilization and transport, particularly with trauma patients. However, during a rescue mission, the desire to achieve speedy transport, as well as to obey the "Golden Hour" rule, may be impossible to fulfill. As a result, you must be able to "shift gears" mentally to an extended-care situation.

In addition to extended field time, you must be prepared to provide more in-depth psychological support for rescue patients than usual. This is especially true when a patient has already been entrapped for a considerable amount of time. Establish a solid rapport with the patient, striking up a constant and reassuring conversation. In quieting the fears, keep in mind the following tips:

- Learn and use the patient's name, and tell the patient your name.
- Be sure other team members know and use the patient's name.
- Be sure the patient knows that you will not abandon him.
- Avoid negative or fearful comments regarding the operation, its cause, or the patient's condition within earshot of the patient.
- Explain all delays to the patient, and identify steps that will be taken to remedy the situation.

Content Review

GOALS OF RESCUE ASSESSMENT
Identify and care for existing patient problem. Anticipate changing patient conditions, and determine in advance the assistance and equipment needed.

✱ **extrication** use of force to free a patient from entrapment.

In responding to rescues, you must be prepared to "shift gears" mentally to an extended-care situation.

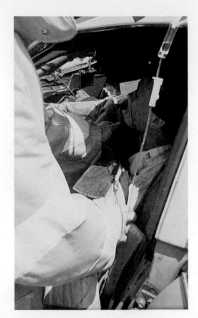

FIGURE 3-15 Disentanglement can be prolonged, as in the case of auto entrapment.

✳ **disentanglement** process of freeing a patient from wreckage to allow for proper care, removal, and transfer.

Disentanglement may be the most technical and time-consuming portion of the rescue.

✳ **active rescue zone** area where special rescue teams operate; also known as the "hot zone" or "inner circle."

It is paramount that the rescuer knows how to properly package the patient to prevent further injury.

- Ask special rescue teams to explain any technical aspects of the operation that could frighten or affect the patient's condition. Translate these operations into clear, simple terms for the patient.

- Do not lie to the patient. If something may hurt, acknowledge it. If the patient suspects an unstable environment, acknowledge that, too. However, be sure to explain what will be done to mitigate the situation.

- Above all else, stay calm and professional. If you don't know the answer to a question, find somebody who does. Remember: Rescues are driven by patient needs.

PHASE 5: DISENTANGLEMENT

Disentanglement involves the actual release from the cause of entrapment, such as the dashboard of a wrecked automobile, a concrete slab from a structural collapse, or the blocked entry to a cave. This phase may be the most technical and time-consuming portion of the rescue (Figure 3-15). If assigned to patient care during this phase of the rescue, you have three responsibilities. They are:

- Confidence and the technical expertise and gear needed to function effectively in the **active rescue zone** ("hot zone" or "inner circle")
- Readiness to provide prolonged patient care
- Ability to call for and use special rescue resources

If you or another member of the rescue team cannot fulfill these requirements, reassess available rescue personnel and call for backup. Disentanglement is not a time for the claustrophobic or the squeamish.

Methods used to disentangle the patient must be constantly analyzed on a risk-to-benefit basis. You and other members of the rescue team must balance the patient's medical needs with such concerns as the time it will take to perform treatment, the safety of the environment, and so on. If a patient has a severely crushed extremity and it will take an inordinate amount of time to release the extremity, the patient may bleed to death without an amputation. This is only one of the hard treatment decisions that may be faced during disentanglement.

PHASE 6: PATIENT PACKAGING

After disentanglement, a patient must be appropriately packaged. You must consider such things as the means of egress—for example, a litter-carry through the woods versus walking a patient out. You must also factor in time based on the patient's medical conditions—for example, rapid extrication techniques versus application of a Kendrick Extrication Device (KED). Some specialized rescue techniques require complex forms of packaging—such as being lifted out of a hole in a Stokes basket by a ladder truck, being vertically hauled through a manhole in a Sked® stretcher, and so on. In situations where the patient may be vertical or suspended in a Stokes, the rescuer must know how to properly package the patient to prevent additional injury.

PHASE 7: REMOVAL AND TRANSPORT

Removal of the patient may be one of the most difficult tasks (Figure 3-16), or it may be as easy as placing the person on a stretcher and wheeling it to a nearby ambulance. Transport to a medical facility should be planned well in advance, especially if you anticipate any delays. Decisions regarding patient transport—by ground vehicle, aircraft, or physical carryout—should be based on advice from medical direction. En route to the hospital, perform ongoing assessment and administer additional therapy per medical direction.

SURFACE WATER RESCUES

Water emergencies are among the most common rescue situations because people are attracted to water in such great numbers and for such a wide variety of activities. Most water rescues are resolved without the involvement of EMS personnel—for example, bystanders jump into a pool to pull out a struggling swimmer, other boaters rescue someone whose canoe has overturned, and so on. However, some water emergencies require special training and equipment. In such cases, the temperature and dynamics of flat or moving water place both the victim and the rescuer at high risk. Although all the possible scenarios for water rescue training cannot be covered here, the following are some general concepts.

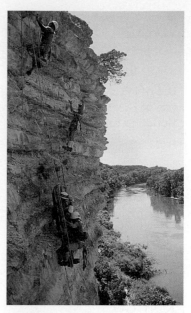

FIGURE 3-16 Packaging and removal can be a time-consuming process, as in the case of a vertical rescue.

GENERAL BACKGROUND

Water rescues may involve pools, rivers, streams, lakes, canals, flooded gravel pits, or the ocean. Some communities have drainage systems that remain dry until flash floods turn them into raging rivers. Most people who get injured or drown in these bodies of water never intended to get into trouble. But one or more factors conspire to create an emergency—the weather changes, swimmers underestimate the water's power, nonswimmers neglect to wear a PFD and fall in, people develop a muscle stitch or cramp while in the water, submerged debris knocks waders off their feet, boats collide, and more.

Nearly all incidents in and around water are preventable. Become familiar with safe aquatic practices. First, know how to swim, and make swimming part of your physical exercise. Second, remember that even the strongest swimmer can get into trouble. Therefore, always carry PFDs aboard your unit, and always wear a PFD whenever you are around water or ice. (Make sure your crew does the same.) Third, consider taking a basic water rescue course.

Water Temperature

Human body temperature is normally 37°C. Almost any body of water is colder and will cause heat loss. Water temperature in smaller bodies of water varies widely with the seasons and the amount of runoff. Yet, even on warm days, water temperatures can be quite cold in most places. As a result, water temperature and heat loss figure in the deaths of most victims and ill-equipped rescuers.

As implied, immersion can rapidly lead to hypothermia, a condition discussed in Chapter 36. As a rule, people cannot maintain body heat in water that is less than 33°C. The colder the water, the faster is the loss of heat. In fact, water causes heat loss 25 times faster than air. Immersion in 2°C water for 15 to 20 minutes is likely to kill a person. Factors contributing to the death of a hypothermic patient include the following:

- Incapacitation and an inability to self-rescue
- Inability to follow simple directions
- Inability to grasp a line or flotation device
- Laryngospasm (caused by sudden immersion in cold water), thus a greater likelihood of drowning

A number of actions can delay the onset of hypothermia in water rescues. The use of PFDs slows heat loss and lessens the energy required for flotation. If people suddenly become submerged, they can also assume the **heat escape lessening position (HELP)**—floating with the head out of water and the body in a fetal tuck. Researchers estimate that someone who has practised HELP can reduce heat loss by almost 60 percent, as compared with the heat expended when treading water. If a group of victims find themselves in the water, researchers also suggest huddling together. This technique not only prevents heat loss, but provides a better target for members of a rescue team.

Basic Rescue Techniques

Basic rescue techniques vary with the dynamics of the water—that is, moving water versus nonmoving (flat) water. If your unit responds to frozen bodies of water, you may also add techniques for ice rescue and include the proper cold water entry dry suits as part of your PPE cache (Figure 3-17).

The water rescue model is REACH-THROW-ROW-GO. All paramedics should be trained in reach-and-throw techniques. A PFD is useless if it is not worn. So, all EMS personnel should put it on, even for shore-based rescues. If at first you are unable to talk the patient into a self-rescue, then reach with a pole or long rescue device. If this is not effective or if the victim is too far out, try throwing a flotation device. All paramedics should become proficient with a water-throw bag for shore-based operations. Remember: Boat-based techniques require specialized rescue training. Water-entry ("go") is the last resort—an action best left to specialized water rescuers.

MOVING WATER

By far the most dangerous water rescues involve water that is moving. Competency at handling the power and dynamics of swift-water rescues comes only with extensive training and experience. The force of moving water can be very deceptive. The hydraulics of moving water change with a number of variables, including water depth, velocity, obstructions to flow, changing tides, and more. Only specially trained rescuers can readily recognize these factors.

To train for swift-water entry, rescuers must develop proficiency in many specialized skills. In preparation for technical rope rescues, they must master the skills required for high-angle rope rescues. They must also become well-practised in such skills as crossing moving water bodies, defensive swimming, use of throw bags and boogy boards, shore-based swimming, boat-based rescue techniques, management of water-specific emergencies, the capability to package the patient with water-related injuries, and more.

Four swift-water rescue scenarios present a special challenge and danger to rescuers. They include recirculating currents ("drowning machines"), strainers, foot/extremity pins, and dams or hydroelectric intakes.

Recirculating Currents

Recirculating currents result from water moving over a uniform obstruction to flow, such as a large rock or low head dam. The movement of currents can create what is known as a "drowning machine" (Figure 3-18).

On first appearance, recirculating currents can look very tame. Anglers, for example, often fish on the downstream portion of a low head dam, casting their lines into the recirculating waters. This is a good place to catch fish because they can often be seen just below the dam. But think about it. If fish with their natural ability to swim get stuck in the recirculating currents, imagine what would

✱ **heat escape lessening position (HELP)** an in-water, head-up tuck or fetal position designed to reduce heat loss by as much as 60 percent.

The water rescue model is REACH-THROW-ROW-GO.

Water entry is a last resort—and is an action best left to specialized water rescuers.

✱ **recirculating current** movement of currents over a uniform obstruction; also known as a "drowning machine."

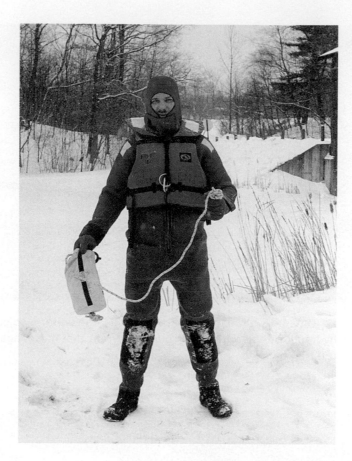

FIGURE 3-17 Safe ice rescue requires proper equipment and protective clothing, particularly a dry suit and water-sealed footwear.

happen to humans if they got too close to the dam. Once caught in the recirculating currents, people find it very difficult to escape. The resulting rescue can be extremely hazardous—even for specially trained rescuers.

Strainers

When moving water flows through obstructions, such as downed trees, grating, or wire mesh, an unequal force is created on the two sides of the so-called "strainers" (Figure 3-19). Currents can literally force a person up against a strainer, making it difficult to be removed due to the power of the current. In some cases, the current might be flowing into a drainage pipe under the surface, which is, in turn, covered by a rebar (metal) grate. Victims can get sucked into the grate and are then pinned against it.

This, too, can be a hazardous rescue. If you are floating downstream and see the potential of getting pinned against a strainer, attempt to swim over the object. Whatever you do, do not put your feet on the bottom—your feet could get stuck, or you could get swept off your feet and slammed into the obstruction.

✱ **strainer** a partial obstruction that filters, or strains, the water, such as downed trees or wire mesh, causing an unequal force on the two sides.

Foot or Extremity Pins

It is always unsafe to walk in fast-moving water over knee depth because of the danger of trapping a foot or extremity. When this occurs, the weight and force of the water can knock you below the surface. To remove the foot or extremity, it must be extracted the same way it went in. Water currents often make this extremely difficult. Again, this is a hazardous rescue because of the need to work below the surface of already dangerous water conditions.

It is always unsafe to walk in fast-moving water over knee depth because of the danger of entrapping a foot or extremity.

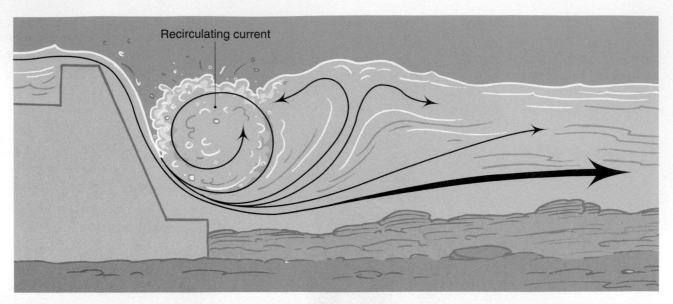

Recirculating current

FIGURE 3-18   When water flows over a large uniform object, it can create a hydraulic or hole with a recirculating current that moves against the river's flow and can trap people.

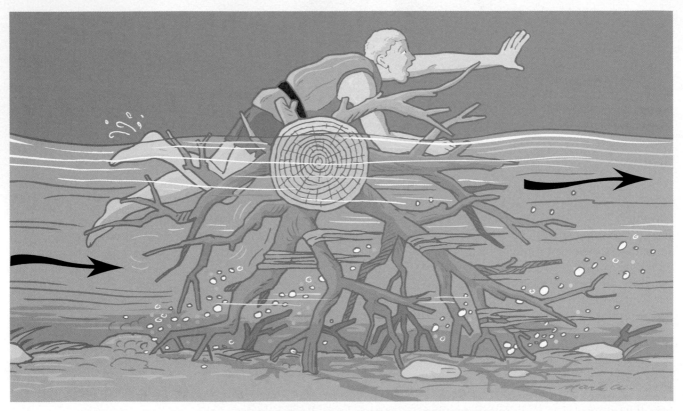

FIGURE 3-19   Strainers are objects that allow water to flow through them but that will trap other objects—and people.

Dams and Hydroelectric Intakes

Yet another dangerous situation involves dams and hydroelectric intakes, such as those often found along rivers. The height of the dam is no indication of the degree of hazard. As already indicated, low head dams can create powerful drowning machines. Assume that all dams have the ability to form recirculating currents. Hydroelectric intakes act as dangerous strainers.

Self-Rescue Techniques

Some water survival techniques have already been mentioned—such as wearing PFDs and the use of HELP. However, if you suddenly fall in swift-running water (or flat for that matter), keep these suggestions in mind:

- Cover your mouth and nose during entry.
- Protect your head and, if possible, keep your face out of the water.
- Do not attempt to stand up in moving water.
- Float on your back, with your feet pointed downstream.
- Steer with your feet, and point your head toward the nearest shore at a 45-degree angle or continue to float downstream until you come to an area where the water slows enough for you to swim to the edge.
- If the water turns a bend, remember that the outside of the curve moves faster that the inside of the curve.
- Look for large objects, such as rocks, that can block the water and cause recirculating currents or strainers.
- Learn to identify **eddies**—water that flows around especially large objects and, for a time, flows upstream around the downside of the obstruction. These back currents move more slowly and can actually sweep you toward the edge—and safety.
- Above all else, take precautions not to fall into the water in the first place. Remember: reach-throw-row-go, with "go" being the absolutely last resort.

* **eddies** water that flows around especially large objects and, for a time, flows upstream around the downside of an obstruction; provides an opportunity to escape dangerous currents.

FLAT WATER

The greatest problem with flat water is that it looks so calm. But a large proportion of drowning or near-drowning incidents take place in flat or slow-moving water. Some of the factors in these deaths were mentioned earlier. In a significant number of cases, alcohol plays a role. Nearly 50 percent of boating fatalities, for example, result from intoxication or impairment by alcohol—a substance that impairs the ability to think, reason, and survive in a water accident.

Factors Affecting Survival

A number of factors help determine the death or survival of a patient. A person's "survivability profile" is affected by age, posture, lung volume, water temperature, and more. Two especially important factors, are the presence of PFDs and what is known as the "cold-protective response."

Personal Flotation Devices Many recreational water users associate "life preservers" with rough water or people who cannot swim. But PFDs should be essential items for all water-related activities. One study, for example, linked nearly 89 percent of all boating fatalities to the lack of PFDs.

Content Review

FACTORS AFFECTING SURVIVAL

Age
Posture
Lung volume
Water temperature
Use of PFDs
Mammalian diving reflex

Every system should have a strict SOP mandating the use of PFDs for all EMS personnel. Even services in arid regions can be involved in water rescues. They can be called to swimming pool accidents or river-rafting accidents. In some places, EMS can respond to flash-flooding in canyons that can trap or kill hikers or "canyoneers." The same flash flooding can overload drainage systems, creating hazardous conditions for the public and the rescuers alike.

Cold Protective Response The same cold water that can kill people also triggers a protective response known as the "mammalian diving reflex." When the face of a human, or any mammal, is plunged into water at less than 20°C temperature, the parasympathetic nervous system is stimulated. The heart rate rapidly decreases to a bradycardic rhythm. Meanwhile, blood pressure drops, and vasoconstriction occurs throughout the body. Blood is shunted from less vital organs to the heart and brain, temporarily delivering life-sustaining oxygen. As a general rule, the colder the water, the more oxygen is diverted.

The mammalian reflex, along with the length of time the head was above water during the cooling process, can significantly delay death. Some patients have been resuscitated after 45 minutes under water. As a rule, the reflex is more pronounced in children than in adults.

Location of Submerged Victims

Because of protective physiological responses, rescuers must make every effort to locate submerged victims. Interview witnesses to establish a relative location. Ask each witness to locate an object across the water to form a line. Repeat this process with each witness. Use the point of convergence among lines to target the most accurate "last seen" location. Start searching from this point, and fan out in larger and larger circles, forming a radius equal to the depth of the water.

Rescue versus Body Recovery

A number of conditions determine when a rescue turns into a body recovery. Some factors are length of time submerged, any known or suspected trauma, age and physical condition of the victim, water temperature and environmental conditions, and estimated time for rescue or removal.

Once a patient is recovered, you should attempt resuscitation on any hypothermic or pulseless, nonbreathing patient who has been submerged in cold water. (Some experts advise providing resuscitation to every drowning patient, regardless of water temperature, even those who have been in the water for some time.) A patient must be rewarmed before an accurate assessment can be made. Remember: Water-rescue patients are never dead until they are warm and dead. (For more on drowning and near-drowning, see Chapter 36.)

Remember: Water-rescue patients are never dead until they are warm and dead.

In-Water Patient Immobilization

In flat water where you are able to stand safely, it is important that you know how to perform in-water immobilization. In general, the procedure mirrors the application of a long board, with the following modifications:

- **Phase One: In-Water Spinal Immobilization**
    1. Apply the head-splint technique. (There are other techniques, but they do not work as well because of the use of PFDs by the rescuers.)
    2. Approach the patient from the side.
    3. Move the patient's arms over the head.

4. Use the patient's arms as a "splint" to hold the head in place.
5. If the patient was found face down, perform steps 1–4, then rotate the patient toward the rescuer in a face-up position.
6. Ensure an open airway.
7. Maintain this position until a cervical collar is applied.

- **Phase Two: Rigid Cervical Collar Application**
  1. A second rescuer determines the proper collar size.
  2. This second rescuer then holds the open collar under the victim's neck.
  3. The primary rescuer maintains immobilization and the patient's airway.
  4. The second rescuer brings the collar up to the back of the patient's neck. The primary rescuer allows the second rescuer to bring the collar around the patient's neck and secure the fastener on the collar while the primary rescuer maintains the airway.
  5. The second rescuer secures the patient's hands at the waist.

- **Phase Three: Back Boarding and Extrication from the Water**
  1. Secure the necessary personnel—two rescuers in the water and additional rescuers at the water's edge—and the correct equipment. It is strongly urged that rescuers use a floating backboard for water rescue.
  2. Submerge the board under the patient's waist.
  3. Never lift the patient to the board. Instead, allow the board to float up to the patient. (If the board does not float, lift it gently to the patient.)
  4. Secure the patient with straps, cravats, or other devices.
  5. Move the patient to an extrication point along the shore or boat.
  6. Always extricate the patient head first so that the body weight does not compress possible spinal trauma.
  7. If possible, avoid extrication of the patient through surf, as the board could capsize and dump the patient back into the water. Consider using bystanders who can swim as a breakwall behind the patient.
  8. Maintain airway management during extrication.

HAZARDOUS ATMOSPHERE RESCUES

Confined-space rescues present any number of potentially fatal threats, but one of the most serious is an oxygen-deficient environment. At first glance, most confined spaces appear relatively safe. Here is where rescue awareness comes in. Nearly 60 percent of all fatalities associated with confined spaces are untrained people attempting to rescue a victim.

According to the Workers' Compensation Board of B.C. Occupational Health and Safety Regulation 9.1, a confined space is as an enclosed area with limited or restricted access that is not designed or intended for human occupancy. Transport Canada notes that the main hazards encountered in confined spaces come from "the presence of hazardous gases, vapours, fumes, dusts or the creation of an oxygen-deficient or oxygen-rich atmosphere." In other words, confined spaces are not safe for people to enter for any sustained period of time. Examples of confined spaces are transport or storage tanks, grain bins and silos, wells and cisterns, manholes and pumping stations, drainage culverts, pits, hoppers, underground vaults, and mine or cave shafts (Figures 3-20A–B).

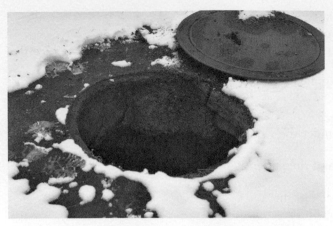

FIGURE 3-20A   Manholes provide access to underground utility vaults. The vault may have a limited or hazardous atmosphere and may offer the potential for entrapment.

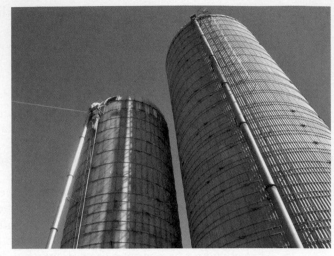

FIGURE 3-20B   Rescuers should never be permitted to enter confined spaces, such as silos, unless they have training, equipment, and experience in this environment.

Confined-space rescues carry a high risk of oxygen deficiency.

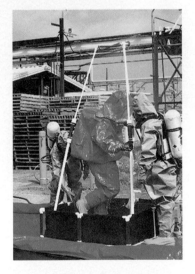

FIGURE 3-21   Rescuers exposed to toxic or hazardous materials will need to go through decontamination.

It only takes one spark to trigger an explosion. Be careful of all potential sources of electricity.

CONFINED-SPACE HAZARDS

Some of the most common risks in confined-space rescues include:

- *Oxygen-deficient atmospheres.* Untrained rescuers may not readily think of oxygen deficiency. It simply is not a "visible" threat. Special entry teams know otherwise. Before going into a confined space, they monitor the atmosphere to determine oxygen concentration, levels of hydrogen sulphide, explosive limits, flammable atmosphere, or toxic contaminants. They are also aware that increases in oxygen content for any reasons—such as a gust of wind—can give atmospheric monitoring meters a false reading.

- *Toxic or explosive chemicals.* Many chemicals found in confined spaces can be toxic, especially if inhaled (Figure 3-21). Some of the poisonous fumes contain gases that displace oxygen in the red blood cells. Other chemicals are highly explosive. Dangerous chemical gases commonly found in confined spaces include hydrogen sulphide (H_2S), carbon dioxide (CO_2), carbon monoxide (CO), exceptionally low or high oxygen concentrations, chlorine (Cl_2), ammonia (NH_3), and nitrogen dioxide (NO_2).

- *Engulfment.* Some confined spaces contain grain, coal, sand, or other substances that can bury a patient or rescuer. Dust from these materials can also create a highly explosive atmosphere.

- *Machinery entrapment.* Confined spaces come with all sorts of machinery or equipment that can entrap a person, including augers or screws.

- *Electricity.* Confined spaces often contain electric-powered equipment. In addition to the risk of shock or electrocution, these machines potentially contain stored energy. To ensure safe entry, it may first be necessary to blank out all power into the site. Second, stored energy should be dissipated, following lock out/tag out procedures. Third, the space may need to be ventilated to ensure against oxygen deficiency or explosive dust particles. Remember: It takes only one spark to trigger an explosion.

- *Structural concerns.* Structure supports and shapes further complicate confined-space rescues. Some confined spaces have "I" beams that can cause injury due to limited light and height. Other confined spaces have noncylindrical shapes that present difficult extrication problems. Confined spaces can be shaped in the form Ls, Ts, Xs, and any combination thereof. Because of limited access, rescuers may find it difficult or even impossible to use standard SCBA. They may have to resort to supplied air breathing apparatus—that is, oxygen lines. They may also need to be lowered into the space with a full-body harness or other system to make retrieval easier in case something goes wrong.

CONFINED-SPACE PROTECTIONS IN THE WORKPLACE

Fortunately, provincial, territorial, and federal laws require most industries to develop a confined-space rescue program. This means that employers must provide a training program for all employees who work in or around confined spaces. These employees may be called on to perform on-site rescues and may indeed be an important part of the emergency response.

Many provincial and territorial occupational health and safety regulations require a permit process before workers may enter a confined space, such as a trench. In addition, most industries must fulfill strict requirements, such as ongoing atmospheric monitoring, posted warnings, and worksite permits with detailed data on hazard management. The area must be made safe, or workers must don PPE. Retrieval devices must also be in place whenever workers enter the spaces. Nonpermitted sites are the most likely locations for emergencies because of inadequate atmospheric monitoring.

The types of confined-space emergencies most commonly encountered in the workplace include falls, medical emergencies (often hazmat-related), oxygen deficiencies or asphyxia, explosions, and entrapment. You should never allow untrained rescuers into a confined space. You will almost always summon outside specialized agencies for support.

CAVE-INS AND STRUCTURAL COLLAPSES

Collapsed trenches or cave-ins can occur almost anywhere. In fact, most trench collapses occur in trenches less than 4.5 m deep and 2 m wide, particularly in trenches that do not comply with safety regulations. To understand the medical magnitude of a collapsed trench, consider these facts. A typical cubic foot of soil weighs 45 kg. As a result, just two cubic feet of soil on the chest or back can weigh between 320 and 455 kg. People are literally buried alive. Unless uncovered quickly, they suffer death by asphyxiation.

Reasons for Collapses and Cave-Ins

Trenches collapse or cave in for a number of reasons:

- Contractors disregard safety regulations. (Federal law requires either shoring or a trench box for excavations deeper than 1.5 m.)
- The lip of one or both sides of the trench caves in.
- The wall shears away or falls in entirely.
- The "spoil pile," or removed dirt, is placed too close to the edge.
- Water seepage, ground vibrations, intersecting trenches, or previously disturbed soil weaken the structural integrity.

Rescue from Trenches and Cave-Ins

If a collapsed trench or cave-in has caused a burial, a secondary collapse is likely.

If a collapse has caused a burial, a secondary collapse is likely. Therefore, your initial actions should be geared toward safety. Secure the scene, establish command, secure a perimeter, and immediately summon a team specializing in trench rescue. Meanwhile, do not allow entry in the area surrounding the trench or cave-in. Safe access can take place only when proper shoring is in place.

HIGHWAY OPERATIONS AND VEHICLE RESCUES

As you know, the most common rescue situations for EMS personnel involve motor vehicle collisions. These generally go through the phases covered earlier. However, certain modifications must be made to meet the special hazards associated with traffic control and the extrication from wrecked vehicles.

HAZARDS IN HIGHWAY OPERATIONS

To prepare for highway rescues, you must assess the scene, identify all hazards, and ensure scene safety. With highway operations, this means reducing traffic-related hazards and identifying hazards related to the vehicle crash itself.

Traffic Hazards

Traffic flow is the largest single hazard associated with EMS highway operations.

Traffic flow is the largest single hazard associated with EMS highway operations. You may have to respond to incidents on roads with limited access and to incidents on highways with unlimited access. In either situation, you will need to work closely with police to avoid unnecessary congestion and further collisions. Remember: Backups impede the flow both to and from the scene.

An even bigger personal danger results from the risk of vehicles hitting EMS apparatus or personnel. Studies have shown that drivers who are tired, drunk, or drugged actually drive right into the emergency lights. Spectators can worsen the situation by getting out of their cars to watch or even "help."

At this point in your career, you probably already know some of the things you can do to reduce traffic hazards. Here are a few tried-and-tested techniques:

Do not rely solely on ambulance lights to warn traffic away.

- *Staging.* Staging is critical at any MCI but has an added importance on limited-access highways. Always consider staging emergency vehicles away from the scene and have command bring the vehicles in whenever there is an appropriate place or assignment for the crews. The staging area should be within a minute or two of the scene, ideally in a large parking area. Some situations simply cannot accommodate the entire response at once.

- *Positioning of apparatus.* When apparatus does arrive, ensure that it causes the minimum reduction of traffic flow. As much as possible, position apparatus to protect the scene. The ambulance loading area should NOT be directly exposed to traffic. Also, DO NOT rely solely on ambulance lights to warn traffic away. These lights are often obstructed when paramedics open the doors for loading.

- *Emergency lighting.* Use only a minimum of warning lights to alert traffic of a hazard and to define the actual size of your vehicle. Too many lights can confuse or blind drivers, causing yet other accidents. Experts strongly advise that you turn off all headlights when parked at the scene and rely instead on amber scene lighting.

- *Redirection of traffic.* Be sure traffic cones and flares are placed early in the incident. If the police are not already on the scene, this is your responsibility. As a first on the scene, you must redirect traffic away from the collision and away from all emergency workers. In other words, you need to create a safety zone. Make sure that you do not place lighted flares too near any sources of fuel or brush, otherwise you risk an explosion or fire. Once you light the flares, allow them to burn out. *Do not* try to extinguish them. Attempting to pick up a flare can cause a very severe thermal burn.

- *High visibility.* Make sure all rescuers are dressed in highly visible clothing. Don a brightly coloured turnout coat or vest with reflective tape. You can apply the tape at the scene.

Other Hazards

Other, nontraffic hazards at highway operations include the following:

- *Fire and fuel.* Spilled fuel increases the chances of fire. Be very careful whenever you smell or see pools of liquid at a collision. Bystanders who are smoking can cause a bigger problem than the original crash if they flick lighted ashes into a fuel leak. *Do not* drive your emergency vehicle over a fuel spill—or worse yet, park on one! Remember that all automobiles manufactured since the 1970s have catalytic converters. They run at a temperature of around 650°C—hot enough to heat fuel to the point of ignition. Be especially careful when a vehicle has gone off the road into dry grass or brush. The debris can be just as dangerous as spilled fuel, especially when brought into contact with a blazing hot catalytic converter.

> *Bystanders who are smoking can cause a bigger problem than the original crash if they flick ashes into a fuel leak.*

- *Alternative fuel systems.* Be equally cautious of vehicles powered by alternative fuel systems. High-pressure tanks, especially if filled with natural gas, are extremely volatile. Even vehicles powered by electricity can be dangerous. The storage cells possess the energy to spark, flash, and more.

- *Sharp objects.* Automobile collisions mean lots of sharp objects— glass, metal, plastic, or fibreglass. Be sure to wear appropriate protective gear, such as heavy leather gloves and eyewear.

- *Electric power.* Contact with downed power lines (Figure 3-22) or underground electrical feeds can be lethal. If a vehicle is in contact with electrical lines, consider it to be "charged," and call the power company immediately. In most newer communities, electric lines run underground. However, a vehicle can still run onto a transformer or an electric feed box. Make sure you look under the car and all around it during your scene assessment. *Do not* touch a vehicle until you have ruled out all electrical hazards.

> *Do not touch a vehicle until you have ruled out all electrical hazards.*

- *Energy-absorbing bumpers.* The bumpers on many vehicles come with pistons and are designed to withstand a slow-speed collision. Sometimes, these bumpers become "loaded" in the crushed position. When exposed to fire or even just tapped by rescue workers, the pistons can suddenly unload their stored energy. Some bumpers have been thrown 30 m from the vehicle when they unload. Therefore, you must examine bumpers for loading. Stay away from a loaded bumper unless you are specially trained to deal with this hazard.

- *Supplemental restraint systems (SRS)/airbags.* Airbags also have the potential to release stored energy. If they have not deployed during

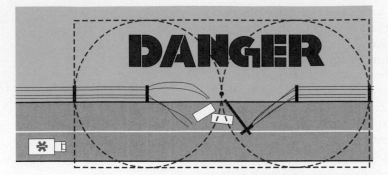

Downed Lines

In accidents involving downed electrical wires and damaged utility poles, the danger zone should extend beyond each intact pole for a full span and to the sides for the distance that the severed wires can reach. Stay out of the danger zone until the utility company has deactivated the wires or until trained rescuers have moved and anchored them.

FIGURE 3-22　Establish a danger zone in motor vehicle collisions involving electrical hazards.

the collision, they may do so during an extrication. These devices must be deactivated prior to disentanglement. Auto manufacturers can provide information about power removal or power dissipation for their particular brand. Also, keep in mind that many new-model vehicles come equipped with side impact bags.

- *Hazardous cargoes.* An incredible amount of hazardous materials travel across the highways of North America. For your personal safety, suspect hazmat at any scene involving commercial vehicles.

- *Rolling vehicles.* As you already know, you must assess the position of a vehicle. You might arrive on the scene and see the vehicle on all four wheels and consider it stable. Then, a crew member jumps into the rear to stabilize the patient's neck manually. Suddenly, the vehicle starts rolling down the street. This situation is not only embarrassing, it is dangerous! So, always check that the transmission is on park. Make sure the parking brake is on, the ignition is off, and any key rings with remote ignition starters are removed.

- *Unstable vehicles.* Motor vehicles can land in all kinds of unstable positions. They can roll onto the side or roof. They can stop on an incline or on unstable terrain. They can be suspended over a cliff or river. They can come to rest on a patch of ice or an on-site spill or leak. In such situations, you need to request the necessary stabilization crew or equipment. You should also know how to apply proper techniques for temporary stabilization, using ropes, chocks, or a come-along. Under no circumstances should you allow rescuers to access the patient until the vehicle is stabilized.

> *For your personal safety, suspect hazmat at any scene involving commercial vehicles.*

AUTO ANATOMY

You must know some basics of automobile construction or "anatomy." Obviously, vehicles can differ greatly, both in terms of manufacture and design. However, most recent automobiles have certain features in common that can guide you in simple access situations.

Basic Constructions

Vehicles can have either a unibody or a frame construction. Most automobiles today have a unibody design, while older vehicles and light-weight trucks have a frame construction. For unibody vehicles to maintain their integrity, all the following features must remain intact: roof posts, floor, firewall, truck support, and windshield.

Both types of construction have roof supports. The support posts are lettered from front to back. The first post, which supports the roof at the windshield, is called the "A" post. The next post is the "B" post. The third post is the "C" post. Station wagons have an additional rear "D" post. If you remove the plastic moulding on the posts, the remaining steel can be easily cut with a hacksaw. Application of power steering fluid helps reduce the heat produced by cutting. Remember that cutting a post will interrupt the unibody vehicle's construction.

Firewall and Engine Compartment

The firewall separates the engine and occupant compartments. Frequently, the firewall can collapse on a patient's legs. Sometimes, a patient's feet may go through the firewall. Movement on other parts of the vehicle, such as cutting a rocker panel or roof support post, can place additional pressure on the feet. The engine compartment usually contains the battery. This can cause a fire hazard, and so many rescue teams cut the battery cables. Before disconnecting the power, it is a good idea to move back power seats and lower power windows.

Glass

Vehicles have two types of glass: safety glass and tempered glass. Safety glass is made from three layers of fused materials: glass–plastic laminate–glass. It is found in windshields and designed to stay intact when shattered or broken. However, safety glass can still produce glass dust or fracture into long shards. These materials can easily get into a patient's eyes, nose, or mouth or create cuts. Therefore, be sure to cover a patient whenever you remove this type of glass.

Tempered glass has high tensile strength. However, it does not stay intact when shattered or broken. It fractures into many small beads of glass, all of which can cause injuries and cuts.

Doors

The doors of most newer vehicles contain a reinforcing bar to protect the occupant in side-impact collisions. They also have a case-hardened steel "Nader" pin. Named after consumer advocate Ralph Nader, these pins help keep the doors from blowing open and ejecting the occupants. If the Nader pin has been engaged, it will be difficult to pry open the door. You must first disengage the latch or use hydraulic jaws.

Before attempting to assist a patient through a door, you should be trained in proper extrication techniques. In general, you should follow these steps:

- Try all four doors first—a door is the easiest means of access.
- Otherwise, gain access through the window farthest from the patient(s).
- Alternatively, use simple hand tools to peel back the outer sheet of metal on the door, exposing the lock mechanism. Unlock the lock and pry the cams from around the Nader pin. Then, pry out the door.

FIGURE 3-23 Modern extrication equipment is essential
for a fast, efficient rescue.

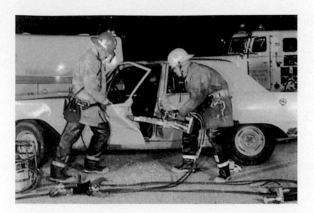

RESCUE STRATEGIES

In managing highway operations or vehicle rescues, you should use the following general strategies:

- *Initial scene assessment.* Establish command, call for appropriate
  backup, locate and triage the patients. Triage may be delayed until
  hazards are controlled.

- *Control hazards.* This topic has already been covered. But always
  remember this point: Traffic can be your worst enemy at a collision.

- *Assess the degree of entrapment and fastest means of extrication.*
  Try all doors. If they cannot be opened, decide whether it is
  advisable or necessary to break the glass. Although you may not
  have the training or responsibility to use extrication equipment, you
  should observe their use so that you know what technical skills are
  available should you need them (Figure 3-23). Be aware of the
  considerations and techniques for door removal, roof removal,
  dashboard or firewall rollup, and construction of a new door.

- *Establish circles of operation.* Set up two circles of operation early in
  the incident. The inner circle is the area where the actual rescue takes
  place. Limit the number of workers in this area to team members
  operating rescue tools or charged with actual patient care. If two
  different units must work in the inner circle—for example, a fire
  department crew and an EMS crew—you will need to maintain a
  good working balance between the crews to avoid "over-rescuing."
  The outer circle is where staging takes place. Hold all additional
  equipment and personnel in this area until they are assigned a duty.

- *Treatment, packaging, removal.* As a rule, the role of EMS
  personnel in vehicle stabilization and removal is that of patient
  care provider. Once specialized rescue personnel assure you that
  the vehicle is stable and the scene is safe to enter, you may
  approach the patient, initiate assessment, and administer
  emergency care. Patient care always precedes removal from the
  vehicle unless delay would endanger the life of the patient, EMS
  personnel, or others. Again, work with rescuers in any way
  possible to minimize risk, both to the patient and to on-scene
  personnel. You should be well-practised in the application of long
  spineboards for rapid removal of the patient through the doors or
  vertical extrication through removed roofs.

*Patient care always precedes
removal from the vehicle
unless delay would endanger
the life of the patient, EMS
personnel, or others.*

RESCUE SKILLS PRACTICE

Depending on local protocols, you should practise or observe the use of the various disentanglement or extrication skills commonly used with vehicle rescues, many of which have already been mentioned. Know how to gain access using hand tools through nondeformed doors, deformed doors, safety and tempered glass, trunks, and floors. Become familiar with the use of heavy hydraulic equipment employed by special rescue teams in your area, and take part in practice scenarios to build agency cooperation.

HAZARDOUS TERRAIN RESCUES

In recent years, outdoor activities—mountain, rock, and ice climbing, mountain biking, cross-country skiing, snowboarding, and hiking—have drawn more and more people into rugged areas. Inevitably, accidents happen in places that can be hard to reach. You do not have to live in the wilderness to take part in a hazardous terrain rescue. For example, a mountain biker can get injured on trails that run along power lines or a rock climber can get injured on an outcropping in a relatively populated area. Some climbers even scale buildings!

As a paramedic, you must know how to take part in rugged terrain rescues. At a minimum, you should know how to perform litter evacuations without causing additional injury to patients. Even more importantly, you should develop a "rescue awareness" so that you know when to call specialized teams and how to work with those teams once they arrive on the scene.

TYPES OF HAZARDOUS TERRAIN

In general, there are three types of hazardous terrain: steep slope or "low-angle" terrain, vertical or "high-angle" terrain, and flat terrain with obstructions. Low-angle terrains typically can be accessed by walking or **scrambling**—climbing over boulders or rocks using both hands and feet. Footing can be difficult, and it may be hazardous to carry a litter even with multiple rescuers. As a result, low-angle teams use ropes to counteract gravity and may set a rope to act as a hand line. Any error can result in a fall or tumble.

High-angle terrain usually involves a cliff, gorge, side of a building, or terrain so steep that hands must be used when scaling it. Crewmembers depend on rope or aerial apparatus for access and litter movement. Errors are likely to cause serious, life-threatening injuries or death.

Flat terrain with obstructions includes trails, paths, or creek beds. Obstructions can take many forms, such as downed trees, rocks, slippery leaves or pine needles, and **scree**—the loose pebbles or rock debris that can form on the slopes or bases of mountains. Although this is the least hazardous type of rugged terrain, it is still possible to slip while carrying a patient, causing injury.

PATIENT ACCESS IN HAZARDOUS TERRAIN

Unless you have been trained in high-angle or low-angle rescue, patient access and removal should be left to specialized teams. Even if you have the skills to perform the rescue, you will in all likelihood need additional resources to provide the necessary balance of technical and medical support for the patient.

High-Angle Rescues

High-angle, or vertical, rescuers must constantly contend with the effects of gravity. Any organization that could be assigned a vertical technical rescue must have

Develop the "rescue awareness" to know when to call specialized rescue teams and how to work with those teams when they arrive on the scene.

Content Review

THREE TYPES OF HAZARDOUS TERRAIN
Steep slope or "low-angle" terrain
Vertical or "high-angle" terrain
Flat terrain with obstructions

✱ **scrambling** climbing over rocks or downed trees on a steep trail without the aid of ropes. This can be especially dangerous when the surface is icy.

✱ **scree** loose pebbles or rock debris that can form on the slopes or bases of mountains; sometimes used to describe debris in sloping dry stream beds.

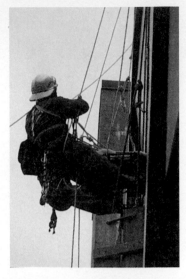

FIGURE 3-24A High-angle rescue is dangerous and difficult and should be deferred to those with special high-angle training and equipment.

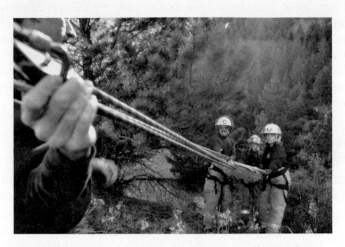

FIGURE 3-24B Low-angle situations are less difficult than high-angle situations. Many EMS agencies have trained their paramedics in the skills of low-angle rescue.

extensive training and top-of-the-line equipment (Figure 3-24A). Each member of a high-angle team must have complete competency in knot tying, use of ladders and ropes to ascend and descend a steep face, ability to rig a hauling system, and the skills for packaging a patient for evacuation by litter and rope.

Low-Angle Rescues

Many EMS systems have trained their paramedics in the skills of low-angle or "off-the-road" rescue. Like high-angle rescues, the rescuers require rope, harnesses, hardware, and the necessary safety systems (Figure 3-24B). Low-angle rescues may be up to 40 degrees, except if the face is overly smooth. Then a high-angle team will be better able to handle the more technical access and evacuation.

Each member of a low-angle crew must know how to assemble a hasty harness tied from two-inch tubular webbing (or don a climbing harness), rappel and ascend by rope, package a patient in a litter, and rig a simple hauling system to assist the litter team up the embankment. Teams must also know how to set up a hasty rope slide to assist with balance and footing on rough terrain. Although low-angle rescues involve less technical skill than high-angle rescues, they still require ongoing practice and proper equipment.

PATIENT PACKAGING FOR ROUGH TERRAIN

The Stokes basket stretcher is the standard litter for rough terrain evacuation (Figures 3-25A and 3-25B). It provides a rigid frame for patient protection and is easy to carry with an adequate number of personnel. Alternative spinal immobilizers can be used in a Stokes basket, such as a clamshell, backboard, and the KED, or the Sked®. As a last resort, the Stokes itself can be used as a spinal immobilizer.

Stokes baskets came in wire, tubular, and plastic styles. The older "military style" wire mesh Stokes will not accept a backboard. Newer models, however, offer several advantages, including greater strength, less expense, better air/water flow through the basket, and better flotation in water rescues.

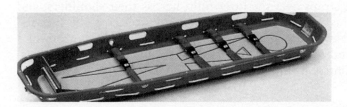

FIGURE 3-25A A basket stretcher.

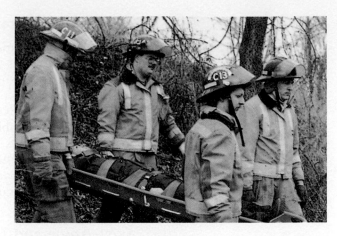

FIGURE 3-25B A basket stretcher is often used to carry patients over rough terrain.

Plastic basket stretchers are usually weaker than wire mesh types. They are often rated for only 136–275 kg. However, they tend to offer better patient protection. In general, Stokes baskets with plastic bottoms and steel frames are best. These versatile units can also be slid in snow when necessary.

Most Stokes baskets, regardless of their style, are not equipped with adequate restraints. As a result, they require additional strapping or lacing for rough terrain. A plastic litter shield can be used to protect the patient from dust and falling objects. When moving across flat terrain, lace the patient into the Stokes basket to limit movement. When using a Stokes basket for high-angle or low-angle evacuation, take the following additional steps:

- Apply a harness to the patient.
- Apply leg stirrups to the patient.
- Secure the patient to a litter to prevent movement.
- Tie the tail of one litter line to the patient's harness.
- Use a helmet or litter shield to protect the patient.
- Administer fluids (IV or orally).
- Allow accessibility for taking BP, performing suction, and assessing distal perfusion.
- Ensure adequate padding—a crucial consideration.
- Consider use of a patient heating/cooling system, especially for prolonged evacuations.
- Provide for an airway clearing system via a gravity "tip line" if necessary.

PATIENT REMOVAL FROM HAZARDOUS TERRAIN

When removing the patient from a hazardous terrain, a nontechnical evacuation is usually faster. In other words, when possible, walk the patient out. Remember: Carrying a patient on a litter can be a strenuous task even under ideal conditions. The rougher the terrain, the more demanding is the litter-carry.

Carrying a patient on a litter over flat ground can be a strenuous task even under ideal conditions.

Flat Rough Terrain

When removing a patient in a litter from a flat rough terrain, make sure you have enough litter carriers to "leapfrog" ahead of each other to save time and to rotate rescuers. An adequate number of litter bearers would be two or three teams of six. Litter bearers of a team should be approximately the same height.

Several devices exist to ease the difficulty of a litter-carry. For example, litter bearers can run webbing straps over the litter rails, across their shoulders, and into their free hands. This will help distribute the weight across the bearers' backs. Another helpful device is the litter wheel. It attaches to the bottom of a Stokes basket frame and takes most of the weight of the litter. Bearers must keep the litter balanced and control its motion.

Low-Angle and High-Angle Evacuation

Before beginning patient removal, rescuers must ensure that all anchors are secure. They must check their own safety equipment and recheck patient packaging. They must also have the necessary lowering and hauling systems in place, again doing the recommended safety checks.

Materials, especially ropes, should never be used if there is any question of their safety. If you see a frayed rope or any stressed or damaged equipment, do not hesitate to point it out to the rescuers in a polite but professional manner. Also, because hauling sometimes requires many "helpers," you may be asked to assist. Make sure you understand all directions given by the rescuers.

Some high-angle units, especially of fire departments, make use of aerial apparatus, such as tower-ladders or bucket trucks, to assist in the removal of a patient in a Stokes basket. These units are usually employed in structural environments but can be adapted to hazardous terrain if there is room for a truck.

When using aerial apparatus, it is necessary to provide a litter relay during movement to a bucket. Litters, of course, must then be correctly attached to the bucket. Use of aerial ladders can be difficult because the upper sections are usually not wide enough to slot the litter. The litter must always be properly belayed if being slid down the ladder. Finally, ladders or other aerial apparatus should *not* be used as a crane to move a litter. They are neither designed nor rated for this work. Serious stress can cause accidents resulting in patient death.

Use of Helicopters

Helicopters can be useful in hazardous terrain rescues, especially when hospitals lie at a distant location. Be aware of the differences in mission, crew training, and capabilities of helicopters that do air medical care versus helicopters that do rescue. You should be familiar with the advantages, disadvantages, and local restrictions for each of the following practices or techniques *before* you summon a helicopter from the field:

- Boarding and deboarding practices
- Restrictions on carrying non-crewmembers
- Use of cable winches for rescues
- Weight restrictions
- Restrictions on hovering rescues
- Use and practice of one-skids and toe-ins
- Use of **short hauls** or sling loads of equipment or personnel, as opposed to the more dangerous rappel-based rescues

Evacuation is a team effort.

Ladders or other aerial apparatus should not be used as a crane to move a litter.

Be aware of the differences in mission, crew training, and capabilities of helicopters that do air medical care versus helicopters that do rescue.

✱ short haul a helicopter extrication technique in which a person is attached to a rope that is, in turn, attached to a helicopter. The aircraft lifts off with the person attached to it. Obviously, this means of evacuation requires highly specialized skills.

Packaging and Evacuation Practice

Depending on local protocols, you should practise the packaging and evacuation techniques expected of EMS personnel in your region. You should familiarize yourself with the specific types of basket stretchers and litters available to your unit and the proper packaging, immobilization, and restraint techniques for use with each type. Also, practise with other equipment used for rough-terrain rescues, including the Sked® and appropriate half-spine devices.

Practise or observe the skills required for low-angle and high-angle rescues. When possible, take part in exercises with the rescue units that you would summon to perform these evacuations. By fully understanding the capabilities of the rescue response teams in your area, you will circumvent any "turf" issues and know how to work together when a multijurisdictional event occurs.

EXTENDED CARE ASSESSMENT AND ENVIRONMENTAL ISSUES

Environmental emergencies can present their own special challenges. For rescue operations, at least some personnel should have formal training in managing patients whose injuries have been aggravated by prolonged lack of treatment, often under extreme conditions. If SOPs do not already exist, procedures adopted from wilderness medical research will prove useful. Position papers written by the Wilderness Medical Society or the National Association for Search and Rescue can serve as guidelines for protocols.

Regardless of the source, you will discover that many protocols for extended care vary substantially from standard EMS procedures. If your agency anticipates involvement in some of the rescue situations described in this chapter, you should consider protocols that at least address the following areas:

- Long-term hydration management
- Repositioning of dislocations
- Cleansing and care of wounds
- Removal of impaled objects
- Nonpharmacological pain management—utilizing proper splinting, distracting the patient by talking or asking questions, scratching or creating sensory stimuli when doing painful procedures
- Pharmacological pain management—utilizing pharmacological agents with isolated trauma, such as amputation or fracture, or with multiple trauma, such as crushing or pinning of more than an extremity
- Assessment and care of head and spinal injuries
- Management of hypothermia or hyperthermia
- Termination of CPR
- Treatment of crush injuries and compartment syndromes.

A number of environmental issues can affect your assessment during a rescue situation. Some of the most important issues include the following:

- *Weather or temperature extremes.* Extreme weather or temperature conditions increase the risk of patient hypothermia or hyperthermia. These conditions also make it difficult or impossible to expose the patient completely for full assessment and treatment.
- *Limited patient access.* Parts of the patient may not be accessible for examination. Cramped spaces and low lighting conditions also make

assessment difficult. For this reason, it is important that you carry a headlamp with extended battery packs.

- *Difficulty transporting street equipment.* Hazardous terrain often makes it difficult to transport typical street equipment to the patient. As a result, equipment usually must be downsized. Often, you will utilize a backpack to keep your hands free for carrying. Essential equipment includes:
  - *Airway*—oral and nasal airways, manual suction, intubation equipment
  - *Breathing*—thoracic decompression equipment, small oxygen tank or regulator, masks or cannulas, pocket mask or bag-valve mask (BVM)
  - *Circulation*—bandages or dressings, triangular bandages, occlusive dressings, IV administration equipment, BP cuff, and stethoscope
  - *Disability*—extrication collars
  - *Expose*—scissors
  - *Miscellaneous*—headlamp/flashlight, space blanket, padded aluminum splint (SAM® splint), PPE (leather gloves, latex gloves, eye shields)

- *Cumbersome PPE.* Necessary, but cumbersome, PPE can restrict rescuer mobility. In certain instances, some of the PPE might be removed to perform care steps. For example, heavy outer gloves might be taken off during administration of an IV but reapplied as soon as possible.

- *Patient exposure.* Patients should be quickly covered to ensure thermal protection. During the extrication, place hard protection, such as a spine board, and take steps to prevent patient contact with sharp objects or debris. For example, use an aluminized blanket to protect against glass shards.

- *Use of ALS skills.* Good BLS skills are mandatory in hazardous terrains, but limit ALS skills to those that are really essential. More wires and tubing complicate the extrication process. Continuous oxygenation, definitive airway control, and volume replacement may be essential. However, rescuers can't carry lots of oxygen tanks into rugged terrains. As a result, you may have to use your tank at a slower flow rate so that it will last longer.

- *Patient monitoring.* Hazardous terrain can alter your use of monitoring equipment. In high-noise areas, for example, you may have to take BP by palpation or use a compact pulse oximetry unit. An ECG monitor can be cumbersome during extrication and more difficult to use than in a street situation.

- *Improvisation.* Improvisation is common in rescue situations. To minimize the amount of equipment carried over hazardous terrain, you may want to consider such techniques as tying upper extremity fractures to the torso or tying lower extremity fractures to the uninjured leg. Lightweight SAM® splints can be very useful in the backwoods and should be part of your downsized medical gear. Whatever you do, continue talking to the patient, and explain exactly what is happening. The patient is already frightened by the entrapment. Don't make the situation worse by making the patient feel even more out of control.

Good BLS skills are mandatory in hazardous terrains, but limit ALS skills to those that are really needed. Do not complicate any already complicated operation.

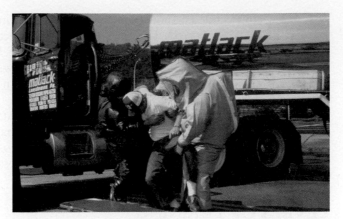

FIGURE 3-26 A hazardous materials emergency can involve any of countless substances and occur in many situations. Warning placards on a truck should immediately alert you to the possible need of a "hazmat" team.

Part 4: Hazardous Materials Incidents

Hazardous materials (hazmats) are all around us. Every day, hazardous materials are transported throughout Canada by truck, pipeline, railroad, tanker, aircraft, and ship (see Figure 3-26). You will learn about some hazardous materials when you study toxicology and environmental emergencies. This chapter deals with hazardous materials that are spilled or released because of an accident, equipment failure, human error, or intentional violation of laws and regulations.

The U.S. Department of Transport (DOT) defines a hazardous material as "any substance which may pose an unreasonable risk to health and safety of operating or emergency personnel, the public, and/or the environment if not properly controlled during handling, storage, manufacture, processing, packaging, use, disposal, or transportation."

ROLE OF THE PARAMEDIC

Even a small-scale hazardous material incident is almost always a multijurisdictional event. All EMS personnel should be trained in how to respond to hazmat incidents and how to interact with other agencies that might respond. Traditionally, paramedics do not perform containment and control functions at a hazmat response. As first on the scene, they may assess the incident, assess the toxicological risk, and activate the incident management system. They will also be called on to evaluate decontamination methods, treatment and transport of exposed patients, and medical monitoring of hazmat teams.

REQUIREMENTS AND STANDARDS

Transport Canada, through the Transportation of Dangerous Good Directorate, developed the Transport of Dangerous Goods Regulations, which establish safety requirements for the transport of hazardous materials in Canada. All provinces and territories have adopted these regulations. Federal, provincial, and territorial legislations regulate an extensive list of dangerous products, substances, and organisms. CANUTEC (the Canadian Transport Emergency Centre), working with the U.S. Department of Transportation and the Secretariat of Communications and Transportation of Mexico, has developed the *Emergency Response Guidebook*. This guide is a primary resource for information on haz-

* **hazardous material (hazmat)** any substance that causes adverse health effects on exposure to humans.

Even a small-scale hazmat incident almost always turns into a multijurisdictional event, thus triggering use of the IMS.

Content Review

EMS HAZMAT EMERGENCY MEDICAL RESPONDER TASKS

Assess incident.
Assess toxicological risk.
Activate the IMS.
Establish command.

ards and recommended responses to hazardous goods incidents. Many Canadian hazmat groups refer to the U.S. National Fire Protection Association (NFPA) publication 473, *Standard for Competencies for EMS Personnel Responding to Hazardous Materials Incidents*. This standard, along with two other NPFA standards for hazmat response, deals with the training standards for EMS personnel assigned to hazmat incidents.

Provincial and territorial agencies may also regulate responses to hazardous materials incidents. For instance, the B.C. Occupational Health and Safety Regulations require written emergency plans for hazardous materials incidents that include an inventory of hazardous materials, risk assessment, evacuation procedures, cleanup and reentry procedures, and training.

Levels of Training

The above documents set forth three levels of training appropriate to EMS response at hazmat incidents—Awareness Level, EMS Level 1, and EMS Level 2. The Awareness Level applies to responders who may arrive first at a scene and discover a toxic substance. Training focuses on recognition of hazmat incidents, basic hazmat identification techniques, and individual protection from involvement in the incident. All EMS personnel, as well as police officers and firefighters, need to be trained to the Awareness Level.

EMS Level 1 training, or the "operations level," is required for those who may perform patient care in the cold zone on patients who do *not* present a significant risk of secondary contamination. This training focuses on hazard assessment, patient assessment, and patient care for previously contaminated patients. EMS Level 2 training, or the "technician level," is required for those who may perform patient care in the warm zone on patients who still present a significant risk of secondary contamination. This training focuses on personal protection, decontamination procedures, and treatment for patients who are beginning or undergoing decontamination.

The level of training required for each individual depends on their role in the hazmat response system. All systems require some individuals trained in both the EMS Level 1 and Level 2 standards. In this way, patient care can begin during decontamination and continue after the patient has been cleaned of contaminants.

INCIDENT ASSESSMENT

Assessing a hazardous materials incident is a very difficult task. You often receive inaccurate or incomplete information, and events tend to develop very quickly. As already indicated, you can also expect a number of agencies to be involved, and you should practise the incident management system regularly with the other agencies that typically respond to a hazmat call.

IMS and Hazmat Emergencies

You should be prepared for the special circumstances surrounding most hazmat emergencies. Some incidents, for example, will require immediate evacuation of patients from a contaminated area. Other incidents will have ambulatory contaminated patients who seek out EMS personnel as soon as you arrive on the scene. Never compromise scene safety during the early phase of a hazmat operation. Otherwise, you risk becoming a contaminated patient yourself.

Quickly determine whether the hazmat emergency is an open or a closed incident—that is, whether it has the potential to generate more patients. As you learned regarding the IMS system, the answer to this question will determine the resources that you request, how you stage them, and how you deploy personnel.

Priorities for a hazmat incident are the same as for any other major incident: life safety, incident stabilization, and property conservation.

Never compromise scene safety during the early phase of a hazmat operation. Otherwise, you risk becoming a patient yourself.

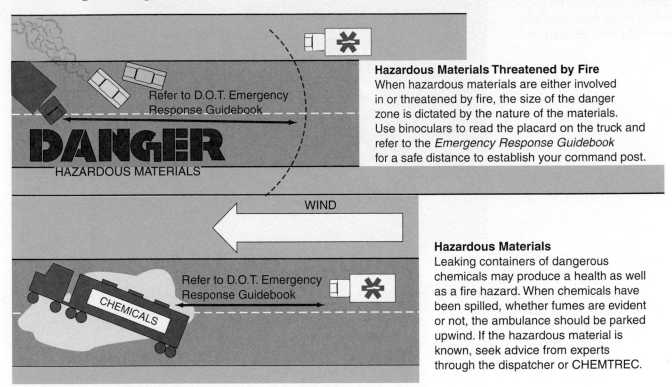

Refer to D.O.T. Emergency Response Guidebook

DANGER
HAZARDOUS MATERIALS

Hazardous Materials Threatened by Fire
When hazardous materials are either involved in or threatened by fire, the size of the danger zone is dictated by the nature of the materials. Use binoculars to read the placard on the truck and refer to the *Emergency Response Guidebook* for a safe distance to establish your command post.

WIND

Refer to D.O.T. Emergency Response Guidebook

CHEMICALS

Hazardous Materials
Leaking containers of dangerous chemicals may produce a health as well as a fire hazard. When chemicals have been spilled, whether fumes are evident or not, the ambulance should be parked upwind. If the hazardous material is known, seek advice from experts through the dispatcher or CHEMTREC.

FIGURE 3-27   Transportation incidents may involve hazardous materials.

In reaching your decision, remember that some chemicals have delayed effects. Triage must be ongoing, as patient conditions can change rapidly.

Finally, keep in mind that the best site for deploying resources will be uphill and upwind. This will help prevent contamination from ground-based liquids, high vapour density gases, runoff water, and vapour clouds (Figure 3-27).

Basic IMS at a hazmat incident will require a command post, a staging area, and a decontamination corridor. Depending on the event, the incident commander may also establish separate areas—such as treatment areas and personnel staging areas—to prevent unnecessary exposure to contamination. A backup plan for areas of operations must be determined early in the event. For example, what would you do if the wind direction suddenly shifted and a cloud of chlorine gas headed toward your staging area?

INCIDENT AWARENESS

Virtually, every emergency site—residential, business, or highway—has the potential for hazardous materials. For example, most households keep ammonia and liquid bleach in the kitchen or laundry. When combined, these substances produce a toxic gas. Homes with kerosene heaters or blocked flues can be filled with carbon monoxide. Always keep the possibility of dangerous substances in mind when you approach the scene. Binoculars can help you survey many scenes from a safe distance (Figure 3-28).

One of the most critical aspects of any hazmat response is the simple awareness that a dangerous substance is present.

Transport

Any transport—automobile, truck, or railroad—accident should raise a suspicion of hazardous materials. Maintain a high degree of hazmat awareness when-

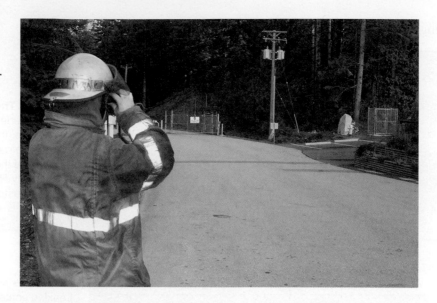

FIGURE 3-28 Don't take any chances. Use binoculars to make a visual inspection of a potentially hazardous situation.

Do not rule out the presence of a hazmat at an MVC just because you do not see a warning placard.

✱ warning placard diamond-shaped graphic placed on vehicles to indicate hazard classification.

✱ weapons of mass destruction (WMD) variety of chemical, biological, nuclear, or other devices used by terrorists to strike at government or high-profile targets, designed to create a maximum number of casualties.

Content Review

POTENTIAL TERRORIST TARGETS

Public buildings
Multinational headquarters
Shopping centres
Workplaces
Sites of assembly

ever you are summoned to collisions involving commercial vehicles, pest control vehicles, tanker trucks, tractor-trailers, or cars powered by alternative fuels. Do not rule out hazardous materials just because you do not see a **warning placard.** Hospitals and laboratories, for example, routinely and legally transport medical radioactive isotopes in unmarked passenger cars. You might look in the back seat and see a container with a label indicating radioactive contents. Railroad accidents merit special attention. A railroad tank car can carry up to 136 000 L of material, and there may be several tank cars hitched together. Fortunately, railroads run along fixed lines, which means you can plan your response.

Fixed Facilities

Hazmat incidents can also take place at fixed facilities. Chemical plants and all manufacturing operations have tanks, storage vessels, and pipelines used to transport products or wastes. Additional fixed sites with possible hazardous materials include warehouses, hardware or agricultural stores, water treatment centres, and loading docks. A farm or ranch may have hazardous materials stored in silos, barns, greenhouses, and other locations. Finally, remember that pipelines can be damaged by earthquakes, construction crew, or, if above ground, vehicle crashes. A ruptured gas or oil line can spell disaster, especially if ignited.

Terrorism

Terrorists can also create hazmat incidents, using a variety of chemical, biological, nuclear, or other devices to strike at government or high-profile targets. These **weapons of mass destruction (WMD)** can be manufactured from materials as simple as those found on most farms, as in the Oklahoma City bombing in 1993, or can be as unexpected as the use of hijacked commercial airliners to attack the World Trade Center and the Pentagon in 2001, with the concomitant release of jet fuel and other substances.

Terrorists usually select their targets by activity, particularly government or industrial, and by the number of people present. Potential targets include public buildings, multinational headquarters, shopping centres, workplaces, and sites of assembly, such as arenas, stadiums, and transport centres, or places of worship. All these locations should be identified in any mass-casualty or disaster plan for your community.

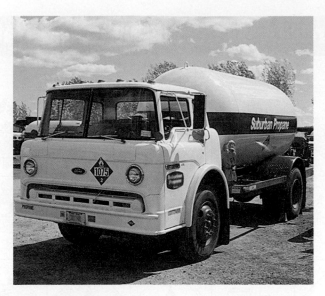

FIGURE 3-29 Vehicles carrying hazardous materials are required to display placards indicating the nature of their contents. You should regularly review the symbols, colour codes, and hazard class numbers so that you can identify dangerous materials.

In responding to a suspected terrorist incident, look for clues. Patients in a closed environment, such as a subway or an office building, will exhibit similar symptoms if they have been exposed to a chemical or biological WMD. In the case of an explosion, remember that a secondary device may exist. Take every precaution not to fall victim to a terrorist attack yourself. Make full use of the Incident Management System and all specialized systems.

At terrorist incidents, remember that a secondary device may be present.

RECOGNITION OF HAZARDS

To aid in the visual recognition of hazardous materials, two simple systems have been developed. CANUTEC, the American DOT, and Mexico have implemented placards to identify dangerous substances in transit, while the National Fire Protection Association (NFPA) has devised a system for fixed facilities.

Placard Classifications

Many vehicles are required by law to carry diamond-shaped placards (Figure 3-29) indicating hazmat classification through a colour code and hazard-class number. Some also carry a four-digit **UN number** specific to the chemical. Placards also use symbols to indicate hazard types. For example, a flame symbol indicates a flammable substance, a ball-on-fire symbol indicates an oxidizer, a propeller symbol indicates a radioactive substance, and a skull-and-crossbones symbol indicates a poisonous substance.

Combined, these colours, numbers, and symbols help you recognize the specific nature of the hazardous material. For instance, a red placard with the number 2 and a flame symbol means that the vehicle is carrying a flammable gas. Over time, you will become more familiar with these and other important symbols, such as a "W" with a line through it, which means "reacts with water."

Keep in mind the several shortcomings of the placard system. Although some substances need to be placarded in all quantities, others need to be placarded only if they are transported in large quantities. This means that there may be hazardous materials on board a truck that fall below the quantity required for placarding. Also, the "Dangerous" placard means that there are two or more substances on board between 455 and 2272 kg total weight. However, the generic placard tells you nothing about the nature of the materials. Finally, people can remove placards or fail to apply them in the first place.

✱ **UN number** a four-digit number specific to a given chemical; some UN numbers are assigned to a group of related chemicals, but with different characteristics, such as the UN 1203 designation for diesel fuel, gasohol, gasoline, motor fuels, motor spirits, and petrol. (The letters *UN* stand for "United Nations." Sometimes the letters *NA* for "North American" appear with or instead of the UN designation.)

Placards may only provide minimal information about a hazardous substance. Some materials, when shipped in smaller quantities, may not require a placard at all.

Hazardous Materials Warning Labels

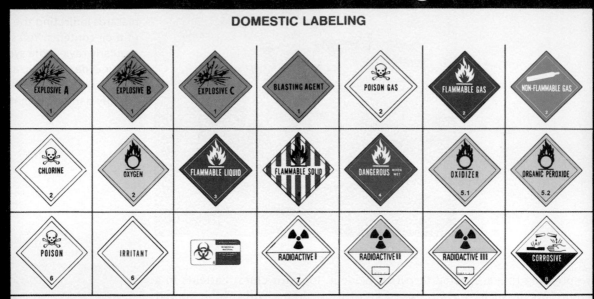

DOMESTIC LABELING

General Guidelines on Use of Labels
(CFR, Title 49, Transportation, Parts 100-177)

- Labels illustrated above are normally for *domestic shipments*. However, some air carriers *may* require the use of International Civil Aviation Organization (ICAO) labels.
- Domestic Warning Labels *may* display UN Class Number, Division Number (and Compatibility Group for Explosives only) [Sec. 172.407(g)].
- Any person who offers a hazardous material for transportation MUST label the package, if required [Sec. 172.400(a)].
- The Hazardous Materials Tables, Sec. 172.101 and 172.102, identify the proper label(s) for the hazardous materials listed.

- Label(s), when required, must be printed on or affixed to the surface of the package near the proper shipping name [Sec. 172.406(a)].
- When two or more different labels are required, display them next to each other [Sec. 172.406(c)].
- Labels may be affixed to packages (even when not required by regulations) provided each label represents a hazard of the material in the package [Sec. 172.401].

Check the Appropriate Regulations
Domestic or International Shipment

Additional Markings and Labels

HANDLING LABELS

Cargo Aircraft Only
172.402(b)

Bung Label
172.402(e)

ORM-E
172.316

INNER PACKAGES
COMPLY WITH
PRESCRIBED
SPECIFICATIONS
173.25(a)(4)

Package Orientation Markings
172.312(a)(c)

Fumigation
173.9

EMPTY
173.427

Here are a few additional markings and labels pertaining to the transport of hazardous materials. The section number shown with each item refers to the appropriate section in the HMR. The Hazardous Materials Tables, Section 172.101 and 172.102, identify the proper shipping name, hazard class, identification number, required label(s) and packaging sections.

Poisonous Materials

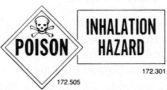

POISON
172.505

INHALATION
HAZARD
172.301

Materials which meet the inhalation toxicity criteria specified in Section 173.3a(b)(2), have additional "communication standards" prescribed by the HMR. First, the words "Poison-Inhalation Hazard" must be entered on the shipping paper, as required by Section 172.203(k)(4), for any primary capacity units with a capacity greater than one liter. Second, packages of 110 gallons or less capacity must be marked "Inhalation Hazard" in accordance with Section 172.301(a). Lastly, transport vehicles, freight containers and portable tanks subject to the shipping paper requirements contained in Section 172.203(k)(4) must be placarded with POISON placards in addition to the placards required by Section 172.504. For additional information and exceptions to these communication requirements, see the referenced sections in the HMR.

Keep a copy of the Transport Canada Emergency Response Guidebook handy!

FIGURE 3–30A   Transport Canada requires packages and storage containers to be marked with specific hazard labels.

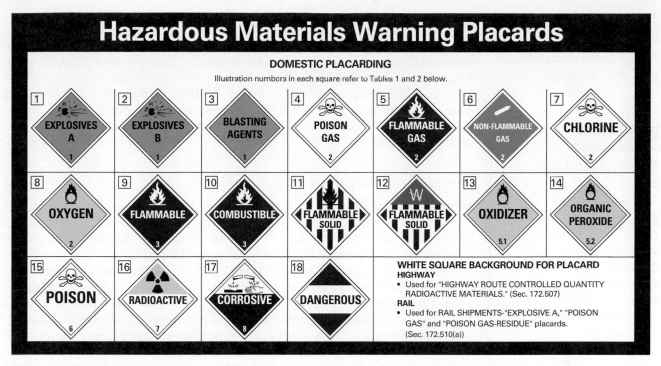

FIGURE 3-30B Transport Canada also requires display placards to be placed on the outside of vehicles.

NFPA 704 System

The NFPA 704 System places placards on tanks and storage vessels at fixed facilities. On these placards, the diamond shape is divided into four colour-coded sections (Figures 3-30A–c). The top, red segment indicates flammability. The left, blue segment indicates health hazard. The right, yellow segment indicates reactivity. The bottom, white segment indicates special information, such as water reactivity, oxidizer, or radioactivity. Flammability, health hazard, and reactivity are measured on a scale of 0 to 4. A designation of 0 indicates no hazard, while a designation of 4 indicates extreme hazard.

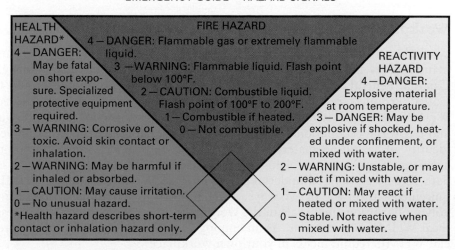

FIGURE 3-30C The NFPA 704 system helps you identify health, reactivity, and fire hazards.

Identification of a specific hazardous substance forms the "crux," or the most problematic part, of a hazmat incident.

Content Review

HAZMAT REFERENCES

Emergency Response Guidebook (ERG)
Shipping papers
Material safety data sheets
Monitors/chemical tests
Databases (CAMEO®)
Hazmat telephone hotlines (CHEMTREC; CHEMTEL, Inc.)
Poison control centres
Toxicologists
Reference books

IDENTIFICATION OF SUBSTANCES

Once you have determined that an incident involves hazardous materials, you must next try to identify the particular substance. This is the crux of dealing with a hazmat incident. You will often lack adequate on-scene information to make a positive identification, or you will get conflicting preliminary information. Therefore, you must be familiar with the resources that can assist you. To prevent dangerous misinterpretations, try to locate two or more concurring reference sources. Do not take action or treat patients until you find this information.

Emergency Response Guidebook (ERG)

Suppose you see a tanker truck bearing a red (3) placard with the UN number 1203 in the middle. Based on what you already know, you can determine that the incident involves a flammable liquid. To identify the specific liquid, you will need the *North American Emergency Response Guidebook*.

The ERG—published by CANUTEC, the U.S. Department of Transportation, and the Secretary of Communications and Transportation of Mexico—should be carried on every emergency vehicle. It lists more than a thousand hazardous materials, along with placards, UN numbers, and chemical names. It also cross-references each identification number to specific emergency procedures related to the chemical. The ERG includes, for example, a list of evacuation distances for the most hazardous substances. It is revised every three years.

When using the ERG, keep in mind two shortcomings. First, the reference provides only basic, generic information on medical treatment. Second, more than one chemical can have the same UN number. For example, UN 1203 may be diesel fuel, gasohol, gasoline, motor fuels, motor spirits, or petrol. The difference between a gasoline leak and a diesel fuel leak is dramatic, highlighting the need to use other methods of positive identification.

Shipping Papers

The most accurate information about a transported substance can be found in the **shipping papers,** or bill of lading. Trucks, boats, airplanes, and trains routinely carry these documents. Ideally, they should list the specific substances and quantities carried. However, drivers, pilots, or engineers may not take these papers when they exit the vehicle or craft, and you may find the scene too unstable to retrieve them. In some cases, the papers may be incomplete or inadequate, requiring location of additional sources of identification.

✱ **shipping papers** documents routinely carried aboard vehicles transporting hazardous materials; ideally should identify specific substances and quantities carried; also known as bills of lading.

Workplace Hazardous Materials Information System

Workplace Hazardous Materials Information System (WHMIS) programs are mandated by provincial occupational health and safety agencies throughout Canada. Federal legislation, including the Hazardous Products Act and Controlled Products regulations, establishes which materials are controlled by WHMIS, and deals with the importation and sale of those materials. Provincial and territorial occupational health and safety regulations mandate employers to identify all hazardous materials in the workplace, provide information on management of accidents involving these hazardous materials (see material safety data sheets below), and undertake worker education and training. WHMIS requirements affect you in two ways. As a paramedic responding to an accident involving hazardous materials in the workplace, you should be able to access the local WHMIS information. As an employee, you must be aware of the provincial WHMIS requirements in your own workplace.

Ensure that you are familiar with the WHMIS regulations and requirements in your jurisdiction. You must be familiar with WHMIS labels and material safety data sheets (see below) and be able to locate information regarding WHMIS materials.

Material Safety Data Sheets (MSDS)

Fixed facility employers are required by law to post **material safety data sheets (MSDS),** containing detailed information about all potentially hazardous substances on site. The sheets typically list the following data: the names and characteristics of the materials; what types of health, fire, and reactivity dangers the materials pose; any specific equipment or techniques required for safe handling of the materials; and suggested emergency first-aid treatment.

✱ material safety data sheets (MSDS) easily accessible sheets of detailed information about chemicals found at fixed facilities.

Monitors and Testing

If you are unable to secure positive identification using the preceding sources, you may have to rely on monitors and other means of testing. If you do not have the training and equipment to do the reconnaissance, leave testing to the hazmat team.

Other Sources of Information

Once you have identified the hazardous substance, you will need to determine its specific chemical or physical properties. You can consult textbooks, handbooks, or technical specialists. You might also make use of a computerized database such as **CAMEO®**—Computer-Aided Management of Emergency Operations. Developed by the Environmental Protection Agency (EPA) and the National Oceanic and Atmospheric Administration (NOAA), this website provides answers to technical questions, opportunities for skills practice, copies of software, links for networking, and more. Yet another source of information is your local or regional poison control centre.

✱ CAMEO® Computer-Aided Management of Emergency Operations; website developed by the EPA and NOAA as a source of information, skills, and links related to hazardous substances.

Two other sources of information are **CHEMTREC**—the Chemical Transportation Emergency Center—and **CHEMTEL, Inc.** Established by the Chemical Manufacturer's Association, CHEMTREC maintains a 24-hour, toll-free hotline. It provides information on the chemical properties of a substance and explains how the material should be handled. If necessary, CHEMTREC will even contact shippers and manufacturers to find out more detailed information about the incident and provide field assistance. In Canada and the United States, the toll-free number for CHEMTREC is 800-424-9300. For collect calls and calls from other points of origin, contact 703-527-3887. CHEMTREC can also refer you to the proper agencies for emergencies involving radioactive materials.

✱ CHEMTREC Chemical Transportation Emergency Center; maintains a 24-hour toll-free hotline at 800-424-9300; for collect calls and calls from other points of origin, dial 703-527-3887.

CHEMTEL, Inc. maintains another 24-hour, toll-free emergency response communications centre for Canada and the United States. In addition to providing support for chemical emergencies, CHEMTEL also supplies the names of state, provincial, territorial, and federal authorities for dealing with radioactive incidents. For toll-free calls, dial 800-255-3024. For collect calls and calls from other points of origin, contact 813-979-0626.

✱ CHEMTEL, Inc. Chemical Telephone, Incorporated; maintains a 24-hour, toll-free hotline at 800-255-3024; for collect calls and calls from other points of origin, dial 813-979-0626.

HAZARDOUS MATERIALS ZONES

As noted, your main priority at a hazmat incident is safety—in order of priority your own safety, then the safety of your crew, patient(s), and the public. Request expert help right away, just as you would under the IMS. Establish command, and hold it until relieved by somebody higher in the chain of command. Keep a bad situation from becoming worse by evacuating people from the area around

While waiting for additional help, keep a bad situation from becoming worse by evacuating uncontaminated people from the area around the incident.

✱ hot zone location at a hazmat incident where the actual hazardous material and highest levels of contamination exist; also called the red zone or the exclusionary zone.

✱ warm zone location at a hazmat incident adjacent to the hot zone; area where a decontamination corridor is established; also called the yellow zone or contamination reduction zone.

✱ cold zone location at a hazmat incident outside the warm zone; area where incident operations take place; also called the green zone or the safe zone.

FIGURE 3-31 The three zones typically established at a hazmat incident.

the incident. Do not risk anyone's safety by allowing "heroic" rescues. The result can only be more contaminated patients. Prepare for the arrival of additional resources by setting up the following control zones (Figure 3-31):

- **Hot (red) zone:** The hot zone, or "exclusionary zone," is the site of contamination. Prevent anyone without appropriate high-level personal protection equipment (PPE) from entering this area. Hold any patients who escape from this zone in the warm zone.

- **Warm (yellow) zone:** The warm zone, also called the contamination reduction zone, abuts the hot zone. It is a "buffer zone" with a decontamination corridor for patients and EMS personnel leaving the hot zone. The corridor has a "hot" end and a "cold" end.

- **Cold (green) zone:** The cold zone, or "safe zone," is the area where the incident operation takes place. It includes the command post, medical monitoring and rehabilitation, treatment areas, and apparatus staging. The cold zone must be free of any contamination. You and your crew should remain inside this zone unless you have the necessary training, equipment, and support to enter other areas.

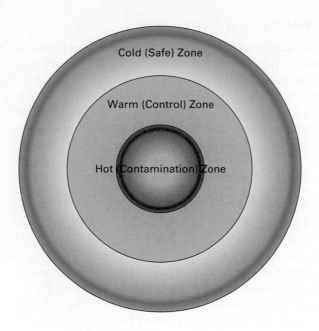

Hot (Contamination) Zone
- Contamination is actually present.
- Personnel must wear appropriate protective gear.
- Number of rescuers limited to those absolutely necessary.
- Bystanders never allowed.

Warm (Control) Zone
- Area surrounding the contamination zone.
- Vital to preventing spread of contamination.
- Personnel must wear appropriate protective gear.
- Life-saving emergency care is performed.

Cold (Safe) Zone
- Normal triage, stabilization, and treatment are performed.
- Rescuers must shed contaminated gear before entering the cold zone.

SPECIALIZED TERMINOLOGY

To prevent conflicts among the personnel or departments working at a hazmat incident, everyone should use the same terminology.

TERMS FOR MEDICAL HAZMAT OPERATIONS

The following are general terms relevant to chemical and/or radioactive materials that you may encounter during a hazmat operation.

- *Boiling point*—temperature at which a liquid becomes a gas.
- *Flammable or explosive limits*—range (upper and lower) of vapour concentration in the air at which an ignition will initiate combustion. The lower explosive limit (LEL) is the lowest concentration of chemical that will burn in the air. Below the LEL, there is not enough chemical to support combustion. The upper explosive limit (UEL) is the highest concentration of chemical that will burn in the air. Above the UEL, there is too much chemical and not enough oxygen to support combustion.
- *Flash point*—lowest temperature at which a liquid will give off enough vapours to ignite.
- *Ignition temperature*—lowest temperature at which a liquid will give off enough vapours to support combustion; slightly higher than the flash point.
- *Specific gravity*—the weight of a volume of liquid compared with an equal volume of water. Chemicals with a specific gravity greater than 1 will sink in water, while chemicals with a specific gravity less than 1 will float on water.
- *Vapour density*—the weight of a vapour or gas compared with the weight of an equal volume of air. Chemicals with a vapour density greater than 1 will fall to the lowest point possible, while chemicals with a vapour density less than 1 will rise.
- *Vapour pressure*—pressure of a vapour against the inside walls of a container. As temperatures increase, so do vapour pressures.
- *Water solubility*—ability of a chemical to dissolve into solution in water.
- *Alpha radiation*—neutrons and protons released by the nucleus of a radioactive substance. This is a very weak particle and will only travel a few inches in the air. Alpha particles are stopped by paper, clothing, or intact skin. They are hazardous if inhaled or ingested.
- *Beta radiation*—electrons released with great energy by a radioactive substance. Beta particles have more energy than alpha particles and will travel 3–4 m in the air. Beta particles will penetrate a few millimetres of skin.
- *Gamma radiation*—high-energy photons, such as x-rays. Gamma rays have the ability to penetrate most substances and to damage any cells within the body. Heavy shielding is needed for protection against gamma rays. Because gamma rays are electromagnetic (instead of particles), no decontamination is required.

TOXICOLOGICAL TERMS

It is equally important to learn the terminology related to the toxic effects of hazardous materials. Here are the most important toxicological terms used in the field:

- *Threshold limit value/time weighted average (TLV/TWA)*—maximum concentration of a substance in the air that a person can be exposed to for eight hours each day, forty hours per week, without suffering any adverse health effects. The lower the TLV/TWA, the more toxic is the substance. The Permissible Exposure Limit (PEL) is a similar measure of toxicity.

- *Threshold limit value/short-term exposure limit (TLV/STEL)*—maximum concentration of a substance that a person can be exposed to for 15 minutes (time-weighted); not to be exceeded or repeated more than four times daily with 60-minute rests between each of the four exposures.

- *Threshold limit value/ceiling level (TLV-CL)*—maximum concentration of a substance that should never be exceeded, even for a moment.

- *Lethal concentration/lethal doses (LCt/LD)*—concentration (in air) or dose (if ingested, injected, or absorbed) that results in the death of 50 percent of the test subjects. Also referred to as the LCt50 or LD50.

- *Parts per million/parts per billion (ppm/ppb)*—representation of the concentration of a substance in the air or a solution, with parts of the substance expressed per million or billion parts of the air or solution.

- *Immediately dangerous to life and health (IDLH)*—level of concentration of a substance that causes an immediate threat to life. It may also cause delayed or irreversible effects or interfere with a person's ability to remove himself from the contaminated area.

CONTAMINATION AND TOXICOLOGY REVIEW

You will study some of the following material in Chapter 34. The following is a preview, highlighting topics relevant to hazmat situations.

TYPES OF CONTAMINATION

When people or equipment come in contact with a toxic substance, they are considered to be contaminated. **Primary contamination** occurs with direct exposure. **Secondary contamination** takes place when a contaminated person or object contacts an uncontaminated person or object. Touching a contaminated patient, for example, can result in a contaminated care provider. Gas exposure rarely results in secondary contamination. Liquid and particulate matter are much more likely to be transferred.

Consider this example. A pipeline ruptures and sprays several people with a hazardous substance. This is primary contamination. One of these patients walks out of the area and calls an ambulance. When this patient climbs into the back of the ambulance, he exposes the paramedics and the ambulance. This is secondary contamination. As a member of the EMS crew, you must make every effort not to become part of the incident through such secondary contamination.

✱ **primary contamination** direct exposure of a person or item to a hazardous substance.

✱ **secondary contamination** transfer of a hazardous substance to a noncontaminated person or item via contact with someone or something already contaminated by the substance.

Although gas exposure rarely results in secondary contamination, liquid and particulate matter can be easily transferred.

ROUTES OF EXPOSURE

There are four routes of exposure to a hazardous substance: inhalation, absorption, injection, and ingestion. The most common is inhalation. Once substances enter the bronchial tree, they can be quickly absorbed, especially in oxygen-deficient atmospheres. The substance then enters the central circulation and is distributed throughout the body. As a result, inhaled substances often trigger a rapid onset of symptoms.

Toxic substances may also be taken in through the skin, by either topical absorption or parenteral injection via a laceration, burn, or puncture. The least common route of exposure to hazardous materials is gastrointestinal. However, in occupations involving hazardous materials, people ingest poisons by eating, drinking, or smoking around deadly substances. People can also forget to wash their hands and introduce the substance into their mouths.

CYCLES AND ACTIONS OF POISONS

Absorption—the rate at which a substance is delivered into the bloodstream—varies with the type and dosage. In general, the higher the dose, the greater is the effect. Resources mentioned earlier provide information on a given substance's actions, distribution to target organs, likely areas of deposit, and so on.

Effects may be acute or delayed. **Acute effects** manifest themselves immediately or shortly after exposure. **Delayed effects** may not become apparent for hours, days, weeks, months, or even years. A person exposed to chlorine gas, for example, immediately develops shortness of breath—an acute effect. A person exposed to a carcinogen may develop a malignancy years later—a delayed effect. Some substances, such as mustard gas, cause immediate damage, but victims do not develop symptoms for many hours.

Once a substance is introduced into the body, it is distributed to target organs. Effects may be local or systemic. **Local effects** involve areas around the immediate site and should be evaluated based on the burn model. You can usually expect some skin irritation (topical) or perhaps acute bronchospasm (respiratory). An acid sprayed on the skin, for example, creates immediate skin damage at the point of contact. **Systemic effects** occur throughout the body. They can affect the cardiovascular, neurological, hepatic, and renal systems. Although hydrofluoric acid may cause local skin burns on contact, for example, it can also trigger hypocalcemia and dysrhythmias, making it potentially fatal.

The organs most commonly associated with toxic substances are the liver and kidneys. The liver metabolizes most substances by chemically altering them, a process known as **biotransformation.** The kidneys can usually excrete the substances through the urine. However, both the liver and kidneys may be adversely affected by chemicals, as are other organs, losing their ability to eliminate the toxic substances and creating a life-threatening situation.

When treating patients exposed to toxic substances, keep in mind that two substances or drugs may work together to produce an effect that neither can produce on its own. This is called **synergism.** Before administering any medication, be sure to consult medical direction or the poison control centre on possible synergistic effects of treatments.

TREATMENT OF COMMON EXPOSURES

After ensuring your own safety, all toxic-exposure patients should receive the necessary supportive measures—airway support and suctioning, respiratory support, supplemental oxygen, circulatory support, and intravenous access. Before you administer specific pharmacological treatment, at least two sources should agree on the medication, and you should confer with medical direction.

The following are several of the most common classifications of chemicals to which patients may be exposed. A brief overview of effects and treatment procedures is provided for each circumstance. This is a generic discussion, not intended to replace the specific resources already described.

Corrosives

Corrosives—acids and alkalis (bases)—can be found in many everyday materials, for example, the alkali sodium hydroxide found in most drain cleaners. Corrosives can be inhaled, ingested, absorbed, or injected. Primary effects include severe skin burns and respiratory burns or edema. Some may have systemic effects.

When decontaminating a patient exposed to solid corrosives, brush off dry particles. In the case of liquid corrosives, flush the exposed area with large quantities of water. Tincture of green soap may help in decontamination. Irrigate eye injuries with water, possibly using a topical ophthalmic anesthetic, such as tetracaine, to reduce eye discomfort. In patients with pulmonary edema, consider the administration of furosemide (Lasix) or albuterol. If the patient has ingested a corrosive, *do not* induce vomiting. If the patient can swallow and is not drooling, you may direct the person to drink 5 mL/kg water up to 200 mL. As with other injuries, maintain and support the ABCs.

Pulmonary Irritants

Many substances can be pulmonary irritants, including fumes from chlorine and ammonia. When inhaled, chlorine mixes with respiratory secretions to produce hydrochloric acid. Ammonia mixes with respiratory secretions to produce ammonium hydroxide, an alkali. In addition to tissue damage, these chemicals can cause pulmonary edema. The substances can also injure intact skin.

Primary respiratory exposure cannot be decontaminated. However, you should remove the patient's clothing to prevent any trapped gas from being contained near the body. You should also flush any exposed skin with large quantities of water. Irrigate eye injuries with water, possibly using tetracaine to reduce eye discomfort. Treat pulmonary edema with furosemide if indicated. Again, treatment includes maintaining and supporting the ABCs.

Pesticides

Toxic pesticides or insecticides primarily include carbamates and organophosphates. Exposure may occur through all four routes of exposure—inhalation, absorption, ingestion, or injection. The substances can act to block **acetylcholinesterase (AChE)**—an enzyme that stops the action of acetylcholine, a neurotransmitter. The result is overstimulation of the muscarinic receptors and SLUDGE syndrome: salivation, lacrimation, urination, diarrhea, gastrointestinal distress, and emesis. Stimulation of the nicotinic receptor may also trigger involuntary muscle contraction and pinpoint pupils.

These chemicals will continue to be absorbed as long as they remain on the skin. As a result, decontamination with large amounts of water and tincture of green soap is essential. Remove all clothing and jewellery to prevent the chemical from being trapped against the skin. Maintain and support the airway, breathing, and circulation. Secretions in the airway may need to be suctioned.

The primary treatment for significant exposure to pesticides is atropinization. The dose should be increased until the SLUDGE symptoms start to resolve. For carbamates, Pralidoxime is *not* recommended. If an adult patient presents with seizures, administer 5–10 mg of diazepam. Do *not* induce vomiting if the patient has ingested the chemical. However, if the patient can swallow and has an intact gag reflex, you can administer 5 mL/kg up to 200 mL of water.

Chemical Asphyxiants

The most common chemical asphyxiants include carbon monoxide (CO) and cyanides, such as bitter almond oil, hydrocyanic acid, potassium cyanide, wild cherry syrup, prussic acid, and nitroprusside. Keep in mind that both CO and cyanides are byproducts of combustion, and so patients who present with smoke inhalation may need to be assessed for these substances as well. Most patients are exposed to CO and cyanides through inhalation. However, keep in mind that cyanides can also be ingested, absorbed, or injected.

These two chemicals have different actions once inhaled. Carbon monoxide has a very high affinity for hemoglobin—approximately 200 times greater than oxygen. As a result, it displaces oxygen in the red blood cells. Cyanides, on the other hand, inhibit the action of **cytochrome oxidase.** This enzyme complex, found in cellular mitochondria, enables oxygen to create the adenosine triphosphate (ATP) required for all muscle energy. Primary effects of CO exposure include changes in mental status and other signs of hypoxia, such as chest pain, loss of consciousness, or seizures. Primary effects of cyanides include rapid onset of unconsciousness, seizures, and cardiopulmonary arrest.

Decontamination of patients exposed to CO and cyanide asphyxiants is usually unnecessary. However, they must be removed from the toxic environment without exposing rescuers to inhalation. Take off the patient's clothing to prevent entrapment of any toxic gases, while maintaining airway, breathing, and circulatory support. Definitive treatment for CO inhalation is oxygenation. In some cases, it may be provided through hyperbaric therapy.

Definitive treatment for cyanide exposure can be provided, if local protocols allow, by several interventions carried in a cyanide kit. First, administer amyl nitrite. This short-acting vasodilator has the ability to convert hemoglobin to methemoglobin, which forms a nontoxic complex with cyanide ions. Wrap an ampule in gauze or cloth and crush it between your fingers. Then, place it in front of a spontaneously breathing patient for 15 seconds. Repeat at one-minute intervals until an infusion of sodium nitrite is ready. Keep in mind that amyl nitrite is volatile and highly flammable when mixed with air or oxygen.

Next, administer the sodium nitrite, 300 mg IV push over five minutes. (Sodium nitrite also produces methemoglobin.) Quickly follow the sodium nitrite with an infusion of sodium thiosulphate, 12.5 g IV push over five minutes. The sodium thiosulphate converts the cyanide/methemoglobin complexes into thiocyanate, which can be excreted by the kidneys. If the signs and symptoms reappear, the process should be repeated at half the original doses.

Hydrocarbon Solvents

Many chemicals can act as solvents, including xylene and methylene chloride. Usually found in liquid form, they give off easily inhaled vapours. Primary effects include dysrhythmias, pulmonary edema, and respiratory failure. Delayed effects include damage to the central nervous system and the renal system. Exposure to these chemicals may be intentional, such as among drug abusers seeking the CNS effects (euphoria) produced by the fumes. If the patient ingests the chemical and vomits, aspiration may lead to pulmonary edema.

Content Review

USE OF CYANIDE KIT

Administer ampule of amyl nitrite for 15 seconds.
Repeat at one-minute intervals until sodium nitrite is ready.
Administer infusion of sodium nitrite, 300 mg IV push over five minutes.
Follow with infusion of sodium thiosulphate, 12.5 g IV push over five minutes.
Repeat at half the original doses if necessary.

Treatment varies with the route of exposure. In cases of topical contact, decontaminate the exposed area with large quantities of warm water and tincture of green soap. If the patient has ingested the solvent, *do not* induce vomiting. If the adult patient presents with seizures, administer 5–10 mg diazepam. In the case of inhalation, maintain and support the ABCs.

APPROACHES TO DECONTAMINATION

Content Review

HAZMAT CHEMICAL CLASSIFICATIONS

Corrosives—acids and bases
Pulmonary irritants—fumes from chlorine and ammonia
Pesticides—carbamates and organophosphates
Chemical asphyxiants—carbon monoxide and cyanides
Hydrocarbon solvents—xylene and methylene chloride

Decontamination (decon) attempts to reduce or remove hazardous substances from people or equipment to prevent adverse health effects. It can be accomplished by physical or chemical means. Physical decontamination involves the removal of chemicals, while chemical decontamination focuses on changing the hazardous substance into something less harmful.

There are several purposes for performing decon. First, decon reduces the dosage of the material to which patients are exposed. Second, it reduces the risk of secondary contamination of rescuers, on-scene personnel, bystanders, hospital personnel, families of rescuers, and the general public.

METHODS OF DECONTAMINATION

There are four methods of decontamination—dilution, absorption, neutralization, and isolation. The method used depends on the type of hazardous substance and the route of exposure. In many instances, rescuers will use two or more of these methods during the decontamination process.

Content Review

METHODS OF DECONTAMINATION

Dilution
Absorption ("blotting")
Neutralization
Isolation/disposal

- *Dilution* involves the application of large quantities of water. Water is considered the universal decon solution, especially for reducing topical absorption. It may be aided by use of a soap, such as tincture of green soap. Note that a few chemicals should never be mixed with water.

- *Absorption* entails the use of pads or towels to "blot" up the hazardous material. The process is usually applied after washing with water to dry the patient or object. Absorption is not usually a primary decon method.

- *Neutralization* occurs when one substance reduces or eliminates the toxicity of another, such as adding an acid to a base. This method is almost never used by EMS personnel because in a field setting, it is difficult to identify the exact substance and proper neutralizing agent. Also, neutralization often produces an exothermic reaction, or release of large quantities of heat, which can be as or more damaging than the original chemical.

- *Isolation* is separating the patient or equipment from the hazardous substance. It begins as hazmat teams remove patients from the hot zone to the warm zone. Further, any items that might contain or trap a hazardous substance are removed, including clothing and jewellery. All contaminated items should be properly disposed of or stored.

Neutralization is almost never used by EMS personnel as a method of decontamination. Be aware of its risks—possible misidentifcation of the chemical or neutralizing agent and potential for exothermic reactions.

DECONTAMINATION DECISION MAKING

The priorities of incident management—life safety, incident stabilization, and property conservation—should guide your decision making throughout a hazmat incident. For example, you should try to prevent any runoff water used for decontamination from damaging the environment. However, environmental considerations form a major concern only when are no life threats—that is, patients are stable and not expected to deteriorate during the decon process. If life threats exist, patients come first, environmental considerations second.

Modes of Operation

In general, there are two modes of EMS operation at hazmat incidents: "fast-break" and long-term decision making. Fast-break decision making occurs when immediate action is needed to prevent contamination and handle life threats. Long-term decision making takes place at extended events with hazmat teams.

Fast–Break Decision Making Contaminated victims will often self-rescue. They will walk themselves from the primary incident site to the EMS units. In such cases, you must make fast-break decisions to prevent rescuer contamination. It may take time for a hazmat team to arrive and set up operations. In the interim, contaminated patients may try to leave the scene entirely. As a result, all EMS units must be prepared for gross decontamination. Basic personal protective equipment should be on board and all personnel should be familiar with the two-step decontamination procedures covered later.

Implement this mode of decision making at all incidents with critical patients and unknown or life-threatening materials. Fire apparatus often respond very quickly and carry large quantities of water that can be used for decon. Remove patient clothing, treat life-threatening problems, and wash with water. Although it is preferable to use warm water to prevent hypothermia, this option is not always available. Please remember that the first rule of EMS is *do not become a patient*! At no time should you or other crewmembers expose yourselves to contaminants—even to rescue a critically injured patient. Instead, contain and isolate the patient as much as possible until the proper support arrives.

When treating critically injured hazmat patients, it is important to perform a rapid risk-to-benefit assessment. Ask yourself these questions: How much risk of exposure will I incur by intubating a patient during decon? Does the patient really need an intravenous line established right now? Few prehospital procedures will truly make a difference if performed rapidly, but one mistake can turn any rescuer into a patient. Take a few moments, and think before you act.

At incidents in which patients are noncritical, rescuers can take a more contemplative approach, especially if they can identify the substance. Decontamination and treatment proceed simultaneously, following the general steps already mentioned. However, depending on whether the substance has been identified and the type of substance involved, you may be able to give special attention to other matters. For example, you might contain runoff water. You might better protect patient privacy, grossly decontaminating ambulatory patients in a more controlled setting. You might also spend time on patient monitoring, reclothing patients, isolating or containing patients, and so on.

Long-Term Decision Making At more extended events, you will engage in long-term decision making. This mode of operation most often occurs when patients remain in the hot zone and have not self-rescued. Traditionally, EMS personnel have not been trained or equipped to enter the hot zone to retrieve these patients. Instead, a hazmat team is summoned promptly, and the EMS crew awaits the team's arrival. The team will not make their entry until you or members of your crew perform the necessary medical monitoring and establish a decontamination corridor. It often takes 60 minutes or more for actual team deployment.

This mode of operation provides a number of advantages: a better opportunity for thorough decontamination, better PPE, less chance of secondary decontamination, greater consideration of the environment, and more detailed research of the actual hazardous substance. Obviously, long-term decision making presents less opportunity for error and is preferable to fast-break decision making. Unfor-

If life threats exist, the patients come first, environmental considerations second.

All EMS units must be prepared for gross decontamination procedures.

At no time should you or other crewmembers expose yourselves to contaminants—even to rescue a critically injured patient.

Content Review

ADVANTAGES OF LONG-TERM DECISION MAKING
More complete decontamination
Better PPE
Less secondary contamination
Greater property conservation
More thorough substance research
Less room for error

tunately, self-rescued patients often decide the mode of operation the minute you arrive on the scene. So, always be prepared for fast-break operations.

FIELD DECONTAMINATION

As mentioned, the decontamination method and type of PPE depend on the substance involved. If in doubt, assume the worst-case scenario. When dealing with unknowns, do not attempt to neutralize. Brush dry particles off the patient before the application of water to prevent possible chemical reactions. Next, wash with great quantities of water—the universal decon agent—using tincture of green soap if possible. Isopropyl alcohol is an effective agent for some isocyanates, while vegetable oil can be used to decon water-reactive substances.

Two-Step Process

Use the two-step decon process for gross decontamination of patients who cannot wait for a more comprehensive decon process, usually patients at a fast-break incident. As noted, remove all clothing, including shoes, socks, and jewellery. (Remember to have some method of accounting for personal effects BEFORE hazmat incidents occur.) Wash and rinse the patients with soap and water, making sure that they do not stay in the runoff. Repeat the process, allowing the fluid to drain away each time. Pay special attention to difficult contamination areas, such as the scalp and hair, ears, nostrils, axilla, fingernails, naval, genitals, groin, buttocks, behind the knees, between the toes, and toenails.

Eight-Step Process

The eight-step process takes place in a complete decontamination corridor and is much more thorough. To leave the hot zone, the rescuers follow these steps:

- **Step 1:** Rescuers enter the decon area at the hot end of the corridor and mechanically remove contaminants from the victims.
- **Step 2:** Rescuers drop equipment in a tool-drop area and remove outer gloves.
- **Step 3:** Decon personnel shower and scrub all victims and rescuers, using gross decontamination. As surface decontamination is removed, the dilution is conducted into a contained area. Victims may be moved ahead to Step 6 or Step 7.
- **Step 4:** Rescuers remove and isolate their SCBA. If reentry is necessary, the team dons new SCBA from a noncontaminated side.
- **Step 5:** Rescuers remove all protective clothing. Articles are isolated, labelled for disposal, and placed on the contaminated side.
- **Step 6:** Rescuers remove all personal clothing. Victims who have not had their clothing removed have it taken off here. All items are isolated in plastic bags and labelled for later disposal or storage.
- **Step 7:** Rescuers and victims receive a full-body washing, using soft scrub brushes or sponges, water, and mild soap or detergent. Cleaning tools are bagged for later disposal.
- **Step 8:** Patients receive rapid assessment and stabilization before being transported to hospitals for further care. EMS crews medically monitor rescuers, complete exposure records, and transport rescuers to hospitals as needed.

These procedures are not set in stone. Small variations may exist from system to system. Know the procedures in your jurisdiction.

Transportation Considerations

No patient who undergoes field decontamination is truly decontaminated. Field-decontaminated patients, sometimes called **semidecontaminated patients,** may still need to undergo a more invasive decon process at a medical facility. Depending on the type of exposure, wounds may need débridement, hair or nails may need to be trimmed or removed, and so on. However, it is always better to deliver a grossly decontaminated living patient to the hospital than a perfectly decontaminated corpse. Just make sure that field-decontaminated patients are transported to facilities capable of performing more thorough decon procedures.

When transporting field-decontaminated patients, always recall that they may still have some contamination in or on them. For example, a patient may have ingested a chemical, which can be expelled if the patient coughs or vomits. As a result, use as much disposable equipment as possible. Keep in mind that any airborne hazard will not only incapacitate the crew in the back of the ambulance but will affect the driver as well. Although it is not practical to line the ambulance in plastic, you can isolate the patient using a stretcher decon pool. The pool can help contain any potentially contaminated body fluids. Plastic can also be used to cover the pool, adding yet another protective barrier.

HAZMAT PROTECTION EQUIPMENT

Personal protective equipment for a hazmat incident is specifically designed for such incidents. There are basically four levels of hazmat protective equipment, from Level A (highest) to Level D (minimum).

- *Level A*—provides the highest level of respiratory and splash protection. This hazmat suit offers a high degree of protection against chemical breakthrough time and fully encapsulates the rescuer, even covering the SCBA. The sealed, impermeable suits are typically used by hazmat teams entering hot zones with an unknown substance and a significant potential for both respiratory and dermal hazards.

- *Level B*—offers full respiratory protection when there is a lower probability of dermal hazard. The Level B suit is nonencapsulating but chemically resistant. Seams for zippers, gloves, boots, and mask interface are usually sealed with duct tape. The SCBA is worn outside the suit, allowing increased manoeuvrability and ease in changing SCBA bottles. The decon team members typically wear Level B protection.

- *Level C*—includes a nonpermeable suit, boots, and gear for protecting eyes and hands. Instead of SCBA, Level C protective equipment uses an **air-purifying respirator (APR).** The APR relies on filters to protect against a known contaminant in a normal environment. The canisters in the APR must be specifically selected and are not usually implemented in a hazmat emergency response. Level C clothing is usually worn during transport of patients with the potential for secondary contamination.

- *Level D*—consists of structural firefighter, or turnout, gear. Level D gear is usually not suitable for hazmat incidents.

The level of hazmat protective gear depends on the substance involved. Ideally, the chemical should be identified so that a permeability chart can be consulted to determine breakthrough time. No single material is suitable to all hazmats. Some materials are resistant to certain chemicals and nonresistant to others.

No patient who undergoes field decontamination is ever truly decontaminated.

✱ semidecontaminated patient another term for field-decontaminated patient.

It is always better to deliver a grossly decontaminated living patient to the hospital than a perfectly decontaminated corpse.

When possible, protect the crew from secondary decontamination by placing a semidecontaminated patient in a stretcher decon pool.

✱ air-purifying respirator (APR) system of filtering a normal environment for a specific chemical substance using filter cartridges.

When chemicals can be identified, consult a permeability chart to determine the breakthrough time on a hazmat suit.

EMS personnel should not become involved in any hazmat situation without PPE. All ambulances carry some level of PPE, even if not ideal. If the situation is emergent and the chemical unknown, use as much barrier protection as possible. Full turnout gear (Level D) or a Tyvek suit is better than no gear at all. HEPA filter masks and double or triple gloves offer good protection against some hazards. Latex gloves are not chemically resistant. Instead, use nitrile gloves, which have a high resistance to most chemicals. Also, leather boots will absorb chemicals permanently, and so be sure to don rubber boots.

MEDICAL MONITORING AND REHABILITATION

One of the primary roles of EMS personnel at a hazmat incident is the medical monitoring of entry personnel. All hazmat team members should undergo regular annual physical examinations, with baseline vital signs placed on file.

ENTRY READINESS

Prior to entry, you or other EMS crew members will assess rescuers and document the following information: blood pressure, pulse, respiratory rate, temperature, body weight, ECG, and mental or neurological status. If you observe anything abnormal, do not allow the hazmat team member to attempt a rescue.

Hazmat team members will enter the hot zone only in groups of two, with two more members in PPE remaining outside as a backup team. The PPE used at hazmat incidents can cause significant stress and dehydration. As a result, entry team personnel should prehydrate themselves with 250–500 mL of water or sport drink.

AFTER-EXIT "REHAB"

After the hazmat entry team exits the hot zone and completes decontamination, they should report back to EMS for postexit monitoring. Measure and document the same parameters as before entry. Rehydrate the team with more water or diluted sport drink. You can use weight changes to estimate any fluid losses. Check with medical direction or protocols to determine fluid replacement PO or IV. Entry team members should not be allowed to reenter the hot zone until they are alert, nontachycardic, normotensive, and within a reasonable percentage of their normal body weight.

HEAT STRESS FACTORS

In evaluating heat stress, primary considerations include temperature and humidity. Prehydration, duration and degree of activity, and the team member's overall physical fitness will also have a bearing on your evaluation. Keep in mind that Level A suits protect a rescuer but prevent cooling. A rescuer essentially works inside an encapsulated sauna. Therefore, place heat stress at the top of your list of tasks for postexit medical monitoring.

IMPORTANCE OF PRACTICE

Practise the skills that you can expect to use at a hazmat incident in most EMS systems. Put on and take off Level B hazmat protective equipment. Set up a rapid two-step decontamination process and an eight-step decontamination process, preferably with the help of the local hazmat team. With a crew member, identify a simulated chemical, determine the correct PPE, and establish the proper decontamination methods. Practise preentry and postexit medical monitoring and documentation. Prepare a patient and ambulance for transport. As these skills may be rarely used except in the busiest EMS systems, you should work closely with your local hazmat team to practise these skills on a regular basis.

Part 5: Crime Scene Awareness

Regardless of where you work as a paramedic—the inner city, suburbs, or rural Canada—you can be affected by violence. It can take all forms, from interpersonal abuse in the home to gang activities in the street and can involve weapons ranging from fists to guns to explosives. People of all ages and backgrounds commit acts of violence. According to the B.C. Ministry of Public Safety and the Solicitor General's *2002 Report on Crime*, 84 percent of violent crimes in B.C. were committed by adults (over 17 years of age), and 84 percent of those were committed by men, mostly between 18 and 35 years of age. Their victims are about evenly split between male and female, and most are between 18 and 35. In approximately 80 percent of violent crimes, the victim and accused knew each other. About half of these incidents occur in the home, and about 10 percent in a restaurant or bar. Assault accounted for approximately 80 percent of violent crimes in B.C. that year.

Approximately one of six victims of violent crimes requires medical attention, often by the emergency medical services. Many victims fail to report the violence to the police. As a result, the EMS may be a victim's only contact with professionals who can intervene to prevent further harm.

EMS providers find it almost impossible to predict exactly when and where a violent incident will occur. Nearly all calls that a paramedic handles on a given day will progress without any threat of danger. In fact, you have a higher risk of being injured by oncoming traffic than by a violent act. Even so, you cannot let down your "crime scene awareness." Otherwise, you risk becoming a victim or hostage of a violent situation. Your most important safety tactic is an ability to identify potentially violent situations as soon as possible. Also, be aware of local issues that hold a potential for violence, such as the presence of street gangs or a known area of drug activity.

Equally importantly, familiarize yourself with standard operating procedures (SOPs) for handling violent situations and the specialized resources that you can call on for backup. Find out, for example, whether your unit has access to a **tactical emergency medical service (TEMS)**—a unit that provides on-site medical support to law enforcement. If so, know how and when to access it. Above all else, remain alert to the signs of danger from the start of a call to the time you return your ambulance to service.

* **tactical emergency medical services (TEMS)** a specially trained unit that provides on-site medical support to law enforcement.

APPROACH TO THE SCENE

Your safety strategy begins with dispatch. Emergency medical dispatchers try to keep callers on the line to obtain as much information as possible, remaining alert to background noises, such as fighting or intoxicated persons, and warn incoming units of these dangers. Modern computer-aided dispatch (CAD) programs provide instant information on previous calls at a location and display "caution indicators" to notify dispatchers when a location has a history of violence.

Even in the age of computers, however, some of your best information can still come from your own experience and that of other crewmembers. Your memory of previous calls can serve as an important indicator of trouble. For example, if a bar or club has a reputation for fights and you are summoned there, you will already have a high suspicion of danger before you arrive.

Your safety strategy begins as soon as you are dispatched on a call.

POSSIBLE SCENARIOS

There are three possible scenarios for violence during a call. The dispatcher may advise you of a potentially violent scene en route to the call and you will be alert to danger from the start. In other cases, you may not spot danger until you arrive on the scene and begin your assessment and approach. In yet another scenario, you may not face danger until the start of patient care or transport.

Advised of Danger en Route

Never follow police units to the scene. To do so might place you at the centre of violence.

When the dispatcher reports possible danger, do not approach the scene until it is secured by law enforcement. Remember that lights and sirens can draw a crowd or alert the perpetrator of a crime, and so use them cautiously or not at all. Never follow police units to the scene. To do so might place you at the centre of violence. If you arrive first, keep the ambulance out of sight so that the rig does not attract the attention of bystanders or parties involved in the incident. While you wait for police to secure the scene, set up a staging area.

Management of the incident requires interagency cooperation. Communicate with the police—you are in this together. Be sure you understand any differences in dispatch terminology. For example, what is a code 1 emergency for police units may be a code 3 emergency for EMS units. Work with police to determine if and when you should approach the scene.

Keep in mind that violence can occur or resume even with the police present. Furthermore, depending on your uniform colours and the use of badges, people might mistake you for the police—especially if you exit from a vehicle with flashing lights and siren. They might expect you to intervene in a violent situation, or they might direct aggression toward you as an authority figure. If the scene cannot be made safe, retreat immediately (Figure 3-32).

Observing Danger on Arrival

Even if dispatch has not alerted you to danger, you must still keep this possibility in mind once you arrive. One of the main purposes of scene assessment is to search for any possible hazards, such as downed power lines or hazardous materials. As you look for these, observe for other signs of trouble, such as crowds gathering on the street, an unusual silence, or a darkened residence. Obviously, you will adopt a different approach for a confirmed medical emergency than that for an "unknown problem, caller hang-up." Even so, do not exit the vehicle until you have ruled out all immediate hazards.

FIGURE 3-32 Never approach the scene until you are advised that the scene is secure. Remember, even if a scene has been declared secure, violence may still erupt.

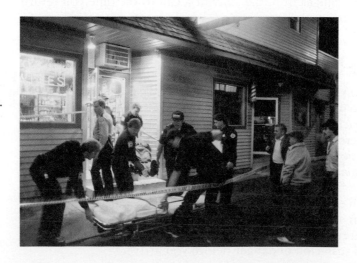

If you have any doubts about a call, park away from the scene. If you must park in view of the location, take an unconventional approach to the door (Figure 3-33). People will expect you to use the sidewalk, and so approach from the side, the lawn, or flush against the house. Avoid getting between a residence and the lighted ambulance so that you do not "backlight" yourself. Hold your flashlight to the side, rather than in front of you (Figure 3-34). Assailants often fire at the light.

Before announcing your presence, observe for signs of danger. If you can, look into windows for evidence of fighting, weapons, or the use of alcohol or drugs. Gradually make your way to the doorknob side of the door or the side opposite the hinges (Figure 3-35). Listen for any signs of danger, such as loud noises, articles breaking, incoherent speech, or the absence of any sounds at all.

If you spot danger at any time during your approach, immediately stop and reevaluate the situation. Decide whether it is in the interest of your own safety to continue or retreat until law enforcement officials can be summoned. Rather than risk becoming injured or killed, err on the side of safety.

Rather than risk becoming injured or killed, err on the side of safety.

Eruption of Danger during Care or Transport

Remain alert throughout a call, especially in areas with a history of violence. You may enter the scene and spot weapons or drugs. Additional combative people may arrive on scene. The patient or bystanders may become agitated or threatening. Even if treatment has begun, you must place your own safety first. You now have two tactical options: (1) Quickly package the patient and leave the scene with the patient, or (2) retreat without the patient.

In most cases, you can legally leave a patient behind when there is a documented danger.

Your choice of action depends on the level of danger. Abandonment is always a concern. However, in most cases, you can legally leave a patient behind when

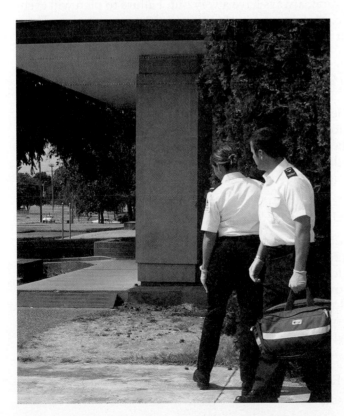

FIGURE 3-33   Approach potentially unstable scenes single file along an unconventional path.

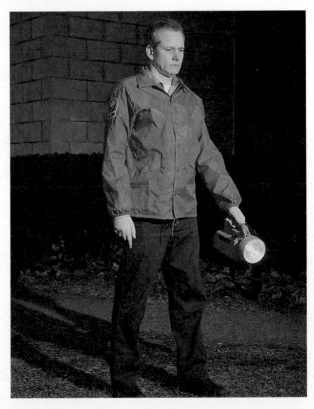

FIGURE 3-34   Hold a flashlight to the side of your body, not in front of it. Armed assailants usually aim at the light.

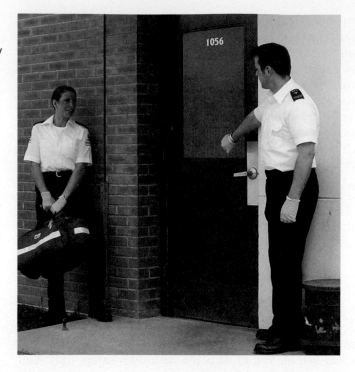

FIGURE 3-35 Stand to the side of the door when knocking. Do not stand directly in front of a door or window, making yourself an unwitting target.

there is a documented danger. As discussed later, keep accurate records of incidents involving violence. If you must defend yourself, use the minimum amount of force necessary. Immediately summon the police, and retreat as needed.

Regardless of the situation, always have a way out. Failure to plan will eventually get you into trouble. Make sure your SOPs include an escape plan. Then, adhere to this plan so that you do not become a victim of violence yourself.

SPECIFIC DANGEROUS SCENES

Most out-of-hospital services were developed to meet the needs of individual patients in controlled situations. However, in recent years, EMS personnel trained for this limited role have been pressed increasingly into service in potentially hazardous situations. The following are some of the known dangers that you may face "on the street." (Tactical safety strategies are discussed later.)

HIGHWAY ENCOUNTERS

The preceding examples of known dangers have focused largely on residences. However, EMS units frequently report to roadside calls involving motor vehicle collisions, disabled vehicles, or sick or unresponsive people inside a car—for example, "man slumped over wheel" calls. Dangers of highway operations and the steps that you should take to protect yourself were discussed earlier in the chapter. However, highway operations also hold the risk of violence from occupants who may be fleeing felons, intoxicated or drugged, or in possession of weapons. Some potential warning signs of danger include the following:

- Violent or abusive behaviour
- An altered mental state
- Grabbing or hiding items inside the vehicle
- Arguing or fighting among passengers

- Lack of activity where activity is expected
- Physical signs of alcohol or drug abuse—for example, liquor bottles, beer cans, or syringes
- Open or unlatched trunks—a potential hiding spot for people or weapons
- Differing stories told by occupants

To make a safe approach to a vehicle at a roadside emergency, follow these steps:

- Park the ambulance in a position that provides safety from traffic.
- Notify dispatch of the situation, location, the vehicle make and model, and the province and number of the licence plate.
- Use a one-person approach. The driver should remain in the ambulance, which is elevated and provides greater visibility.
- The driver should remain prepared to radio for immediate help and to back or drive away rapidly once the other medic returns.
- At nighttime, use the ambulance lights to illuminate the vehicle. However, do not walk between the ambulance and the other vehicle. You will be backlighted, forming an easy target.
- Since the police approach vehicles from the driver's side, you should approach from the passenger's side—an unexpected route.
- Use the A, B, and C door posts for cover.
- Observe the rear seat. Do not move forward of the C post unless you are sure there are no threats in the rear seat or foot wells.
- Carefully watch the occupants of the vehicle. Use the side mirrors to look inside the vehicle.
- Retreat to the ambulance (or another strategic position of cover) at the first sign of danger.
- Make sure you have mapped out your intended retreat and escape with the ambulance driver.

VIOLENT STREET INCIDENTS

The following are some of the dangerous street situations that you may face at some point in your EMS career.

Murder, Assault, Robbery

Violent acts take place at residences, schools, and commercial establishments. However, the most common location is on the streets. In order of occurrence, the most frequent crimes are simple assaults, aggravated assaults, rapes and sexual assaults, robberies, and homicides. In one-quarter of violent crimes, offenders used or threatened the use of a weapon. Homicides are most commonly committed with handguns, but knives, blunt objects, and other types of guns or weapons may also be used. About one in five violent victimizations involve the use of alcohol.

Although motives vary, there has been a recent rise in **hate crimes**—crimes committed against a person solely on the basis of the individual's actual or perceived race, colour, national origin, ethnicity, gender, disability, or sexual orientation. A number of jurisdictions have passed legislation on the management of hate crimes, including the steps to be taken on the scene. Determine whether these laws exist in your area, and establish protocols that your agency should follow. Crew assignments, for example, should be well thought out in advance of

* **hate crimes** crimes committed against a person wholly on the basis of the individual's actual or perceived race, colour, national origin, ethnicity, gender, disability, or sexual orientation.

Crew assignments should be well thought out in advance of the response to a hate crime.

the response to a hate crime. You should also know the specific type of information that must be documented for later use by the courts.

In responding to the scene of any violent crime, keep these points in mind:

- Dangerous weapons may have been used in the crime.
- Perpetrators may still be on the scene or could return to the scene.
- Patients may sometimes exhibit violence toward EMS personnel, particularly if they risk criminal penalties as a result of the original incident.

Dangerous Crowds and Bystanders

Crowds can quickly become large and volatile, especially in the case of a hate crime. Violence can be directed against anyone or anything in the path of an angry crowd. Your status as an EMS provider does not give you immunity. Whenever a crowd is present, look for these warning signs:

- Shouts or increasingly loud voices
- Pushing or shoving
- Hostilities toward anyone on the scene, including the perpetrator of a crime, the victim, the police, and so on
- Rapid increase in the crowd size
- Inability of law enforcement officials to control bystanders

Constantly monitor the crowd and retreat if necessary. If possible, take the patient with you. Rapid transport may require limited or tactical assessment at the scene with more in-depth assessment done inside the safety of the ambulance. Be sure to document reasons for the quick assessment and transport.

Street Gangs

Street gangs can be found in big cities, suburban towns, and lately in rural areas. In fact, some organized gangs have purposely branched out into smaller towns in an effort to escape surveillance and expand their illicit businesses. Gangs account for a disproportionate amount of youth violence. Gang activity is associated with high levels of delinquency, illegal drug use, physical violence, and weapons possession. Young people from all demographic backgrounds report some knowledge of gangs or gang activity.

Commonly observed gang characteristics include the following:

- *Appearance*—Gang members frequently wear unique clothing specific to the group. Because the clothing is often a particular colour or hue, it is referred to as the gang's "colours." Wearing a colour, even a bandana, can signify gang membership. Within the gang, members sometimes wear different articles to signify rank.
- *Graffiti*—Gangs have territories, or "turfs." Members often mark their turf with graffiti of the gang's logo, warning away intruders, bragging about crimes, insulting rival gangs, or taunting the police.
- *Tattoos*—Many gang members wear tattoos or other body markings to identify their gang affiliation. Some gangs even require these tattoos. The tattoos will be in the gang's colours and often contain the gang's motto or logo.
- *Hand signals or language*—Gangs commonly create their own methods of communication. They give gang-related meanings to everyday words or create codes. Hand signs provide quick identification among gang members, warn of approaching law enforcement, or

show disrespect to other gangs. Gang members often perform signals so quickly that an uninformed outsider may not spot them, much less understand them.

EMS units venturing into gang territory must be extremely cautious. Danger is increased if your uniform looks similar to the uniform worn by the police. Gangs with a history of arrest may, in fact, make every effort to prevent you from transporting one of their members to a hospital or any other place beyond the reach of the gang. Do not force the issue if your safety is at stake.

EMS uniforms should not resemble law enforcement uniforms.

DRUG-RELATED CRIMES

The sale of drugs goes hand-in-hand with violence. Hundreds of people die each year in drug deals gone bad. In addition, drug dealers protect their drug stashes and "shooting galleries" with booby traps, weapons, and attack dogs. The combination of a high cash flow, addiction, and automatic weapons threatens anyone who unwittingly walks onto the scene of a drug deal or threatens to uncover an illicit drug operation.

Signs that can alert you to the involvement of drugs at an EMS call include the following:

- Prior history of drugs in the neighbourhood of the call
- Clinical evidence that the patient has used drugs of some kind
- Drug-related comments by bystanders
- Drug paraphernalia visible at the scene, such as the following:
  – Tiny zip-top bags or vials
  – Sandwich bags with the corners torn off (indicating drug packaging) or untied corners of sandwich bags (indicating drug use)
  – Syringes or needles
  – Glass tubes, pipes, or homemade devices for smoking drugs
  – Chemical odours or residues

Whenever you observe any of the preceding items, assume the use or presence of drugs at the scene. Even if the patient is not involved, others at the scene may still pose a danger. Keep in mind that not all patients who use drugs will be seeking to harm you. Some may, in fact, be looking for help. Evaluate each situation carefully. Above all else, remember to retreat or request police backup at the earliest sign of danger.

CLANDESTINE DRUG LABORATORIES

Drug dealers often set up "laboratories" to manufacture controlled substances or to otherwise refine or convert a substance to another more profitable or useable form, such as tablets. One of the most common substances manufactured in drug laboratories is methamphetamine, also known by such street names as "crank," "speed," or "crystal." Other drugs include LSD, "crack," and more.

Clandestine drug laboratories, or "clan labs," have three requirements: privacy, utilities, and such equipment as glassware, chemical containers, and heating mantles or burners. Most clan labs are uncovered by neighbours who report suspicious odours or activities. Raids on clan labs have a way of turning into hazmat operations. All too often, the labs contain toxic fumes and volatile chemicals. The people on the scene complicate matters by fighting or shooting at the rescuers who come to extricate them from the toxic environment. As they retreat, drug dealers may also trigger booby traps or wait for police or EMS personnel to trigger them. If you ever come on a clan lab, take these actions:

- Leave the area immediately.

- Do not touch anything.
- Never stop any chemical reactions already in progress.
- Do not smoke or bring any source of flame near the lab.
- Notify the police.
- Initiate ICS and hazmat procedures.
- Consider evacuation of the area.

Laboratories can be found anywhere—on farms, in trailers, in city apartments, and more. They may be mobile, roaming from place to place in campers or trucks. Or they may be disassembled and stored in a variety of locations. The job of raiding clan labs belongs to specialized personnel—not EMS crews.

Grow Operations

Illegal indoor marijuana grow operations are an increasing problem in many communities. Houses are turned into "greenhouses" using hydroponic lighting and fans. These "grow ops" share many characteristics with clandestine drug laboratories and may be found in rural or urban settings. The operations are often connected with organized crime. Specific hazards from grow ops include toxic fumes and the potential for fires from unsafe electrical bypass wiring. In addition, there is a significant potential for violence associated with these operations.

Signs of a grow op may include the following:

- Windows that are covered over (provide privacy and to prevent escape of high-intensity light) or heavy condensation on windows
- Occupants are rarely visible, and there are no signs of normal daily activity (e.g., garbage and recycling not put out)
- Evidence of discarded equipment, such as PVC pipes, wiring, pots, nutrient containers, or soil
- Humming noises from fans and lights
- Odd odours (often pungent or skunky)
- Frequent vehicular and pedestrian traffic at odd hours

If you encounter a grow operation, follow the same procedures as you would for a clandestine lab: Leave immediately, notify the police, and initiate ICS and hazmat procedures.

DOMESTIC VIOLENCE

Domestic violence may be physical, emotional, sexual, verbal, or economic. It may be directed against a spouse or partner, or it may involve children and/or older relatives. When you go to the scene of domestic violence, the abuser may turn on you or other crewmembers. You have two main concerns: the safety of yourself and your crew and protection of the patient from further harm.

TACTICAL CONSIDERATIONS

As mentioned on several occasions, your best tactical response to violence is observation. Know the warning signs, and stay out of danger in the first place. If the dispatcher alerts you to hazards, resort to staging until the appropriate authorities can resolve the situation. That said, you still may find yourself in situations with a potential for danger. In such instances, you must have a "game plan" in place. This section presents some of the actions you can take to protect your own safety while attempting to provide tactical patient care.

SAFETY TACTICS

Content Review

SAFETY TACTICS
Retreat
Cover and concealment
Distraction and evasion
Contact and cover
Warning signals and communication

Dangerous situations mean extreme stress. As a result, your response to danger will be most effective if you practise tactical options frequently. Even on routine calls, think about safety, contact and cover, escape routes, and other strategies that can help you make a better decision when you are faced with actual danger. Borrowing a phrase from professional sports: "You will play the game the way you practise." If you have rehearsed the responses to danger before you actually need them, you will be more likely to use them successfully. The following sections describe some proven methods for EMS safety in dangerous situations.

Retreat

The prudent strategy is to retreat whenever you spot indicators of violence or potential physical confrontations, particularly with fleeing criminals or emotionally disturbed people. Retreat in a calm but decisive manner. Be aware that the danger is now at your back, and integrate cover into your retreat. Ideally, you will retreat to the ambulance so that you can summon help. However, if a dangerous obstacle—such as a crowd—blocks access to your rig, retreat by foot or by any means possible. Nothing in the ambulance is worth your life.

Nothing in the ambulance is worth your life. Retreat by foot or by whatever means possible to avoid violence that threatens your life.

In deciding how far to retreat, your primary goal is to protect. You must be out of the immediate line of sight. You must also seek cover from gunfire. Finally, you must allow enough distance to react if a person or crowd attempts to move toward you again. You need time and space to respond to changing situations. As soon as possible, notify other responding units and agencies of the danger. Activate appropriate codes, SOPs, and interagency agreements, particularly with law enforcement. Be sure to document your observations of danger and your specific responses. Include such information as:

- Actions taken while on scene
- Reasons you retreated
- Time at which you left or returned to the scene
- Personnel or agencies contacted

Keep in mind that retreat does not mean the end of a call. As already mentioned, you should seek to stage at a safe area until the police secure the scene and you can respond again. Staging, along with thorough documentation, will reduce liability and provide evidence to refute charges of abandonment.

Cover and Concealment

When faced with danger, two of your most immediate and practical strategies are cover and concealment (Figures 3-36A and 3-36B). **Concealment** hides your body, such as when you crouch behind bushes or vehicle doors. However, most common objects do not stop bullets. During armed encounters, seek **cover** by hiding your body behind solid and impenetrable objects, such as brick walls, rocks, large trees or telephone poles, or a vehicle engine block.

In applying these safety tactics, keep in mind these general rules:

- As you approach any scene, remain aware of the surroundings and any potential sources of protection in case you must retreat or are "pinned down."

✳ **concealment** hiding the body behind objects that shield a person from view but that offer little or no protection against bullets or other ballistics.

✳ **cover** hiding the body behind solid and impenetrable objects that protect a person from bullets.

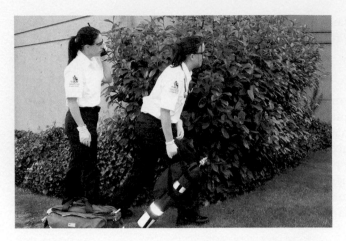

FIGURE 3-36A Concealing yourself means placing your body behind an object that can hide you from view.

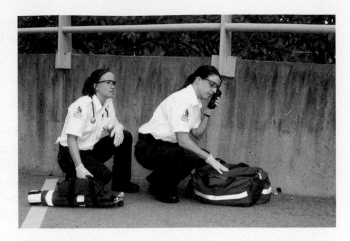

FIGURE 3-36B Taking cover is finding a position that both hides you and protects your body from projectiles.

- Choose your cover carefully. You may have only one chance to pick your protection. Select the item that hides your body adequately while shielding you against ballistics.
- Once you have made your choice of cover, conceal as much of your body as possible. Be conscious of any reflective clothing that you may be wearing. Armed assailants can use it as a target, especially at night.
- Constantly look to improve your protection and location.

Distraction and Evasion

Distraction and evasion can be integrated into any retreat. Some specific techniques to avoid physical violence include the following:

- Throwing equipment to trip, slow, or distract an aggressor
- Wedging a stretcher in a doorway to block an attacker
- Using an unconventional path while retreating
- Anticipating the moves of the aggressor and making countermoves
- Overturning objects in the path of the attacker
- Using planned tactics with your partner to confuse or "throw off" an aggressor

Key to the success of these tactics is your own physical condition. Regular exercise and good health ensure that you will have the strength to outrun or, if necessary, defend yourself against an attacker. Some units provide basic training in self-defence or have protocols on its use. Make sure you take advantage of the training and know the protocols related to application of force.

Contact and Cover

The concept of contact and cover comes from a police procedure developed in San Diego, California, where several officers were injured or killed while interviewing suspects. Studies of the incidents revealed that the officers focused directly on the suspect, reducing their ability to observe the "big picture." This left them exposed to violence. To solve this problem, the San Diego police adopted an interview approach in which one officer "contacts" the suspect while another stands 90 degrees to the side. By standing at a different angle, the second officer can provide "cover" to the officer dealing with the suspect.

When adapted to EMS practice, the procedure assigns the roles shown in Table 3-1. As with any tactic adopted from another discipline, contact and cover has obvious correlations and drawbacks for EMS. The tactic is ideal for street encounters with intoxicated persons or subjects acting in a suspicious manner. An obvious drawback is that two medics working on a cardiac arrest patient will not be able to designate one person to act solely as a "cover" medic.

Perhaps the best application of this police procedure to EMS is its emphasis on the importance of observation and teamwork. A crew that works well together will assign roles—formally or informally—to guarantee safety and patient care. In its most basic form, contact and cover means that you will watch your partner's back while your partner watches yours.

Warning Signals and Communication

In the case of "street survival," communication is an invaluable tool. Every team or crew should develop methods of alerting other providers to danger without alerting the aggressor. Devise prearranged verbal and nonverbal clues, and then practise them. Be sure to involve dispatch in the process. Choose signals that will indicate a variety of circumstances while sounding harmless to an attacker. This can be a life-saving technique in situations where you find yourself, the crew, or the patient held hostage. Your so-called "routine" radio reports can spell out the nature of the trouble and summon help from a **Special Weapons and Tactics (SWAT) Team**—a trained police unit equipped to handle hostage holders or other difficult law enforcement situations.

* Special Weapons and Tactics (SWAT) Team a trained police unit equipped to handle hostage holders and other difficult law enforcement situations.

TACTICAL PATIENT CARE

The increased involvement of care providers in violent situations has raised discussion and debate over the tactical training and protection offered to the EMS community. Interagency planning is essential, especially for clarifying the duties and roles of EMS and law enforcement agencies at crime scenes, riots, or terrorist events. Other aspects of tactical patient care include the use of body armour by EMS providers and the training of special tactical EMS personnel.

Body Armour

Several years ago few EMS providers would have considered wearing **body armour,** or bullet-proof vests, while on duty. Today, more and more providers are taking "tactical patient care" seriously. An increasing number of EMS agencies have chosen to supply body armour or to provide cash toward its purchase. Body armour manufacturers have responded by designing and marketing vests specifically for the EMS community.

Unlike conventional armour, body armour is soft. Fibres, such as Kevlar®, are woven tightly together to form the vest. The tight weave and strength of the

* body armour vest made of tightly woven, strong fibres that offers protection against handgun bullets, most knives, and blunt trauma; also known as "bullet-proof vests."

Table 3-1 CONTACT AND COVER	
Contact Provider	**Cover Provider**
Initiates and provides direct patient care.	Observes the scene for danger while the "contact" provider cares for the patient.
Performs patient assessment.	Generally avoids patient care duties that would prevent observation of the scene.
Handles most interpersonal scene contact.	In small crews, may perform limited functions, such as handling equipment.

material offer protection from many handgun bullets, most knives, and blunt trauma. The number of layers of fibre determine the rating or "stopping power" of a vest. Most body armours are rated from level 1 (least protective) to level 3 (most protective). Specialty vests with steel inserts and other materials are available for use by the military or by SWAT teams.

Some critics of body armour claim that wearers may feel a false sense of security. They point out that body armour offers reduced protection when wet and that it provides little or no protection against high-velocity bullets, such as those fired by a rifle, or from thin or dual-edged weapons. An ice pick, for example, can penetrate between the fibres of most vests. Supporters of body armour feel it should be viewed just like any other PPE. They point to the new threats faced by emergency responders, such as paramilitary groups, terrorists, drug-related violence, and the widespread possession of handguns.

Whether you purchase or wear body armour is a personal decision. However, for it to be effective, you must follow several guidelines:

- Keep in mind the limitations of body armour. Never do anything you would not do without it.

- Remember that body armour does not cover the whole body. You can still get seriously injured or killed.

- Even though body armour can prevent many types of penetration, you can still experience severe cavitation.

- For body armour to work, it must be worn. The temptation not to wear it—especially in hot temperatures—can render even the best body armour useless.

Tactical EMS

As already mentioned, the provision of care in violent or tactically "hot" zones, such as sniper situations, necessitates risks far beyond those found on most EMS calls. Medical personnel assigned to such incidents require special training and authorization. Like hazmat teams, they must don special equipment, function with compact gear, and, in most cases, work as medical adjuncts to the police or military.

The patient care offered by a tactical emergency medical service (TEMS) differs from routine EMS care in several ways:

- A major priority is extraction of the patient from the hot zone.
- Care may be modified to meet tactical considerations.
- Trauma patients outnumber medical patients.
- Treatment and transport interventions must almost always be coordinated with an incident commander.
- Patients must be moved to tactically cold zones for complete assessment, care, and transport.
- Metal clipboards, chemical agents, and other tools may be used as defensive weapons.

✱ **EMT-Tacticals (EMT-Ts)** EMS personnel trained to serve with a Technical Emergency Medical Service or a law enforcement agency.

Local protocols, standing orders, and issues of medical direction must be resolved before employment of a TEMS unit, which comprises EMTs, paramedics, and physicians who operate as part of a tactical law enforcement team. The training required of **EMT-Tacticals (EMT-Ts)** or SWAT-Medics involves strenuous physical activity under a variety of conditions. In a TEMS program, paramedics may be exposed to scenarios or skills, such as:

- Raids on clandestine drug laboratories
- Emergency medical care in barricade situations
- Wounding effects of weapons and booby traps
- Special medical gear for tactical operations
- Use of CS, OC, or other riot-control agents
- Blank-firing weapons
- Helicopter operations
- Pyrotechnics (smoke and distraction devices)
- Operation under extreme conditions, darkness, and psychological stress
- Fire fighting and hazmat operations

In summoning or working with a TEMS unit, follow the same general approaches and procedures recommended in Parts 2, 3, and 4 of this chapter. If you have not had exposure to such a unit, find out more about SWAT-Medics from local law enforcement officials or from sites sponsored by **CONTOMS** on NTOA on the internet.

✱ CONTOMS Counter-Narcotics Tactical Operations; program that manages the training and certification of EMT-Ts and SWAT-Medics.

EMS AT CRIME SCENES

The goal of performing EMS at a crime scene is to provide high-quality patient care while preserving evidence. NEVER jeopardize patient care for the sake of evidence. However, do not perform patient care with disregard for the criminal investigation that will follow.

Never jeopardize patient care for the sake of evidence.

EMS AND POLICE OPERATIONS

Often, police and EMS personnel respond to the same crisis but for different purposes. The EMS crew is there to treat patients and save lives. Law enforcement officers have come to protect the public and to solve a crime. These two goals sometimes create tensions between the two teams. For example, the police and the paramedics often work under different time constraints. As a paramedic, you have a limited time at the scene. The police, however, spend much more time at the location of a crime. In some major cases, the police can remain on the scene for days or weeks as they methodically look for evidence.

The key to cooperation between EMS and law enforcement personnel is communication. You should become aware of the nature and significance of physical evidence at a crime scene and, if possible, keep that evidence intact. Police, conversely, should be aware that your responsibility is to save lives. However, the police and the paramedics can usually reach a common ground. By preserving evidence, you can help the police to lock up a criminal before the person hurts or kills someone else. Remember: EMS personnel and law enforcement are really on the same side. Talk to each other.

Remember: EMS personnel and law enforcement are really on the same side. Talk to each other.

PRESERVING EVIDENCE

Be aware that anything on and around the patient may be evidence. You never know when a seemingly unimportant item may, in fact, be evidence that could help solve a crime. Whenever in doubt, save or treat an object as evidence.

Anything you touch, walk on, pick up, cut, wipe off, or move could be evidence. Developing an awareness of evidence can affect the way you treat patients. For example, if clothing must be removed, never cut through a gunshot or knife hole. Instead, try to cut as far away from the wound as possible. Instead of

Whenever in doubt, save or treat an object as evidence.

* **blood spatter evidence** the pattern that blood forms when it is splattered or dropped at the scene of a crime.

placing the cut cloth or garment in a plastic bag, put it in a brown paper bag so condensation does not build up and destroy body fluid evidence.

Also, when examining a patient, remember that you may be at risk. The victim may have a concealed weapon, such as a knife or gun. Or the person who committed the crime may be intent on finishing it and reappear to attack the patient. As always, your first responsibility is to protect yourself. If you have any suspicions at all about the patient or the safety of the scene, wait for the police to frisk the patient or secure the scene.

Types of Evidence

Although it is unrealistic to train EMS personnel in the details of police work, it is not unrealistic to ask them to develop an awareness of the general types of evidence that they may expect to encounter at a crime scene. Some of the main categories of evidence include: prints, blood and body fluids, particulate evidence, and your own observations at the scene.

Prints Prints include fingerprints, footprints, and tire prints. Of the three, fingerprints can be the most valuable source of evidence. As a paramedic, try not to disturb any fingerprint evidence that may be present. Second, do not leave behind your own fingerprints at a crime scene. The only way to achieve that is simply not to touch anything. Of course, this is impossible when treating a patient. However, you can and should minimize what you touch. If you must touch or move an item, remember to tell the police.

You will be wearing disposable gloves as part of infection control. These gloves prevent you from leaving your own fingerprints, but they will not prevent you from smudging existing prints. Again, touch as little as possible. Bring in only necessary equipment. The more equipment you have, the more evidence you have to disturb, including fingerprints. Also, scan the approach to the scene and the scene itself for footprints or tire prints and avoid disturbing them.

Blood and Body Fluids Blood and body fluids also give police a lot of information about a crime. Matching the DNA found in blood samples or other body fluids to the DNA of a suspect is nearly 100 percent accurate. Technologists need only a small sample to ascertain the genetic code. The way in which blood is splattered or dropped at the scene (called **blood spatter evidence**) provides yet other clues for police.

Preserving blood evidence can be performed in the following ways:

* Avoid mixing samples of blood whenever possible. Cross-contamination of blood will render blood evidence useless.
* Avoid tracking blood on your shoes. You will leave your own footprints, plus risk contaminating other blood evidence.
* If you must cut bloody clothing from a victim, place each piece in a separate brown paper bag. If the garment is wet, gently roll it in the paper bag to layer it. Place the entire contents in a second paper bag and then in a plastic bag for body fluid protection.
* Do not throw clothes stained with blood or other body fluids in a single pile or in a puddle of blood.
* Do not clean up or smudge blood spatters left at a scene.
* If you leave behind blood from a venipuncture, notify the police.
* Because blood can be a biohazard, ask the police whether the scene should be secured for evidence collection.

Particulate Evidence Particulate evidence, also known as microscopic or trace evidence, refers to evidence that cannot be readily seen by the human eye, such as hairs or carpet and clothing fibres. Minimal handling of a victim's clothes by EMS personnel may help preserve this evidence.

* particulate evidence such evidence as hairs or fibres that cannot be readily seen with the human eyes; also known as microscopic or trace evidence.

On-Scene Observations Everything that you and other members of the EMS crew see and hear can serve as evidence. Your observations of the scene will become part of the police record—and ultimately part of the court record. Be sure to look for and record the following information:

Everything that you and other members of the EMS crew see and hear can serve as evidence.

- Conditions at the scene—absence or presence of lights, locked or unlocked doors, open or closed curtains, and so on
- Position of the patient or victim
- Injuries suffered by the patient or victim
- Statements of persons at the scene
- Statements by the patient or victim
- Dying declarations
- Suspicious persons at, or fleeing from, the scene
- Presence and location of any weapons

If the victim is deceased by the time you arrive, any staff not immediately needed on the scene should leave to minimize the risk of disturbing evidence. If a gun is seen or found on the deceased victim, do not touch or move it unless it must be secured for the safety of others. Pick it up only as a last resort, and only touch it by the side grips or handles. The grips are coarse and will not generally leave good fingerprints. *Never* put anything into the barrel of the gun to lift or move it. The barrel of a gun can house the majority of the evidence used by the police—traces of gun powder, rifling patterns, and even flesh or blood.

Never put anything into the barrel of a gun to lift or move it.

Documenting Evidence

Record only the facts at the scene of a crime, and record them accurately. Use quotation marks to indicate the words of bystanders and any remarks made by the patient. Avoid opinions not relevant to patient care. If the patient has died, do not offer any judgments that might contradict later findings by the medical examiner. For example, a knife wound is not a knife wound until it is proven that a knife caused the laceration. Instead, describe the shape and anatomical location of the puncture or cut.

Record only the facts at the scene of a crime, and record them accurately.

Also, keep in mind the protocols, local laws, and ethical considerations in reporting certain crimes, such as child abuse, rape, elder abuse, or domestic violence. (For more on reporting abuse and assault see Chapter 44.) Finally, follow local policies and regulations regarding confidentiality surrounding any criminal case. Any offhand remarks that you make might later become testimony in a courtroom along with documents that you prepare at the scene.

SUMMARY

As a paramedic, you should be familiar with standards that influence ambulance design, equipment requirements, and staffing. You should also regularly complete all checklists regarding onboard equipment and essential supplies. Be aware of items that require routine maintenance or calibration as well as the expiration dates on all drugs. Keep in mind local safety requirements, and know how to report equipment problems or failures. Be familiar with the profile of a typical ambulance collision and to develop strategies for preventing it from occurring. Also, be aware of the issues and policies surrounding the staging and staffing of ambulances. Appreciate the conditions or situations that merit air medical transport and the safety issues involved in packaging the patient, selecting a landing site, and approaching the aircraft.

Every paramedic should be thoroughly familiar with the procedures used in a typical incident management system. You should be able follow these procedures at every multipatient, multiunit response—from the smallest incident to the largest. Expect to respond to several MCIs during your EMS career. A good preplan, regular use of the IMS, and MCI training will allow you to handle each event calmly and professionally.

Whenever you function in any phase of a rescue, you must be properly outfitted with protective equipment. You must also have training specific to the type of rescue. During the operational phases of a rescue, you must provide direct patient care and work with technical teams to ensure optimal patient management. Any paramedic assigned to rescue duties should have training in the care of patients who may require prolonged management.

Every member of an EMS team should be prepared to face the challenges of the hazmat incident. As with any EMS operation, the primary consideration is your own safety. You become useless at a hazmat incident if you become contaminated yourself.

Similarly, your first priority at any crime scene is your own safety. To protect your life and the lives of others, you need to develop a "crime scene awareness." Do not needlessly expose yourself to dangers better left to professional emergency medical personnel, such as SWAT-Medics. When you do treat the victim(s) at a crime scene, keep in mind that police and EMS personnel must work together to preserve the evidence. Touch only those items or objects that pertain directly to patient care.

DIVISION 2
PATIENT ASSESSMENT

CHAPTER 4

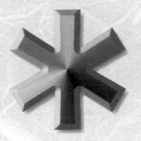

Therapeutic Communications

Objectives

After reading this chapter, you should be able to:

1. Define communication. (p. 219)
2. Identify internal and external factors that affect a patient interview. (pp. 219–221, 226–227)
3. Identify strategies for developing a rapport with the patient. (pp. 219–220)
4. Discuss open-ended and closed questions. (pp. 224–225)
5. Discuss common errors made when interviewing patients. (pp. 226–227)
6. Identify the nonverbal skills used in patient interviewing. (pp. 222–223)
7. Identify interview methods used to assess mental status. (pp. 224–225)
8. Discuss strategies for interviewing a patient who is not motivated to talk. (pp. 225, 227–228)
9. Describe the use of, and differentiate among, facilitation, reflection, clarifica-

tion, empathetic responses, confrontation, and interpretation. (p. 226)
10. Differentiate among strategies used for interviewing hostile and uncooperative patients. (pp. 225, 231)
11. Summarize developmental considerations that influence patient interviewing. (pp. 222, 225, 228–229)
12. Define the unique interviewing techniques for patients with special needs. (pp. 227–233)
13. Discuss cross-cultural interviewing considerations. (pp. 230–231)
14. Describe the basic principles of conflict resolution. (pp. 231–233)
15. Given several preprogrammed simulated patients, provide a patient interview using therapeutic communication. (pp. 219–233)

INTRODUCTION

Communication should be easy. After all, **communication** is only a matter of exchanging common symbols—written, spoken, or other kinds, such as signing and body language. However, as you know, even in the best circumstances, communication can be a challenge. EMS providers have a particularly difficult job of it because they must communicate with strangers who are in crisis.

As a paramedic, you must learn how to use every available strategy to make sure that you understand your patients and they, in turn, understand you. You also must be able to communicate well with the patient's relatives, bystanders, and other EMS providers. Strategies you will use include persistently paying attention to word choices, tones of voice, facial expressions, and body language. You will learn to minimize external and internal distractions and to adjust your personal communication style to fit each new situation, especially when dealing with children, elderly people, people of different cultures, and hostile people.

Helpful core traits for effective communication in EMS include a genuine liking for people, a sincere desire to be part of a helping profession, an understanding of human strengths and weaknesses, and **empathy,** or the ability to view the world through another's eyes while remaining true to yourself.

BASIC ELEMENTS OF COMMUNICATION

Communication consists of a sender, a message, a receiver, and feedback. First, the sender has to **encode,** or create a message; that is, she must write, speak, or otherwise place symbols common to both parties in an understandable format. Encoding may mean translating the message into another language, using words a child can understand, or writing the words on paper. The receiver then must **decode,** or interpret, the message, ideally with the same meaning the sender intended to convey. Finally, the receiver gives the sender **feedback** (a response to the message). If by way of this response, the sender believes the message was received accurately, both parties can congratulate themselves on communicating successfully.

Unfortunately, partial or complete failure to communicate occurs often. There are abundant reasons for this. In EMS, those reasons include the following:

- Prejudice, or lack of empathy, particularly in the paramedic toward the patient or situation
- Lack of privacy, which inhibits a patient's responses to questions
- External distractions, such as traffic, crowds, loud music, EMS radios, or TVs
- Internal distractions, or thinking about things other than the situation at hand

One way to minimize failure is to keep in mind that patience and flexibility are hallmarks of a good communicator.

TRUST AND RAPPORT

As a representative of EMS, you are granted a certain amount of the public's trust at each new emergency scene. You have to earn the rest by putting the patient and others at ease and by letting them know that you are on their side, you respect their comments, and you want to help. Little courtesies, such as asking the

---

✱ communication the exchange of common symbols—written, spoken, or other kinds, such as signing and body language.

Helpful core traits for effective communication in EMS include a genuine liking for people, a sincere desire to be part of a helping profession, an understanding of human strengths and weaknesses.

✱ empathy identification with and understanding of another's situation, feelings, and motives.

✱ encode to create a message.

✱ decode to interpret a message.

✱ feedback a response to a message.

Content Review

REASONS FOR FAILING TO COMMUNICATE
- Prejudice
- Lack of privacy
- External distractions
- Internal distractions

Patience and flexibility are hallmarks of a good communicator.

Effective communication begins and ends with trust and rapport.

patient her name and thereafter pronouncing it correctly, can help to accomplish this goal. So can recognizing and responding with compassion to signs of discomfort or suffering. Once trust is established, rapport follows.

With good rapport, the people you are serving will follow your lead, even if that means some pain (such as with a needle stick) and inconvenience (such as cancelling a trip to have a medical evaluation at the hospital). The people with whom you work also will be more motivated to do difficult and sometimes dangerous tasks. Remember that effective communication begins and ends with trust and rapport. Without them, your safety could be at risk.

PROFESSIONAL BEHAVIOURS

First impressions are crucial. What others see in you during the first few seconds of an encounter can lay the foundation for success or failure. The patient relies almost exclusively on visual input, and so your physical presentation—from facial expression to the appearance of your clothing—matters. Even though encounters with patients are typically brief, patients usually remember them for a very long time. Make sure your first impression is a positive one.

The elements of a good first impression involve all conventional professional standards:

- A clean, neat uniform that allows you to be easily identifiable as a paramedic
- Good personal hygiene, including clean, cut fingernails and inoffensive breath; avoiding use of colognes and perfumes
- Physical fitness
- An overall professional demeanour that is calm, capable, and trustworthy
- A facial expression that is open, interested, caring; avoiding expressions of disdain or disgust
- A confident (not arrogant) stance
- An appropriate gait; avoiding running or strolling
- Consideration for the patient, such as wiping your feet on the doormat before entering the residence

The next period of interaction with your patient is the time for obtaining in-depth information about the emergency and the patient's medical history. This may be called the **patient interview**. A good starting point is always to ensure the patient's privacy, which also minimizes inhibitions and distractions. It helps to be sure that lighting is adequate and noise is minimized. Equipment that might be alarming (such as needles) should be placed out of the patient's sight.

Other ways to help build the trust and rapport you need to conduct a patient interview include the following:

- *Introduce yourself, your partner, and other rescuers.* By introducing yourself and other rescuers, you break down barriers to communication. You are no longer a stranger but someone with a name who has come to help.
- *Get to the level of the patient.* After you introduce yourself, move so that you are in a position to talk with the patient eye to eye. When the patient is at a lower level than you, a barrier to communication exists; you are in a superior position. By moving to the patient's level (by sitting on a chair or kneeling, for example), you break down that barrier.

Make sure your first impression is a positive one.

Maintain professional behaviour not only on a call with a patient, but when you stop for a coffee as well!

Content Review

WAYS TO BUILD TRUST AND RAPPORT

- Use the patient's name.
- Address the patient properly.
- Modulate your voice.
- Use a professional but compassionate tone.
- Explain what you are doing and why.
- Keep a kind, calm expression.
- Use an appropriate style of communication.

patient interview interaction with a patient for the purpose of obtaining in-depth information about the emergency and the patient's pertinent medical history.

Content Review

HOW TO REMEMBER A NAME

- Say the name out loud three times.
- "See" the name in bold capital letters.
- "Feel" yourself writing the name.

- *Address your patient properly.* Use formal forms of address, such as "Mr." and "Mrs." or "Ms." as appropriate. Never call patients "honey," "dude," or any name other than their own. Also, be careful about shortening children's names. If a child is introduced to you as "Matthew," use that name, or ask the child if he goes by a nickname, such as "Matt."

- *Use your patient's name.* It is a powerful tool for forming a quick bond. A technique for remembering a name involves three steps: First, say the patient's name out loud three times in the first minute. Then, "see" the patient's name in your mind in bold capital letters. Finally, "feel" yourself writing the name in your imagination. Some people actually write the name on their paperwork, but this does not work as well as the mental imagery.

- *Modulate your voice.* Pay attention to your volume. Speak quietly and in low tones. If the patient is hard of hearing or difficult to control, speak up. Check your pitch; some people find it hard to hear high voices. Also, check your rate of speaking. Be especially aware that people in crisis may have difficulty taking in information at a normal rate, and so slow down.

- *Use a professional but compassionate tone of voice.* Avoid tones that portray sarcasm, irritation, anger, or other emotions that fail to serve the patient.

- *Explain what you are doing and why.* This helps ease your patient's anxiety, especially if she is in pain. For example, if you must immobilize a broken bone, explain that a splint will help prevent movement and more pain. Tell the patient that applying a splint may be painful, but once it is applied, the broken limb should be more comfortable. (Note: Never make false promises or false assurances. They violate your patient's trust.)

- *Keep a kind, calm facial expression.* Remember that facial expressions can reflect a wide variety of emotions and conditions, including relaxation, relief, pain, fear, anger, sorrow, and so on. No matter what the emergency, maintain a kind-looking poker face. It will convince others that you can handle things.

- *Use the appropriate style of communication.* There is a wide range to choose from. In general, patients will respond well to a calm, reassuring demeanour, but be prepared to use a tough, authoritative approach when needed. Also, if a situation requires you to be firm, be completely firm. Do not let your facial expression, for example, ruin the effect (such as one that says, "Gosh, I hope they believe me!").

At the end of a call, a final word or two can be very helpful, particularly after emotional calls. A "goodbye and good luck" can help bring the event to a close for the patient and family.

COMMUNICATION TECHNIQUES

GENERAL GUIDELINES

Patients generally respond to questioning in one of three ways: (1) They may pour out information easily, (2) they may reveal some things and conceal others that might be embarrassing or shameful, or (3) they may resist, hiding information from themselves and, therefore, from you. The patient who conceals infor-

Content Review

RESPONSES TO QUESTIONING

Patients may
- Pour out information easily.
- Reveal some things and conceal others.
- Resist responding.

To get the information you need, you must be consistently professional, nonjudgmental, and willing to talk about any concern the patient may have.

mation or resists giving it may be trying to maintain a certain image or may be fearful about how others will respond (perhaps with ridicule or rejection). To get the information you need, you must be consistently professional, nonjudgmental, and willing to talk about any concern the patient may have.

Nonverbal Communication

* **nonverbal communication** gestures, mannerisms, and postures by which a person communicates with others; also called *body language*.

Nonverbal communication, or body language, consists of gestures, mannerisms, and postures by which a person communicates with others. Your position within the environment and in relation to your patient is part of that language. Examples include the following:

Content Review

ELEMENTS OF NONVERBAL COMMUNICATION
• Distance
• Relative level
• Stance

* **open stance** a posture or body position that is relaxed and suggests confidence, ease, warmth, and attentiveness.

* **closed stance** a posture or body position that is tense and suggests negativity, discomfort, fear, disgust, or anger.

- *Distance* (Table 4-1). The socially acceptable distance between strangers is 1.2–3.5 m. A "comfortable" distance may be described as twice the length of a patient's arm. In most cases, paramedics are able to break social convention and quickly enter a patient's "intimate space" (0.5 m or less) because people intuitively understand the need for medical personnel to get "hands on" with them. However, if the patient stiffens or backs away from you, the best strategy may be to linger at a less threatening distance until you have built more trust and rapport.

- *Relative level.* A different message is sent to the patient each time you stand at her eye level, above it, or below it. Remaining at eye level indicates equality. Standing above or over the patient imparts an air of authority, but it also can be intimidating. Dropping below eye level indicates a willingness to let the patient have some control of the situation, a strategy that can be especially helpful when your patient is an elderly adult or a child.

- *Stance* (Figure 4-1). Arms extended, open hands, relaxed large muscles, and a nodding head characterize an **open stance**. A paramedic who has an open stance sends the message that she is confident and at ease. When it is safe to do so, use this stance to communicate warmth and attentiveness.

  A **closed stance** is just the opposite. In this position, arms are flexed or crossed tightly over the chest. The fists are clenched or a

Table 4-1 INTERPERSONAL ZONES

Zone	Distance	Characteristics
Intimate zone	0–0.5 m	Visual distortion occurs.
		Best for assessing breath and other body odours.
Personal distance, or "personal space"	0.5–1.2 m	Perceived as extension of self.
		No visual distortion.
		Body odours are not apparent.
		Voice is moderate.
		Much of patient assessment, and sometimes patient interviewing, may occur at this distance.
Social distance	1.2–3.5 m	Used for impersonal business transactions.
		Perceptual information is much less detailed than at personal distance.
		Patient interview may occur at this distance.
Public distance	3.5 m or more	Allows impersonal interaction with others.
		Voices must be projected.

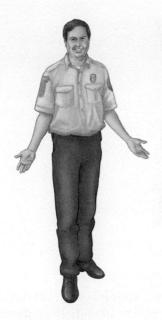

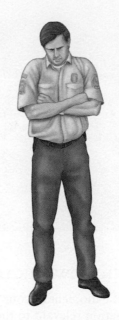

FIGURE 4-1A   An open stance.

FIGURE 4-1B   A closed stance.

finger may be pointing. The head may be shaking negatively. The body is square to the patient or, in some cases, may turn slightly away. This posture suggests disinterest, discomfort, disgust, fear, or anger and sends negative signals to the patient.

Watch your patient's body language, too. It can tell you how well communication is going. If the patient has a closed stance, you may need to change your approach.

Eye Contact

A powerful source of effective communication comes with eye contact. While you are interviewing the patient, use it as much as possible. (Always remove your sunglasses while working with patients.) Even when you are taking notes, look at the patient frequently. Eye contact is one way to send a message to your patient, whether it is a compassionate "I care about you" or a stern "settle down now." With eye contact, you can hold the attention of a patient so powerfully that your patient can feel you are helping her hang on in desperate circumstances.

Of course, using eye contact means that the other person is looking at you, too, which can be unnerving, especially if you are unfamiliar with this technique. If you feel uncomfortable, look at the bridge of the other person's nose for a bit of relief. Then, try direct eye contact again. Build this skill over time, and it will serve you well.

Compassionate Touch

Another communication skill is touching (Figure 4-2). The ability to hold a hand, touch an arm or shoulder, or even give a hug, in the right circumstances can yield information that would otherwise not be given. Some paramedics need to learn this skill the way they learn how to use an IV. That is, it can be awkward at first, but it is worth the effort. Nothing builds trust and rapport, or calms patients, faster than the power of touch. How effective it is depends on the patient's age, gender, cultural background, past experience, and current setting. Be careful to touch appropriately. There is a line between compassion and improper intimacy. Remember that as a paramedic, you must always carefully guard the integrity of the public's trust in you.

Nothing builds trust and rapport, or calms patients, faster than the power of touch.

FIGURE 4-2   Use an appropriate compassionate touch to show your concern and support.

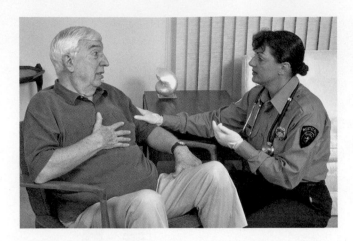

INTERVIEW TECHNIQUES

From the moment of your first contact with the patient, your job is to find out all information relevant to the present emergency. You need to identify the patient's chief complaint (the reason that 911 was called), find out the circumstances that caused the emergency, and determine the patient's condition. Much of this is accomplished by asking questions, observing the patient, and listening effectively.

Questioning Techniques

An important part of patient assessment is gathering information that is accurate, complete, and relevant to the present emergency. To begin, you must identify the patient's chief complaint. Although dispatch probably will have given you an idea of what the emergency is about, it is important for you to let the patient state the chief complaint in her own words. If you were to ask **leading questions** (ones that guide the patient's replies), such as "Are you having chest pain?" or "I see you've injured your arm. How does it feel?" you could easily miss a serious problem. Instead, ask **open-ended questions**: "What happened that led you to call 911?" or "What seems to be the problem?" They will allow your patient to respond in an unguided, spontaneous way. They also encourage patients who are reluctant to speak to describe their complaint in a way that might not be possible otherwise.

The patient's chief complaint should then drive the evolution of all other questions to be asked. For example, if your patient's chief complaint is chest pain, you are required to obtain answers to a specific set of questions. But instead of asking them as if you were reading a shopping list, individualize the process. For example, you would have to find out whether a patient with chest pain takes any medications. If your patient tells you that the chief complaint is "chest pain so bad even the nitroglycerine tablets aren't helping," your question about medications might be worded thus: "What medications do you take in addition to nitroglycerine?" This tells the patient you have been listening, which can yield a greater rapport. Other questioning techniques include the following:

* *Continue to ask open-ended questions.* They do not limit the patient's responses, which can help to reveal unexpected but important facts. For example, instead of asking a patient with abdominal pain "Did you have breakfast today?" which can be answered with either a "yes" or a "no," ask: "What have you eaten today?"
* *Use direct questions* when necessary. Direct questions, or **closed questions,** ask for specific information. ("Did you eat lunch? Does the

* **leading questions** questions framed to guide the direction of a patient's answers.

* **open-ended questions** questions that permit unguided, spontaneous answers.

* **closed questions** questions that ask for specific information and require only very short or yes-or-no answers. Also called *direct questions*.

abdominal pain come and go like a cramp, or is it constant?") These questions are good for three reasons: They fill in information generated by open-ended questions. They help answer crucial questions when time is limited. And they can help control overly talkative patients, who might want to tell you about their gall-bladder surgery in 1949 when the chief complaint now is a sprained ankle.

- *Do not ask leading questions.* Avoiding them means avoiding being taken down a path unrelated to the current emergency.

- *Ask only one question at a time, and allow for complete answers.* If you ask more than one question, the patient may not know which one to answer and may leave out portions of information or become confused.

- *Listen to the patient's complete response before asking the next question.* By doing so, you might find that you need to ask a question that is different from the one you were expecting to ask.

- *Use language the patient can understand.* In general, people do not understand medical terms. For example, you may need to use "pee" instead of "urine," or "breaths" instead of "respirations." However, be careful to avoid jargon and slang. Also, keep in mind that children are very literal and concrete minded. Never tell a child, for example, that you are going to "take" her blood pressure. Say instead that you are going to "measure" it.

- *Do not allow interruptions, if possible,* unless your partner or other EMS personnel need to give you patient care information of a critical nature. Interruptions will interfere with your patient's and your trains of thought. Interruptions also can cause you to miss information important to the patient's medical care.

Ask only one question at a time, and allow for complete answers.

Observing the Patient

Observe the patient during the interview. External signs, such as overall appearance (including clothing and jewellery) and other physical signs, may give you some indication of the patient's condition. Other clues you pick up may offer you a way to explore the patient's internal experiences, or mental status.

While you are interacting with the patient, observe her level of consciousness and body movements. Assess her rate and clarity of speech, her thinking, and her ability to pay attention, concentrate, and comprehend. You may be able to check the patient's orientation to person, place, and time, and her remote, recent, and immediate memories. Explore her mood and energy level, too. Watch for evidence of autonomic responses (sweating, trembling, and so on) and for unusual facial movements, such as a tic around the mouth, nose, or eyes. Note that lack of eye contact can suggest that the patient is shy, withdrawn, confused, bored, intimidated, apathetic, or depressed.

Many people do not cope well with being the centre of attention. Be aware of various defence mechanisms people may use so that you can be prepared to deal with them if necessary. For example, if your patient is self-grooming (fixing hair or straightening clothes), it may be that she needs some reassurance. If the patient keeps shifting focus away from your questions, back off for a bit and then return to the topic from a different angle.

If the patient is acting out and hostile, point out the behaviour in a professional manner, ask if the behaviour is intentional, let the patient know that such behaviour defeats the purpose of calling for help, and then name behaviours you would rather see. If there is any indication that the patient's hostility may threaten your safety or that of your crew, maintain distance and an exit path. (Additional information about hostile patients appears later in this chapter.)

Effective Listening and Feedback

Few people practise the art of listening well. Usually, they think about what they are going to say next while others are still talking to them. There may be less than a one-half second gap between speakers, and many people cannot even wait that long and instead finish others' sentences for them.

Listening is an active skill, not a passive one. It requires your complete attention, and it requires constant practice. In order to listen well, you must focus on the messenger. Stop doing other things. Discipline yourself to cease any internal dialogue that can distract or interrupt you mentally. Never finish the other person's sentences, and do not consider your response until the speaker has finished speaking. Allow some silence when the speaker has stopped.

Once the speaker has stopped talking, provide feedback to confirm that you have understood his message correctly. Feedback techniques include the following:

Content Review

FEEDBACK TECHNIQUES
- Silence
- Reflection
- Facilitation
- Empathy
- Clarification
- Confrontation
- Interpretation
- Explanation
- Summarization

- *Silence.* Give the patient time to gather her thoughts and add to what has been said.
- *Reflection.* To check your understanding and to reassure the speaker, echo her message back to her using your own words.
- *Facilitation.* Encourage the speaker to provide more information.
- *Empathy.* Let your body language show that you understand so that the patient feels accepted and more open to talking.
- *Clarification.* Ask the speaker to help you understand, when you need to eliminate confusion about what has been said.
- *Confrontation.* Help the patient focus on one particular factor of the interview.
- *Interpretation.* State your interpretation of the information; that is, link events, make associations, identify an implied cause, or draw conclusions.
- *Explanation.* Share factual or objective information related to the message.
- *Summarization.* Briefly review the interview and your interpretation of the situation. Ask open-ended questions, if needed, to allow the patient to clarify details.

Traps of interviewing, or common errors made when listening and providing feedback to patients, include the following:

- *Providing false assurances.* Never make any promises you cannot keep. For example, saying "everything will be all right" is a false reassurance.
- *Giving advice.* People call 911 because they are seeking advice, but the paramedic must be careful how it is conveyed. Saying "my opinion is that your chest pain should be evaluated at the hospital" is acceptable advice. Saying "I think you would be crazy not to be seen by a doctor" is not.
- *Authority.* Remember that EMS is not a power trip. Although paramedics are imbued with the power to do a difficult job, that power must never be used inappropriately. A paramedic provides a vital public service. Doing so correctly requires constant attention to protecting the public's trust and avoiding behaviours that might be interpreted as abuse of power.

- *Using avoidance language.* Avoidance language is "an unproductive conflict strategy in which a person takes mental or physical flight from the actual conflict," according to communication expert Joseph DeVito.[1] For example, a person who chooses to change the conversation rather than get into a discussion about something difficult may use avoidance language. If a paramedic does this, the patient's whole story may not be revealed.

- *Distancing.* When the paramedic is insensitive to distancing, she may stand too close or too far from patient to attain optimal rapport. Noticing the effects of distancing and adjusting accordingly is a hallmark of a good communicator.

- *Professional jargon.* Although it is necessary to make sure the patient knows what you are doing and why, it is unnerving for her to hear that you are going to "slip a line and jam a tube." Watch your language, and make sure you are speaking at your patient's comprehension level.

- *Talking too much.* Remember that listening is also a part of communication.

- *Interrupting.* As already discussed, good listening skills require you to wait until your patient answers you fully.

- *Using "why" questions.* The question "why" often steers a conversation toward blame: "Why did you put your hand in the lawn mower while it was running?" or "Why didn't you call for help three hours ago?" This type of question is counterproductive.

Demonstrating good listening and feedback skills on an emergency call is challenging. So many things are happening it can seem like a whirlwind. It may be necessary to apply monitoring equipment to the patient while you ask questions, for example. If this happens, reassure the patient by saying something like, "I know it seems overwhelming to you, but please understand that I am listening to your answers while I work."

PATIENTS WITH SPECIAL NEEDS

Patients generally are more than willing to answer your questions, though some will require more time and a variety of techniques. Note that difficult interviews stem from several sources. The patient's condition, including a developing cognitive impairment, may impact her ability to talk. The patient may be afraid to talk to you because of a psychological disorder, language or cultural difference, or even the difference between your ages. Or the patient intentionally may want to deceive you (to hide illegal drug abuse, for example).

Use the same techniques on a patient who is reluctant to talk to you as you would on any other patient, but use them in a slightly different way. For example, start your interview in the usual manner. If the patient does not respond to your questions, take time to develop a rapport by reviewing the reason that dispatch gave for the call. Ask open-ended questions. If unsuccessful, try direct questions, including ones that require only a yes-or-no response. Accept that you may not be able to obtain any elaboration or details about the facts. Provide positive feedback to any response the patient provides.

If the patient continues to be reluctant, be sure she understands your questions. Rule out language barriers and hearing difficulties. Once you know the patient can understand you, continue to ask questions about the critical information you need to know to progress with treatment. If you cannot get even

> **Content Review**
>
> **SOURCES OF DIFFICULT INTERVIEWS**
> - Patient's physical condition
> - Patient's fear of talking
> - Patient's intentions to deceive

---

[1] J. DeVito, *Essentials of Human Communication,* Third Edition (New York City: Longman, 1999).

this much, attempt to rule out pathology (disease) by asking family members or others at the scene how long the patient has been uncommunicative.

If you determine that pathology is not the cause, you may need to continue to build trust and rapport with the patient. One way to do this is to encourage the patient to ask you questions about your equipment, profession, medical care, or any topic that might start conversation. Model how you would like the patient to respond to your questions by answering her fully.

Further information on communicating with patients who require a special effort on your part follows. These patients include children and their parents, elderly people, people who are blind or deaf, people from other cultures, and people who are hostile or uncooperative.

Children

Effective communication with pediatric patients (infants, children, and adolescents) depends on their age. Have a good idea of what to expect at each stage of development so that your efforts to communicate can be appropriate.

In general, you can start by talking to the caregivers, then gradually approach the patient. Remember your body language. When dealing with younger children especially, it will help to get down to their eye level (Figure 4-3). Children pick up on anxiety easily and often take cues from what they observe, and so it is very important to stay calm. Introduce yourself, and use the child's name often. Be careful not to work silently.

Even if your own anxieties and the pressure of the medical requirements of the call are taxing your limits, talk! Tell the child everything: what you are looking at ("Now let's look at this arm . . .") and why it is important (". . . so we can be sure it's okay, too."). Explain your equipment, and if there is time, let the child see how the equipment works. Above all, explain what you intend to do, even to very young children. For example, you might say, "Alexander, I am going to make your leg hurt less by putting on this splint. I will need to make the leg move first, which might hurt some. But after that, it should be a lot better. Okay?" Never tell a child that something will not hurt when, in actuality, it will. Once you have lost the trust of a child, it is very difficult to regain it.

Most importantly, you must build trust. Once you have that, a child will put up with a lot. Giving a child a stuffed toy may be helpful. Also, be sure to move slowly, talk gently, explain everything, and be honest. To engage children, ask questions, and when you answer their questions, be sure not to talk down. Use straightforward language. Never try to hide the fact that something is wrong.

Never tell a child that something will not hurt when it will. Once you have lost the trust of a child, it is very difficult to regain it.

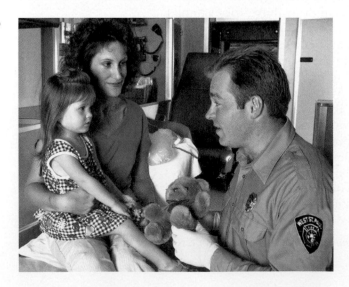

FIGURE 4-3 Getting down to patient's level can help improve communications on a pediatric call.

When something will hurt or will be at all uncomfortable, tell them. The more matter-of-fact and informative you can be, the better it is. If you are fair about the difficult parts and avoid springing nasty surprises, you will find greater overall co-operation. The need to be gentle whenever possible should be obvious.

Never try to hide the fact that something is wrong.

If a child is especially fearful, let her play with a toy or other object and then gradually increase contact. Do not be in a hurry to touch a child unless the situation is critical. Use plenty of eye contact and compassionate touch, too. Keep in mind that even if the child cannot understand you, your tone of voice is reassuring and your words and actions will be meaningful to the family and bystanders. Ask the child for feedback frequently, wait for an answer, and acknowledge that answer. Involve the child in decision making whenever possible. If the child is crying, do not take it personally, and do not tell her to stop. Instead, try saying, "Go ahead and cry until you don't want to cry any more." Lending control in this way can work wonders.

Be aware that young children are very literal. Word choice is important. As noted earlier, do not "take" a pulse, "measure" it. A blood-pressure cuff does not "squeeze," it "hugs." When one child was told that she would fly to the hospital, she started to cry. "I don't know how to fly," she wailed. Think about what you will say.

With pediatric patients, it is important to understand that caregivers, especially parents, may be very concerned and upset. Remember that you must manage them as well as your patient. Common responses include crying, emotional outbursts, anger, guilt, and confusion, which may be directed at you. Do not take it personally. You must build trust and rapport with the parents as well as with the child.

Sometimes, parents interfere with emergency care and must be separated from the child. Usually, however, it is most effective to let the parents stay and, if appropriate, even hold the child. No matter how parents behave, always treat them with courtesy, respect, and understanding. Avoid raising your voice. Tell them that you know they want help for their child. They need your support and understanding, too.

When possible, allow parents to remain with the pediatric patient.

Note that with younger children (ages one to six), most of your conversation will be with caregivers. Be aware that you are collecting information about the child's history from an adult's point of view, but do not put the caregiver on the defensive. Be careful to be nonjudgmental, especially if it appears that the child has not been provided with proper care or safety before your arrival. Be observant but not confrontational.

Elderly Patients

Be careful of your own prejudices with all special populations, but particularly with the elderly. Be respectful of them. Always use a formal mode of address, such as "Mr." and "Mrs." or "Ms." Speak slowly and clearly. Interviews might take longer because many older patients cannot process a lot of information quickly due to interfering physical disabilities and the fact that they can fatigue easily. Remember that the use of compassionate touch can be a welcome and important means of nonverbal support.

Always treat elderly patients with respect.

Give the elderly patient choices whenever possible. Take along their "living assists," such as walkers, hearing aids, and eyeglasses, and their books of phone numbers to facilitate reaching family or friends. Many elderly people are set in their ways and can be stubborn, but if you respect their dignity and do not rush them, you usually can build enough rapport to work with them effectively.

Patients with Sensory Impairment

Blind people as well as sighted patients whose injuries may require covering the eyes benefit from verbal communication. Tell them everything you are going to do before doing it. If you need to have them walk, lead them by letting them hold onto your bended arm. Use touch as a form of contact for reassurance.

Ask hearing-impaired and deaf patients about their preferred method of communication: lip reading, signing, or writing. Writing often is necessary—and the best method of communication—in the out-of-hospital environment. Always be sure your face is illuminated when you speak to patients who cannot hear. At night, also be sure that the deaf person who is trying to lip-read is not blinded by a flashlight. If the patient has some hearing, speak normally, and do not exaggerate your enunciation of words or use too much volume, which can distort sound. Be aware that many hearing-impaired patients will nod "yes," even if they do not hear what is said or asked, possibly in a misguided effort to be agreeable.

Language and Cultural Considerations

An emergency situation in which people of different cultures and languages must interact requires you to be especially compassionate. To accomplish this, you must understand that cultures vary. **Ethnocentrism,** or viewing your own life as the most desirable, acceptable, or best, and acting in a superior manner, will only hinder communication. You must imagine the additional fear and frustration a patient in crisis feels when trying to explain the emergency to a paramedic who cannot speak her language or understand her attitudes. To really empathize, you must be able to avoid **cultural imposition;** that is, avoid imposing on the patient your own beliefs, values, and patterns of behaviour.

In a transcultural situation in which your patient does not speak your language, you have the opportunity to make the experience less stressful by being caring and calm—and by finding an interpreter. Some important principles when using an interpreter are as follows:

* Allow children of immigrants to act as interpreters. If this occurs, remember to keep what you are saying at the appropriate age level.
* Recognize that the emergency may cause distressing emotions in the interpreter, especially if the interpreter is a child.
* Speak slowly.
* Phrase questions carefully and clearly.
* Address both the patient and the interpreter.
* Ask only one question at a time, and wait for a complete response.
* Understand that the information you receive may not be reliable.
* Have patience.

Cultural differences include more than just language differences. People of some cultures are more comfortable at a different distance when communicating than you are; some expect health-care workers to have all the answers to their illnesses; some treat ill or injured family members in different ways than yours. Asian, Aboriginal, Indochinese, and Arab people may consider direct eye contact impolite or aggressive and may therefore demonstrate respect to you by averting their eyes. The welts on a feverish Southeast Asian child may not be from abuse but rather from a folk practice known as "coin rubbing" or "coining," which many believe will draw out fever.

Understand that both you and the patient may bring cultural stereotyping to the situation. If either of you acts as if one culture is superior to the other, the situation could be ripe for problems. As with any call, create an appropriate professional relationship, but keep in mind that the rules about interpersonal space, eye contact, and touching may all be very different from those you know. As you can see, it is a good idea to study the various cultures typical to your area. Be open to the different ways of people, and do not act as if your way is the only correct way to manage things. There is no reason to impose your beliefs, values, and patterns of behaviour on others.

* **ethnocentrism** viewing your own life as the most desirable, acceptable, or best, and acting in a superior manner to another culture's way of life.

* **cultural imposition** the imposition of your beliefs, values, and patterns of behaviour on people of another culture.

Many cultures have established and accepted folk-medicine beliefs. Although these may be new to you, they are very important to those who believe in and practise them. If you work in an area with a concentration of a particular ethnic group, try to learn about the folk-medicine beliefs and practices of that group.

Hostile or Uncooperative Patients

There are times when you will need to build a rapport with someone who cannot or does not want you to. If this is the case, be sure you do not seem threatening. Avoid confrontation, but keep trying until you are successful. Use the same questioning techniques you usually use. Sometimes, patients open up if you clearly explain the benefits and advantages of cooperation. You also may be able to obtain the information you need from observing the scene and from questioning the patient's family, bystanders, or even law enforcement officers.

Set limits and establish boundaries with an uncooperative patient if necessary. If the patient is sexually aggressive, for example, clarify your professional role to the patient. Tell the patient in a way that you are certain she understands that you are there to provide emergency medical care. Be sure to document unusual situations, and ask witnesses to document their observations as well. In extreme cases, consider having a same-sex witness ride in the back of your ambulance or tape record all interactions.

If a patient is blatantly hostile or there is any hint that your safety is jeopardized, be sure to stay far enough away from the patient to be safe. Monitor her closely, and never leave the patient alone without adequate assistance. To prevent a hostile situation from getting worse, be sure to have an appropriate show of force (enough personnel to overpower the patient) if necessary. Remember, your personal safety is paramount. Always be sure you have a clear path to the nearest exit, and always position yourself so you can observe others entering or exiting the area. Know local protocols regarding the use of restraints and psychotropic medications. Do not hesitate to call for law enforcement backup if necessary.

Conflict Resolution

The Centre for Conflict Resolution at the Justice Institute of British Columbia defines conflict as the "actual or perceived opposition of needs, values, and interest between people resulting in unwanted stress or tension and negative feelings between disputants."

Consider the following situation:

> You arrive at a scene involving an assault. Police have secured the scene. Two young men are sitting on the ground, several metres from each other, both in handcuffs, and still yelling at each other. One has a large laceration over his left ear. The other has a black eye and is bleeding from the nose. You see a blood covered baseball bat three or four metres away. An officer tells you that they had a hard time separating the two of them. Your partner moves to the closer patient, and you assess the other. As you try to work, the two patients continue to yell and struggle. A police officer is anxious to separate the men and asks if one of the men could be moved to the ambulance to settle things down. Your partner tells the officer to back off, that she is in charge of this scene, and that her patient is not going anywhere. In moments, their voices are competing with the ongoing argument between the patients.

You may encounter conflict in many forms. Your call may be the result of conflict between your patient and others at the scene. You may find that your desired course of action is in conflict with what your patient wants to do. Your goals and protocols in dealing with a situation on a call may differ from the priorities of other responding agencies. Or you may disagree with your partner over stocking the kit or performing station duties. You may encounter stressful situations in crowded emergency departments or during implementation of new protocols that you have concerns about. In fact, conflict is an inevitable experience, as we all have different needs, values, and interests. Whether conflict develops into a negative condition depends on our emotional reactions to situations.

Conflict can come from a variety of sources that include structural issues, such as social concerns and policy constraints, or issues involving communication, relationships, interests, and values. The degree of conflict can be influenced by your approach and attitude, the nature of the conflict and the context in which it occurs, as well as the nature, approach, and previous relationships of the individuals who are involved.

The Centre for Conflict Resolution identifies five basic styles for approaching conflict (Figure 4-4). These approaches can be cooperative or adversarial and differ in their focus:

1. *Competing/Controlling:* The most adversarial approach, characterized by a focus on your own interests
2. *Avoiding:* Can be either cooperative or adversarial and is characterized by a focus away from conflict
3. *Accommodating:* Can be either cooperative or adversarial; is most focused on the other person and least on the self
4. *Compromising:* Also cooperative or adversarial, this style focuses on satisfying both parties, with a preference toward the self
5. *Collaborating:* Most cooperative style, it focuses on satisfying both parties to the greatest degree possible

We each have learned styles or preferences for dealing with conflict, but we can adapt our approach based on the situation in which we find ourselves. However, most people tend to use a dominant style when pressured.

In a conflict, we take a position that is at odds with the position of the other parties in the dispute. These positions represent our preconceived ideas of how the situation should be resolved. When conflict focuses on positions, the discussion tends to be framed in terms of who is "right" or "wrong" and is generally adversarial. Another way of approaching conflict is to identify what the conflict is really about. Discussion focused on issues rather than on positions is more likely to become collaborative. When the discussion explores the interests, or the reasons and rationale that support this position, the parties are more likely to achieve understanding and outcomes that are favourable to both parties.

FIGURE 4-4 Approaches to conflict resolution.

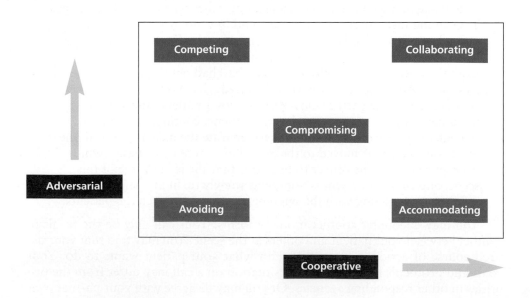

In general, collaborative approaches are best for meeting the needs of all parties. However, there are times and situations, such as during a technical extrication or in the middle of a complicated cardiac arrest when collaborative approaches are not suitable. Conflict is a part of many of our interactions; it is how we react to these situations that determine whether conflict escalates and becomes negative or moves toward resolution. Our own responses and approaches to conflict have a significant impact on how the situation develops.

Resolving conflict involves initiating efforts; framing the discussion; exploring the positions, issues, and interests involved with the goal of reaching understanding; and achieving closure. Closure may include agreeing to disagree, coming to a common understanding, developing a plan for next actions, or apologizing.

Within a prehospital setting, this process may occur quickly or over longer periods, depending on the situation. In the earlier scenario, obvious conflicts existed between the two patients and between your partner and the police officer. Your partner's position was that the patients had to be assessed and packaged before being moved. The police officer's position was that the two men had to be separated as quickly as possible. At issue was whether to move the patients before spinal precautions were in place. Your partner's interests were based on the history and mechanism of injury and the risk of moving a patient with potential spinal injuries. The police officer's interests were based on the potential for further violence while the two men remained near each other.

Your approach to the situation could be either adversarial (one or the other could "take control" of the scene and impose her position) or cooperative (finding a way to keep the two men from interacting with each other while assessment and treatment are completed). Resolving this particular situation is easier if you have previously established mutual trust and a rapport with the other emergency agencies in your area. Remember the importance of maintaining professional behaviour and effectively employing your full range of communication skills.

TRANSFERRING PATIENT CARE

When you arrive at the scene of an emergency, emergency medical responders (EMRs) may already be there. Before they transfer patient care to you, be sure to listen to their report carefully. Integrate the information they give you into the questions you ask your patient; she will trust you more if you show you have listened to your colleagues. Say something like: "The emergency medical responder said you felt dizzy before you fell today. Were there any other sensations you can remember?"

Once you arrive at the hospital, if the emergency department is busy, the receiving nurse or doctor may appear to be distracted. If this is true, important medical information could get lost. In noncritical circumstances, therefore, respectfully wait until the nurse or doctor looks at you. Then say, "Are you the person who will be listening to my handoff report?" If so, follow up with, "Are you ready to listen, or would you rather wait a moment?" Be sure to introduce the patient by name and to say goodbye to the patient before you leave.

∫UMMARY

The skills required to manage medical situations are obviously an important part of emergency care. Remember, much of the information you will gather from all your patients is extremely personal. You will need an enormous degree of sensitivity to recognize and respond to the signs of suffering in order to create an ideal, individualized process of communication.

CHAPTER 5

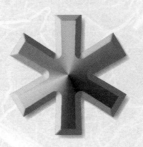

History Taking

Objectives

After reading this chapter, you should be able to:

1. Describe the techniques of history taking. (pp. 235–238)

2. Describe the structure and purpose of a comprehensive health history, and describe how to obtain one. (pp. 235–251)

3. List the components of a comprehensive history of an adult patient. (pp. 238–246)

INTRODUCTION

In the majority of medical cases, you will base your field diagnosis on patient history. Clearly, how you conduct the patient interview and the questions you ask will determine how much relevant medical information your patient reveals. In medical cases, obtaining an adequate history of your patient's **chief complaint,** recent illnesses, and significant past medical history is as important as, if not more important than, the secondary assessment. The information you gather will direct the secondary assessment and reveal clues to your patient's problem. Although we present the history by itself in this chapter, you will most likely conduct it simultaneously with parts of the secondary assessment.

The ability to elicit a good history is the foundation for providing good care to patients you have never met before. To conduct a good interview, you must gain your patient's trust in a very short time. Then, you must ask the right questions, listen intently to your patient's answers, and respond accordingly. In this chapter, we will discuss both the verbal and nonverbal components of taking a comprehensive medical history.

We present the medical history in its entirety, as a well-structured, yet flexible tool having several component procedures that are conducted in order. In reality, your patient's answers will alter the sequence of your questioning, and some of the information in this chapter is not readily adaptable to prehospital emergency medicine. As you gain clinical experience, you will learn which components of the history are appropriate to the particular situations you encounter. Whether your patient is critical or stable, the situation determines the length and completeness of the interview. For example, complicated medical cases require a close investigation of your patient's chief complaint and past history. Trauma cases are generally sudden events not precipitated by medical conditions and require a modified approach to history taking.

The interview is the focal point of your relationship with your patients. It establishes the bonding necessary for effective and efficient patient care. By asking a series of well-designed questions, you begin to build a profile of your patient. You also should have a good understanding of their problems and a list of causes (**differential field diagnosis**) to explain their signs and symptoms. Often, learning about your patient's history, medications, and even lifestyle will reveal clues to your final field diagnosis.

✱ chief complaint the reason the ambulance was called.

You must ask the right questions, listen intently to your patient's answers, and respond accordingly.

✱ differential field diagnosis the list of possible causes for your patient's symptoms.

ESTABLISHING PATIENT RAPPORT

Your patients will form an opinion about you within the first minute, and so you must establish a positive rapport quickly. This is not always easy. The situation, the patient, and the conditions will affect your ability to establish rapport. You can do several things, however, to improve patient rapport. By asking the patient the right questions, you will discover their chief complaint and their symptoms. By responding to them with empathy, you will win their trust and encourage them to discuss their problems with you. Their answers will also help you decide which areas require in-depth investigation and on which body systems to focus.

SETTING THE STAGE

Sometimes, you will assess a patient at a long-term care facility. If your patient's chart is available, as in a nursing home or extended care facility, review it before conducting the interview. Quickly note the patient's age, sex, race, marital status, address, and occupation. The insight into your patient's life experiences that you begin developing with this information may provide subtle clues to help steer your questioning. Determine any past medical problems or previous referrals for the same condition. Note any treatments rendered and their effects. On emergency scenes, review the emergency medical responder's call sheet. Look for the chief complaint, a brief history including a current medication list, and vital signs. Be careful not to let your patient's chart or past medical history, or someone else's first impression, bias your possible field diagnoses. Always accept such information gratefully, but briefly reconfirm it with the patient, and conduct your interview with an open mind.

If possible, conduct the interview in a quiet room, alone, with no distractions. Since you are asking your patient to divulge very intimate information, privacy encourages open communication. It should be a place where you and your patient can comfortably talk about his current problem and past experiences. Unfortunately, on emergency calls, you conduct the patient interview in a variety of settings beyond your control, from the kitchen floor to a busy street corner or a crowded bus. Often, the back of your ambulance is where your patient will disclose important personal information to you. Some patients, however, will still be reluctant to reveal intimate information to a nonphysician in the emergency setting. Paramedics are often surprised at the hospital when their patients tell a different story to the physician in the emergency department. To maximize your chances of obtaining a good history, practise the following techniques for developing better patient rapport.

LANGUAGE AND COMMUNICATION

Use appropriate language. Nothing distances you from your patient more quickly than sophisticated medical terminology. "Have you ever had a heart attack?" is better than "Have you ever had an MI?" Effective communication means connecting with your patient. Most of your patients will not understand medical terms. Use an appropriate level of questions, but do not appear condescending. Other barriers to communication include cultural differences, language differences, deafness, speech impediments, and even blindness. When you encounter such obstacles, try to enlist someone who can communicate with your patient and act as an interpreter. An alternative is to adopt a conservative approach toward assessment, field diagnosis, and treatment.

Listening is an important part of the interview. The old saying, "Listen to your patients; they will tell you what is wrong," explains why it is crucial for a skilled clinician to be a good listener. Listen closely to what your patients tell you. Be careful not to develop tunnel vision based on dispatch information. Begin your assessment without any preconceived notions about your patient's injuries or illnesses. Also, watch for subtle clues that your patient may not be telling the truth. For example, your patient tells you that the chest pain went away, but his facial expressions and body language suggest otherwise. Developing good communication skills takes time and practice.

Avoid working your way in strict order down any prearranged list of questions (such as those in this chapter). Use these lists as a guide only. Listen to your patients, and watch for clues to important signs, symptoms, emotions, or other factors. Then modify your questions to follow those clues. The following practices promote **active listening**.

Facilitation Maintain sincere eye contact, use concerned facial gestures, and lean forward while you listen. Such cues as "Mm-hmm," "Go on," or "I'm listening" all help your patient open up. Sometimes, strategic silence is also helpful.

Be careful not to let your patient's chart or past medical history, or someone else's first impression, bias your possible field diagnoses.

✱ active listening the process of responding to your patient's statements with words or gestures that demonstrate your understanding.

Content Review

ACTIVE LISTENING SKILLS
Facilitation
Reflection
Clarification

Reflection Repeat your patient's words. This encourages him to provide more details. Just make sure not to disturb his train of thought. For example:

> *Patient:* I can't breathe.
> *You:* You can't breathe?
> *Patient:* No, it feels like I can't take in a full breath because my chest hurts.
> *You:* Your chest hurts, too?
> *Patient:* Yes, it started this morning when I was working in the yard. I usually take a Nitro but I'm all out.

This simple reflection encouraged the patient to reveal facts about a history of heart disease. If the paramedic had merely investigated the chief complaint of dyspnea, discovering its true cause may have taken longer. Since the primary problem is not always the chief complaint, allowing your patient to take the lead is sometimes advantageous.

Clarification In crises, patients often cannot clearly describe what they feel. They will use vague, general words. Do not hesitate to ask for clarification. For example:

> *You:* Do you have any allergies?
> *Patient:* Yes, the last time I took penicillin I had a bad reaction.
> *You:* Can you describe the reaction?
> *Patient:* Well, I got itchy all over with a rash.
> *You:* Did you have any difficulty breathing or feel as if you were choking?
> *Patient:* Oh, no, just the itching and rash.

By asking for clarification you distinguish between a simple allergic reaction and life-threatening anaphylaxis.

TAKING A HISTORY ON SENSITIVE TOPICS

Paramedic students normally have difficulty questioning their patients about embarrassing, sensitive, or very personal topics, such as sexual activities, death and dying, physical deformities, bodily functions, and domestic violence. Even though you may feel uneasy discussing these matters, you may learn important information about your patient's illness. To become more comfortable dealing with these subjects, watch experienced clinicians discuss them with their patients. Familiarize yourself with and practise some opening questions on sensitive topics that both put your patient at ease and encourage him to talk about it. If a particular area makes you most uncomfortable, attend a lecture or seminar and learn how professionals deal with this subject daily. Make the unfamiliar familiar, and it will seem less imposing.

Let us look at two sensitive topics—physical violence and sexual history. Your patient may not want to reveal a history of physical abuse. You should consider it when any of the following conditions are present:

- Injuries that are inconsistent with the story given
- Injuries that embarrass your patient
- A delay between the time of the injury and seeking help
- A past history of "accidents"
- Suspicious behaviour of the supposed abuser

To earn your patient's trust, try to make him feel that the problem is common and that you understand the reasons. For example, you can ask your female patient, "Sometimes when husbands and wives argue a lot, it leads to physical fighting. I noticed you have some bruises. Can you tell me what happened? Did someone hit you?" With active listening techniques, such questioning will help establish a rapport that encourages open communication.

Taking a sexual history can be the most embarrassing and uncomfortable experience for an inexperienced health-care provider. The sexual history is normally taken later during the history but can be a part of the present illness or past history, depending on your patient's chief complaint. For example, if your patient complains of a genitourinary problem, the sexual history becomes important during questioning about the present illness. If your patient has a history of a sexually transmitted disease, then the sexual history is relevant to the past history. Whenever you begin the sexual history, it is helpful to prepare your patient with introductory statements and questions like, "Now I need to ask you some questions about your sexual health and activity. It may help me determine the cause of your problem and provide better care for you. This information will be strictly confidential. May I begin?" If your patient consents, proceed as follows: "Are you sexually active? Have you had sex with anyone in the last six months? Do you have more than one partner? Do you have sex with men, women, or both? Do you take precautions to avoid infection or unwanted pregnancy? Do you have any problems or concerns about your sexual function?" This may seem very uncomfortable for the beginning paramedic, but with time and clinical experience, you will develop a sense of where and when these questions are appropriate. It is critical that you remain calm, objective, and nonjudgmental, regardless of how your patient answers.

THE COMPREHENSIVE PATIENT HISTORY

This section presents the components of a comprehensive patient history in a systematic order. In practice, you will ultimately select only those components that apply to your patient's situation and status. For example, if you conduct preemployment secondary assessment for a company, you may use the entire form. However, if you respond to a gasping patient with acute pulmonary edema, you will focus on the present illness. Common sense and clinical experience will determine how much of the following history to use.

PRELIMINARY DATA

For documentation, always record the date and time of the assessment. Determine your patient's age and gender. This provides a starting point for the interview and establishes you as the interviewer. Who is the source of the information you receive about your patient? Is it the competent patient, a spouse, a friend, or a bystander? Are you receiving a report from an emergency medical responder (EMR), the police, or another health-care worker? Do you have the medical record from a transferring facility? After you have gathered the information, you should establish its reliability, which will vary according to the source's knowledge, memory, trustworthiness, and motivation. Again, reconfirm the information with the patient if possible. This is a judgment call based on your experience. For example, if the patient information you received from a particular EMR has been accurate in the past, you probably will trust him again. Conversely, if the nurse at a physician's office has repeatedly provided you with erroneous information, you probably will doubt his accuracy.

THE CHIEF COMPLAINT

The history begins with an open-ended question about your patient's chief complaint. The chief complaint is the pain, discomfort, or dysfunction that caused your patient to request help. In a medical case, it may be a woman's call for help because she has chest pain. In a trauma case, it may be a bystander's call for assistance to a "man down" or a police officer's reporting an injury in an auto collision. Your patient may have called because of more than one symptom. It is important to begin with a general question that allows your patient to respond freely. For example, "Why did you call us today?" or "What seems to be the problem?" Avoid the tunnel vision that often biases paramedics who focus on dispatch information that may or may not accurately describe the situation. As you interview and assess your patient, the chief complaint becomes more specific.

The chief complaint differs from the **primary problem**. Although the chief complaint is a sign or symptom noticed by the patient or a bystander, the primary problem is the principal medical cause of the complaint. For example, your patient's chief complaint may be leg pain, while the primary problem is a tibia fracture. When possible, report and record the chief complaint in your patient's own words. For example, "I am having a hard time breathing" is better than "the patient has dyspnea." For the unconscious patient, the chief complaint becomes what someone else identifies or what you observe as the primary problem. In some trauma situations, for instance, the chief complaint might be the mechanism of injury, such as "a gunshot to the chest," or "a fall from 10 m."

THE PRESENT ILLNESS

Once you have determined the chief complaint, explore each of your patient's complaints in greater detail. Be naturally inquisitive when exploring the events surrounding these complaints. A practical template for exploring each complaint follows the mnemonic OPQRST-ASPN, an acronym for *Onset, Provocation, Quality, Region/Radiation, Severity, Time, Associated Symptoms,* and *Pertinent Negatives*. This line of questioning provides a full, clear, chronological account of your patient's symptoms.

Onset Did the problem develop suddenly or gradually? What was your patient doing when the symptoms started? In medical emergencies, investigate your patient's activities at the time of, or shortly before, the signs or symptoms developed. In some cases, especially trauma, you may have to gather information from a few weeks before the onset of symptoms. For example, the signs and symptoms of a subdural hematoma may not appear until weeks following an injury. Was the patient exercising or exerting himself, or at rest or sleeping? Was he eating or drinking? If so, what? In trauma cases, ensure that a medical problem did not cause the accident. For example, the sudden onset of an illness, such as a seizure or syncope, may have caused a fall.

Provocation/Palliation What provokes the symptom (makes it worse)? Does anything palliate the symptom (make it better)? In many illnesses, certain factors such as motion, pressure, and jarring may increase or decrease pain, discomfort, or dysfunction. Does eating, movement, exertion, stress, or anything else provoke the current problem? Positioning may also be a factor. Your patient may want to curl up and lie on his side to reduce abdominal pain. Your congestive heart failure patients will sit straight upright to ease respiration. They also may sleep with several pillows raising their upper body to relieve paroxysmal nocturnal dyspnea (PND), a sleep-disturbing breathing difficulty caused by fluid that accumulates in the lungs when they are supine. Ask your patient how breathing affects the discomfort. Deep breathing may increase the pain in a patient with acute abdomen pain. A patient with pleuritic or rib-fracture pain will not breathe deeply, whereas breathing may not affect the pain of angina. Any patient with respiratory pain will breathe with shallower but more frequent breaths.

If your patient took a medication shortly before you arrived, its effect or lack of effect may help determine the problem. Such drugs as bronchodilators, hypoglycemic agents, antihypertensives, and anticonvulsants are commonly prescribed and taken at home. Investigate any medication used to relieve a problem, and note its effectiveness. Ask about any activity, medication, or other circumstance that either alleviates or aggravates the chief complaint.

Quality How does your patient perceive the pain or discomfort? Ask him to explain how the symptom feels, and listen carefully to the answer. Does your patient call the pain crushing, tearing, oppressive, gnawing, crampy, sharp, dull, or otherwise? Quote the descriptors in your report.

Region/Radiation Where is the symptom? Does it move anywhere else? Identify the exact location and area of pain, discomfort, or dysfunction. Does your patient complain of pain "here," while holding a clenched fist over the sternum, or does he grasp the entire abdomen with both hands and moan? If your patient has not done so, ask him to point to the painful area. Identify the specific location, or the boundary of the pain if it is regional.

✱ **tenderness** pain that is elicited through palpation.

Determine if the pain is truly pain (occurring independently) or **tenderness** (pain on palpation). Also, determine if the pain moves or radiates. Localized pain occurs in one specific area, while radiating pain travels away from the source, in one, many, or all directions. Evaluate moving pain's initial location and progression and any factors that affect its movement.

✱ **referred pain** pain that is felt at a location away from its source.

Note any pain that may be referred from other parts of the body. **Referred pain** is felt in a part of the body away from the source of the disease or problem. The heart and diaphragm are two areas that most commonly produce referred pain. Cardiac problems, such as myocardial infarction or anginal pain, are usually referred to the left arm, with occasional referral to the neck, jaw, and back. Pain associated with irritation of the diaphragm (most commonly blood in the abdomen of the supine patient) generally is referred to the clavicular region.

Severity How bad is the symptom? Severity is the intensity of pain or discomfort felt by your patient. Ask the patient how bad the pain feels, and then have him compare it with other painful problems he has experienced. Sometimes, a patient can describe the severity of the pain on a scale of 1 to 10, with 10 being the worst pain he has ever felt. Also, notice the amount of discomfort your patient's condition causes. How easy is it to distract your patient from his concern over the pain? Is your patient very still and resistive to your touch? Is he writhing about? The answers should give you a good idea of the intensity of your patient's pain.

Time When did the symptoms begin? Is a symptom constant or intermittent? How long does it last? How long has this symptom affected your patient? For several days, hours, or just a few minutes or seconds? When did any previous episodes occur? How does this episode's length vary from earlier ones?

Associated Symptoms Other symptoms commonly associated with the chief complaint in certain diseases can help in your field diagnosis. For example, if the chief complaint is chest pain, ask, "Are you short of breath? Are you nauseated? Have you vomited? Are you dizzy or lightheaded?" The presence of these symptoms would help support a field diagnosis of cardiac chest pain.

Pertinent Negatives Are any likely associated symptoms absent? Their absence is as important to the field diagnosis as their presence because they help rule out a particular disease or injury. Note any element of the history or secondary assessment that does not support a suspected or possible field diagnosis. For example, it is significant if your patient who complains of chest pain denies shortness of breath, nausea, and lightheadedness.

THE PAST HISTORY

The past medical history may provide significant insights into your patient's chief complaint and your field diagnosis.

The past medical history may provide significant insights into your patient's chief complaint and your field diagnosis. Look in-depth at your patient's general state of health, childhood and adult diseases, psychiatric illnesses, accidents or injuries, surgeries, and hospitalizations. They may reveal general or specific clues that will help you correctly assess the current problem. Your patient's condition, the situation, and time constraints will determine how much information you can and should gather on the scene. For example, asking about childhood diseases may not be relevant for your acute cardiac or trauma patient.

General State of Health How does your patient perceive his general state of health?

Childhood Diseases What childhood diseases did your patient have? Did he have mumps, measles, rubella, whooping cough, chickenpox, rheumatic fever, scarlet fever, or polio? Again, this line of questioning's relevance depends on the patient and the situation.

Adult Diseases Does your patient have diabetes? Does he have a history of heart disease, breathing problems, high blood pressure, or similar conditions? A preexisting medical problem may contribute to your patient's current problem or influence his care during the next few hours. To discover significant preexisting medical problems, ask if your patient has recently seen a physician or been hospitalized. If so, for what conditions? If you discover a preexisting problem, investigate its effects on your patient. When did the problem last affect him? Is your patient on any special diets or prescribed medications or restricted in activity? Even with the trauma patient, do not forget that a medical problem may have led to an accident or may complicate the effects of trauma. Obtain the name of your patient's physician, since it may be helpful to the emergency department staff.

Psychiatric Illnesses Does your patient have a history of mental illness? Has he ever been diagnosed with depression, mania, schizophrenia, or other problems? Is your patient being treated for a mental illness? If so, what medications is he taking? Has your patient ever had thoughts of suicide or attempted suicide? Tailor these questions for patients you suspect have a mental illness.

Accidents or Injuries Has your patient ever had a serious accident or injury requiring hospitalization? Has he had a previous injury that could be a factor in the current problem? For example, a seemingly minor head injury one week ago may now present as a subdural hematoma in your unconscious elderly patient. Keep this line of questioning to relevant information only. An old football injury or childhood laceration is probably not influencing your patient's chest pain and respiratory distress today. But his pneumonectomy (surgical removal of a lung) probably is the reason for the absence of lung sounds on the right side.

Surgeries or Hospitalizations Has your patient had any other hospitalizations or surgeries not already mentioned? Again, these may offer some insight into your probable field diagnosis. For example, your patient is an 85-year-old man with a long history of congestive heart failure and no history of chronic lung disease. He suddenly presents with severe difficulty in breathing and with audible wheezing. You should suspect the obvious—a cardiac problem.

CURRENT HEALTH STATUS

The current health status assembles all the factors in your patient's present medical condition. Here, you try to gather information that completes the puzzle surrounding your patient's primary problem. Look for clues and correlations among the various sections of this part of the history. For example, your patient is a heavy smoker, has many allergies to inhaled particles, works in a coal mine, and frequently uses bronchodilating medications. Your patient now complains of shortness of breath and expiratory wheezing. He is probably having an exacerbation of his chronic lung disease.

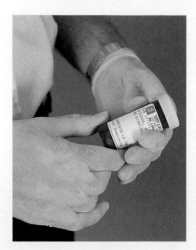

FIGURE 5-1   You should take your patient's medications with you to the hospital when practical.

Current Medications Is your patient taking any medications? These include over-the-counter drugs, prescriptions, home remedies, vitamins, and minerals. If so, why? Your patient's explanation may not be medically accurate, but it may help determine underlying conditions. For example, your 65-year-old patient tells you she takes a "water pill." You can safely assume she takes a **diuretic** and has a history of renal or cardiac problems. A medication not taken as prescribed may be responsible for the current medical problem—possibly due to under- or overmedication. A recently prescribed medication may cause an allergic or untoward (severe and unexpected) reaction. It also may be out of date and no longer effective. Even for trauma, emergency department personnel will need to know what medications your patient is taking. For example, if your patient takes warfarin, an anticoagulant, it would interfere with the normal clotting process and actually promote bleeding. If practical, bring your patient's medications to the hospital (Figure 5-1).

Allergies Does your patient have any known allergies, especially to penicillin, the "caine" family (local anesthetics), tetanus toxoid, and narcotics? These agents are occasionally given in emergency situations. What type of reaction did your patient have to the medication? For example, was it just a mild allergic reaction with a rash and itching or localized swelling, or was it anaphylactic shock? Knowledge of your patient's allergies may prevent additional complications during the emergency department visit, especially if your patient becomes disoriented or unconscious during transport. If your patient is short of breath with wheezing, ask about environmental allergies. In cases of possible anaphylaxis, ask about allergies to drugs, to such foods as shellfish, nuts, and dairy products, and to insect bites and stings.

Last Oral Intake Knowing what your patient has eaten or drunk may help explain the present problem. For example, an altered level of consciousness in a patient with diabetes is explained when you find out that the patient has forgotten to eat after taking insulin. You may also find out with this line of questioning that the patient has taken too little or too much of a medication. For the patient who may require surgery, this is important information for the hospital.

Tobacco Does your patient use tobacco? If so, how (cigarettes, cigars, pipe, smokeless, or other), how much, and for how long? To quantify a smoking history, note the number of packs smoked per day and the number of years the patient has been smoking.

Alcohol, Drugs, and Related Substances Alcohol and drugs are often contributing factors in, if not the primary cause of, your patient's medical problems. Your job is not to pass judgment but to gather data that will help direct your patient's medical treatment. Remaining nonjudgmental will aid you in your questioning. Start with a general question, such as "How much alcohol do you drink?" If you suspect a drinking problem may be a factor, you can use the CAGE questionnaire (an alcoholism screening instrument) to determine the presence of alcoholism. Reserve this line of questioning for the chronic patient in a controlled setting. It would be inappropriate in a bar with an unruly, intoxicated patient.

The CAGE Questionnaire

Have you ever felt the need to **c**ut down on your drinking?

Have you ever felt **a**nnoyed by criticism of your drinking?

Have you ever had **g**uilty feelings about drinking?

Have you ever taken a drink first thing in the morning as an **e**ye-opener?

Two or more "yes" answers suggest alcoholism and further lines of inquiry.

Ask about blackouts, accidents, or injuries that happened while drinking. Also, ask about alcohol-related job losses, marital problems, and arrests while under the influence of alcohol. Similarly, ask about drug use. For example, "Do you use marijuana, cocaine, heroin, sleeping pills, or painkillers? How much do you take? How do these drugs make you feel? Have you had any bad reactions?" As your patients realize that you are not judging their substance abuse, they may feel more comfortable telling you about their patterns of use.

Diet Ask about your patient's normal daily intake of food and drink. Perhaps your 78-year-old retiree just moved to a home without air conditioning and underestimated the increased fluid loss due to sweating. He did not realize he needed to increase his daily fluid intake, and now he presents weak and dizzy from dehydration. Are there any dietary restrictions or supplements? Ask specifically about his use of foods with stimulating effects, such as coffee, tea, cola drinks, and other beverages containing caffeine. For example, your 23-year-old patient with a rapid heart beat (200 beats per minute) drinks continuous cups of coffee each morning at his highly stressful job.

Screening Tests Ask about certain screening tests that may have been done for your patient. Some examples include a purified protein derivative (PPD) test for suspected tuberculosis, Pap smears and mammograms for female problems, stool testing for occult blood, and cholesterol tests. Record the dates of the tests and their results.

Immunizations Ask your patient about immunizations for such diseases as tetanus, pertussis, diphtheria, polio, measles, rubella, mumps, influenza, hepatitis B, and pneumonia. For example, ask the parent of a child suspected of epiglottitis whether the child had the hemophilus influenza B vaccine. The H-flu is a common cause of epiglottitis in children.

Sleep Patterns Ask your patient what time he normally goes to bed and arises. Does your patient take daytime naps? Does he have problems falling asleep or staying asleep?

Exercise and Leisure Activities Does your patient exercise regularly or lead a sedentary existence? Sometimes, your patient's lifestyle will support your field diagnosis.

Environmental Hazards Ask about possible hazards in the home, in school, and at the workplace. For example, your patient may live or work in an area with high levels of toxic substances. Many health problems can be traced to these environmental causes.

Use of Safety Measures In a motor-vehicle accident, did your patient use a seat restraint system? Was it a lap and shoulder belt, or a lap belt only? Were all passengers belted in? Did the air bag deploy? Such information aids you and the emergency department staff in determining the extent of damage caused by a particular mechanism of injury. For bicycle, in-line skate, and skateboard injuries, ask about the use of helmets and knee and elbow pads.

Family History Since many disease processes are hereditary, the medical history of immediate family members is important. In the nonemergency setting, you may explore deep into the family tree and chart the medical history of grandparents, parents, aunts, and uncles. In the emergency setting, learning that your 45-year-old patient with chest pain had a father and brother who both died of heart attacks in their late forties is important information. Look for a family history of diabetes, heart disease, hypercholesterolemia, high blood pressure, stroke, kidney disease, tuberculosis, cancer, arthritis, anemia, allergies, asthma, headaches, epilepsy, mental illness, alcoholism, drug addiction, and any symptoms like your patient's.

Since many disease processes are hereditary, it is important to learn the medical history of immediate family members.

Home Situation and Significant Others Who lives at home with your patient? Ask him about his home life—or lack of one. Ask about friends, family, support groups, and loved ones. Find out if your patient has a support network and whom it includes. Who takes care of your patient when he needs help? Loneliness and isolation may complicate your patient's physical symptoms.

Daily Life Ask your patient to describe a typical day. When does he get up? What does he do first? Then what? Such questions reveal a lot about your patient's state of mind and general wellness. Is he busy, active, and motivated to get up in the morning? Does the patient merely exist from the time he awakens and go through life with no purpose or direction? Is he under high levels of stress from morning to night in a job that requires him to take his problems home with him? Find out what kind of life your patient leads. It may reveal a lot about the illness.

Important Experiences Ask about your patient's upbringing and home life growing up. How much schooling does he have? Was he in the military? What kinds of jobs has he held? What is his financial situation? Is your patient married, single, divorced, or widowed? What does he do for fun and relaxation? Is your patient retired or looking forward to retirement? Again, the answers give you a broader picture of your patient.

Religious Beliefs Some religions forbid certain treatments and have guidelines regarding the management of illness and injury. For example, some forbid whole blood transfusions. Knowing your patient is guided by these beliefs can help you understand and care for him better. These questions require some expression of sensitivity, or it might be best to ask broadly if your patient has any limitations in medical care.

The Patient's Outlook Find out what your patient thinks and how he feels about the present and future.

REVIEW OF SYSTEMS

* **review of systems** a list of questions categorized by body system.

The **review of systems**, sometimes called a functional inquiry, is a series of questions designed to identify problems your patient has not already mentioned. It is a system-by-system list of questions that are more specific than those asked during the basic history. Again, the patient's chief complaint, condition, and clinical status determine how much, if any, of the review of systems you will use. For example, if your patient complains of chest pain, you may want to review the respiratory, cardiac, gastrointestinal, and hematological systems. If your patient complains of a headache, you may want to review the **HEENT** (head, eyes, ears, nose, and throat), neurological, peripheral vascular, and psychiatric systems. Let your patient lead you through the history. The following sampling includes a few of the many questions that you might ask.

* **HEENT** head, eyes, ears, nose, and throat.

General What is your patient's usual weight, and have there been any recent weight changes? Has he had weakness, fatigue, or fever?

Skin Has your patient noticed any new rashes, lumps, sores, itching, dryness, colour change, or changes in nails or hair? Could cosmetics or jewellery have caused these problems?

Head, Eyes, Ears, Nose, and Throat (HEENT) Has your patient had headaches or recent head trauma? How is his vision? Does he wear glasses or contact lenses? When was his last eye exam? Has your patient experienced any of the following: pain, redness, excessive tearing, double vision, blurred vision, spots, specks, flashing lights? Has he ever had glaucoma or cataracts? How is his hearing? Does he use hearing aids? Has your patient ever experienced ringing in the ears (**tinnitus**),

* **tinnitus** the sensation of ringing in the ears.

vertigo, earaches, infection, or discharge? Does he have frequent colds, nasal stuffiness, nasal discharge, hay fever, nosebleeds, sinus problems? Does he wear dentures? When was his last dental exam? Describe the condition of the teeth and gums. Do his gums bleed? Does he get a sore tongue, dry mouth, frequent sore throats, or hoarseness? Does your patient have lumps or swollen glands? Has he ever had a goitre, neck pain, difficulty swallowing, or stiffness?

Respiratory Has your patient ever had wheezing, coughing up blood (**hemoptysis**), asthma, bronchitis, emphysema, pneumonia, TB, or pleurisy? When was his last chest x-ray? Is he coughing now? If so, can you describe the sputum?

✱ **hemoptysis** coughing up blood.

Cardiac Has your patient ever had heart trouble, high blood pressure, rheumatic fever, heart murmurs, chest pain or discomfort, palpitations, shortness of breath (**dyspnea**), shortness of breath while lying flat (**orthopnea**), or peripheral edema? Has he ever been awakened from sleep with shortness of breath (**paroxysmal nocturnal dyspnea**)? Has he ever had an ECG or other heart tests?

✱ **dyspnea** the sensation of having difficulty in breathing.

✱ **orthopnea** difficulty in breathing while lying supine.

✱ **paroxysmal nocturnal dyspnea** sudden onset of shortness of breath at night.

Gastrointestinal Has your patient ever had trouble swallowing, heartburn, loss of appetite, nausea/vomiting, regurgitation, vomiting blood (**hematemesis**), indigestion? How often does he move his bowels? Describe the colour and size of his stools. Have there been any changes in his bowel habits? Has he had rectal bleeding or black, tarry stools, hemorrhoids, constipation, diarrhea? Has your patient had abdominal pain, food intolerance, excessive belching, or passing of gas? Has he had jaundice, liver or gallbladder problems, or hepatitis?

✱ **hematemesis** vomiting blood.

Urinary How often does your patient urinate? Has he ever had excessive urination (**polyuria**), excessive urination at night (**nocturia**), burning or pain while urinating, blood in the urine (**hematuria**), urgency, reduced calibre or force of urine flow, hesitancy, dribbling, or incontinence? Has he ever had urinary tract infection or stones?

✱ **polyuria** excessive urination.

✱ **nocturia** excessive urination at night.

✱ **hematuria** blood in the urine.

Reproductive—Male Has your patient ever had a hernia, discharge from or sores on the penis, testicular pain or masses? Has he ever had a sexually transmitted disease? If so, how was it treated?

Reproductive—Female At what age did your patient have her first menstrual period? Describe the regularity, frequency, duration, and amount of bleeding of her periods. When was her last menstrual period? Does she bleed between periods or after intercourse? Has she ever had difficulty with her period (**dysmenorrhea**) or premenstrual tension? At what age did she become menopausal? Were there symptoms or bleeding? Has she ever had any vaginal discharge, lumps, sores, or itching? Has she ever had a sexually transmitted disease? If so, how was it treated? How many times has she been pregnant? How many deliveries? Any abortions (spontaneous or induced)? Some health-care personnel use the G-P-A-L system to document a patient's history of pregnancy:

✱ **dysmenorrhea** menstrual difficulties.

Gravida	How many times pregnant?
Para	How many viable births?
Abortions	How many abortions?
Living	How many living children?

Has she ever had complications of pregnancy? Does she use birth control? If so, what type? If postmenopausal, is she on hormone replacement therapy?

Peripheral Vascular Has your patient ever had intermittent calf pain while walking (**intermittent claudication**), leg cramps, varicose veins, or blood clots?

✱ **intermittent claudication** intermittent calf pain while walking that subsides with rest.

Musculoskeletal Has your patient ever experienced muscle or joint pain, stiffness, arthritis, gout, or backache? Describe the location or symptoms.

Neurological Has your patient ever experienced any of the following: fainting, blackouts, seizures, speech difficulty, vertigo, weakness, paralysis, numbness or loss of sensation, tingling, "pins and needles," tremors, or other involuntary movements?

Hematological Has your patient ever been anemic? Has he ever had a blood transfusion? If so, did he have a reaction to it? Does your patient bruise or bleed easily?

Endocrinological Has your patient ever had thyroid problems? Did he ever experience heat or cold intolerance, or excessive sweating? Does he have diabetes? Has your patient ever had excessive thirst, hunger, or urge to urinate?

Psychiatric Is your patient nervous? Is he under much stress and tension? Has he ever been depressed? Has he ever thought of committing suicide?

SPECIAL CHALLENGES

No matter how long you practise as a paramedic, some patients will present with special circumstances that challenge your skills. Your ability to deal with them will improve with time and practice.

SILENCE

Silence can become very uncomfortable if you are impatient. Why has your patient suddenly become silent? This question has no single answer. Silence can have many meanings and many uses. It may result from an organic brain condition that prevents the patient from forming thoughts. Or it may be due to dysarthria (difficulty in speaking due to muscular impairment). Maybe he is just collecting his thoughts or trying to remember details. Or maybe the patient is deciding whether he trusts you. He might be clinically depressed, or perhaps, he simply deals with situations by being quiet.

What do you do during the silence? Stay calm, and observe your patient's nonverbal clues. Is he in pain? Is he scared? Is your patient on the verge of becoming hysterical or combative, or is he about to cry? You can encourage him to continue speaking by confronting him with your perceptions. For example, "I see you are obviously very upset about this. Do you want to talk about it?" If you sense your patient is not responsive to your questions, perform a brief orientation exam. Speak to him in a loud voice, and call him by name. Shake the patient gently if he does not respond. If this does not elicit a response, assume a neurological problem, and proceed accordingly.

Sometimes, your behaviour might have caused the silence. Are you asking too many questions too quickly? Have you offended your patient? Have you frightened him? Have you been insensitive? Have you failed to respond to your patient's needs? If your patient suddenly becomes silent, try to determine why, what is happening, and what you should do about it.

OVERLY TALKATIVE PATIENTS

The patient who rambles on can be just as frustrating to deal with as the one who will not talk at all. Why is your patient talking so fast and so much? Some patients react to stress this way. Maybe he has a lot to say. Maybe he needs someone to talk to; some lonely patients will take any opportunity to communicate with another human being. What can you do in the emergency setting when time is scarce? This problem has no perfect solution. You can lower your goals and accept a less comprehensive history. You can briefly give your patient free rein.

You can focus on the important areas and ask closed-ended questions about them. You can interrupt him frequently and summarize what he says. Above all, try not to become impatient.

PATIENTS WITH MULTIPLE SYMPTOMS

Patients often present with multiple complaints. For example, your elderly patient may present you with a barrage of symptoms from an extensive medical history. Your challenge is to discover the chief complaint and why he called you today. If he complains of symptoms that suggest multiple disease states, the challenge is compounded. In these types of cases, you must sort through a multitude of information quickly and recognize patterns that lead you to a correct field diagnosis.

Some patients will answer "Yes" to every question you ask. They have every symptom you mention; although possible, this phenomenon is not probable. Your patient might simply misunderstand or be trying hard to cooperate; it is more than likely he has an emotional problem and requires a psychosocial assessment. Document your findings on your prehospital care report and request a psychological referral. Asking the patient what single complaint led him to call for help today often helps.

ANXIOUS PATIENTS

Anxiety is a natural reaction to stress. People who face serious illness or injury can be expected to exhibit some degree of anxiety. Sometimes, this manifests itself as simple nervousness, tenseness, sweating, or trembling. Some patients will fall silent, while others will ramble. Still others may exhibit anxiety attacks marked by a rapid heart rate, nausea and vomiting, chest pain, and shortness of breath. When you detect signs of anxiety, encourage your patient to speak freely about it. For example, you can say, "I see you are concerned about this. Do you want to talk about it?"

PATIENTS NEEDING REASSURANCE

Appropriate reassurance is a cornerstone of patient care. You must be careful, however, not to be overly reassuring or to prematurely reassure your anxious patient. It is natural to say, "Relax, everything is going to be all right. We are going to take care of you and get you to the hospital. Just relax and you will be all right." But your patient may have anxiety about something of which you are not aware. For instance, if your chest pain patient is anxious, you might naturally assume he is apprehensive about dying. In reality, he may be anxious about something entirely different. Your patient may be embarrassed about these anxieties, and instead of helping him deal with them, you have helped him cover them up. Now he may decide you are not interested in what is really bothering him and block further communication. Listen carefully to your patient before offering reassurance.

ANGER AND HOSTILITY

You will often encounter angry patients or their families. They might be angry for many reasons. Your patient is sick, perhaps dying. The family is anticipating a loss. Often, family members will lash out at the easiest target—you. Sometimes, you cannot do anything quickly enough or well enough for them. Understand that their anger is a natural part of the grieving process and they may be merely venting their frustration. Unfortunately, you find yourself at the receiving end of their outbursts. Try to accept their feelings without getting defensive or angry in return.

INTOXICATION

Dealing with belligerent, intoxicated patients challenges even the most experienced paramedic. These patients are irrational, they disrupt your control of the scene, and they rarely allow you to examine them. First and foremost, make sure your environment is safe. If your patient acts violently, call for the police before attempting any interaction. As you approach your patient, introduce yourself and offer a handshake. Avoid any challenging body language or remarks. Appear friendly and nonjudgmental, but always stay alert for a potential violent outburst. If your patient is shouting or cursing, do not try to get him to stop or to lower his voice. Listen to what your patient says, not how he says it, and try to understand the situation before making a clinical judgment. Sometimes, a genuine offer of a place to sit will help calm an agitated, intoxicated person. Then, you can begin your assessment.

CRYING

Sometimes, your patients will cry. This can make any paramedic uncomfortable. Crying is just another form of venting, an important clue to your patient's emotions. Accept it as a natural release, and do not try to suppress it. Be patient, allow your patient to cry, and then offer a supportive remark. Quiet acceptance and supportive remarks will open the lines of communication once your patient composes himself.

DEPRESSION

* **depression** a mood disorder characterized by hopelessness and malaise.

Depression is a common problem in medicine. It is also commonly misdiagnosed or ignored. It often presents with such symptoms as insomnia, fatigue, weight loss, or mysterious aches and pains. Depression is potentially lethal, and so you must recognize its signs and evaluate its severity just as you would chest pain or shortness of breath. Ask whether your patient has ever thought about committing suicide, is currently thinking about suicide, has the means to commit suicide, and has ever attempted it. The more exact and precise the suicide plan, the more apt your patient is to carry it out.

SEXUALLY ATTRACTIVE OR SEDUCTIVE PATIENTS

Occasionally, you will encounter a patient who is attracted to you or to whom you are attracted. These feelings are natural. The key is not to allow these feelings to affect your behaviour. Always keep your relationship professional. If necessary, clearly tell any patient who behaves seductively that you are there on a professional basis, not a personal one. Afterward, determine if how you dressed, what you did, or what you said led your patient to get the wrong impression about your relationship. Did you send the wrong signals? Whenever possible, always have a partner or another trustworthy person with you to avoid any accusations of improper behaviour or touching.

CONFUSING BEHAVIOURS OR HISTORIES

* **dementia** a deterioration of mental status that is usually associated with structural neurological disease.

* **delirium** an acute alteration in mental functioning that is often reversible.

You may encounter a patient whose story you just cannot follow. No matter what you ask, the answers leave you confused and frustrated. You cannot seem to develop a clear picture about your patient's problems. In fact, the answers do not even seem to make any sense. For example, you ask, "When did your headache begin?" and he answers, "My head feels like a squirrel." In these cases, the problem is most likely psychotic (mental illness) or organic (**dementia** or **delirium**). Also, consider head injury or other physiological conditions, such as stroke.

Many psychotic patients live and function in their communities, with varying degrees of success. Some will provide an accurate past history, while others will not. If your patient's behaviour seems distant, aloof, inappropriate, or even bizarre, suspect a mental illness, such as schizophrenia. It may be helpful to focus your assessment on this patient's mental status, with special emphasis on thought, perceptions, and mood.

Delirium and dementia are disorders relating to cognitive function. Delirium is common in the acutely ill or intoxicated patient; dementia occurs more frequently in the elderly. These patients often cannot provide clear, accurate histories. Their descriptions of their symptoms and their accounts of how things happened will be vague and inconsistent. They may appear inattentive to your questions and hesitant in their answers. They may even make up stories to fill in the gaps in their memories. In these cases, do not spend too much time trying to get a detailed history because you will only become more frustrated. Focus on the mental status assessment, with special emphasis on level of response, orientation, and memory. For a more detailed discussion of these problems, see Chapter 38 on psychiatric and behavioural emergencies.

LIMITED INTELLIGENCE

You can usually obtain an adequate history from a patient with limited intelligence. Do not assume that he will not be able to provide accurate information concerning his current or past medical status. Also, do not overlook obvious omissions because your patient appears to be giving you a good story. Try to evaluate your patient's education and mental abilities. If you suspect severe mental retardation, obtain the patient's history from family or friends. Above all, show a genuine interest in your patient, and try to establish a positive relationship. Communication can still happen.

LANGUAGE BARRIERS

Few things are more frustrating than responding to an automobile accident with several patients who speak a language you do not understand. It is almost impossible to get an accurate history of the event. In these cases, try to locate an interpreter. Sometimes, a family member speaks both languages and is willing to translate for you. Often, however, family members cause more confusion by paraphrasing what the patient and you are saying. Instead of hearing your patient's exact words, you hear the translator's version, and the true meanings become vague. Do not waste time using your broken foreign language from high school because you will invariably confuse everyone involved.

HEARING PROBLEMS

The challenge of communicating with a hearing-impaired person is much like that of overcoming a language barrier. Some options, however, afford a degree of flexibility. You can try handwritten questions, but they can be time consuming. Sign language is effective if the patient practises it and you find a proficient interpreter. If your patient reads lips, you must modify your communication techniques accordingly. Always face him directly in a well-lit setting, and speak slowly in a low-pitched voice. Avoid covering your mouth and trailing off the end of your sentences. If your patient has one good ear, use that to your advantage. If he wears a hearing aid, make sure it is working. If he has eyeglasses, make sure he wears them. Augment your speech with hand gestures and facial expressions.

FIGURE 5-2 If the patient cannot provide useful information, gather it from family members or bystanders.

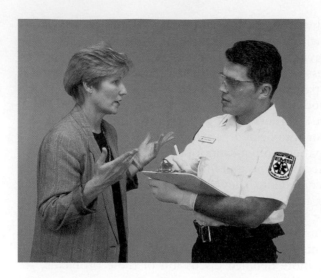

BLINDNESS

Blind patients present special problems. They need you to identify yourself immediately, since they cannot see your uniform. Always announce yourself, and explain who you are and why you are there. If possible, take your patient's hand to establish a personal contact and to show him where you are. Remember that nonverbal communications, such as hand gestures, facial expressions, and body language, are useless in these cases. Your voice is your only tool for effective communication.

TALKING WITH FAMILIES OR FRIENDS

You will often encounter patients who cannot give you any useful information. In these cases, find a third party who can augment the patient history and offer a useful adjunct to the patient's answers (Figure 5-2). The typical case is the postictal patient who cannot describe his seizure activity to you. Another example is learning from a friend that your patient's spouse died in an automobile accident just three weeks ago. Now you better understand why your patient appears depressed and suicidal. Make sure that patient confidentiality is a priority when you accept personal information from a family member, friend, or bystander. Patient assessment is a process of comprehensive history and secondary assessement.

SUMMARY

This chapter dealt with taking a good history. Although it presented the patient history in its entirety, common sense will determine which parts are appropriate for a given situation. Most of a paramedic's work is patient contact. It is making a connection with people in crisis. Patients most often comment on the attitudes of their paramedics. How well did they relate to them? Did they make them feel at ease? Did they care for them? Patients rarely comment on a paramedic's technical skills. Top-notch paramedics are technically skillful and treat all their patients with dignity and compassion. This begins with the history taking.

Good patient interaction can lead to good patient outcomes, improved patient satisfaction, and better adherence to treatment. As a paramedic, you have the first opportunity to treat your patient when he enters the health-care world. Let the first impression of the health-care industry be your caring, compassionate, professional demeanour. Conducting effective and efficient interviews and communicating with your patient are essential to good medical practice. Medical interviewing is a basic clinical skill that must be learned and practised, much like airway management.

CHAPTER 6

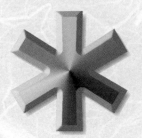

Physical Assessment Techniques

Objectives

After reading this chapter, you should be able to:

1. Define and describe the techniques of inspection, palpation, percussion, and auscultation. (pp. 254–258)
2. Describe the evaluation of mental status. (pp. 319–321)
3. Evaluate the importance of a general survey. (pp. 266–273)
4. Describe the examination of the following body regions, differentiate between normal and abnormal findings, and define the significance of abnormal findings:
   - skin, hair, and nails (pp. 274–279)
   - head, scalp, and skull (p. 280)
   - eyes, ears, nose, mouth, and pharynx (pp. 280–289)
   - neck (pp. 289–291)
   - thorax (anterior and posterior) (pp. 291–296)
   - arterial pulse, including rate, rhythm, and quality (pp. 296–300)
   - jugular venous pressure and pulsations (pp. 296–300)
   - heart and blood vessels (pp. 296–300)
   - abdomen (pp. 300–301)
   - male and female genitalia (pp. 301–303)
   - anus and rectum (pp. 303–304)

Continued

Objectives Continued

- peripheral vascular system (pp. 314, 316–318, 301–305)
- musculoskeletal system (pp. 304–305)
- nervous system (p. 318)
- cranial nerves (pp. 321–324)

5. Describe the assessment of visual acuity. (pp. 280, 282)
6. Explain the rationale for the use of an ophthalmoscope and an otoscope. (pp. 264, 283–284)
7. Describe the survey of respiration. (pp. 259–261, 292–296)
8. Describe percussion of the chest. (pp. 293, 294, 296)
9. Differentiate the percussion notes and their characteristics. (pp. 256–257)
10. Describe the special examination techniques related to the assessment of the chest. (pp. 291–296)

11. Describe the auscultation of the chest, heart, and abdomen. (pp. 293–299, 300–301)
12. Distinguish between normal and abnormal auscultation findings of the chest, heart, and abdomen and explain their significance. (pp. 293–299, 300–301)
13. Describe the special techniques of cardiovascular examination. (pp. 296–300)
14. Describe the general guidelines of recording examination information. (pp. 338–339)
15. Discuss the examination considerations for an infant or child. (pp. 333–338)

PHYSICAL ASSESSMENT APPROACH AND OVERVIEW

Although patient assessment formally starts with the history, the physical assessment actually begins when you first set eyes on your patient.

Patient assessment approaches differ from one EMS system to another. Generally, you perform an initial, or primary assessment, followed by a more in-depth secondary assessment. The secondary assessment consists of the history, which is covered in the previous chapter, vital signs, and a physical assessment. Although assessment of a medical patient formally starts with the history, the physical assessment actually begins when you first set eyes on your patient. On meeting her, you immediately assess her general appearance (degree of distress), level of consciousness, breathing effort, and skin colour. If you initially use touch as a reassuring gesture, you can also assess skin condition and peripheral pulses. Your physical assessment continues throughout the history as you ask questions and observe your patient's body language, facial expressions, and general demeanour. Thus, you cannot draw an exact dividing line between the history and the physical assessment. In emergency street medicine, the two usually occur simultaneously.

The purpose of the physical assessment is to investigate areas that you suspect are involved in your patient's primary problem.

The purpose of the physical assessment is to investigate areas that you suspect are involved in your patient's primary problem. As we covered the entire history in the previous chapter, we present the entire physical assessment in this one. Again, if you practise in a setting other than the prehospital setting, such as conducting preemployment physicals for a company, you might perform the entire physical assessment outlined here. On an emergency run, you limit the assessment to only those aspects that you decide are appropriate. Practice and clinical experience will dictate your ability to apply the skills you learn in this section to real situations.

ASSESSMENT TECHNIQUES

Four techniques—inspection, palpation, auscultation, and percussion—are the foundation of the formal physical assessment. Each can reveal information essential to a comprehensive patient assessment.

Inspection

★ inspection the process of informed observation.

Inspection is the process of informed observation (Figure 6-1). A simple, noninvasive technique that clinicians often take for granted, it is also one of their most valuable tools in appraising patient condition. With a keen eye, you can evaluate your patient's condition in great detail.

FIGURE 6-1 Inspect your patient's body for signs of injury or illness.

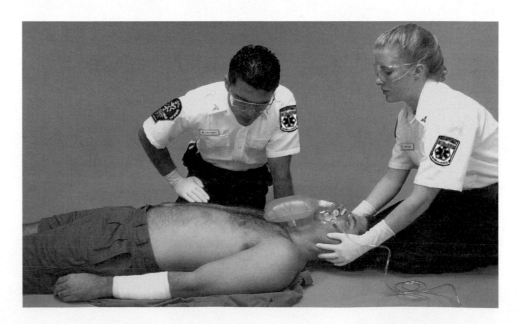

Inspection begins when you first meet your patient and continues while you take the history. Often, this first impression forms the basis for your history because you will judge your patient's clinical status immediately. Note how she presents herself. Is your patient conscious and alert or unconscious and flaccid? What is the level of distress: mild, moderate or severe? Is she lying on the floor, sitting upright, or limping badly on one foot? Is she breathing normally or gasping for each breath? You can learn a great deal about your patient's neurological, musculoskeletal, and respiratory systems just by careful observation. Watch for changes in emotional and mental status throughout the history and physical assessment.

During the formal physical assessment, consciously evaluate each body area, looking for discoloration, unusual motion, or deformity. Pay special attention to areas where you most expect to find signs and where the patient complains of symptoms. For example, if your patient struck her chest against a bent steering wheel, you would expect to see chest wall abnormalities. Remember that you may not notice the skin colour changes that follow a significant contusion until after your patient arrives at the emergency department.

Effective inspection depends on good lighting, adequate time, and a curiosity for looking beyond the obvious. During your inspection, draw on your past clinical experiences to identify the signs of illness and injury. Knowing what you are looking for is essential. Do not hurry. Give yourself enough time to inspect and then to process what you see. Inspection is an ongoing process that should not end until you transfer your patient to emergency department staff. Finally, while respecting your patient's modesty and dignity, never allow clothing to obstruct your assessment.

Palpation

Palpation is usually the next step in assessing your patient, although sometimes you will inspect and palpate your patient simultaneously. **Palpation** involves using your sense of touch to gather information. With your hands and fingers, you can determine a structure's size, shape, and position. You also can evaluate its temperature, moisture, texture, and movement. You can check for growths, swelling, tenderness, spasms, rigidity, pain, and crepitus (Figure 6-2). When you become skilled at this procedure, you can detect a distended bladder, an enlarged liver, a laterally pulsating abdominal aorta, or the position of a fetus.

Certain parts of your hands and fingers are better than others for specific types of palpation. For example, the pads of your fingers are more sensitive than

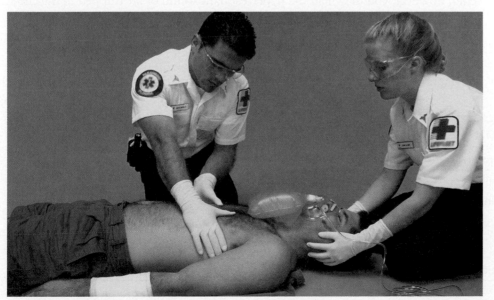

FIGURE 6-2 Palpate with the pads of your fingers to detect masses, fluids, and crepitus.

Content Review

PHYSICAL ASSESSMENT TECHNIQUES
- Inspection
- Palpation
- Percussion
- Auscultation

the tips for detecting position, size, consistency, masses, fluid, and crepitus; therefore, you would use them to palpate lymph nodes or rib fractures. The palm of your hand is better for sensing vibrations, such as fremitus. Because its skin is thinner and more sensitive, the back of your hand or fingers is better for evaluating temperature.

Palpation may be either deep or light. You control its depth by applying pressure with your hand and fingers. Since deep palpation may elicit tenderness or disrupt tissue or fluid, you should always perform light palpation first. Use light palpation to assess the skin and superficial structures. Press in approximately 1 cm. Apply the same gentle pressure you use to feel a pulse. Too much pressure dulls your sensitivity and can injure your patient.

To assess visceral organs, such as those in the abdomen, use deep palpation. Apply pressure by placing the fingers of the opposite hand over the sensing fingers and gently pressing in about 4 cm. This will increase your sensitivity to any masses, guarding, or other abdominal pathology. Feel for areas of warmth that might reflect injury before significant edema or discoloration occurs. Observe how your patient responds with facial expressions when you palpate tender areas. Even if your patient is unconscious, she may respond to pain with facial expressions or with purposeful or purposeless motion.

Palpation begins your physical assessment of your patient. Three common sense tips will help make it therapeutic and respectful. Keep your hands warm, keep your fingernails short, and be gentle to avoid discomfort or injury to your patient.

Percussion

Percussion is the production of sound waves by striking one object against another. In this technique, you strike a knuckle on one hand with the tip of a finger on the opposite hand. The impact causes vibrations that produce sound waves from 4 to 6 cm deep in the underlying body tissue. We hear these sound waves as percussion tones. The density of the tissue through which the sound must travel determines the degree of percussion. The denser the medium, the quieter is the tone. The tone's resonance or lack of resonance indicates whether the underlying region is filled with air, air under pressure, fluid, or normal tissue. Listen to each sound and evaluate its meaning (Table 6-1).

Move across the area that you are percussing and compare sounds with what you know to be normal. For example, in the chest, you expect to hear the resonant sound of a healthy lung filled with air and tissue. In a pneumothorax or emphysema, however, you may hear the hyperresonant sound of air trapped in the chest. In a hemothorax, you may hear the dull sound of blood in the same area.

Percussion is simple. Place one hand on the area of the body you want to percuss. Use a finger of that hand (usually the middle finger) as the striking surface. Sharply tap the distal knuckle of that finger with the tip of your other middle finger (Figure 6-3). The tap should come from snapping the wrist, not the forearm or

---

To make palpation therapeutic and respectful, keep your hands warm, keep your fingernails short, and be gentle.

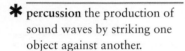

✱ percussion the production of sound waves by striking one object against another.

Table 6-1 PERCUSSION SOUNDS

Sound	Description	Intensity	Pitch	Duration	Location
Tympany	Drum-like	Loud	High	Medium	Stomach
Hyperresonance	Booming	Loud	Low	Long	Hyperinflated lung
Resonance	Hollow	Loud	Low	Long	Normal lung
Dull	Thud	Medium	Medium	Medium	Solid organs—liver
Flat	Extremely dull	Soft	High	Short	Muscle, atelectasis

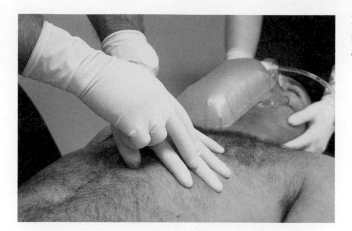

FIGURE 6-3 Percuss your patient to evaluate vibrations and sounds.

shoulder. Snap the finger back quickly to avoid dampening the sound. When percussing the chest, make sure your finger lies between the ribs and parallel to them. In this way, you will percuss the tissue underneath the ribs, not the ribs themselves.

A wall in your home is a good place to practise your percussion skills. As you percuss the air-filled area between studs, you will hear a hollow, resonant sound. Wall spaces filled with insulation will sound less resonant. When you percuss over a wall stud, you will notice a flatter, dull sound. You can apply this principle to the percussion of body cavities. Compare the sounds on the affected side with those on the unaffected side. The key is knowing what is normal, and so above all, you must practise percussion on healthy people in order to recognize abnormalities in sick or injured patients.

Unfortunately, at most emergency scenes, especially those in the street, noise prevents percussing your patient effectively. Your clinical experience and common sense will tell you when to use this valuable assessment technique.

You must practise percussion on healthy people in order to recognize abnormalities in sick or injured patients.

Auscultation

Auscultation involves listening for sounds produced by the body, primarily the lungs, the heart, the intestines, and the major blood vessels. It is difficult to master. You may hear some sounds clearly, such as stridor, the high-pitched squeal of a partially obstructed upper airway. Most, however, require a stethoscope. You should perform auscultation in a quiet environment. Unfortunately, this is not always practical in emergency services. Hearing the low amplitude heart and lung sounds against on-scene noise or in-transit background noise may be especially difficult.

For your patient's comfort, warm the end piece of your stethoscope with your hands before auscultating. To auscultate, hold the end piece of your stethoscope between your second and third fingers and press the stethoscope's diaphragm firmly against your patient's skin (Figure 6-4). If you are using the bell side, place it evenly and lightly on the skin. Avoid touching the tubing with your hands or allowing it to rub any surfaces. Make sure the earpieces point anteriorly before you put them in your ears.

Listen for the presence of sound and its intensity, pitch, duration, and quality. When reporting and recording lung sounds, always note abnormal sounds (crackles, wheezes), their locations (bilateral, right lower lobe, bases), and their timing during the respiratory cycle (inspiratory, end-expiratory). Sometimes, closing your eyes helps you concentrate on the sounds by eliminating visual stimuli. Try to isolate and concentrate on one sound at a time. Generally, auscultate after you have used other assessment techniques. The only exception is the abdomen, which

* **auscultation** listening with a stethoscope for sounds produced by the body.

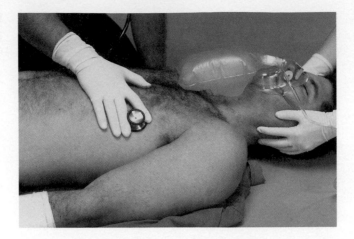

FIGURE 6-4 Auscultate body sounds with the stethoscope.

you should auscultate before palpation and percussion. A paramedic should be proficient in auscultating blood pressure, lung sounds, heart sounds, bowel sounds, and arterial bruits. As with any other physical assessment tool, you cannot detect abnormalities unless you know what is normal. Take every opportunity to auscultate lung, heart, and bowel sounds regularly.

Measurement of Vital Signs

The four basic vital signs in medicine are pulse, respiration, blood pressure, and body temperature. Although any complete physical assessment should include all four, the first three are most important in prehospital care. They are the primary indicators of your patient's health. Measure them early in the physical assessment, and in emergency situations, repeat them often and look for trends. For example, in a serious head injury, watch for your patient's systolic blood pressure to rise, her pulse pressure to widen, and her pulse rate to fall. These trends suggest an increase in intracranial pressure, a serious medical emergency. Conversely, a falling blood pressure with an increasing pulse rate may indicate shock. As a paramedic, you should become an expert at taking vital signs on patients of every age.

Pulse As the heart ejects blood through the arteries, a pulse wave results. Each pulse beat corresponds to a cardiac contraction and results from the ejected blood's impact on the arterial walls. The pulse is a valuable indicator of circulatory function. Your patient's pulse rate, rhythm, and quality indicate her hemodynamic (circulatory) status and the critical nature of the condition. **Pulse rate** refers to the number of pulsations felt in one minute. It can be slow (bradycardic), normal, or fast (tachycardic). **Pulse rhythm** refers to the pulse's pattern and the equality of intervals between beats. It can be regular, regularly irregular, or irregularly irregular. **Pulse quality** refers to the pulse's strength. Terms such as weak, strong, or bounding are used to describe the pulse's quality.

The normal pulse rate for an adult is 60–100 beats per minute. Rates below 60 are bradycardic; rates above 100 are tachycardic. **Bradycardia** may indicate an increase in parasympathetic nervous system stimulation. It might also be the result of a head injury, hypothermia, severe hypoxia, or drug overdose. Bradycardia is sometimes a normal finding in the well-conditioned athlete. Treat bradycardia only if it compromises your patient's cardiac output and general circulatory status. **Tachycardia** usually indicates an increase in sympathetic nervous system stimulation with which the body is compensating for another problem, such as blood loss, fear, pain, fever, or hypoxia. It is an early indicator of shock and may indicate ventricular tachycardia, a life-threatening cardiac dysrhythmia.

Measure vital signs early in the physical assessment and, in emergency situations, repeat them often, and look for trends.

✻ **pulse rate** number of pulses felt in one minute.

✻ **pulse rhythm** pattern and equality of intervals between beats.

✻ **pulse quality** strength, which can be weak, thready, strong, or bounding.

✻ **bradycardia** pulse rate slower than 60.

✻ **tachycardia** pulse rate faster than 100.

The pulse's rhythm, when present, may be regular, regularly irregular, irregularly irregular, or grossly chaotic. Irregular pulse rates may be due to extra beats, skipped beats, or pacemaker problems and usually indicate a cardiac abnormality. The rhythm's effect on cardiac output determines whether intervention is necessary.

The pulse's quality can be weak, strong, or bounding. Weak, thready pulses may indicate a decreased circulatory status, such as shock or circulation compromise. Strong, bounding pulses may indicate high blood pressure, heat stroke, or increasing intracranial pressure. The pulse location may be another indicator of your patient's clinical status. The presence of a carotid pulse generally means that her systolic blood pressure is at least 60 mmHg. The presence of peripheral pulses indicates a higher blood pressure; their absence suggests circulatory collapse. Practise finding each of the pulse locations (Figure 6-5). As with other vital signs, take your patient's pulse frequently in the emergency setting and note any trends.

Respiration Since oxygen and carbon dioxide exchange is essential to sustain life, **respiration** must occur continuously and must be effective. The lungs supply the arteries with oxygen and maintain the blood's pH by eliminating or retaining carbon dioxide. These two functions occur during respiration. Continuously observe your patient's respiratory rate, effort, and quality. Look for subtle signs of distress. Recognize when your patient requires rapid intervention, such as aggressive airway management, positive pressure ventilation, and oxygenation. These interventions, some invasive, often will make the difference between life and death.

 respiration exchange of oxygen and carbon dioxide in the lungs and at the cellular level.

Recognizing when your patient's respiration requires rapid intervention often will make the difference between life and death.

Peripheral Pulse Sites

Temporal – lateral to eye orbit

Carotid – medial to and below angle of jaw

Brachial – just medial to biceps tendon

Radial – thumb side of wrist

Ulnar – little finger side of wrist

Femoral – just below inguinal ligament

Popliteal – just behind knee

Dorsalis pedis – top of foot

Posterior tibial – behind medial malleolus

FIGURE 6-5   Know each pulse location.

✱ respiratory rate number of times patient breathes in one minute.

✱ tachypnea rapid breathing.

✱ bradypnea slow breathing.

Very rapid or very slow breathing rates require rapid intervention to ensure that the adequate exchange of gases continues.

✱ respiratory effort how hard the patient works to breathe.

✱ quality of respiration depth and pattern of breathing.

✱ tidal volume amount of air one breath moves into and out of lungs.

✱ blood pressure force of blood against arterial walls as the heart contracts and relaxes.

✱ systolic blood pressure force of blood against arteries when ventricles contract.

✱ diastolic blood pressure force of blood against arteries when ventricles relax.

✱ Korotkoff sounds sounds of blood hitting arterial walls.

Your patient's **respiratory rate** is the number of times of breaths in one minute. In general, the normal respiratory rate for a healthy adult at rest is 12 to 20 breaths per minute. Rapid breathing (**tachypnea**) can be the result of hypoxia, shock, head injury, or anxiety. Slow breathing (**bradypnea**) can be caused by drug overdose, severe hypoxia, or central nervous system insult. Very rapid or very slow breathing rates require rapid intervention to ensure that the adequate exchange of gases continues.

Your patient's **respiratory effort** is how hard she works to breathe. Normal inhalation involves using the respiratory muscles (diaphragm and intercostals) to increase the chest's inner diameter. It is an active process that requires energy. The increasing space creates negative pressure, like a vacuum, that draws air into the lungs. Exhalation is the passive process of the respiratory muscles' elastic recoil. This normally effortless process can become difficult with some respiratory conditions. For example, an airway obstruction may compromise inhalation. The resultant increased breathing effort is evident in accessory muscle use, retractions, and possibly abnormal breath sounds.

Diseases like asthma and emphysema, in which the smaller airways collapse and trap air in the distal airways, may obstruct exhalation. Exhalation then becomes an active process that leads to respiratory distress and failure. Some injuries can decrease the respiratory effort. Rib fractures, for example, will cause a decrease in chest wall expansion because it hurts to breathe. A pneumothorax decreases effective gas exchange because the air enters the pleural space instead of the alveoli. Children become tired and decrease their respiratory effort, making their condition even worse. Evaluating your patient's respiratory effort will provide invaluable information about her respiratory status.

The **quality of respiration** refers to its depth and pattern. The depth, or **tidal volume,** of respiration is the amount of air your patient moves into and out of the lungs in one breath. The normal depth for a healthy adult at rest should be approximately 500 mL, just enough to cause the chest to rise. The tidal volume may increase during exercise or anxiety. It may decrease in the presence of a rib injury when every breath hurts.

Assess your patient's respiratory depth by inspecting and palpating the chest wall for symmetrical chest expansion, by feeling and listening for air movement and noise from the nose and mouth, and by auscultating for lung sounds. The depth may be shallow, normal, or deep. Once again, to recognize inadequate respiratory depth, you must know what is normal. The respiratory pattern should be regular. Variations in respiratory pattern can be associated with specific diseases (Table 6-2). Some irregular patterns, such as Cheyne-Stokes, may indicate serious brain or brain stem problems.

Blood Pressure Blood pressure is the force of blood against the arterial walls as the heart contracts and relaxes. It is equal to cardiac output times the systemic vascular resistance. Any alteration in the cardiac output or the vascular resistance will alter the blood pressure. An important indicator of your patient's condition, blood pressure is measured during both systole and diastole. **Systolic blood pressure** (the higher numeric value) measures the maximum force of blood against the arteries when the ventricles contract. **Diastolic blood pressure** (the lower numeric value) measures the pressure against the arteries when the ventricles relax and are filling with blood. The diastolic blood pressure is a measure of systemic vascular resistance and correlates well with changes in vessel size. The sounds of blood hitting the arterial walls are called the **Korotkoff sounds.**

Many factors may influence your patient's blood pressure. Anxiety, for example, may cause it to rise. Your patient's position (sitting, lying, standing) also may affect the measurement. If your patient has recently been smoking, exercising, or eating, you must wait at least 5 to 10 minutes to allow her blood pressure

Table 6-2 BREATHING PATTERNS

	Condition	Description	Causes
	Eupnea	Normal breathing rate and pattern	
	Tachypnea	Increased respiratory rate	Fever, anxiety, exercise, shock
	Bradypnea	Decreased respiratory rate	Sleep, drugs, metabolic disorder, head injury, stroke
	Apnea	Absence of breathing	Deceased patient, head injury, stroke
	Hyperpnea	Normal rate, but deep respirations	Emotional stress, diabetic ketoacidosis
	Cheyne-Stokes	Gradual increases and decreases in respirations with periods of apnea	Increasing intracranial pressure, brain stem injury
	Biot's	Rapid, deep respirations (gasps) with short pauses between sets	Spinal meningitis, many CNS causes, head injury
	Kussmaul's	Tachypnea and hyperpnea	Renal failure, metabolic acidosis, diabetic ketoacidosis
	Apneustic	Prolonged inspiratory phase with shortened expiratory phase	Lesion in brain stem

to return to a resting level before you measure it. Because of these many intangibles, you should never use blood pressure as the single indicator of your patient's condition. Always correlate it with other clinical signs of end-organ **perfusion**, such as level of response, skin colour, temperature, and condition, and peripheral pulses.

The average blood pressure in the healthy adult is 120/80. Females usually will have a lower blood pressure until menopause. **Pulse pressure** is the difference between the systolic and diastolic pressures. For example, a blood pressure of 120/80 represents a pulse pressure of 40 mmHg. A normal pulse pressure is generally 30–40 mmHg. In certain conditions, such as pericardial tamponade or tension pneumothorax, the pulse pressure will narrow. In others, such as increasing intracranial pressure or fever, the pulse pressure will widen. Again, take your physiologically unstable patient's blood pressure as often as every five minutes to chart trends.

What is normal? This question has no easy answer. Generally, systolic blood pressure in adults ranges from 100 to 135 mmHg, diastolic from 60 to 80 mmHg. **Hypertension** in adults is defined as a pressure higher than 140/90. A blood pressure of 130/70, however, may represent hypertension if a patient's usual pressure is 90/60 or **hypotension** if the usual pressure is 170/90. The numbers are not as important as detecting trends and assessing end-organ perfusion. Do not define hypotension by numbers but by whether perfusion is adequate to sustain life.

Hypertension can result from cardiovascular disease, kidney disease, stroke, or head injury, where it is a classic sign of increasing intracranial pressure. It may be a predisposing factor to, and preexist in, stroke or cardiovascular disease. Did the hypertension occur before or after the condition? Hypotension usually indicates shock due to cardiac insufficiency (cardiogenic shock), low blood volume (hypovolemic shock), or massive vasodilation (vasogenic shock). Orthostatic hypotension is a decrease in your patient's blood pressure when she stands or sits up.

If you suspect shock due to blood or fluid volume loss and you do not suspect a spinal injury, perform a tilt test. Take your patient's pulse and blood pressure while she is supine. Then, have your patient sit up and dangle her feet and then stand. In 30–60 seconds, retake her vital signs. The healthy patient's vital signs should not change. The tilt test is positive if either pulse rate increases 10–20 beats per minute or if the systolic blood pressure drops 10–20 mmHg. (Research

Never use blood pressure as the single indicator of your patient's condition; always correlate it with other clinical signs of end-organ perfusion.

✱ **perfusion** passage of blood through an organ or tissue.

✱ **pulse pressure** difference between systolic and diastolic pressures.

✱ **hypertension** blood pressure higher than normal.

✱ **hypotension** blood pressure lower than normal.

has found that an increase in heart rate is a more sensitive indicator of hypovolemia than a decrease in systolic blood pressure.) This finding is common in patients suspected of hypovolemia.

Body Temperature The body works hard to maintain a temperature of approximately 37°C. This temperature reflects the balance between heat production and heat loss through the skin and respiratory system. Even a slight variance can mean that significant events are happening within the body or on the body from environmental factors. Assess your patient's temperature to approximate her internal core temperature.

An increase in body temperature (**hyperthermia**) can result from environmental extremes, infections, drugs, or metabolic processes. Ordinarily, the body's cooling mechanisms maintain a steady core temperature. In an extremely hot and humid environment or in cases like heat stroke, the cooling mechanisms can fail and the core temperature will rise despite an internal thermostat that wants to maintain a normal temperature. Fever results when the body tries to make its internal environment inhospitable to invading organisms. It often presents with a history of illness. The skin is somewhat dry until the fever breaks and the body's cooling mechanisms begin to take effect. As the body temperature rises, it begins to threaten body processes, specifically those of the brain. A temperature of up to 38°C increases metabolism markedly. As body temperature rises above 39°C, the neurons of the brain may denature. At temperatures above 41°C, brain cells die and seizures may occur.

Extreme cold also affects body temperature. When peripheral vasoconstriction and shivering mechanisms can no longer balance heat production and loss, core temperature drops (**hypothermia**). At a body temperature of 34°C, normal body-warming mechanisms begin to fail. As the core temperature drops below 31°C, shivering stops, heart sounds diminish, and cardiac irritability increases. If the temperature drops much below 22°C, your patient will present with a death-like appearance and, possibly, irreversible asystole (absence of heartbeat).

A variety of methods can provide accurate temperature readings. You can use glass thermometers to take oral, rectal, or axillary temperatures. A rectal thermometer is the preferred device for children younger than six years old and for patients with an altered level of consciousness. An axillary temperature reading is the least accurate of the three methods.

EQUIPMENT

To conduct a comprehensive physical assessment, you will need a stethoscope, a sphygmomanometer, an ophthalmoscope, an otoscope, a scale, and other equipment. The ophthalmoscope, otoscope, and scale are not considered prehospital assessment tools.

Stethoscope The **stethoscope** is a basic paramedic tool used to auscultate most sounds (Figure 6-6). It transmits sound waves from the source through an end piece and along rubber tubes to the ear. One side of the end piece is a rigid diaphragm that best transmits high-pitched sounds, such as heart sounds and blood pressure sounds. The diaphragm also screens out low-pitched sounds, such as lung sounds and bowel sounds. The other side of the end piece is a bell that uses the skin as a diaphragm. The sounds that the bell transmits vary with the amount of pressure exerted. For example, with light pressure, the bell picks up low-pitched sounds; with firm pressure, it acts like the diaphragm and transmits high-pitched sounds. Whether you use the bell or the diaphragm depends on which sounds you are auscultating. To hear blood pressure or heart sounds, for instance, use the diaphragm; to hear lung or bowel sounds, use the bell side.

Even a slight variance in body temperature can mean that significant events are happening within the body.

✳ **hyperthermia** increase in body's core temperature.

✳ **hypothermia** decrease in body's core temperature.

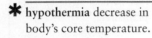

Content Review

PHYSICAL ASSESSMENT EQUIPMENT

- Stethoscope
- Sphygmomanometer
- Ophthalmoscope
- Otoscope
- Scale
- Tongue blades
- Thermometer
- Penlight
- Visual acuity chart/card
- Reflex hammer

✳ **stethoscope** tool used to auscultate most sounds.

Accurate auscultation depends in part on the quality of your instrument. Your stethoscope should have the following important characteristics:

- A rigid diaphragm cover
- Thick, heavy tubing, which conducts sound better than thin, flexible tubing
- Short tubing (30–40 cm) to minimize distortion
- Earpieces that fit snugly—large enough to occlude the ear canal—and are angled toward the nose to project sound toward the eardrum
- A bell with a rubber-ring edge to ensure good contact with the skin

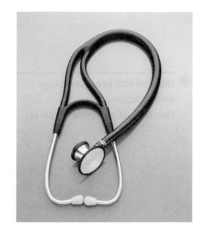

FIGURE 6-6 Use a stethoscope to auscultate most sounds.

Sphygmomanometer The circumstances and the patient care setting determine what type of equipment you use to measure blood pressure (Figure 6-7). Intensive care unit staff commonly use intra-arterial pressure devices for critically ill patients who need continuous monitoring. When a noisy environment makes auscultation difficult or when the sounds are especially weak, a doppler device that amplifies the sounds is useful. You will see these devices in the emergency department, newborn nursery, emergency vehicles, and labour and delivery suites. The most familiar blood-pressure measuring device is the aneroid **sphygmomanometer.** You will use it with your stethoscope to auscultate the sounds of the blood moving through an artery, usually the brachial artery. Because your patient's blood pressure is important in evaluating her condition, you must be able to measure it accurately.

✱ **sphygmomanometer** blood pressure measuring device comprising a bulb, a cuff, and a manometer.

Because your patient's blood pressure is important in evaluating her condition, you must be able to measure it accurately.

A sphygmomanometer includes a bulb, a cuff, and a manometer. The cuff has an airtight, flat, rubber bladder enclosed within a fabric cover. Cuffs are available

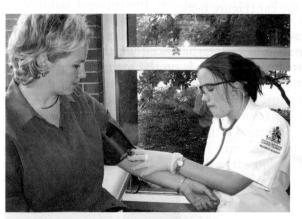

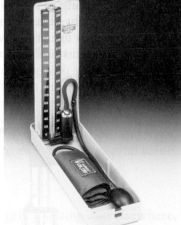

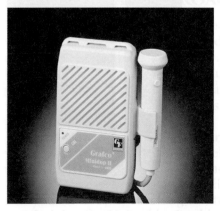

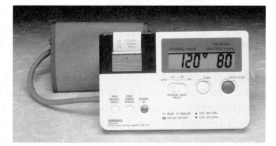

FIGURE 6-7 Use a blood pressure device suited to the circumstances. Clockwise from upper left: aneroid sphygmomanometer, mercury sphygmomanometer, digital electronic, and doppler device.

illness. In the emergency setting, no matter how nervous and apprehensive you may be, never let your patient see anything but a calm, professional, confident demeanour. This will help alleviate anxiety about disclosing personal information to, and being examined by, a nonphysician. Try to remain objective, even when confronted by alarming or disgusting information. A bad bedsore, a perverted sexual incident, or black tarry stools (melena) can test even the most experienced clinician's composure. Simply thinking about how embarrassed your patient must be may help you keep your own poise.

OVERVIEW OF A COMPREHENSIVE PHYSICAL ASSESSMENT

This section gives an overview of the comprehensive physical assessment. Later in the chapter, we will discuss each component in detail. The key to an effective, comprehensive assessment is to integrate each individual section into a unified patient assessment. Chapter 7 provides a template for conducting a problem-oriented patient assessment on both medical and trauma patients.

As a paramedic, you will determine which elements of the comprehensive assessment to use. You will base your decision on your patient's presenting problem and clinical status. For example, if you are conducting comprehensive physicals for your fire department, you may choose to use the entire assessment. If you are assessing a child just struck by an automobile and lying unconscious in the street, you will narrow your focus to the child's injuries. A comprehensive assessment should include a general survey and a detailed assessment of anatomical regions.

THE GENERAL SURVEY

A general survey is the first part of a comprehensive assessment. It begins with noting your patient's appearance and goes on to include vital signs and other assessments.

Appearance

A thorough evaluation of your patient's appearance can provide a great deal of valuable information about her health. Note her level of consciousness and posture, and any obvious signs of distress, such as sitting upright gasping for each breath or slumped to one side. Is her motor activity normal or does your patient have noticeable tremors or paralysis? Observe her general state of health, dress, grooming, and personal hygiene. Obvious odours can also furnish significant information.

Level of Consciousness Is your patient awake? Is she alert? Does she speak to you in a normal voice? Are her eyes open, and does she respond to you and others at the scene? If your patient is not apparently awake, speak in a loud voice. If she does not respond to your verbal cues, shake your patient gently. If she still does not respond, apply a painful stimulus, such as pinching a tendon, rubbing her sternum, or rolling a pencil across a nail bed. Note the response.

Signs of Distress Is your patient in distress? For example, does she have a cardiac or respiratory problem, as evidenced by laboured breathing, wheezing, or a cough? Is your patient in pain, as evidenced by wincing, sweating, or protecting the painful area? Is she anxious, as evidenced by facial expression, cold moist palms, or nervous fidgeting? What is the level of distress? Mild, moderate, or severe?

The key to an effective, comprehensive assessment is integrating each individual section into a unified patient assessment.

Apparent State of Health Is your patient healthy, robust, and vigorous? Or is she frail, ill-looking, or feeble? Does she have an obvious abnormality? Base your evaluation of the general state of health on your observations throughout the interview and physical assessment.

Vital Statistics Vital statistics, height and weight, are used widely in clinical medicine. Accurately measuring your patient's weight and height with a scale, however, is not a practical prehospital assessment procedure. You will occasionally estimate your patient's weight to administer medications for which the dose is weight dependent. You also may use a **Broselow Tape** to measure your infant patient's length. The Broselow tape provides information concerning drug dosages, airway management adjuncts, and intravenous calculations based on your patient's height.

Note your patient's general stature. Is she lanky and slender, short and stocky, muscular and symmetrical? Does she have any obvious deformities or disproportionate areas? Is she extremely thin or obese? If obese, is the fat evenly distributed or is it concentrated in the trunk? Has your patient gained or lost weight recently?

Sexual Development Is your patient's sexual maturity appropriate for her age and gender? Consider such indicators as voice, facial and body hair, and breast size.

Skin Colour and Obvious Lesions Is your patient's skin pale, suggesting decreased blood flow or anemia? Does she have central (lips, oral mucosa) or peripheral (nail beds, hands) cyanosis, the bluish colour resulting from decreased oxygenation of the tissues? Does she have the yellow colour of jaundice or high carotene levels? Note any rashes, bruises, scars, or discoloration.

Posture, Gait, and Motor Activity Observe your patient's posture and presentation. Is she sitting straight up and forward, bracing her arms (tripodding)? This suggests a serious breathing problem, such as acute pulmonary edema or airway obstruction. Does one side of her body droop and seem immobile, suggesting a stroke? Does she sit quietly or seem restless? Does your patient have tremors or other involuntary movements?

Dress, Grooming, and Personal Hygiene Does your patient dress appropriately for the climate and situation? Are the clothes clean and properly fastened? Are they conventional for her age and social group? Abnormalities in dress might suggest the cold intolerance of hypothyroidism or the hiding of a skin rash or needle marks, or they might simply reflect personal preference. Look at her shoes. Are they clean? Do they have holes, slits, open laces, or other alterations to accommodate painful foot conditions, such as gout, bunions, or edema? Does your patient wear slippers instead of shoes? Is she wearing unusual jewellery, such as a copper bracelet for arthritis or a medical information tag? Do grooming and hygiene seem appropriate for her age, lifestyle, occupation, and social status? Does her lack of concern over appearance (overgrown nails and hair, for instance) suggest a long illness or depression?

Odours of Breath or Body Does your patient have any unusual or striking body or breath odour? The acetone breath of a diabetic, the bitter-almond breath of cyanide poisoning, the putrid smell of bacterial infection, or the obvious smell of alcohol may give important clues to the underlying problem. Avoid tunnel-vision when you smell alcohol, which often masks other serious illnesses, such as liver failure, or injuries, such as a subdural hematoma.

Facial Expression Watch your patient's facial expressions throughout your interaction. Her face should reflect her emotions during the interview and physical assessment. The patient with hyperthyroidism may stare intently. The Parkinson's patient's face may appear immobile.

* **vital statistics** height and weight.

* **Broselow Tape** a measuring tape for infants that provides important information regarding airway equipment and medication doses based on your patient's length.

Vital Signs

Take a complete set of vital signs to include pulse, respiration, blood pressure, and temperature. Note that different EMS systems include various elements in their vital signs assessment. You may encounter systems that also include level of consciousness; pupil size and reaction; skin colour, temperature, and condition; or other assessment components.

Pulse To take the pulse of a conscious adult or large child, the most accessible and commonly used location is the radial artery. With the pads of your first two or three fingers, compress the radial artery onto the radius, just below the wrist on the thumb side (Procedure 6-1a). In the unconscious patient, begin by checking her carotid pulse. To locate the carotid pulse, palpate medial to and just below the angle of the jaw. Locate the thyroid cartilage (Adam's apple) and slide your fingers laterally until they are between the thyroid cartilage and the large muscle in the neck (sternocleidomastoid). In infants and small children, use the brachial artery or auscultate for an apical pulse. Remember that auscultating an apical pulse does not provide information about your patient's hemodynamic status. To locate the brachial artery, feel just medial to the biceps tendon. Auscultate the apical pulse just below the left nipple. First, note your patient's pulse rate by counting the number of beats in one minute. If the pulse is regular, you can count the beats in 15 seconds and multiply that number by four. If the pulse is irregular, you must count it for a full minute to obtain an accurate total. Note also the pulse's rhythm and quality.

Respiration To measure your patient's respiratory rate, place one hand on your patient's chest and count the breaths taken in 30 seconds (Procedure 6-1b). Multiply that number by two. Because your patient may consciously or subconsciously control her breathing, try to evaluate it without her knowing. Also, assess respiratory effort and quality of respiration.

Blood Pressure To measure your patient's blood pressure, first, choose the arm you will use. Remove any clothing that covers the upper arm; do not take the blood pressure over clothing if possible. Look for a dialysis shunt in patients with renal failure. Do not take a blood pressure in that arm. Place the arm in a slightly flexed position, palm up and fingers relaxed. Support the upper arm at the level of your patient's heart.

Use the correct size cuff to obtain an accurate measurement. Its width should be one-half to one-third the circumference of your patient's arm. For most adults, unless they are obese or extremely slim, the large-size cuff (15 cm wide) will suffice. If your patient has an obese arm, use a larger cuff. If the larger cuff is still too small, use your patient's forearm and place your stethoscope over the radial artery. For all patients, use a cuff that covers approximately two-thirds of the upper arm or thigh. Using a cuff that is too wide, too narrow, too long, or too short will result in an inaccurate measurement.

Turn the control valve counterclockwise to open it; squeeze all the air out of the bladder before applying the cuff. Locate the brachial artery by palpating on the medial side of the antecubital space until you feel a pulse. Place the lower edge of the cuff one inch above the antecubital space. Find the centre of the bladder (usually marked on the cuff with an arrow), and place it directly over the artery. Fasten the cuff so that it is smooth and fits tightly enough to obtain an accurate reading. If you have difficulty inserting a finger between the cuff and your patient's arm, it is snug enough. Also make sure the rubber tubing is clear of the cuff. Check the placement of the manometer so that you can see it easily.

Now, palpate the radial artery. With your other hand, turn the control valve completely clockwise and squeeze the bulb rapidly to inflate the cuff to approximately 30 mmHg over the point where the radial pulse disappears. Place your stethoscope directly over the brachial artery and hold it firmly in place without pressing on the artery (Procedure 6-1c). Turn the control valve counterclockwise slowly and steadily to deflate the cuff at a rate of 2–3 mmHg per heart beat. Deflating too slowly or too rapidly will cause an inaccurate reading.

As you slowly deflate the cuff, watch the manometer and listen for the Korotkoff sounds. When you hear the first pulse beat, note the reading on the manometer dial or mercury column. This is the systolic pressure. Continue deflating the cuff until the pulsations diminish or become muffled. This is the diastolic pressure.

If you do not obtain a reading, wait 30 seconds to allow the blood pressure to normalize before inflating the cuff again. Sometimes you can palpate the artery during the deflation. The point at which you feel the pulse return marks the systolic reading. You cannot evaluate the diastolic pressure with the palpation method. To take your patient's blood pressure with a doppler, follow the same procedure as for the palpation method, but instead of palpating for the return of the pulse, place the doppler device over the palpated artery and listen for the "whoooosh" of flowing blood indicating the systolic measurement (Procedure 6-1d). Record the blood pressure on your patient's chart. Include the systolic and diastolic pressures (for instance, 134/78), the arm used (right/left), and your patient's position (lying, sitting, standing).

Temperature The type of glass thermometer you use determines how long you must leave it in place to get an accurate reading. To take your patient's temperature orally with a glass thermometer, place the thermometer under her tongue for at least 3–4 minutes. It may provide a false reading if your patient has swallowed liquid or smoked within 15–30 minutes. To use a rectal thermometer, lubricate it well and then insert it 3.75 cm into the rectum; leave it in place for at least 2–3 minutes. If you use an axillary thermometer, it must remain under your patient's armpit at least 10 minutes. If your service uses battery-operated devices, become familiar with them and follow the manufacturer's instructions for their use (Procedure 6-1e). Many services are now using a battery-operated tympanic thermometer. When using the tympanic membrane device, place the speculum into the ear canal, push the button and hold it for two to three seconds, then remove the device (Procedure 6-1f). The temperature is then displayed on a digital readout.

Additional Assessment Techniques

Additional assessment techniques include pulse oximetry, cardiac monitoring, and blood glucose determination.

Pulse Oximetry The **pulse oximeter** is a noninvasive device that measures the oxygen saturation of your patient's blood. It can reliably indicate your patient's cardiorespiratory status because it may tell you how well she is oxygenating the most peripheral vessels of the circulatory system. It also quantifies the effectiveness of your interventions, such as oxygen therapy, medications, suctioning, and ventilatory assistance. For example, on room air, your patient's reading is 92 percent; after two minutes of high-flow oxygen therapy, it is 99 percent, showing a definite improvement.

The pulse oximeter has a probe-sensor and a monitoring unit with digital readouts. Attach the probe-sensor clip to your patient's finger, toe, or earlobe (Figure 6-12). The probe directs two lights (one red and one infrared) through a small area of tissue. The lights penetrate the tissue and are absorbed. Since saturated and desaturated hemoglobin absorb the lights differently, the sensors can determine their individual concentrations. The result is a measurement of your patient's oxygen saturation, or SaO_2.

Normal oxygen saturation at sea level should be between 96 and 100 percent. Generally, if the reading is below 95 percent, suspect shock, hypoxia, or

✴ pulse oximeter noninvasive device that measures the oxygen saturation of blood.

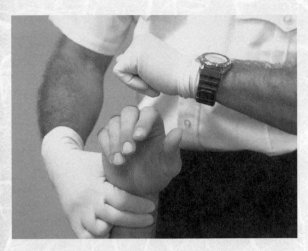

6-1a   Assess the pulse and count the rate as an indicator of circulatory function. Note the rhythm and strength.

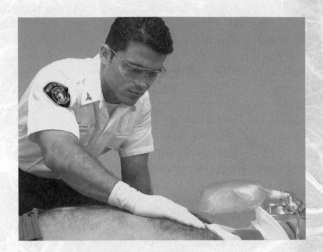

6-1b   Assess your patient's respirations and count the rate. Also, note depth and effort.

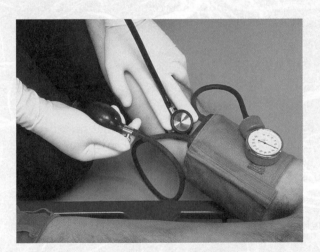

6-1c   Assess blood pressure with a sphygmo-manometer and stethoscope.

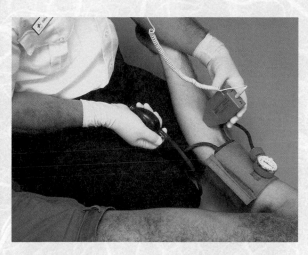

6-1d   If you cannot hear blood pressure with a stethoscope, use an ultrasonic doppler.

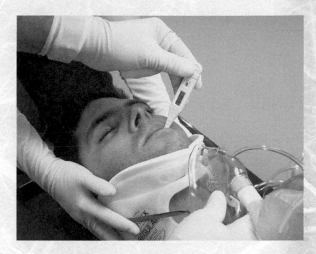

6-1e   Use a battery-operated oral thermometer to take your patient's temperature.

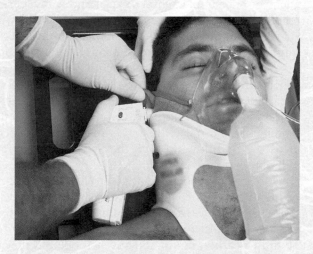

6-1f   Use a specially designed, battery-operated thermometer to measure temperature inside the ear.

FIGURE 6-12 Pulse oximetry allows you quickly and accurately to determine your patient's oxygenation status.

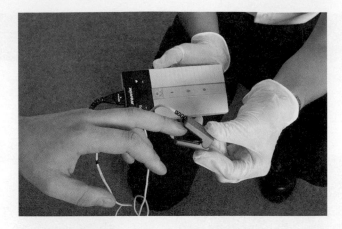

FIGURE 6-13 The cardiac monitor is essential to managing advanced cardiac life support.

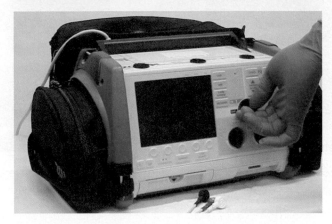

respiratory compromise. Provide your patient with the appropriate airway management and supplemental oxygen and watch carefully for further changes. Any reading below 90 percent requires aggressive airway management, positive pressure ventilation, or oxygen administration. The unresponsive patient may require invasive airway management and positive pressure ventilation.

Several factors affect the accuracy of a pulse oximetry reading. The sensors can accurately measure the oxygen saturation only if blood flow through the tissue is adequate. Most pulse oximeters display a digital readout of the pulse rate; others display a pulsation wave. In either case, if the display does not match your patient's actual pulse, the SaO_2 reading will be erratic. If your patient has decreased blood flow through the tissue, as in hypovolemia or hypothermia, you will obtain a false reading.

In cases of carbon monoxide (CO) poisoning, your saturation readings will be high while your patient's tissues are severely ischemic. This is because the CO molecule saturates the hemoglobin molecule 200 times more easily than does oxygen and the pulse oximetry probe cannot distinguish between hemoglobin that is bound to carbon monoxide and hemoglobin that is bound to oxygen. Your patient's hemoglobin is, in fact, saturated, but with carbon monoxide, not oxygen. Other than these limitations, the pulse oximeter, when teamed with other patient assessment techniques, can be a useful tool in the prehospital setting.

Cardiac Monitoring The **cardiac monitor** is essential in assessing and managing the patient who requires advanced cardiac life support (ACLS) (Figure 6-13). The most simple prehospital machines monitor the electrical activity of the heart in three "leads" or positions. These "limb leads" adequately identify

✱ **cardiac monitor** machine that displays and records the electrical activity of the heart.

life-threatening cardiac rhythms. Also available for prehospital use are 12-lead ECGs. They are essential in gathering data to confirm a myocardial infarction.

Other features of cardiac monitors include pacing capabilities and the "quick-look" paddles and the "hands-off" defibrillation pads used in cardiac arrest. The paddles, which you place on your patient's chest, allow you to check the cardiac rhythm and deliver a rapid electrical countershock. The hands-off defibrillation pads have two large electrodes that you attach to the chest wall. These replace the paddles and allow you to deliver a countershock without risk of injuring yourself.

All monitor-defibrillators can deliver a synchronized countershock in the presence of an unstable tachycardia. Most have a transcutaneous pacemaker that is placed externally on the chest and provides an electrical impulse to stimulate cardiac contraction in cases of bradycardia and heart blocks. This is a temporary measure until a permanent pacemaker can be implanted. Finally, some ECG machines have a "code summary" feature that prints out the electrical record of events and their times. This helps you document your patient's progress while in your care. Some devices also incorporate BP, SaO_2, and CO_2 monitoring.

The cardiac monitor is a useful tool for measuring electrical activity, but it has one major disadvantage. It cannot tell you if the heart is pumping efficiently, effectively, or at all. The ECG reading does not necessarily correlate with the mechanical function of the heart. Electrical activity can exist with no mechanical contraction. Always assess your patient and compare what you see on the monitor with the rate and quality of the pulse.

Always compare what you see on a cardiac monitor with what you feel for a pulse.

Blood Glucose Determination In cases of altered mental status due to diabetic emergencies, seizures, and strokes, you will want to measure your patient's blood glucose level. The arrival of inexpensive, handheld **glucometers** makes this test easy to perform in the field. Most diabetic patients do it several times each day at home by themselves.

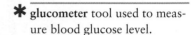

✱ **glucometer** tool used to measure blood glucose level.

To perform this procedure you will need a glucometer with test strips, a finger stick device with sterile lancets, alcohol wipe, and tissue or gauze pads. Simply place a drop of your patient's capillary blood from a finger stick onto a chemical reagent strip (Figure 6-14). Following the manufacturer's instructions, place the test strip in the glucometer and wait for the reading to appear. This procedure takes less than one minute to perform.

Since all glucometers work differently, you must read the manufacturer's instructions carefully. The slightest mistake can alter the measurement's accuracy. Do not allow alcohol to contaminate the blood. Glucometers are moderately accurate when used properly and calibrated daily.

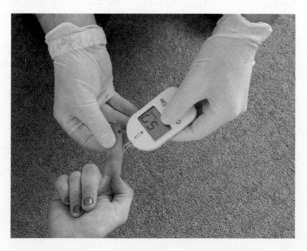

FIGURE 6-14 Use a glucometer to determine your patient's blood glucose.

ANATOMICAL REGIONS

Content Review

ANATOMICAL REGIONS

- Skin
- Head, eyes, ears, nose, throat
- Neck
- Chest
- Abdomen
- Extremities
- Posterior body
- Neurological

After you complete the general survey, you will examine the body regions and systems in more detail. Again, the specific situation and your experience and common sense will determine whether you conduct a thorough assessment, as you would when performing physicals for an insurance company, or narrow the focus of your assessment, as you might in an emergency setting.

THE SKIN

Although you will observe your patient's skin throughout your assessment, a comprehensive physical assessment must also include a concentrated inspection of all areas of the skin. The skin provides data on a variety of systemic problems in addition to skin-related disorders. Examining the skin requires good light and a keen eye. The characteristics of normal skin vary with your patients' racial, ethnic, and familial backgrounds. Evaluate its colour, moisture, temperature, texture, mobility and turgor, and any lesions. Always wear protective gloves especially if your patient has any areas of open skin, exudative lesions, or rashes.

Colour Normal skin colour in light-skinned people is pink, indicating adequate cardiorespiratory function and vascular integrity. This means that the capillaries in the skin are well oxygenated. The bright red oxyhemoglobin in the oxygen-rich blood circulating through the capillary beds gives the epidermis its pink appearance. A pale colour suggests decreased blood flow through the skin. This is typical in hypothermia, hypovolemia, and compensatory shock, where blood flow through the distal capillary beds is severely diminished. It also is common in anemia, in which your patient's red blood cell count is low. As the hemoglobin loses its oxygen to the tissues, it changes to the darker, blue deoxyhemoglobin. Increased deoxyhemoglobin causes cyanosis, a bluish skin colour. Cyanosis means that less oxygen is available at the tissue level.

Content Review

SKIN CHARACTERISTICS TO ASSESS

- Colour
- Moisture
- Temperature
- Texture
- Mobility and turgor
- Lesions

Evaluate skin colour where the epidermis is thinnest. This includes the fingernails and lips and the mucous membranes of the mouth and conjunctiva. In dark-skinned people, evaluate the sclera, conjunctiva, lips, nail beds, soles, and palms. Note any discoloration caused by vascular changes underneath the skin. Petechiae are small, round, flat, purplish spots caused by capillary bleeding from a variety of etiologies. Ecchymosis is a blue-black bruise resulting from trauma or bleeding disorders. Jaundice first appears in the sclera and then, in the late stages of liver disease, all over the skin. If only your patient's palms, soles, and face are yellow, she may have carotanemia, a harmless nutritional condition caused by eating a diet high in carrots and yellow vegetables or fruits.

Moisture Inspect and palpate the skin for dryness, increased sweating, and excessive oiliness. Dry skin, common during the cold winter months and in the elderly, may be the result of other conditions. Excessive oiliness, especially where the sebaceous glands are concentrated in the face, neck, back, chest, and buttocks, may suggest acne or hyperthyroidism. Increased sweating may indicate a sympathetic nervous system response to anxiety, fear, or exertion.

Temperature Use the backs of your fingers to feel the skin temperature in several different locations. Compare symmetrical body areas. Generalized warming or cooling suggests an environmental, infectious, or thyroid problem. Localized warmth may indicate bleeding or swelling.

Texture Feel your patient's skin. Is it rough or smooth? Are there large patches or small areas of scaling? Observe the skin's thickness. Thin and fragile skin is a sign of debilitating disease in the elderly. Thick skin often occurs with eczema and psoriasis. Inspect the palms and soles for calluses.

Mobility and Turgor Test the skin's **turgor** and elasticity by picking up a fold of skin over a bony prominence and then releasing it. Normal skin immediately returns to its original state. Poor turgor (tenting) results from dehydration. Test the skin's mobility by moving it over the bony prominence. Decreased mobility suggests edema or scleroderma, a progressive skin disease.

✱ **turgor** normal tension in the skin.

Lesions A skin **lesion** is any disruption in normal tissue. Skin lesions are classified as vascular, involving a blood vessel (Figure 6-15); primary, arising from previously

✱ **lesion** any disruption in normal tissue.

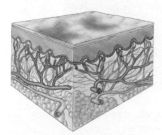
Purpura – Reddish-purple blotch, diameter more than 0.5 cm

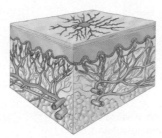
Spider angioma – Reddish legs radiate from red spot

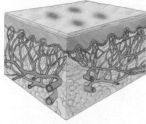
Petechiae – Reddish-purple spots, diameter less than 0.5 cm

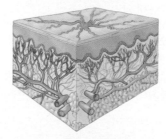
Venous star – Bluish legs radiate from blue centre

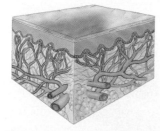
Ecchymosis – Reddish-purple blotch, size varies

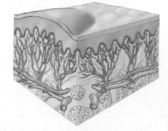
Capillary hemangioma – Irregular red spot

FIGURE 6-15 Vascular skin lesions.

normal skin (Figure 6-16); or secondary, resulting from changes in primary lesions (Figure 6-17). Skin lesions can take any shape, colour, or arrangement. Note their anatomical location and distribution. Are they generalized or localized? Do they involve exposed surfaces or areas that fold over? Do they relate to possible irritants, such as wristbands, bracelets, necklaces? Are they linear, clustered, circular, or dermatomal (following a sensory nerve pathway)? What type are they? Inspect and feel all skin lesions carefully. Skin tumours are another variety of skin lesion. These include basal cell and squamous cell carcinomas, malignant melanomas, Kaposi's sarcoma in AIDS, actinic keratosis, and seborrheic keratosis.

When you detect a skin lesion, use anatomical landmarks to describe its exact location on the skin's surface. Describe its shape in such terms as oval, spherical, irregular, or tubular. Sometimes, sketching an outline of the lesion is helpful. Record the size of the mass in centimetres, carefully measuring its length, width, and depth.

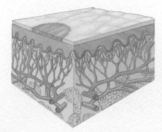

Macule – Flat spot, colour varies from white to brown or from red to purple, diameter less than 1 cm

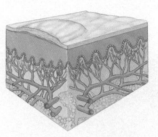

Plaque – Superficial papule, diameter greater than 1 cm, rough texture

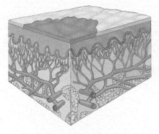

Patch – Irregular flat macule, diameter greater than 1 cm

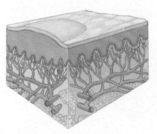

Wheal – Pink, irregular spot varying in size and shape

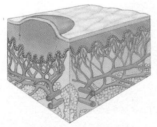

Papule – Elevated firm spot, colour varies from brown to red or from pink to purplish red, diameter less than 1 cm

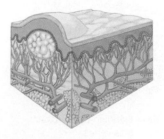

Nodule – Elevated firm spot, diameter 1–2 cm

FIGURE 6-16   Primary skin lesions.

Describe the consistency of the mass exactly as it feels to you (for instance, soft, firm, edematous, cystic, or nodular). Of particular concern is its mobility. If the mass is affixed to a specific structure, suspect a malignancy. Note any pain or tenderness surrounding the mass on palpation. Pulsation in the mass is another significant finding. For example, a mass that pulsates in all directions suggests an aneurysm.

THE HAIR

Inspect and palpate the hair, noting its colour, quality, distribution, quantity, and texture. Is there hair loss? Is there a pattern to the loss? Patients undergoing chemotherapy for cancer may experience generalized hair loss. Failure to develop normal hair growth during puberty may indicate a pituitary or hormonal problem. Abnormal facial hair growth in women (hirsutism) also may indicate

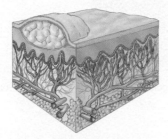

Tumour – Elevated solid, diameter greater than 2 cm, may be same colour as skin

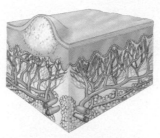

Pustule – Elevated area, diameter less than 1 cm, contains purulent fluid

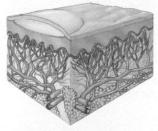

Vesicle – Elevated area, diameter less than 1 cm, contains serous fluid

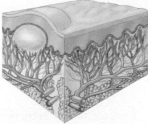

Cyst – Elevated, palpable area containing liquid or viscous matter

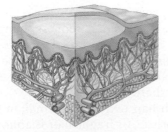

Bulla – Vesicle with diameter greater than 1 cm

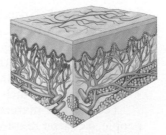

Telangiectasia – Red, thread-like line

FIGURE 6-16 (CONTINUED) Primary skin lesions.

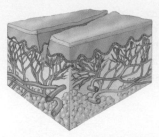

Fissure – Linear red crack ranging into dermis

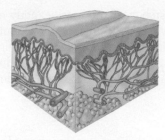

Scar – Fibrous, depth varies, colour ranges from white to red

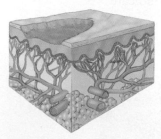

Erosion – Depression in epidermis, caused by tissue loss

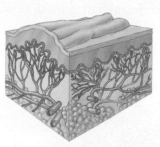

Keloid – Elevated scar, irregular shape, larger than original wound

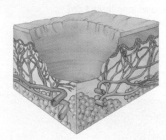

Ulcer – Red or purplish depression ranging into dermis, caused by tissue loss

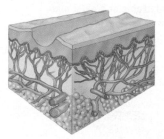

Excoriation – Linear, may be hollow or crusted, caused by loss of epidermis leaving dermis exposed

FIGURE 6-17   Secondary skin lesions.

a hormonal imbalance. Part the hair in several places and palpate the scalp (Figure 6-18). A normal scalp is clean with no scaling, lesions, redness, lumps, or tenderness. Dandruff is characterized by mild flaking, psoriasis by heavy scaling, and seborrheic dermatitis by a greasy scaling. Try to differentiate the flaking of dandruff from the nits (eggs) of lice. Dandruff flakes off the hair easily, while nits firmly attach themselves to the hair shaft.

Feel the hair texture. In white people, a soft hair texture is normal; in black people, a coarser texture is normal. Very dry, brittle, or fragile hair is abnormal. Inspect and palpate the eyebrows. Note the quality and distribution of the hair and any scaling of the underlying skin. When assessing hair, remember that the normal quantity and distribution of hair is related to sex and racial group. For instance, men have more trunk and body hair than do women. Aboriginal men have less facial and body hair than do white men. In addition, white people have more abundant and coarser body hair than do Asians.

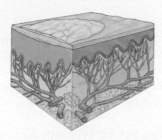

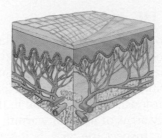

Scale – Elevated area of excessive exfoliation, varies in thickness, shape, and dryness and ranges in colour from white to silver or tan

Lichenification – Thickening and hardening of epidermis with emphasized lines in skin, resembles lichen

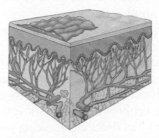

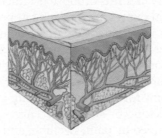

Crust – Reddish, brown, black, tan, or yellowish dried blood, serum, or pus

Atrophy – Skin surface thins and markings disappear, semitransparent parchment-like appearance

FIGURE 6-17 (CONTINUED)   Secondary skin lesions.

THE NAILS

Inspect and palpate the fingernails and toenails. Observe the colour beneath the transparent nail. Normally, it is pink in white people and black or brown in blacks. Note whether the nails appear blue-black or purple, brown, or yellow-grey. Look for lesions, ridging, grooves, depressions, and pitting. Depressions that appear in all nails are usually caused by a systemic disease. Gently squeeze the nail between your thumb and forefinger to test for adherence to the nail bed. A boggy nail suggests the clubbing seen in systemic cardiorespiratory diseases. The condition of the fingernails also can provide important insight into your patient's self-care and hygiene. Check the toenails for any deformity or injury, such as being ingrown.

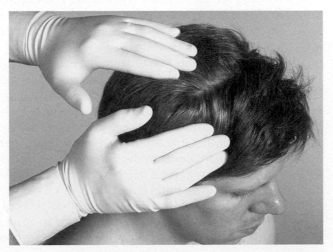

FIGURE 6-18   Inspect and palpate your patient's hair and scalp.

THE HEAD

You can also examine the skull when you inspect and palpate the scalp and hair. Look for any wounds or active bleeding. Observe the general size and contour of the skull. Palpate the cranium from front to back (Procedure 6-2a). It should be symmetrical and smooth. Note any tenderness or deformities (depressions or protrusions). An indentation in the skull may suggest a depressed skull fracture. Note any areas of unusual warmth.

Inspect the face. Is it symmetrical? Are there any involuntary movements? Note any masses or edema. Observe the bony orbits of the eye for periorbital ecchymosis, a bluish discoloration also known as "raccoon eyes." Also, check the mastoid process for discoloration (Procedure 6-2b). These are classic signs of a basilar skull fracture. They normally will not appear immediately but will present hours after the injury occurs. Palpate the facial bones for stability and note any crepitus or loose fragments (Procedure 6-2c). Note whether your patient's facial expressions change appropriately with her mood.

Evaluate the temporomandibular joint (TMJ). Place the tip of your index finger into the depression in front of the tragus (the cartilaginous projection just in front of the ear's outer opening) and ask your patient to open her mouth (Procedure 6-2d). The tips of your fingers should drop into the joint space. Palpate the joint for tenderness, swelling, and range of motion. Sometimes, you may hear a clicking or snapping. This is neither unusual nor problematic unless it is accompanied by pain, swelling, and crepitus. Test for range of motion by asking your patient to open and close her mouth, jut and retract the jaw, and move it from side to side. Finally, assess the skin of the face for colour, pigmentation, texture, thickness, hair distribution, and lesions.

THE EYES

✱ visual acuity wall chart/card wall chart or handheld card with lines of letters used to test vision.

The ideal environment for an eye assessment is a quiet room, free from distractions, in which you can control the lighting and make your patient comfortable. First, test for visual acuity. Place your patient 6 m from a **visual acuity wall chart** or have her hold a **visual acuity card** 35 cm from her face. Ask her to cover one eye with a card and begin reading the lines (Procedure 6-3a). Record the visual acuity grade next to the smallest line in which your patient can read at least one-half of the letters. The result is written as a fraction. The first number represents the distance away from the chart. The second number is the distance from which a normal eye could read the line. Normal is 20/20. A result of 20/70 means that a normal eye could read the line from 70 feet away but your patient could only read it from 20 feet. If no chart is available, you can have your patient count your raised fingers, read from a distance something printed, or distinguish light from dark. This type of exam is routinely conducted as part of a comprehensive physical assessment in a clinic setting.

Test the visual fields by confrontation. Sit directly in front of your patient. Have her cover the left eye while you cover your right eye. Ask her to look at your nose. Extend your left arm to the side and slowly bring it toward you. Ask your patient to say when she first sees your finger. Use your own peripheral vision as a guide. If your patient sees your finger when you do, her visual field is grossly normal in that direction. Do this test in all four quadrants (left and right, up and down). Then, perform the same test with the other eye (Procedure 6-3b). Any abnormalities suggest a defect in peripheral vision. Some common abnormalities include a horizontal defect (loss of vision in the upper or lower half of an eye), a blind eye, bitemporal hemianopsia (loss of vision in the outside half of each eye), left or right homonymous hemianopsia (loss of vision in the right half of both eyes or the left half of both eyes), or homonymous quadrantic de-

VISUAL FIELD ABNORMALITIES

Horizontal defect

Blind eye

Bitemporal hemianopsia

Homonymous hemianopsia

Homonymous quadrantic defect

Left Right

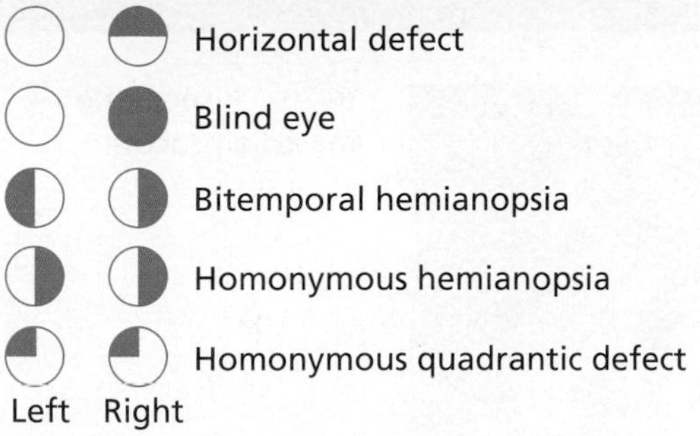

FIGURE 6-19 Visual field abnormalities.

fect (loss of vision in the same quadrant of both eyes). Record the area of defect as illustrated in Figure 6-19.

Now, examine the external part of the eyes. Place yourself directly in front of your patient. Inspect the eyes for symmetry in size, shape, and contour. Do they look alike? Do they protrude (proptosis)? Are they properly aligned? Note the eyelids' position relative to the eyeballs. They should cover the upper quarter of the iris. Are the eyes totally exposed or do the eyelids droop (ptosis)? Have your patient close her eyes. Do they close completely? Do you see any edema, inflammation, or mass? Note the eyelid's colour. It should be pink, indicating good central oxygenation. If the lid is pale, your patient could be in shock or anemic. If cyanotic, she could have central hypoxemia. Are there any lesions?

Carefully observe the eyelids' shape and inspect their contours for any growths. If you see any drainage, note its colour and consistency. Do the eyelashes turn inward to scrape against the eyeball or outward to prevent the complete closure of the eye? Are the eyelashes clean and free from debris? Is there a stye (reddened swelling of the inner eyelid)? Quickly assess the regions of the lacrimal sacs and glands for swelling, excessive tearing, or dryness of the eyes.

Now, ask your patient to look up while you pull down both lower eyelids to inspect the sclera and conjunctiva (Procedure 6-3c). Be careful not to put pressure on the eyeball. Ask your patient to look left and right, up and down. The conjunctiva should be clear and transparent, with no redness or cloudiness. Redness or a cobblestone appearance suggests an allergic or infectious conjunctivitis. Bright red blood in a sharply defined area surrounded by normal tissue, not extending into the iris, indicates a hemorrhage under the conjunctiva. Look for any nodules, swelling, or discharge. The normal sclera is white. A yellow sclera suggests the jaundice of liver disease.

With an oblique light source, inspect each cornea for opacities. Also, check the lens for opacities that you may see through the pupil. Inspect the iris when you inspect the cornea. Shine the light directly from the lateral side and look for a crescent-shaped shadow on the medial side of the iris. Since the iris is flat, the light should cast no shadow. A shadow could suggest glaucoma, caused by a blockage that restricts aqueous humor from leaving the anterior chamber. This increases intraocular pressure and threatens your patient's eyesight.

Inspect the size, shape, and symmetry of the pupils. Are they unusually large (excessive dilation) or unusually small (excessive constriction)? Are they equal? Some patients (20 percent) have unequal pupils, a condition known as anisocoria; if the difference in the pupil's size is less than 2 mm and they react normally to light, anisocoria is benign. To test the pupils, first shine a light into one eye and observe that eye's reaction (Procedure 6-3d). This tests the eye's direct response. The pupil should constrict. Repeat this test for the other eye. Now, shine

Procedure 6-2 Examining the Head

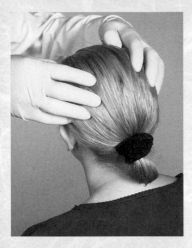

6–2a Palpate the cranium from front to back.

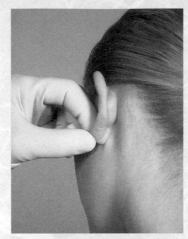

6–2b Inspect the mastoid process.

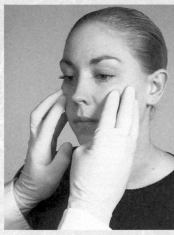

6–2c Palpate the facial bones.

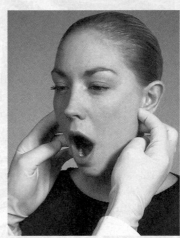

6–2d Palpate the TMJ.

Procedure 6-3 Examining the Eyes

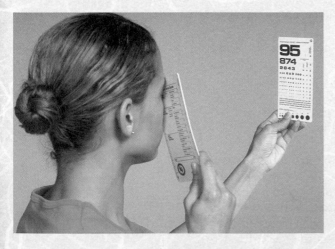

6-3a Use a visual acuity chart to test visual acuity.

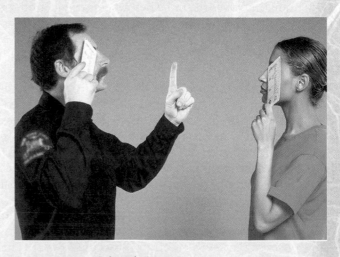

6-3b Test peripheral vision.

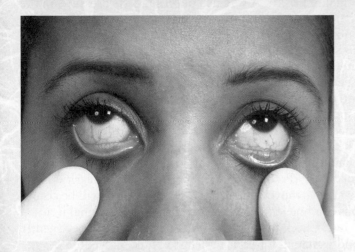

6-3c Inspect the external eye.

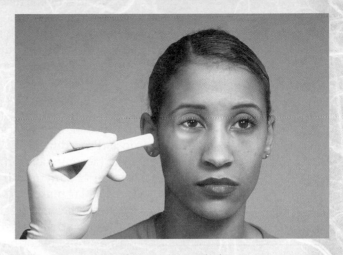

6-3d Test the pupil's reaction to light.

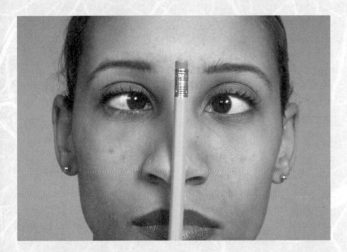

6-3e Test for accommodation.

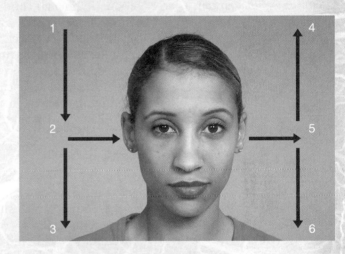

6-3f Move your finger in an *H* pattern to test your patient's extraocular muscles.

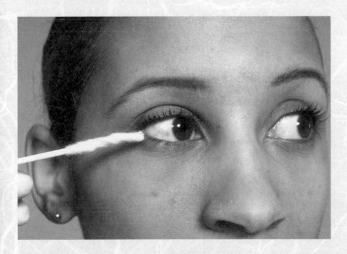

6-3g Check the corneal reflex.

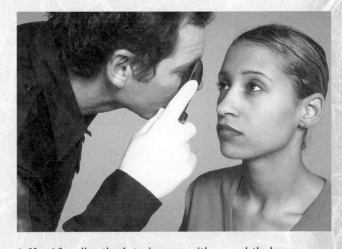

6-3h Visualize the interior eye with an ophthalmoscope.

a light into one eye and observe the other eye's reaction. This tests the eye's consensual response. Both eyes should react simultaneously to the light. Repeat this test for the other eye.

Normal pupils react to light briskly. A sluggish pupil suggests pressure on the oculomotor nerve (CN-III) from increased intracranial pressure. Bilateral sluggishness may indicate global hypoxia to the brain tissue or an adverse drug reaction. Constricted pupils suggest an opiate overdose, whereas fixed and dilated pupils usually mean brain death.

Now, have your patient focus on an object in the distance. Ask her to focus on an object right in front. As your patient focuses on the near object, the pupils should constrict (near response). Now, have your patient follow your finger or a pen, pencil, or similar object as you move it from a distance to the bridge of her nose (Procedure 6-3e). The eyes should converge on the object as the pupils constrict (accommodation). Finally, have your patient follow your finger as you move it in an *H* pattern in front of her (Procedure 6-3f). This tests the integrity of the extraocular muscles. Normal eye movements to follow your finger will be conjugate (together). Nystagmus is a fine jerking of the eyes; it may be normal if noted at the far extremes of the test. Check the corneal reflex by touching the eye gently with a strand of cotton and watching for your patient to blink (Procedure 6-3g).

Examining the eye's interior with an ophthalmoscope is a detailed process that is very difficult to master and requires skill and practice.

Using an ophthalmoscope, visualize the eye's anterior chamber for cells, blood (hyphema), and pus (hypopyon) (Procedure 6-3h). Also, visualize the retina, blood vessels, and optic nerve. Look for foreign bodies under the eyelid or in the cornea; check the cornea for lacerations, abrasions, and infection; and examine the vitreous humor. Look also for cataracts, papilledema caused by increased intracranial pressure, arterial and venous occlusions, and retinal hemorrhages, common clinical conditions you can visualize with an ophthalmoscope. Examining the eye's interior with an ophthalmoscope is a detailed process that is very difficult to master; it requires skill and practice.

THE EARS

Begin examining the external ears facing your patient. Are they symmetrical? Then, examine each ear separately. Inspect the auricles for size, shape, symmetry, landmarks, colour, and position on the head. Observe the surrounding area for deformities, lumps, skin lesions, tenderness, and erythema (redness). Pull the helix upward and outward and note any tenderness or discomfort (Procedure 6-4a). Press on the tragus and on the mastoid process (Procedure 6-4b). Pain or tenderness in any of these areas suggests infection such as otitis or mastoiditis. Discoloration in this area is known as Battle's sign, a common, but late, finding in a basilar skull fracture. An earache may arise from the ear itself or be referred from another place through adjoining and shared sensory nerve pathways. Sources of referred pain may include sinus problems, a bad tooth, temporomandibular joint pain, the common cold, a sore throat, and the cervical spine.

Inspect for discharge (otorrhea) from the ear canal (Procedure 6-4c). The discharge may contain mucus, pus, blood, or cerebrospinal fluid that may have leaked from the skull through a fracture in its base. Injuries to the ear itself can result from blunt trauma to the side of the head, causing temporary or permanent damage to the outer or middle ear. A ruptured eardrum can result from sticking a sharp object into the ear canal or from a pressure wave caused by an explosion.

Check hearing acuity by having your patient close one ear. Test the open ear by whispering, then speaking, in its direction (Procedure 6-4d). Repeat this test for the other ear. Hearing loss can result from many causes. These include trauma, accumulation of debris (particularly cerumen, or "wax") in the ear canal, tympanic membrane rupture, certain drugs, previous surgery, or even prolonged exposure to loud noise. Tinnitus is the perception of abnormal noise in the ear. It usually presents as a buzzing or ringing and is associated with some degree of hearing loss.

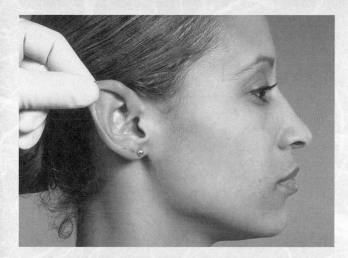

6-4a   Examine the external ear.

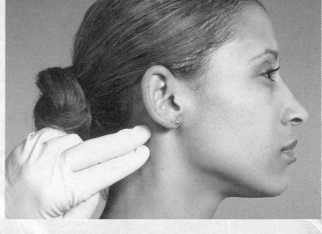

6-4b   Press on the mastoid process.

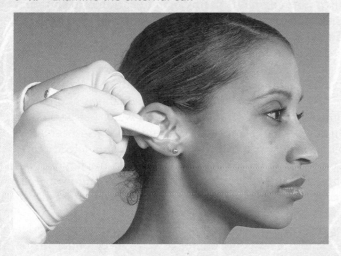

6-4c   Inspect the ear canal for drainage.

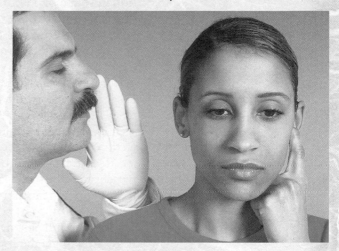

6-4d   Whisper in your patient's ear.

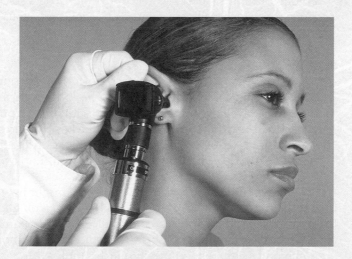

6-4e   Visualize the inner ear canal and tympanic membrane.

Visualize the inner ear canal and tympanic membrane using an otoscope. Attach to the otoscope the largest speculum that will fit into your patient's ear canal. Hold the otoscope either upward or downward. To enter the canal, first tilt your patient's head slightly away from you. Grasp the auricle gently and pull slightly up and backward to straighten the external canal (Procedure 6-4e). Insert the speculum gently and examine the ear canal for cerumen, discharge, redness, lesions, perforations, and foreign bodies.

Now, focus farther back on the eardrum itself and note its colour. The tympanic membrane should be a pearly, translucent grey. A change in colour suggests a middle ear or tympanic membrane abnormality, such as fluid or infection behind the eardrum. Observe the landmarks of the drum. You will need to move the scope around to visualize the drum's entirety. Begin with the light reflection in the anterior inferior quadrant. It should be sharp and bright. Then, check the centre of the drum for bulging or protractions. Note the long process of the malleus. Finally, move to the rim of the drum. Follow along the drum's perimeter and look for perforations from a ruptured tympanic membrane.

THE NOSE

Check your patient's nose from the front and from the side and note any deviation in shape or colour. Also, note any nasal flaring, an indication of respiratory distress. Palpate the external part of the nose for depressions, deformities, and tenderness (Procedure 6-5a).

To inspect the nose's internal structures, tilt your patient's head back slightly. Insert the speculum of your otoscope and check the nasal septum for deviation and perforations (Procedure 6-5b). Erosions suggest intranasal cocaine use. Examine the nasal mucosa for evidence of drainage and note the colour, quantity, and consistency of the discharge. Rhinitis (a runny nose) may produce a watery, clear fluid, as seen in seasonal allergies. If the discharge appears thick and yellow, suspect an infection. Epistaxis (a nosebleed) may be caused by trauma or a septal defect.

Test for nasal obstruction by occluding one side of the nose and having your patient breathe through the other side (Procedure 6-5c). It is normal for one side to be more patent than the other. A deviated septum, foreign body, excessive secretions, or mucosal edema may cause abnormal obstructions.

Inspect and palpate the frontal and maxillary sinuses for swelling and tenderness. To palpate the frontal sinus, press your thumbs upward, deep under the orbital ridges (Procedure 6-5d); to palpate the maxillary sinuses, press up under the zygomatic arches (cheeks) (Procedure 6-5e). You also can tap on each area for similar symptoms. Swelling or tenderness suggests a sinus infection or obstruction.

THE MOUTH

Assess the mouth from anterior to posterior, starting with the lips. Note their condition and colour. They should be pink, smooth, and symmetrical and devoid of lesions, swelling, lumps, cracks, or scaliness. Gently palpate the lips with the jaw closed and note any lesions, nodules, or fissures, especially at the corners (Procedure 6-6a). Observe the undersurfaces of the upper and lower lips (Procedure 6-6b). They should be wet and smooth. Look for any of the lip abnormalities in Table 6-3.

To examine the mouth you will need a bright light and a tongue blade. Holding the tongue blade like a chopstick will give you good downward leverage. Examine the oral mucosa for colour, ulcers, white patches, and nodules. The oral mucosa should appear pinkish-red, smooth, and moist. Note the colour of the gums and teeth. The gums should be pink with a clearly defined margin surrounding each tooth. Inspect the teeth for colour, shape, and position. Are any

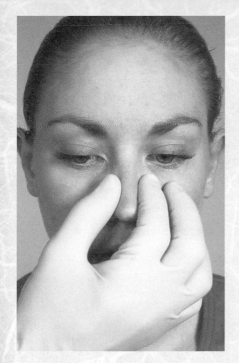

6-5a Palpate the external part of the nose.

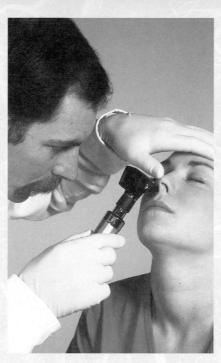

6-5b Inspect the internal part of the nose with an otoscope.

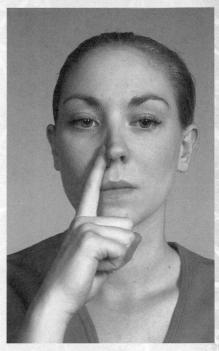

6-5c Inspect the nose for nasal obstruction.

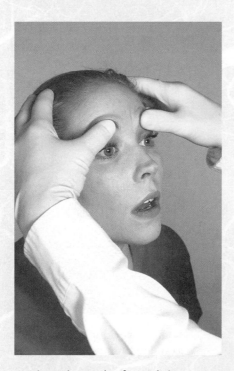

6-5d Palpate the frontal sinus.

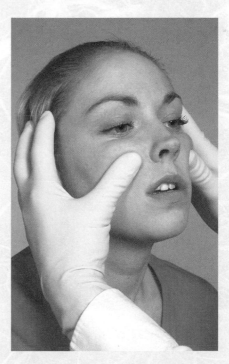

6-5e Palpate the maxillary sinus.

Anatomical Regions **287**

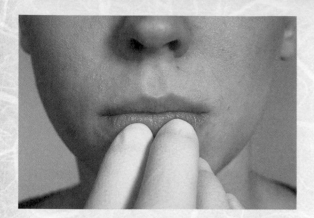

6-6a   Palpate the lips.

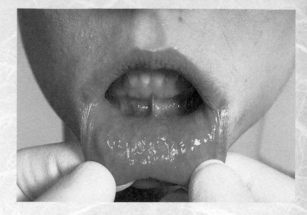

6-6b   Inspect the lips' undersurfaces.

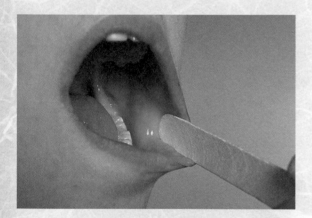

6-6c   Examine the buccal mucosa.

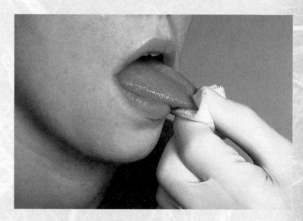

6-6d   Inspect the tongue using a gauze pad and a gloved hand.

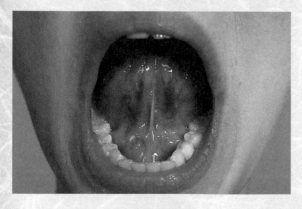

6-6e   Inspect under the tongue.

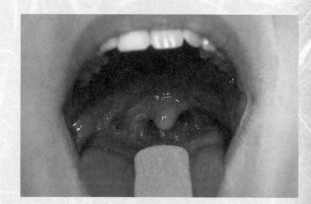

6-6f   Have your patient say "aaahhh" while you examine the soft palate and uvula.

Table 6-3	LIP ABNORMALITIES	
Lips	**Cause**
Dry, cracked lips	Dehydration, wind damage
Swelling/edema	Infection, allergic reaction, burns
Lesions	Infection, irritation, skin cancer
Pallor	Anemia, shock
Cyanosis	Respiratory or cardiac insufficiency

missing or loose? Suspect periodontal disease if the gums are swollen, bleed easily, and are separated from the teeth by large crevices that trap food. Use a tongue blade to move the lateral lip to one side while you examine the buccal mucosa and parotid glands (Procedure 6-6c). Note the buccal mucosa's colour and texture.

Ask your patient to stick her tongue straight out and then to move it from side to side. Coating of the tongue indicates dehydration. Note its colour and normally velvety surface. Hold the tongue with a gauze pad and a gloved hand to manipulate it for inspection (Procedure 6-6d). Make sure to inspect the sides and bottom of the tongue because malignancies are more likely to develop there, especially in patients over age 50 who smoke, chew tobacco, or drink alcohol (Procedure 6-6e). The undersurface should be smooth and pink; often, you can see the bluish discoloration of dilated veins or the yellowish tint of early jaundice. Inspect the floor of the mouth, the submandibular ducts, and the fold over the sublingual gland.

Now, examine the normally white hard palate and the normally pink soft palate (Procedure 6-6f). Check them for texture and lesions. Observe the posterior pharyngeal wall. Press the blade down on the middle third of the tongue and have your patient say "aaaaahhhh." Examine the posterior pharynx, the palatine tonsils, and the movement of the uvula. Inspect the tonsils for colour and symmetry. Look for exudate (pus), swelling, ulcers, or drainage. The uvula should move straight up with no deviation.

Note any odours from your patient's mouth. The smell of alcohol, feces (bowel obstruction), acetone (diabetic ketoacidosis), gastric contents, or the bitter-almond smell of cyanide poisoning may all provide important clues to your patient's problem. Also, look for any fluids or unusual matter in your patient's mouth. For example, coffee-grounds-like material suggests an upper gastrointestinal (GI) bleed. Pink-tinged sputum indicates acute pulmonary edema, whereas green or yellow phlegm suggests respiratory infection. Pay special attention to anything in your patient's mouth that can eventually obstruct her upper airway, including dentures or missing teeth.

Pay special attention to anything in your patient's mouth that can eventually obstruct her upper airway.

THE NECK

If necessary, maintain spinal precautions while assessing the patient's head and neck. Briefly inspect your patient's neck for general symmetry and visible masses. Note any obvious deformity, deviation, tugging, masses, surgical scars, gland enlargement, or visible lymph nodes. Examine any penetrating injuries to the neck closely for damage to the trachea or major blood vessels; handle gently to avoid dislodging a clot that has halted bleeding. Immediately cover any open wounds with an occlusive dressing to prevent air from entering a lacerated jugular vein during inspiration. Look for jugular vein distention while your patient is sitting upright and at a 45-degree incline.

Palpate the trachea for midline position (Procedure 6-7a). Then, gently palpate the carotid arteries and note their rate and quality of their pulses (Procedure 6-7b). Now, palpate the butterfly-shaped thyroid gland from behind your patient.

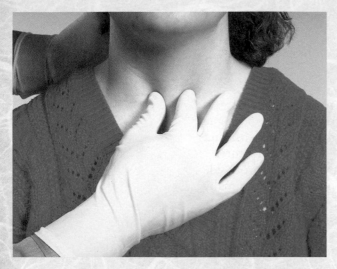

6-7a   Assess the trachea for midline position.

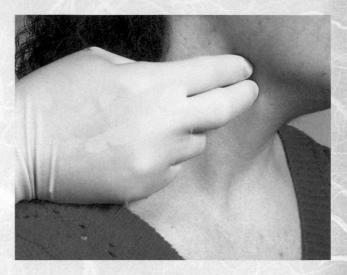

6-7b   Palpate the carotid arteries.

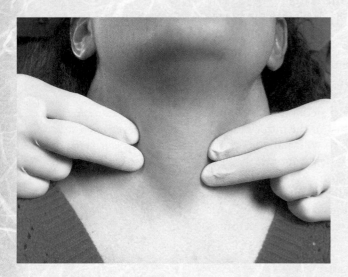

6-7c   Palpate the thyroid gland.

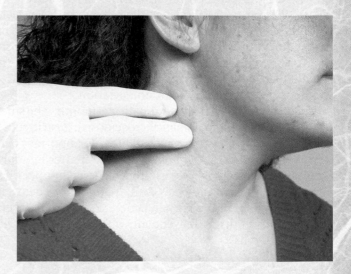

6-7d   Palpate the lymph nodes.

Table 6-4 LYMPH NODE EXAM

Node	Exam
Preauricular	Press on the tragus and "milk" anteriorly.
Postauricular	Palpate on or under the mastoid process.
Occipital	Palpate at the base of the skull lateral to the thick bands of muscle.
Submental	Palpate at the base of the mandible under the chin.
Submaxillary	Palpate along the underside of the jawline.
Anterior cervical	Palpate anterior to the sternocleidomastoid muscle.
Posterior cervical	Palpate posterior to the sternocleidomastoid muscle.
Deep cervical	Encircle and palpate the sternocleidomastoid muscle.
Supraclavicular	Palpate just above the clavicle in the deep groove.

Rest your thumbs on her trapezius muscles and place two fingers of each hand on the sides of the trachea just beneath the cricoid cartilage (Procedure 6-7c). Have your patient swallow and feel for the movement of the gland. If you can feel it, it should be small, smooth, and free of nodules. Examining the lymph nodes requires a systematic approach (Table 6-4). Using the pads of your fingers, palpate the nodes by moving the skin over the underlying tissues in each area (Procedure 6-7d). When swollen, the nodes are palpable, sometimes even visible. Note their size, shape, mobility, consistency, and tenderness. Tender, swollen, and mobile nodes suggest inflammation, usually from infection. Hard or fixed nodes suggest a malignancy. Inspect and palpate for subcutaneous emphysema, the presence of air just below the skin. This generally suggests a tear in the tracheobronchial tree or a pneumothorax.

THE CHEST AND LUNGS

To assess the chest and thorax you will need a stethoscope with a bell and diaphragm, a marking pen, and a centimetre ruler. Have your patient sit upright, if possible, and expose her entire chest. At the same time, try to maintain your female patient's modesty when assessing her thorax and lungs by keeping her breasts covered. Perform your assessment in the standard sequence—inspect, palpate, percuss, auscultate—and compare the findings from each side. Always try to visualize the underlying lobes of the lungs during your assessment.

Observe your patient's breathing. Look for signs of acute respiratory distress. Now, count the respiratory rate and note the breathing pattern. Obviously prolonged inhalation or exhalation indicates difficulty moving air in or out of the lungs. Do you hear sounds of an upper airway obstruction (inspiratory stridor) or a lower airway obstruction (expiratory wheezing, rhonchi)? Any gross abnormalities in the respiratory rate or pattern require rapid emergency intervention.

Inspect the anterior chest wall and assess its symmetry. Funnel chest (pectus excavatum) is a condition in which the lower portion of the sternum is depressed (Figure 6-20). With a pigeon chest (pectus carinatum), the sternum curves outward. Do both sides of your patient's chest wall rise in unison? Note whether she is using neck muscles during inhalation or abdominal muscles during exhalation. If the skin retracts in the area above her clavicles (supraclavicular), at the notch above the sternum (suprasternal), and between the ribs (intercostal), suspect a ventilation problem. If multiple ribs are fractured, creating a "floating segment" or "traumatic flail chest," you may find paradoxical (opposite) movement of that part of the chest wall during breathing.

Any gross abnormalities in the respiratory rate or pattern require rapid emergency intervention.

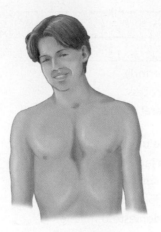

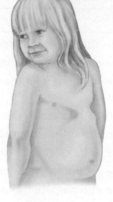

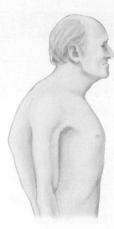

Funnel chest   Pigeon chest   Barrel chest

FIGURE 6-20   Chest wall abnormalities.

Now, look at the chest from the side. Normally, an adult's thorax is twice as wide as it is deep. That is, the transverse diameter of the chest wall is usually twice the anteroposterior diameter. In infants, the elderly, or patients with chronic pulmonary disease, however, the anteroposterior diameter is increased, giving them a barrel chest appearance.

Posterior Chest Examination

Next, examine the posterior chest. Ask your patient to fold her arms across her chest and breathe normally during the exam. This moves the scapulae out of the way and allows you more access to the posterior lung fields. Inspect her posterior chest for deformities and symmetrical movement as she breathes. Some patients may exhibit thoracic kyphoscoliosis, an abnormal spinal curvature that deforms the chest and makes your lung exam more challenging. Inspect the intercostal spaces for retractions or bulging; both are abnormal. Retractions may appear when airflow is impeded during inspiration. Bulging may appear when airflow is impeded during exhalation. Respiratory movement should be smooth and effortless. When it is not, suspect underlying respiratory disease or structural impairment.

Palpate the rib cage for rigidity. Feel for tenderness, deformities, depressions, loose segments, asymmetry, and crepitus. Then, evaluate for equal expansion. First, locate the level of the posterior 10th rib. To do this, find the lowest rib and simply move up two more ribs. An alternative method for locating the posterior 10th rib is to palpate the spinous processes. Ask your patient to touch her chin to her chest. The most prominent spinous process is the 7th cervical vertebra. Locate it and count down to T-10 in the midline. Now, place your hands parallel to the 10th rib on your patient's back with your fingers spread. Lightly grasp her lateral rib cage with your spread hands (Procedure 6-8a). Ask your patient to inhale deeply. Normally, the distance between your thumbs will increase symmetrically by 3–5 cm during deep inspiration. If you detect decreased thoracic expansion or feel unilateral delay, suspect a disorder of the underlying lung, pleura, or diaphragm.

When your patient speaks, you can feel vibrations on the chest wall. This is known as tactile fremitus. Place the palm of your hand on your patient's chest wall and have her say "ninety-nine or one-on-one." As she does, palpate the posterior chest; feel the vibrations in different areas of the chest wall and compare symmetrical areas of the lungs (Procedure 6-8b). Identify and note any

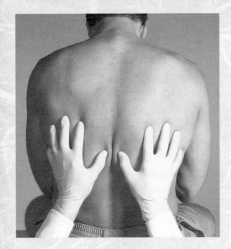

6-8a   Palpate the posterior chest for excursion.

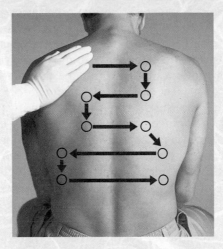

6-8b   Palpate the posterior chest for tactile fremitus.

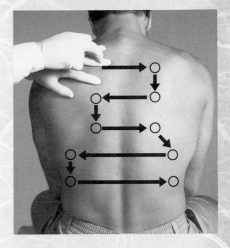

6-8c   Percuss the posterior chest.

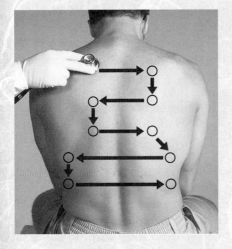

6-8d   Auscultate the posterior chest.

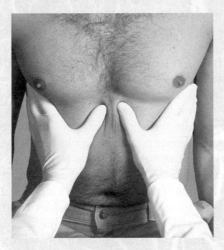

6-8e   Palpate the anterior chest for excursion.

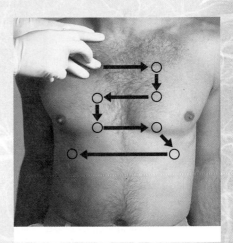

6-8f   Percuss the anterior chest.

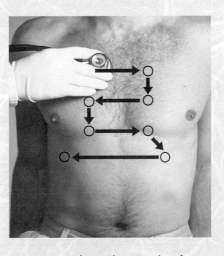

6-8g   Auscultate the anterior chest.

areas of increased, decreased, or absent vibrations. You will feel increased fremitus when sound transmission is enhanced through areas of consolidated lung tissue, such as in a tumour, pneumonia, or pulmonary fibrosis. You will feel decreased or absent fremitus when sound transmission is diminished in a certain area, as may occur with a pleural effusion, emphysema, or pneumothorax.

Percuss your patient's posterior chest to determine whether the underlying tissues are air filled, fluid filled, or solid. Also, percuss to determine the position and boundaries of the diaphragm and underlying organs. Percuss both sides of the chest symmetrically from the apex to the base at 5-cm intervals, avoiding bony areas, such as the scapulae (Procedure 6-8c). Percuss at least twice in each area and compare both sides of the thorax. Identify and note any area of abnormal percussion. For example, a hyperresonant sound in the right chest may indicate a pneumothorax, whereas a dull sound in the same area may indicate a hemothorax. Assess the percussion sounds according to their quality, intensity, pitch, and duration. Practise percussing the chest so that you will become familiar with the normal resonance of the lungs and be able to identify abnormal sounds.

Next, assess for diaphragmatic excursion. Identify the level of the diaphragm during quiet breathing by percussing for dullness as the diaphragm moves during the respiratory cycle. Percuss at the lower rib margin on one side and note when dullness (muscle) replaces resonance (air). With a pen, mark the location of the diaphragm at the end of inhalation and at the end of exhalation. The distance between the marks is the diaphragmatic excursion. In the normal healthy adult at rest, the diaphragmatic excursion should be approximately 6 cm. Now, measure diaphragmatic excursion on the opposite side and compare the marks. If you find asymmetrical diaphragmatic levels, a paralyzed phrenic nerve may be the problem. Here, reevaluate your patient's respiratory depth for adequacy and provide the appropriate intervention as needed.

Auscultate your patient's chest for normal breath sounds, adventitious breath sounds, and voice sounds. Auscultate all lung fields and compare each side. Evaluate the normal breath sounds produced by airflow through the upper and lower airways. These include tracheal, bronchial, bronchovesicular, and vesicular breath sounds (Table 6-5).

Besides the normal breath sounds already mentioned you also may hear adventitious sounds. These include crackles, wheezes, rhonchi, stridor, and pleural rubs.

Also known as "rales," **crackles** are light crackling, popping, nonmusical sounds heard usually during inspiration. They are produced by air passing through moisture in the bronchoalveolar system or from the abrupt opening of closed alveoli. Early inspiratory crackles, associated with chronic bronchitis and heart failure, begin shortly after inspiration starts, and they stop soon thereafter. These are coarse crackles—loud, low pitched, and long, similar to the sound of water boiling. They are often audible at the mouth.

✱ **crackles** light crackling, popping, nonmusical sounds heard usually during inspiration.

Table 6-5	NORMAL BREATH SOUNDS		
Sound	Description	Location	Duration
Tracheal	Very loud, harsh	Over the trachea	Nearly equal inspiratory and expiratory phases
Bronchial	Loud, high pitch, hollow	Over the manubrium	Prolonged expiratory phase
Bronchovesicular	Soft, breezy, lower pitch	Between the scapulae/ 2nd–3rd ICS lateral to the sternum	Approximately equal inspiratory and expiratory phases
Vesicular	Soft, swishy, lowest pitch	Lung periphery	Prolonged inspiratory phase

Late inspiratory crackles, associated with congestive heart failure and interstitial lung diseases, begin in the first half of the inspiratory phase and continue into late inspiration. They are fine crackles—soft, high pitched, and very brief, similar to the sound of Rice Krispies crackling. They commonly appear first at the base of the lungs and move upward as your patient's condition worsens. Usually, you can expect them to shift to dependent regions with changes in your patient's position. For example, if your heart failure patient is sitting up, expect to hear crackles first in the bases. If she is bedridden, expect to hear crackles first in the back.

Wheezes are continuous, high-pitched musical sounds similar to a whistle. They result when air moves through partially obstructed smaller airways. Their causes include asthma, bronchospasm, and foreign bodies. You may hear them without a stethoscope or by auscultating the chest during any or all phases of the respiratory cycle. They often originate in the small bronchioles and first appear at the end of exhalation. The closer to the end of inspiration they appear, the worse your patient's condition is.

✱ **wheezes** continuous, high-pitched musical sounds similar to a whistle.

Rhonchi are continuous sounds with a lower pitch and a snoring quality. They are caused by secretions in the larger airways, a common finding in bronchitis (diffuse) and pneumonia (localized). Rhonchi usually appear in early exhalation but may occur in early inspiration as well.

✱ **rhonchi** continuous sounds with a lower pitch and a snoring quality.

Stridor is a predominantly high pitched inspiratory sound. It indicates a partial obstruction of the larynx or trachea.

✱ **stridor** predominantly inspiratory wheeze associated with laryngeal obstruction.

Pleural friction rubs are the squeaking or grating sounds of the pleural linings rubbing together. They occur where the pleural layers are inflamed and have lost their lubrication. Pleural rubs are common in pneumonia and pleurisy (inflammation of the pleura). Because these sounds occur whenever your patient's chest wall moves, they appear during the entire respiratory cycle.

✱ **pleural friction rub** the squeaking or grating sound of the pleural linings rubbing together.

You may hear no breath sounds in some areas. This may result from effusion (fluid in the pleural space causing a decrease in functional lung tissue) or consolidation (infectious pus causing collapsed alveoli). In either case, note the area's size and intervene appropriately to ensure adequate ventilation and oxygenation of your patient.

Auscultate the posterior chest systematically. Have your patient fold her arms across her chest and breathe through her mouth more deeply and slowly than usual. Auscultate the same areas you percussed and compare the bilateral findings (Procedure 6-8d). Listen for at least one full breath at each location. Be alert for patient discomfort or hyperventilation. Note the pitch, intensity, and duration of each inspiratory and expiratory sound. If the sounds are decreased, suspect impaired airflow or poor sound transmission. If the sounds are absent, suspect no airflow. Note whether you hear sounds where you normally should. For example, when you auscultate over the peripheral lung fields, you should not hear tracheal, bronchial, or bronchovesicular breath sounds. Listen carefully and note what you hear, where you hear it, and when you hear it during the respiratory cycle. Also note whether the sounds change when your patient coughs or changes position.

If you hear abnormally located tracheal, bronchial, or bronchovesicular breath sounds, assess your patient's transmitted voice sounds. Ask her to repeat the words "ninety-nine" as you auscultate her chest wall. Normally, you should hear muffled, indistinct sounds. Hearing the words clearly is an abnormal finding known as **bronchophony**. Bronchophony occurs when fluid (water, blood) or consolidated tissue (pus, tumour) replaces the normally air-filled lung. After you check your patient for bronchophony, assess her for **whispered pectoriloquy** and **egophony**. For pectoriloquy, ask your patient to whisper "ninety-nine" while you auscultate. As with bronchophony, the words will be clear and distinct if sound transmission through an area is abnormally enhanced. For egophony, ask her to repeat the long *e* sound while you auscultate. You should hear a muffled long *e*. If vocal resonance is abnormally increased, you will hear an *a* sound instead. This is known as "*e* to *a* egophony."

✱ **bronchophony** abnormal clarity of patient's transmitted voice sounds.

✱ **whispered pectoriloquy** abnormal clarity of patient's transmitted whispers.

✱ **egophony** abnormal change in tone of patient's transmitted voice sounds.

Anterior Chest Examination

Your examination of the anterior chest will be similar to your examination of the posterior chest. Begin by having your patient lie supine with her arms relaxed but slightly abducted at her sides. Look for any gross deformities or asymmetrical movements. Does the chest wall rise symmetrically? Is there accessory muscle use? Look for abnormal retractions in the suprasternal, supraclavicular, and intercostal areas. Also, check for callused elbows from tripodding (leaning with elbows on a table or chair arms), and finger clubbing—both common signs of chronic lung disease. Is the trachea midline or deviated; does it tug during inhalation? In cases of tension pneumothorax, the trachea will deviate away from the affected side. In cases of pulmonary fibrosis and atelectasis, it will tug toward the affected side during inhalation.

Palpate the anterior chest for deformities and areas of tenderness. Check for chest expansion by placing your thumbs along the costal margins on both sides and gently grasping the lateral rib cage (Procedure 6-8e). Ask your patient to inhale deeply. Normally, your thumbs will separate symmetrically, and the distance between them will increase from 3 to 5 cm. If you detect decreased thoracic expansion or feel unilateral delay, suspect a disorder of the underlying lung, pleura, or diaphragm.

As with the posterior chest, test for tactile fremitus, bronchophony, whispered pectoriloquy, and egophony if you detect abnormal breath sounds.

Percuss your patient's anterior chest to help determine whether the underlying tissues are air filled, fluid filled, or solid and to determine the position and boundaries of the diaphragm and underlying organs. Percuss each side of your patient's anterior chest from its apex to its base at 5-cm intervals at the midclavicular lines (Procedure 6-8f). Percuss at least twice in each area, and compare both sides of the thorax. Identify and note any area of abnormal percussion. Remember that when percussing the right chest, you will hear dullness at the upper border of the liver. On the left side, you will hear the normal resonance of the lung change to tympany when you reach the stomach. You also will percuss an area of cardiac dullness from the 3rd to the 5th intercostal spaces.

Finally, auscultate the anterior and lateral thoraces systematically. Have your patient breathe through her mouth more deeply and slowly than usual. Auscultate the same areas you percussed and compare symmetrical areas (Procedure 6-8g). Listen for at least one full breath at each location. Be alert for patient discomfort or hyperventilation. As with posterior chest auscultation, note the pitch, intensity, and duration of each inspiratory and expiratory sound and whether you heard sounds where you should normally expect them. Listen for adventitious sounds. If you hear abnormally located tracheal, bronchial, or bronchovesicular breath sounds, assess for bronchophony, whispered pectoriloquy, and egophony.

THE CARDIOVASCULAR SYSTEM

✱ **diastole** phase of cardiac cycle when ventricles relax.

✱ **systole** phase of cardiac cycle when the ventricles contract.

To assess cardiac function, you must understand the cardiac cycle. During **diastole,** the heart's resting period, the ventricles relax. The pressure in the atria is greater than the pressure in the ventricles. This opens the tricuspid valve on the right side and the mitral valve on the left, allowing blood from the atria to fill the ventricles. During **systole,** the ventricles contract and the tricuspid and mitral valves close, preventing backflow into the atria. The vibrations of these valves' closings generate the first heart sound—S_1, or the "lub." The increased pressure in the right ventricle opens the pulmonic semilunar valve, sending deoxygenated blood to the lungs. The increased pressure in the left ventricle opens the aortic semilunar valve, sending freshly oxygenated blood to the body. At the end of systole, as pressure in the ventricles falls, the pulmonic and aortic semilunar valves

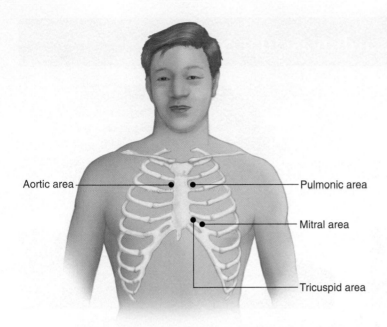

FIGURE 6-21   Sites for cardiac auscultation.

In the figure: Aortic area, Pulmonic area, Mitral area, Tricuspid area

close tightly to prevent backflow. These vibrations generate the second heart sound—S_2, or the "dub." This cycle repeats approximately 60–100 times per minute in the healthy adult at rest. Extra sounds known as heart murmurs result when valves do not fully open or close, causing turbulent flow that an experienced clinician can detect.

You must auscultate for heart sounds at the proper places on the chest wall (Figure 6-21). Always listen downstream. For example, since the tricuspid and mitral valves direct blood flow to the ventricles, which are toward your patient's feet, listen for S_1 at the apex of the heart. This is found near the lower left sternal border. Since the aortic and pulmonic valves direct blood flow to the lungs and aorta, which are toward your patient's head, listen for S_2 at the base of the heart. This is found at the 2nd intercostal space near the sternum.

Begin your cardiovascular assessment by inspecting for signs of arterial insufficiency or occlusion in your patient's trunk and extremities. Look for skin pallor and other signs of decreased perfusion. Now, assess the arterial pulses. Inspect the carotid arteries for visible pulsations just medial to the sternocleidomastoid muscles. Palpate the carotid arteries at the level of the cricoid cartilage to avoid pressing on the carotid sinus (Procedure 6-9a). Never palpate both carotids simultaneously; doing so may decrease cerebral blood flow. Assess the carotid pulse for rate, rhythm, and quality. Does its quality vary? Do the variations correspond to respiration? For example, in pulsus paradoxus, the amplitude of the pulse diminishes with inspiration and increases with exhalation. Do you feel a vibration or humming (**thrills**) when you palpate the carotid artery? If so, auscultate the area with your stethoscope for **bruits,** the sounds of turbulent blood flow around a partial obstruction (Procedure 6-9b).

If you have not already taken your patient's blood pressure, do so now. Also, check for jugular venous pressure, which approximates your patient's right atrial pressure. Position your patient supine, with her head elevated to about 30 degrees. Turning your patient's head away from the side you are assessing, identify the external jugular veins on both sides and locate the pulsations of the internal jugular veins. Look for the pulsation in the area around the suprasternal notch and where the sternocleidomastoid muscle inserts on the clavicle and manubrium.

Content Review

HEART SOUNDS
- S_1—"lub"
- S_2—"dub"
- Split S_1—"la-lub"
- Split S_2—"da-dub"
- S_3—"lub-dub-dee" (Kentucky)
- S_4—"dee-lub-dub" (Tennessee)
- Click
- Snap
- Pericardial friction rub
- Murmur

✱ **thrill** vibration or humming felt when palpating the pulse.

✱ **bruit** sound of turbulent blood flow around a partial obstruction.

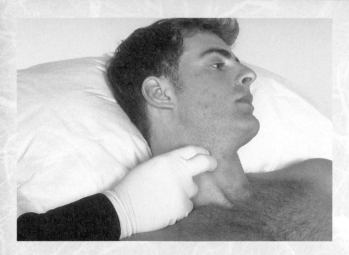

6-9a   Assess the carotid pulse.

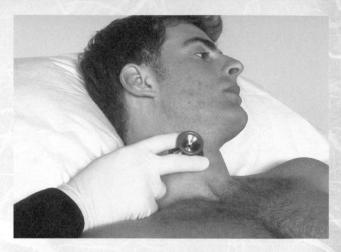

6-9b   Auscultate for bruits.

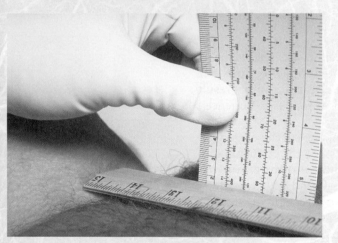

6-9c   Measure jugular venous pressure.

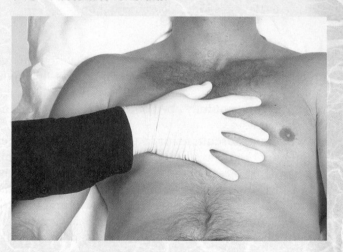

6-9d   Palpate for the apical impulse (PMI).

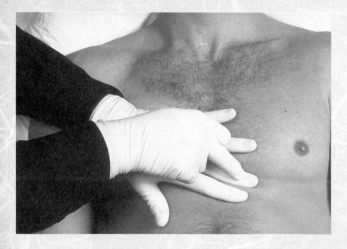

6-9e   Percuss for the PMI.

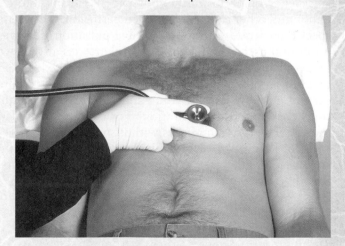

6-9f   Auscultate for heart sounds.

Now, identify the internal jugular vein's highest point of pulsation (the point at which the pulse diminishes) and measure its vertical distance from the sternal angle (midline at the 2nd costal cartilage). To do this, place a ruler perpendicular to the chest at the sternal angle and position a straight edge at a right angle to the ruler (Procedure 6-9c). Lower the straight edge until it rests atop the jugular vein pulsation. The corresponding ruler mark is your measurement. Normal venous pressure is 1–2 cm. If you cannot visualize the pulsations, observe the point at which the external jugular veins collapse and use the same measuring parameters.

Examine the external jugular veins for equality of distention. Abnormal bilateral distention indicates fluid volume overload or that something, such as congestive heart failure or cardiac tamponade, is blocking venous return to the heart. Unilateral distention suggests a localized problem.

With your patient's head still raised to about 30 degrees, inspect and palpate the chest for the apical impulse, or PMI (point of maximal impulse) (Procedure 6-9d). When examining a woman with large breasts, gently displace the left breast upward and laterally if needed, or ask her to do this for you. First, look for a pulsation at the cardiac apex, normally at the 5th intercostal space just medial to the midclavicular line. This pulsation represents the PMI. It helps you locate the left ventricle's apex.

If you cannot see the pulsation, ask your patient to exhale and stop breathing for a few seconds. Lateral displacement of the PMI indicates an enlarged right ventricle. The PMI may be displaced upward and to the left in pregnant women. If your patient is obese or has a very muscular chest wall or a barrel chest, you may not detect the PMI. Percussion may help if you have difficulty palpating the PMI. Start lateral and work your way toward the midline (Procedure 6-9e). When you hear a change from resonance (lung) to dullness (heart), you have located the PMI.

Using the diaphragm of your stethoscope, auscultate your patient's anterior chest for normal heart sounds and for abnormal or extra heart sounds (Procedure 6-9f). Listen for the high-pitched sounds of S_1 at the 5th intercostal space at the left sternal border (tricuspid valve) and at the PMI (mitral valve) using the diaphragm of your stethoscope. Listen for the high-pitched sounds of S_2 at the 2nd intercostal space at the right sternal border (aortic valve) and 2nd intercostal space at the left sternal border (pulmonic valve). For a comprehensive auscultation of heart sounds, you should also listen at the 3rd and 4th intercostal spaces. Although there is nothing specific behind those spaces, you may hear something there that you will not hear in the other places if the heart is not anatomically perfect.

Because the mitral and aortic valves (left side) close slightly before the tricuspid and pulmonic valves (right side), you may hear two sets of sounds instead of one. This is known as splitting. A split S_1 sounds like "la-lub" and a split S_2 like "da-dub." Instead of "lub-dub," you will hear "la-lub—da-dub." Splitting of S_2 during inspiration is normal in healthy children and young adults. Expiratory or persistent splitting suggests an abnormality.

You also may hear extra or abnormal heart sounds, depending on your patient's age and condition. A third heart sound, S_3, is sometimes called the ventricular gallop. It is the "dee" of "lub-dub-dee" and has the same cadence as the word "Kentucky." This extra heart sound develops from vibrations that result when blood fills a dilated ventricle. Commonly heard in children and young adults, an S_3 is usually considered pathological in patients over age 30. It generally develops with ventricular failure and ventricular volume overload and disappears when the problem is resolved. S_3 is a low-pitched sound heard in early to mid-diastole. Listen for S_3 at the apex using the bell of your stethoscope with your patient lying on her left side.

Atrial gallop is the fourth heart sound, S_4. It is the "dee" of "dee-lub-dub" and has the same cadence as the word "Tennessee." An S_4 develops from vibrations produced in late diastole when atrial contraction forces blood into a ventricle that has decreased compliance or that resists filling and causes volume overload. It usually disappears when the problem is resolved. Listen for the low-pitched S_4 at the apex using the bell of your stethoscope with your patient lying on her left side.

Experienced cardiologists can also detect clicks, snaps, friction rubs, and murmurs. An ejection click results from a stiff or stuck valve. An opening snap results when a stenotic mitral or tricuspid valve's leaflets recoil abruptly after ventricular diastole. A pericardial friction rub occurs when inflammation causes the heart's visceral and parietal surfaces to rub together at each heartbeat. A murmur is a rumbling or vibrating noise that results from turbulent blood flow through the heart valves, a large artery, or a septal defect.

THE ABDOMEN

To examine the abdomen, you need good lighting, a relaxed patient, and exposure from above the xiphoid process to the symphysis pubis. Make sure your patient does not have a full bladder. Make your patient comfortable in the supine position with one pillow under the head and another under the knees. Have her place her hands at the sides. This helps relax the abdominal muscles, making the examination easier for you and more comfortable for your patient.

Ask your patient to point out any areas of pain or tenderness. Examine these areas last. Use warm hands and a warm stethoscope, and keep your fingernails short. If your hands are cold, palpate your patient through her clothes until your hands warm up. Begin your exam slowly and avoid any quick, unexpected movements. Monitor your patient's facial expressions for pain and discomfort. During the exam, distract her with conversation or questions. Use inspection, auscultation, percussion, and palpation to perform the exam. Always auscultate before percussing or palpating because these manipulations may alter your patient's bowel motility and resulting bowel sounds.

When you examine the abdomen, you will assess the gastrointestinal organs and other nearby organs and structures. Inspect the skin of the abdomen and flanks for scars, dilated veins, stretch marks, rashes, lesions, and pigmentation changes. Look for discoloration over the umbilicus (**Cullen's sign**) or over the flanks (**Grey-Turner's sign**); these are late signs suggesting intra-abdominal bleeding. Assess the size and shape of your patient's abdomen to determine whether it is scaphoid (concave), flat, round, or distended. Ask the patient if it is its usual size and shape. Note its symmetry. Check for bulges, hernias, or distended flanks. **Ascites** appears as bulges in the flanks and across the abdomen and indicates edema caused by congestive heart failure. A distended bladder or pregnant uterus can cause a suprapubic bulge. Bulges in the inguinal or femoral areas suggest a hernia.

Now, look at your patient's umbilicus. Note its location and contour and observe for any signs of herniation or inflammation. Check for any visible pulsation, peristalsis (the wave-like motion of organs moving their contents through the digestive tract), or masses. You may see the normal pulsation of the aorta just lateral to the umbilicus. If you notice a bounding or exaggerated pulsation, suspect an aortic aneurysm. Visible peristalsis may indicate a bowel obstruction.

Next, auscultate for bowel sounds and other sounds, such as bruits, throughout the abdomen. To auscultate for bowel sounds, first warm your stethoscope's diaphragm in your hand because a cold diaphragm might cause abdominal tension. Gently place the diaphragm on your patient's abdomen and proceed systematically, listening for bowel sounds in each quadrant. Note their location, frequency, and character.

Normal bowel sounds consist of a variety of high-pitched gurgles and clicks that occur every 5–15 seconds. More frequent sounds indicate increased bowel motility in conditions like diarrhea or an early intestinal obstruction. Occasionally, you may hear loud, prolonged, gurgling sounds known as **borborygmi**. These indicate hy-

✱ **Cullen's sign** discoloration around the umbilicus (occasionally the flanks) suggestive of intra-abdominal hemorrhage.

✱ **Grey-Turner's sign** discoloration over the flanks suggesting intra-abdominal bleeding.

✱ **ascites** bulges in the flanks and across the abdomen, indicating edema caused by congestive heart failure.

✱ **borborygmi** loud, prolonged, gurgling bowel sounds indicating hyperperistalsis.

perperistalsis. Decreased or absent sounds suggest a paralytic ileus or peritonitis. Listen at least two minutes for bowel sounds if the abdomen is silent. Bruits are swishing sounds that indicate turbulent blood flow. To confirm bruits, use the bell of your stethoscope to listen in areas over abdominal blood vessels, such as the aorta and renal arteries (Procedure 6-10a). If you hear a bruit, suspect an arterial disorder, such as an abdominal aortic aneurysm or renal artery stenosis.

Percussing the abdomen produces different sounds based on the underlying tissues. These sounds help you detect excessive gas and solid or fluid-filled masses. They also help you determine the size and position of solid organs, such as the liver and spleen. Percuss the abdomen in the same sequence you used for auscultation. Note the distribution of tympany and dullness. Expect to hear tympany in most of the abdomen; expect dullness over the solid abdominal organs, such as the liver and spleen.

Palpate the abdomen last to detect tenderness, muscular rigidity, and superficial organs and masses. Before you begin palpation, ask your patient if she has any pain or tenderness. If your patient does, ask her to point to the area with one finger. Palpate that area last, using gentle pressure with a single finger. Ask your patient to cough and tell you if and where she experiences any pain. If coughing causes pain, suspect peritoneal inflammation.

Now, ask your patient to take slow, deep breaths with her mouth open, and have her flex the knees to relax the abdominal muscles. Perform light palpation by moving your hand slowly and just lifting it off the skin (Procedure 6-10b). Palpate all areas in the same sequence you used for auscultation and percussion. Watch your patient's face for signs of discomfort. Identify any masses and note their size, location, contour, tenderness, pulsations, and mobility. Abdominal pain on light palpation suggests peritoneal irritation or inflammation. If you feel rigidity or guarding while palpating, determine whether it is voluntary (patient anticipates the pain or is not relaxed) or involuntary (peritoneal inflammation).

Next, palpate the abdomen deeply to detect large masses or tenderness. Use one hand on top of another and push down slowly (Procedure 6-10c). Assess for rebound tenderness by pushing down slowly and then releasing your hand quickly off the tender area. If the peritoneum is inflamed, your patient will experience pain when you let go. Alternatively, hold your hand 1 cm above your patient's abdomen at rest. Then, ask your patient to push her abdomen out to touch your hand. Limitation by pain suggests peritoneal irritation.

If you note a protruding abdomen with bulging flanks and dull percussion sounds in dependent areas, you might perform two tests for ascites. First, assess for areas of tympany and dullness while your patient is supine. Then, ask her to lie on one side. Percuss again, noting once more any areas of tympany and dullness. If your patient has ascites, the area of dullness will shift down to the dependent side and the area of tympany will shift up. To test for fluid wave, ask an assistant to press the edge of her hand firmly down the midline of your patient's abdomen (Procedure 6-10d). With your fingertips, tap one flank and feel for the impulse's transmission to the other flank through excess fluid. If you detect the impulse easily, suspect ascites.

THE FEMALE GENITALIA

Except in cases of imminent childbirth, trauma, or abuse, you rarely would be expected to examine the female genitalia. Before examining the external female genitalia, make sure that the room is warm and quiet and that your patient's bladder is empty. Be sure to maintain privacy during this examination. To reduce any anxiety or embarrassment your patient may feel, explain what you are doing during the exam. Expose her body areas only as necessary, be sensitive to her feelings, and project a professional demeanour. Place a pillow under her head and shoulders to help relax her abdominal muscles.

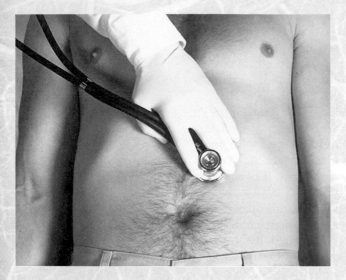

6-10a   Auscultate for renal bruits.

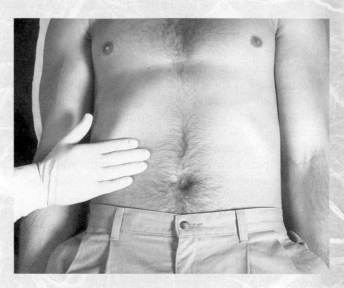

6-10b   Light abdominal palpation.

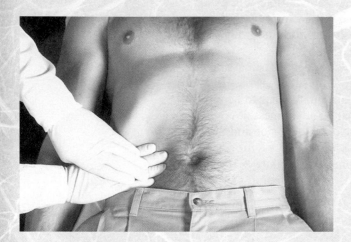

6-10c   Deep abdominal palpation.

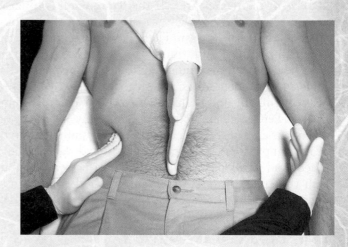

6-10d   Test for ascites.

Begin your assessment by inspecting your patient's external genitalia. Look at the mons pubis, labia, and perineum for abnormalities, such as inflammation, swelling, or lesions. These abnormalities may signal a sebaceous cyst or a sexually transmitted disease, such as syphilis or herpes simplex virus infection. Check the bases of the pubic hair for signs of lice, such as excoriation or small, itchy, red maculopapules.

Assess for vaginal discharge. The normal discharge is clear or cloudy and has little or no odour. A white, curd-like discharge with no odour or a yeasty, sweet odour may suggest a fungal infection (candidiasis). A yellow, green, or grey discharge with a foul or fishy odour may suggest a bacterial infection (gonorrhea or *Gardnerella*). Examining the external female genitalia can be an embarrassing, uncomfortable experience, especially for male clinicians. Remember, it is probably twice as awkward for your patient. If possible, a female clinician should perform the inspection. If a male clinician performs the examination, another female (for example, a partner or a family member) should be present.

THE MALE GENITALIA

Except for trauma, you rarely would be expected to inspect the male genitalia. Before examining the male genitalia, make sure that the room is warm and quiet and that your patient's bladder is empty. If possible, a male clinician should perform the inspection. Be sure to maintain privacy during this examination. To reduce any anxiety or embarrassment your patient may feel, explain what you are doing during the exam. Expose his body areas only as necessary, be sensitive to his feelings, and project a professional demeanour.

Begin your assessment by inspecting your patient's penis and scrotum. Note any inflammation, and inspect the skin around the base of the penis for abnormalities, such as lesions that may be caused by sexually transmitted diseases. Also, check the bases of the pubic hair for signs of lice, such as excoriation or small, itchy, red maculopapules. Next, inspect the glans for signs of degeneration or other abnormalities. If the foreskin is present, ask your patient to retract it. Note any abnormalities and the location of the urethral meatus. Inspect the anterior surface of the scrotum and note its contour. Then, lift the scrotum to inspect its posterior surface and note any swelling or lumps. Expect acute epididymitis or testicular torsion if your patient has scrotal swelling and lower abdominal pain. Testicular torsion requires immediate intervention.

Assess any discharge from the urethral meatus. Normally, no discharge is present. A profuse, yellow discharge may be a sign of gonorrhea. A scant, clear or white discharge may suggest a nongonococcal urethritis. Examining the male genitalia can be an embarrassing, uncomfortable experience, especially for female clinicians. Remember, it is probably twice as awkward for your patient. It is customary for female clinicians to have a male partner present during the examination.

THE ANUS

Examining the anus is normally not a prehospital assessment practice. Unless your patient presents with rectal bleeding, there will be no reason for you to examine this area. Because routine internal rectal and prostate examinations are beyond the scope of this course, this section will focus on the external anal exam. As always, your aim is gentleness, a calm demeanour, and talking to your patient about what you are doing.

Before examining the anus, make sure the room is warm and quiet. Be sure to maintain privacy during this examination. To reduce any anxiety or embarrassment your patient may feel, explain what you are doing during the exam. Drape your patient appropriately and expose body areas only as necessary; be sensitive to your patient's feelings and project a professional demeanour. Place your patient on her left side with legs flexed and the buttocks near the edge of the examination table. Glove your hands and spread the buttocks apart. Inspect the sacrococcygeal and perianal areas for lumps, ulcers, inflammations, rashes, or excoriation. Palpate any abnormal areas carefully and note any tenderness or inflammation. If appropriate, obtain a fecal sample and test it for occult blood. Simply smear a small sample onto a special test slide and add a couple drops of developer onto the sample. If it turns blue, there is blood in the stool.

THE MUSCULOSKELETAL SYSTEM

An examination of the musculoskeletal system must include a detailed assessment of function and structure. Inspect and palpate your patient's joints, their structure, their range of motion, and the surrounding tissues. Begin your assessment with a general observation of posture, build, and muscular development. Watch how your patient's body parts move, and observe their resting positions. Begin the exam with your patient sitting, to evaluate the head, neck, shoulders, and upper extremities. Then, have your patient stand, to assess the chest, back, and ilium; ask her to walk so that you can assess her gait. Finally, ask your patient to lie down to examine the hips, knees, ankles, and feet.

Inspect for swelling in or around joints, changes in the surrounding tissue, redness of the overlying skin, deformities, and symmetry of impairment. Swelling may be caused by trauma to the area or by excess synovial fluid in the joint space or tissues surrounding the joint. Tissue changes may include muscle atrophy, skin changes, and subcutaneous nodules resulting from rheumatoid arthritis or rheumatic fever. Skin redness may suggest inflammation or arthritis. Deformities may be produced by restricted range of motion, misalignment of the articulating bones, dislocation (complete separation of bone ends), or subluxation (partial dislocation). Symmetrical impairment is usually associated with a disorder, such as rheumatoid arthritis.

Inspect and palpate each body part, then test its range of motion and muscle strength as explained in the "Motor System" section later in this chapter. Examine each joint and compare joints on opposite sides for equal size, shape, colour, and strength. Swelling in a joint usually involves the synovial membrane or a bursa, which will feel spongy on deep palpation within the joint space. It also may involve the surrounding structures, such as ligaments, cartilage, tendons, or the bones themselves. Redness of the overlying skin suggests a nontraumatic joint inflammation, such as arthritis, gout, or rheumatic fever. Palpate for tenderness in and around the joint. Try to identify the specific structure that is tender, such as a ligament or tendon. Some common causes of a tender joint include arthritis, tendinitis, bursitis, or osteomyelitis. With the back of your hand, feel over the tender area for increased heat, which suggests arthritis.

After you have inspected and palpated each body part with your patient at rest, assess range of motion. Test each joint for passive range of motion, range of motion against gravity, and range of motion against resistance. First, test the joint's passive range of motion by moving it in the directions that it normally allows. For example, test the elbow, a hinge joint, for flexion and extension. Note any resistance and whether the range of motion is within normal limits. Now, test range of motion against gravity by asking your patient to perform the same movements by herself. Again, note the range of motion and any difficulties. Finally, test range of motion against resistance. Have your patient perform the same movements while you apply resistance.

Passive and active range should be equal. A discrepancy indicates either a muscle weakness or a joint problem. If your patient has difficulty with passive and active tests, suspect a joint problem. If she has difficulty only with active tests, suspect a weakened muscle or nerve disorder. A decreased range of motion could indicate arthritis or injury, while an increased range of motion suggests a loosening of the structures that support the joint.

Listen for **crepitation** (or **crepitus**), the crunching sounds of unlubricated parts rubbing against each other, while you manipulate the joint. Crepitus may indicate an inflamed joint or osteoarthritis. An obvious traumatic deformity could indicate a sprained ligament, a bone fracture, or a dislocation. In these cases, modify your manipulation and range of motion exam accordingly. Non-traumatic deformities are caused by arthritis or the misalignment of bones. Avoid manipulating a painful joint.

* **crepitation** (or **crepitus**) crunching sounds of unlubricated parts in joints rubbing against each other.

The Extremities

Wrists and Hands Begin by inspecting your patient's hands and wrists. Next palpate them by feeling the medial and lateral aspects of the distal interphalangeal (DIP) joints and then the proximal interphalangeal (PIP) joints with your thumb and forefinger (Procedure 6-11a). Note any swelling, sponginess, bony enlargement, or tenderness. Then, palpate the tops and bottoms of these joints in the same manner. Now, ask your patient to flex the hand slightly so you can examine each metacarpophalangeal (MCP) joint. Compress the MCP joints by squeezing the hand from side to side between your thumbs and fingers and note any swelling, tenderness, or sponginess (Procedure 6-11b). Finally, palpate each wrist joint with your thumbs and note any swelling, sponginess, or tenderness (Procedure 6-11c). If your patient has had swelling of both wrists or finger joints for several weeks, suspect an inflammatory condition, such as rheumatoid arthritis.

To assess range of motion, ask your patient to make a fist with each hand and then open the fist and extend and spread her fingers. She should be able to make a tight fist and spread the fingers smoothly and easily. Next, ask your patient to flex and then extend her wrist. Normal flexion is 90 degrees, extension 70 degrees (Procedure 6-11d). Check for radial and ulnar deviation by asking your patient to flex the wrist and move her hands medially and laterally. Normal radial movement is 20 degrees, ulnar movement 45 degrees (Procedure 6-11e).

If your patient complains of hand pain and numbness, especially at night, suspect carpal tunnel syndrome, the painful inflammation of the median nerve. To detect additional signs of this disorder, hold your patient's wrists in acute flexion for 60 seconds (Procedure 6-11f). In carpal tunnel syndrome, she will develop numbness or tingling in the areas innervated by the median nerve—the palmar surface of her thumb, index, and middle fingers, and part of the ring finger. Throughout these manoeuvres watch for deformities, redness, swelling, nodules, or muscular atrophy.

Elbows To examine the elbow, support your patient's forearm with your hand so that her elbow is flexed about 70 degrees (Procedure 6-12a). Inspect the elbow joint and note any deformities, swelling, or nodules. Palpate the joint structures for tenderness, swelling, or thickening. Press on the medial and lateral epicondyles (Procedure 6-12b). Inflammation of either the medial epicondyle (tennis elbow) or of the lateral epicondyle (golfer's elbow) suggests tendinitis at those muscle insertion sites. To assess range of motion, ask your patient to flex and extend the elbow (Procedure 6-12c). Normally, she will flex her elbow up to 160 degrees and return it back to the neutral position. Then, ask her to keep the elbows

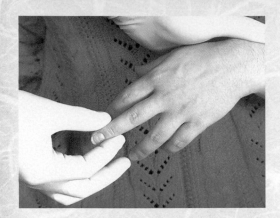

6-11a   Palpate the DIP and PIP joints.

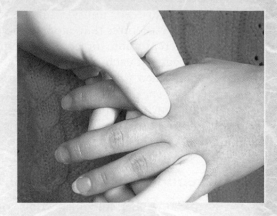

6-11b   Palpate the MCP joint.

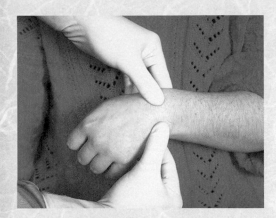

6-11c   Palpate the wrist.

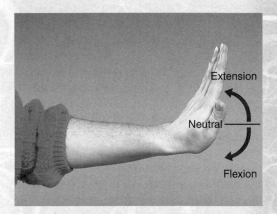

6-11d   Assess wrist flexion and extension.

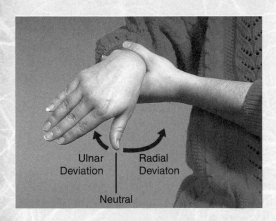

6-11e   Assess radial and ulnar deviation.

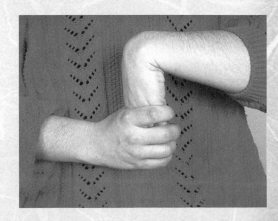

6-11f   Test for carpal tunnel syndrome.

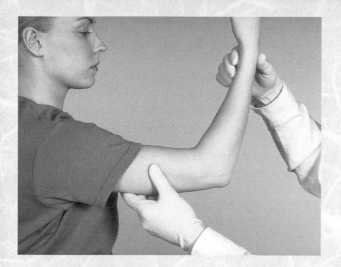

6-12a   Inspect the elbow.

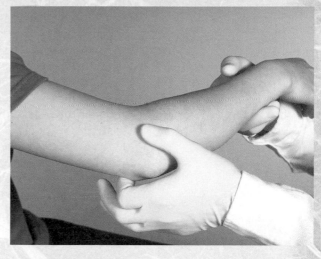

6-12b   Palpate the lateral and medial epicondyles.

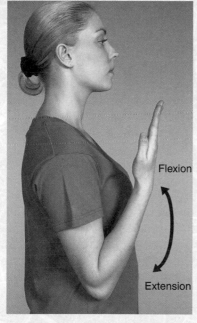

Flexion

Extension

6-12c   Assess elbow flexion and extension.

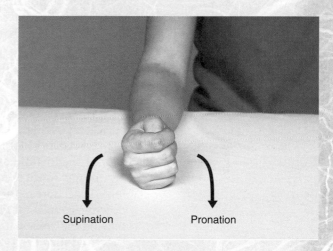

Supination   Pronation

6-12d   Assess supination and pronation of the wrist.

flexed and arms at her sides. Now, have your patient turn her palms up and then down. Normally both supination and pronation are 90 degrees (Procedure 6-12d).

Shoulders To assess your patient's shoulders, look at them from the front and then look at the scapulae from the back. Inspect the entire shoulder girdle for swelling, deformities, or muscular atrophy. Before you palpate, ask your patient if she has any pain in the shoulders. If so, have her point to it with one finger; palpate this area last. Palpate the shoulders with your fingertips, moving along the clavicles out toward the humerus (Procedure 6-13a). Palpate the sternoclavicular joint, acromioclavicular joint, subacromial region, and the bicipital groove for tenderness (biceps tendinitis) or swelling (bursitis). Now, palpate over the greater tubercle of the humerus as you abduct the arm at the shoulder. Then, palpate the scapulae.

To assess range of motion, ask your patient to raise both arms forward and then straight overhead (flexion) (Procedure 6-13b). Expect to see forward flexion of 180 degrees. Next ask your patient to extend both arms behind her back (extension). Normal extension is 50 degrees. Now, have your patient raise both arms overhead from the side (abduction) (Procedure 6-13c). Normal abduction is 180 degrees. Then, ask her to lower her arms and swing them as far as possible across her body (adduction). Normal shoulder adduction is 75 degrees. Finally, have your patient adduct her shoulders to 90 degrees, pronate, and flex her elbows 90 degrees to the front of her body. Now, ask your patient to rotate her shoulders to the "goal post" position (external rotation) (Procedure 6-13d). Normal external rotation is 90 degrees. Finally, ask your patient to place both hands behind the small of her back (internal rotation). Normal internal rotation is 90 degrees. During these motions, cup your hands over your patient's shoulders and note any crepitus.

Ankles and Feet Inspect the foot and ankle for obvious deformities, nodules, swelling, calluses, or corns. Palpate the anterior aspect of each ankle joint with your thumbs and note any sponginess, swelling, or tenderness (Procedure 6-14a). Feel along the Achilles tendon for tenderness or nodules. Exert pressure between your thumbs and fingers on each metatarsophalangeal joint (Procedure 6-14b). Acute inflammation of these joints suggests gout. Tenderness is an early sign of rheumatoid arthritis.

To test range of motion, ask your patient to bring her foot upward (dorsiflexion) (Procedure 6-14c). Normal dorsiflexion is 20 degrees. Then, have her point it downward (plantar flexion). Normal plantar flexion is 45 degrees. Next, while stabilizing the ankle with one hand, grasp the heel with the other hand and invert the foot, and then evert it (Procedure 6-14d). Normal inversion is 30 degrees, normal eversion 20 degrees. These four movements test the ankle joint's stability. A sprained ankle will cause your patient pain when the injured ligament is stretched or torn. Since the lateral ligaments are smaller and weaker than the medial ligaments, lateral sprains are more common, causing severe pain on inversion and plantar flexion. In arthritis, pain and tenderness will accompany movement in any direction. Finally, flex and extend the toes (Procedure 6-14e). Expect a great range of motion in these joints, especially the big toes.

Knees Inspect your patient's knees for alignment and deformities. Look for the concave areas that usually appear on each side of the patella and just above it. The absence of these concavities indicates swelling in the knee or the surrounding structures. If swelling is present, milk the medial aspect of the knee firmly upward two or three times to displace the fluid. Then, press the knee just behind the lateral margin of the patella and watch for a return of fluid (a positive sign

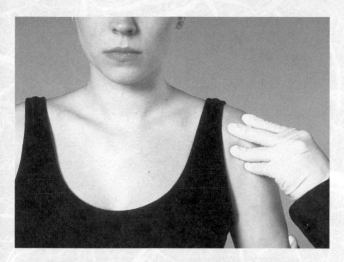

6-13a   Palpate the shoulder with your fingertips.

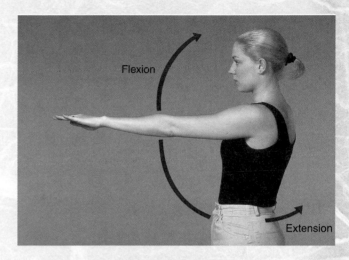

6-13b   Assess shoulder flexion and extension.

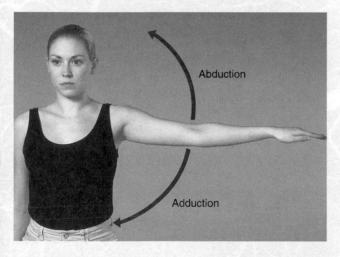

6-13c   Assess shoulder abduction and adduction.

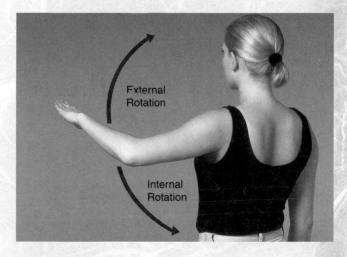

6-13d   Assess internal and external shoulder rotation.

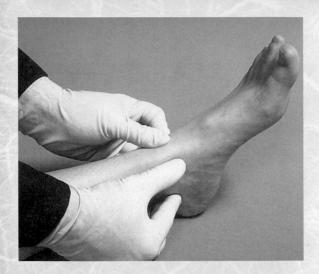

6-14a   Palpate the ankle and foot.

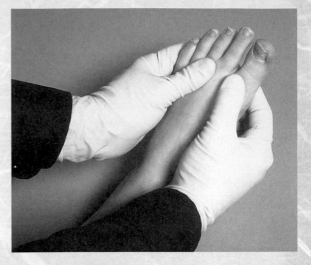

6-14b   Palpate the metatarsophalangeal joints.

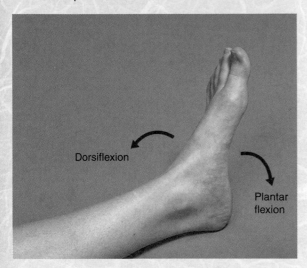

6-14c   Assess dorsiflexion and plantar flexion.

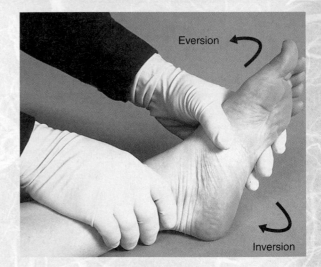

6-14d   Assess inversion and eversion of the foot.

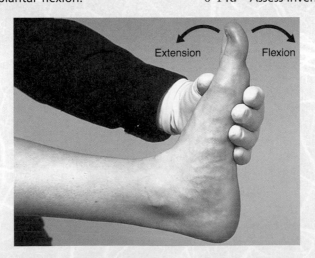

6-14e   Test flexion and extension of the toes.

for effusion) (Procedure 6-15a). Feel for any thickening or swelling around the patella; these suggest synovial thickening or effusion. Compress the patella and move it against the femur (Procedure 6-15b). Note any pain or tenderness.

To test for range of motion, have your patient flex the knee to 90 degrees. Press your thumbs into the joint and palpate along the tibial margins from the patellar tendon laterally. Palpate along the course of each ligament and note any points of tenderness. If your patient has tenderness, expect damage to the meniscus or to the lateral ligaments. If you feel irregular bony ridges, suspect osteoarthritis. Now, test for stability of the medial and collateral ligaments by moving the knee joint from side to side with the knee flexed to 30 degrees (Procedure 6-15c). There should be little movement if the joint is stable. Evaluate the anterior and posterior cruciate ligaments by using the "drawer" test. Try to move the knee joint anteriorly and posteriorly, much like opening and closing a drawer (Procedure 6-15d). Again, if the ligaments are strong, there should be little movement.

Now, have your patient sit at the edge of the exam table with her lower legs dangling. Ask her to extend her leg. Normal extension is 90 degrees (Procedure 6-15e). Ask her to roll over and try to touch her foot to her back. Normal flexion is 135 degrees. With your patient standing, inspect the posterior surface of the legs, especially the popliteal region behind the knees. Note any deformity or abnormalities, such as bowlegs, knock-knee, or flexion contracture, the inability to fully extend the knee.

Hips Inspect the hips for deformities, symmetry, and swelling. Palpate for tenderness all around the joint, including the three bursa and greater trochanter of the femur (Procedure 6-16a). Test the hip's range of motion with your patient supine. Ask her to raise her knee to the chest and pull the knee firmly against the abdomen. Observe the degree of flexion at the knee and hip (normally 120 degrees) (Procedure 6-16b). Now, flex the hip at 90 degrees, and stabilize the thigh with one hand while you grasp the ankle with the other. Swing the lower leg medially to evaluate external rotation and laterally to evaluate internal rotation (Procedure 6-16c). Normal external rotation is 40 degrees, normal internal rotation 45 degrees. Arthritis restricts internal rotation. To test for hip abduction, have your patient extend her legs. Then, while you stabilize the anterior superior iliac spine with one hand, abduct the other leg until you feel the iliac spine move. This marks the degree of hip abduction, which is normally 90 degrees (Procedure 6-16d). If your patient complains of hip pain or if range of motion is limited, palpate the three bursa for swelling (bursitis) and tenderness.

The Spine

To assess your patient's spine, first inspect the head and neck for deformities, abnormal posture, and asymmetrical skin folds. The head should be erect and the spine straight. Ask your patient to bend forward slightly while you visually identify the spinous processes, the paravertebral muscles, the scapulae, the iliac crests, and the posterior iliac spines (usually marked by dimples). Draw imaginary horizontal lines across the shoulders and iliac crests. Now, draw an imaginary vertical line from T1 to the space between the buttocks (gluteal cleft). Any deviations suggest a variety of pathologies.

Next, observe your patient from the side. Evaluate the curves of the cervical, thoracic, and lumbar spine, and note any irregularities. Common abnormalities

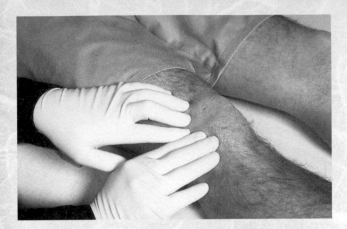

6-15a   Palpate the knee.

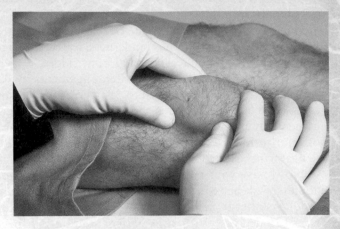

6-15b   Palpate the patella.

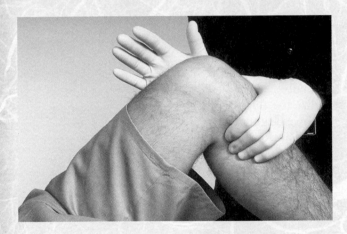

6-15c   Test the collateral ligaments of the knee.

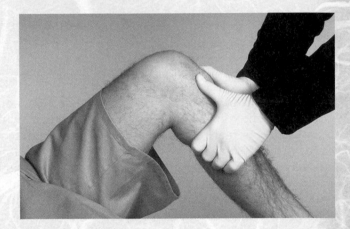

6-15d   Test the cruciate ligaments of the knee.

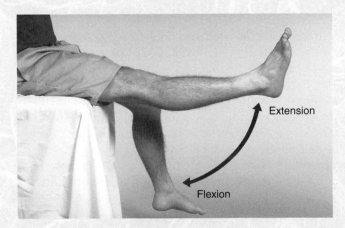

Extension

Flexion

6-15e   Assess knee flexion and extension.

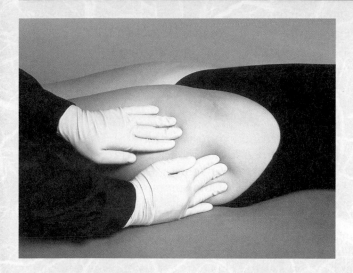

6-16a   Palpate the hip.

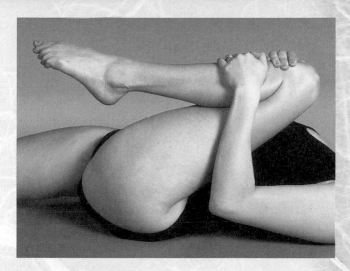

6-16b   Assess hip flexion with the knee flexed.

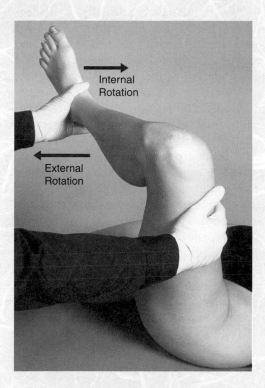

Internal
Rotation

External
Rotation

6-16c   Assess external and internal rotation of the hip.

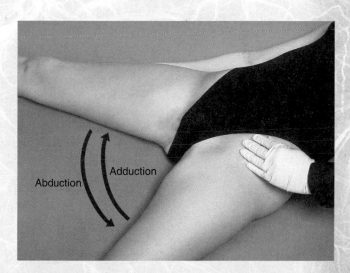

Adduction

Abduction

6-16d   Assess hip abduction and adduction.

Table 6-6	SPINAL CURVATURES
Condition	**Description**
Normal	Concave in cervical and lumbar regions, convex in thorax
Lordosis	Exaggerated lumbar concavity (swayback)
Kyphosis	Exaggerated thoracic concavity (hunchback)
Scoliosis	Lateral curvature

of the spine include lordosis, scoliosis, and kyphosis (Table 6-6). Using the pads of your fingers, palpate the spinous processes for tenderness (Procedure 6-17a). Feel the supporting structures for muscle tone, symmetry, size, and tenderness or spasms. If your patient exhibits tenderness of the spinous processes and paravertebral muscles, suspect a herniated intervertebral disc, most commonly found between L4 and S1.

Now, test range of motion. First, test for flexion by asking your patient to touch her chin to her chest (Procedure 6-17b). Flexion is normally 45 degrees. Next, ask her to bend her head backward. This tests extension, which normally is up to 55 degrees. Now, test for rotation by asking your patient to touch her chin to each shoulder (Procedure 6-17c). Normal rotation is 70 degrees on each side. Finally, ask your patient to touch her ears to her shoulders without raising the shoulders. This assesses lateral bending, which normally is 40 degrees on each side (Procedure 6-17d). Now, test for flexion of the lower spine with your patient standing. Ask your patient to bend and touch her toes (Procedure 6-17e). Note the smoothness and symmetry of movement, the range of motion, and the curves in the lumbar region. Normal flexion ranges from 75–90 degrees. If the lumbar area remains concave or appears asymmetrical during this exam, your patient may have a muscle spasm. Next, stabilize your patient's pelvis with your hands and have her bend sideways; normal lateral bending is 35 degrees on each side (Procedure 6-17f). To assess hyperextension, ask her to bend backward toward you; normal hyperextension is 30 degrees (Procedure 6-17g). Finally, test spinal rotation by asking your patient to twist her shoulders one way and then the other. Normally, they will rotate 30 degrees to each side (Procedure 6-17h).

If your patient complains of lower back pain radiating down the back of one leg, assess it by having her lie supine on the table. Ask your patient to raise her straightened leg until she feels pain. Note the angle of elevation at which the pain occurs, as well as the quality and distribution of the pain. Now, dorsiflex your patient's foot. If this causes a sharp pain that radiates from your patient's back down the leg, suspect compression of the nerve roots of the lower lumbar region. Repeat this test with the other leg. Increased pain in the affected leg when the opposite leg is raised confirms the finding.

THE PERIPHERAL VASCULAR SYSTEM

To assess your patient's peripheral vascular system, inspect both arms from the fingertips to the shoulders. Note their size and symmetry. Observe swelling, venous congestion, the colour of the skin and nail beds, and the skin texture. Yellow or brittle nails or poor colour in the fingertips indicates chronic arterial insufficiency. Palpate the peripheral arteries to evaluate pulsation and capillary refill and to assess skin temperature (Procedure 6-18a and 6-18b). To palpate a

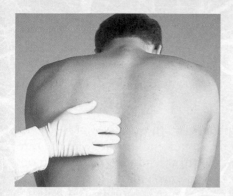

6-17a   Palpate the spine.

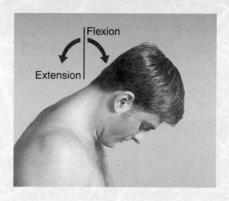

6-17b   Test flexion and extension of the head and neck.

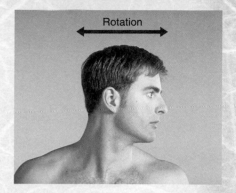

6-17c   Test rotation of the head and neck.

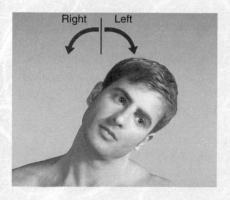

6-17d   Assess lateral bending of the head and neck.

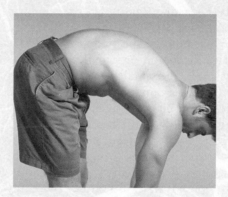

6-17e   Assess flexion of the lower spine.

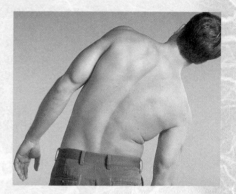

6-17f   Assess lateral bending of the lower spine.

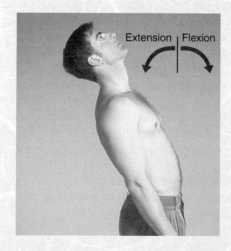

6-17g   Assess spinal extension.

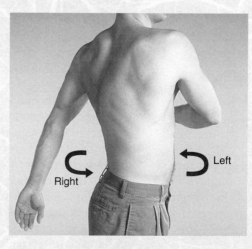

11-17h   Assess spinal rotation.

Table 6-7	ASSESSING A PERIPHERAL PULSE
Score	**Description**
0	Absent pulse
1+	Weak or thready
2+	Normal
3+	Bounding

peripheral pulse, lightly place your fingerpads over the artery's pulse point. Slowly increase the pressure until you feel a maximum pulsation. Note the rate, regularity, equality, and quality of the pulses. Count the number of beats in one minute. Then, determine whether the pulse is regular, regularly irregular, or irregularly irregular. Finally, assess the quality of the pulse by noting its amplitude and contour; rate its quality from 0 to 3+ as shown in Table 6-7. Determine if it is absent, normal, weak, or bounding, and note any thrills, humming vibrations that feel similar to the throat of a purring cat. Thrills suggest a cardiac murmur or vascular narrowing. Expect the pulse of a normal adult to range between 60 and 100 beats per minute with a regular rhythm and normal amplitude.

Compare peripheral pulses bilaterally. If you detect a weak or absent pulse in one extremity, suspect an arterial occlusion proximal to the pulse point. Also, compare distal and proximal pulses for equality. If you cannot palpate a distal artery, move proximally to another artery. For example, if you cannot palpate the radial artery, move to the the brachial artery in the antecubital area. While you are at the elbow, you can also assess the epitrochlear lymph nodes; they will be palpable only if inflamed.

Next, assess the feet and legs. Have your patient lie down and remove her socks. Inspect the legs from the feet to the groin. Note their size and symmetry. Evaluate the presence of swelling, venous congestion, the colour of the skin and nail beds, and the skin texture. Note any venous enlargement. Evaluate scars, pigmentation, rashes, and ulcers. Palpate and compare the femoral pulses (Procedure 6-18c). Note the rate, regularity, equality, and quality of the pulses. Palpate the popliteal pulse behind the knee, the dorsalis pedis pulse on top of the foot, and the posterior tibial pulse just behind the medial malleolus (Procedure 6-18d through 6-18f). Feel the temperature of the legs, feet, and toes with the back of your fingers and compare both sides. Unilateral coldness indicates an arterial occlusion. Bilateral coldness is due to an environmental problem, bilateral occlusion (saddle embolus), or a general circulatory problem (shock). Palpate the superficial inguinal lymph nodes for enlargement and tenderness.

Observe the legs for edema, the presence of an abnormal amount of fluid in the tissues. Compare one leg and foot with the other. Note their relative size and symmetry. Are veins, tendons, and bones easily visible under the skin? Edema will usually obscure these structures. Palpate for pitting edema by pressing firmly with your thumb for five seconds over the top of the foot, behind each medial ankle, and over the shins (Procedure 6-18g). **Pitting** is a depression left by the pressure of your thumb. Normally, there should be no depression. If edema is present, evaluate the degree of pitting that can range from slight to marked (Figure 6-22). You can grade the depth of the pitting according to the appropriate scale in Table 6-8. Expect the pit to disappear within 10 seconds after you release the pressure. Bilateral edema suggests a central circulatory problem, such as congestive heart failure or renal failure; unilateral edema suggests a lower extremity circulation abnormality, such as deep vein thrombosis or venous occlusion. Note the extent of the edema. How far up the leg does it spread? The higher the edema, the more severe is the problem.

* **pitting** depression that results from pressure against skin when pitting edema is present.

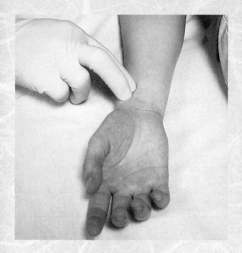

6-18a   Palpate the radial artery.

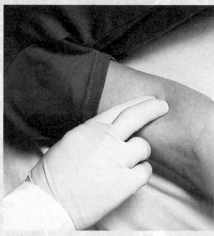

6-18b   Palpate the brachial artery.

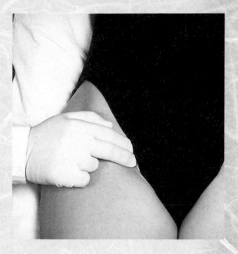

6-18c   Palpate and compare the femoral arteries.

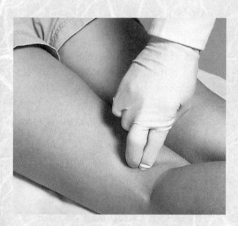

6-18d   Palpate the popliteal pulse.

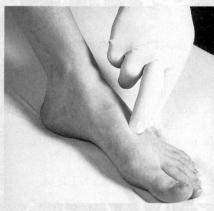

6-18e   Palpate the dorsalis pedis pulse.

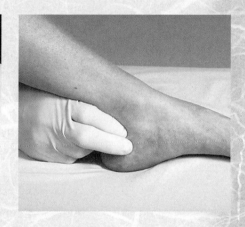

6-18f   Palpate the posterior tibial pulse.

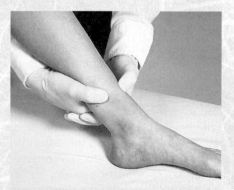

6-18g   Palpate for edema.

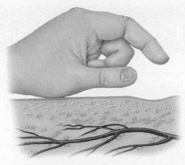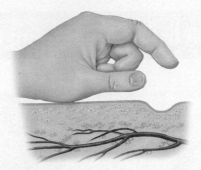

+1 Slight pitting edema   +4 Deep pitting edema

FIGURE 6-22 Assessing for edema.

Table 6-8	PITTING EDEMA SCALE
Score	**Description**
1+	0.5 cm (0.25 in.) or less
2+	0.5–1.25 cm (0.25–0.5 in.)
3+	1.25–2.5 cm (0.5–1 in.)
4+	2.5 cm (1 in.) or more

During your assessment, look for visible venous distention. An associated swollen, painful leg suggests deep vein thrombosis (DVT). Palpate the femoral vein just medial to the femoral artery. If you detect a tender femoral vein, flex the knee and palpate the calf for tenderness, another classic sign of DVT. Is there a local redness or warmth? Feel for a cord-like vessel. Evaluate the skin for discoloration, ulcers, and unusual thickness. Finally, ask your patient to stand. Evaluate the legs for varicose veins, and if present, palpate them for signs of thrombophlebitis (redness, swelling, pain, and tenderness).

THE NERVOUS SYSTEM

A comprehensive physical assessment includes a thorough evaluation of your patient's mental status and thought processes. On the scene of an emergency, you would limit your mental exam to level of consciousness and basic orientation questions, such as "What is your name?" "Where are you right now?" "What day is it today?" If you are conducting a full physical assessment or evaluating someone with altered mentation, some or all of the following techniques will be useful.

When you conduct a neurological exam, you are attempting to answer two vital questions. First, are the findings symmetrical or unilateral? Second, if the signs are unilateral, is the site of origin in the central nervous system (brain and spinal cord) or in the peripheral nervous system (everything else)? You will conduct many parts of the neurological exam while you assess other anatomical areas and systems. For example, you can examine the cranial nerves while evaluating the head and face. You can note any weaknesses or abnormal neurological findings while evaluating the arms and legs during the musculoskeletal exam.

A nervous system exam covers five areas: mental status and speech, the cranial nerves, the motor system, the reflexes, and the sensory system. This section presents the complete neurological exam. The chief complaint, clinical condition of your patient, and time constraints will determine which parts you actually use.

A neurological exam attempts to answer two vital questions: Are the findings symmetrical or unilateral, and if unilateral, where do they originate?

Content Review

FIVE AREAS OF NEUROLOGICAL EXAM
- Mental status and speech
- Cranial nerves
- Motor system
- Sensory system
- Reflexes

Mental Status and Speech

Generally, you will evaluate your patient's mental status and speech when you begin your interview. During this time, you will assess her level of response, general appearance and behaviour, and speech. If you detect abnormalities, continue your assessment with more specific questioning or testing as presented here.

Appearance and Behaviour First, assess your patient's level of response. Is she alert and awake? Does your patient understand your questions? Are the responses appropriate and timely, or does she drift off the topic easily or lose interest? If you detect an abnormality, continue with more specific questions. Is your patient lethargic (drowsy, but answers questions appropriately before falling asleep again)? Is she obtunded (opens her eyes and looks at you but gives slow, confused responses)? Sometimes, you must arouse your patient repeatedly by gently shaking her or shouting her name. If your patient does not respond to your verbal cues, assess her with painful stimuli for coma or stupor. The stuporous patient is arousable for short periods but is not aware of her surroundings. The comatose patient is in a state of profound unconsciousness and is totally unarousable.

If your patient is awake and alert, observe her posture and motor behaviour. Does she lie in bed or prefer to walk around? Your patient's posture should be erect and she should look at you. A slumped posture and a lack of facial expression may indicate depression. Excessive energetic movements or constantly watchful eyes suggest tension, anxiety, or a metabolic disorder. Watch the pace, range, and character of the movements. Are they voluntary? Are any parts immobile? Do her posture and motor activity change with the environment? Some possible findings are listed in Table 6-9.

Observe your patient's grooming and personal hygiene. How is she dressed? Are her clothes clean, pressed, and properly fastened? Is her appearance appropriate for the season, climate, and occasion? A deterioration in grooming and personal hygiene in a previously well-groomed person may suggest an emotional problem, a psychiatric disorder, or an organic brain disease. Patients with obsessive-compulsive behaviour may exhibit excessive attention to their appearance. Note your patient's hair, teeth, nails, skin, and, in male patients, the beard. Are they well groomed? Compare one side to the other. One-sided neglect may suggest a brain lesion.

Also, observe your patient's facial expressions. Are they appropriate? Do they vary when she talks with others and when the topic changes, or is her face immobile throughout the interaction? Can your patient express happiness, sadness, anger, or depression? Patients with Parkinson's disease often have facial immobility, producing a mask-like appearance.

Speech and Language Note your patient's speech pattern. Normally, a person's speech is inflected, clear and strong, and fluent and articulate, and it varies in volume. It should express thoughts clearly. Is your patient excessively talkative or silent? Does she speak spontaneously or only when you ask her a direct question? Is her speech slow and quiet, as in depression? Is it fast and loud, as in a manic episode? Does your patient speak clearly and distinctly? Does she

Table 6-9	POSTURE AND BEHAVIOUR	

Motor Activity	Meaning
Tense posture, restlessness, fidgeting	Anxiety
Crying, hand wringing, pacing	Agitation, depression
Hopeless, slumped posture, slowed movements	Depression
Singing, dancing, expansive movements	Manic

have dysarthria (defective speech caused by motor deficits), dysphonia (voice changes caused by vocal cord problems), or aphasia (partial or complete loss of speech caused by neurological damage to the brain)? With expressive aphasia, her words will be garbled; with receptive aphasia, her words will be clear but unrelated to your questions. A patient with aphasia may have such difficulty talking that you mistakenly suspect a psychotic disorder.

Mood Observe your patient's verbal and nonverbal behaviour for clues to her mood. Note any mood swings or behaviours that suggest anxiety or depression. Is your patient sad, elated, angry, enraged, anxious, worried, detached, or indifferent? Assess the intensity of your patient's mood. How long has she been this way? Is this behaviour normal for the circumstances? For example, anxiety is normal for someone having a heart attack; if your heart attack patient did not act frightened and concerned, that would be abnormal. If your patient is depressed, is she suicidal? If you suspect the possibility of suicide, ask directly, "Have you ever thought of committing suicide? Are you currently thinking of committing suicide?"

Thought and Perceptions Assess how well your patient organizes her thoughts when speaking. Is she logical and coherent? Does your patient shift from one topic to an unrelated topic without realizing that the thoughts are not connected? These "loose associations" are typical in schizophrenia, manic episodes, and other psychiatric disorders. Does she speak constantly in related areas with no real conclusion or end-point? Such "flight of ideas" is most often associated with mania. Does your patient ramble with unrelated, illogical thoughts and disordered grammar? You may see this "incoherence" in severe psychosis. Does she make up facts or events in response to questions? You may see this "confabulation" in amnesia. Does your patient suddenly lose her train of thought and stop in midsentence before completing an idea? Such blocking occurs in normal people but is pronounced in schizophrenia.

Assess the thought content of your patient's responses as they occur during the interview. For example, "You said you thought you were allergic to your mother. Can you tell me why you think that way?" In this way, you can ask about your patient's unpleasant or unusual comments. Allow her the freedom to explore these thoughts with you. Is your patient driven to try to prevent some unrealistic future result (compulsion)? Does she have a recurrent, uncontrollable feeling of dread and doom (obsession)? Does she sense that things in the environment are strange or unreal (feelings of unreality)? Does your patient have false personal beliefs that other members of her group don't share (delusions)? Compulsions and obsessions are neurotic disorders, while delusions and feelings of unreality are psychotic disorders.

Determine whether your patient perceives imaginary things. Does she see visions, hear voices, smell odours, or feel things that aren't there? Ask about these false perceptions just as you would ask about anything else. For example, "When you see the pink elephants, what are they doing?" Decide whether your patient is misinterpreting what is real (illusions) or seeing things that are not real (hallucinations). Both illusions and hallucinations may occur in schizophrenia, posttraumatic stress disorders, and organic brain syndrome. Auditory and visual hallucinations are common in psychedelic drug ingestion, while tactile hallucinations suggest alcohol withdrawal.

Insight and Judgment During the interview, you will most likely evaluate your patient's insight and judgment. Does she understand what is happening to her? Does your patient realize that what she thinks and feels is part of the illness? Patients with psychotic disorders may not have insight into their illness. Judgment refers to your patient's ability to reason appropriately. Does your mature patient respond appropriately to questions concerning her family and personal life? Ask her what she would do if she cut herself. Proper judgment means that your patient can evaluate the data and provide an adequate response. Impaired judgment is common in emotional problems, mental retardation, and organic brain syndrome.

Memory and Attention Assess your patient's orientation. Does she know her name? Person disorientation suggests trauma, seizures, or amnesia. Does she know the time of day, day of the week, month, season, and year? Time disorientation may suggest anxiety, depression, or organic brain syndrome. Does your patient know where she is, where she lives, the name of the city and province or territory? Place disorientation suggests a psychiatric disorder or organic brain syndrome. Your patient should be oriented to person, time, and place and respond appropriately to your questions.

Your patient should be oriented to person, time, and place and respond appropriately to your questions.

To assess your patient's ability to concentrate, use the following three exercises. First, have her repeat a series of numbers back to you (digit span). Normally, a person can repeat at least five numbers forward and backward. Then, ask your patient to start from 100 and subtract seven each time (serial sevens). A normal person can complete this in 90 seconds with fewer than four errors. Finally, ask your patient to spell a common five-letter word backward (spelling backward). Poor performance in these tests may suggest delirium, dementia, mental retardation, loss of calculating ability, anxiety, or depression.

Memory can be divided into three grades: immediate, recent, and remote. First, test your patient's immediate memory. Ask her to repeat three or four words that have no correlation, such as "desk," "toothbrush," "six," and "blue." This tests immediate recall and is similar to digit span. Next, test your patient's recent memory by asking her what she had for lunch or to repeat something she told you earlier in the interview. Make sure the information you ask for is verifiable. Finally, test for remote memory by asking about such facts as the spouse's name, child's birthday, or social insurance number. Ask your patient to describe the house in which she grew up or the schools she attended. Long-term and short-term memory problems may be due to amnesia, anxiety, or organic causes. Finally, test your patient's ability to learn new things. Give her the names of three or four items, such as "man, chair, grass, and hot dog." Ask her to repeat them. This tests registration and immediate recall. About five minutes later, ask your patient to repeat them again. Normally, people will be able to name all four. Note the accuracy and awareness of whether she is correct or if she tries to confabulate by making up new words.

The Cranial Nerves

The 12 pairs of cranial nerves originate from the base of the brain and provide sensory and motor innervation, mostly to the head and face. Each pair bears the name of its function and carries either sensory fibres, motor fibres, or both. Table 6-10 lists the cranial nerves' names, their specific functions, and the areas they innervate.

Most likely you will conduct parts of the cranial nerve exam when you assess other areas, such as the eyes, ears, throat, and musculoskeletal system. The following is the cranial nerve exam in its entirety.

CN-I Test your patient's olfactory nerve by having her close her eyes and compress one nostril while you present a variety of common, nonirritating odours (Procedure 6-19a). Repeat the test with each nostril. Ask your patient to identify the odour. Most people will do so easily. If your patient cannot, several causes are possible. Bilateral loss of smell suggests head trauma, nasal stuffiness, smoking, cocaine use, or a congenital defect. A unilateral loss of smell without nasal disease suggests a frontal lobe lesion.

	Table 6-10	CRANIAL NERVES		

CN	Name	Function	Innervation
I	Olfactory	Sensory	Smell
II	Optic	Sensory	Sight
III	Oculomotor	Motor	Pupil constriction; superior rectus, inferior rectus, inferior oblique muscles
IV	Trochlear	Motor	Superior oblique muscles
V	Trigeminal	Sensory	Opthalmic (forehead), maxillary (cheek), and mandibular (chin) regions
		Motor	Chewing muscles
VI	Abducens	Motor	Lateral rectus muscle
VII	Facial	Sensory	Tongue
		Motor	Face muscles
VIII	Acoustic	Sensory	Hearing balance
IX	Glossopharyngeal	Sensory	Posterior pharynx, taste to anterior tongue
		Motor	Posterior pharynx
X	Vagus	Sensory	Taste to posterior tongue
		Motor	Posterior palate and pharynx
XI	Accessory	Motor	Trapezius muscles Sternocleidomastoid muscles
XII	Hypoglossal	Motor	Tongue

CN-II Test the optic nerve with the visual acuity and visual field tests described earlier in this chapter in the section on the eyes.

CN-III Test the oculomotor nerve with the optic nerve when you perform pupil reaction tests. Inspect the size and shape of your patient's pupils and compare one side to the other. A slight inequality may be normal. Usually, the pupil is midpoint. Constricted or dilated pupils may result from medications, drug abuse, glaucoma, and neurological disease. Darken the room, if possible, to test for pupillary reaction. Ask your patient to look straight ahead. Shine a bright light obliquely into one of her pupils. Watch for direct reaction (pupillary constriction in the same eye) and for consensual reaction (pupillary constriction in the opposite eye). Repeat this test on the other side. Now, assess for the near-response, asking your patient to follow your finger as you move it in toward the bridge of her nose. Watch for the pupils to constrict and the eyes to converge.

CN-III, IV, VI Test the oculomotor, trochlear, and abducens nerves by evaluating your patient's extraocular movements (EOM). Ask her to follow your finger with only her eyes as you move it through the six cardinal positions of gaze (Procedure 6-19b). Make a wide "H" in the air with your finger. Observe for conjugate (together) movements of your patient's eyes in each direction. Normally, your patient can follow your finger with no strabismus (deviation) or nystagmus (involuntary movements). Inability to move in any direction can be the result of a problem with a cranial nerve, an ocular muscle, or an eye orbit that may be fractured and impinging on the muscle or nerve. Finally, look for ptosis (a droopy eyelid) that may be the result of CN-III palsy or myasthenia gravis.

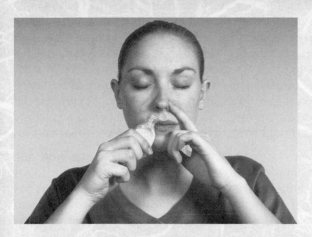

6-19a   Test the olfactory nerve by having your patient identify common odours.

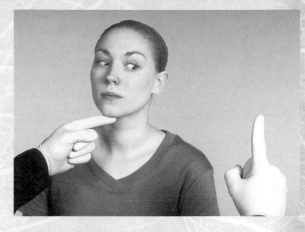

6-19b   Test the oculomotor, trochlear, and abducens nerves by evaluating your patient's extraocular movements.

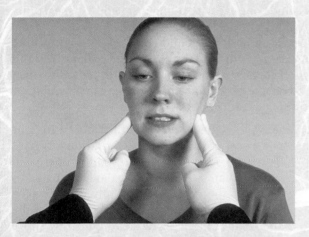

6-19c   Test motor function of the trigeminal nerve by palpating the temporal and masseter muscles.

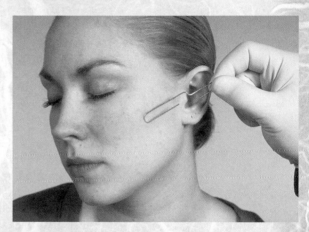

6-19d   Test sensory function of the trigeminal nerve with sharp and dull objects.

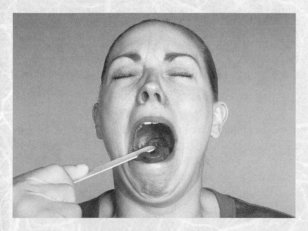

6-19e   Test the glossopharyngeal and vagus nerves with a tongue blade.

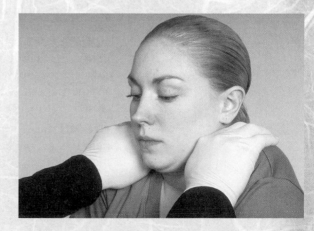

6-19f   Test the spinal accessory nerve by having your patient shrug her shoulders against resistance.

CN-V Test motor function by asking your patient to clench her teeth while you palpate the temporal and masseter muscles (Procedure 6-19c). Note the strength of the muscle contraction. Unilateral weakness or the inability to contract suggests a trigeminal nerve lesion. Bilateral dysfunction suggests motor neuron involvement.

To test for sensory function in the three main divisions of the trigeminal nerve, first, ask your patient to close her eyes. Using something sharp and something dull, lightly scrape the objects across the forehead, cheek, and chin on both sides, and ask your patient to distinguish the sensations (Procedure 6-19d). The two ends of a paper clip work well for this procedure; straighten one end and use its tip as the sharp object. Unilateral loss of sensation suggests a trigeminal nerve lesion. Finally, test the corneal reflex. Ask your patient to look up and away as you touch her cornea lightly with some fine cotton fibres. She should blink. Repeat this test on the other eye.

CN-VII First, assess your patient's face at rest and during conversation. Note any asymmetry, eyelid drooping, or abnormal movements, such as tics. Test the facial nerve by having your patient assume a variety of facial expressions. Ask your patient to raise her eyebrows, frown, show the upper and lower teeth or smile, and puff out her cheeks. Also, ask your patient to close her eyes tightly so that you cannot open them; then, to test muscle strength, try to open them. Bell's palsy is an inflammation of CN-VII. Your patient will present with unilateral facial drooping from paralysis of this nerve.

CN-VIII Ask your patient to occlude one ear with a finger. Then, whisper something softly into the other ear. Ask her to repeat what you said. Any loss of hearing warrants further testing to detect air and bone conduction problems. Test the acoustic nerve for the senses of hearing and balance. Ask your patient to stand erect and close her eyes. Now, evaluate her balance, and ask your patient to open her eyes. If your patient doesn't become dizzy and opens her eyes to your command, the eighth nerve is functioning appropriately.

CN-IX, X Test the glossopharyngeal and vagus nerves together. Listen to your patient's voice. Hoarseness suggests a vocal cord problem; a nasal quality suggests a palate problem. Ask your patient to swallow; note any difficulties. Ask her to open her mouth and say "aaahhh"; watch for the soft palate and uvula to rise symmetrically. The posterior pharynx should move medially. If the vagus nerve is paralyzed, the soft palate and uvula will deviate toward the side of the lesion. Test the gag reflex with a tongue blade on the posterior tongue (Procedure 6-19e). Absence of a gag reflex suggests a lesion in one of these nerves.

CN-XI Inspect the upper portions of your patient's trapezius muscles and sternocleidomastoid muscles for symmetry at rest. To test the trapezius muscles, place your hands on your patient's shoulders and ask her to raise the shoulders against resistance (Procedure 6-19f). Now, test the sternocleidomastoid muscles. Place your hands along your patient's face and ask her to turn her head to each side as you apply resistance. Note any bilateral or unilateral weaknesses. A supine patient with bilateral weakness of the sternocleidomastoids will have trouble lifting her head.

CN-XII First, evaluate your patient's speech articulation. Then, ask your patient to stick out her tongue; watch for a midline projection. A CN-XII lesion will make the tongue deviate away from the affected side. Have your patient move her tongue from side to side as you watch for symmetry.

You may conduct a cranial nerve exam according to this sequence. More likely, you will develop your own efficient system of testing these nerves.

The Motor System

Inspect your patient's general body structure, muscle development, positioning, and coordination. What is your patient's position at rest? Is she erect or does she slump to one side, suggesting unilateral paralysis or weakness? Note any obvious asymmetries, deformities, or involuntary movements. Are there tremors, tics, or fasciculations (twitches)? If so, note their location, rate, quality, rhythm, amplitude, and relation to your patient's posture, activity, fatigue, emotion, and other factors. For example, if your patient's hand begins to shake only when you ask her to perform a task with it, such as writing her name or lifting a spoon, this suggests a postural tremor. Conversely, a tremor at rest that may disappear with voluntary movement suggests Parkinson's disease. To assess involuntary movement, observe your patient throughout the exam.

To determine your patient's muscle bulk, observe the size and contour of the muscles. Look for atrophy, a decrease in bulk and strength; hypertrophy, an increase in bulk and strength; or pseudohypertrophy, an increase in bulk and decrease in strength, as in muscular dystrophy. Flattened or concave contours, especially with fasciculations, may result from lower motor neuron disease. Some degree of muscle atrophy may be a normal part of the aging process or may result from the effects of diabetes on the peripheral nervous system. Look for signs of general muscle atrophy by checking for flattening of the thenar (thumb) muscle and for furrowing between the metacarpals. Unilateral muscle atrophy in the hands suggests median or ulnar nerve paralysis.

To assess muscle tone, feel the muscle's resistance to passive stretching in the extremities. Ask your patient to relax one arm. Then, put the arm, wrists, and hands through a moderate range-of-motion exam (Procedure 6-20a). Repeat the exam for the lower extremities. If you detect decreased resistance, shake the hand loosely back and forth. It should move freely, but it should not be floppy (flaccid). Increased resistance may be caused by tension. Does the resistance persist throughout the motion (lead-pipe rigidity), or does it vary? If the resistance increases at the extreme limits of the movement, it is called spasticity. A ratchet-like jerkiness in the resistance is known as "cog-wheel rigidity," a common finding in a patient faking the symptoms or trying to resist your examination. Table 6-11 describes some common muscle tone findings.

Now, focus on your patient's muscle strength. First, assess the strength of her grip. Test both grips simultaneously and compare them. Cross your middle finger over the top of your index finger to prevent your fingers from being hurt; then, ask your patient to squeeze them as hard as possible (Procedure 6-20b). Normally, you will have difficulty removing your fingers from your patient's grip. Continue testing all of the muscle groups listed in Table 6-12. While assessing muscle strength, remember that each patient's age, gender, size, and muscular training will affect

Table 6-11 MUSCLE TONE

Finding	Description
Spasticity	Increased tone when passive movement applied, especially at the end of range. Common in stroke.
Rigidity	Increased rigidity throughout movement (lead-pipe). Common in Parkinson's disease and extrapyramidal reactions. Cog-wheel motion is a patient-applied resistance.
Flaccidity	Loss of muscle tone causing limb to be loose. Common in stroke, spinal cord lesion, and Guillain-Barré syndrome.
Paratonia	Sudden changes in tone with passive movement. Can be increased or decreased resistance. Common in dementia.

Table 6-12	MUSCLE STRENGTH TESTS		
Muscles	**Nerves**		**Test**
Biceps	C5, C6		Flexion of the elbow
Triceps	C6, C7, C8		Extension of the elbow
Wrist extensors	C6, C7, C8, radial nerve		Extension of the wrist
Fingers	C8, T1, ulnar nerve		Finger abduction
Thumb	C8, T1, median nerve		Thumb opposition
Iliopsoas	L2, L3, L4		Hip flexion
Hip extensor	S1		Hip extension
Hip abductors	L4, L5, S1		Hip abduction
Hip adductors	L2, L3, L4		Hip adduction
Quadriceps	L2, L3, L4		Knee extension
Hamstrings	L4, L5, S1, S2		Knee flexion
Feet	L4, L5		Dorsiflexion
Calf muscles	S1		Plantar flexion

your exam results. When comparing sides, your patient's dominant side will be stronger. Test for muscle strength by having your patient move actively against your resistance (Procedure 6-20c). If the muscle is too weak to perform against resistance, have your patient try the movement against gravity or with gravity eliminated (you support the limb). Grade muscle strength on a scale from 0 to 5 (Table 6-13).

To assess your patient's position sense and coordination, first, observe her gait. Ask your patient to walk across the room, turn, and come back. Normally, a person will be able to maintain balance, swing the arms at the side, and turn easily. If your patient's gait is ataxic—uncoordinated, reeling, or unstable—suspect cerebellar disease, loss of position sense, or intoxication. Next, ask her to walk heel to toe in a straight line. This "tandem walking" may reveal an ataxia not previously seen. Now, ask your patient to walk first on her toes and then on her heels. This will assess plantar flexion and dorsiflexion of the ankle as well as balance. Next, ask her to hop in place on each foot in turn. Difficulty hopping may result from leg muscle weakness, lack of position sense, or cerebellar dysfunction. Now, ask her to do a shallow knee bend on each leg in turn. Difficulty doing this suggests muscle weakness in the pelvic girdle and legs. If your patient is old and unable to hop or do knee bends, have her rise from a sitting position without arm support, or step up onto a stool.

Next, perform the Romberg test. Ask your patient to stand with feet together and her eyes open. Now, have her close her eyes for 20 to 30 seconds. Observe the ability to remain upright with minimal swaying and no support.

Table 6-13	MUSCLE STRENGTH SCALE
Score	**Description**
5	Active movement against full resistance with no fatigue
4	Active movement against some resistance and gravity
3	Active movement against gravity
2	Active movement with gravity eliminated
1	Barely palpable muscle contraction with no movement
0	No visible or palpable muscle contraction

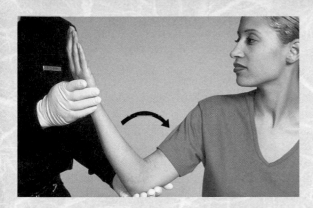

6-20a   Assess the elbow's range of motion.

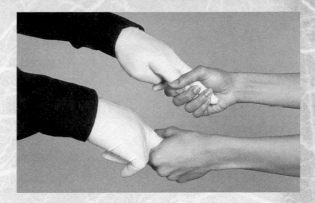

6-20b   Test your patient's grip.

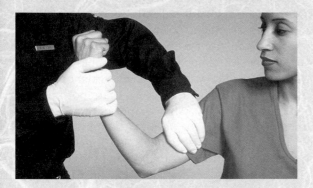

6-20c   Test arm strength.

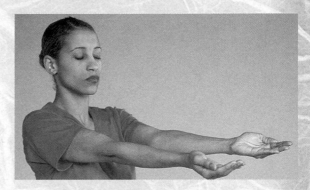

6-20d   Test for pronator drift.

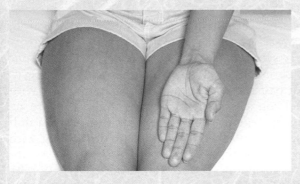

6-20e   Test for coordination with rapid alternating movements.

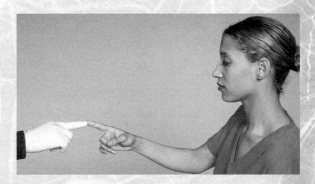

6-20f   Test coordination with point-to-point testing.

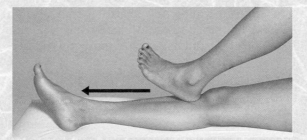

6-20g   Assess coordination with heel-to-shin testing.

Losing the balance indicates a positive Romberg test caused by ataxia from a loss of position sense. An inability to maintain balance with her eyes open and feet together represents a cerebellar ataxia. Now, check your patient for pronator drift. Ask your patient to stand with the arms straight out in front with the palms up and her eyes closed (Procedure 6-20d). Ask her to maintain this position for 20 to 30 seconds. Normally, your patient can do this easily. If one forearm pronates, suspect a mild hemiparesis. If it drifts sideways or upward, suspect a loss of position sense.

To assess your patient's coordination, test for rapid alternating movements. These manoeuvres can be difficult to describe, and so you should always demonstrate them to your patient. Ask her to repeat them as rapidly as possible while you observe for speed, rhythm, and smoothness. Your patient should repeat all movements with both sides of the body. Keep in mind that the dominant hand usually will perform better than the nondominant hand. If the movements are slow, irregular, and clumsy, suspect cerebellar or extrapyramidal tract disease or upper motor neuron weakness.

First, have your patient tap the distal joint of her thumb with the tip of the index finger as rapidly as possible. Then, ask her to place her hand, palm up, on the thigh, quickly turn it over palm down, and return it palm up (Procedure 6-20e). Have your patient repeat this movement as quickly as possible for 15 seconds; evaluate both hands. Next have her perform point-to-point testing. Ask your patient to alternate touching your index finger and her nose several times while you observe for accuracy and smoothness (Procedure 6-20f). Note any tremors or difficulty performing this task, indicating cerebellar disease; evaluate both hands. Now, assess for point-to-point testing in the legs. Ask your patient to touch her heel to the opposite knee and then run it down the shin to the big toe (Procedure 6-20g). Note the smoothness and accuracy of the actions. Repeat the test with the other leg. To test your patient's position sense, have her close her eyes and repeat this test for both legs. Abnormalities suggest cerebellar disease.

The Sensory System

To assess the sensory system, test for pain, light touch, temperature, position, vibration, and discriminative sensations. Remember to compare distal areas with proximal areas, to compare symmetrical areas bilaterally, and to scatter the stimuli to assess most of the dermatomes. Ask your patient to close her eyes for each of these tests. To test for pain sensation, touch your patient's skin with a sharp object and ask her to tell you whether it is sharp or dull. Compare areas as you move along the different regions, intermittently substituting a dull object for the sharp one. To test for light touch, softly touch your patient with a fine piece of cotton. Ask her to tell you whenever she feels the cotton. An abnormality suggests a peripheral neuropathy. Test for temperature sensation by touching her skin with a vial filled with either hot or cold liquid. Then, test for position sense by pulling one of her toe's upward and asking your patient to tell you whether it is up or down. Test for vibration sense by placing the stem of a vibrating tuning fork against a bony prominence (Figure 6-23). Finally, test for discriminative sensation by putting a familiar object, such as a key, in your patient's hand and asking her to identify it.

Reflexes

The sensory pathways manage conscious sensation and participate in the reflex arc. The reflex arc connects some sensory impulses directly to motor neurons, triggering immediate responses to noxious stimuli, such as touching your hand to a flame. Deep tendon reflexes are a similar involuntary response to direct muscu-

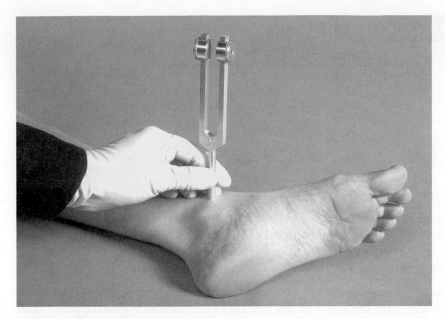

FIGURE 6-23   Test vibration sense with a tuning fork.

lar stretch. Striking a slightly flexed tendon with a reflex hammer sends an impulse to the spinal cord, where a reflex arc occurs (Figure 6-24). This immediately sends a motor response back to the tendon, which begins the muscle contraction.

When you perform a nervous system exam, also test your patient's superficial and deep tendon reflexes. Always compare one side with the other. Grade the reflexes on a scale of 0 to 4+ (Table 6-14) and record your findings on a stick figure diagram. A hyperactive response suggests upper motor neuron disease. A diminished response or no response suggests damage to the lower motor neurons or spinal cord.

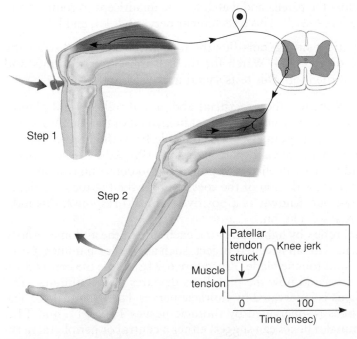

FIGURE 6-24   A reflex arc depicts muscle tension over time.

Table 6-14	REFLEX SCALE
Grade	**Description**
0	No response
+	Diminished, below normal
++	Average, normal
+++	Brisker than normal
++++	Hyperactive, associated with clonus

Deep tendon reflexes can be tested at several places on the body. Use the pointed end of a reflex hammer for striking small areas, the flat end for striking larger areas. First, ask your patient to relax. Then, properly position the limb you are testing. Quickly strike the tendon using wrist motion only.

Biceps Support your patient's arm in the slightly flexed position with your thumb directly over the distal biceps tendon in the antecubital space (Procedure 6-21a). Strike your thumbnail with the point of the reflex hammer and watch for contraction of the biceps muscle and the resulting flexion of the elbow. This tests for spinal nerves C5 and C6.

Triceps Flex your patient's arm at a right angle. With the point of your reflex hammer, strike the triceps tendon along the posterior aspect of the distal humerus (Procedure 6-21b). Watch for triceps contraction and the resulting elbow extension. This tests spinal nerves C6, C7, and C8.

Brachioradialis Support your patient's arm with the forearm slightly pronated (Procedure 6-21c). Now, strike her radius about 5 cm above the wrist. Watch for contraction of the brachioradialis and the resulting flexion and supination of the forearm. This tests cervical nerves C5 and C6.

Quadriceps Have your patient sit with her leg hanging off the end of the exam table. Tap the tendon just below the patella and watch for the quadriceps to contract and extend the knee (Procedure 6-21d). This tests lumbar nerves L2, L3, and L4.

Achilles With your patient sitting, dorsiflex the foot at the ankle and strike the Achilles tendon (Procedure 6-21e). Watch for the calf muscles to contract and cause plantar flexion of the foot. This tests sacral nerves S1 and S2.

Abdominal/Plantar Now, test the superficial abdominal reflexes and plantar response. These are initiated by stimulating the skin instead of muscle. Assess the plantar reflex by stroking the lateral aspect of the sole from the heel to the ball of your patient's foot, curving medially across the ball (Procedure 6-21f). Begin with the lightest stimulus that will elicit a response. If you detect no response, be more firm. Watch for plantar flexion of the toes. Note if the big toe dorsiflexes while the other toes fan out. Known as a positive **Babinski response,** this indicates a central nervous system lesion.

Test the abdominal reflex by lightly stroking each side of the abdomen above and below the umbilicus with an irregular object, such as a reflex hammer, a broken cotton swab, or a split tongue blade (Procedure 6-21g). Note the contraction of the abdominal muscles and how the umbilicus deviates to the stimulus. The area above the umbilicus is innervated by thoracic nerves T8, T9, and T10. The area below the umbilicus is innervated by thoracic nerves T10, T11, and T12. The absence of abdominal reflexes can suggest either a central or peripheral nervous system disorder.

✱ **Babinski response** big toe dorsiflexes and the other toes fan out when sole is stimulated.

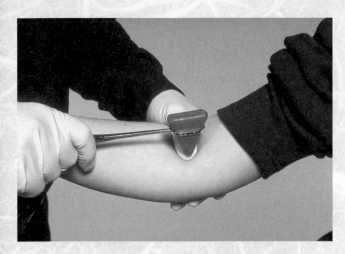

6-21a   Test the biceps reflex (cervical nerves C5 and C6).

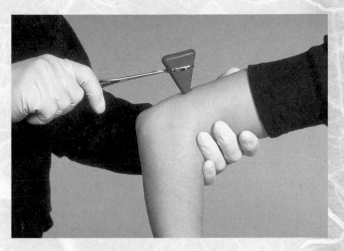

6-21b   Test the triceps reflex (cervical nerves C6, C7, and C8).

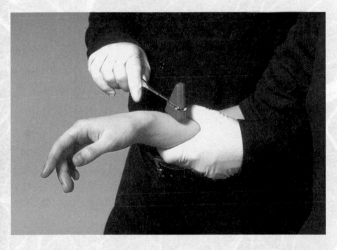

6-21c   Test the brachioradialis reflex (cervical nerves C5 and C6).

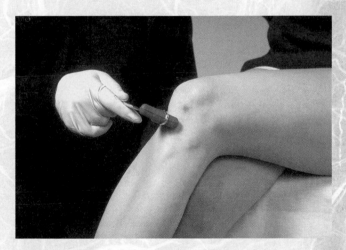

6-21d   Test the quadriceps reflex (lumbar nerves L2, L3, and L4).

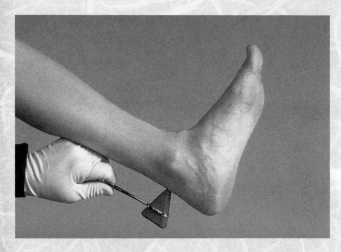

6-21e   Test the Achilles reflex (sacral nerves S1 and S2).

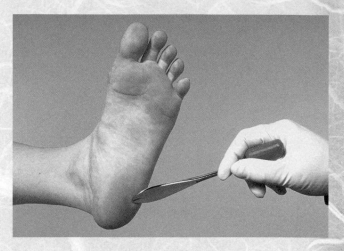

6-21f   Test the plantar reflex (central nervous system).

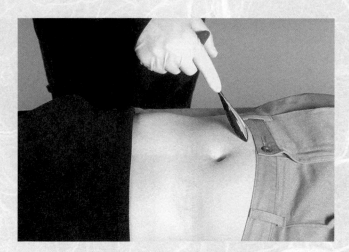

6-21g   Test abdominal reflexes (thoracic nerves T8, T9, T10, T11, and T12).

PHYSICAL ASSESSMENT OF INFANTS AND CHILDREN

Conducting a physical assessment of a sick or injured child can challenge any clinician. Your success will depend on several factors. First, you must be familiar with the anatomical differences between children and adults. Second, you must understand the physical and psychological developmental stages of the different age groups. Most importantly, you must practise these skills daily.

BUILDING PATIENT AND FAMILY RAPPORT

Children are not just small adults, and you cannot treat them as if they were. Children are naturally apprehensive of strangers and new things. A sick or injured child is a frightened child. She fears pain, separation from her family, and unfamiliar surroundings. Dealing with these fears paves the way for a successful encounter with the child and the parents. You are a stranger. In uniform, you become even more ominous. Gaining your pediatric patient's trust becomes a vital part of your assessment. Unless the child requires emergency critical care, take time to establish a rapport. This will help ensure continuous cooperation.

Although different age groups have specific fears and characteristics, the following general rules apply to pediatrics as a whole. Remain calm and confident. Be direct and honest about what you are doing, especially if you are performing a painful procedure. If possible, do not separate the child from the parents. Instead, elicit their help in obtaining the history and allow them to help hold the child while you conduct your assessment. The more invasive the procedure, the later in the assessment you should perform it—unless, of course, your patient is critically ill or injured. (Never delay important procedures or techniques on the critically ill or injured child.) Once your patient begins crying and carrying on, the rest of your assessment will be more difficult, if not impossible. Finally, provide continuous reassurance and feedback to your patient and the family members. This helps reduce everyone's anxiety over what is wrong, what you are doing, and what comes next.

Position yourself at the child's eye level, use a soft voice, and smile a lot. Often, a small toy, such as a teddy bear, can distract your patient while you assess her. If you are using diagnostic equipment, allow the child to handle it while you explain how it works. Make sure your movements are slow and deliberate, and explain everything you are doing.

ANATOMY AND THE PHYSICAL ASSESSMENT

To assess a child properly, you must understand her unique anatomy (Figure 6-25). The anatomical differences among age groups will alter your interpretation of physical findings. For example, since an infant's skin is thinner and contains less subcutaneous fat, you can expect environmental temperature extremes to affect an infant more severely.

This section deals with examining infants and children in the clinical situation. The pediatric chapter, Chapter 42, discusses a more detailed pediatric assessment.

General Appearance

Especially in the emergency setting, note whether your patient looks toxic, or sick. A toxic child appears not to recognize or respond to the parents. She may look tired, have a decreased respiratory effort, and may have mottled skin or a generalized rash. She may be grey or cyanotic and just look very sick, usually from some type of bacterial process. These children, who present with the signs and symp-

Children are not just small adults, and you cannot treat them as if they were.

The more invasive the procedure, the later in the assessment you should perform it.

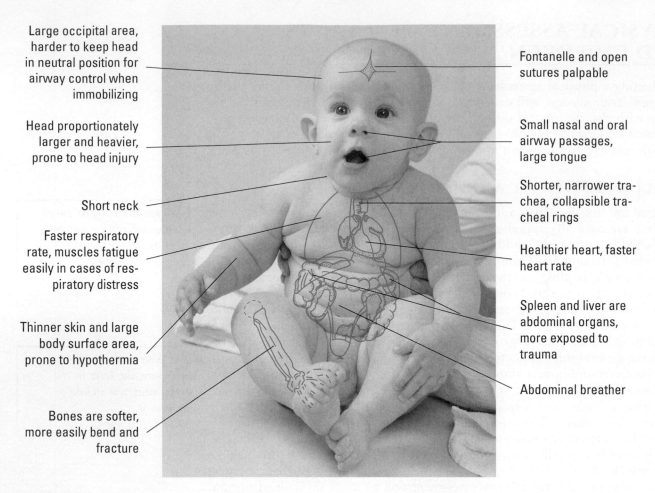

Large occipital area, harder to keep head in neutral position for airway control when immobilizing

Head proportionately larger and heavier, prone to head injury

Short neck

Faster respiratory rate, muscles fatigue easily in cases of respiratory distress

Thinner skin and large body surface area, prone to hypothermia

Bones are softer, more easily bend and fracture

Fontanelle and open sutures palpable

Small nasal and oral airway passages, large tongue

Shorter, narrower trachea, collapsible tracheal rings

Healthier heart, faster heart rate

Spleen and liver are abdominal organs, more exposed to trauma

Abdominal breather

FIGURE 6-25   Pediatric anatomy and physiology. You must understand a child's unique anatomy to assess him properly.

toms of respiratory failure or shock, usually require rapid transport while you provide aggressive resuscitation procedures (advanced airway management, oxygenation and ventilation, intravenous access, and rapid fluid administration).

Head and Neck

The bones of the skull are soft, and the fontanelles ("soft spots," spaces between a child's cranial bones) stay open until about 18 months of age (Figure 6-26). From this time until about age five, cartilage connects the sutures. This allows the skull to expand as the brain grows. Check the sutures for bulging (increased intracranial pressure) or sunkenness (dehydration). In infants, a soft bulging spot following a history of trauma suggests a head injury with increasing intracranial pressure. The same finding associated with a fever suggests meningitis.

Because a child's airways are so much smaller than an adult's, a minor obstruction can create an acute respiratory problem. Watch the child's face for signs of distress and increased respiratory effort, such as nasal flaring. Children in acute respiratory distress will appear anxious and not interested in their surroundings. Also, watch for retractions and head bobbing. Listen for stridor, wheezing, and grunting as further signs of severe breathing problems. As the child speaks, listen for hoarseness (upper airway obstruction) or moaning (decreasing level of consciousness). These findings always require appropriate

Hoarseness, suggesting an upper airway obstruction, or moaning, suggesting decreased consciousness, requires intervention and rapid transport.

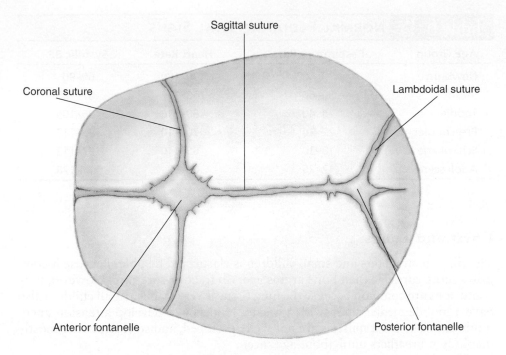

Coronal suture

Sagittal suture

Lambdoidal suture

Anterior fontanelle

Posterior fontanelle

FIGURE 6-26　Fontanelle of the infant skull.

intervention and rapid transport. Remember, a crying or screaming child has a patent airway.

Observe the child's face for signs of pain and discomfort as you continue your examination. Inspect the eyes as you would an adult's. Assess the outer ear for position. The top of the ear should be on a horizontal line with the outer corner of the eye. As a child grows, the anatomy of the external ear canal changes. In infancy, the canal curves downward, and so you should pull down the auricle to see the tympanic membrane at the distal end of the canal. As the child grows, the canal starts to move up and backward, and the ear is relatively higher and farther back on the head. Remember to pull the auricle upward and backward to afford the best view with the otoscope. Brace your hand against the child's skull to prevent injury from sudden movement.

Choose the largest speculum that will fit comfortably into the child's ear. Tilt the child's head away from you. Hold the otoscope firmly in one hand and, with your free hand, pull the ear appropriately to straighten the ear canal. Slowly insert the speculum 0.5–1.25 cm into the canal. Observe the amount, texture, and colour of wax and the presence of foreign bodies. Inspect the tympanic membrane for colour, light reflex, and bony landmarks. Repeat the same steps for the other ear.

Inspect the child's mouth much the same as you would for the adult. A young child's mouth is small, while the tongue is relatively large, and so examining the oral cavity will be a challenge. Examine the nose using the nasal speculum and penlight or the appropriate attachment to the otoscope. To examine the mucous membrane, tip the child's head back and use the otoscope to inspect for colour or swelling.

Evaluate the child's neck for stiffness, which—when associated with a fever—suggests meningitis. Evaluate for lymphadenopathy (enlarged lymph nodes) in the neck by assessing the nodes' size, warmth, tenderness, and mobility. Certain infectious diseases, such as mononucleosis, rubella, and mumps, are associated with lymphadenopathy. Nodes commonly feel enlarged due to recurrent upper respiratory infection.

Table 6-15	NORMAL PEDIATRIC VITAL SIGNS		
Age Group	**Respiratory Rate**	**Heart Rate**	**Systolic BP**
Newborn	30–60	100–180	60–90
Infant	30–60	100–160	87–105
Toddler	24–40	80–110	95–105
Preschooler	22–34	70–110	95–110
School age	18–30	65–110	97–112
Adolescent	12–26	60–90	112–128

Chest and Lungs

The rib cage in infants and small children is elastic and flexible. Because it comprises more cartilage than bone at this age, rib fractures are rare. However, lung contusions are common because the lung tissue is very fragile. Small children also have a mobile mediastinum with a greater tendency to develop a tension pneumothorax. The chest muscles are not well developed, and so children are mostly diaphragm breathers until about age seven.

The chest muscles are considered accessory muscles in the young child; to evaluate breathing, observe both the chest and abdomen for movement. A child in severe respiratory distress may exhibit a "see-saw" pattern in which the sternum and abdomen rise and fall in opposition to each other. Count the respiratory rate without touching your patient if possible. Assess the rate, quality, and depth of the respirations. Normal respiratory rates vary with age, but generally they decrease as the child grows older. Table 6-15 gives normal vital signs for the various pediatric age groups. Auscultate for breath sounds with the bell of your stethoscope at the midaxillary lines (Figure 6-27). Use this location to avoid hearing transmitted breath sounds from the opposite lung fields.

Cardiovascular System

Unless the child has a congenital defect, the heart will be strong and healthy. The heart rate will vary with age, but generally it will decrease as the child gets older. If the child is alert and uncooperative, measure the pulse rate by listening to the heart. Place your stethoscope between the sternum and nipple on your patient's left side. Children have thin chest walls, and so you will usually be able to observe the apical

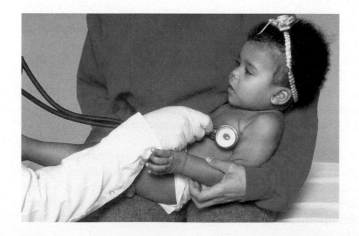

FIGURE 6-27 Place your stethoscope along your young patient's midaxillary line.

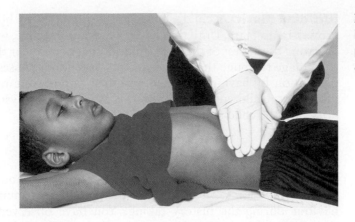

FIGURE 6-28 Gradually increase the pressure when palpating a young patient's abdomen.

impulse of the heart. Remember that tachycardia or bradycardia can both be a response to hypoxia in infants and young children. Bradycardia is the initial response to this condition in the newborn; without aggressive intervention, cardiopulmonary arrest will soon follow. Blood pressure will vary in children, but generally it will rise as they grow older. Children respond to hypovolemia by increasing cardiac function.

Tachycardia or bradycardia can both be a response to hypoxia in infants and young children; without aggressive intervention, cardiopulmonary arrest will soon follow.

Abdomen

A child's liver and spleen are proportionally larger and more vascular than an adult's. Thus, they extend beyond the rib cage and are more exposed. Likewise, the child's immature abdominal muscles provide less protection than an adult's. Inspect the abdomen first for movement. Normally, only respiratory movements should be visible; peristalsis is not normally observable. Next, assess contour. The abdomen normally bulges by the end of inspiration. Note any asymmetry. Inspect the groin area for inguinal hernias, common in male children. Finally, look at the umbilicus for any hernias, common in children under three years. Percuss and auscultate the abdomen as in an adult.

Before you begin palpating the abdomen, make sure the child is comfortable. Bend her knees to relax the abdominal muscles and make palpation easier. Your hands should be warm. If the child is ticklish, cover her hands with yours as you palpate. Begin with light palpation and gradually increase the pressure (Figure 6-28). Palpate all four quadrants. Deep palpation is performed next. You are feeling for masses and tenderness. The child's facial expression is a better guide to pain than are words, since she may interpret your pressure as pain.

Musculoskeletal System

Evaluate pulses, sensation, movement, and warmth in all four extremities. Check for capillary refill and feel for peripheral pulses (Figure 6-29). Evaluate the skin, which reveals important clues in children. Its colour, turgor, moisture, and temperature are key indicators of the cardiovascular system's condition. Unlike the adult's, the child's capillary refill time accurately reflects her peripheral perfusion status. When examining the musculoskeletal system, remember the growth and posture at different stages of the child's development. For example, a toddler walks with a broad base for support and is likely to appear bowlegged. A teenager with poor posture may suffer from a skeletal problem, such as scoliosis.

Palpate the upper and lower extremities for swelling, tenderness, and contractions. Next, have the child demonstrate the range of motion of her joints while you feel for smoothness of movement. Examine all joints. Check muscle strength in all muscle groups by asking the child to prevent you from moving a

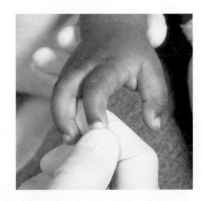

FIGURE 6-29 Pressing a child's fingernail is one of several ways to assess capillary refill. The child's capillary refill time is a good indicator of the child's peripheral perfusion status.

part of her body. A child's bones are more likely to break at the ends, where growth takes place. Until the child reaches adolescence, when these areas become as strong as the rest of the bone, injuries that occur near the joints are more likely to damage the bone than the ligaments or tendons. Assess the child's muscle coordination by having her stand and then hop on one foot. Repeat this for the other foot. Children usually enjoy this aspect of the physical assessment. You can also have the child skip or jump.

Nervous System

The child's general behaviour, level of consciousness, and orientation are signs of cerebral function. You have asked the parents to comment on their child's behaviour during the history taking. You have observed the child's behaviour throughout the examination and already have learned much about her cerebral function by interacting with the child. Now, test specific functions, such as language and recall. You will have checked most of the 12 cranial nerves during your head and neck exam.

You can test for cerebellar function with several games that children usually enjoy. First, as you move your finger, ask the child to touch her nose and then your finger. Consistent past-pointing should arouse your suspicion. An alternative test is to have the child pat her knees alternately with the palms and backs of the hands. Check for sensation over the child's face, trunk, arms, and leg. Check for hot and cold sensation by alternately touching the skin with warm and cold test tubes. Ask the child to close her eyes and tell you which temperature she feels. Be sure to test for reflexes on both sides of the body, just as with an adult. If the child has difficulty relaxing, test a parent's reflexes to show that it does not hurt.

Remember, the most important characteristic of a physical assessment is thoroughness. Be systematic in your approach, and with practice, you will be able to do a complete and accurate physical assessment.

The most important characteristic of a physical assessment is thoroughness.

RECORDING ASSESSMENT FINDINGS

After you perform the history and physical assessment, it is time to record the findings on your patient's chart, or permanent medical record. The information you enter enables you and other members of the health-care team to identify health problems, make a diagnosis, plan the appropriate care, and monitor your patient's response to treatment. The patient record is only as good as the accuracy, depth, and detail you provide.

The patient record is only as good as the accuracy, depth, and detail you provide.

All health-care clinicians follow a standard format when charting patient information. Using it and appropriate medical terminology will allow everyone to easily read and understand your assessment findings. Although your first attempts at writing a complete history and physical assessment will be lengthy and possibly disorganized, clinical experience will eventually lead to a more efficient and organized record.

Your patient's chart is a legal document, and any information you enter may be used in court. Proper documentation is vital to your protection. Present the data legibly, accurately, and truthfully. They should represent your findings of history and physical assessment—no more, no less. State your assessment, your analysis of the problem, and your management plan clearly and exactly. No question should ever arise about your assessment or care of your patient if you document it properly.

Be sure to include all data about your assessment. You cannot formulate an impression unless you have clearly spelled out the positive and negative details on which it was made. Remember that the absence of a sign or symptom (pertinent negative) may be just as important as its presence. Record everything in writing. If you do not document a neurological exam, you will never convince anyone that you performed it, especially not a plaintiff's lawyer or a jury. Be complete, but avoid unnecessary words. For example, say "pale," not "pale in colour." Also, avoid lengthy repetitive phrases, such as "patient states." Use accepted abbreviations and symbols whenever possible. Avoid using vague adjectives, such as *good, normal,* and *poor,* because they are open to interpretation by other providers. Document what your patient tells you, not what you infer or interpret. Use direct quotes whenever possible.

The universally accepted organization for patient charts follows the SOAP format. SOAP stands for subjective, objective, assessment, and plan. Use this format when writing your patient's chart. Subjective information is what your patient tells you. It comprises the chief complaint, the history of present illness, the past history, the current health status, and the review of systems. Objective information includes the data collected from the general survey, vital signs, head-to-toe anatomical exam, systems-oriented exam, and neurological exam, including the mental status. These are the data you gathered by inspection, palpation, percussion, auscultation, and other techniques of physical assessment. Objective information also includes the results of any laboratory tests. The assessment summarizes the relevant data for each problem identified in the history and physical assessment. The plan outlines your management strategy in three categories: diagnostic (how you will assess progress), therapeutic (any treatments), and educational (what you need to teach your patient). Chapter 9, "Documentation," deals with prehospital documentation in detail.

Record everything in writing.

> **Content Review**
>
> **SOAP**
> - Subjective
> - Objective
> - Assessment
> - Plan

SUMMARY

This chapter has presented both a regional and a systems approach to physical assessment. The setting, chief complaint, and clinical status of your patient will dictate how much of the physical assessment you actually use. For example, if you are hired to conduct preemployment physicals, you may decide to conduct a complete assessment. If you are at the scene of a critically ill or injured patient, you will assess only those areas relevant to the situation. If your patient presents with a minor, isolated musculoskeletal injury, you may focus your assessment on that area and system. As you become more experienced, making these decisions will become easier.

CHAPTER 7

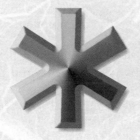

Patient Assessment in the Field

Objectives

After reading this chapter, you should be able to:

1. Recognize hazards/potential hazards associated with the medical and trauma scene. (pp. 343–349)
2. Identify unsafe scenes and describe methods for making them safe. (pp. 343–349)
3. Discuss common mechanisms of injury and the nature of illness. (pp. 350–352)
4. Predict patterns of injury based on the mechanism of injury. (pp. 350–352, 363–364)
5. Discuss the reason for identifying the total number of patients at the scene. (pp. 349–350)
6. Organize the management of a scene following assessment. (pp. 343–349)
7. Explain the reasons for identifying the need for additional help or assistance during the scene assessment. (pp. 343, 345–349)
8. Summarize the reasons for forming a general impression of the patient. (p. 353)
9. Discuss methods of assessing mental status or levels of consciousness in the adult, infant, and child patients. (pp. 354–355)

Continued

INTRODUCTION

✳ **patient assessment** problem-oriented evaluation of patient and establishment of priorities based on existing and potential threats to human life.

Content Review

COMPONENTS OF PATIENT ASSESSMENT

Primary assessment
Focused history and
   secondary assessment
Ongoing assessment
Detailed secondary
   assessment

Patient assessment means conducting a problem-oriented evaluation of your patient and establishing priorities of care based on existing and potential threats to human life. In the previous two chapters, you studied the techniques of performing a comprehensive history and physical assessment. Such all-inclusive evaluations are best suited for patients without a chief complaint. They also establish a baseline health evaluation for patients admitted to the hospital. As a paramedic, however, you will certainly never perform a comprehensive assessment in the acute setting. It is too time consuming and yields too much irrelevant information. Instead, you will use your foundation of knowledge, skills, and tools to assess the acutely ill or injured patient. With time and clinical experience, you will learn which components of the comprehensive assessment apply to your particular patient.

Now, you can use the pertinent components of the comprehensive history and physical assessment to perform patient assessments—problem-oriented assessments based on your patient's chief complaint. The basic components of patient assessment include the primary assessment; the focused history and seconday assessment, including vital signs; an ongoing assessment; and in some cases, a detailed secondary assessment. In many EMS systems, the initial assessment is known as the primary survey or primary assessment, and the physical exam is called the secondary survey (or secondary assessment).

Your patient's condition will determine which components you use and how you use them. For example, for trauma patients with a significant mechanism of injury, you will perform a primary assessment followed by a rapid trauma assessment (a head-to-toe assessment aimed at identifying traumatic signs and symptoms) and, if time allows, a detailed secondary assessment en route to the hospital. For patients with minor, isolated trauma, a primary assessment followed by a focused secondary assessment is warranted. For the responsive medical patient, you will conduct a primary assessment followed by a focused history and secondary assessment. Finally, for the unresponsive medical patient, you will perform a primary assessment followed by a rapid medical assessment (a head-to-toe assessment aimed at identifying medical signs and symptoms). In all cases, you will perform an ongoing assessment en route to the hospital to detect changes in patient condition.

The primary assessment's goal is to identify and correct immediately life-threatening conditions. These include airway compromise, inadequate ventilation, and major hemorrhage. During this rapid evaluation you use a variety of manoeuvres and special equipment to manage any life threats as you find them. Immediately following the primary assessment, you will establish the priorities of care. People such as the trauma patient with unstable vital signs and the unresponsive medical patient require a rapid head-to-toe asessment and immediate transport to the hospital. Patients with minor, isolated trauma and most medical emergencies allow time to perform further assessments and provide care before transport.

Your proficiency in performing a systematic patient assessment will determine your ability to deliver the highest quality of prehospital care to sick and injured people. Paramedic patient assessment is a straightforward process. Your assessment must be thorough because many prehospital care procedures are potentially dangerous. Safely and appropriately performing advanced procedures, such as administration of drugs, defibrillation, synchronized cardioversion, needle decompression of the chest, or endotracheal intubation, will depend on your assessment and correct field diagnosis. If your assessment does not reveal your patient's true problem, the consequences can be devastating.

As always, common sense dictates how you proceed in the field. When you assess the responsive medical patient, the history reveals the most important diagnostic information and takes priority over the secondary assessment. For the trauma patient and the unresponsive medical patient, the reverse is true. Yet,

If your assessment does not reveal your patient's true problem, the consequences can be devastating.

trauma may cause a medical emergency, and conversely, a medical emergency may cause trauma. Only by performing a thorough patient assessment can you discover the true cause of your patient's problems. This chapter provides problem-oriented patient assessment templates based on the information and techniques presented in the previous two chapters. You will need to refer to those chapters for the details of taking a history and conducting a physical assessment.

SCENE ASSESSMENT

Scene assessment is the essential first step at any emergency. Before you enter a scene, take the necessary time to judge the situation. Fire fighters drive just past a burning house so that they can see three of its sides before they make strategic decisions. Follow their lead. Never rush into any situation; first stop and look around (Figure 7-1).

On arrival, determine whether the scene is safe. What body substance isolation precautions are required? Is the mechanism of injury or the nature of illness obvious? Are there multiple patients? Do you need immediate additional resources? After an initial scene assessment, if necessary, report to your dispatcher what you have, what you need, and what you are doing. This way, you keep everyone informed and your dispatcher can send any necessary additional support.

Although scene assessment is your initial responsibility, remember that it is also an ongoing process. Emergency scenes are dynamic and can change suddenly. An injury to a child call can erupt into a violent domestic dispute if one parent blames the other. A hazardous material spill can ignite. An improperly stabilized car can shift. Always be alert for subtle signs of danger, and avoid becoming a patient yourself.

Assessment of the scene gives you important information that will guide your actions. In trauma, a brief assessment of the accident scene reveals the mechanism of injury. From this, you can estimate the degree of energy transfer and possible seriousness of injuries. In a medical emergency, you can sometimes

Only by performing a thorough patient assessment can you discover the true cause of your patient's problems.

Never rush into any situation; first stop and look around.

Always be alert for subtle signs of danger.

Assessment of the scene gives you important information that will guide your actions.

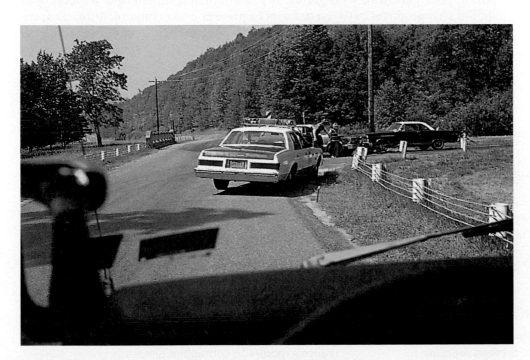

FIGURE 7-1   Always stop to assess the scene before going in.

determine the nature of your patient's illness from clues at the scene. The smell of a lower gastrointestinal bleed, the sound of a hissing oxygen tank, or the sight of drug paraphernalia provides clues and an initial insight into your patient's situation. Learn to use all your senses when assessing the scene.

The components of a scene assessment include:

- Body substance isolation (personal protective equipment)
- Scene safety
- Location of all patients
- Mechanism of injury
- Nature of the illness

BODY SUBSTANCE ISOLATION

Body fluids frequently contain health-threatening pathogens. The best defence against bloodborne, body-fluid-borne, and airborne agents is to take appropriate body substance isolation precautions. Your goal is to prevent infectious disease from spreading to you or to others. Make sure that personal protective equipment, such as gloves, masks, gowns, and eye protection, is available on every emergency vehicle, and take the appropriate precautions on every emergency call (Figure 7-2). Your patient's clinical condition and the procedures you perform will determine the required precautions.

Most body substance isolation procedures are simply common sense. Wash your hands thoroughly before and after treating each patient whenever possible (Figure 7-3). This simple technique is the most effective method of preventing disease transmission between patients and their health-care workers. Wear latex or vinyl gloves anytime you expect to contact blood or other body fluids or if you are unsure of any risk. This includes the mucous membranes, any areas with broken skin, or items soiled with blood or body fluids. Since you often cannot wash your hands before examining your patient, you should wear gloves to avoid exposing your patient to your germs. If you are managing multiple patients, you should change gloves between patients to prevent cross-contamination. Discard all contaminated gloves in the appropriate biohazard bag (Figure 7-4).

Always use all the equipment recommended for a particular procedure or patient to maximize your protection against communicable diseases. If blood, vomit, or secretions might splash near your eyes, nose, or mouth, wear a face mask and protective eyewear. Such situations may include arterial bleeding, childbirth,

Content Review

COMPONENTS OF SCENE ASSESSMENT
Body substance isolation (personal protective equipment)
Scene safety
Location of all patients
Mechanism of injury
Nature of the illness

The best defence against bloodborne, body-fluid-borne, and airborne pathogens is to take body substance isolation precautions.

Washing your hands is the most effective method of preventing disease transmission between you and your patients.

Always use all the equipment recommended for a particular procedure or patient to maximize your protection against communicable diseases.

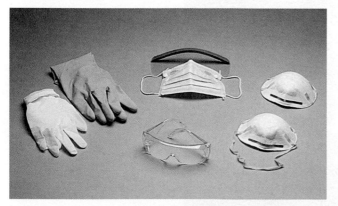

FIGURE 7-2   Always wear the appropriate personal protective equipment (PPE) to prevent exposure to contagious diseases.

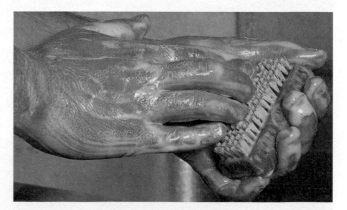

FIGURE 7-3   Careful, methodical hand washing helps reduce exposure to contagious disease.

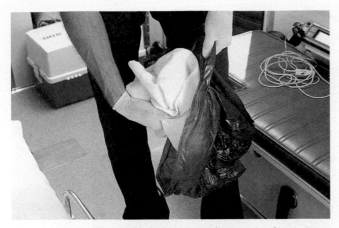

FIGURE 7-4   Place all contaminated items in the appropriate biohazard bag.

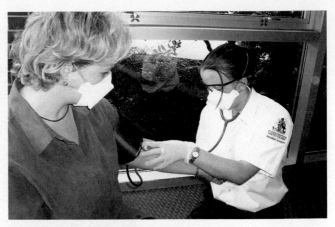

FIGURE 7-5   With a suspected tuberculosis patient, you may place a surgical-type mask on the patient while you wear a NIOSH-approved respirator. Monitor the patient's airway and breathing carefully.

invasive procedures, such as endotracheal intubation, and oral suctioning, as well as during cleanup when heavy scrubbing is necessary. If you expect large blood splashes, such as in emergency childbirth, wear a gown to protect your clothing.

Consider masking both yourself and your patient whenever the potential for airborne transmission of disease exists (Figure 7-5). High-efficiency particulate air (HEPA) respirators filter out the tuberculosis (TB) bacillus. Always wear a properly fitted HEPA mask if you are managing a patient with suspected TB, especially when performing procedures like endotracheal intubation, oral suctioning, and administering nebulized medications. Follow local protocols regarding the use of personal protective equipment for specific situations (e.g., possible SARS patients). These procedures present a high risk for the transmission of airborne particles.

SCENE SAFETY

Scene safety simply means doing everything possible to ensure a safe environment for you, your crew, other responding personnel, your patient, and any bystanders—in that order. Your personal safety is the top priority at any emergency scene. Make sure you are not injured while providing care. If you become a patient yourself, you will do your own patient little good. You must determine that no hazards may endanger the lives of people on the scene. If your scene is unsafe, either make it safe or wait until someone else does (Figure 7-6).

As the first unit on the scene, you may overestimate your capability to manage a rescue situation. Do not attempt a hazardous rescue unless you are properly clothed, equipped, and trained. Individual acts of courage are sometimes necessary, but modern rescue operations emphasize safety first, not heroics. Foolish heroics often end in tragedy. If in doubt, it is better to err on the side of caution than to risk personal harm.

Many factors can make an emergency scene unsafe. Through experience you will learn to identify those factors quickly. Do not become complacent. Sometimes even the most nonthreatening, harmless-looking scene can turn into a disaster (Figure 7-7). If you are not sure the scene is safe, do not enter. As you approach a scene, immediately evaluate the surrounding area. Is it as your dispatcher's information has led you to expect, or does something just not look right? What do the bystanders' faces tell you? Are they angry, scared, or panicked? Be alert for situations that look or feel suspicious. If necessary, wait until law enforcement personnel secure the scene. Use all your senses to evaluate a

FIGURE 7-6 Look for potential hazards during scene assessment.

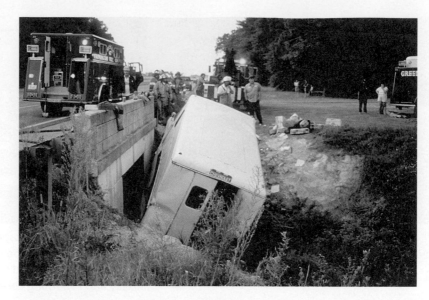

scene and learn to trust your intuition. If your instincts tell you not to enter or to get out, follow them. They are the subconscious sum of your experiences. Listen to your instincts; they are probably correct.

Carefully look for and identify on-scene hazards before even attempting to reach your patient. To do otherwise places you, other rescuers, and your patient at risk. Remember that you may find such dangers at either medical or trauma scenes. These hazards may be violent patients or aggressive bystanders. Other potential hazards include fire, structural collapse, traffic, unstable surfaces, and broken glass or jagged metal. Other risks involve hazardous materials—chemical spills, radiation, or gas leaks that might ignite or explode. A simple spark can set off a gas leak or oil spill. Electric wires threaten both fire and electric shock. Look

FIGURE 7-7 Even the most peaceful-looking scene can pose potential dangers.

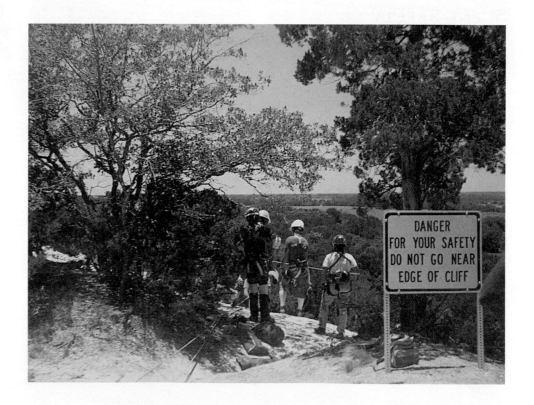

around to determine the possibility of lightning, avalanche, rock slides, cave-ins, or similar dangers. Other potential hazards include poisonous or caustic substances; biological agents; germ-infested materials; confined spaces, such as vessels, trenches, mines, silos, or caves; and extreme heights. In every case, let common sense dictate scene management.

Crime scenes pose a special threat. When responding to a call in which the initial dispatch includes words like *shooting, stabbing,* or *domestic dispute,* wait for law enforcement personnel to secure the scene before entering (Figure 7-8). In fact, do not even enter the neighbourhood, as sitting in your ambulance on the scene may undermine an already unstable environment. If possible, turn off your lights and siren and stage your vehicle a few blocks away where it cannot be seen from the scene. Refer to the crime scene awareness section of Chapter 3 for more information on this topic.

Crash scenes requiring heavy-duty rescue procedures, scenes where toxic substances are present, crime scenes with a potential for violence, or scenes with such unstable surfaces as slippery slopes, ice, or rushing water all call for specialized crews, additional medical supplies, and sophisticated equipment (Figure 7-9). Do not even consider entering such situations unless you have the proper clothing, equipment, and training to work in them. Because getting backup requires extra time, this phase is critical. A prompt call to your dispatch centre can save critical minutes in a life-threatening situation.

Without the appropriate protective gear, you will jeopardize your safety and your patient's. To participate in a rescue operation, you should have at least the following equipment immediately available: four-point suspension helmets, eye goggles or industrial safety glasses, high-quality hearing protection, leather work gloves, high-top steel-toed boots, insulated coveralls, and turnout gear (Figure 7-10). Only personnel thoroughly trained in using hazardous material (hazmat) suits or self-contained breathing apparatus (SCBA) should use them (Figure 7-11). These items are often supplied on specialty support vehicles, such as hazmat response units and heavy-rescue trucks (Figure 7-12).

In every case, let common sense dictate scene management.

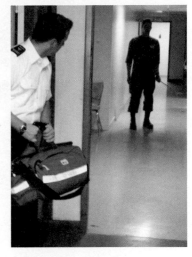

FIGURE 7-8   Wait for the police before entering a potentially hazardous scene.

Do not even consider entering hazardous scenes unless you have the proper clothing, equipment, and training to work in them.

A prompt call for backup can save critical minutes in a life-threatening situation.

Content Review

MINIMUM RESCUE OPERATION EQUIPMENT

Four-point suspension helmets
Eye goggles and industrial safety glasses
High-quality hearing protection
Leather work gloves
High-top steel-toed boots
Insulated coveralls
Turnout gear

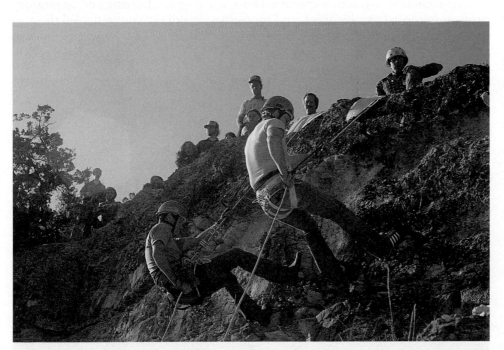

FIGURE 7-9   Never enter a specialized rescue situation without proper training and equipment.

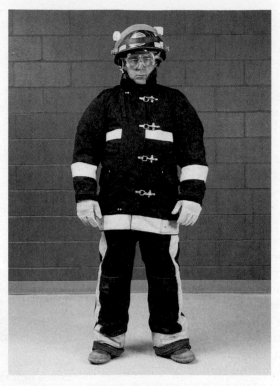

FIGURE 7-10 Full protective gear, including eye protection, helmet, turnout gear, and gloves.

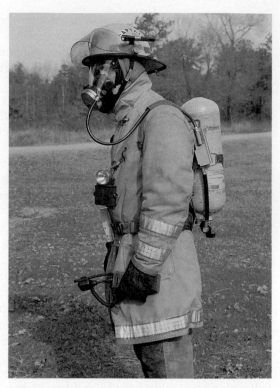

FIGURE 7-11 Self-contained breathing apparatus (SCBA).

After you ensure that responding personnel have adequate safety equipment to manage the rescue scene, consider patient safety. Many considerations for rescuer safety also apply to patients. Additionally, patient safety equipment should at least include construction-type hard hats, eye goggles, hearing and respiratory protection, protective blankets, and protective shielding. You will need these to protect your patient during rescue operations (Figure 7-13). Patient safety also

Safe, orderly, and controlled incident management is essential for everyone's safety.

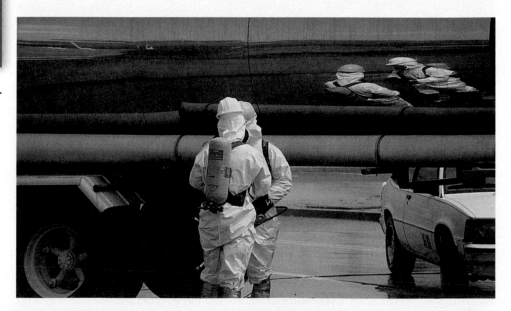

FIGURE 7-12 Hazardous materials responses require special training and equipment.

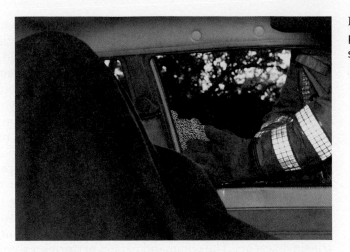

FIGURE 7-13 Protect the patient from hazards at the scene.

includes simple measures like removing them from unstable environments, such as temperature extremes, smoky rooms, or hostile crowds. For example, the simplest way to begin managing a patient suffering from hypothermia is to move him into a warm environment.

Safe, orderly, and controlled incident management is essential for everyone's safety. Call for specialty personnel to stabilize wreckage or turn off electrical power. Make sure someone routes traffic safely around a vehicle collision. Control bystanders and spot potential human hazards. Be certain that a hostile crowd or someone who assaulted your patient is not ready to attack you. Scenes involving toxic exposures, environmental hazards, and violent patients are especially worrisome. When possible, have law enforcement personnel establish a tape line to cordon off the hazard zone to protect bystanders who do not realize the potential dangers of watching operations (Figure 7-14).

LOCATION OF ALL PATIENTS

Scene assessment also includes a search of the area to locate all of the patients. Ask yourself if other persons could be involved in the accident or affected by the medical problem. Determine where you are most likely to find the most seriously affected patients and how many patients will need transport. The mechanism of injury or the nature of the illness can help you determine the number of patients. For example, a two-car collision must include at least two drivers. Clues, such as diaper bags, child auto seats, toys, colouring books, clothing, or twin spider-web impact

Search the area to locate all patients.

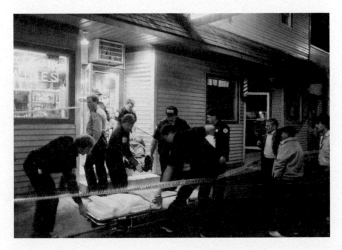

FIGURE 7-14 Tape lines help keep bystanders out of hazardous scenes.

marks in the windshield, should lead you to search for more patients, especially children, than those who may be readily apparent. Some medical situations, such as carbon monoxide poisoning, can affect an entire household. A hazardous liquid spill in the chemistry lab can affect students and staff in an entire wing of a school.

If you find more patients than you can safely and effectively manage, call for assistance early. If possible, you should do this before you make contact with any patients because you are less likely to call for help once you become involved with patient care. Often, as you proceed into a scene, more patients become apparent. It is wise to overestimate when asking for help at the scene.

Initiate the mass-casualty plan according to your local protocols (Figure 7-15). Again, try not to become involved in patient care, for two important functions must occur in the initial stages of any mass-casualty incident—command and triage. If you and your partner find yourselves in a situation that overwhelms your resources, one of you should establish command, while the other begins triaging patients. The command person performs a scene assessment, determines the needs of the incident, makes a radio report requesting the necessary additional help, and directs oncoming crews to their duties (Figure 7-16). The triage person performs a triage exam on every patient and prioritizes them for immediate or delayed transport (Figure 7-17). He may perform simple life-saving procedures, such as opening the airway or controlling bleeding, but as a rule, the triage person should not stop to provide intensive care for any one patient.

> *Call for assistance early; it is wise to overestimate when asking for help.*

MECHANISM OF INJURY

The **mechanism of injury** is the combined strength, direction, and nature of forces that injured your patient. It is usually apparent through careful evaluation of the trauma scene and can help you anticipate both the location and the seriousness of injuries. Identify the forces involved, the direction from which they came, and the bodily locations affected (Figure 7-18). For example, in a fall injury, how high was the patient, what did he land on, and what part of his body hit first? If your patient jumped from a height and landed on his feet, expect lower extremity, pelvic, and lumbar spine injuries.

In an automobile collision, the mechanism of injury is the process by which forces are exchanged between the automobile and what it struck, between your patient and the automobile's interior, and among the various tissues and organs as they collide with one another within the patient. Close inspection of the automobile and the forces, or various collisions, can lead to an **index of suspicion** (a prediction of injuries based on the mechanism of injury) for possible injuries. What does the car look like? If the windshield is cracked, expect head and neck

* **mechanism of injury** combined strength, direction, and nature of forces that injured your patient.

* **index of suspicion** your anticipation of possible injuries based upon your analysis of the event.

FIGURE 7-15 Follow local protocols when you respond to a mass-casualty incident.

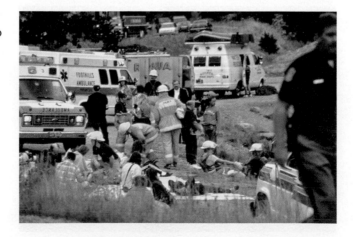

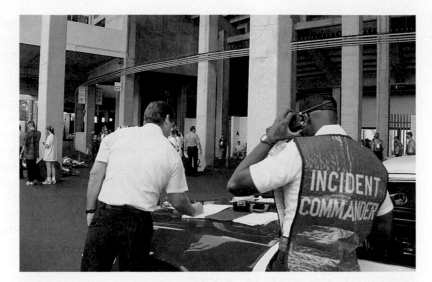

FIGURE 7-16 The incident commander directs the response and coordinates resources at a multiple-casualty incident.

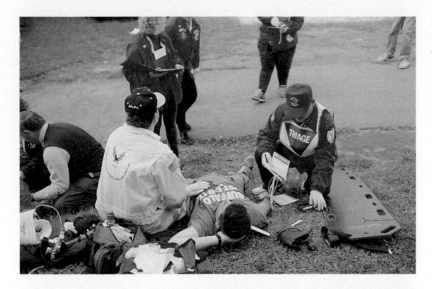

FIGURE 7-17 The triage person examines and prioritizes patients.

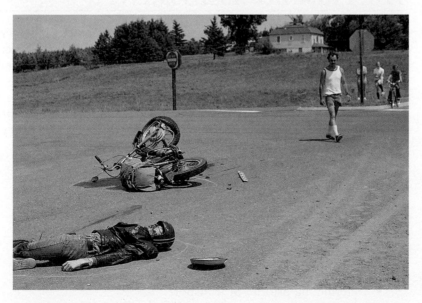

FIGURE 7-18 With trauma, try to determine the mechanism of injury during scene assessment.

injuries. If the steering wheel is bent, expect chest and abdominal injuries. With a major intrusion into the passenger compartment, expect major trauma.

Expect a pedestrian struck by a car to have fractures of the lower extremities. If the auto was moving at 30 km/h, expect less severe fractures than if it were moving at 90 km/h. Internal injuries are also less likely at lower speeds than at higher speeds. By evaluating the strength and nature of impact, you can anticipate which organs are injured and the degree of their damage.

For a gunshot patient, determine the type of gun used, the range of the shot, and whether an exit wound exists. This information will enable you to estimate the damage along the bullet's path and to formulate an index of suspicion for your patient's possible injuries. Expect the internal injuries from serious blunt trauma to be more extensive and severe than those you see externally. Often, the mechanism of injury is the only clue to the possibility of serious internal injury. Chapters 17 and 18 on blunt and penetrating traumas describe the mechanisms of these injuries in depth.

NATURE OF THE ILLNESS

Determine the nature of the illness from bystanders, family members, or your patient. If he is alert and oriented, he is usually the best source of information about his problem. If he is unresponsive, disoriented, or otherwise unable to provide information, rely on family members, bystanders, or visual cues for this information.

The scene can give additional clues to your patient's condition. How is he positioned? Does he sit straight upright gasping to breathe? Are pill bottles or drug paraphernalia nearby? Is there medical-care equipment, such as an oxygen tank, a nebulizer, or a glucometer, in the room? For example, if you respond to a "difficulty breathing" call and your patient is using his nebulizer when you arrive, suspect a history of pulmonary disease, such as asthma, emphysema, or chronic bronchitis. If your patient is an agitated 17-year-old with a rapid pulse and you notice crack cocaine ampules on the floor, suspect a substance abuse problem.

Sometimes, the nature of the illness is not readily apparent. Your patient with severe difficulty breathing, for instance, may be suffering from respiratory disease, a cardiac problem, an allergic reaction, or a toxic exposure. Remember that the nature of your patient's illness may be very different from the chief complaint.

THE PRIMARY ASSESSMENT

The **primary assessment** exemplifies the basis of all prehospital emergency medical care. Its goal is to identify and correct immediately life-threatening patient conditions of the <u>a</u>irway, <u>b</u>reathing, or <u>c</u>irculation (ABCs). If you find these conditions during this part of your assessment, treat them at once. For example, open a closed airway, provide ventilation, or control hemorrhage before moving on. Immediately following the primary assessment, decide priority regarding immediate transport or further on-scene assessment and care. The primary assessment consists of the following steps:

- Forming a general impression
- Stabilizing the cervical spine as needed
- Assessing a baseline mental status
- Assessing the airway
- Assessing breathing
- Assessing circulation
- Determining priority or transport

Often, the mechanism of injury is the only clue to the possibility of serious internal injury.

Remember that the nature of your patient's illness may be very different from the chief complaint.

* primary assessment prehospital process designed to identify and correct life-threatening airway, breathing, and circulation problems.

Content Review

STEPS OF PRIMARY ASSESSMENT

1. Form general impression.
2. Stabilize cervical spine as needed.
3. Assess baseline level of response.
4. Assess airway.
5. Assess breathing.
6. Assess circulation.
7. Assign priority.

The primary assessment should take less than one minute unless you have to intervene with life-saving measures. Perform the primary assessment as part of your ongoing assessment throughout the patient contact, especially after any major intervention or whenever your patient's condition changes.

FORMING A GENERAL IMPRESSION

The **general impression** is your initial, intuitive evaluation of your patient. It will help you determine his general clinical status (stable versus unstable) and priority for immediate transport. Base your first impression on the information you gather from the environment, the mechanism of injury, the nature of the illness, the chief complaint, the initial presentation of the patient, and your instincts.

Your patient's age and gender often influence your index of suspicion. Very old and very young patients are more apt to have severe complications from injury or illness. For example, age is a factor in burn mortality, along with degree and body percentage. A 25-year-old patient with third-degree burns over 50 percent of his body will have a 75 percent chance of mortality. A 45-year-old patient with the same burns will have a 95 percent chance of mortality. Suspect a female of child-bearing age with lower abdominal pain and vaginal bleeding to have a life-threatening gynecological emergency known as ruptured ectopic pregnancy.

Determine whether your patient's problem results from trauma or from a medical problem. Sometimes, this will not be readily apparent. For example, did your patient slip and fall or get dizzy and fall? Note your patient's face and posture, and decide whether rapid intervention or a more deliberate approach is warranted. With experience you will be able to recognize even the most subtle clues of a patient in critical condition. Generally, the more serious the condition, the quieter your patient will be. Look at, listen to, and smell the environment. Gather as many clues as possible as you enter the scene. Qualify the patient's level of distress: none, mild, moderate, or severe.

Take the necessary body substance isolation precautions with every patient. Then, if your patient is alert, identify yourself and begin to establish a rapport. For example, "Hello, I'm Jen Stevens, a paramedic with the ambulance service. I'm here to help you." This establishes your level of training, authority, and reason for being at your patient's side. It also allows your patient to refuse care. As discussed in Chapter 2 on medical-legal aspects of advanced prehospital care, you cannot provide care without either implied or informed consent.

Reassure your patient. Listen and do not trivialize his complaints. Frequently, we forget how significant an injury or illness, even a minor one, seems to a patient. With your experience, the problem may seem small, but for your patient it is a real concern. The ill or injured patient may worry about the long-term consequences for work, childcare, and finances. Understand these fears and support your patient psychologically as well as physiologically.

If the mechanism of injury is significant or if your patient is unresponsive and you cannot rule out a cervical-spine injury, have your partner manually stabilize your patient's head and neck (Figure 7-19a). Do this before establishing his mental status and continue manual stabilization until you fully immobilize him to a long spine board. If your patient is awake, explain what you are doing and ask him not to move his neck. You do not want him to turn his head when you try to assess mental status. Ask your partner to maintain your patient's head in a neutral position as you begin your assessment. If your patient is a small child, place a small towel or pad beneath the shoulders to maintain proper alignment of the cervical spine (Figure 7-19b). This will compensate for the large occiput of the child's head, which normally would flex the neck if the child was placed on a flat surface.

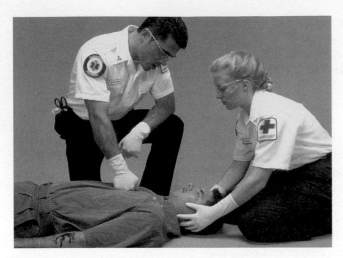

FIGURE 7-19a Manually stabilize the head and neck on first patient contact.

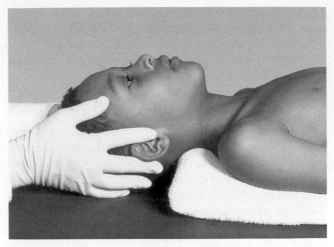

FIGURE 7-19b Place a folded towel under your young patient's shoulders to keep the airway aligned.

MENTAL STATUS

Your assessment of baseline mental status is crucial for all patients. For example, when you deliver your head injury patient to the emergency department, the neurosurgeon will want a chronological report of your patient's mental status from the time you arrived on the scene. This vital information helps the surgical team diagnose a deteriorating brain injury. If the patient was alert and oriented when you arrived, then became sleepy en route, and within 30 minutes was responsive only to deep pain stimuli, the suspicion for epidural hematoma is high. Rapid surgical intervention can save lives in most cases if the diagnosis is made quickly. Your baseline mental status documentation is critical to these patients' emergency care. Establishing a baseline mental status is also crucial in assessing the variety of medical situations that cause altered levels of response. Drug overdoses, poisonings, diabetic emergencies, sepsis, hypoxia, and hypovolemia are just a few of the many conditions that result in altered mentation. For the stroke patient, identifying the time of the symptoms' onset is critical for the emergency physician to consider administering clot-dissolving drugs within the three-hour window of opportunity. This is possible only with your accurate assessment of your patient's change in mental status.

To record your patient's mental status, use the acronym *AVPU*. Your patient is **a**lert, responds to **v**erbal stimuli, responds only to **p**ainful stimuli, or is **u**nresponsive. Perform this exam by starting with verbal and then moving to painful stimuli only if he fails to respond to your verbal cues.

Alert An alert patient is awake, as evidenced by open eyes. He may be oriented to person (who he is), place (where he is), and time (day, month, and year) and give organized, coherent answers to your questions. He also may be disoriented and confused. For example, the patient with a suspected concussion will often present as dazed and confused. The hypoxic or hypoglycemic patient may present as combative. The shock patient may be restless and anxious. If his eyes are open and he appears awake, he is categorized as alert. Children's responses to your questions will vary with their age-related physical and emotional development. Infants and young children usually will be curious but cautious when a stranger approaches. Their level of response may not indicate the gravity of their conditions. In fact, the quiet child is usually the seriously injured or ill child.

Verbal If your patient appears to be sleeping but responds when you talk to him, he is responsive to verbal stimuli. This patient can respond by speaking, opening his eyes, moaning, or just moving. Note the level of his verbal response. Does he speak clearly, mumble inappropriate words, or make incomprehensible sounds? Children may respond to your verbal commands by turning their heads or stopping activity. For infants, you may have to shout to elicit a response.

Pain If your child or adult patient does not respond to verbal stimuli, try to elicit a response with painful stimuli. Pinch his fingernails or rub your knuckles on the sternum, and watch for a response. Again, he may respond by waking up, speaking, moaning, opening his eyes, or moving. Note the type of motor response to the painful stimuli. Is his response purposeful or nonpurposeful? If your patient tries to move your hand away or to move away from the pain, it is purposeful. **Decorticate** (arms flexed, legs extended) or **decerebrate** (arms and legs extended) posturing is nonpurposeful and suggests a serious brain injury. For the infant, flick the soles of the feet and expect crying as the appropriate response.

 decorticate arms flexed, legs extended.

✻ decerebrate arms and legs extended.

Unresponsive The unresponsive patient is comatose and fails to respond to any painful stimulus. The AVPU scale describes your patient's general mental status. Avoid using terms like *semi-conscious, lethargic,* or *stuporous,* since they are broadly interpreted and you have not had a chance to conduct a comprehensive neurological exam at this point. Your patient's response to stimulation will tell you a great deal about his condition. Any alteration or deterioration in mental status may indicate an emergent or already serious problem. A patient with an impaired mental status may have lost, or be in danger of losing, the ability to protect his airway. Take immediate steps to protect your patient's airway by proper positioning, use of airway adjuncts, or intubation as appropriate. Provide oxygen to any patient with diminished mental status and seek out its cause.

Any alteration in mental status may indicate an emergent or already serious problem.

AIRWAY ASSESSMENT

If your patient is responsive and can speak clearly, you can assume that his airway is patent. If your patient is unconscious, however, his airway may be obstructed. The supine unconscious patient's tongue often obstructs his upper airway. Because the mandible, tongue, and epiglottis are all connected, gravity allows these structures to block your patient's upper airway as his facial muscles relax.

You can open your patient's airway with one of two simple manual manoeuvres, the jaw thrust and the head-tilt/chin-lift. For the trauma patient with a suspected cervical-spine injury or any patient for whom you cannot rule out a cervical-spine injury, use the jaw thrust to avoid movement of the cervical spine. Place your thumbs on your patient's cheeks and lift up on the angle of the jaw with your fingers. For all other patients, use the head-tilt/chin-lift. Place one hand on your patient's forehead and lift up under the chin with the fingers of your other hand. To open the airways of infants and young children, apply a gentle and conservative extension of the head and neck. These patients' upper airway structures are very flexible and are easily kinked when their necks are flexed or hyperextended. You must constantly readjust their airways to maximize patency.

You must constantly adjust infants' and young children's airways to maximize patency.

To assess your patient's airway, look for the chest to rise while you listen and feel for air movement. Look for fluid or obvious obstructions in the patient's mouth. If the airway is clear, you should hear quiet air flow and feel free air movement. A noisy airway is a partially obstructed airway. Snoring occurs when the tongue or epiglottis partially blocks the upper airway. In this case, reposition the head and neck and reevaluate. Gurgling indicates that fluid, such as blood, secretions, or gastric contents, is blocking the upper airway. Gently open and examine the mouth for foreign bodies you can remove easily and quickly. Use aggressive suctioning to remove blood, vomitus, secretions, and other fluids (Figure 7-20).

FIGURE 7-20 Suction fluids
from your patient's airway.

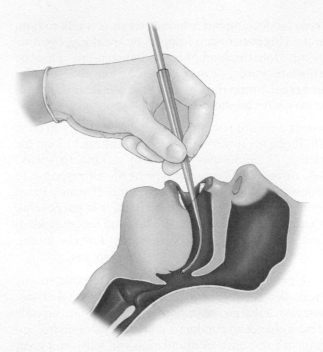

*Stridor signals a potentially
life-threatening airway
obstruction.*

The high-pitched inspiratory screech of stridor is caused by a life-threatening
upper airway obstruction that may be due to a foreign body, severe swelling, allergic reaction, or infection. If you suspect a foreign body obstruction and your
patient exhibits poor air movement, a weak cough, or a diminishing mental status, immediately deliver abdominal thrusts (Heimlich manoeuvre) to dislodge the
object. If your patient is less than one year old, use back blows and chest thrusts
instead of abdominal thrusts. If these manoeuvres are ineffective, remove the object under direct laryngoscopy with Magill forceps.

Other causes of stridor require vastly different approaches. Upper respiratory infections, such as croup or epiglottitis, call for blow-by oxygen and a quiet
ride to the hospital; respiratory burns demand rapid endotracheal intubation;
and anaphylaxis necessitates vasoconstrictor medications. Since these vastly different management techniques are potentially life threatening when applied inappropriately, your correct field diagnosis is critical. If your patient presents with
stridor, take time to evaluate the history and clinical signs and symptoms for foreign body obstruction (sudden onset while eating), epiglottitis (fever, illness,
drooling, inability to swallow), respiratory burns (history of facial burns, hoarseness), and anaphylaxis (hives, history of allergies).

The softer, expiratory whistle of wheezing is caused by constricted bronchioles, the smaller, lower airways. You will hear it in such cases as asthma, bronchitis, emphysema, or other causes of bronchospasm. Bronchiolitis, a lower respiratory infection, often causes these sounds in infants and young children.
Wheezing patients require a bronchodilator medication to dilate the bronchioles
and reduce airway resistance.

If your patient is not moving air, he is in respiratory arrest. Immediately provide
ventilation with a bag-valve mask. Ventilate adult patients at a minimum of 12
breaths per minute and all children at a minimum of 20 breaths per minute. If you
cannot ventilate the lungs, reposition the head and neck and try again. If there is still
no air movement, assume a complete obstruction and begin measures to correct it.

*Once you have cleared the
airway, keeping it open may
require constant attention.*

Once you have cleared the airway, keeping it open may require constant attention. In these cases, insert a basic airway adjunct to help keep the tongue from
blocking the upper airway. If your patient is unconscious and lacks a gag reflex, insert an oropharyngeal airway. If he has a gag reflex or significant orofacial trauma,

insert a nasopharyngeal airway. Be cautious using a nasopharyngeal airway if you suspect a basilar skull fracture. If your patient has no gag reflex and cannot protect his airway, you will need to use advanced techniques to maintain airway patency. These include endotracheal intubation, multilumen airways, such as the Pharyngotracheal Lumen (PL) airway and the Esophageal Tracheal CombiTube (ETC), and transtracheal techniques, such as needle or surgical cricothyrostomy. The multilumen airways are not appropriate for use in children. All these devices for maintaining upper airway patency are described in detail in Chapter 27 on airway management and ventilation. If your patient has an airway problem or an altered mental status, administer high-concentration oxygen by nonrebreather mask.

BREATHING ASSESSMENT

Assess your patient for the presence and adequacey of breathing. Immediately note any signs of inadequate breathing:

- Altered mental status, confusion, apprehension, or agitation
- Shortness of breath while speaking
- Retractions (supraclavicular, suprasternal, intercostal)
- Asymmetric chest wall movement
- Accessory muscle use (neck, abdominal)
- Cyanosis
- Audible sounds
- Abnormally rapid, slow, or shallow breathing
- Nasal flaring

Content Review

SIGNS OF INADEQUATE BREATHING
Altered mental status
Shortness of breath
Retractions
Asymmetric chest wall movement
Accessory muscle use
Cyanosis
Audible sounds
Abnormal rate or pattern
Nasal flaring

Assess the approximate respiratory rate and quality. Normal respiratory rates vary according to your patient's age. Abnormally fast or slow rates (Table 7-1) actually decrease the amount of air that reaches the alveoli for gas exchange. For patients with abnormally fast or slow respiratory rates and decreased tidal volumes, provide positive pressure ventilation with, for example, a bag-valve mask and supplemental oxygen, to ensure full lung expansion and maximum oxygenation. Note the respiratory pattern. Rapid (tachypneic), deep (hyperpneic) respirations are a compensatory mechanism and suggest the body is attempting to rid itself of excess acids. They may indicate a diabetic problem, severe acidosis, or head injury. They also may result from hyperventilation syndrome or from simple exertion. Kussmaul's respirations (deep, rapid breathing) accompanied by a fruity breath odour are a classic sign of a patient in a diabetic coma. In either case, always ensure an adequate inspiratory volume and administer high-flow oxygen. Cheyne-Stokes respirations, a series of increasing and decreasing breaths

Table 7-1 RESPIRATORY RATES

Age	Low Rate	High Rate
Newborn	30	60
Infant (< 1 year)	30	60
Toddler (1–2 years)	24	40
Preschooler (3–5 years)	22	34
School age (6–12 years)	18	30
Adolescent (13–18 years)	12	26
Adult (> 18 years)	12	20

followed by a period of apnea, most likely result from a brain stem injury or increasing intracranial pressure. Biot's respirations, identified by short, gasping, irregular breaths, may signify severe brain injury. Again, ensure adequate inspiratory volume and provide ventilation with supplemental oxygen as needed.

If your trauma patient's breathing is inadequate, immediately conduct a rapid trauma assessment of the neck and chest before moving on to circulation. Identify and correct any life-threatening conditions, such as a sucking chest wound, a flail chest, or a tension pneumothorax. If your patient exhibits adequate breathing, move directly to circulation.

CIRCULATION ASSESSMENT

The **circulation assessment** consists of evaluating the pulse and skin and controlling hemorrhage. Go directly to the wrist and feel for a radial pulse (Procedure 7-1a). Its presence suggests a systolic blood pressure of at least 90 mmHg. If the radial pulse is absent, check for a carotid pulse (Procedure 7-1b). The carotid pulse's presence suggests a systolic blood pressure of at least 60 mmHg. In the infant, palpate the brachial pulse (Procedure 7-1c), or if necessary, auscultate the apical pulse. If the pulse is absent in the adult patient, begin chest compressions immediately, evaluate the cardiac rhythm, and provide prompt defibrillation as needed. In the child, immediately begin cardiopulmonary resuscitation (CPR).

Assess your patient's pulse for rate and quality as detailed in Chapter 6. The normal heart rate varies with your patient's age (Table 7-2). Very fast rates (tachycardia) and very slow rates (bradycardia) may indicate a life-threatening cardiac dysrhythmia. Note the quality of the pulse. The normal pulse should be regular and strong. An irregular pulse may indicate a cardiac dysrhythmia requiring advanced cardiac life support procedures. In head injury, heat stroke, or hypertension, you will often find a strong, bounding pulse. A weak, thready pulse usually indicates poor perfusion due to fluid loss, pump failure, or massive vasodilation.

Stop your patient's bleeding if you haven't already done so (Procedure 7-1d). Major bleeding usually originates with trauma, but it also can result from a medical emergency. For example, vaginal bleeding, rectal bleeding, and even a nosebleed associated with hypertension can result in life-threatening blood loss. For external bleeding, employ any appropriate measures for hemorrhage control, including direct pressure and elevation, pressure dressings, pressure points, and the last-resort tourniquet. Internal bleeding is not easily controlled in the prehospital setting and demands initiating transport as soon as possible.

Assess the skin for temperature, moisture, and colour (Procedure 7-1e). Peripheral vasoconstriction decreases peripheral perfusion to the skin early in shock. The skin may appear mottled (blotchy), cyanotic (bluish), pale, or ashen. It may also feel cool and moist (clammy). This often indicates that warm, circulating blood has been shunted away from the skin to the core of the body to maintain perfusion of vital organs. If you find any of these signs, suspect conditions related to or caused by poor perfusion. In infants and young children, capillary refill is a reliable indicator of circulatory function (Procedure 7-1f). In adults, smoking, medications, cold weather, or chronic conditions of the elderly may affect capillary refill, and so you should always also consider the other indicators of circulatory function.

If your patient shows signs of circulatory compromise, place the patient supine and consider elevating the legs to support venous return to the vital organs (Procedure 7-1g) and keep him warm. Chapter 19 on hemorrhage and shock explains this procedure fully. Consider starting large-bore intravenous lines en route to the hospital and infusing fluids to augment your patient's circulating blood volume (Procedure 7-1h). Also, consider using vasoconstricting drugs and antidysrhythmic medications for other specific causes of poor perfusion.

If your patient's breathing is inadequate, immediately conduct a rapid trauma assessment of the neck and chest and provide positive pressure ventilation with supplemental oxygen.

* **circulation assessment** evaluating the pulse and skin and controlling hemorrhage.

Internal bleeding is not easily controlled in the prehospital setting and demands initiating transport as soon as possible.

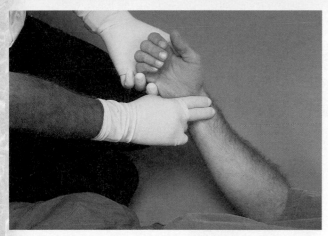

7-1a   To assess an adult's circulation, feel for a radial pulse.

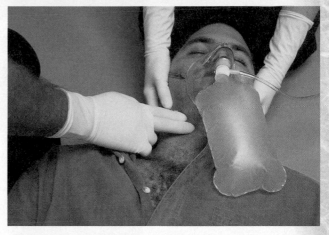

7-1b   If you cannot feel a radial pulse, palpate for a carotid pulse.

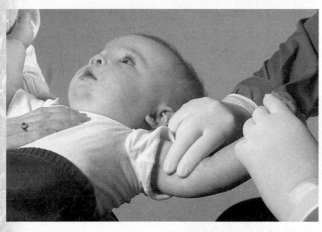

7-1c   To assess an infant's circulation, palpate the brachial pulse.

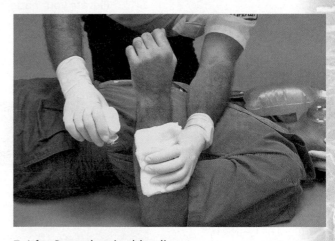

7-1d   Control major bleeding.

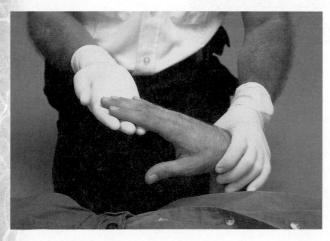

7-1e   Assess the skin.

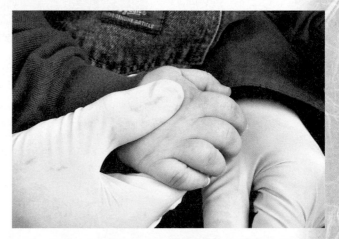

7-1f   Capillary refill time provides important information about the circulatory status of infants and young children.

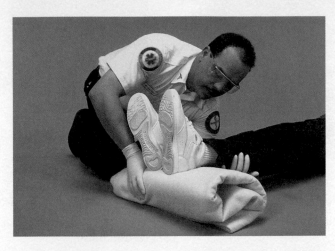

7-1g   Elevate your patient's feet if you suspect circulatory compromise.

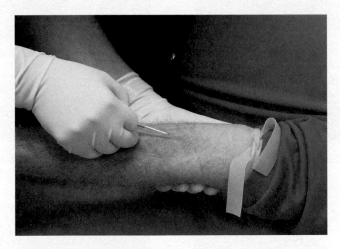

7-1h   En route to the hospital, establish an IV.

Table 7-2	NORMAL PULSE RATE RANGES	
Age	Low Rate	High Rate
Newborn	100	180
Infant (< 1 year)	100	160
Toddler (1–2 years)	80	110
Preschooler (3–5 years)	70	110
School age (6–12 years)	65	110
Adolescent (13–18 years)	60	90
Adult (> 18 years)	60	100

PRIORITY DETERMINATION

Once you have conducted a primary assessment, determine your patient's priority. If the primary assessment suggests a serious illness or injury, conduct a rapid head-to-toe assessment to identify other life threats and transport your patient immediately to the nearest appropriate facility that can deliver definitive care (Figure 7-21). Do not delay transport for detailed assessments and procedures that you can provide en route to the hospital. Consider top priority and rapid transport for the following patients:

Do not delay transport for detailed assessments and procedures that you can provide en route to the hospital.

- Patients with a poor general impression
  - Apnea
  - Pulselessness
  - Obvious severe distress
- Patients with altered mental status
- Patients with unresolved airway compromise
  - Obstructive sounds, such as gurgling, snoring, or stridor
  - Vomitus, secretions, blood, or foreign bodies obstructing the airway
  - Inability to protect the airway (absence of a gag reflex)

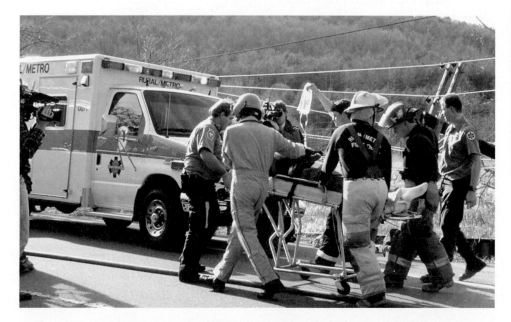

FIGURE 7-21 Expedite transport for a high-priority patient and continue assessment and care en route.

Content Review

TYPES OF PATIENTS

Trauma patient with
  significant mechanism
  of injury
Trauma patient with
  isolated injury
Responsive medical patient
Unresponsive medical patient

- Patients with abnormal breathing
  - Rates less or greater than normal for age
  - Absent or diminished air movement and breath sounds
  - Retractions
  - Accessory muscle use
- Patients with poor circulation
  - Weak or absent peripheral pulses
  - Pulse rates less or greater than normal for age
  - Irregular pulse
  - Pale, cool, diaphoretic skin
  - Uncontrolled bleeding
- Obvious serious or multiple injuries
- Mechanism of injury suspicious of shock

In these cases, expedite transport and initiate advanced life support procedures en route. For unstable trauma patients, use minimum immobilization and transport, with further assessment and procedures en route. On the way to the hospital, you can conduct a detailed secondary assessment and provide additional care as time allows. If your patient is stable, you may choose to conduct a **focused and problem-oriented secondary assessment** at the scene. You may then complete a more detailed assessment either at the scene or during transport if necessary.

The primary assessment is the crucial first step in providing life-saving measures to seriously ill or injured patients. It should take you less than one minute to perform, and yet it will provide you with enough vital information to confirm your priority determination.

✱ focused and problem-oriented secondary assessment a process based on primary assessment and chief complaint.

THE SECONDARY ASSESSMENT

The secondary assessment (or secondary survey) consists of the focused history, vital signs, and physical assessment. It is a problem-oriented process based on your primary assessment and your patient's chief complaint. How you conduct the secondry assessment will depend on which of four general categories your patient's initial presentation falls under:

- Trauma patient with a significant mechanism of injury or altered mental status
- Trauma patient with an isolated injury
- Responsive medical patient
- Unresponsive medical patient

Each type of patient requires a different approach.

Content Review

ORDER OF FOCUSED
HISTORY AND SECONDARY
ASSESSMENT FOR MAJOR
TRAUMA PATIENTS

Primary assessment
Rapid trauma assessment
Packaging
Rapid transport and
  ongoing assessment

THE MAJOR TRAUMA PATIENT

The **major trauma patient** is one who has sustained a significant mechanism of injury or has an altered mental status from the incident. For serious trauma patients, you will conduct a primary assessment followed by a rapid trauma assessment, package your patient, provide rapid transport to the emergency department, and perform a ongoing assessment en route, in that order. If time allows, you can also perform a secondary assessment.

✱ major trauma patient person who has suffered significant mechanism of injury.

Mechanism of Injury

Begin the focused history and secondary assessment for major trauma patients by reconsidering the mechanism of injury (Figure 7-22). Although trauma poses a serious threat to life, its appearance often masks your patient's true condition. Extremity injuries, for example, are frequently obvious and grotesque, and yet they rarely cause death. Conversely, life-threatening problems, such as internal bleeding and rising intracranial pressure, often occur with only subtle signs and symptoms. Your assessment of trauma patients must look beyond obvious injuries to the mechanism of injury for evidence that suggests life-threatening situations. Certain mechanisms predictably cause serious internal injury:

- Ejection from a vehicle
- Fall from higher than 6 m
- Rollover of vehicle
- High-speed vehicle collision with resulting severe vehicle deformity
- Vehicle-pedestrian collision
- Motorcycle crash
- Penetration of the head, chest, or abdomen

Additional considerations for infants and children include the following:

- Fall from higher than 3 m
- Bicycle collision
- Medium-speed vehicle collision with resulting severe vehicle deformity

These mechanisms' presence suggests a high index of suspicion for serious injury. Quickly transport patients to a trauma centre when either the mechanism of injury or your patient's clinical presentation indicates a likelihood of internal injury.

Your assessment of trauma patients must look beyond obvious injuries to the mechanism of injury.

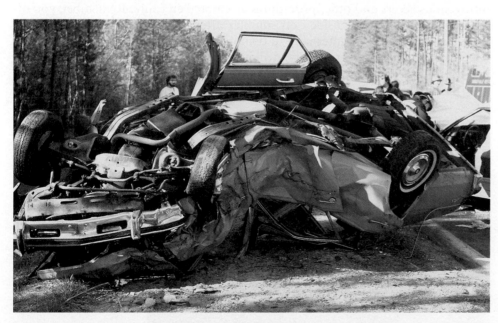

FIGURE 7-22 Evaluate the trauma scene to determine the mechanism of injury.

Other significant mechanisms of injury can result from seat belts, airbags, and child safety seats. Do not rule out serious injury just because your patient wore a seat belt. Seat belts can actually cause injuries, even when worn properly. Always ask your patient if he wore a seat belt and look for bruises across the chest or around the waist. If present, expect hidden internal injuries.

In general, airbags have been effective devices in preventing serious injury by protecting passengers from hitting the windshield, steering wheel, and dashboard. They deploy when the car hits another object. But they are not without complication. For example, they are designed to cushion the chests of large adults. If the passenger is a child or a short adult, the airbag will hit him in the face, causing injury. Also, airbags are designed to deflate automatically within seconds after inflation, which may allow passengers to be propelled into the steering wheel or dashboard. For this reason, they may not be effective without the seat belt. Always lift the deployed bag and inspect the steering wheel for deformity. If you discover a bent steering wheel, suspect serious internal injury (Figure 7-23).

A child safety seat, when used appropriately, also can save a life. But if the safety seat is not securely fastened to the car seat, it can come loose and be thrown when the collision occurs, causing severe head, neck, and body cavity trauma to its occupant. If the safety seat is used in the car's front seat, the child can suffer a serious injury when the airbag deploys.

If your primary assessment rules out any immediate life threat, examine the suspected area of trauma. Physical signs of trauma, such as abrasions or contusions, confirm your index of suspicion. If you do not identify any physical evidence, reexamine the mechanism of injury and evaluate your patient's vital signs. You will miss many serious injuries if your index of suspicion is too low.

Usually, you will distinguish between those patients who need on-the-scene stabilization and those who need rapid transport after your primary assessment and rapid trauma assessment. Whether to transport your patient immediately or to attempt more extensive on-the-scene assessment and care is among your most difficult decisions, but the care you provide will be more effective if you decide quickly. As a rule, patients who experience the mechanisms of injury listed earlier or who display serious clinical findings should be transported quickly with intravenous access and other procedures attempted en route. Remember, you often arrive at the patient's side only minutes after the accident. He may not yet have lost enough blood internally to demonstrate signs of shock or progressive head injury. If in doubt, transport to an appropriate medical facility without delay. It is always best to err on the side of caution.

FIGURE 7-23 A bent steering wheel signals potentially serious injuries.

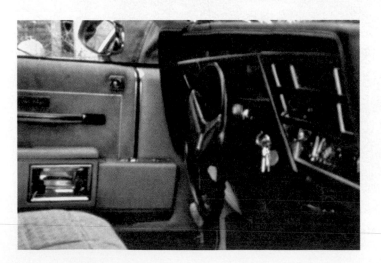

Rapid Trauma Assessment

After you finish your primary assessment, conduct a rapid trauma assessment to identify all other life-threatening conditions. Every trauma patient with a significant mechanism of injury, altered mental status, or multiple body-system trauma should receive a rapid trauma assessment. If your patient is responsive, ask about symptoms as you proceed with your exam. Do not, however, focus totally on the areas your patient identifies as the chief problem. A patient with multiple injuries usually complains about the most painful injury. Sometimes, this may not be the most serious problem. Assess your patient systematically and avoid the tunnel-vision invited by dispatch information, emergency medical responders' reports, and your patient's chief complaint.

Assume that any trauma patient has a spinal injury if he has injuries above the shoulders, has a significant mechanism of injury, or complains of weakness, numbness, or spinal pain. Maintain spinal immobilization throughout your rapid trauma assessment.

As you proceed through the assessment and discover additional information about your patient, reconsider your decision to transport. Things can change unexpectedly, especially with children. For example, your child patient who appeared stable suddenly deteriorates, requiring you to expedite transport to the closest appropriate facility. The hallmark of an experienced paramedic is the ability to improvise, adapt to new situations, and overcome obstacles that hinder good patient care.

The **rapid trauma assessment** is not a detailed secondary assessment but a fast, systematic assessment for other life-threatening injuries. Since you perform it before packaging your patient for transport, you must conduct it quickly. First, reassess your patient's mental status using the AVPU mnemonic and compare your findings with the baseline mental status from your primary assessment. Pay special attention to the head, neck, chest, abdomen, and pelvis. Injuries in these areas can occur with limited signs and symptoms, and yet they may rapidly lead to patient deterioration and death. When inspecting an area for injury, keep in mind that the discoloration of contusions will develop over time and may not be apparent at first. Remember, your major concern may not be the injury you see but the internal injuries beneath the superficial wounds. Palpate to identify other signs like tenderness, deformity, crepitation, symmetry, subcutaneous emphysema, or paradoxical movement. Compare muscle tone and tissue compliance from one side of the body or from one limb to another.

The mnemonic DCAP-BTLS may be helpful. The letters represent the eight common signs of injury for which you are looking during most of this assessment: <u>d</u>eformities, <u>c</u>ontusions, <u>a</u>brasions, <u>p</u>enetrations, <u>b</u>urns, <u>t</u>enderness, <u>l</u>acerations, and <u>s</u>welling.

Head Assess the head for DCAP-BTLS and crepitation (Procedure 7-2a). The scalp is extremely vascular and lacks the protective vasospasm mechanism that helps control bleeding. Thus, even the most minor lacerations tend to bleed profusely. Inspect the scalp for lacerations that are hidden under hair matted with clotted blood. Look for blood flowing into the hair, and examine your gloved fingers periodically for blood or other body fluids (Procedure 7-2b). If you detect uncontrolled bleeding from the scalp, apply a direct pressure dressing immediately. A simple scalp laceration can cause a life-threatening hemorrhage.

Quickly palpate the skull for open wounds, depressions, protrusions, lack of symmetry, and any unusual warmth. Use cupped hands and do not probe with your fingers. If you feel a depression, stop palpating it, as this risks pushing a broken piece of bone into the brain. If you find an impaled object, stabilize it in place with bulky dressings. If your patient presents with an altered mental status and any abnormality in the structure of the skull, consider this a serious emergency and expedite transport while you continue your assessment and treatment.

Avoid the tunnel vision invited by dispatch information, emergency medical responders' reports, and your patient's chief complaint.

✳ **rapid trauma assessment** quick check for signs of serious injury.

Content Review

DCAP-BTLS
Deformities
Contusion
Abrasions
Penetration
Burns
Tenderness
Lacerations
Swelling

**Immediately cover any neck
lacerations that may involve
the major blood vessels.**

✱ **semi-Fowler's position** sitting
up at 45 degrees.

✱ **subcutaneous emphysema**
crackling sensation caused by
air just underneath the skin.

Neck Inspect and palpate the neck for DCAP-BTLS and crepitation (Proce-dure 7-2c). Immediately cover any lacerations that may involve the major blood vessels, such as the carotid arteries and jugular veins, with an occlusive dressing. This is a high-pressure area, and your patient can suffer significant blood loss quickly. Because inspiration generates negative pressures in the chest, the jugular veins may draw in air. This can result in a massive air embolus that prevents the heart from pumping blood.

Examine the jugular veins for abnormal distention. In a patient lying supine without circulatory compromise, these veins should distend slightly. If they do not, your patient may be hypovolemic. In the **semi-Fowler's position** (sitting up at 45 degrees), the veins should not distend. Distention beyond 45 degrees is sig-nificant because something is inhibiting blood return to the chest. In the trauma patient, this may be the result of cardiac tamponade or tension pneumothorax.

Inspect and palpate the position of the trachea. It should lie midline and re-main fixed during the breathing cycle. Tugging to one side during inspiration suggests a pneumothorax on that side. Displacement to one side may indicate a tension pneumothorax on the opposite side as the entire mediastinum is pushed away from the injury.

Finally, inspect and palpate the neck for **subcutaneous emphysema,** the crackling sensation caused by air just underneath the skin. This condition is the result of air leaking from the respiratory tree into the tissues of the neck. It strongly indicates a serious neck or chest injury.

Now, palpate the posterior neck for evidence of spinal trauma (Procedure 7-2d). Gently feel the spinous processes and note any deformities, swelling, and ten-derness. If you feel a muscle spasm, consider it a reflex sign following injury somewhere along the spinal column. When a corroborating mechanism of injury is present, suspect a significant spinal injury requiring immobilization. At this point, you can apply a cervical spinal immobilization collar (CSIC). Have some-one maintain head and neck stabilization even after applying the collar until your patient is fully fastened to the long board.

Chest Look for signs of acute respiratory distress. If your patient has an upper airway obstruction, he may need to create tremendous negative pressures within his chest just to draw in air. To do so, he will use accessory muscles in his neck and chest to help lift the chest wall. These negative pressures may cause suprasternal, supraclavicular, and intercostal retractions. A patient with a lower airway obstruction may have difficulty moving air out. To do so, he may use his abdominal muscles to force the diaphragm upward and inward. He also may purse his lips during exhalation in an attempt to maintain a back pressure to keep the airways open. Infants and small children grunt to maintain this back pres-sure. Accessory muscle use always indicates a patient in respiratory distress due to a difficulty in moving air. Assist these patients with positive pressure ventila-tion and supplemental oxygen as needed.

Quickly inspect and then palpate the chest. Begin palpating at the clavicles and work down and around the rib cage, checking for stability. Palpate the clavicles over their entire length, bilaterally (Procedure 7-3a). These bones, which fracture more frequently than any other bone in the human body, are located directly over the subclavian artery and vein and the superior-most aspect of the lung. Their frac-ture and displacement may lacerate the vessels or puncture lung tissue, leading to hemothorax, pneumothorax, hypovolemia, or all three.

Be especially careful when palpating the ribs. Beneath each rib lie an artery, a vein, and a nerve that overaggressive palpation can easily damage. Classical soft-tissue injury signs may not be present because the ecchymotic coloration of bruising likely will not have had time to develop. Look for erythema caused by impact to the ribs. The first three ribs are well supported by muscles, ligaments, and tendons.

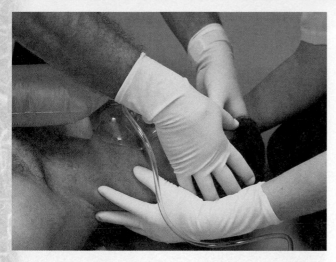

7-2a   The first step in the rapid trauma assessment is to palpate the head.

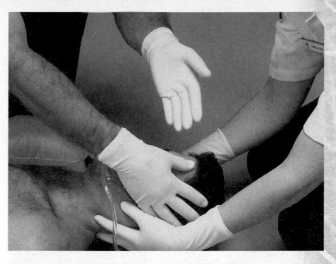

7-2b   Periodically examine your gloves for blood.

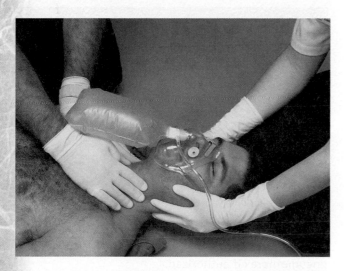

7-2c   Inspect and palpate the anterior neck. Pay particular attention to tracheal deviation and subcutaneous emphysema.

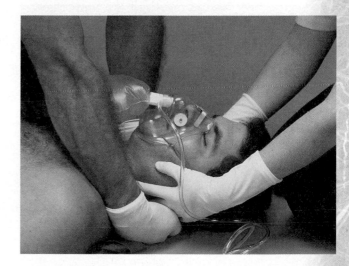

7-2d   Inspect and palpate the posterior neck. Note any tenderness, irregularity, or edema.

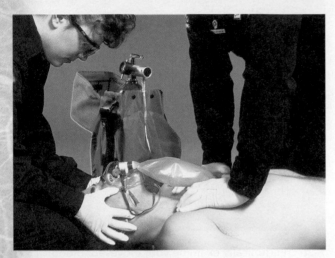

7-3a   Palpate the clavicles.

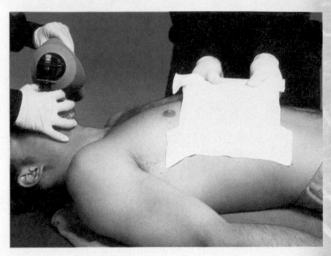

7-3b   Stabilize flail chest.

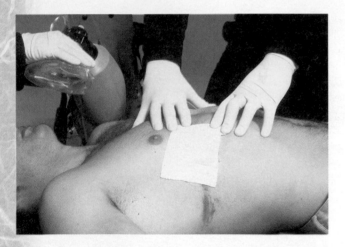

7-3c   Seal any sucking chest wound with tape on three sides.

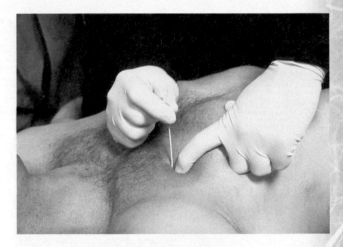

7-3d   Perform needle decompression to relieve tension pneumothorax if authorized.

Because of the energy required to fracture them, you should suspect major damage to the underlying organs, especially vascular structures, when they are broken.

If you notice the crackling of subcutaneous emphysema during chest palpation, suspect pneumothorax or a tracheobronchial tear. This condition results when air collects in the soft tissues. Subcutaneous air will normally flow from the upper chest to the neck and head. In some cases, it will drastically change your patient's facial features before your eyes.

Observe for equal, symmetrical, effortless chest rise. The chest should rise with inhalation and fall with exhalation. An abnormality in the chest wall may inhibit this process. For example, a patient with a rib fracture hesitates to expand his chest because it hurts. The fracture of two or more adjacent ribs in two or more places causes an unstable flail (floating) segment, which may be evidenced by paradoxical chest wall movement. Paradoxical movement may not appear early in a flail segment because the muscles surrounding the fractured ribs may contract spasmodically, securing the ribs in place. As the muscles fatigue and relax, the flail segment becomes obvious in the paradoxical movement. A flail chest greatly reduces air movement. The underlying lung contusion and subsequent decreased tidal volume limit the air available for gas exchange. To ensure enough air movement for adequate gas exchange, assist ventilation with a bag-valve mask and supplemental oxygen. If the flail segment is loose, stabilize it to the chest wall with a large pad and tape (Procedure 7-3b).

Inspect your patient's chest front and back for open wounds. The lungs expand because they adhere to the inner chest wall. This adherence is made possible by the presence of two thin membranes, the visceral pleura, which covers the lungs, and the parietal pleura, which covers the inner chest wall. A film of liquid between these two layers creates a negative-pressure bond that forces the lungs to expand with the chest wall. Any opening in this system can disrupt adherence and cause the lung to collapse. Since air follows the path of least resistance, it may enter the chest cavity through the hole instead of through the respiratory tract. Thus, you should seal any open wounds with an occlusive dressing at the end of exhalation. Tape the dressing on three sides only to create a "one-way valve" effect, allowing air to escape but not be drawn in (Procedure 7-3c). Remember to check carefully under the armpits and back for knife and small-calibre gunshot wounds. You can easily miss these because the elastic skin closes quickly over the wound and limits external bleeding.

Auscultate both lungs quickly at each midaxillary line for equal and adequate air movement. Unequal air movement may indicate the presence of a collapsed lung from a pneumothorax or hemothorax. Absent sounds on one side and diminished sounds on the other may suggest a life-threatening condition known as tension pneumothorax. This condition also presents with severe respiratory distress, accessory muscle use, retractions, tachycardia, hypotension, narrowing pulse pressure, and distended neck veins. Tracheal deviation may be a late sign of tension pneumothorax. If authorized, perform needle decompression immediately. Insert a large-bore IV catheter into the pleural space at the second intercostal space over the tip of the rib, midclavicular line, allowing the trapped air to escape and release the tension (Procedure 7-3d). Only through practice and repetition will you gain the confidence to recognize the difference between adequate and diminished lung sounds. Again, for patients with inadequate lung sounds, administer 100 percent oxygen and assist ventilation with a bag-valve mask as needed.

Abdomen Inspect and palpate the abdomen for DCAP-BTLS and crepitation. Note any areas of bruising and guarding. Exaggerated abdominal-wall motion to assist respiration may result from spinal injury, airway obstruction, or respiratory muscle failure. Solid organs, such as the kidneys, liver, and spleen, can bleed enough blood into the abdominal cavity to cause profound shock.

Avoid spending time needlessly trying to make a specific diagnosis during rapid trauma assessment of the abdomen.

Two characteristic areas for bruising are over the umbilicus (**Cullen's sign**) and over the flanks (**Grey-Turner's sign**). Both signs indicate intra-abdominal hemorrhage but usually will not occur until hours after the injury. Perform deep palpation over each quadrant and note any tenderness, rigidity, and guarding. Be careful, because deep palpation sometimes can aggravate the problem. Avoid spending time needlessly trying to make a specific diagnosis. You need only to recognize the possibility that an intra-abdominal hemorrhage exists and that your patient requires immediate transport to an appropriate medical facility for surgery.

Hollow organs, such as the stomach and intestines, when injured, spill their toxic contents into the abdomen, irritating the peritoneum, the inner abdominal lining. Testing for rebound tenderness will help you determine if your patient's peritoneum is irritated. Gently palpate an area, and release your hand quickly. If your patient experiences pain with this release, it is likely due to peritoneal irritation. If you suspect intra-abdominal hemorrhage, provide oxygen and expedite transport. Intra-abdominal hemorrhage can cause the abdomen to be rigid and distended. En route to the hospital, provide IV fluid resuscitation as needed.

Pelvis Examine the pelvis for DCAP-BTLS and crepitation. The importance of a stable pelvic ring cannot be overemphasized. A patient with a pelvic fracture or dislocation risks lacerating the iliac arteries and veins, major blood vessels running through that area. He can easily lose a significant amount of blood into the pelvic cavity.

Evaluate the pelvic ring at the iliac crests and symphysis pubis. With the palms of your hands, direct pressure medially and posteriorly (Procedure 7-4a and 7-4b). Then, press posteriorly on the symphysis pubis, being careful not to entrap the penis or cause injury to the urinary bladder. Any pain, instability, or crepitus suggests a pelvic fracture. Always immobilize the pelvis before transport to prevent movement and a possible circulatory catastrophe.

Do not spend time splinting an unstable patient's fractures on the scene.

Extremities Inspect and palpate all four extremities for DCAP-BTLS and crepitation (Procedure 7-4c and 7-4d). Splint fractures en route to the hospital if your patient is unstable. Do not spend time splinting fractures on the scene.

Before placing your patient on a backboard and immobilizing his spine, evaluate distal neurovascular function by checking for pulses, sensation, and the ability to move (Procedure 7-4e and 7-4f). If you cannot locate a pulse, determine the adequacy of perfusion by assessing the temperature, colour, and condition of the skin of the extremity. Assume vascular compromise if pulse is absent, the extremity is cool, or the skin is ashen or cyanotic. The inability to feel and move both legs indicates complete spinal cord disruption. Diminished sensation or diminished motor ability may indicate a partial disruption. Weakness or disability on only one side of the body suggests brain injury due to a stroke or head injury. Evaluate these functions again after spinal immobilization to make certain they have not changed. Report and record all extremity function tests. Check for Medic Alert tags, which will identify a medical condition that may complicate the injury (Figure 7-24).

Posterior Body Carefully maintain manual stabilization of the head and spine as you log-roll the patient onto his side. The back should be inspected for injury even if you do not suspect a spinal injury. Inspect and palpate the posterior trunk for DCAP-BTLS and crepitation (Figure 7-25). Particularly note any tenderness in the spinal area. Palpate the buttocks to rule out hemorrhage, contusion, or other injury. Though predominantly soft tissue, this area is a large mass and can conceal considerable internal blood loss. Next place the long spine board snugly against your patient's body and maintain alignment of the head and spine as you log-roll him into a supine position on the spine board. He is now ready to be secured to the spine board and transported.

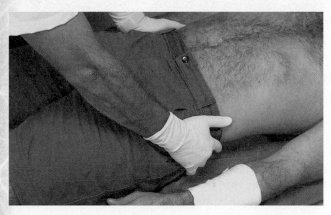

7-4a   Assess the integrity of the pelvis by gently pressing medially on the pelvic ring.

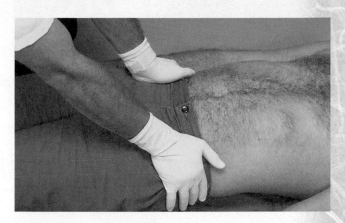

7-4b   Compress pelvis posteriorly.

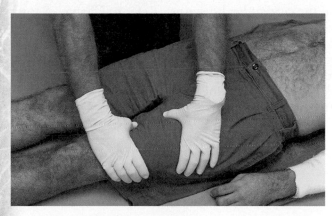

7-4c   Palpate the legs.

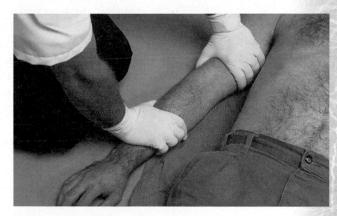

7-4d   Palpate the arms.

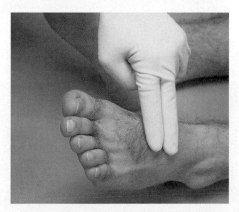

7-4e   Palpate the dorsalis pedis pulse to evaluate distal circulation in the leg.

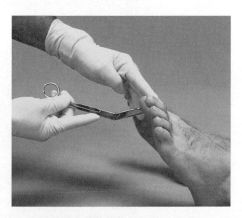

7-4f   Assess distal sensation and motor function.

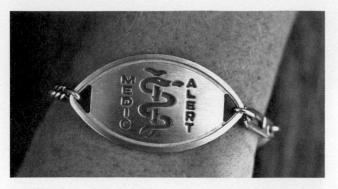
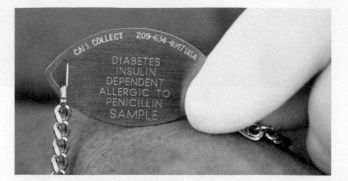

FIGURE 7-24   Medic Alert tags can give important information about the patient's condition and medical history.

Content Review

BASELINE VITAL SIGNS

Pulse rate and quality
Blood pressure
Respiration rate and quality
Skin condition

Vital Signs

Take a baseline set of vital signs, either at the scene or during transport, as your patient's condition and circumstances allow. These vital signs include pulse rate and quality, blood pressure, respiration rate and quality, and skin temperature and condition. Inspect the pupils for equality and reaction to light.

History

The history consists of four elements: the chief complaint, the history of present illness, the past history, and the current health status. (Refer to Chapter 5 for a detailed description of taking a history.) For major trauma cases, when time is critical, use an abbreviated format that forms the acronym SAMPLE: **s**ymptoms, **a**llergies, **m**edications, **p**ast medical history, **l**ast oral intake, and **e**vents preceding the incident. This handy mnemonic is especially useful for eliciting a quick history from your trauma patient. If your patient cannot provide this information, elicit it from family, friends, and bystanders.

Content Review

SAMPLE HISTORY

Symptoms
Allergies
Medications
Past medical history
Last oral intake
Events preceding the
    incident

THE ISOLATED-INJURY TRAUMA PATIENT

Some trauma patients sustain an isolated injury, such as a cut finger or sprained ankle. These patients have no significant mechanism of injury and show no signs

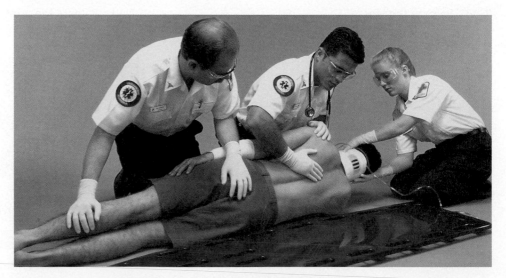

FIGURE 7-25   Inspect and palpate the posterior body.

of systemic involvement, such as poor peripheral perfusion, altered mental status, tachycardia, or breathing problems. They do not require an extensive history or comprehensive secondary assessment. To treat the trauma patient with an isolated injury, first ensure his hemodynamic status via the primary assessment. Then, conduct your focused history and secondary assessment on the specific isolated injury. Use the mnemonic DCAP-BTLS to evaluate the injured area and take a full set of vital signs. Then, if time allows, this is an excellent opportunity to use some of the advanced assessment techniques you learned in Chapter 6. After your assessment of the isolated injury, take a SAMPLE history. Remember that some trauma patients may complain of an isolated problem but actually have more significant injuries. Avoid tunnel vision and develop a low threshhold for suspecting other injuries based on the mechanism of injury and your patient's story.

Focus your minor-trauma assessment on the specific injury, and conduct a DCAP-BTLS assessment in that area.

IN THE FIELD

1. Your patient sustains a laceration to the palm of his hand from a breadknife. After you have controlled the bleeding and ensured no systemic involvement or major loss of blood, you decide to examine the hand further before bandaging it. You conduct a DCAP-BTLS assessment and note that distal neurovascular function is intact. Knowing that the flexor tendons all run through the palm of the hand, you examine each tendon's function through a full range of motion exam. You ask your patient to make a fist, then open his hand and extend all of his fingers. You note any abnormalities, pain, or limitations in the range of motion.

2. Your patient is a teenager who was punched in the eye during a minor altercation with a classmate. After determining that he had no loss of consciousness and that he is alert and oriented with stable vital signs, equal and reactive pupils, and no signs or symptoms of serious head injury, you may conduct a more detailed exam of the injured eye. First you inspect the external structures for discoloration, deformity, or swelling and find all three. You palpate the orbit of the eye for tenderness and deformity. You look for evidence of hyphema (blood in the anterior chamber), indicating severe blunt trauma.

THE RESPONSIVE MEDICAL PATIENT

Assessing the responsive patient with a medical emergency is entirely different from assessing the trauma patient for two reasons. First, the history takes precedence over the secondary assessment. This is because in the majority of cases, you will formulate your field diagnosis from your patient's story. The secondary assessment serves mostly to support your diagnostic impression. Second, your secondary assessment is aimed at identifying signs of medical complications, such as inflammation, infection, and edema, rather than signs of injury. The focused secondary assessment evaluates pertinent areas suggested by the history. Remember that you will begin treatment as you conduct your assessment. For example, while interviewing your patient who complains of chest pain, simultaneously take vital signs, administer oxygen, provide cardiac monitoring, administer ASA and nitro and start an IV if appropriate (Figure 7-26). The following focused history and secondary assessment pertains to the responsive medical patient. For a more detailed description of the information and techniques outlined here, refer to Chapters 5 and 6.

Listen to your patient; he will tell you what is wrong.

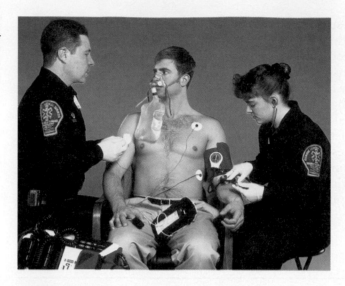

The History

Conscious, alert patients can usually tell you a great deal about their illness. Remember the old medical adage, "Listen to your patient; he will tell you what is wrong." Ask questions and then listen intently to your patient's answers. Since children may not be able to describe their illness and medical history clearly, look to their parents for this information. Elderly patients may pose several obstacles to the clear communication of medical information. They are more likely to be confused, to have poor short-term and long-term memories, and to have hearing, speech, or sight difficulties. Obtaining an accurate history from such patients requires patience, empathy, and outstanding communication skills.

The history consists of four elements: the chief complaint, the history of the present illness, the past history, and the current health status.

The Chief Complaint The **chief complaint** is the pain, discomfort, or dysfunction that caused your patient to request help. Ask your patient, "What seems to be the problem?"

The History of Present Illness Discover the circumstances surrounding the chief complaint, following the acronym OPQRST-ASPN:

Onset	What was your patient doing when the problem/pain began? Did emotional or environmental factors contribute to the problem?
Provocation/**P**alliation	What makes the problem/pain worse or better?
Quality	Can your patient describe the problem/pain?
Region/**R**adiation	Where is the problem/pain and does it radiate anywhere?
Severity	How bad is the problem/pain? Can your patient rate it on a scale of 10?
Time	When did the problem/pain begin? How long does the pain last?
Associated **S**ymptoms	Is your patient having any other problems?
Pertinent **N**egatives	Are any likely associated symptoms absent?

Content Review

ELEMENTS OF THE HISTORY FOR RESPONSIVE MEDICAL PATIENTS
Chief complaint
History of present illness
Past history
Current health status

✱ **chief complaint** the pain, discomfort, or dysfunction that caused your patient to request help.

Content Review

OPQRST-ASPN
Onset
Provocation/Palliation
Quality
Region, radiation
Severity
Time
Associated symptoms
Pertinent negatives

Past Medical History The past medical history may provide significant insights into your patient's chief complaint and your field diagnosis. It includes your patient's general state of health, childhood and adult diseases, psychiatric illnesses, accidents and injuries, and surgeries and hospitalizations. If your history taking reveals significant medical problems, investigate in more detail. Note when your patient first recognized the problem and how it affected him. How frequently did it happen, and what medical care did he seek? Was the treatment effective, or did the problem recur?

Current Health Status The current health status assembles all of the factors regarding your patient's medical condition. It tries to gather information that will complete the puzzle surrounding your patient's primary problem. The elements of the current health status include current medications, allergies, tobacco use, alcohol and substance abuse, diet, screening exams, immunizations, sleep patterns, exercise and leisure activities, environmental hazards, the use of safety measures, and any pertinent family or social history. Look for clues and correlations among the various sections of this part of the history. If your patient is critical and your time is limited, use the abbreviated SAMPLE format to elicit the history.

Patient Chart Another valuable source of information is your patient's medical chart. You may have access to this information through the patient's family physician or when transporting a patient between institutions. In particular, review admission forms and recent radiological or laboratory data.

Medical tests can be used for screening, to diagnose conditions, or to monitor the patient's response to treatment over time. Tests fall into several categories. Some tests, such as vital sign or ECG monitoring, check body functions. Others analyze body fluids or genetic material. And imaging technologies and endoscopies are used to view structures and organs within the body.

Many tests provide results and a comparative value. "Normal values" represent the range of results found in 95 percent of a healthy population. Note that these values may differ between women and men or with age.

Focused Secondary Assessment

Once you have obtained the history, begin a focused secondary assessment based on the information you have elicited from your patient. Let the diagnostic impression you formed during the history guide your examination. For example, if you suspect a myocardial infarction, examine areas pertinent to a patient having a heart attack—cardiac and respiratory systems, chest, neck, and peripheral perfusion. It would be pointless and impractical to test deep tendon reflexes, extraocular movements, or the elbow's range of motion. Use those exam techniques presented in Chapter 6 that pertain to your patient's special situation and clinical status.

Three common presentations among your responsive medical patients will be cardiac chest pain or respiratory distress, altered mental status, and acute abdomen. The following sections outline problem-oriented secondary assessments for those complaints. Note that for each of these cases, the focused secondary assessment is different. As you gain clinical experience, you will be able to quickly assess your patient's pertinent areas according to your suspected field diagnosis. Likewise, clinical judgment and the seriousness of your patient's condition will determine which assessment techniques you use on the scene and which you use en route to the hospital.

Chest Pain or Respiratory Distress For a patient complaining of chest pain or respiratory distress, assess the following.

HEENT (head, eyes, ears, nose, and throat) Note the colour of the lips. Lip cyanosis is an ominous sign of central circulatory hypoxia. Examine the oral mu-

Let the diagnostic impression you formed during the history guide your examination of a responsive medical patient.

cosa for pallor suggesting decreased circulation as in shock. Inspect any fluids in the mouth. Pink, frothy sputum (the result of plasma proteins' mixing with air and red blood cells in the alveoli) is a classic sign of acute pulmonary edema. Always keep the mouth clear of any fluids that may block the upper airway by aggressive suctioning. Note any swelling, redness, or hives, suggesting an allergic reaction.

Neck Observe the neck for accessory muscle use and retractions, signs of acute respiratory distress. Retractions in the supraclavicular (above the clavicles) and suprasternal (above the sternum) notches indicate your patient is having difficulty inhaling. Palpate the carotid arteries for rate, quality, and equality; if you detect weak or unequal pulses, auscultate for bruits. Examine the jugular veins for abnormal distention. In a patient lying supine without circulatory compromise, these veins should distend slightly. This is normal. If the jugular veins do not distend in the supine position, your patient may be hypovolemic. In the semi-Fowler's position (sitting up at 45 degrees), the veins should disappear. Distention beyond 45 degrees is significant because something is inhibiting blood return to the chest. This may be the result of cardiac tamponade, tension pneumothorax, or right heart failure. Inspect and palpate the position of the trachea. It should lie midline and remain fixed during the breathing cycle. Tugging to one side during inspiration suggests a pneumothorax on that side. Displacement to one side may indicate a tension pneumothorax on the opposite side as the entire mediastinum is displaced.

Chest Assess the respiratory rate and pattern again and administer oxygen or ventilation as needed. Note the length of the inspiratory and expiratory phases. A prolonged inspiratory phase suggests an upper airway obstruction. A prolonged expiratory phase suggests a lower airway obstruction, such as in asthma and emphysema. Inspect and palpate the chest wall for symmetry of movement and intercostal retractions. A barrel chest suggests a history of emphysema. Look for the classic midline scar from open heart surgery or the typical bulge of an implanted pacemaker or defibrillator.

Auscultate all lung fields (anterior to posterior, apices to bases) and compare sides. Report and record the sounds you hear (crackles, wheezes), where you hear them (in the bases, apices, diffuse), and when they occur during the respiratory cycle (inspiratory, expiratory). For example, if your patient has bilateral inspiratory rales, you might suspect congestive heart failure or pulmonary edema. If he has diffuse expiratory wheezing, you might suspect the bronchospasm associated with asthma or chronic obstructive pulmonary disease. The presence of both would suggest acute pulmonary edema. A localized wheeze might indicate a pulmonary embolism, a foreign body aspiration, or an infection. Patients with unilateral (one-sided) decreased breath sounds require further testing, such as tactile fremitus, bronchophony, egophony, or whispered pectoriloquoy. Percuss the chest and back for hyperresonance (asthma, emphysema, pneumothorax) and dullness (pulmonary edema, pleural effusion, pneumonia).

Cardiovascular Inspect for signs of arterial insufficiency or occlusion in your patient's trunk and extremities. Look for skin pallor and other signs of decreased perfusion. Inspect and palpate the chest for the PMI. Assess central and peripheral pulses for equality, rate, regularity, and quality. Auscultate for heart sounds, identifying S1, S2, and any additional sounds.

Abdomen Look for exaggerated abdominal muscle use during exhalation, a sign of lower airway obstruction as seen in asthma and emphysema. Inspect and palpate the abdomen for distention due to air or fluid. Ascites is an accumulation of fluid within the abdominal cavity caused by increased pressure in the systemic circulation as seen in patients with right heart failure. It is also common in patients with cirrhosis of the liver, where portal circulation (to and from the liver) is increased. Inspect and palpate the flanks and presacral area for edema in bedridden patients suspected of having congestive heart failure. Check for unusual pulsation of the descending aorta, just left of the umbilicus. Palpate for liver enlargement or upper quadrant tenderness suggesting ulcer disease, gall bladder disease, or pancreas problems, all of which can be confused as chest pain.

Extremities Perform neurovascular checks on both hands and feet. These consist of checking for pulses, sensation, and the ability to move. Pay special attention to the equality of pulses in all extremities. Unequal pulses in the upper extremities suggest a thoracic aneurysm; unequal pulses in the lower extremities suggest an abdominal aneurysm. Assume vascular compromise if the pulse is absent, the limb is cool, or the skin is cyanotic or ashen. In cardiac and respiratory emergencies, evaluate the lower extremities for pitting edema. Depress the skin on the tibial plateau (Figure 7-27). If the depression remains after you remove your finger, pitting edema exists. This is a sign of chronic fluid retention as seen in heart and renal failure. Examine the fingernails for pitting. Check the wrists for Medic Alert identification.

Altered Mental Status For a patient with an altered mental status, assess the following:

HEENT Inspect and palpate the head to rule out any evidence of trauma. For example, your stroke patient may have suffered a skull fracture from falling on the floor. Palpate the fontanelles of the infant for sunkenness (dehydration) and bulging (increasing intracranial pressure). Examine the face for symmetry. Unilateral facial drooping may indicate a stroke or inflammation of the facial nerve (Bell's palsy). Examine the pupils for direct and consensual response to light. One pupil's getting larger or reacting more slowly to light could indicate a deteriorating brain pathology, such as a stroke. A small portion of the population, however, has unequal pupils, a benign condition known as anisocoria. Bilaterally sluggish pupils usually suggest decreased blood flow to the brain and hypoxia. Fixed and dilated pupils indicate severe brain anoxia. Your patient's pupils also may dilate from sympathomimetic or anticholinergic drug use. Pinpoint pupils suggest a narcotic drug overdose or pontine hemmorhage (bleeding within the pons). Next, test for near response and accommodation. Test the integrity of the extraocular muscles with the "H" test. Normally, your patient will move his eyes conjugately (together) to follow your finger. He may exhibit a nystagmus, a fine jerking of the eyes. At the far extremes of the test, nystagmus may be normal, but if you observe it during all extraocular movements, it suggests a pathology. Examine the conjunctiva for redness (irritation), pallor (hypoperfusion), or cyanosis (hypoxia). Inspect the sclera for jaundice.

Chest Inspect, palpate, and auscultate the chest for any signs of cardiorespiratory involvement.

Abdomen Look for evidence of trauma or internal bleeding. Listen for bowel sounds that are absent in anticholinergic drug ingestions.

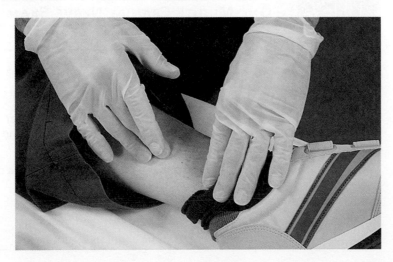

FIGURE 7-27 Check for peripheral edema.

Pelvis   Look for evidence of incontinence and check the stability.

Extremities   Perform neurovascular checks on both hands and feet. These consist of checking for pulses, sensation, and the ability to move. Assume vascular compromise if the pulse is absent, the limb is cool, or the skin is cyanotic or ashen. Since the motor and sensory nerves run along different pathways in the spinal cord, you must check your patient's extremities both for mobility and for sensation of light touch and pain. As with trauma patients, the inability to feel and move both legs indicates complete spinal cord disruption. Diminished sensation or diminished motor ability indicates a partial disruption. Weakness or disability on only one side suggests brain dysfunction, such as a stroke. Report and record all extremity function tests.

Posterior Body   Inspect the posterior body for deformities of the spine. Also, check for evidence of incontinence. In the supine patient, inspect the flanks for presacral edema.

Neuro   Reassess your patient's level of consciousness and compare his response to your earlier findings. Note his speech pattern and any deficits in speech or language. Observe mood swings or behaviours that suggest anxiety or depression. Determine your patient's person, time, and place orientation. Does he know his name, the day of the week, and where he is? Perform the one-minute cranial nerve exam outlined in Table 7-3. Inspect general body structure, muscle development, positioning, and coordination. Note any obvious asymmetries, deformities, or involuntary movements. Assess muscle tone by feeling the muscle's resistance to passive stretching in the extremities. Note the degree of resistance. Test for muscle strength by applying resistance during the range of motion evaluation. Check for pronator drift and watch for any drifting sideways or upward. Assess for coordination and cerebellar function, using rapid alternating movements and point-to-point testing. Note seizure activity tremors.

Acute Abdomen   For a patient complaining of abdominal pain, assess the following:

HEENT   Note any unusual odours coming from your patient's mouth. The smell of alcohol does not rule out a serious medical condition. The sweet smell of ketones suggests diabetes. A fecal odour may indicate a lower-bowel obstruction. The acidic smell of gastric contents means that your patient has vomited and may again. Inspect any fluids in the mouth. Coffee-ground emesis (vomiting) results from blood's mixing with stomach acids and suggests an upper GI bleed. Fresh blood usually means recent hemorrhage from the upper GI tract.

Chest   Listen to breath sounds. Crackles may indicate pneumonia, a cause of upper abdominal pain.

Table 7-3	ONE-MINUTE CRANIAL NERVE EXAM
Cranial Nerves	**Test**
I	Normally not done.
II, III	Direct response to light.
III, IV, VI	"H" test for extraocular movements.
V	Ask patient to clench teeth; palpate massiter and temporal muscles. Test sensory to forehead, cheek, and chin.
VII	Ask patient to show teeth.
IX, X	Ask patient to say "aaaahhhh"; watch uvula movement. Test gag reflex.
XII	Ask patient to stick out tongue.
VIII	Test balance (Romberg test) and hearing.
XI	Ask patient to shrug shoulders, turn head.

Abdomen Look for discoloration over the umbilicus (Cullen's sign) or over the flanks (Grey-Turner's sign) suggesting intra-abdominal bleeding. Check for any visible pulsation, peristalsis, or masses. If you notice a bounding or exaggerated pulsation, suspect an aortic aneurysm. Visible peristalsis may indicate a bowel obstruction. Auscultate for bowel sounds and renal bruits. Percussing the abdomen produces different sounds based on the underlying tissues. Percuss the abdomen in the same sequence you used for auscultation. Note the distribution of tympany and dullness. Expect tympany in most of the abdomen; expect dullness over the solid abdominal organs, such as the liver and spleen.

Palpate the abdomen last to detect tenderness, muscular rigidity, and superficial organs and masses. The normal abdomen is soft and nontender. Abdominal pain on light palpation suggests peritoneal irritation or inflammation. If you feel rigidity or guarding while palpating, determine whether it is voluntary (patient anticipates the pain or is not relaxed) or involuntary (peritoneal inflammation). Then, palpate the abdomen deeply to detect large masses or tenderness. If the peritoneum is inflamed, your patient will experience pain when you let go.

Posterior Body Inspect the posterior body for evidence of rectal bleeding.

Baseline Vital Signs

Prehospital medicine employs four basic vital signs: blood pressure, pulse, respiration, and temperature. You may add level of consciousness and a basic pupil assessment to this list. Your patient's vital signs are your windows to what is happening inside his body. They provide a unique, objective capsule assessment of his clinical status. Vital signs indicate severe illness and the urgency to intervene. Subtle alterations in these vital signs are often the only indication that your patient's condition is changing. They can warn you that your patient is deteriorating, or they can reassure you that he is responding to therapy.

Of the secondary assessment techniques, taking accurate sets of vital signs reveals the most important information. As a paramedic, you must assess these signs on every patient you evaluate. If your patient is with you for an extended time, measure and record his vital signs at intervals as his clinical condition dictates. Always reevaluate the vital signs after invasive procedures, such as endotracheal intubation or fluid resuscitation, and after any sudden change in your patient's condition. Accurate records of these numbers are invaluable when documenting your patient assessment.

Always reevaluate vital signs after invasive procedures and after any sudden change in your patient's condition.

If you suspect your patient of being hypovolemic, consider performing an orthostatic vital sign assessment, commonly known as the tilt test. Take your patient's pulse and blood pressure while he is supine. Then, have him sit up and dangle his feet. Finally, tell him to stand. Then, in 30–60 seconds, retake the vital signs. They should not change in the healthy patient. An increase in the pulse rate of 10–20 beats per minute or a drop in blood pressure of 10–20 mmHg is a positive tilt test. This is a common finding in patients suspected of hypovolemia. Chapter 6 describes vital sign evaluation in detail.

Additional Assessment Techniques

Additional techniques include pulse oximetry, cardiac monitoring, and blood glucose determination. Refer to Chapter 6 for detailed descriptions of these techniques.

Pulse Oximetry The pulse oximeter is a noninvasive device that measures the oxygen saturation of your patient's blood. It is usually a good indicator of cardiorespiratory status because it tells you how well your patient is oxygenating the most distal ends of his circulatory system. It also quantifies the effectiveness of your interventions, such as oxygen therapy, medications, suctioning, and

Content Review

ADDITIONAL ASSESSMENT TECHNIQUES
Pulse oximetry
Cardiac monitoring
Blood glucose
  determination

ventilatory assistance. Normal oxygen saturation at sea level should be between 96 percent and 100 percent. Generally, if the reading is below 95 percent, suspect shock, hypoxia, or respiratory compromise. Provide your patient with the appropriate airway management, supplemental oxygen, and watch carefully for further changes. Any reading below 90 percent requires aggressive airway management, positive pressure ventilation, or oxygen administration.

Cardiac Monitoring The cardiac monitor, which measures electrical activity, is essential in assessing and managing the patient who requires advanced cardiac life support (ACLS) measures. You should apply it to any patient you suspect of having a serious illness or injury. Its one major disadvantage, however, is that it cannot tell you if the heart is pumping efficiently, effectively, or at all. When assessing your patient, always compare what you see on the monitor with what you feel for a pulse. If available, perform 12-lead ECG monitoring to identify the presence and location of a possible myocardial infarction.

Blood Glucose Determination In cases of altered mental status, such as diabetic emergencies, seizures, and strokes, measure your patient's blood sugar level. Inexpensive, hand-held glucometers make this test simple and easy to perform in the field.

Emergency Medical Care

After conducting your secondary assessment, provide the necessary emergency medical care authorized by your medical director via standing orders. Then, as required, contact the online medical direction physician to request further orders. For example, you may administer 50 percent dextrose to an adult patient (25 percent dextrose to a pediatric patient) with documented hypoglycemia (Figure 7-28), intubate a patient in severe respiratory distress, or apply external cardiac pacing to a patient with third-degree heart block. Always base your emergency care on your patient's signs and symptoms as obtained through a thorough focused history and secondary assessment. Finally, en route to the hospital, conduct an ongoing assessment as described later in this chapter.

Again, if time allows, in certain situations you may want to selectively use some of the advanced assessments described in Chapter 6. For example, en route to the hospital, you might conduct a complete neurological exam for your patient who complains of stroke-like symptoms. This would comprise a full mental status assessment including orientation, appearance and behaviour, speech and language, mood, thoughts and perceptions, insight and judgment, and memory and attention; a cranial nerve exam; a motor system assessment, including

Apply the cardiac monitor to any patient you suspect of having a serious illness or injury.

Always base care of responsive medical patients on your patient's signs and symptoms as obtained through a thorough focused history and secondary assessment.

FIGURE 7-28 Administer 50 percent dextrose to a patient in insulin shock.

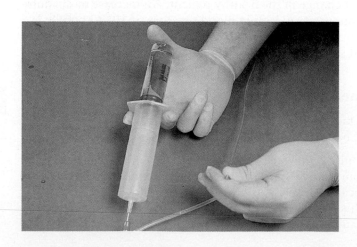

muscle bulk, tone, and strength; a sensory exam including sharp and dull identification, temperature discrimination, position and vibration sense, and discriminative sensation; and deep tendon, as well as superficial, reflex tests. For your patient with upper respiratory distress and flu symptoms, you may decide to examine the posterior pharynx and tonsils for redness and exudate; palpate the cervical lymph nodes for presence and tenderness; and thoroughly assess the lungs for tactile fremitus, egophony, bronchophony, and whispered pectoriloquoy. For your patient suspected of having acute appendicitis, you may want to use the psoas test. Ask your patient to bring the right knee to his chest, contracting the iliopsoas muscle group. This motion usually causes pain as the muscles rub against the inflamed appendix. Your clinical experience and judgment will guide these types of decisions. The scope of paramedic practice is changing, not in procedures but in assessment capabilities. You will learn much more than your predecessors about anatomy and physiology, pathophysiology, and patient assessment. In time, you will learn which assessment techniques yield the most relevant information and use them in your daily practice.

THE UNRESPONSIVE MEDICAL PATIENT

Since he cannot tell you what is wrong, the unresponsive medical patient requires an entirely different approach than does the responsive patient. Assess the unresponsive medical patient much as you would a trauma patient. Begin with the primary assessment; then conduct a rapid head-to-toe assessment known as the rapid medical assessment; and finally, take a brief history from family or friends. This approach to the unresponsive medical patient also will help you to detect whether trauma may be involved.

After conducting the primary assessment, position your patient so that his airway is protected. If the cervical spine is not involved, place your patient in the recovery position—laterally recumbent. This will prevent secretions from obstructing his airway. Now, begin the rapid medical assessment. The rapid medical assessment is similar to the rapid trauma assessment, except that you will look for signs of illness, not injury. Assess the head, neck, chest, abdomen, pelvis, extremities, and posterior aspect of the body. Perform the entire assessment with the unresponsive patient. Then, assess baseline vital signs: pulse, blood pressure, respiration, and temperature. Finally, obtain a history from bystanders, family members, friends, or medical identification devices or services. If possible, it should include the chief complaint, history of the present illness, past medical history, and current health status.

Evaluate your data, and provide emergency medical care while performing additional tests, such as cardiac monitoring, blood glucose determination, and pulse oximetry as needed. Consider your unresponsive patient unstable and expedite transport to the hospital, performing an ongoing assessment every five minutes en route.

Expedite transfer of unresponsive medical patients to the hospital and perform an ongoing assessment every five minutes en route.

IN THE FIELD

The rapid assessment is not a comprehensive history and secondary assessment, but a practical, systematic assessment aimed at quickly identifying the cause of your patient's unresponsive condition. Your care for a patient with a coma of unknown origin, for example, might go something like this.

You are dispatched to an "unresponsive person" in a residential neighbourhood. Your patient is an elderly man who presents laterally recumbent on the floor of his bathroom. You conduct a primary assessment while your partner elicits information from the patient's wife:

General:	Your patient appears pale and diaphoretic, moaning unintelligibly. You find no apparent signs of trauma, and he appears to have slumped to the floor from the toilet.
Mental Status:	You establish your patient's mental status with the AVPU mnemonic. He responds to your voice but cannot answer your questions.
Airway:	You open your patient's airway with a head-tilt/chin-lift manoeuvre and observe his breathing. His airway is clear. His breathing is rapid and shallow, but not laboured. You ask your partner to administer positive pressure ventilation with supplemental oxygen while you continue with your assessment.
Circulation:	You palpate his radial pulse and note its absence. His carotid pulse is slow, irregular, and weak. His skin is pale, cool, and clammy, indicating poor peripheral perfusion.

You prioritize this patient high because of his altered mental status; his rapid, shallow breathing; and his poor peripheral perfusion. You suspect shock and begin a rapid medical assessment.

HEENT:	You note lip cyanosis, a sign of central hypoxia. You see no lip pursing, nasal flaring, or other signs of increased breathing effort, such as retractions or accessory muscle use. You smell no unusual odours or fluids from the mouth. The face is symmetrical; the pupils are equal and round but react to light sluggishly. The trachea is midline, and there is no JVD.
Chest:	You note symmetrical chest wall movement and an equal and adequate rise and fall of the chest with each ventilation. You note some crackles in the lung bases. Your patient has no surgical scars.
ABD:	You see no ascites or abdominal distention, no rigidity or guarding, no rebound tenderness, no renal or carotid bruits, no needle marks, no surgical scars or pulsating masses.
Pelvis:	You see no evidence of bladder or bowel incontinence or of rectal bleeding.
Extremities:	No finger clubbing, no medical identification, no needle marks. Peripheral circulation is poor with no radial or pedal pulses. You note some pitting edema in lower extremities.
Posterior:	You note some edema in your patient's flanks.
Vitals:	Heart rate, 46 and regular; BP, 78/38; respirations, 36 and shallow.
Additional:	ECG monitor shows third-degree AV block; pulse oximetry, 92% on room air, 99% with oxygen; blood glucose, 6.1 mmol/L.

Your patient's wife reveals his long history of heart disease and a long list of cardiac medications. Your field diagnosis is cardiogenic shock due to the bradycardic rate of the third-degree block. While your partner initiates an IV, you set up for immediate external cardiac pacing.

THE DETAILED SECONDARY ASSESSMENT

The **detailed secondary assessment** uses many components of the comprehensive evaluation presented in the previous two chapters. It is a careful, thorough process of eliciting the history and conducting a physical assessment. The detailed secondary assessment is a luxury, designed for use en route to the hospital, if time allows, for patients with significant trauma or serious medical illnesses. Ironically, with critical patients you usually will not have time to perform this in-depth assessment because you will be preoccupied with performing ongoing assessments and providing emergency care. So, you will seldom, if ever, perform a complete assessment in the field. In fact, physicians in the emergency department rarely perform a detailed assessment on their critical patients. It is too comprehensive and time consuming and yields little relevant information.

In the emergency setting, use a modified approach. You can individualize the assessment to your patient's particular situation in many ways. For example, for the multitrauma patient, perform a head-to-toe assessment that is more detailed and slower than the rapid trauma assessment yet focuses on injury. For the 17-year-old football player who presents with shoulder pain, you may perform the entire portion of the shoulder exam. Palpating the abdomen and auscultating heart sounds would yield little useful information. For your stable patient who complains of abdominal pain, you may conduct an extensive history as detailed in Chapter 5, instead of the abbreviated SAMPLE history. Often, you will elicit vital information from a seemingly obscure question during the review of systems. Again, clinical experience and your patient's condition will determine how you proceed with the detailed assessment.

When you conduct the detailed assessment you will use components of the comprehensive assessment presented in Chapters 5 and 6. Refer to those chapters for a complete description of the components outlined in this section. Interview your patient to ascertain the history, and then conduct a systematic head-to-toe physical assessment. Place special emphasis on those areas suggested by your patient's chief complaint and present problem. Remember that the secondary assessment can be an anxiety-provoking experience for both the patient and the examiner. Using a professional, calm demeanour will minimize this anxiety. The following example illustrates how you might conduct a secondary assessment for a multitrauma patient en route to the hospital.

Head Palpate the cranium from front to back for symmetry and smoothness (Procedure 7-5a). Note any tenderness, deformities, and areas of unusual warmth. Inspect and palpate the facial bones for stability and note any crepitus or loose fragments (Procedure 7-5b). Any instability or asymmetry of the eye orbits, nasal bones, maxilla, or mandible suggests a facial bone fracture. In these cases, pay careful attention to the upper airway for obstruction from blood, bone chips, and teeth. Suction these patients aggressively to keep the upper airway clear.

When the base of the skull is fractured, blood and fluid from the brain can seep into the soft tissues around the eyes and ears and can drain from the ears or nose. Observe the bony orbits of the eye and the mastoid process behind the ears for discoloration. **Periorbital ecchymosis** (raccoon eyes) is a black and blue discoloration surrounding the eye sockets. **Battle's sign** is a similar discoloration over the mastoid process just behind the ears (Procedure 7-5c). They are both late signs and usually are not visible on the scene unless a previous injury exists. Evaluate the temporomandibular joint for tenderness, swelling, and range of motion.

Eyes Examine the external structure of the eyes for symmetry in size, shape, and contour. Inspect the sclera and conjunctiva for discoloration, swelling, and exudate. Inspect the eyes for discoloration, foreign bodies, or blood in the anterior chamber (hyphema). Hyphema suggests that a tremendous blunt trauma to the

---

✱ detailed secondary assessment careful, thorough process of eliciting the history and conducting a physical assessment.

In the emergency setting, individualize the assessment to your patient's particular situation.

Aggressively suction patients with facial fractures to keep the upper airway clear.

✱ periorbital ecchymosis black and blue discoloration surrounding the eye sockets.

✱ Battle's sign black and blue discoloration over the mastoid process.

anterior part of the eye has occurred. Check the pupils for equality in size and reaction to light (Procedure 7-5d). Bilaterally sluggish pupils usually suggest decreased cerebral perfusion and hypoxia. Fixed and dilated pupils indicate severe cerebral anoxia. Unequal pupils may indicate a variety of pathologies, including brain lesions, meningitis, drug poisoning, third-nerve paralysis, and increasing intracranial pressure.

Examine the eyes for conjugate movement, their ability to move together. Muscle or nerve damage to the eyes and certain drugs can cause dysconjugate gaze, in which the eyes seem to look in different directions. Check for extraocular movements. Note any inability of the eyes to follow your finger as you draw a large imaginary "H" in front of them; this indicates either nerve damage or an orbital fracture impinging on the extraocular muscles (Procedure 7-5e). Test for visual acuity and peripheral vision if appropriate.

Ears Examine the external ears, and observe the surrounding area for deformities, lumps, skin lesions, tenderness, and erythema. Examine the ear canal for drainage (Procedure 7-5f). A basilar skull fracture can cause blood and clear cerebrospinal fluid to leak into the auditory canals and flow to the outside. Do not try to block this flow; just cover it with sterile gauze to prevent an easy route for infection. Check for hearing acuity as appropriate.

Nose and Sinuses Check your patient's nose from the front and from the side and note any deviation in shape or colour. Palpate the external part of the nose for depressions, deformities, and tenderness. Examine the nares for flaring, a sign of respiratory distress, especially in small children. Pay special attention to infants less than three months old. They are mainly nose breathers and need a clear, unobstructed nasal cavity for respiration. Examine the nasal mucosa for evidence of drainage and note the colour, quantity, and consistency of the discharge (Procedure 7-5g). A clear, runny discharge may indicate leaking cerebrospinal fluid (CSF) from a basilar skull fracture. Test for nasal obstruction.

The nasal cavity has a rich blood supply to warm the inspired air. Unfortunately, this can make bleeding in the nasal cavity severe and very difficult to control. If unconscious, these patients require aggressive suctioning. The patient who swallows this blood may complain later of nausea and vomiting.

Lip cyanosis is an ominous sign of central circulatory hypoxia.

Mouth and Pharynx Note the condition and colour of the lips. Lip cyanosis is an ominous sign of central circulatory hypoxia. Examine the oral mucosa for pallor suggesting poor perfusion as in shock (Procedure 7-5h). Ask your patient to extend his tongue straight out and then move it from side to side. Press a tongue blade down on the middle third of the tongue and have your patient say "aaaahhhh." Examine the movement of the uvula. Asymmetrical movement of the uvula suggests a cranial nerve lesion. Note any odours or fluids coming from your patient's mouth; they can provide clues to infection, poisoning, and metabolic processes, such as diabetic ketoacidosis.

Neck Briefly inspect the neck for general symmetry. Note any obvious deformity, deviation, tugging, masses, surgical scars, gland enlargement, or visible lymph nodes. Examine any penetrating injuries to the neck closely for injury to the trachea or major blood vessels. Look for jugular vein distention while your patient is sitting up and at a 45-degree incline. Palpate the trachea for midline position (Procedure 7-5i). Then, palpate the carotid arteries and note their rate and quality.

Chest and Lungs Observe your patient's breathing. Look for signs of acute respiratory distress. Count his respiratory rate and note his breathing pattern. Inspect the anterior and posterior chest walls for symmetrical movement. Note the use of neck muscles (sternocleidomastoids, scalene muscles) during inhalation or abdominal muscles during exhalation. Accessory muscle use suggests partial

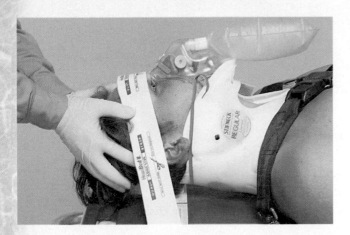

7-5a   Inspect and palpate the cranium from front to back.

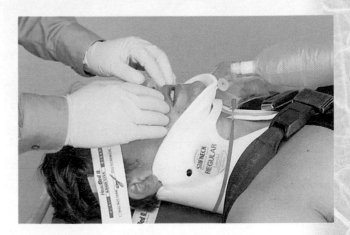

7-5b   Inspect and palpate the facial bones.

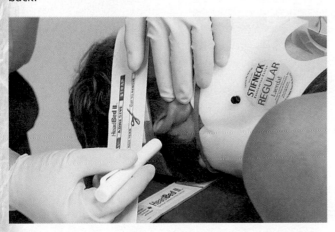

7-5c   Inspect the mastoid process for Battle's sign.

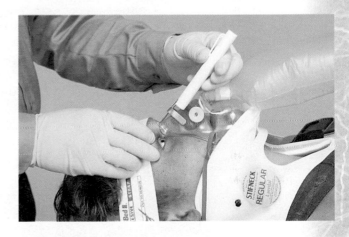

7-5d   Check the pupils for reaction to light.

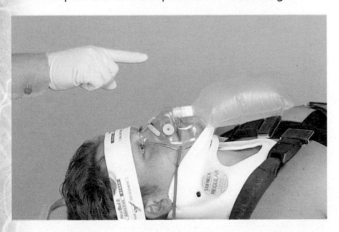

7-5e   Check for extraocular movement.

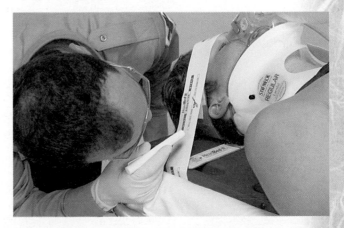

7-5f   Inspect the ear canal for drainage.

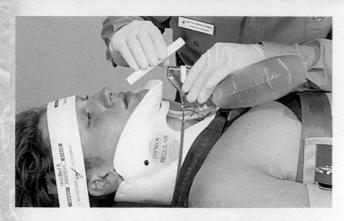

7-5g   Examine the nasal mucosa for drainage.

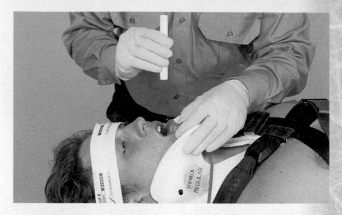

7-5h   Examine the oral mucosa for pallor.

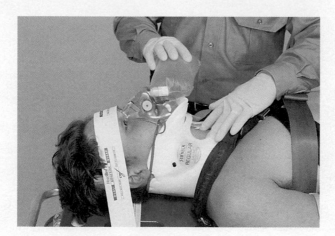

7-5i   Palpate the trachea for midline position.

airway obstruction and difficulty moving air. Inspect the intercostal spaces for retractions or bulging.

Palpate the rib cage for rigidity (Procedure 7-6a). Feel for tenderness, deformities, depressions, loose segments, asymmetry, and crepitus. Evaluate for equal expansion. Percuss the chest symmetrically from the apices to the bases. Identify and note any area of abnormal percussion. Auscultate all lung fields and compare sides (Procedure 7-6b).

Percussion can also provide evidence regarding chest pathology. If the region is hyperresonant, the thorax may contain air under pressure (tension pneumothorax). If the region is dull to percussion, it may be filled with blood (hemothorax) or other fluid (pleural effusion). Be sure to compare the sounds left to right and, during examination of the posterior body, front to back to confirm your evaluation.

Cardiovascular System Look for skin pallor and other signs of decreased perfusion. Inspect and palpate the carotid arteries for rate, rhythm, and quality or amplitude. Inspect and palpate the chest for the PMI. Auscultate for normal, abnormal, and extra heart sounds.

Abdomen Inspect the skin of the abdomen and flanks for scars, dilated veins, stretch marks, rashes, lesions, and pigmentation changes. Look for Cullen's sign or Grey-Turner's sign suggesting intra-abdominal bleeding. Assess the size and shape of your patient's abdomen and note its symmetry. Palpate the abdomen last to detect tenderness, muscular rigidity, and superficial organs and masses (Procedure 7-6c). Assess for rebound tenderness, a classic sign of peritoneal irritation, by pushing down slowly and then releasing your hand quickly off the tender area.

Pelvis Reevaluate the pelvic ring at the iliac crests and symphysis pubis (Procedure 7-6d). With the palms of your hands, direct pressure medially and posteriorly. Then, press posteriorly on the symphysis pubis, being careful not to entrap the penis or cause injury to the urinary bladder. Any pain, instability, or crepitus suggests a pelvic fracture. Always immobilize the pelvis before transport to prevent movement and a possible circulatory catastrophe.

Genitalia The external genitalia are extremely vascular and can bleed profusely when lacerated. Control hemorrhage in this area with direct pressure. Examine the male organ for priapism, a painful, prolonged erection usually caused by spinal cord injury or blood disturbances. Suspect a major spinal cord injury in any patient with a priapism. The female genitalia are somewhat well protected from all but penetrating injury.

If you suspect your patient may have been raped or sexually abused, limit your assessment and management to only those techniques that are essential to patient stabilization. If possible, have a member of the same sex treat these patients. This may relieve any hostilities and anxiety that might be directed toward a caregiver of the opposite sex. Discourage the patient from bathing. One of your most important tasks is to provide emotional support and reassurance. (For more on this subject, see Chapter 44 on abuse and assault.)

One of your most important tasks for possible victims of rape or sexual abuse is to provide emotional support and reassurance.

Anus and Rectum Examining the anus is normally not a prehospital assessment practice. If your patient presents with severe rectal bleeding, apply direct pressure to the area with sterile pads, and be prepared to treat him for shock. You will have no other reason to examine this area.

Peripheral Vascular System Inspect all four extremities, noting their size and symmetry. Palpate the peripheral arteries for pulse rate and quality. Assess the skin for temperature, moisture, colour, and capillary refill.

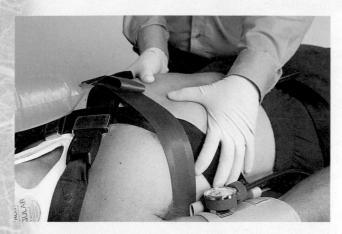

7-6a   Palpate the ribcage.

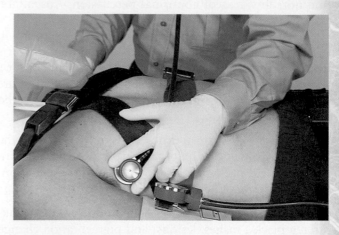

7-6b   Auscultate the lungs.

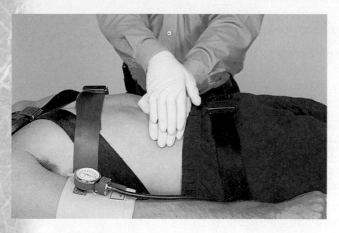

7-6c   Palpate the abdomen.

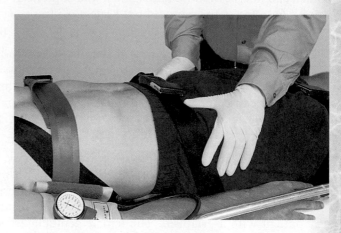

7-6d   Evaluate the pelvis.

Musculoskeletal System Reinspect and palpate all four extremities. Inspect and palpate your patient's joints, their structure, their range of motion, and the surrounding tissues. Inspect for swelling in or around joints, changes in the surrounding tissue, redness of the overlying skin, deformities, and symmetry of impairment. Compare both sides for equal size, shape, colour, and strength. Palpate for tenderness in and around the joint. Try to identify the specific structure that is tender, such as a ligament or tendon.

Test for range of motion passively and against gravity and resistance. Difficulty during passive range of motion tests suggests a joint problem. Difficulty with gravity or against resistance suggests a muscular weakness or nerve problem. Listen for crepitation, the crunching sounds of unlubricated parts rubbing against each other, while you manipulate the joint. Perform distal neurovascular checks.

Nervous System A nervous system exam covers five areas: mental status and speech; the cranial nerves; the motor system; the reflexes; and the sensory system.

Mental Status and Speech First, assess your patient's level of consciousness and compare his response with your earlier findings. Observe his posture, motor behaviour, grooming, and personal hygiene. Note speech pattern and use of language. Observe your patient's mood from his verbal and nonverbal behaviours. Assess his thought content, perceptions, insight and judgment, memory, attention, and learning ability.

Cranial Nerves Test any cranial nerves that you have not already checked. (Review Table 7-3 for a quick, reliable, practical, cranial nerve exam that should take no longer than one minute to perform.)

Motor System Inspect your patient's general body structure, muscle development, positioning, and coordination. Note any obvious asymmetries, deformities, or involuntary movements. Assess muscle tone by feeling the muscle's resistance to passive stretching in the extremities. Test for muscle strength by applying resistance during the range of motion evaluation. Check for pronator drift and watch for any drifting sideways (laterally) or upward (superiorly). Assess for coordination and cerebellar function, using rapid alternating movements and point-to-point testing.

Reflexes Test your patient's deep tendon reflexes with a reflex hammer and note any hyperactive or diminished response. Check the biceps, triceps, brachioradialis, quadriceps, and Achilles reflexes. Test the superficial abdominal reflexes and plantar response.

Sensory System Test for pain, light touch, temperature, position, vibration, and discriminative sensations. Compare distal areas to proximal areas and symmetrical areas bilaterally, and scatter the stimuli to assess most of the dermatomes. Assess your patient's ability to distinguish sharp from dull sensations.

VITAL SIGNS

Take another set of vital signs and compare them with earlier sets to detect any trends, patterns that indicate either an improvement or deterioration in your patient's condition. These trends include a rising or falling pulse rate and blood pressure; an increasing or decreasing respiratory rate and effort; changing skin temperature, colour, and condition; and changing pupillary equality and response to light. Such trends may suggest specific pathologies that you will learn in Chapters 16 to 26 on trauma emergencies and Chapters 27 to 40 on medical emergencies.

RECORDING ASSESSMENT FINDINGS

Record all assessment findings on the appropriate call sheet or chart. Remain objective and nonjudgmental when recording the data. Chapter 9, "Documentation," gives detailed instructions on writing patient care reports.

Content Review

AREAS OF NERVOUS SYSTEM EXAM
Mental status and speech
Cranial nerves
Motor system
Reflexes
Sensory system

Content Review

REFLEX TESTS
Biceps
Triceps
Brachioradialis
Quadriceps
Achilles
Abdominal plantar

Content Review

SENSORY SYSTEM TESTS
Pain
Light touch
Temperature
Position
Vibration
Discrimination

En route to the hospital, conduct an ongoing series of assessments to detect trends, determine changes in your patient's condition, and assess the effectiveness of your interventions. Patient condition can change suddenly. You must steadfastly reassess mental status, airway patency, breathing adequacy, circulation, and any deterioration in areas already compromised (Procedure 7-7a). Conduct your ongoing assessment every 15 minutes for stable patients, every 5 minutes for unstable patients. Compare your findings with the baseline findings and note any trends. Consider this ongoing assessment as frequently repeating the primary assessment.

You must steadfastly reassess mental status, ABCs, and any areas already compromised.

Any deterioration in mental status is cause for great concern.

MENTAL STATUS

Recheck your patient's mental status by performing the AVPU assessment frequently during transport. Any deterioration in mental status is cause for great concern. The brain demands a constant supply of oxygen and glucose and a constant elimination of waste products. When it is deprived of either, even briefly, expect rapid mental status changes. A falling level of response indicates either a direct or indirect brain pathology. For example, following a head injury, your patient who was alert and oriented at the scene gradually becomes sleepy and eventually unarousable. You should suspect a life-threatening increase in intracranial pressure (pressure inside the enclosed skull) and expedite transport to the appropriate medical facility. Or your patient with an intra-abdominal hemorrhage becomes increasingly less arousable due to the decreased oxygenated blood flow to the brain (indirect pathology). Or sometimes patients improve following your interventions. After you administer 50 percent dextrose to your hypoglycemic patient with diabetes, for instance, he becomes alert and begins talking.

AIRWAY PATENCY

The patency of your patient's airway can change instantly. Bleeding, vomiting, and even secretions can suddenly obstruct the upper airway. Be prepared to open your patient's airway and suction quickly. Respiratory burns and anaphylaxis can cause life-threatening swelling in a matter of minutes. Croup and epiglottitis also can quickly deteriorate into total upper airway occlusion.

Endotracheal intubation is the best way to secure the airway in patients with no gag reflex. But endotracheal tubes can become dislodged easily during transport. Recheck for tube placement frequently during transport and every time you move your patient onto a back board, onto the stretcher, or onto the hospital gurney.

The path of proper airway management is eternal vigilance and a pessimistic outlook— anything that can go wrong will go wrong. Be prepared for the worst.

BREATHING RATE AND QUALITY

A change in respiratory rate or quality might indicate improvement or deterioration. A sudden increase in rate or respiratory effort suggests deterioration. For example, if your patient suddenly begins to gasp for air, has retractions, and uses the accessory neck muscles, he has a serious problem. Sometimes, the signs are not so obvious. Subtle increases in respiratory rate can suggest a developing problem. A decrease in rate and effort could mean that your treatments are effective and your patient is improving. For example, after you administer a salbutamol treatment, your patient breathes easier and his lung sounds improve. In infants and young children, however, a decrease in rate and effort may mean that your patient is exhausted and requires aggressive intervention. If while assisting ventilation with a bag-valve mask, your partner suddenly complains that squeezing the bag is becoming more difficult, consider the possibility that a tension pneumothorax is developing or that bronchospasm or laryngospasm may be occurring. Airway and breathing management require constant reevaluation.

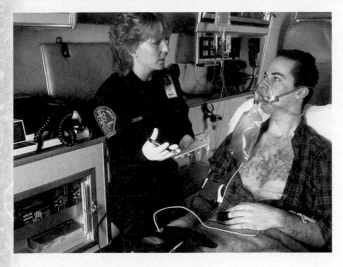

7-7a   Reevaluate the ABCs.

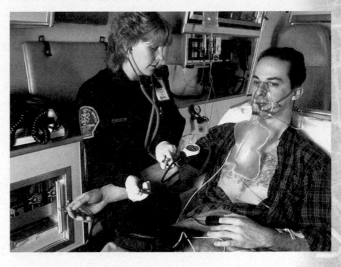

7-7b   Take all vital signs again.

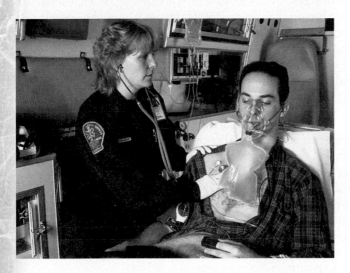

7-7c   Perform your focused assessment again.

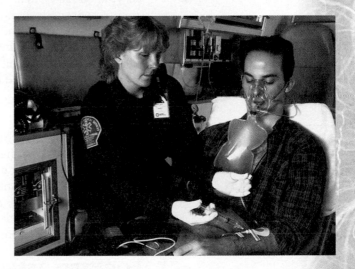

7-7d   Evaluate your interventions' effects.

PULSE RATE AND QUALITY

Check central and peripheral pulses and compare the findings with earlier measurements. A rising pulse rate could indicate shock, hypoxia, or cardiac dysrhythmia. A falling rate could mean the terminal stage of shock or a rise in intracranial pressure. A sudden change in rate or regularity may suggest a cardiac dysrhythmia. The loss of peripheral pulses could mean decompensating shock.

SKIN CONDITION

Similar to mental status, the skin quickly reflects the body's hemodynamic status. Reevaluate your patient's skin colour, temperature, and condition. Cyanosis suggests decreased oxygenation. Lip cyanosis indicates central hypoxia (overall oxygen status), while peripheral cyanosis indicates decreased oxygen to the tissues. Pallor and coolness suggest decreased circulation to the skin, as seen in shock. If your patient suddenly develops hives after you administer a medication, suspect an allergic reaction. A localized redness and warmth could indicate bleeding under the skin or vasodilation. Cyanosis and coolness in a lower extremity suggest a peripheral vascular problem, such as an arterial occlusion. A deep vein thrombosis will result in redness, swelling, and warmth in the lower leg.

TRANSPORT PRIORITIES

Sometimes, stable patients suddenly deteriorate en route to the hospital. For example, the formerly conscious and alert head-injury patient now responds only to pain. Or your stable cardiac patient suddenly develops a life-threatening dysrhythmia. Or your patient suddenly cannot breathe because a simple pneumothorax has developed into a tension pneumothorax. In these cases, while you provide life-saving treatments, change your transport decision to a higher priority. If your unstable patient becomes stable, you might want to downgrade your priority transport decision and decrease the danger and liability of driving with lights and siren on.

VITAL SIGNS

Reevaluate your critical patient's vital signs every five minutes.

Reassessing vital signs reveals trends clearly (Procedure 7-7b). A rising pulse rate combined with a falling blood pressure indicates shock. A decreasing pulse rate combined with a rising blood pressure, associated with an irregular respiratory pattern, suggests a rise in intracranial pressure. Any change in heart rate could indicate a cardiac dysrhythmia. A narrowing pulse pressure with a weakening pulse indicates cardiac tamponade, a tension pneumothorax, or hypovolemic shock. Reevaluate your critical patient's vital signs every five minutes and look for changes.

FOCUSED ASSESSMENT

Elicit your patient's chief complaint again to determine whether the problem still exists or if other problems have arisen. Often, following trauma, your patient will develop more complaints en route to the hospital as the excitement of the incident begins to wear off. Patients often focus on their major injuries and might not even be aware of other problems. Repeat your focused assessment as your patient's chief complaint dictates (Procedure 7-7c).

EFFECTS OF INTERVENTIONS

Evaluate the effects of any interventions (Procedure 7-7d). Did the salbutamol treatment help open the lower airways? Did the oxygen and nitroglycerine relieve the chest pain? What are the effects of the fluid challenge? Did your intervention help or harm your patient? Is he getting better or worse? Know the expected therapeutic benefits of your interventions, and then evaluate whether they worked. For example, you administer lidocaine to convert ventricular tachycardia. Following administration, observe your patient's electrocardiogram for changes while noting any harmful side effects, such as nausea, vomiting, or seizures.

MANAGEMENT PLANS

Evaluate whether your care is working. If it is not, consider another management plan. Develop the courage to admit when your plan is not working and the flexibility to change your course of action. For example, your patient, an elderly man with a history of congestive heart failure (CHF) and chronic obstructive pulmonary disease (COPD), presents with severe difficulty breathing and audible wheezing. You suspect he is having an exacerbation of his COPD and administer two nebulizer treatments and begin transporting. En route, however, he is not improving, and now you also can hear crackles bilaterally. At this point, you suspect he is in CHF and change your management to administering nitroglycerine, furosemide, and morphine.

Patients often present with multiple complaints, symptoms, and histories. Formulating a definitive diagnosis is difficult without the hospital's labs, x-rays, and other assessment tools. Your ability to reassess your patient, reevaluate your field diagnosis, and alter your management plan will optimize patient care.

Have the courage to admit it if your plan is not working and the flexibility to change it.

Your ability to reassess your patient, reevaluate your field diagnosis, and alter your management plan will optimize patient care.

SUMMARY

Patient assessment is the key to providing effective prehospital emergency medical care. Its components include the primary assessment, the focused history and secondary assessment, vital signs, ongoing assessment, and the detailed secondary assessment. The primary assessment is designed to identify life-threatening airway, breathing, and circulation problems. The secondary assessment is designed to identify the signs and symptoms surrounding your patient's chief complaint. It is a problem-oriented approach that is easily modified to match your patient's clinical situation. The ongoing assessment is designed to reevaluate your patient for changes in status en route to the hospital. The detailed secondary assessment is a comprehensive head-to-toe evaluation designed to identify any conditions not already found. Although more suited to a clinical setting, it is intended to be done en route to the hospital if time allows.

The four general types of patients require distinctly different assessment approaches. The trauma patient with a significant mechanism of injury should receive an primary assessment, a rapid trauma assessment, and rapid transport. The patient with isolated, minor trauma, such as a cut finger or sprained ankle, should receive a secondary assessment focused on the particular problem or area. The responsive medical patient requires a primary assessment, a history and physical assessment that focuses on the chief complaint, and vital signs. The unresponsive medical patient requires a primary assessment, followed by a rapid head-to-toe medical assessment and rapid transport. You will perform a detailed secondary assessment en route to the hospital if time and your patient's condition allow.

The assessment templates in this chapter are only guidelines. They do not dictate an exact procedure for assessing every patient. Instead, they provide general chronological guides to help you make critical transport and management decisions. As a paramedic, you will be expected to use clinical judgment when deciding which assessment tools to use for your particular patient and situation. With time and experience, you will become adept at assessing real patients in crises. The more effective and efficient you become with this process, the better your patient care will be.

CHAPTER 8

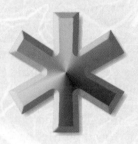

Communications

Objectives

After reading this chapter, you should be able to:

1. Identify the role and importance of verbal, written, and electronic communications in the provision of EMS. (pp. 397–402)

2. Describe the phases of communications necessary to complete a typical EMS response. (pp. 399–402)

3. List factors that impede and enhance effective verbal and written communications. (pp. 397–398)

4. Explain the value of data collection during an EMS response. (pp. 398; 406)

5. Recognize the legal status of verbal, written, and electronic communications related to an EMS response. (pp. 397–398, 409–410)

6. Identify current technology used to collect and exchange patient or scene information electronically. (pp. 403–406)

7. Identify the various components of the EMS communications system and describe their functions and uses. (pp. 396, 399–402)

Continued

Objectives Continued

8. Identify and differentiate among the following communications systems:

   - Simplex (p. 403)
   - Multiplex (p. 403)
   - Duplex (p. 403)
   - Trunking (p. 403)
   - Digital communications (pp. 403–404)
   - Cellular telephone (p. 404)
   - Facsimile (p. 404)
   - Computer (p. 405)

9. Describe the functions and responsibilities of Industry Canada. (pp. 409–410)

10. Describe the role of emergency medical dispatch and the importance of prearrival instructions in a typical EMS response. (pp. 399–402)

11. List appropriate caller information gathered by the emergency medical dispatcher. (p. 400)

12. Describe the structure and importance of verbal patient information communication to the hospital and medical direction. (pp. 406–409)

13. Diagram a basic communications system. (pp. 397–398)

14. Organize a verbal radio report for electronic transmission to medical direction for several narrative patient scenarios. (pp. 406–409)

INTRODUCTION

Knowledge of communications plays an important role in your paramedic training. All aspects of prehospital care require effective, efficient communications. During a routine transfer or a life-threatening emergency run, you will communicate with a wide variety of people:

- The emergency medical dispatcher (EMD) whose job it is to manage an entire system of EMS response and readiness, not just your call. You will transmit administrative information, such as "responding," "arrived," "transporting," and "back in service." The EMD must know the location of all her resources to manage the system effectively. On a serious emergency call, the EMD can be your best ally by securing for you the resources you need to manage your incident.

- Your patient, her family, bystanders, and others who may, at times, not understand what you are doing and become obstructive. Quite often, people misconstrue your actions and words. You must try to keep them well informed.

- Personnel from other responding agencies, such as the police department, fire department, or mutual aid ambulances, who may not share your priorities at the scene. You must communicate effectively with other responders to coordinate and implement your treatment plan. You will accomplish this face-to-face and via the radio. These communications require you to exhibit confidence and authority.

- Health-care staff from physicians' offices, health-care facilities, and nursing homes, who usually do not understand the extent of your training or abilities. Often, uninformed staff will call you "ambulance drivers." In these cases, you must exhibit professionalism and a calm demeanour while you ask pertinent questions and discuss the case intelligently.

- The medical direction physician who has extended her licence to you in the field. The physician's expertise and advice can be a tremendous resource for you during the call. You will need to communicate patient information and scene assessment effectively to her. She can prepare for your arrival if you have communicated the needs of your patient. For example, you are transporting a patient with a serious head injury who exhibits a decreasing level of consciousness. By reporting this information, the emergency department (ED) can arrange for the trauma team, including a neurosurgeon, to meet you in the ED on arrival. In such cases, good communication results in good patient care.

You must interact effectively with everyone involved in the call to coordinate a unified effort resulting in top-quality patient care. EMS is the ultimate team endeavour. Your performance as a paramedic is just one component in a series of interactions that ensures continuous first-rate care. From the call taker to the rehabilitation specialist, every player is equally important—only the roles differ. Communication is not merely one aspect of an EMS response; it is the key link in the chain that results in the best possible patient outcome. Effective communication optimizes patient care during every phase of the EMS response.

Communication is the key link in the chain that results in the best possible patient outcome.

VERBAL COMMUNICATION

Factors that can enhance or impede effective communication may be either **semantic** (the meaning of words) or technical (communications hardware). Communication requires a mutual language. For example, an urban unit and a rural unit that use different **10-code** systems will find it difficult to communicate effectively. A 10-10 may mean a working fire in one system and a cardiac emergency in another. Thus, many EMS systems have changed from using 10-codes to using plain English.

When reporting your patient's condition to the medical direction physician, you should use terminology that is widely accepted by both the medical and the emergency services communities. Using a 10-code system with which the ED staff are unfamiliar would be inappropriate. Telling the medical direction physician that you have a victim of a 10-21-Golf (assault with a gun) may be meaningless. Conversely, if the medical direction physician asks you for your pregnant patient's EDC (due date) or her LMP (last menstrual period) and you do not know those abbreviations, you have failed to communicate. The receiver must be able to decode the sender's message.

Your communication network must consist of reliable equipment designed to afford clear communication among all agencies within the system. This becomes a challenge in systems that cover large geographical areas or where the terrain interferes with transmission and reception. If you want to communicate with a unit clear across the county but your radio is not powerful enough to transmit that far, communication will be difficult, if not impossible. A system that covers a large geographical expanse can place repeaters strategically throughout its service area. These devices receive transmissions from a low-powered source and rebroadcast them at a higher power (Figure 8-1).

 semantic related to the meaning of words.

 10-code radio communications system using codes that begin with the word *ten*.

Many EMS systems have changed from using 10-codes to using plain English.

Your communication network must consist of reliable equipment designed to afford clear communication among all agencies within the system.

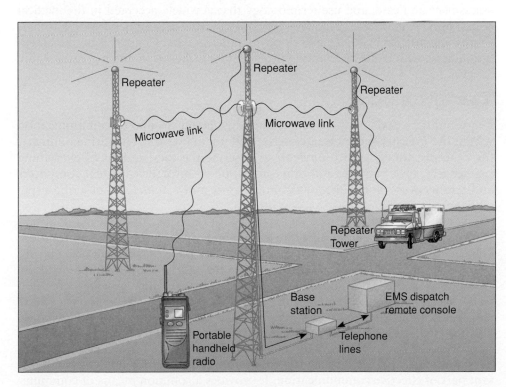

FIGURE 8-1 Example of an EMS system using repeaters.

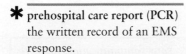

✳ radio band a range of radio frequencies.

✳ radio frequency the number of times per minute a radio wave oscillates.

✳ ultrahigh frequency radio frequency band from 300 to 3000 megahertz.

✳ prehospital care report (PCR) the written record of an EMS response.

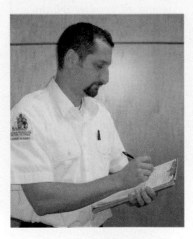

FIGURE 8-2 The prehospital care report is as important as the call itself. Complete it promptly, accurately, and legibly.

Using industry terminology appropriately provides a common means of communicating with other emergency care professionals.

Your regional EMS system may consist of many agencies that have conducted business for decades on different **radio bands** and **frequencies.** Urban units may transmit on **ultrahigh frequency** (UHF) radio waves because they penetrate concrete and steel well and are less susceptible to interference. Rural units may use a low-band frequency because those waves travel farther and better over varied terrain. In any event, communication between agencies will be difficult unless all units share a common frequency. This is rarely the case. The spectrum of communications equipment currently ranges from antiquated radios to mobile data terminals mounted inside emergency vehicles. Geographically integrating communications networks would enable routine and reliable communication among EMS, fire, law enforcement, and other public safety agencies. This would, in turn, facilitate coordinated responses during both routine and large-scale operations. Developing the necessary hardware (equipment and network) and software (language) will be essential to improving emergency communications.

WRITTEN COMMUNICATION

Written records are another important aspect of EMS communications. Your **prehospital care report (PCR)** is a written record of events that includes administrative information, such as times, location, agency, and crew, as well as medical information. It will be used by hospital staff, medical control, agency administrators, system quality-assurance/improvement committees, insurance and billing departments, researchers, educators, and lawyers. The data collected from your PCR can help monitor and improve patient care through medical audits, research, education, and system policy changes. Furthermore, your written documentation becomes a legal record of the incident and may become part of your patient's permanent medical record. All legal rules regarding confidentiality and disclosure pertain to your PCR.

The same factors that influence verbal communication also affect written communication. Be objective, write legibly, thoroughly document your patient's assessment and care, and use terminology that is widely accepted in the medical community (Figure 8-2). Finally, your PCR illustrates your professionalism. A sloppy, incomplete PCR suggests sloppy, inefficient care. Chapter 9 on documentation deals with PCRs and other written communications in much greater detail.

TERMINOLOGY

Every industry develops its own terminology. Doing so makes communication within the industry more clear, concise, and unambiguous. The airline industry, for example, uses the term *payload* to describe the total weight of everything (passengers, fuel, luggage, and other items) on an airplane. Musical composers and arrangers use words like *fortissimo, allegro,* and *a cappella* to describe a specific tempo or style.

The medical field also uses an extensive list of terms, acronyms, and abbreviations that allow quick, accurate communication of complex information. (The documentation chapter includes an extensive table of standard charting abbreviations.) An emergency physician may request a CBC (complete blood count), ABGs (arterial blood gases), or a CIP (cardiac injury profile)—common terms describing diagnostic tests run on acutely ill patients. The emergency services industry has further developed its own terms for radio communication (Table 8-1). These words or phrases shorten airtime and transmit thoughts and ideas quickly. For example, *copy, 10-4,* and *roger* mean "I heard you and I understand what you said." Using industry terminology appropriately is an important part of effective communication. It provides a common means of communicating with other emergency care professionals.

Table 8-1 COMMON RADIO TERMINOLOGY

Term	Meaning
Copy, 10-4, roger	I understand
Affirmative	Yes
Negative	No
Stand by	Please wait
Repeat, say again	Please repeat what you said
Land line	Telephone communications
Rendezvous	Meet with
LZ	Landing zone (helicopter)
ETA	Estimated time of arrival
Over	I am finished with my transmission
Mobile status	On the air, driving around
Stage	Wait before entering a scene
Clear	End of transmission
Unfounded	We cannot find the incident/patient
Be advised	Listen carefully to this

THE EMS RESPONSE

Your ability to communicate effectively during a stressful EMS response will determine the success or failure of your efforts. A brilliant assessment or management plan will be futile if you cannot communicate it to others. Dealing effectively with your patient and bystanders requires a variety of communication skills, such as empathy, confidence, self-control, authority, and patience. Your clinical experience will suggest which skills to use in any particular situation. For example, you might use confidence and an authoritative demeanour when dealing with unruly bystanders, while you would need to be gentle and empathetic with a child or an elderly grandmother. If you were in charge of an incident, you would have to communicate your authority within the structure of the emergency scene to providers from other responding agencies. Delegating tasks, listening to initial reports, and coordinating the scene require effective communication and interpersonal skills.

The sequence of an EMS response illustrates the importance of communications in prehospital care. A typical EMS response includes the following chain of events.

Detection and Citizen Access To begin the response to any emergency once it has occurred, someone must detect the problem and summon EMS (Figure 8-3). Any citizen with an urgent medical need should have a simple and reliable mechanism for accessing the EMS system. In Canada, most people access EMS by telephone; thus, a well-publicized universal telephone number, such as 911, provides direct citizen access to the communications centre. At enhanced 911 (E-911) communication centres, a computer displays the caller's telephone number and location. The centres also have instant callback capabilities, should the caller hang up too soon. The 911 system has been available since the late 1960s. The majority of the population in Canada has a 911 system. Highway call boxes, citizens' band (CB) radio, and amateur radio also provide alternative means of accessing emergency help in some regions.

A call to 911 usually connects the caller to a **public safety answering point** (**PSAP**), which then directs the caller to the appropriate agency for dispatch and response. In some systems, the PSAP call taker will elicit the information and

A brilliant assessment or management plan will be futile if you cannot communicate it to others.

* **PSAP** public safety answering point.

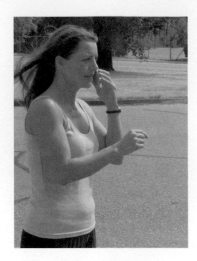

FIGURE 8-3 The response begins when someone detects an emergency and summons EMS support.

✱ **EMD** emergency medical dispatcher.

✱ **priority dispatching** system using medically approved questions and predetermined guidelines to determine the appropriate level of response.

✱ **prearrival instructions** dispatcher's instructions to caller for appropriate emergency measures.

FIGURE 8-4 Priority dispatching and prearrival medical instruction have enhanced the efficiency of the EMS system.

determine the nature of the response. In others, she will simply answer with the question, "Is this a police, fire, or medical emergency?" and transfer the caller to the appropriate dispatcher, who will then elicit the information. Many systems use computerized technology at the PSAP to connect the caller automatically with the appropriate agency. Some even provide language translation. Global positioning systems allow specialized communication services to pinpoint a vehicle's location. Additionally, automakers are installing communications computers in some automobiles. When involved in an accident, these "black boxes" automatically provide the dispatcher with the location, speed, type of collision, projected damage, and suspected severity of injury.

In some systems, all public safety agencies are located within the same facility. In others, they are connected electronically. No one way is best. If the public receives timely, appropriate responses to all emergency calls, the system is effective.

Call Taking and Emergency Response The **emergency medical dispatcher** (**EMD**) is the public's first contact with the EMS system and plays a crucial role in every EMS response. The most important information the call taker must obtain is the address of the incident, the caller's name, the call-back number, and other pertinent factors. Ideally, she also will ascertain the nature of the emergency and other pertinent factors.

In a coordinated system known as **priority dispatching,** medical dispatchers interrogate a distressed caller using a set of medically approved questions to elicit essential information about the chief complaint (Figure 8-4). Then, the dispatcher follows established guidelines to determine the appropriate level of response (Figure 8-5). These predetermined guidelines are based on criteria approved by the medical director. For example, an elderly man with a history of heart problems who is complaining of chest pain radiating to his left arm may indicate a high-priority response (life-threatening emergency, lights and siren). In some systems, the appropriate response may include an emergency medical responder (EMR) in a first-responder role, a primary care paramedic (PCP) ambulance, and an advanced care paramedic (ACP) unit. Other systems may require only a paramedic ambulance. This form of call-screening, when done appropriately, saves time and money because only the necessary resources are sent. It also limits the liability associated with a lights and siren response to possible life-threatening incidents. Many private and public EMS systems throughout Canada use the priority dispatching system.

Prearrival Instructions Many EMS systems provide **prearrival instructions,** a service that is considered the standard of care. Prearrival instructions complement the

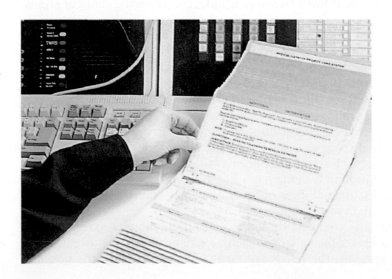

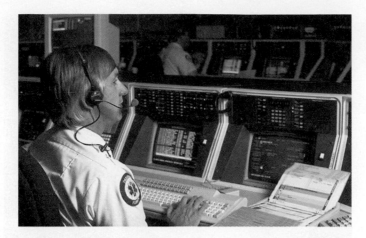

call-screening process in a priority dispatch system. As the dispatcher sends the appropriate response, the caller remains on the line and receives prearrival instructions for suitable emergency measures, such as choking, cardiopulmonary resuscitation, or hemorrhage control. During prearrivals, the dispatcher also can obtain further information for the responding units. In the case of cardiac arrest, the dispatcher can relay information concerning the presence of a living will, a "do not resuscitate" (DNR) form, or other advance directives. In another case, a unit en route to a baby who had stopped breathing could reduce their response speed if they learned that the child had started breathing and was conscious. Prearrival instructions have saved many lives since 1974. They also are useful for comforting a distressed caller or providing emotional support to bystanders, family members, or the patient.

Call Coordination and Incident Recording After sending the appropriate response and providing prearrival instructions, the emergency medical dispatcher's main duties are support and coordination. The dispatcher will provide the responding units with any additional resources needed and record such information about the call as times, locations, and units involved. Your dispatcher can be your best friend. She can assign the resources you need to manage an incident—additional medical personnel to help with a cardiac arrest, for instance, or the fire department to provide specialized rescue. Your dispatcher also may facilitate communication with other agencies, hospitals, communication centres, and support services.

Discussion with Medical Direction Physician After conducting your assessment and initiating care as outlined by your local protocols, you may contact the medical direction physician to discuss the case. Following consultation, the physician may give you further orders for such interventions as medications or other medical procedures. The many ways to conduct this communication include the radio, telephone, and cellular phone. Taping these communications for use later is advisable. For example, if a discrepancy arose as to your orders, you could always refer to the tape. At this point, you continue treatment and prepare your patient for transport. You will contact your dispatcher, who will record when you leave the scene and when you arrive at your destination.

Your professional relationship with your medical direction physicians must be based on trust. Transmitting clear, concise, controlled reports will encourage your medical direction physicians to accept your assessments and on-scene treatment plans. Your ability to communicate effectively on the radio will create a large part of your professional reputation. The general radio procedures and standard format sections later in this chapter offer guidelines for communicating with your medical direction physician and transmitting patient information (Figure 8-6).

Transmitting clear, concise, controlled reports will encourage your medical direction physicians to trust your assessments and on-scene treatment plans.

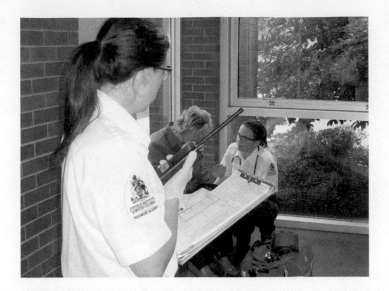

FIGURE 8-6 You will discuss each case with the medical direction physician and follow instructions for patient care.

Transfer Communications As you transfer care of your patient to advanced care crews on to the receiving hospital staff, you must give a formal verbal briefing (Figure 8-7). This report should include your patient's vital information, chief complaint and history, secondary assessment findings, and any treatments rendered. Do not assume that the receiving nurse heard your radio report and knows about your patient. Some systems require the receiving nurse to sign the prehospital care report (PCR) to verify and document the transfer of care. In any case, never leave your patient until you have completed some type of formal transfer of care, as this may be a form of abandonment. Many systems likewise require the medical direction physician to sign the PCR for any medications administered by paramedics, especially if they included controlled substances, such as morphine or diazepam. In all cases, end your documentation with transfer of care information on your PCR.

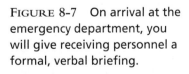

Never leave your patient until you formally transfer responsibility for her care.

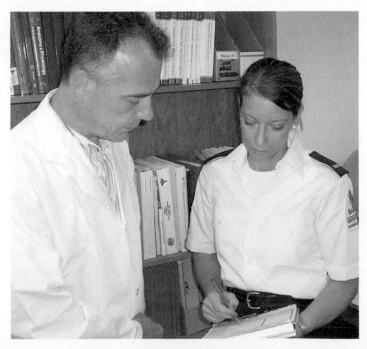

FIGURE 8-7 On arrival at the emergency department, you will give receiving personnel a formal, verbal briefing.

COMMUNICATION TECHNOLOGY

EMS systems can use all of today's various communication technologies. These include the more traditional forms of radio communication as well as innovations in radio technology and other media.

RADIO COMMUNICATION

Many types of radio transmission are possible, with new technologies being developed every day. Usage may vary from system to system. This section discusses some of the more common technologies in use today.

Simplex The most basic communications systems use **simplex** transmissions. These systems transmit and receive on the same frequency and thus cannot do both simultaneously. After you transmit a message, you must release the transmit button and wait for a response. This slows communication because you have to wait for all traffic to stop before you can speak. It also makes the system more formal and prevents open discussion. Simplex communication systems are most effective on the scene, when the incident commander or EMS dispatcher must transmit orders or directions without interruption. Most dispatch systems and on-scene communications use simplex transmissions.

* simplex communication system that transmits and receives on the same frequency.

Duplex **Duplex** transmissions allow simultaneous two-way communications by using two frequencies for each channel. Each radio must be able to transmit and receive on each channel. For example, on channel one, a hospital base station might transmit on 468.000 megahertz (MHz) and receive on 478.000 MHz. Field radios would then transmit on 478.000 MHz and receive on 468.000 MHz—just the opposite. Either party could then transmit and receive on the same channel simultaneously.

* duplex communication system that allows simultaneous two-way communications by using two frequencies for each channel.

Duplex systems work like telephone communications. Many areas use them for communications between the field paramedic and the medical direction physician. The duplex system's major advantage is that one party does not have to wait to speak until the other party finishes a transmission. This allows a much freer discussion and consultation between physician and paramedic. For example, the medical direction physician can interrupt your report with an important question or concern. However, this ability to interrupt can be a disadvantage when abused.

Duplex systems all allow the transmission of either voice messages or data such as ECG strips.

Multiplex **Multiplex** systems are duplex systems with the additional capability of transmitting voice and data simultaneously. This enables you to carry on a conversation with the medical direction physician while you are transmitting an ECG strip. Speaking while you are transmitting the ECG strip, however, causes much interference on the ECG strip.

* multiplex duplex system that can transmit voice and data simultaneously.

Trunking Many communications systems operating in the 800 MHz range use **trunking** to hasten communications. Trunked systems pool all frequencies. When a radio transmission comes in, a computer routes it to the first available frequency. The computer routes the next transmission to the next available frequency, and so on. When a transmission terminates, that frequency becomes available and reenters the pool of unused frequencies. Trunking thus frees the dispatcher or field unit from having to search for an available frequency.

* trunking communication system that pools all frequencies and routes transmissions to the next available frequency.

Digital Communications Voice transmission can be time-consuming and difficult to understand. The trend toward combining radio technology with computer technology has encouraged a shift from voice (analog) to **digital communications.** Digital radio equipment is becoming increasingly popular in emergency services communication systems. This technology translates, or en-

* digital communications data or sounds are translated into a digital code for transmission.

codes, sounds into digital code for broadcast. Digital transmission is much faster and much more accurate than analog transmission. Since the messages are transmitted in condensed form, they help ease the overcrowding of radio frequencies. Also, because you need a decoder to translate digital transmissions back into voice, scanners cannot monitor them. Your communications, therefore, are considerably more secure than over the radio. Many cellular phone companies now use digital transmissions. Future technology will link patient-monitoring devices to a small computer equipped with a radio for transmission.

The **mobile data terminals** in many emergency vehicles are a basic form of digital communications. They are mounted in the vehicle cab and wired to the radio. When a data transmission, such as the address of the incident, comes in, the terminal displays the message on a screen or prints it in hard copy. Responders can reply by punching a button to send a message, such as "en route," "arrived," or "transporting to the hospital." Though somewhat restrictive and primitive, these terminals have reduced on-air time to a minimum even in the busiest systems. It is important to remember, however, that voice communications will always have a place in emergency services. Crew members will always need to speak to one another, to physicians and nurses, or to dispatchers.

ALTERNATIVE TECHNOLOGIES

Among the more common alternatives to radio communications are the cellular telephone, the facsimile machine, and the computer.

Cellular Telephone Many EMS systems have found that **cellular telephones** are a cost-effective way to transmit essential patient information to the hospital (Figure 8-8). Cellular technology is available in even the most remote areas of the country. A cellular telephone service is divided into regions called cells. These cells are radio base stations, with which the mobile telephone communicates. When the transmission leaves one cell's range, another cell picks it up immediately, without interruption.

Like duplex radio transmissions, cellular phones make communication less formal, promote discussion, and reduce online times. They further allow the medical direction physician to speak directly with the patient and offer the advantages of being widely available and highly reliable. Because the ECG signal is digitized, the hospital receives a better signal than if it were transmitted over radio waves. The telephones themselves are inexpensive, but cellular telephone systems charge a monthly fee for their use. Their major disadvantage is that each cell can handle only a limited number of calls. Geography can interfere with the cellular telephone's signals, and in large metropolitan areas, the cells often fill up and become unavailable, especially during peak hours. Another disadvantage is that anyone with a scanner can monitor conversations on analog cellular phones. Despite their limitations, cellular telephones have become a popular medium for dispatching, on-scene, and medical direction communications.

Facsimile A **facsimile machine** (fax) provides a quick way to send printed information. This machine "reads" the printed information, digitizes it line-by-line, and transmits it to another machine, which then decodes it and prints a facsimile of the original. A fax machine enables health-care agencies to exchange medical information immediately. Future systems will allow EMS responders to access a patient's medical record from a general database; responders or database operators will be able to send the same information to the receiving facility. With some electronic call sheet systems, you will be able to transmit your patient information to the receiving hospital long before you arrive. This technology's one obvious limitation is that both the sending and the receiving agency must have access to a fax machine and a telephone line.

* **mobile data terminal** vehicle-mounted computer keyboard and display.

* **cellular telephone system** telephone system divided into regions, or cells, that are served by radio base stations.

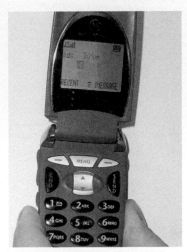

FIGURE 8-8   Cellular telephones allow direct contact with the medical direction physician.

* **facsimile machine** device for electronically transmitting and receiving printed information.

Computer Computers have entered every aspect of our daily lives. In emergency services communications, they have revolutionized system management and incident data collection. Most dispatchers no longer enter data via pen and pencil, time stamping machines, or typewriters. They can make a permanent record of any incident's events in real time. Computers also make research faster and easier. For example, if you wanted to determine the day of the week when most cardiac calls happen, what time of day is busiest, or which area of a city needs more coverage, you could retrieve the pertinent data from your computerized records immediately. You can program your system to provide whatever type of data you want, in whatever format you desire. Computers also eliminate the need to enter retrospective data when conducting research. For example, the times, locations, and particulars of a call already will be in the computer files for immediate retrieval during a research project. A computer's limitations include its own power, speed, and capacity, as well as its operator's ability. Also, rigidly programmed machines that function only in certain restrictive ways can limit your flexibility.

NEW TECHNOLOGY

New technology is being developed every day. The U.S. National Aeronautics and Space Administration (NASA) has pioneered communications that allow television viewers to hear and see astronauts in space. Ground crews can monitor each astronaut's biological function and maintain a permanent record throughout the trip. And they have been doing this for decades.

In comparison with other professions, public safety communication systems are nearly archaic. Most EMS agencies still document patient assessment and care with handwritten call sheets, and some use radio equipment so old that replacement tubes are no longer available. But times are changing rapidly. Time constraints, storage space, and congested radio traffic necessitate developing new systems that will allow paramedics to transmit, receive, and store vital patient information quickly and reliably. Computer-based technology, digital satellite transmission, and electronic storage and retrieval of patient information are replacing radio communications, written documentation, and file cabinets filled with EMS call sheets.

Current documentation systems already allow you to record all aspects of your EMS response electronically, by use of a **touch pad** (see Figure 8-9). With pen-based reporting systems, you can record patient information on a handheld computer. These systems do away with written documentation and capture information in real time, eliminating your need to estimate times after the call. Some systems integrate diagnostic technology and enable you to transmit ECG and pulse oximetry readings to the hospital before arrival. Such advanced knowledge of diagnostic test results from the field may radically change a medical direction physician's decisions and reduce the time needed to make an in-hospital diagnosis and begin therapy. Transmitting a 12-lead ECG, for example, will reduce the time before paramedics in transit or receiving emergency department personnel can begin cardiac muscle–saving thrombolytic therapy for the patient with a suspected myocardial infarction. In some cases, paramedics will be able to start therapy en route. Other systems allow you to receive important medical information from your patient's permanent record while on the scene or in transit (see Figure 8-10). For instance, at the home of a patient with an altered mental status and no family to relate her history, you might access her medical records and attain her history via a computerized database. In this type of system, the transferring facility, the receiving hospital, and you can all access this information simultaneously.

A disadvantage of electronic recording systems is the absence of a "paper record" of the incident, should the information be accidentally erased or destroyed.

✱ touch pad computer on which you enter data by touching areas of the display screen.

> *One of your most important skills will be gathering essential patient information, organizing it, and relaying it to the medical direction physician.*

The legal guidelines that apply to written and spoken communication also apply to electronic reporting. You must maintain patient confidentiality, you must be objective, and you must not **slander** or **libel** another person.

REPORTING PROCEDURES

As a paramedic, you must effectively relay all relevant medical information to the receiving hospital staff. Initially, you might do this over the radio or by cellular telephone. Later, when you deliver your patient to the emergency department, you can give additional information in-person to the appropriate receiving hospital personnel.

One of your most important skills will be gathering essential patient information, organizing it, and relaying it to the medical direction physician. The medical direction physician will then issue appropriate orders for patient care. The amount and type of information you relay to the medical direction physician will depend on the type of technology you use, your patient's priority, and your local communication **protocols**. For example, if communications in your region are not secure (private), you must limit the type of information you can communicate without breaching patient confidentiality. The acuteness of your patient's clinical status and the amount of local radio traffic also may determine the length of your report. For a critical patient, you may give a brief report while you tend to your patient's medical needs. For a complicated medical emergency, you may want to communicate a greater share of the results of your history and physical assessment to the medical direction physician.

STANDARD FORMAT

Communicating patient information to other EMS crews, to the hospital, or to the medical direction physician is a crucial function within the EMS system. Verbal communications, which may occur via radio or land line, give the hospital enough information on your patient's condition to prepare for her care. These

FIGURE 8-9 Tablet computers are used to create an electronic PCR.

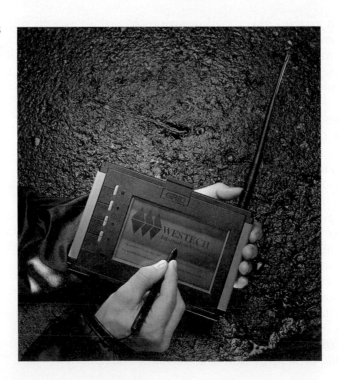

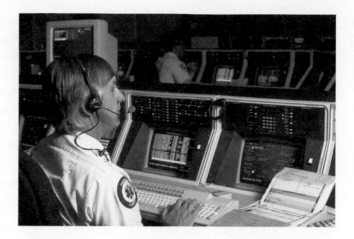

FIGURE 8-10 Computer-assisted dispatch systems (CAD) automate many data-collection tasks.

communications also should initiate the medical orders you need to treat your patient in the field. A standard format for transmitting patient assessment information helps achieve those goals in several ways. First, it adds to the medical communications system's efficiency. Second, it helps the physician assimilate information about the patient's condition quickly. Third, it ensures that medical information is complete. In general, your verbal reports to medical direction should include the following information:

- Identification of unit and provider
- Description of scene
- Patient's age, sex, and approximate weight (for drug orders)
- Patient's chief complaint and its severity
- Brief, pertinent history of the present illness or injury (e.g., OPQRST)
- Pertinent past medical history, medications, and allergies (e.g., SAMPLE)
- Pertinent secondary assessment findings
- Treatment given so far/request for orders
- Response to treatment
- Estimated time of arrival at the hospital
- Other pertinent information

The formats and contents of reports for medical and trauma patients include only the information relevant to either type of emergency. Reports for medical patients emphasize the history in the beginning of the report; reports for trauma patients emphasize the injuries and the secondary assessment.

After transmitting your report, you will await further questions and orders from the medical direction physician. On arrival, your spoken report will give essential patient information to the provider assuming care. It should include a brief history, pertinent physical findings, treatment, and responses to that treatment.

GENERAL RADIO PROCEDURES

Using the radio properly will make your communications skillful and efficient. All your transmissions must be clear and crisp, with concise, professional content (Figure 8-11). Always follow these guidelines for effective radio use:

1. Listen to the channel before transmitting to ensure that it is not in use.
2. Press the transmit button for one second before speaking.

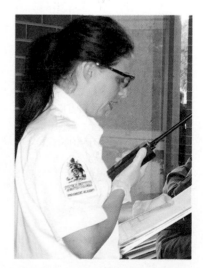

FIGURE 8-11 The professionalism of your communications reflects the professionalism of your patient care.

3. Speak at close range, approximately 5–8 cm from the microphone, directly into, or across the face of, the microphone.

4. Speak slowly and clearly. Pronounce each word distinctly, avoiding words that are difficult to understand.

5. Speak in a normal pitch, keeping your voice free from emotion.

6. Be brief. Know what you are going to say before you press the transmit button.

7. Avoid codes unless they are part of your EMS system.

8. Do not waste airtime with unnecessary information.

9. Protect your patient's privacy. When appropriate:
   - Use a telephone rather than the radio.
   - Turn off external speaker.
   - Do not use your patient's name.

10. Use proper unit or hospital numbers and correct names or titles.

11. Do not use slang or profanity.

12. Use standard formats for transmission.

13. Be concise in order to hold the attention of the person receiving your radio report.

14. Use the **echo procedure** when receiving directions from the dispatcher or orders from the physician. Immediately repeating each statement will confirm accurate reception and understanding.

15. Always write down addresses, important dispatch communications, and physician orders.

16. When completing a transmission, obtain confirmation that your message was received and understood.

* **echo procedure** immediately repeating each transmission received during radio communications.

Occasionally, communications equipment will not function properly. Even a weak battery can disrupt clear communication. If you are far from the base station, particularly if you have a portable radio, try to broadcast from higher terrain. Structures that contain steel and concrete can interfere with radio transmission. Simply moving outside the building or near a window may improve communications. If that does not work, try to telephone.

MODEL VERBAL REPORTS

The following examples demonstrate professional verbal reports for a medical patient and for a trauma patient. Neither report takes more than 45 seconds, and each gives the medical direction physician enough information to make an initial diagnosis and prepare for arrival. As you read them, consider how they follow the principles of effective communication discussed throughout this chapter, and note their differences in format and information.

Medical Patient

Paramedic Identification: This is Medic 4, Paramedic Smith.

Patient Identification: We have a 63-year-old, 70-kg alert male.

Subjective Data: He complains of sudden onset of substernal chest pain radiating to the neck for the past half hour. He also complains of shortness of breath and nausea. He has a past history of cardiac problems and takes nitroglycerine, Isordil, and Adalat XL.

Content Review

ELEMENTS OF MEDICAL PATIENT REPORT
- Paramedic identification
- Patient identification
- Subjective data
- Objective data
- Plan

Objective Data: He appears in moderate distress at this time, clutching his chest but able to speak in full sentences. Vitals: BP—138/80; pulse—88 and regular; respirations 24 and slightly laboured; skin warm and dry. He has clear lung sounds bilaterally, no JVD, peripheral edema, or ascites. ECG shows sinus rhythm with an occasional unifocal PVC. Pulse oximetry is 92 percent on room air.

Plan: We have him on oxygen at 15 litres per minute via nonrebreather mask, we have a saline lock in place, and have given him 2 baby aspirin and 3 nitro with no relief. Request permission to administer 2.5 milligrams of morphine IV until relief of pain. Our ETA is 20 minutes.

Trauma Patient

Paramedic Identification: This is Rescue 7, Paramedic Jones.

Patient Identification: We have a 23-year-old unresponsive female.

Mechanism of Injury: She was the unbelted driver in a high-speed, head-on one-car versus telephone pole accident with severe damage to the car and intrusion into the passenger compartment.

Injuries: She has major head and chest trauma and shows signs of decompensated shock. Vitals are BP—76 by palpation; pulse—120 weak and regular, carotid only; respirations 40 and shallow; skin cool, pale, and clammy. She has a depressed skull fracture in the left parietal region and a right-sided flail chest. Her pupils are unequal and slow to react, no drainage from the ears or nose, no Battle's sign or raccoon eyes. Trachea is midline, no JVD. She shows paradoxical chest wall movement and is cyanotic with diminished lung sounds on the right side. Pulse oximetry is 88 percent on room air.

Plan: We have the patient fully immobilized, have stabilized the flail segment, and are assisting ventilation with a bag-valve mask and supplemental oxygen. We have an IV of normal saline running wide open and are starting a second line. Our ETA is 20 minutes.

REGULATION

Radio communications and procedures are regulated by Industry Canada. The Spectrum Management branch establishes radio frequency guidelines and technical specifications for the use of radio communications. Public safety frequencies generally are assigned operating frequencies in the **very high frequency** band

✻ **very high frequency** radio frequency band from 30 to 300 megahertz

(VHF) and the ultrahigh frequency band (UHF). EMS communications must follow all appropriate governmental regulations and laws. Individual EMS operators may establish additional policy and procedures for radio communications. Ensure that you are familiar with federal and local policies and regulations.

SUMMARY

As one of the fundamental aspects of prehospital care, accurate communications help ensure an EMS system's efficiency. Communications begin when the citizen accesses the EMS system and end when you complete your patient report. Your spoken messages must be understandable, and your written messages must be legible. All your communications must be concise and complete and conform to national and local protocols. The more sophisticated and advanced your EMS system grows, the more sophisticated and advanced its communications—and, accordingly, your communications skills—must become.

CHAPTER 9

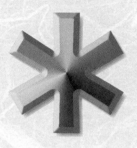

Documentation

Objectives

After reading this chapter, you should be able to:

1. Identify the general principles regarding the importance of EMS documentation and ways in which documents are used. (pp. 412–414)
2. Identify and properly use medical terminology, medical abbreviations, and acronyms. (pp. 415, 417–420)
3. Explain the role of documentation in agency reimbursement. (p. 413)
4. Identify and eliminate extraneous or nonprofessional information. (p. 425)
5. Describe the differences between subjective and objective elements of documentation. (pp. 425–427)
6. Evaluate a finished document for errors and omissions and proper use and spelling of abbreviations and acronyms. (pp. 422, 424–425)
7. Evaluate the confidential nature of an EMS report. (p. 435)
8. Describe the potential consequences of illegible, incomplete, or inaccurate documentation. (pp. 422, 424–425)

Continued

Objectives Continued

9. Describe the special documentation considerations concerning patient refusal of care or transport. (pp. 431–432)
10. Demonstrate how to properly record direct patient or bystander comments. (p. 421)
11. Describe the special considerations concerning mass-casualty incident documentation. (p. 433)
12. Demonstrate proper document revision and correction. (p. 424)
13. Identify the types and describe the key elements of other professional correspondence. (p. 434)
14. Given a prehospital care report and a narrative patient care scenario, record all pertinent administrative information, using a consistent format; identify and record the pertinent, reportable clinical data for each patient; correct errors and omissions, using proper procedures; and note and record "pertinent negative" clinical findings. (pp. 412–435)

INTRODUCTION

Document exactly what you did, when you did it, and the effects of your interventions.

Your PCR reflects your professionalism.

Treating your patient and documenting your findings and actions are separate but equally important duties. The written prehospital care record (PCR) is known by many names, including the ambulance call report (ACR), call report, and crew report. Your PCR is often the only documented record of what happened on your call. When completed correctly, it describes your assessment and treatment throughout the call. It documents what you did on the call, what you found, what actions you took, and the results of your interventions. It can be your best friend or your worst enemy in a court proceeding.

Your PCR is your sole permanent, complete written record of events during the ambulance call. The dispatch centre may have a record of the call times and audio tapes of radio transmissions, and your patient will have his memory of the call. You and other responders also may have some recollections about the call. Your PCR, however, will always be considered the most comprehensive and reliable record of the event. In addition, it reflects your professionalism. A well-written, thorough PCR suggests a thorough, efficient assessment and quality care. A sloppy, incomplete PCR suggests sloppy, inefficient care.

USES FOR DOCUMENTATION

Your PCR will be a valuable resource for a variety of people. They include medical professionals, EMS administrators, researchers, and occasionally, lawyers.

MEDICAL

Hospital staff (nurses and physicians) may need more information from you than they can get before you have to take another call. For example, they may want a chronological account of your patient's mental status from the time you arrived on the scene. Your PCR can tell the emergency department staff of your patient's condition before he arrived at the hospital. It serves as a baseline for comparing assessment findings and detecting trends that indicate improvement or deterioration. The surgical staff will want to know the mechanism of injury and other pertinent findings during your primary assessment of your patient and the scene.

If your patient is admitted to the hospital, the floor or intensive care unit staff may need more information about his original condition than he can remember. In addition, your PCR provides staff with information from people at the scene to whom they might not have access—family, bystanders, emergency medical responders, or other witnesses. Knowing about the circumstances that led to the event or the mechanism of injury may also help rehabilitation specialists to provide better therapy. Your PCR becomes an important document that helps ensure your patient's continuous effective care (Figure 9-1).

ADMINISTRATIVE

EMS administrators must gather information for quality improvement and system management. Information regarding **response times,** call location, the use of lights and siren, and date and time is vital to evaluating your system's readiness to respond to life-threatening emergencies. It also is essential to evaluating community needs. The quality improvement or quality assurance committee will use PCRs to identify problems with individual paramedics or with the EMS system. In some agencies, the billing department will need to determine which services are billable. Insurance carriers may need to know more about the illness or injury to process the claim. Some provinces and territories may use your PCR data to allocate funding for regional systems.

RESEARCH

Your PCR may give researchers useful data about many aspects of the EMS call. For example, researchers may analyze your recorded data to determine the efficacy of medical devices or such interventions as drugs and invasive procedures.

Your PCR is an important document that helps ensure your patient's continuity of care.

* response time time between when a unit is alerted until it arrives on the scene.

RESPONSE INFORMATION		TIMES					KILOMETERS				
RESPONSE NUMBER	GEOCODES	CALL RECEIVED	0	8	1	0	START	1 6		1 6 5	
1 5 5 2 4 5	D 45	EN ROUTE	0	8	1	1	SCENE	1 6		1 6 8	
RESPOND TO:		ARRIVAL SCENE	0	8	1	5	DESTINATION	1 6		1 7 4	
95946 117A STREET		TO DESTINATION	0	8	2	9	QUARTERS	1 6		1 7 8	
AT THE REAR		AT DESTINATION	0	8	4	3	RESPONSE MODE				
NATURE OF CALL		CLEAR	0	9	0	2	TO SCENE ② Ⓧ CHANGED ② ③				
CHEST PAIN, CARDIAC		QUARTERS	0	9	1	0	TO DESTINATION Ⓧ ③ CHANGED ② ③				
RESEARCH CODES		Ⓧ CARDIAC ○ COLLAPSE ○ TRAUMA	○ RESPIRATORY ○ FOUND DOWN ○ MVA	○ ABDOMINAL ○ ANAPHYLAXIS ○ ASSAULT	○ NEURO ○ DIABETIC ○ OTHER TRAUMA	○ OD/ETOCH ○ OBS/GYN ○ OTHER					

FIGURE 9-1   The information in a prehospital care report is vital to your agency's efforts to improve patient care.

FIGURE 9-2 The handheld electronic clipboard enables you to enter your prehospital care report directly into a computer.

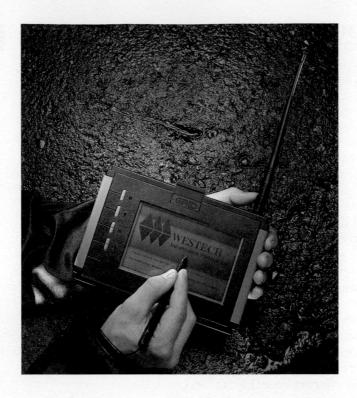

FIGURE 9-2 The handheld electronic clipboard enables you to enter your prehospital care report directly into a computer.

They also may use the data to cut costs, alter staffing, and shorten response times. Some systems use computerized or electronic PCRs and a computerized database to analyze the data (Figure 9-2). Regardless of the method you use, your written documentation provides the basis for continually improving patient care in your EMS system.

LEGAL

Your PCR becomes a permanent part of your patient's medical record. Lawyers may refer to it when preparing court actions, and in a legal proceeding, it might be your sole source of information about the case. You may be called on to testify in a case in which your PCR becomes the central piece of evidence in your testimony. Or your PCR may serve as evidence in a criminal case and help determine the accused's innocence or guilt. Each province or territory has its own laws regarding the length of time records must be kept.

Always write your PCR as if you knew you would have to refer to it someday in a court proceeding. Describe your patient's condition when you arrived and during your care, and note his status on arrival at the hospital. Always document your patient's condition before and after any interventions, and avoid writing any subjective opinions, such as "the patient is intoxicated, obnoxious, and looks like a crack-addict." After your PCR is written, ask your partner to review it for completeness and accuracy. A complete, accurate, and objective account of the emergency call may be your best and only defence against a plaintiff's attorney who will try to find inconsistencies and ambiguities in your account.

GENERAL CONSIDERATIONS

Every EMS system has its own specific requirements for documentation. The type of call record used also varies from system to system. Some systems use re-

Your PCR provides the basis for continually improving patient care in your EMS system.

A complete, accurate, and objective account of the emergency call may be your best and only defence in court.

ports with check boxes, and some use **bubble sheets,** computer-scannable reports on which you record patient information by filling in boxes or "bubbles" (Figure 9-3). Still others may use computerized documentation. The particular type of operational data collected, such as time intervals, will also differ among systems. For example, proprietary EMS agencies may require more billing information than do community-based volunteer agencies. The general characteristics of a well-written PCR, though, remain constant among all agencies and systems.

MEDICAL TERMINOLOGY

An essential component of good documentation is the appropriate use of medical terminology. Medical terms, though sometimes difficult to spell, transform your report into a universally accepted medical document. Learning the meanings and correct spellings of the medical terms that you will use in your PCRs is essential. Misused or misspelled words reflect poorly on your professionalism and may confuse the report's readers.

If you do not know how to spell a word, look it up or use another word. Many paramedics carry pocket-size medical dictionaries in their ambulances for this purpose. Using "plain English" is acceptable when you do not know the appropriate medical term or its correct spelling. "Chest" is just as accurate as "thorax" and better than "thoracks." "Belly" is not as professional as "abdomen," but it is still better than "abodemin."

ABBREVIATIONS AND ACRONYMS

Medical abbreviations and acronyms allow you to increase the amount of information you can write quickly on your report (Table 9-1 on pages 417–420). They also pose problems, however, because they can have multiple meanings. For instance, their meanings can vary in different areas of medicine. Is "CP" chest pain, cardiovascular perfusion, or cerebral palsy? Is "CO" cardiac output or carbon monoxide? Is "BLS" basic life support or burns, lacerations, and swelling? These are all common abbreviations for more than one accepted term. Furthermore, many abbreviations are specific to one community. You must be familiar with those used in your local EMS system.

Abbreviations and acronyms can cause considerable confusion when someone unfamiliar with the call reads your report. Health-care professionals who are not familiar with local customs or with emergency medicine might not understand them. One way to clarify the meaning of a new abbreviation or acronym is to write it out the first time you use it, followed by the abbreviation or acronym in parenthesis. After that, you can use only the abbreviation throughout the report. The following examples illustrate how abbreviations and acronyms can shorten your narratives. In standard English, the report might be written as follows:

> The patient is a 54-year-old conscious and alert male who complains of sudden onset of chest pain and shortness of breath which started 20 minutes ago. He has taken 2 nitroglycerine with no relief. He denies any nausea, vomiting, or dizziness. He has a past history of coronary artery disease, a heart attack 3 years ago, and high blood pressure. He takes nitroglycerine as needed, Adalat XL, hydrochlorothiazide, and potassium. He has no known drug allergies.

Using abbreviations and acronyms, the same report might be written as:

> Pt. is 54 y/o CAO male c/o sudden onset CP/SOB × 20 min. Pt took NTG × 2 s̄ relief. ∅ n/v, dizziness. PH: CAD, AMI × 3y, HTN. Meds: NTG prn, Adalat XL, HCTZ and K^+; NKDA.

Content Review

CHARACTERISTICS OF A WELL-WRITTEN PCR

- Appropriate medical terminology and correct spelling
- Correct abbreviations and acronyms
- Accurate, consistent times
- Thoroughly documented communications
- Pertinent negatives
- Relevant oral statements of witnesses, bystanders, and patient
- Complete identification of all additional resources and personnel

bubble sheet scannable call sheet on which you fill in boxes or "bubbles" to record assessment and care information.

If you do not know how to spell a word, look it up or use another word.

You must be familiar with your local EMS system's acronyms and abbreviations.

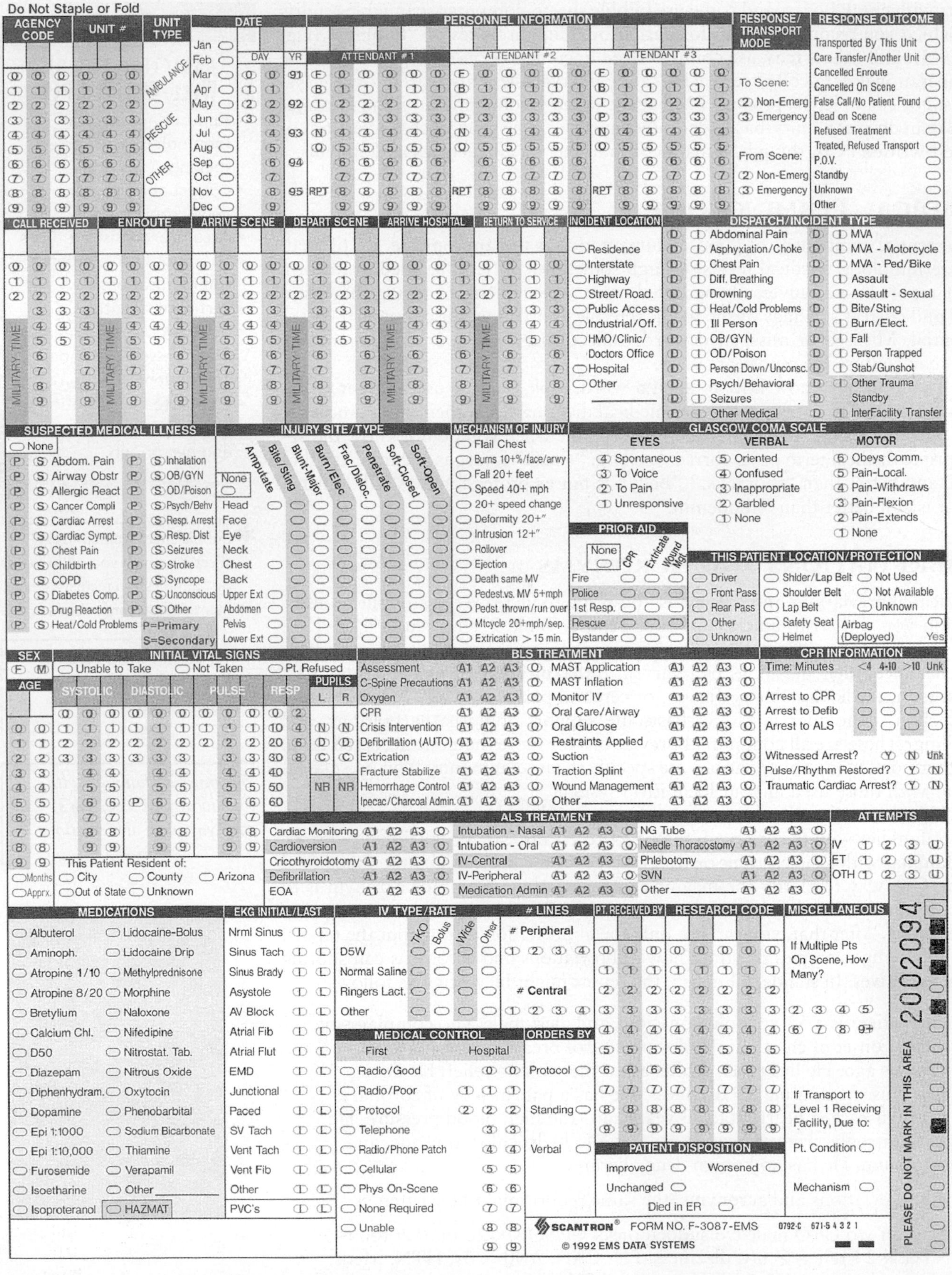

FIGURE 9-3   This prehospital care report's format allows a computer to scan its information.

Table 9-1   STANDARD CHARTING ABBREVIATIONS

Patient Information/Categories

Asian	A	Medications	Med, Rx
Black	B	Newborn	NB
Chief complaint	CC	Occupational history	OH
Complains of	c/o	Past history	PH
Current health status	CHS	Patient	Pt
Date of birth	DOB	Physical exam	PE
Differential diagnosis	DD	Private medical doctor	PMD
Estimated date of confinement	EDC	Review of systems	ROS
Family history	FH	Signs and symptoms	S/S
Female	♀	Social history	SH
Hispanic	H	Visual acuity	VA
History	Hx	Vital signs	VS
History and physical	H&P	Weight	Wt
History of present illness	HPI	White	W
Impression	IMP	Year-old	y/o
Male	♂		

Body Systems

Abdomen	Abd	Gynecological	GYN
Cardiovascular	CV	Head, eyes, ears, nose, and throat	HEENT
Central nervous system	CNS	Musculoskeletal	M/S
Ear, nose, and throat	ENT	Obstetrical	OB
Gastrointestinal	GI	Peripheral nervous system	PNS
Genitourinary	GU	Respiratory	Resp

Common Complaints

Abdominal pain	abd pn	Lower back pain	LBP
Chest pain	CP	Nausea/vomiting	n/v
Dyspnea on exertion	DOE	No apparent distress	NAD
Fever of unknown origin	FUO	Pain	pn
Gunshot wound	GSW	Shortness of breath	SOB
Headache	H/A	Substernal chest pain	sscp

Diagnoses

Abdominal aortic aneurysm	AAA	Infectious disease	ID
Abortion	Ab	Inferior wall myocardial infarction	IWMI
Acute myocardial infarction	AMI	Insulin-dependent diabetes mellitus	IDDM
Adult respiratory distress syndrome	ARDS	Intracranial pressure	ICP
Alcohol	ETOH	Mass-casualty incident	MCI
Atherosclerotic heart disease	ASHD	Mitral valve prolapse	MVP
Cerebral vascular accident (stroke)	CVA	Motor-vehicle collision	MVC
Chronic obstructive pulmonary disease	COPD	Multiple sclerosis	MS
Chronic renal failure	CRF	Non-insulin-dependent diabetes mellitus	NIDDM
Congestive heart failure	CHF	Organic brain syndrome	OBS
Coronary artery bypass graft	CABG	Otitis media	OM
Coronary artery disease	CAD	Overdose	OD
Cystic fibrosis	CF	Paroxysmal nocturnal dyspnea	PND
Dead on arrival	DOA	Pelvic inflammatory disease	PID
Delirium tremens	DTs	Peptic ulcer disease	PUD
Deep vein thrombosis	DVT	Pregnancies/Births *(gravida/para)*	G/P
Diabetes mellitus	DM	Pregnancy-induced hypertension	PIH
Dilation and curettage	D&C	Pulmonary embolism	PE
Duodenal ulcer	DU	Rheumatic heart disease	RHD
End-stage renal failure	ESRF	Sexually transmitted disease	STD
Epstein-Barr virus	EBV	Transient ischemic attack	TIA
Foreign body obstruction	FBO	Tuberculosis	TB
Fracture	Fx, #	Upper respiratory infection	URI
Hepatitis B virus	HBV	Urinary tract infection	UTI
Hiatal hernia	HH	Venereal disease	VD
Hypertension	HTN	Wolff-Parkinson-White syndrome (disease)	WPW

Table 9-1 STANDARD CHARTING ABBREVIATIONS (continued)

Medications

Angiotensin-converting enzyme	ACE	Lactated Ringer's, Ringer's Lactate	LR, RL
Aspirin	ASA	Magnesium sulphate	Mg^{++}
Bicarbonate	HCO_3^-	Morphine sulphate	MS
Birth control pills	BCP	Nitroglycerine	NTG
Calcium	Ca^{++}	Nonsteroidal anti-inflammatory agent	NSAID
Calcium channel blocker	CCB	Normal saline	NS
Calcium chloride	$CaCl_2$	Penicillin	PCN
Chloride	Cl^-	Phenobarbital	PB
Digoxin	Dig	Potassium	K^+
Dilantin (phenytoin sodium)	DPH	Sodium bicarbonate	$NaHCO_3$
Diphendydramine	DPHM	Sodium chloride	NaCl
Diphtheria-Pertussis-Tetanus	DPT	Tylenol	APAP
Hydrochlorothiazide	HCTZ		

Anatomy/Landmarks

Abdomen	Abd	Lymph node	LN
Antecubital	AC	Medial collateral ligament	MCL
Anterior axillary line	AAL	Metacarpalphalangeal (joint)	MCP
Anterior cruciate ligament	ACL	Metatarsalphalangeal (joint)	MTP
Anterior-posterior	A/P	Midaxillary line	MAL
Distal interphalangeal (joint)	DIP	Posterior axillary line	PAL
Dorsalis pedis (pulse)	DP	Posterior cruciate ligament	PCL
Gallbladder	GB	Proximal interphalangeal (joint)	PIP
Intercostal space	ICS	Right lower lobe	RLL
Lateral collateral ligament	LCL	Right lower quadrant	RLQ
Left lower lobe	LLL	Right middle lobe	RML
Left lower quadrant	LLQ	Right upper lobe	RUL
Left upper lobe	LUL	Right upper quadrant	RUQ
Left upper quadrant	LUQ	Temporomandibular joint	TMJ
Left ventricle	LV	Tympanic membrane	TM
Liver, spleen, and kidneys	LSK		

Physical Assessment/Findings

Arterial blood gas	ABG	Hemoglobin	Hgb
Bilateral breath sounds	BBS	Inspiratory	Insp
Blood sugar	BS	Jugular venous distention	JVD
Breath sounds	BS	Laceration	lac
Cardiac injury profile	CIP	Level of awareness	LOA
Central venous pressure	CVP	Level of consciousness	LOC
Cerebrospinal fluid	CSF	Moves all extremities (well)	MAEW
Chest X-ray	CXR	Nontender	NT
Complete blood count	CBC	Normal range of motion	NROM
Computerized tomography	CT	Palpation	Palp
Conscious, alert, and oriented	CAO	Passive range of motion	PROM
Costovertebral angle	CVA	Point of maximal impulse	PMI
Deep tendon reflexes	DTR	Posterior tibial (pulse)	PT
Dorsalis pedis (pulse)	DP	Pulse	P
Electrocardiogram	EKG, ECG	Pupils equal and reactive to light	PEARL
Electroencephalogram	EEG	Pupils equal, round, reactive to light	
Expiratory	Exp	and accommodation	PERRLA
Extraocular movements (intact)	EOMI	Range of motion	ROM
Fetal heart tones	FHT	Respirations	R
Full range of motion	FROM	Tactile vocal fremitus	TVF
Full-term normal delivery	FTND	Temperature	T
Heart rate	HR	Unconscious	unc
Heart sounds	HS	Urinary incontinence	UI
Heel-to-shin (cerebellar test)	H→S		

Table 9-1 STANDARD CHARTING ABBREVIATIONS (continued)

Miscellaneous Descriptors

After (post-)	$\bar{p}$	Not applicable	n/a
After eating	pc	Number	No or #
Alert and oriented	A/O	Occasional	occ
Anterior	ant.	Pack per years	pk/yrs, p/y
Approximate	≈	Per	/
As needed	prn	Positive	+
Before (ante-)	$\bar{a}$	Posterior	post.
Before eating (*ante cibum,* before meal)	ac	Postoperative	PO
Body surface area (%)	BSA	Prior to arrival	PTA
Celsius	C°	Radiates to	→
Change	Δ	Right	®
Decreased	↓	Rule out	R/O
Equal	=	Secondary to	2°
Fahrenheit	F°	Superior	sup.
Immediately	stat	Times (for 3 hours)	× (×3h)
Increased	↑	Unequal	≠
Inferior	inf.	Warm and dry	W/D
Left	Ⓛ	While awake	WA
Less than	<	With (*cum*)	$\bar{c}$
Moderate	mod.	Within normal limits (*or* we never looked)	WNL
More than	>	Without (*sine*)	$\bar{s}$
Negative	−	Zero	0
No, not, none	Ø		

Treatments/Dispositions

Advanced cardiac life support	ACLS	Nasogastric	NG
Advanced life support	ALS	Nasopharyngeal airway	NPA
Against medical advice	AMA	No transport—refusal	NTR
Automated external defibrillator	AED	Nonrebreather mask	NRM
Bag-valve mask	BVM	Nothing by mouth	NPO
Basic life support	BLS	Occupational therapy	OT
Cardiopulmonary resuscitation	CPR	Oropharyngeal airway	OPA
Carotid sinus massage	CSM	Oxygen	O_2
Continuous positive airway pressure	CPAP	Per square inch	psi
Do not resuscitate	DNR	Physical therapy	PT
Endotracheal tube	ETT	Positive end-expiratory pressure	PEEP
Estimated time of arrival	ETA	Short spine board	SSB
External cardiac pacing	ECP	Therapy (drug)	Rx
Intermittent positive-pressure ventilation	IPPV	Treatment	Tx
Long spine board	LSB	Turned over to	TOT
Nasal cannula	NC	Verbal order	VO

Medication Administration/Metrics

Centimetre	cm	Kilogram	kg
Cubic centimetre	cc	Litre	L
Decilitre	dL	Litres per minute	LPM, L/min
Drop(s)	gtt(s)	Microgram	µg
Drops per minute	gtts/min	Milliequivalent	mEq
Every	q	Milligram	mg
Grain	gr	Millilitre	mL
Gram	g, gm	Millimetre	mm
Hour	h, hr, or °	Millimetres of mercury	mmHg
Hydrogen-ion concentration	pH	Minute	min
Intracardiac	IC	Orally	po
Intramuscular	IM	Subcutaneous	SC, SQ
Intraosseous	IO	Sublingual	SL
Intravenous	IV	To keep open	TKO
Intravenous push	IVP	To keep vein open	TKVO
Joules	j		
Keep vein open	KVO		

| Table 9-1 | STANDARD CHARTING ABBREVIATIONS (continued) |

Cardiology

Atrial fibrillation	AF	Paroxsysmal atrial tachycardia	PAT
Atrial tachycardia	AT	Paroxsysmal supraventricular tachycardia	PSVT
Atrioventricular	AV	Premature atrial contraction	PAC
Bundle branch block	BBB	Premature junctional contraction	PJC
Complete heart block	CHB	Premature ventricular contraction	PVC
Electromechanical dissociation	EMD	Pulseless electrical activity	PEA
Idioventricular rhythm	IVR	Supraventricular tachycardia	SVT
Junctional rhythm	JR	Ventricular fibrillation	VF
Modified chest lead	MCL	Ventricular tachycardia	VT
Normal sinus rhythm	NSR	Wandering atrial pacemaker	WAP

The times you record on your PCR are considered the official times of the incident. For medical and legal purposes, you must ensure their accuracy.

TIMES

Incident times are another important but tricky part of the PCR. The times you record on your PCR are considered the official times of the incident. For medical and legal purposes, you must ensure their accuracy.

The PCR typically has spaces for the time the call was received, the dispatch time, the time of arrival at the scene, time of departure from the scene, time of arrival at the hospital, and time back in service. Other time intervals are important, as well. The time you and your crew arrived at the patient's side is often very different from the time the ambulance arrived at the scene—when your patient is on the fourth floor of a building without an elevator, for example, or in a field several hundred metres from the road. Whatever the reason, document in your report any significant discrepancies between your arrival at the scene and your arrival at the patient's side. The times of vital signs assessment, medication administration, certain medical procedures as local protocols require, and changes in patient condition are also important and require accurate documentation.

One common problem with documenting times is inconsistencies among the dispatch centre clock, the ambulance clock, and your watch. Imagine a report that documents that the ambulance arrived on scene at 20:32 according to the dispatch time, that CPR was started at 20:29 according to your watch, and the first defibrillation was administered at 20:43 according to the defibrillator's internal clock. Although we may recognize this phenomenon and tend to discount the accuracy of the recorded times, they are nonetheless the official, legal times. Whenever possible, therefore, record all times from the same clock. When that is not possible, be sure that all the clocks and watches you use are synchronized. If they cannot be synchronized and the documented times seem to conflict with each other, explain this in your narrative. A simple statement, such as "All time intervals on the scene were documented using my watch, all other times are those reported by the dispatch centre" will suffice.

Whenever possible, record all times from the same clock.

COMMUNICATIONS

Your communications with the hospital are another important item to document. Though your system may make voice recordings of those communications, the recordings are usually not kept indefinitely. Again, the PCR will likely be the only permanent record of your discussion with the medical direction physician. Specifically, you should document any medical advice or orders you receive and the results of implementing that advice and those orders. In some situations, you might need to document what you reported to the physician or discussed with him so that the reader will be able to understand the decision-making process.

Document any medical advice or orders you receive and the results of implementing the advice or orders.

Finally, always document the physician's name on your PCR, and, if possible, have him sign it to verify your treatments.

PERTINENT NEGATIVES

The patient assessment and medical interventions are the essence of the EMS event and become the core of your PCR. We will discuss specific approaches to documenting assessment and interventions later in this chapter, but some general rules apply regardless of the method used.

Document all findings of your assessment, even those that are normal. Although the positive findings are usually of most interest, some negative findings—known as pertinent negatives—are also important. For example, if your respiratory distress patient does not have swollen ankles or crackles, that helps rule out a field diagnosis of congestive heart failure. Or if your patient with a broken leg does not have loss of sensory or motor function, it suggests he has no serious neurological injury. You should include such information in your report.

The pertinent negatives vary for each chief complaint. In general, if a positive assessment finding for any given chief complaint would be important, a negative finding probably is pertinent. Even though these findings do not warrant medical care or intervention, your seeking them demonstrates the thoroughness of your assessment and history of the event.

Document all findings of your assessment, even those that are normal.

ORAL STATEMENTS

Also essential to every PCR, regardless of approach, are the statements of witnesses, bystanders, and your patient. These statements help document the mechanism of injury, your patient's behaviour, the events leading up to the emergency, and any first aid or medical care others rendered before you arrived. The statements also may include information regarding the disposition of personal items, such as wallets or purses. At crime scenes, document safety-related information, such as weapons disposition. Your PCR may be the only written report of what happened to a murder weapon. Other details, such as where you first saw a victim, what position he was in, and the time you arrived on the scene, may be crucial evidence someday in a criminal proceeding.

Whenever possible, quote the patient—or other source of information—directly. Clearly identify the quotation with quotation marks, and identify its source. For example:

> Bystanders state the patient was "acting bizarre and threatening to jump in front of the next passing car."

ADDITIONAL RESOURCES

Document all the resources involved in the event. If an air-medical service transported your patient, your documentation should include your assessment and all interventions up to the point at which you transferred care. Identify the air-medical service and your patient's ultimate destination, if you know it. If other EMS, fire, rescue/extrication, or law enforcement agencies were involved in the call, document their roles. This can be particularly important in mutual aid calls, when many different agencies cooperate in your patient's care. Also, include personnel from the coroner's or medical examiner's office for dead-on-arrival (DOA) scenes.

If a physician stops to help, document his name and qualifications. If one of your medical direction physicians is on the scene and directs care, document his activities. Likewise, document the names, credentials, and activities of any other medically qualified personnel present who offer to help. Your clinical experience and local protocols will determine how you integrate qualified health-care workers into your emergency scene. Document that integration carefully.

ELEMENTS OF GOOD DOCUMENTATION

Content Review

ELEMENTS OF GOOD DOCUMENTATION

• Accuracy
• Legibility
• Timeliness
• Absence of alterations
• Professionalism

A well-written PCR is accurate, legible, timely, unaltered, and professional. Each of these traits is essential.

COMPLETENESS AND ACCURACY

The accurate PCR should be precise but comprehensive. Include all the relevant information that anyone might be expected to want later, and exclude superfluous information. For example, if your patient's foot was run over by a lawn mower, reporting that his great toe on that foot had been amputated six years ago would be important; documenting that he had his tonsils removed when he was three years old probably would not. That you applied direct pressure to the bleeding foot is pertinent; that the lawn mower was a John Deere model 6354 is not.

Many PCRs provide check boxes and a space for written codes narratives (Figure 9-4). You should complete both the narrative and the check-box sections of every PCR. All check-box sections of a document must show that you attended to them, even if you did not use a given section on a call. The check boxes can help ensure that routine, common information is recorded for every call, but no PCR has a check box for every possible chief complaint, assessment finding, or intervention. Some PCRs use codes to document common findings and actions.

The narrative is the core of the documentation. Even if you document something in a check box, repeating that information in the narrative might be worthwhile. By doing so, you can expand on the yes-or-no limitations of the check box to explain the timing, the assessment findings, the circumstances, or the changes in patient condition associated with the indicated action.

Remember that proper spelling, approved abbreviations, and proper acronyms also affect your PCR's accuracy. Misspelled words lose their meaning; many abbreviations are not universally recognized; and several acronyms have more than one meaning. Make sure that the meaning of any abbreviation or acronym is clear.

LEGIBILITY

Poor penmanship and illegible reports lead to poor documentation. Some EMS providers say, "I wrote it, and I can read it. That's all that matters." This is simply not true. The PCR does not exist solely for its author's reference. It is a permanent record that many different people may use, including hospital staff, quality assurance personnel, and medical control. Your handwriting must be neat enough that other people can read and understand the report—especially the narrative. It must also be neat enough that you can read and understand it yourself many years from now, long after the event has faded from your memory. Your writing must be firm enough to transfer through multi-copy forms. Using a ball-point pen whenever possible makes carbon copies more legible and makes it difficult for someone to tamper with the document. Clearly mark the check boxes to eliminate any doubt that a check mark is not just a meaningless scratch. Always remember that other members of the health-care team may use the report for medical information, research, or quality improvement.

Your handwriting must be neat enough that other people can read and understand the report.

Prehospital Care Report

FOR BLS FR USE ONLY

M	D	Y		RUN NO.		AGENCY CODE	VEH. ID.
DATE OF CALL							

Name		Agency Name	MILEAGE		USE MILITARY TIMES

Name

Address

Ph #

Agency Name		MILEAGE	
Dispatch Information		END	
Call Location		BEGIN	
		TOTAL	

CHECK ONE: ☐ Residence ☐ Health Facility ☐ Farm ☐ Indus. Facility ☐ Other Work Loc. ☐ Roadway ☐ Recreational ☐ Other

LOCATION CODE

	CALL REC'D	
	ENROUTE	
	ARRIVED AT SCENE	
	FROM SCENE	
	AT DESTIN	
	IN SERVICE	
	IN QUARTERS	

AGE | **DOB** M D Y | **SEX** ☐ M ☐ F

Physician

CALL TYPE AS REC'D.
☐ Emergency
☐ Non-Emergency
☐ Stand-by

COMPLETE FOR TRANSFERS ONLY
Transferred from ☐☐☐
☐ No Previous PCR
☐ Unknown if Previous PCR
Previous PCR Number ☐–☐☐☐☐☐

CARE IN PROGRESS ON ARRIVAL:
☐ None ☐ Citizen ☐ PD/FD/Other First Responder ☐ Other EMS

MECHANISM OF INJURY
☐ MVA (✓ seat belt used →) ☐ Fall of ___ feet ☐ GSW ☐ Machinery
☐ Struck by vehicle ☐ Unarmed assault ☐ Knife ☐

☐ Extrication required ___ minutes

Seat belt used? ☐ Yes ☐ No ☐ Unknown

Seat Belt Use Reported By ☐ Crew ☐ Patient ☐ Police ☐ Other

CHIEF COMPLAINT | **SUBJECTIVE ASSESSMENT**

PRESENTING PROBLEM
If more than one checked, circle primary

☐ Airway Obstruction
☐ Respiratory Arrest
☐ Respiratory Distress
☐ Cardiac Related (Potential)
☐ Cardiac Arrest

☐ Allergic Reaction
☐ Syncope
☐ Stroke/CVA
☐ General Illness/Malaise
☐ Gastro-Intestinal Distress
☐ Diabetic Related (Potential)
☐ Pain

☐ Unconscious/Unresp.
☐ Seizure
☐ Behavioral Disorder
☐ Substance Abuse (Potential)
☐ Poisoning (Accidental)

☐ Other ___

☐ Shock
☐ Head Injury
☐ Spinal Injury
☐ Fracture/Dislocation
☐ Amputation

☐ Major Trauma
☐ Trauma-Blunt
☐ Trauma-Penetrating
☐ Soft Tissue Injury
☐ Bleeding/Hemorrhage

☐ OB/GYN
☐ Burns
Environmental
☐ Heat
☐ Cold
☐ Hazardous Materials
☐ Obvious Death

PAST MEDICAL HISTORY	TIME	RESP	PULSE	B.P.	LEVEL OF CONSCIOUSNESS	GCS	R	PUPILS	L	SKIN	STATUS
☐ None		Rate:	Rate:		☐ Alert		☐ Normal		☐ Unremarkable	☐ C
☐ Allergy to ___		☐ Regular	☐ Regular		☐ Voice		☐ Dilated		☐ Cool ☐ Pale	☐ U
☐ Hypertension ☐ Stroke		☐ Shallow	☐ Irregular		☐ Pain		☐ Constricted		☐ Warm ☐ Cyanotic	☐ P
☐ Seizures ☐ Diabetes		☐ Labored			☐ Unresp.		☐ Sluggish		☐ Moist ☐ Flushed	☐ S
☐ COPD ☐ Cardiac							☐ No-Reaction		☐ Dry ☐ Jaundiced	
☐ Other (List) ☐ Asthma		Rate:	Rate:		☐ Alert		☐ Normal		☐ Unremarkable	☐ C
		☐ Regular	☐ Regular		☐ Voice		☐ Dilated		☐ Cool ☐ Pale	☐ U
Current Medications (List)		☐ Shallow	☐ Irregular		☐ Pain		☐ Constricted		☐ Warm ☐ Cyanotic	☐ P
		☐ Labored			☐ Unresp.		☐ Sluggish		☐ Moist ☐ Flushed	☐ S
							☐ No-Reaction		☐ Dry ☐ Jaundiced	
		Rate:	Rate:		☐ Alert		☐ Normal		☐ Unremarkable	☐ C
		☐ Regular	☐ Regular		☐ Voice		☐ Dilated		☐ Cool ☐ Pale	☐ U
		☐ Shallow	☐ Irregular		☐ Pain		☐ Constricted		☐ Warm ☐ Cyanotic	☐ P
		☐ Labored			☐ Unresp.		☐ Sluggish		☐ Moist ☐ Flushed	☐ S
							☐ No-Reaction		☐ Dry ☐ Jaundiced	

(left margin: VITAL SIGNS)

OBJECTIVE PHYSICAL ASSESSMENT

COMMENTS

TREATMENT GIVEN

☐ Moved to ambulance on stretcher/backboard
☐ Moved to ambulance on stair chair
☐ Walked to ambulance
☐ Airway Cleared
☐ Oral/Nasal Airway
☐ Esophageal Obturator Airway/Esophageal Gastric Tube Airway (EOA/EGTA)
☐ EndoTracheal Tube (E/T) ☐☐
☐ Oxygen Administered @ ☐☐ L.P.M., Method ___
☐ Suction Used
☐ Artificial Ventilation Method ___
☐ C.P.R. in progress on arrival by: ☐ Citizen ☐ PD/FD/Other First Responder ☐ Other
☐ C.P.R. Started @ Time ▶ ☐☐☐ Time from Arrest Until C.P.R. ▶ ☐☐☐ Minutes
☐ EKG Monitored (Attach Tracing) [Rhythm(s) ___]
☐ Defibrillation/Cardioversion No. Times ☐ ☐ Manual ☐ Semi-automatic

☐ Medication Administered (Use Continuation Form)
☐ IV Established Fluid ___ Cath. Gauge ☐☐
☐ Mast Inflated @ Time ___)
☐ Bleeding/Hemorrhage Controlled (Method Used: ___)
☐ Spinal Immobilization Neck and Back
☐ Limb Immobilized by ☐ Fixation ☐ Traction
☐ (Heat) or (Cold) Applied
☐ Vomiting Induced @ Time ___ Method ___
☐ Restraints Applied, Type ___
☐ Baby Delivered @ Time ___ In County ___
  ☐ Alive ☐ Stillborn ☐ Male ☐ Female
☐ Transported in Trendelenburg position
☐ Transported in left lateral recumbent position
☐ Transported with head elevated
☐ Other ___

DISPOSITION (See list) | **DISP. CODE** | **CONTINUATION FORM USED** YES ←

CREW	IN CHARGE	DRIVER'S NAME	NAME	NAME
	☐ EMT ☐ AEMT #	☐ CFR ☐ EMT ☐ AEMT #	☐ CFR ☐ EMT ☐ AEMT #	☐ CFR ☐ EMT ☐ AEMT #

AGENCY COPY/WHITE

EMS 100 (11/86) provided by NYS-EMS PROGRAM
DOH 3822 (6/94)

FIGURE 9-4   Complete both the narrative and check-box sections of every PCR.

TIMELINESS

As a rule, you should avoid writing your report in the ambulance during transport of your patient for two reasons. First, the bumpy ride makes it difficult to write neatly. More importantly, your time is better spent communicating with your patient and conducting ongoing assessments. Most hospitals have an area where you can sit and complete your paperwork.

Ideally, you should complete your report immediately after you complete the emergency call, when the information is fresh in your mind and you can check with your partner or patient if you have any questions about the events. At times, you may be too busy to complete the entire documentation immediately following a call. If so, make notes on scratch paper, and write enough of the report that you will be able to finish it completely and accurately later. The sooner you finish it, the more details you are likely to recall and the better the report will be.

ABSENCE OF ALTERATIONS

Mistakes happen. During a busy shift or in the middle of the night, you will check the wrong box, misspell a word, or omit important information. You will be thinking of one medication and write another's name on your report. If you make a mistake writing your report, simply cross through the error with one line and initial it (Figure 9-5). Some systems may expect you to date the correction, as well. Do not scribble over or blacken out any area of the call report. Never try to hide an error. Such foolish tactics only raise the reader's curiosity about what you wrote originally. After crossing out the error, continue with the correct information. If you find the error after you have already written several more sentences, submit an **addendum.**

Whenever possible, have everyone involved in the call read or reread the PCR before you submit it. Make all corrections before you submit the report to the hospital or to the EMS administrative offices. Do not make changes on the original report after you have submitted it. If for any reason you need to make corrections after you have submitted the report, or some portion of it, use an addendum. Simply note on the original report, "See addendum," and attach the addendum to the original report. Write the addendum on a separate sheet of paper or on an official form if one exists. Likewise, if more information comes to your attention after you have submitted the report, write a supplemental narrative on a separate report form.

Write any addendum to your report as soon as you realize that you made an error or that additional information is needed. Note the purpose of the revision and why the information did not appear on your original report. The addendum should document the date and time that it was written, the reason it was written, and the pertinent information. Only the original author of a report should attach an addendum, as it is part of the official call record. Agencies should have separate forms for other EMS personnel, supervisors, or citizens who, for some reason, want to contribute to the documentation.

Ideally, you should complete your report immediately after you complete the emergency call.

Never try to hide an error.

addendum addition or supplement to the original report.

The ~~left~~ right pupil was fixed and dilated

FIGURE 9-5   The proper way to correct a prehospital care report is to draw a single line through the error, write the correct information beside it, and initial the change.

PROFESSIONALISM

Write your report in a professional manner. Remember that someday it may be scrutinized by hospital staff, medical control, quality improvement committees, supervisors, lawyers, and the news media. Your patient's family may request, and is entitled to, a copy of your report from your agency. Write cautiously, and avoid any remarks that might be construed as derogatory. **Jargon** can be confusing and does little to enhance your image. Do not describe a patient well known to EMS providers as a "frequent flyer." Never include slang, biased statements, or irrelevant opinions. Include only objective information. "The patient smelled of beer and had slurred speech and difficulty walking" are factual statements. "The patient was very drunk" is an inference; even if accurate, it is still just your opinion. Libel and slander are, respectively, writing or speaking false and malicious words intended to damage a person's reputation. Always write and speak carefully.

> *Write cautiously, and avoid any remarks that might be construed as derogatory.*
>

＊ **jargon** language used by a particular group or profession.

NARRATIVE WRITING

The narrative is the part of the written report in which you depict the call at length. Less structured than the check-box or fill-in sections of your report, the narrative allows you the freedom to describe your assessment findings in detail. When other people read your report, they usually will rely on your written narrative for the most relevant information. For example, as you transfer care to the emergency department nurse, he will usually scan your PCR for information concerning your patient's history, vital signs, and secondary assessment.

NARRATIVE SECTIONS

Any patient documentation includes three sections of importance: the subjective narrative, the objective narrative, and the assessment/management plan.

Subjective Narrative

The subjective part of your narrative typically comprises any information that you elicit during your patient's history. This includes the chief complaint (CC), the history of present illness (HPI), the past history (PH), the current health status (CHS), and the review of systems (ROS). In trauma, this also includes the mechanism of injury, as told to you by your patient or bystanders. The following is a typical subjective narrative on a patient complaining of shortness of breath:

CC: The patient is a 74-year-old conscious black male who complains, "I can't catch my breath."

HPI: Gradual onset of severe shortness of breath for the past 3 hours; began while sitting in living room watching television; nothing provokes or relieves the dyspnea; his son states this is worse than usual. He has had a 3-day history of some vague chest discomfort. He denies any chest pressure, nausea, or dizziness.

PH: He has a 5-year history of heart problems and congestive heart failure; hospitalized for this problem 3 times in the past 5 years; no surgeries.

CHS: Meds: Isosorbide, nitroglycerine, furosemide, digoxin, potassium; No known drug allergies; 50 pack/year smoker; nondrinker; non–drug abuser.

ROS: Resp: Unproductive cough for 1 day; audible wheezing; no hx of COPD or asthma; last chest X-ray 1 year ago. Card: no palpitations, pressure, or pain; + orthopnea; + paroxysmal

nocturnal dyspnea; + edema for past few days; past ECG 1 year ago.
GU: No changes in urinary patterns. Per. Vasc: + pitting edema for few
days; cold feet.

Objective Narrative

<table>
<tr><td>**Content Review**</td></tr>
</table>

The objective part of your narrative usually includes your general impression and
any data that you derive through inspection, palpation, auscultation, percussion,
and diagnostic testing. This includes vital signs, secondary assessment, and such
tests as cardiac monitoring, pulse oximetry, and blood glucose determination.

Content Review

**APPROACHES TO THE
SECONDARY ASSESSMENT**
• Head to toe
• Body systems

Vital Signs Vital signs are often documented in a separate table on the your PCR
(see Figure 9-6). You will generally have rows to document several sets of vital
signs. Ensure that you record your patient's initial vital signs (including the time
taken) and the last set of vital signs taken on arrival at hospital. Document additional sets of vital signs in the narrative section of your PCR or on an addendum.
Note that different EMS systems include different findings in their vital sign sets.

To document your secondary assessment, you can use either of two approaches—head-to-toe or body systems. Although the medical community accepts both extensively, emergency medical services more often uses the head-to-toe approach.

Head to Toe The head-to-toe approach is well suited for any call for which you
perform an entire secondary assessment because you document your findings in
the same order that you conducted the assessment—from head to toe. Remember that even though you may have conducted your pediatric assessment from
toe to head, you should document it in head-to-toe order. This style encourages
you to be systematic and thorough. It is appropriate for major trauma and serious medical emergencies, when you assess every body area and system. Include
all circulatory and neurological findings within the body area you are documenting. For example, when recording findings in the extremities, include distal
neurovascular function. When documenting the head, include the results of cranial nerve testing. The following illustrates the head-to-toe approach for a patient from an automobile collision:

General: The patient presents in the front seat of the car, in moderate
distress with bruises to his forehead and some facial
lacerations. Pt. is alert and oriented to self, time, and place.

HEENT: Depression to right frontal bone, minor bleeding
controlled before arrival; no drainage from ears, nose.
No periorbital ecchymosis or Battle's sign; pupils equal
and reactive to light; extraocular movements intact,
cranial nerves II—XII intact.

Neck: Trachea midline; no jugular vein distention; + cervical
spine tenderness.

Chest: Equal expansion; bruises across the chest wall; no
deformities; equal bilateral breath sounds.

FIGURE 9-6 Vital signs are
often documented in a
separate section of your PCR.

Time	Level of Consciousness				Pulse		Resp		BP		Skin	
	E	V	M	Ttl	Rate	Char	Rate	Char	Systolic	Diastolic	Colour	Condition
0715	4	5	6	15	88	irreg	18	easy	156	92	pale	clammy
0722	3	5	6	14	96	irreg	20	shallow	136	90	pale	diaph.

Abdomen:	Soft, nontender.
Pelvis:	Unstable pelvic ring; pain upon palpation.
Extremities:	+ Circulation, sensory, and motor function in all four extremities; no deformities noted.
Posterior:	No injuries noted.
Labs:	Sinus tachycardia no ectopy, pulse oximetry 97% on supplemental oxygen.

Body Systems The body systems approach focuses on body systems instead of body areas. It is best suited to screening and preadmission assessments in which you conduct a comprehensive assessment involving all body systems. Each body system has different key components that you should assess and document.

When you use the body systems approach in emergency medicine, you usually will focus only on the system, or systems, involved in the current illness or injury. For example, a patient having an asthma attack would require an in-depth evaluation of the respiratory system. Another patient with lower abdominal pain would need a close assessment of the gastrointestinal system. Neither patient would require a full head-to-toe secondary assessment but, instead, intensive documentation of the affected body system or systems. The body systems approach can be one of the most comprehensive approaches to documentation.

The following illustrates a body systems approach for a patient with chest pain and shortness of breath:

General:	Patient is a healthy-looking male who presents sitting upright in his chair, able to speak in phrases only.
HEENT:	+ Lip cyanosis and pursing; some nasal flaring; pink, frothy sputum; jugular veins distended.
Respiratory:	Good respiratory effort; accessory neck muscle use; trachea midline; + intercostal, supraclavicular, suprasternal retractions; = chest expansion; diffuse crackles and wheezing in all lung fields, decreased breath sounds.
Per. Vasc.:	+ Ascites fluid wave; + 2 pitting edema in lower extremities; strong peripheral pulses.
Labs:	Sinus tachycardia with occasional unifocal premature ventricular contractions. Pulse oximetry—92% room air; 97% on supplemental oxygen.

Assessment/Management

In the assessment/management section, you document what you believe to be your patient's problem. This is called your **field diagnosis,** working assessment, or impression. For example, your field diagnosis for a patient with chest pain may be "possible angina or rule out myocardial infarction." You do not have to make an exact diagnosis. When you are not sure, simply document what you suspect is the general problem. Sometimes, for instance, your field impression might be "rule out acute abdomen, or seizures." *Rule out* identifies possible diagnoses that you believe the emergency physician should evaluate.

Record your complete management plan from start to finish. This includes how you packaged and moved your patient to the ambulance. Did you carry him on a stair chair or on a backboard fully immobilized, or did he walk? List any interventions you completed before contacting your medical control physician. For example, did you control bleeding with direct pressure? Did you start an IV? Then, describe any orders from the medical control physician, and always include his

* **field diagnosis** prehospital evaluation of the patient's condition and its causes, based on your history and physical assessment.

Record your complete management plan from start to finish.

name. Describe how you transported your patient and the effects of any interventions, such as drug administration or other invasive procedures. Include the results of ongoing assessments and any changes in your patient's condition. Finally, describe your patient's condition when you transferred care to the emergency department staff. The following example is a management plan for a trauma patient with a pelvic fracture whose condition deteriorates en route to the hospital.

On-Scene

Extrication:	Rapid extrication from vehicle, placed supine on backboard
Airway:	Airway cleared with suctioning, nasopharyngeal airway inserted
Breathing:	Oxygen @ 15 litres/min via nonrebreather mask
Circulation:	Foot of stretcher raised 30°; bleeding from arm laceration controlled with dry sterile dressing and direct pressure; IV—60 L left antecubital area—normal saline run TKVO per standing order.

Transport

Transported by ground ambulance to University Hospital with full body immobilization supine on long spine board; ETA 10 minutes.

Ongoing:	Patient becomes restless and anxious; VS: pulse—120 weak carotid only, BP—50 palpated, Resp—28, skin: cool, pale, clammy with some mottling; initial IV run wide open; second IV 60 L right antecubital normal saline—run wide open.

Arrival

Patient transferred to ED staff restless; VS: pulse 120, BP—80 palpated, Resp—26, skin—mottled and cool.

GENERAL FORMATS

The mnemonics SOAP and CHART identify two common patterns for organizing a narrative report. These acronyms provide templates for most medical and trauma reports. They help you arrange your history, secondary assessment, and management plan into a logical, readable structure. They are widely used because they group information in categories that differentiate between subjective and objective information. For example, someone wanting only to determine your patient's medications can find that list easily in either the SOAP or the CHART format. Either pattern is acceptable and effective when used consistently.

SOAP

SOAP stands for *s*ubjective, *o*bjective, *a*ssessment, and *p*lan. The detailed SOAP format includes the following:

Subjective:	• Chief complaint
	• History of present illness
	• Past history
	• Current health status
	• Family history
	• Psychosocial history
	• Review of systems

Objective:	• Vital signs
	• General impression
	• Secondary assessment
	• Diagnostic tests
Assessment:	• Field diagnosis/working assessment
Plan:	• Standing orders
	• Physician orders
	• Effects of interventions
	• Mode of transport
	• Ongoing assessment

CHART

CHART stands for *c*hief complaint, *h*istory, *a*ssessment, *r*x (treatment), and *t*ransport. The detailed CHART format includes the following:

Content Review

CHART
• Chief complaint
• History
• Assessment
• Rx (treatment)
• Transport

Chief Complaint

History:	• History of present illness
	• Past history
	• Current health status
	• Review of systems
Assessment:	• Vital signs
	• General impression
	• Secondary assessment
	• Diagnostic tests
	• Field diagnosis
Rx:	• Standing orders
	• Physician orders
Transport:	• Effects of interventions
	• Mode of transport
	• Ongoing assessment

Other Formats

Like patient assessment itself, documentation is not "one-size-fits-all." No one narrative format is ideal for all situations. Two additional formats—patient management and call incident—are appropriate in certain circumstances.

Patient Management The patient management format is preferred for some critical patients, such as those in cardiac arrest, when you focus on immediately managing a variety of patient problems and not on conducting a thorough history and secondary assessment. This format is a chronological account from the time you arrived on the scene until you transferred care to someone else. It emphasizes your assessment and management of the conditions you found. Simply begin your chart with a description of the event and any other pertinent information, and then document your management, starting with your airway, breathing, and circulation (ABCs) assessment. Record everything in real time and in absolute chronological order, and always include the results of your interventions. A patient management chart would look like this:

No single narrative format is ideal for all situations.

Use the patient management format for critical patients when you focus on immediately managing a variety of patient problems.

Patient is an 89-year-old Asian male who was found by his wife unconscious on the floor immediately after collapsing. He presents pulseless and apneic.

Time	Intervention
1320	Airway cleared with suctioning; quick look—ventricular fibrillation.
1321	Defibrillation @ 200, 300, 360 joules—no change.
1322	CPR begun; oropharyngeal airway inserted, ET tube inserted, lung sounds bilaterally with BVM ventilation with BVM @ 12/min with supplemental oxygen.
1324	IV 18-gauge left antecubital area—normal saline TKVO; epinephrine 1:10 000 1 mg IVP.
1325	Defibrillation @ 360 joules—no change.
1327	Defibrillation @ 360 joules—patient converts to normal sinus rhythm rate of 72 with strong peripheral pulses, BP—110/76, no spontaneous respirations.
1328	Ventilation continued @ 12/min via BVM.
1332	Patient transferred to ambulance on stretcher—transported to University Hospital.
1335	Patient has spontaneous respirations @ 20/min, + bilateral breath sounds; becoming more awake; HR—72, BP—120/76.
1340	Arrived at UH—Patient is conscious, alert, and oriented with retrograde amnesia.

Call Incident The call incident approach simply emphasizes the mechanism of injury, the surrounding circumstances, and how the incident occurred. Use this approach to begin documenting a trauma call with a significant mechanism of injury. It is most suitable when the events surrounding the call might be significant. It would be inappropriate for a man sitting in his living room with chest pain or for someone who simply cut his finger with a carving knife. You may use this style in both the subjective and the objective sections of your PCR. The following example shows call incident documentation for a motor-vehicle collision:

Use the call incident approach to begin documenting a trauma call with a significant mechanism of injury.

Subjective: The patient is a 46-year-old conscious and alert white male who was an unrestrained driver in a low-speed, head-on, two-car motor-vehicle collision, moderate front-end damage, no passenger compartment intrusion, deformity to windshield, dashboard, and steering wheel. Patient states he "reached for cigarette on floor and when he looked up, there was another vehicle in front of him." He denies any loss of consciousness and can recall all details before and immediately following the crash. Patient complains of pain to the head, neck, chest, and hip from being thrown against the dashboard and windshield.

Objective: The patient presents in the front seat of the car, appears in moderate distress with bruises to his forehead, facial lacerations, and a deformed left leg. His left leg is pinned underneath the dashboard with his left foot hooked around the brake pedal. On arrival, fire department rescue personnel were holding manual stabilization of his head and neck and stabilizing the vehicle.

These are not the only systems of documentation. Indeed, you may use some combination of these systems or develop a unique format for your regional system. The important thing is for your documentation to be complete, accurate, and consistent. By using the same system to document every call, you will be less likely to accidentally overlook or omit something.

SPECIAL CONSIDERATIONS

Some circumstances create special problems for EMS documentation. Patient refusals, calls for which transport is unnecessary, multiple patients, and mass casualties are among the more common examples. In these and other unusual circumstances, take extra care to document everything that happened during the call.

PATIENT REFUSALS

Two types of patients might refuse care. The first type is the person who is not seriously ill or injured and simply does not want to go to the hospital. For example, the belted driver of a minor automobile collision has an abrasion on his knee from striking the dashboard. He is alert and oriented, has no other injuries, and claims he will seek medical attention if it bothers him later. This type of patient usually signs your PCR in a special place marked "Refusal of Care," and you return to service.

The second type of patient is more worrisome. This patient refuses care even though you feel he needs it. This is known as **against medical advice**, or **AMA.** Some legal experts regard AMA as your failure to convince your patient to accept necessary treatment and transport. Such patient refusals are particularly troublesome because they have the most potential to end badly. Still, patients retain the right to refuse treatment or transport if they are competent to make that decision and are not actively suicidal. Although you cannot make a legal determination of competence (sometimes it takes a court decision), document that you believe your patient was competent to refuse care. Though specific laws vary among provinces and territories, your patient will demonstrate competence by his understanding of the circumstances and the risks associated with refusing care and by accepting those risks and the responsibility for refusing care. Assess your patient as thoroughly as possible, with special emphasis on mental status and behaviour. Pay extra attention to any patient suspected of being under the influence of drugs or alcohol. Clearly document that your patient has an adequate mental status and understands your field diagnosis, alternative treatments, and the consequences of refusing care. Also, record the reason given for refusing care (Table 9-2).

Even after you document your patient's competence, most patient refusals require more thorough documentation than the typical EMS call because the opportunity for and consequences of abandonment charges are tremendous. Simply having your patient sign your PCR is not sufficient. Again, document that you described your pa-

* **against medical advice (AMA)** your patient refuses care even though you feel he needs it.

Patients retain the right to refuse treatment or transport if they are competent to make that decision.

Table 9-2 REFUSAL OF CARE DOCUMENTATION CHECKLIST

❑ Thorough patient assessment

❑ Competency of patient

❑ Your recommendation for care and transport

❑ Explanation to the patient about possible consequences of refusing care, including possibility of death, if appropriate

❑ Other suggestions for accessing care

❑ Willingness to return if patient changes mind

❑ Patient's understanding of statements and suggestions and apparent competence to refuse care based on that understanding

---

tient's injuries to him and that he understood the risks of refusing treatment and transport. Inform your patient of potential complications from injuries that might not be obvious. Discuss those associated risks, and document this discussion. Also, document any involvement of your patient's family or friends. Since ruling out serious injury is all but impossible in the field, you may need to make clear the possibility of your patient's dying. Although this might seem extreme, it plainly conveys that the risks are serious. A patient who was informed that he was at risk of dying, refused care, and subsequently had his leg amputated because of an infection would have a hard time convincing a jury that he did not think the risks were serious.

In many systems, you must contact the medical direction physician before allowing a patient to refuse transport. If you confer with a physician, document any information, advice, or orders that the physician gives you. If your patient speaks directly to the physician, document that as well. Once more, document that your patient understands the circumstances and the risks and still chooses to refuse transport. Note that you instructed him to call an ambulance or go to the emergency department if his condition worsens, or if he just changes his mind. You can ask a bystander or law enforcement officer to witness the patient refusal, although this is not always required.

Your documentation also should include a complete narrative with quotations and statements from others on the scene. For example, if your patient's wife and son plead with him to go to the hospital, include their comments in your report. If your system uses a specific form for patient refusals, complete that paperwork as well (Figure 9-7). The additional form, however, is not a substitute for a complete documentation of the circumstances.

RELEASE FROM RESPONSIBILITY

DATE _____ 19 _____ TIME _____ □ a.m. □ p.m.

This is to certify that _____

is refusing ☐ TREATMENT ☐ TRANSPORT

against the advice of the attending Emergency Medical Technician and of the Phoenix Fire Department, and when applicable, the base hospital and the base hospital physician.

I acknowledge that I have been informed of the following:

1. The nature and potential of the illness or injuries.
2. The potential risks of delaying treatment and transportation, up to and including death.
3. The availability of ambulance transportation to a hospital for treatment.

Nevertheless, I assume all risks and consequences of my decision, including further physical deterioration, loss of limb, paralysis, and even death, and hereby release the attending Emergency Medical Technician and the Phoenix Fire Department, and when applicable, the base hospital and the base hospital physician from any ill effects which may result from my refusal.

Witness _____ Signed: **X** _____

Witness _____ Relationship to Patient _____

Refusal must be signed by the patient; or by the nearest relative or legal guardian in the case of a minor, or when patient is physically or mentally incompetent.

☐ Patient refuses to sign release despite efforts of attending Emergency Medical Technician to obtain such signature after informing patient of concerns listed in numbers 1, 2, and 3 above.

GUIDELINES — Patient Refusal Documentation

In addition to those items normally documented (chief complaint, history of present illness, mechanism of injury, physical assessment, etc.) the following items should be recorded, regardless of patient's cooperation:

- Mental Status (orientation, speech, etc.)

- Suspected presence of alcohol or drugs

- Patient's exact words (as much as possible) in the refusal of care OR the signing of the release form

- Circumstances or reasons (including exact words of patient, if possible) for INCOMPLETE ADVISEMENT (risk of injury, abusiveness, unruliness, risk of injury other than from patient, etc.)

- Advice given to patients' guardian(s)

FIGURE 9-7   One example of a refusal of care form.

SERVICES NOT NEEDED

Some systems allow you to determine that your patient does not need ambulance transport. Although such policies help reduce ambulance utilization rates, the risks of denying transport are even greater than those of patient refusals. In these cases, the documentation must clearly demonstrate that transport was unnecessary. As with patient refusals, document any discussion you have with the emergency department physician and any advice you give to your patient.

The risks of denying transport are even greater than those of patient refusals.

Transport may not be needed for other reasons as well. Ambulances are often called to minor accidents in which no injuries have occurred. When this happens, emergency medical responders, such as the fire department rescue unit or a police agency, might cancel the ambulance. If the ambulance is cancelled en route, document the cancelling authority and the time of notification. If you arrive on the scene and find no patients, document that. If, when you arrive, you are cancelled by on-scene personnel, document that you made no patient contact, and record the person and agency who cancelled you. The difference is considerable between "no patients found" and "only minor injuries, patients refusing transport." Although they might refuse transport, evaluate people with even the most minor injuries. Consider them patients, and document them accurately.

MASS-CASUALTY INCIDENTS

Multiple patients, mass casualties, and disasters all present special documentation problems. The number of patients needing care and transport during such situations may overwhelm you. Often, more than one ambulance crew cares for the many patients. Some EMS personnel may fill support roles and never actually provide patient care. Obtaining complete patient information might be impossible, and completing documentation for one patient before going on to care for others might be impractical.

In these situations, you must weigh your patients' needs against the demand for complete documentation. Document as much as possible—as quickly as possible—on your PCR. You can complete the documentation later as an addendum. If you cannot remember the particulars of a specific patient or transport, do not guess. Document only what you know to be factual and accurate. A simple note at the end of the documentation explaining the circumstances will account for any missing information.

Some EMS agencies use special forms for multiple-patient events, and most provide a general incident report form or record that anyone connected with the call may complete. You should become familiar with local policies and procedures for documenting these situations. Many systems use **triage tags** to record vital information on each patient quickly. A triage tag has just enough room for your patient's vital information—name, major injuries, vital signs, treatment, and priority (urgent, nonurgent). You affix it to your patient, and it remains there throughout the event; you can transfer its information to your PCR later. Whatever your local policies, document as completely and accurately as possible without detracting from patient care.

✱ **triage tags** tags containing vital information, affixed to your patient during a multi-patient incident.

Whatever your local policies regarding multiple patients and mass casualties, document as completely and accurately as possible without detracting from patient care.

CONSEQUENCES OF INAPPROPRIATE DOCUMENTATION

Inappropriate documentation can have both medical and legal consequences. The medical consequences of inadequate documentation are potentially the most serious. Health-care providers across several disciplines may refer to your PCR in planning their care for a patient. Do not guess about your patient's medical problems

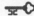

if you are not certain. An inaccurate or incomplete report can affect patient care for many hours, even days, after the ambulance call ends. Failing to document a medication allergy or documenting an incorrect medical history could have grave effects. If no one can read your sloppy report, it is useless despite the importance of its information. Good documentation now enables good care later.

The potential legal consequences of inadequate documentation are enormous. If poor documentation results in inappropriate care, you may be held responsible. Or if the documentation does not make it clear that you informed a patient of the risks when he refused transport, you may be legally accountable for any harmful consequences. If the documentation does not explicitly say that the patient in ventricular fibrillation was defibrillated immediately, you might be accused of providing inadequate care. Even though you did everything appropriately, poor, incomplete, or inaccurate documentation will encourage a frivolous lawsuit. Good documentation discourages such actions. Always remember that if it is not documented, you did not do it.

Inaccurate, incomplete, illegible documentation also reflects poorly on the EMS provider writing the report. Missing information, misspelled words, and poor penmanship give the impression of a sloppy, incompetent provider. Good documentation, conversely, enhances the EMS provider's professional stature.

PROFESSIONAL CORRESPONDENCE

As a paramedic, you may be called on to communicate using a variety of documents, including forms, reports, records, letters, and articles.

In the normal course of your work, you will routinely complete various forms and reports: your patient care record, personal notebooks, occurrence reports, accident investigation reports, and illness/injury forms. In addition, you will use a number of administrative documents, which may include payroll forms, personnel records, and scheduling documents. You may also be required to write letters, reports, proposals, articles for local papers or journals, and other forms of professional communication.

Use the following guidelines whenever you must create professional correspondence:

- Plan your document. Consider the purpose of the document, who your intended audience is, and what your intended outcome is. List your key ideas, and organize them in a way that best makes your point.
- Write concisely. Use appropriate language, terminology, abbreviations, and grammar.
- Use the appropriate format. Many organizations have templates or formats for common documents, such as memos, letters, and reports. Use a style guide or manual, such as *Canadian Manual of Style* or the *Canadian Press Style*.
- Ensure that your writing has a beginning, a middle, and an ending. Use your introduction to outline the purpose of the document, your objectives, and your intent. Use the body of the document to present and develop your ideas or points. Summarize the document by restating your conclusions in a way that shows you have met your stated purpose or objectives.
- Edit your work. Check spelling, punctuation, and language.

CLOSING

As a paramedic, you will assume responsibility for your documentation. Although documentation is often a begrudged task, it is one of the most important parts of an EMS call. Ensuring that your documentation is complete, accurate, legible, and appropriate is one of your professional responsibilities. As a professional, you should recognize this responsibility and set a positive example for others as you fulfill it.

Your report's confidentiality cannot be overemphasized. Confidentiality is your patient's legal right. Do not discuss your report with anyone not medically connected directly with the case. Generally, you are allowed to share patient information with another health-care provider who will continue care, with third-party billing companies, with the police if it is relevant to a criminal investigation, and with the court if it issues a subpoena. Your report also may be used for quality assurance or research. In these cases, information that could indentify the patient should be removed or blocked out.

Computer charting will certainly become common in the future. Several systems now on the market allow you to enter data electronically, transmit that information to the receiving facility, and immediately receive a printed report. When you use such systems, remember that the principles of effective documentation still apply.

SUMMARY

Regardless of the system you use for documentation, all EMS records should possess the same basic attributes. Appropriate terminology, proper spelling, accepted abbreviations and acronyms, and accurate times are essential. A description of the patient assessment and interventions, including pertinent negatives and communications with online physicians, is equally important. Finally, all the personnel and resources involved in a call must be documented. The record must be accurate and precise, free of jargon, and neatly written. Corrections should be made properly, including the use of an addendum when appropriate.

Prehospital care providers may use many systems of documentation, including the CHART and SOAP formats. Whatever system you use, it is best if you use the same one consistently. This results in more reliable, complete documentation and reduces the chances of omitting important information. Any of the existing documentation systems can incorporate a head-to-toe assessment of the patient. Special situations, such as multiple patients and refusals of transport, require extra attention. They are often the most difficult calls to document, and yet they are also the calls for which good documentation can be most valuable. A complete narrative—in addition to any check boxes or filled-in "bubbles"—is the best way to ensure that all the necessary information is documented.

Although EMS providers frequently dislike documentation, it is one of the most important parts of the EMS call. Ensuring that the documentation is complete, accurate, legible, and appropriate is one of an EMS provider's professional responsibilities. Your PCR is the only permanent record of the ambulance call and the only permanent reflection of your professionalism.

CHAPTER 10

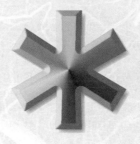

Clinical Decision Making

Objectives

After reading this chapter, you should be able to:

1. Compare the factors influencing medical care in the prehospital environment with those in other medical settings. (p. 438)

2. Differentiate between critical life-threatening, potentially life-threatening, and non-life-threatening patient presentations. (pp. 438–439)

3. Evaluate the benefits and shortfalls of protocols, standing orders, and patient care algorithms. (pp. 439, 440)

4. Define the components, stages, and sequences of the critical thinking process for paramedics. (pp. 439–443)

5. Apply the fundamental elements of critical thinking for paramedics. (pp. 445–447)

6. Describe the effects of the "fight or flight" response and its positive and negative effects on a paramedic's decision making. (p. 444)

7. Summarize the "six Rs" of putting it all together: *R*ead the scene, *R*ead the patient, *R*eact, *R*eevaluate, *R*evise the management plan, *R*eview performance. (p. 447)

8. Given several preprogrammed and moulaged trauma and medical patients, demonstrate clinical decision making. (pp. 437–447)

INTRODUCTION

As a paramedic, you eventually will face a situation that requires you to make a critical decision. Often, you will have several options, but choosing the best one may mean the difference between life and death. And you will be all alone. Others may be at the scene, but as the paramedic, you will be responsible for that decision. That you someday will have to make a decision on which your patient's life hinges is a sobering thought.

In the 1970s, with rare exceptions, the first paramedics made few critical decisions. They usually worked under rigidly written protocols developed by their medical director. Mostly, they were required to contact the medical direction physician who, after hearing their report, would diagnose the patient's problem and order treatment. They were no more than technicians who needed only good psychomotor skills to conduct patient assessments and follow orders. As prehospital care evolved, paramedics began to do much more than collect data for the physician to evaluate. You not only will have to gather information but also analyze it, form a field diagnosis, and devise a management plan. In most cases, you will do these things before contacting your medical direction physician.

Twenty-first-century paramedics are prehospital practitioners of emergency medicine—not field technicians. To fill this role, you will need to develop your critical-decision-making skills—to be able to think rationally about what you are doing. Because patients seldom present with the classic textbook signs and symptoms, you will encounter situations that appear totally unfamiliar. These cases will call for you to use sound judgment in devising a management plan that meets your patient's needs. Making such decisions requires **clinical judgment,** the use of your knowledge and experience to make critical decisions regarding patient care. No one can teach you clinical judgment; you must develop it from experience. Unfortunately, experience often includes making bad decisions. We learn from our mistakes, if someone points them out and explains them to us. Throughout your career as a paramedic, you will be evaluated, and your calls will be reviewed by many professionals, including hospital staff, medical control staff, and your partner, and through your service's quality assurance (QA)/quality improvement (QI) program.

Your instructors also will place you in as many problem-solving situations as possible to begin developing your clinical judgment. The number and type of supervised patient contacts you make during this program will determine how much clinical judgment you develop as a student. The more types of cases you see during your clinical rotations, the more clinically competent you will be when you complete your education.

PARAMEDIC PRACTICE

As a paramedic, you must gather, evaluate, and synthesize much information in very little time. You will obtain this information using your senses (sight, smell, hearing, and touch) during the history and secondary assessment. Analyzing these data will involve the total of your education, training, and clinical experience. For example, as you enter a patient's home, the sound of her gasping for breath with audible wheezes startles you. Having heard wheezing before and having learned in class that it results from a variety of problems will help you make what is called a differential diagnosis. The differential diagnosis is a preliminary list of possible causes for your patient's problem. For example, a differential diagnosis for diffuse wheezing might include asthma, emphysema, bronchitis, and acute pulmonary edema. Now, you conduct a history and secondary assessment and arrive at a field diagnosis, or impression.

Your next step will involve applying your clinical experience and exercising independent decision making as you develop and implement a management plan.

As a paramedic you inevitably will face a critical decision that can mean the difference between life and death.

Twenty-first-century paramedics are prehospital practitioners of emergency medicine—not field technicians.

✱ **clinical judgment** the use of knowledge and experience to diagnose patients and plan their treatment.

For example, your gasping and wheezing patient is an elderly female who presents with severe difficulty breathing. She has a history of cardiac and pulmonary disease, and you are not sure which problem precipitates this episode. You gather information and make an initial field diagnosis of congestive heart failure. You immediately administer medications (nitroglycerine, furosemide, morphine) to reduce cardiac preload, ease the workload of the heart, and increase urine production. You also decide to intubate and ventilate your patient to ease her respiratory effort. This decision to administer potentially life-threatening drugs requires you to think clearly and work effectively under pressure. Few prehospital situations create more pressure than a patient struggling to breathe.

The prehospital emergency medical setting is unlike any other medical care environment. Paramedics carry out the same tasks as other clinicians. They assess patients, obtain vital signs, start IVs, manage airways, and perform many other invasive procedures. The difference is that paramedics perform these procedures in various uncontrolled and unpredictable environments under circumstances that do not exist in other clinical settings and without information gathered from laboratory results and x-ray. For example, starting an IV line in a well lit, quiet hospital room is not a major challenge. Starting one while balancing yourself in the back of a rapidly moving ambulance is. Often, you will use your skills in seemingly unmanageable circumstances. The key is to block out the distractions and focus on the task. Experienced paramedics do this better than anyone.

PATIENT ACUITY

* **acuity** the severity or acuteness of your patient's condition.

Not everyone who calls 911 has a life-threatening emergency. Just the opposite is true. The vast majority of patients are people who want transport to the hospital for non-life-threatening problems. For some, the emergency department is their only health-care option, even for a sore throat. The spectrum of care in the prehospital setting includes three general classes of patient **acuity**: those with obvious critical life threats, those with potential life threats, and those with non-life-threatening presentations. Patients with obvious life-threatening conditions include major multisystem trauma; devastating single-system trauma; end-stage disease presentations, such as liver or renal failure, when the patient is in the last days of terminal illness and is close to death; and acute presentations of chronic diseases, such as asthma or emphysema. These patients present with serious airway, breathing, circulation, or neurological problems and often require aggressive resuscitation. Potential life-threatening conditions include serious multisystem trauma and multiple disease etiologies, such as a diabetic with cardiac complications. Non-life-threatening presentations include isolated minor illnesses and injuries. You will be expected to manage cases in all three categories. In a typical 12-hour shift, you may manage a patient in cardiac arrest; deliver a baby; control a lacerated, spurting artery; and transfer an elderly woman back to her nursing home. The wide range of patient types, degrees of severity, and complicating environmental factors make out-of-hospital care a unique form of emergency medicine.

Arriving at a management plan for patients with minor medical and traumatic events requires little critical thinking or clinical judgment. For example, if your patient has a fractured tibia, you will splint the leg and transport her to the emergency department for x-rays and casting. You have no real life-saving decisions to make. On the opposite end of the acuity spectrum, patients with obvious life threats, such as cardiac arrest and major trauma, also require few critical decisions because caring for them is largely rote and standardized. For cardiac arrest, you perform CPR and work through the protocol associated with your patient's cardiac rhythm. For major trauma, you manage the ABCs while providing rapid transport to a trauma centre.

Content Review

CLASSES OF PATIENT ACUITY
- Critically life threatening
- Potentially life threatening
- Not life threatening

Patients who fall between minor medical and life-threatening on the acuity spectrum pose the greatest challenge to your critical thinking abilities. These patients might become unstable at any moment. For example, if your patient is an infant with signs of respiratory distress, you must recognize the signs of early respiratory failure and take precautionary measures to keep her from deteriorating to respiratory arrest. In these cases, you use your knowledge of pediatric respiratory assessment, your skills in airway and breathing management, and your clinical judgment to determine how and when to intervene. You will constantly reassess and revise your interventions as needed.

PROTOCOLS AND ALGORITHMS

Paramedics function in an emergency medical services system under the licence of a medical director. Every province and territory has enacted legislation allowing paramedics to practise medicine in the field and describing the scope of their practice. Within these laws, provinical, territorial, and local EMS medical directors devise **protocols** that detail exactly what paramedics can do. Protocols are standards that include general and specific procedures for managing certain patient conditions. For example, every system will develop standards for managing asthma, congestive heart failure, and tension pneumothorax. Each will also develop protocols or policies for special situations, such as physician on scene, radio failure, and termination of resuscitation. **Standing orders** authorize you to perform certain procedures before contacting your medical direction physician. For example, you may administer oxygen, start an IV, and administer Aspirin and nitroglycerine to a patient with cardiac chest pain. For repeat nitroglycerine orders, you may have to consult the physician. Patient care **algorithms** are flow charts with arrows, lines, and boxes arranged schematically (Figure 10-1). To use them, you simply start at the top and follow wherever your patient's signs and symptoms lead.

* **protocol** standard that includes general and specific principles for managing certain patient conditions.

* **standing orders** treatments you can perform before contacting the medical direction physician for permission.

* **algorithm** schematic flow chart that outlines appropriate care for specific signs and symptoms.

Protocols, standing orders, and patient care algorithms provide a standardized approach to emergency patient care. However, they address only "classic patients." Unfortunately, many patients present with atypical signs and symptoms, often requiring you to use clinical judgment and instinct to develop a management plan. Patients frequently present with nonspecific complaints that do not match any specific algorithm. Sometimes, your patients just do not clearly describe what is bothering them. Another limitation of protocols is that they cannot adequately cover multiple disease etiologies, such as the patient with chronic obstructive pulmonary disease and congestive heart failure. When your patient with this multiple history presents with severe difficulty breathing, you must quickly identify the underlying condition that is causing the present problem and follow the appropriate protocol. Nor do protocols deal with managing more than one patient problem at a time in possible multiple treatment situations. For example, your stroke patient also presents with shock and with bilateral Colles' fractures and a fractured hip from the fall. Protocols are standards designed to promote consistent patient care in common situations. They are written to allow you, in consultation with the medical direction physician, to use clinical judgment to provide optimum care in unusual situations. The linear thinking, or "cookbook medicine," that protocols promote should not restrict you from consulting with your medical direction physician in difficult or unusual cases.

CRITICAL THINKING SKILLS

The ability to think under pressure and make decisions cannot be taught; it must be developed. As a paramedic, you will be a team leader on emergency scenes. In

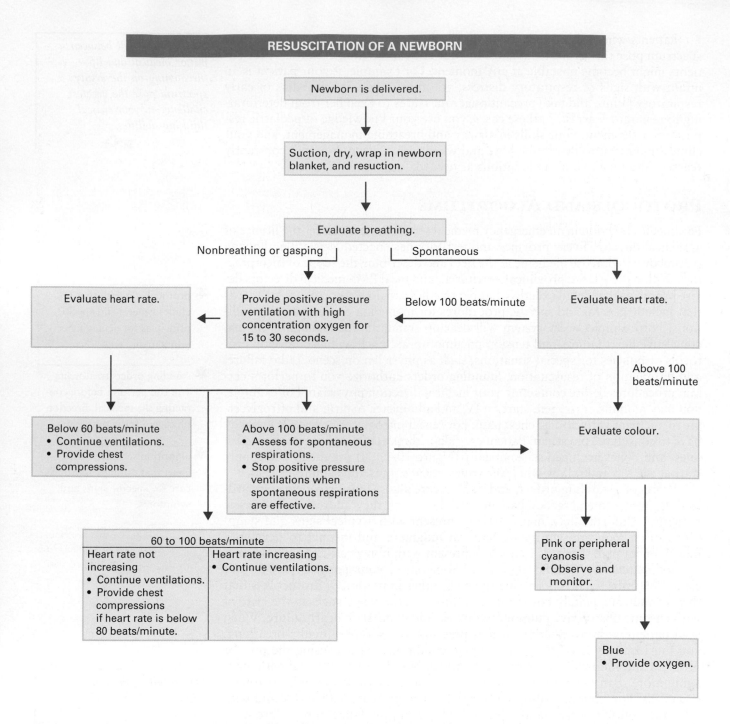

FIGURE 10-1 To use a patient care algorithm, follow the arrows to your patient's symptoms, and provide care as indicated.

that role you must make sound, reasonable decisions regarding your patient's care. Your training will help you develop this essential skill. In the classroom, you will work on case histories. In the labs, you will practise patient scenarios on moulaged victims. In the hospital, you will assess and help manage real patients in the emergency department and critical care units. In the field internship, you will assess and manage patients on the streets. In all of these settings, you will begin developing clinical judgment.

FUNDAMENTAL KNOWLEDGE AND ABILITIES

First, you must have an excellent working knowledge of anatomy and physiology and of the pathophysiology of your patient's disease or injury. To assess and manage a patient with difficulty breathing, for instance, you must know which organs and body systems are involved in breathing. You must understand the process of normal breathing and each body system's role in that effort. You must recall the factors that inhibit normal breathing and recognize the signs and symptoms of respiratory distress. For example, a patient might wheeze because of lower airway obstruction from secretions, bronchoconstriction, edema, or any combination of these conditions. All reduce the inner diameter of the airways, restricting airflow and making moving air in to and out of the lungs difficult. Managing this patient would require a knowledge of the respiratory and cardiovascular causes of wheezing because their treatments are vastly different. Respiratory causes for generalized wheezing include asthma and bronchitis, which you would manage with bronchodilators. Cardiac causes for wheezing include congestive heart failure, which you would manage with vasodilators and diuretics. Without a good working knowledge of these diseases, you might make an incorrect and potentially devastating field diagnosis.

You also must be able to focus on many specific data. When you conduct a patient assessment, you will evaluate all relevant information while focusing on specific important findings. You will be inundated with information requiring you to establish relationships and form conclusions. Your patient who presents with difficulty breathing and wheezing in the previous example would require an in-depth history and focused assessment of her cardiac and respiratory systems. You also would assess other systems relative to her chief complaint (HEENT, musculoskeletal, neurological, and lymphatic) while remaining focused on the primary problem (cardiorespiratory). Although her chief complaint is difficulty breathing, her primary problem might be cardiac, muscular, infectious, allergic, or neurological.

You must be able to organize the information you obtain and form concepts from it. Initially, you elicit your patient's chief complaint and begin to formulate a **differential field diagnosis.** As you conduct the history and a clearer picture of your patient's problem emerges, you narrow your differential field diagnosis to the most probable disease. For example, your patient has severe difficulty breathing and inspiratory stridor. Your differential field diagnosis might include foreign body obstruction, epiglottitis, respiratory burns, anaphylaxis, laryngeal trauma, and throat cancer. Then, you learn that she is hoarse and febrile, has had a sore throat for two days, and in the past six hours has had increasing difficulty swallowing. You now suspect epiglottitis. This ability to formulate a working field diagnosis is essential for paramedics.

You must be able to identify and deal with medical ambiguity. Many patients present with vague signs and symptoms. It is not unusual for a patient to complain of "just not feeling right." She will provide you with an imprecise story and you will be unable to arrive at a specific field diagnosis. In these cases, your field diagnosis will have to be generalized: "abdominal pain" or "general illness." Often, it will be almost impossible to definitively diagnose your patient without laboratory results, x-rays, and other tests.

You must be able to differentiate between relevant and irrelevant data. You will have to sift the important data from the many bits of information you receive during your patient assessment. A positive family history for sudden cardiac death is relevant for your patient with chest pain; for your patient with a fractured arm, it is not. Pupil and extraocular movement assessments are relevant for trauma and for patients with an altered mental status; for a patient with asthma or arthritis, they are not. When you radio the medical direction physician, you will report

DECISION-MAKING REQUIREMENTS

- Knowing anatomy, physiology, and pathophysiology
- Focusing on large amounts of data
- Organizing information
- Identifying and dealing with medical ambiguity
- Differentiating between relevant and irrelevant data
- Analyzing and comparing similar situations
- Explaining decisions and constructing logical arguments

✳ **differential field diagnosis** the list of possible causes of your patient's symptoms.

critical information only. Likewise, in your written documentation, you will record relevant information and pertinent negatives, while omitting the rest.

You must be able to analyze and compare similar and contrasting situations. What were the similarities among your last three stroke patients? Did all three have facial drooping, slurred speech, and unilateral paralysis? Did they all have a history of hypertension? Can you depend on any patterns of presentation for future calls like this? Have some patient presentations been unusual? Have any patients presented with signs of stroke but had a different diagnosis? For example, your patient is a 45-year-old woman who presents with right-sided facial drooping. Your initial impression may be stroke, but further investigation reveals no other neurological deficits. You now change your impression to Bell's palsy, caused by inflammation of the facial nerve (CN-VII). You must be able to recall the factors that help rule in or rule out a particular disease or injury.

You must be able to explain your decisions and construct logical arguments. Often, the emergency physician will want to know what you were thinking when you made your field diagnosis. You must be able to express yourself rationally while you make your case. These are the times when you demonstrate your professionalism to other health-care providers. Consider the following conversation:

Physician: Why did you think your patient had Bell's palsy and not a stroke? How can you rule out a stroke in the field?

Paramedic: Well, she had paralysis on the entire right side of her face, indicating a lesion of the seventh cranial nerve, rather than the lower facial paralysis of a stroke. All other neuro tests were negative.

Physician: OK, I agree. Good job!

Through interactions such as this, you establish credibility with the emergency physician. The next time you contact her regarding a patient, she is more apt to trust your assessment and judgment.

USEFUL THINKING STYLES

As a paramedic, you will face confusing emergencies that would challenge even the most knowledgeable, analytical care provider. You must be able to stay calm and not panic. Your self-control in the face of extreme chaos will set the example for other team members to follow. Even when you are struggling to maintain your composure—especially then—never let others know. The key is focusing on the task and blocking out the distractions. Be like the duck—cool and calm on the water's surface while paddling feverishly underneath.

Assume and plan for the worst, and always err on the side of benefitting your patient. For example, if you are deliberating whether to immobilize your patient, initiate advanced life support procedures, or administer oxygen, just do it! It is better to err by providing care than by withholding it. Be pessimistic. Anticipate all potential bad side effects of your treatments and prepare "plan B." For example, as you deliver a bronchodilating drug to your severe asthmatic patient, anticipate that it will not work, and mentally prepare to intubate her and perform positive pressure ventilation. Or while you are administering atropine to your patient with symptomatic bradycardia, plan ahead for external cardiac pacing and dopamine, if atropine therapy fails to restore adequate circulation.

Establish and maintain a systematic assessment pattern. Practise your assessments until they become second nature, and you will avoid skipping and missing steps. Be disciplined, and stay focused, especially when you are confronted with a complex emergency scene. For example, your patient lies moaning

Content Review

FACILITATING BEHAVIOURS
- Stay calm.
- Plan for the worst.
- Work systematically.
- Remain adaptable.

Be like the duck—cool and calm on the water's surface while paddling feverishly underneath.

on the ground in a pool of blood. Bystanders are screaming at you to help her; others are trying to tell you what happened. The police are gathering the story and trying unsuccessfully to talk with your patient. You must gain control of this scene. You do so by focusing on your patient and performing a systematic assessment. Use common acronyms (MS-ABC, OPQRST, SAMPLE), or make up your own to help you remember the key elements of your assessment. Except for safety concerns, never allow anything to distract you from your most important job—assessing and caring for your patient.

Except for safety concerns, never allow anything to distract you from your most important job—assessing and caring for your patient.

The different situations you encounter will require a variety of management styles. Adapting your styles of situation analysis (reflective versus impulsive), data processing (convergent versus divergent), and decision making (anticipatory versus reactive) to each situation will enable you to provide the best possible care in every case.

Reflective versus Impulsive Some situations call for you to be **reflective**, take your time, and figure out what is wrong with your patient. You have a patient who complains of "not feeling well." She has a long history of cardiac, renal, respiratory, and diabetic problems. Since she is in no real distress and is hemodynamically stable, you can take your time to determine her primary problem. Other situations call for immediate action. They require you to make an instinctive, **impulsive** decision and manage your patient's life-threatening condition. For example, if your patient presents apneic and pulseless, you will immediately begin CPR and prepare for rapid defibrillation. If she presents with a spurting artery, you will at once take measures to control the hemorrhage. If she is choking and has a weak, ineffective cough, you will quickly perform the Heimlich manoeuvre. You have to think fast in these situations.

∗ reflective acting thoughtfully, deliberately, and analytically.

∗ impulsive acting instinctively without stopping to think.

Divergent versus Convergent To process the data you receive from your patient and the scene, you can use either a divergent approach or a convergent approach. The **divergent** approach considers all aspects of a situation before arriving at a solution. It is insightful and works well when you are confronted with complex scenarios. For example, your emotionally distraught, stable patient presents with multiple problems and a long, complicated medical history. You need to consider the physical, emotional, and psychological aspects of her condition before making a field diagnosis and management plan. Likewise, extricating a victim from a wooded scene requires you to weigh a variety of environmental and medical factors before selecting a mode of transport.

∗ divergent taking into account all aspects of a complex situation.

The **convergent** approach focuses narrowly on a situation's most significant aspects. This technically oriented approach relies heavily on step-by-step problem solving and is best suited for simple, uncomplicated situations that require little thought or reflection. For example, you have an unresponsive, apneic, pulseless patient who presents in ventricular fibrillation. Your immediate concern is simple and straightforward—you manage the ABCs and defibrillate her as quickly as possible. Experienced paramedics employ both approaches effectively in the appropriate situations.

∗ convergent focusing on only the most important aspect of a critical situation.

Anticipatory versus Reactive Your decision-making process can be either anticipatory or reactive. You either anticipate the possible ramifications of your actions in a proactive way or you react to events as you encounter them. For example, your patient presents with a deep laceration and severe blood loss. The bleeding is controlled. Now, you can either anticipate her going into shock and begin measures before it happens or you can wait until she shows signs of shock and then act. Unfortunately, by then, it is often too late to do anything about it. Whenever possible, it is best to anticipate problems and act before they occur.

Whenever possible, anticipate problems, and act before they occur.

THINKING UNDER PRESSURE

* **autonomic nervous system** part of the nervous system that controls involuntary actions.

When you must make a critical decision, physical influences may help or hinder your ability to think clearly. Your **autonomic nervous system,** which controls your involuntary actions, may respond by secreting "fight or flight" hormones. These hormones will enhance your visual and auditory acuity and will improve your reflexes and muscle strength. However, they may also impair your ability to think critically and diminish your ability to assess and concentrate. In these instances, you will revert to your most basic instincts. Many an inexperienced paramedic has been "mentally paralyzed" by a complicated, critical call. With experience, you will learn to manage your nervousness and maintain a steadfast, controlled demeanour.

* **pseudo-instinctive** learned actions that are practised until they can be done without thinking.

One way to enhance your ability to remain in control is to raise your technical skills to a **pseudo-instinctive** level. This means that you do not have to concentrate on them to perform them. For example, you do not think about tying your shoelaces, you just tie them. Such "muscle memory" is essential when performing emergency medical skills. When you set up for an salbutamol nebulizer treatment, for instance, you automatically fit together the pieces of the device and administer the treatment without hesitation. This way you can concentrate on your patient's condition, controlling the scene, and managing the multitude of items that usually complicate any emergency call. Concentrating on more than one thing simultaneously is difficult, if not impossible.

Maintaining your composure, especially during a chaotic, complicated call, is key to developing a management plan for the best patient outcome.

MENTAL CHECKLIST

Thinking under pressure is not easy. Maintaining your composure, especially during a chaotic, complicated call is key to developing a management plan for the best patient outcome. Developing a routine mental checklist is a good way to stay focused and systematic. Pilots work through their preflight checklists routinely before turning over their engines. Medical clinicians develop acronyms and mnemonics to remember critical elements during stressful incidents. For example, when conducting a primary assessment, use the acronym MS-ABC. Use OPQRST to elicit your patient's present history, or use SAMPLE when time is critical. You can adopt the following checklist any time you must make a critical decision.

Scan the Situation Stand back, and scan the situation. Sometimes, you can miss subtle signs if you focus too narrowly on one aspect of your patient's problem. Look for environmental factors and other not-so-obvious clues. For example, your patient lies unconscious and cyanotic on the floor. You rule out any airway, breathing, or circulation problems. No medical history is available and no medication bottles are present. When you detect a fruity odour on your patient's breath, you suspect diabetic ketoacidosis.

Content Review

MENTAL CHECKLIST
- Scan the situation.
- Stop and think.
- Decide and act.
- Maintain control.
- Reevaluate.

Stop and Think Do not do anything without stopping and weighing your actions. Consider all of your options before you act. Remember that for every action, there is a reaction. Know what reactions to expect, and anticipate their possible harmful effects. For example, after administering amiodarone, monitor your patient closely for the expected benefits (eradication of ventricular tachycardia) and early signs of toxicity (numbness and tingling to the lips, drowsiness, nausea).

Decide and Act Once you have assessed the situation, make your decision, and act confidently. Announce your management plan to your crew with a combination of authority, confidence, and respect. Convey the feeling that you know your actions are correct and will work. This confidence helps reassure your patient, her family, your crew, and other responders even in the most stressful situations.

Maintain Control To maintain clear, efficient control of the scene and everyone involved, you must first control yourself. Many situations will challenge your inner strength and self-control. You will eventually be in charge of a scene in which everyone seems out of control. These chaotic incidents can occur anywhere and any time. Your job is to remain steadfast under fire.

Reevaluate Regularly reevaluate your plan's effects, and revise it accordingly. Never assume that your plan is working to perfection. Anticipate ways your patient might deteriorate, and devise alternative plans. Conduct an ongoing assessment en route to the hospital, and be prepared to revise your management plan. For example, if you note increased lung congestion after administering fluids, stop the infusion.

THE CRITICAL DECISION PROCESS

Understanding the **critical-thinking** process is essential for a paramedic. Your ability to analyze data effectively and devise a practical management plan optimizes patient care. You can conduct the most comprehensive history and secondary assessment, but if you cannot analyze the data and devise the proper management plan, your efforts will be fruitless. The critical-thinking process has five steps: forming a concept, interpreting the data, applying the principles, evaluating the results, and reflecting on the incident. To explain the critical decision-making process, we will consider a 19-year-old female patient with a sudden onset of sharp pain to her right lower quadrant with some vaginal bleeding.

✱ **critical thinking** thought process used to analyze and evaluate.

FORM A CONCEPT

The first step in critical decision making is to gather information and form a concept of your patient and the scene. You will get this information by assessing the general environment and the immediate surroundings. Note the mechanism of injury, if applicable. Then, observe your patient's mental status, skin colour, and positioning, and note any deformities or asymmetry. In our sample case, your patient presents at home, sitting on a sofa. At first glance, she appears pale, diaphoretic, and anxious. Next, you conduct a primary assessment, focusing on the MS-ABCs. Your initial goal is to identify and manage critical life threats. In this case, your general impression is of an alert and oriented but anxious young woman in moderate distress who presents with a clear airway; good air movement, as evidenced by her ability to converse in complete sentences; a strong, rapid, regular pulse; and cool, moist skin.

Now, you ascertain your patient's chief complaint, history of present illness, past history, and current health status while observing her affect (her general demeanour and attitude) and her degree of distress. You determine that her chief complaint is lower right quadrant pain that began suddenly 30 minutes ago. She also states she began bleeding about the same time. She denies any nausea, vomiting, or diarrhea. You learn she has a past history of pelvic inflammatory disease and an active, unprotected sex life with multiple partners. Her last menstrual period was six weeks ago. She has had four pregnancies but no viable births. She appears in moderate distress.

> **Content Review**
>
> **STEPS IN CRITICAL DECISION MAKING**
> - Form a concept.
> - Interpret the data.
> - Apply the principles.
> - Evaluate.
> - Reflect.

Finally, you conduct a focused secondary assessment of the appropriate areas. This includes any diagnostic testing, such as an electrocardiogram, pulse oximetry, and blood glucose testing. You take a full set of vital signs, which can help you identify most life-threatening conditions. Remember that your patient's age, underlying physical or medical condition, and current medications can influence her vital signs. For example, the use of beta blockers could cause a general decrease in her pulse and blood pressure. Your patient has some deep palpation tenderness in the lower right quadrant but no rebound tenderness, and the rest of her abdomen is soft and nontender. She has minor bleeding at this time and has used only one sanitary pad since the bleeding began. Her vital signs are HR—110 and regular; respirations—20, not laboured; BP—120/86.

INTERPRET THE DATA

After you assess the patient, you will interpret all the data in light of your knowledge and experience. In this case, your knowledge base includes female reproductive anatomy, the physiology of a normal pregnancy, and the pathophysiology of pregnancy complications along with their classic signs and symptoms. It also involves the anatomy, physiology, and pathophysiology of the cardiovascular system and the signs and symptoms of shock. Your experience base includes every patient you have assessed and managed with a similar presentation. Your attitude toward managing patients with these symptoms also becomes a factor because your experience may prejudice you. Consider all the data and determine the most common and statistically probable conditions that fit your patient's initial presentation. This is your differential field diagnosis. Then, consider the most serious condition that fits your patient's situation. In our example, a field diagnosis of a ruptured ectopic pregnancy is obvious. When a clear medical diagnosis is elusive, base your treatment on the presenting signs and symptoms.

APPLY THE PRINCIPLES

With your field diagnosis in mind, you devise a management plan that covers all contingencies. You will use written protocols, standing orders, and all the interventions at your disposal to manage your patient's particular problem. Sometimes, patients present with atypical signs and symptoms. For example, a patient who presents with a sore throat and cough may actually be having a heart attack and congestive heart failure. Other times, a protocol for your patient's problem simply may not exist. For example, your system may not have a protocol for facilitated intubation in head injuries. In these cases, consult with your medical direction physician for guidance in providing optimum care to your patient. The physician's emergency medical expertise and experience can be invaluable to you and your patient in unusual and difficult cases.

In our example, although your patient presents with relatively normal vital signs and is fully alert and oriented, you are very concerned. A basic principle of medicine is that all females of child-bearing age with lower abdominal pain are pregnant until proven otherwise. You initiate advanced life support precautions en route to the hospital, including high-flow oxygen and two large-bore intravenous lines. Her presentation has led you to expect the worst. If her fallopian tube ruptures and begins to hemorrhage, she will need rapid fluid resuscitation and general shock management. Your experience includes similar patients who suddenly suffered a life-threatening hemorrhage from a ruptured fallopian tube. Again, your attitude becomes a factor in that you will not allow her stable presentation to undermine your initial instinct—that she is potentially in serious trouble.

EVALUATE

During the ongoing assessment, you reassess your patient's condition and the effects of your standing order/protocol interventions. In other words, you determine whether your treatment is improving your patient's condition and status. For example, has the salbutamol helped your patient's breathing? Did the nitro and oxygen relieve the chest pain? Is the hemorrhage under control? Reflect on your actions, and continue your original plan, discontinue treatment, or take a completely different approach. You may alter your initial impression if your patient's condition worsens or if you discover new information. If time and circumstances allow a detailed assessment, you may discover less obvious problems.

In our sample case, your patient remains in potentially unstable condition. Your repeat assessment shows her vital signs are holding with the infusion of IV fluids. She is alert and not as anxious as before, and her skin is becoming warm and normal in colour. You deliver her to the emergency department in stable, but guarded, condition.

REFLECT

After the call, discuss your field diagnosis and care with the emergency physician. Compare your field diagnosis with her diagnosis. Conduct a call critique with your crew and discuss ways to improve your assessment and management of this case and future cases. Add these data to your information and experience base for future calls. Make every patient contact a learning experience. In this case, the emergency physician confirms your field diagnosis with lab tests and an ultrasonogram.

Make every patient contact a learning experience.

PUTTING IT ALL TOGETHER

A helpful mnemonic for the critical decision making process is the "six *R*s":

1. *R*ead the scene—Observe the general environmental conditions, the immediate surroundings, and any mechanism of injury.

2. *R*ead the patient—Observe your patient's level of consciousness, skin colour, position, location, and any obvious deformity or asymmetry. Talk to your patient to determine the chief complaint and whether it is a new problem or a worsening of a preexisting condition. Use touch to evaluate skin temperature and condition, and pulse rate and quality. Auscultate for problems with the upper and lower airways. Identify any life threats with the ABCs, and take a full set of vital signs.

3. *R*eact—Address any life threats found, determine the most common and serious existing conditions, and treat accordingly.

4. *R*eevaluate—Conduct a focused and detailed secondary assessment, note any response to your initial management interventions, and discover other less obvious problems.

5. *R*evise the management plan—Change or stop interventions that are not working or are causing your patient's condition to worsen, or try something new.

6. *R*eview your performance at call critique—Be honest, and critically evaluate your performance, always looking for better ways to manage a particular case presentation.

> ## Content Review
> ### THE SIX *R*s
> 1. *R*ead the scene.
> 2. *R*ead the patient.
> 3. *R*eact.
> 4. *R*eevaluate.
> 5. *R*evise the management plan.
> 6. *R*eview your performance.

SUMMARY

Clinical decision making is an essential paramedic skill that you will develop with time and experience. The prehospital environment is unlike any other medical care setting, and you will have to make decisions in less-than-optimal and sometimes dangerous conditions. Most times, you will have the benefit of consulting with your medical direction physician in difficult and unusual situations; other times, you may not. Your ability to gather information, analyze it, and make a critical decision may some day be the difference between your patient's life and death. This is inevitable. How well you prepare for that challenge will determine your ultimate success. The process begins in your paramedic training program. You must develop a good working knowledge of anatomy, physiology, pathophysiology, and the principles of emergency medicine. In time, through repeated patient contacts, you will develop the clinical judgment you need to make effective patient care decisions.

The critical-decision-making process involves a series of steps that experienced clinicians do almost unconsciously. First, you gather information (history and secondary assessment) to form an initial impression and then interpret it against your knowledge and experience to develop a working field diagnosis. You next apply the principles of emergency medicine to devise and implement a management plan and evaluate the effects of your treatments. Then, you reevaluate and revise your plan as necessary. Finally, you compare your findings with the emergency physician's diagnosis and discuss alternative ways to manage similar patients. With every patient contact, your experience grows and your clinical judgment improves. This is the essence of paramedic practice.

CHAPTER 11

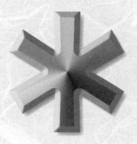

Assessment-Based Management

Objectives

After reading this chapter, you should be able to:

1. Explain how effective assessment is critical to clinical decision making. (pp. 451–453)
2. Explain how the paramedic's attitude and uncooperative patients affect assessment and decision making. (pp. 453–455)
3. Explain strategies to prevent labelling, tunnel vision, and decrease environmental distractions. (pp. 453–456)
4. Describe how personnel considerations and staffing configurations affect assessment and decision making. (pp. 455–456)
5. Synthesize and apply concepts of scene management and choreography to simulated emergency calls. (pp. 455–456)
6. Explain the roles of the team leader and the patient care provider. (pp. 455–456)
7. List and explain the rationale for bringing the essential care items to the patient. (pp. 456–457)

Continued

8. When given a simulated call, list the appropriate equipment to be taken to the patient. (pp. 456–457)
9. Explain the general approach to the emergency patient. (pp. 457–461)
10. Explain the general approach, patient assessment differentials, and management priorities for patients with various types of emergencies that may be experienced in prehospital care. (pp. 457–461)

11. Describe how to effectively communicate patient information face to face, over the telephone, by radio, and in writing. (pp. 461–462)
12. Given various preprogrammed and moulaged patients, provide the appropriate scene assessment, primary assessment, focused assessment, and detailed assessment, then provide the appropriate care, ongoing assessments, and patient transport. (pp. 450–463)

INTRODUCTION

A paramedic does more than just follow a standard sequence of assessment steps—scene assessment, primary assessment, focused history and secondary assessment, ongoing assessment, and detailed assessment. While carrying out the assessment in a systematic way, a paramedic is constantly thinking and reasoning.

The kind of reasoning a paramedic needs to do has been described as an "inverted pyramid"—with the broad end at the top and the narrow point at the bottom (Figure 11-1). As soon as you receive the dispatch and the patient's chief complaint, you try to form a mental list of all the possible causes of the patient's problem. (Such a list is often called a "differential diagnosis.") You want to keep your mind wide open, avoiding tunnel vision.

For example, the victim of a motor-vehicle collision has an obvious open extremity fracture with associated external blood loss. Serious as it is, the paramedic should resist being distracted by this injury. Suppose the patient had suffered a heart attack or cardiac arrest before or following the crash. Suppose the patient had other, more serious injuries, such as blunt abdominal trauma and internal bleeding. What if the paramedic fails to consider these other possibilities, focuses on the obvious leg injury, and spends on-scene time splinting the fracture instead of completing the assessment and initiating rapid transport?

It is far better if the paramedic uses inverted-pyramid reasoning skills (which may also be called critical thinking, problem solving, or clinical decision making) to assess the patient and prioritize emergency care. The paramedic begins by considering a wide variety of possible medical conditions and injuries. Then, while working through the standard sequence of assessment steps, the paramedic uses the information gathered at each step of the assessment to eliminate some possibilities and support other possibilities. The paramedic considers pertinent negatives (signs that are *not* present, such as paralysis or an erratic pulse) as well as

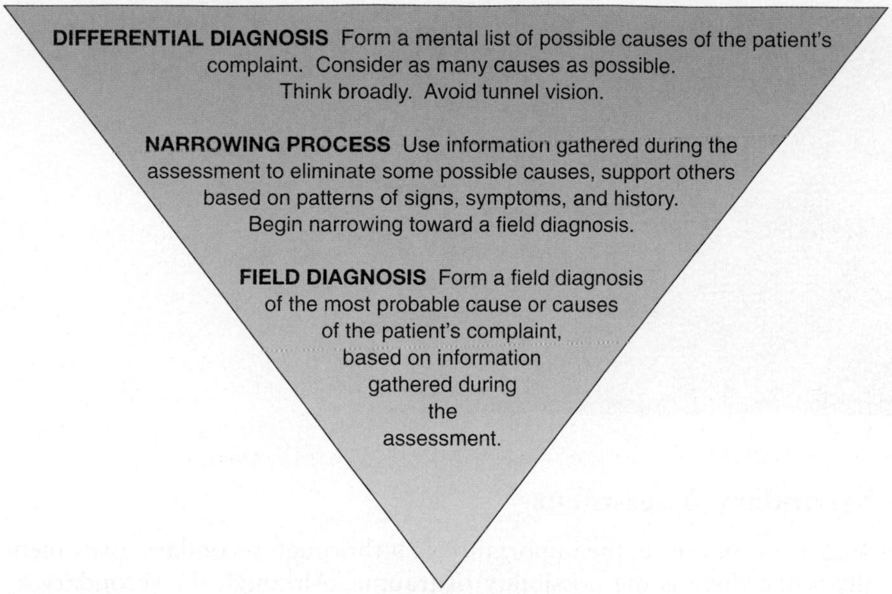

DIFFERENTIAL DIAGNOSIS Form a mental list of possible causes of the patient's complaint. Consider as many causes as possible. Think broadly. Avoid tunnel vision.

NARROWING PROCESS Use information gathered during the assessment to eliminate some possible causes, support others based on patterns of signs, symptoms, and history. Begin narrowing toward a field diagnosis.

FIELD DIAGNOSIS Form a field diagnosis of the most probable cause or causes of the patient's complaint, based on information gathered during the assessment.

FIGURE 11-1 Follow an inverted pyramid format to avoid tunnel vision while working toward a field diagnosis.

findings that are present (such as reddening and tenderness in one abdominal quadrant) to narrow in on a field diagnosis.

EFFECTIVE ASSESSMENT

Assessment forms the foundation for patient care. You can't treat or report a problem that is not found or identified. To find a problem, you must gather, evaluate, and synthesize information. Based on this process, you can then make decisions and take appropriate actions—formulate a management plan and determine the priorities for patient care.

A paramedic is entrusted with a great deal of independent judgment and responsibility for performing the correct actions for each individual patient, including such advanced skills as electrocardiogram (ECG) interpretation, rapid sequence intubation, and medication administration. Additionally, the medical director and hospital staff must rely on your experience and expertise as you describe the patient's condition and your conclusions about it. Consequently, the ability to reason and to reach a field diagnosis is critical to paramedic practice.

Assessment forms the foundation for patient care.

IMPORTANCE OF ACCURATE INFORMATION

The decisions that you make as a paramedic will only be as good as the information that you collect. To make accurate decisions, you need to gather accurate information.

The decisions you make as a paramedic will only be as good as the information you collect.

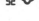

The History

A patient's history is a crucial part of the medical record, especially in medical conditions (as contrasted with trauma, where the secondary assessment takes precedence over the history). Very often, doctors will base 80 percent of their diagnosis on the history. As a result, it is important for you to question the patient, family members, and bystanders (Figure 11-2). However, you must not allow your knowledge of the disease—or your suspicion of the underlying problem—to affect the quality of the history you gather. Just because a patient has had a heart attack in the past does not mean that the person is having one now. Focus your questioning on the present complaint and associated problems.

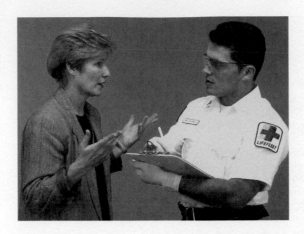

FIGURE 11-2 If the patient is unable to provide a history, gather information for the patient history from family members or bystanders.

The Secondary Assessment

Never forget, or minimize, the importance of a thorough secondary assessment, especially when there is the possibility of trauma. Although the secondary assessment may be compromised by field conditions, it should never be done in a cursory manner. Even when you are dealing with angry family members or are in a bad physical environment, you must perform an effective assessment. If field conditions make the assessment difficult or nearly impossible, you may have to move the patient into the ambulance or some other controlled environment to perform the assessment. If the patient is unresponsive or if there is a significant mechanism of injury, perform a complete head-to-toe assessment. If a patient is a responsive medical patient or has suffered minor trauma, focus your assessment on the systems associated with the patient's chief complaint.

Pattern Recognition

In assessing a patient, remain alert to patterns. Compare the information that you gather with your knowledge base—what you have learned about the pathophysiology and presentation of various diseases and injuries. For example, a trauma patient with decreased mental status, unequal pupils, swelling or discoloration around the eyes, and bleeding from the ear is presenting a pattern typical of basilar skull fracture. A patient who complains of a cough, gradual onset of breathing difficulty, sharp chest pain, and shaking chills with an elevated temperature is displaying a pattern typical of pneumonia. There may be times when you do not recognize a pattern. Obviously, the greater your knowledge base, the greater the likelihood you will recognize patterns. The ability to recognize patterns also increases with experience, which is why new paramedics are generally assigned to work with experienced paramedics for a time.

Assessment/Field Diagnosis

Sometimes, your field diagnosis will be based on a combination of pattern recognition and intuition, which is also based on experience. Once you have determined the problem, your next step is to formulate a plan of action, based on the patient's condition and the environment.

BLS/ALS Protocols

All EMS systems have protocols devised by medical direction that guide both BLS and ALS patient care. However, protocols and standing orders do not replace the paramedic's judgment. For example, you must exercise judgment, based on your assessment and field diagnosis, to know which protocol to use. You must exercise judgment to know when and how to follow a protocol—and you must also exercise judgment about when to deviate from a protocol. If a patient is allergic to a medication, for example, you do not administer it, even though a protocol calls for its use.

FACTORS AFFECTING ASSESSMENT AND DECISION MAKING

A number of factors—both internal (for example, your personal attitudes) and external (for example, the patient's attitude, distracting injuries, or environmental factors at the scene)—can affect your assessment of the patient and ultimately your decisions on how to manage treatment. By keeping these factors in mind, you can avoid the limitations that they impose on your collection and evaluation of patient information.

Personal Attitudes

Your attitude is one of the most critical factors in performing an effective assessment. You must be as nonjudgmental as possible to avoid "short circuiting" accurate data collection and pattern recognition by leaping to conclusions before completing a thorough assessment. Remember the popular computer mnemonic GIGO—garbage in/garbage out. You cannot reach valid conclusions about your patient based on a hasty or incomplete assessment. You will be unable to provide good medical management if, for example, you base decisions on the patient's social standing or "likability."

> *You must be as non-judgmental as possible to avoid "short circuiting" accurate data collection and the recognition of patterns.*

Seek to identify any preconceived notions that you may have about a group, and then work to eliminate them. As mentioned in Chapter 43, for example, a number of signs and symptoms have been mistakenly ascribed to aging when, in fact, they may point to serious medical conditions. A preconception that decreased mental acuity in an elderly patient is "normal" may lead you to miss what is really wrong with this patient and cause you to provide inadequate care.

Uncooperative Patients

Admittedly, uncooperative patients make it difficult to perform good assessments. All too often, these patients are perceived as being "high," either on alcohol or drugs. However, you must remember that there are many other possible causes for patient belligerence.

When assessing an uncooperative or restless patient, consider medical causes—hypoxia, hypovolemia, hypoglycemia, or a head injury, such as a concussion or a subdural hematoma. Be careful not to jump to the conclusion that this patient is "just another drunk" or a "frequent flyer." The "frequent flyer" that you have transported for alcoholic behaviour in the past may, this time, be suffering from trauma or a medical emergency.

If the person is a substance abuser, keep in mind that abuse or addiction is an illness. A substance abuser is often unwell to begin with and may present with other medical conditions that require medical intervention. No matter how difficult these patients are to manage, they still deserve the best care that you can provide (Figure 11-3). If you treat every patient in the manner in which you would want your loved ones treated, you will seldom go wrong.

> *If you treat every patient in the manner in which you would want your loved ones treated, you will seldom go wrong.*

Patient Compliance

Not all patients welcome the sight of a paramedic. Cultural and ethnic barriers—as well as prior negative experiences—may cause a patient to lack confidence in the rescuers. Such situations make it difficult for you to be effective at the scene,

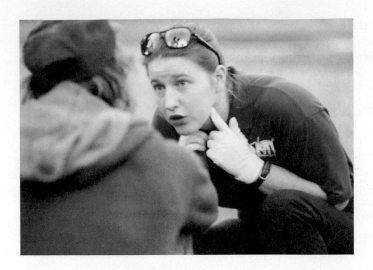

and the patients, in fact, may refuse to provide expressed consent for treatment or transport. It is your job to treat the patients in a way that will increase their confidence. If language is a barrier, try to speak through a friend, relative, or bystander who understands the patient's language or, in the case of deafness, signs. If you live in a community with a large ethnic population, try to become familiar with body language and customs of that culture. For example, some groups consider it rude to make eye contact. (For more on culturally diverse patients, see Chapter 45.) Again, do not permit yourself to make snap judgments about the patient.

Distracting Injuries

Yet another factor that can affect your assessment and decisions involves obvious but distracting injuries. A nasty-looking tibial fracture might cause the paramedic to overlook the less obvious signs of internal bleeding. Scalp lacerations usually look worse than they really are and could divert your attention from more serious injuries, such as an open chest wound. You must resist the temptation to form a field diagnosis too early. Although paramedics often have to rely on their "gut instinct," it may also lead them to make snap judgments. An open, bleeding fracture of the femur may be so distracting that a paramedic rushes to treat it, missing the fact that the patient is also having difficulty breathing. Always take a systematic approach to patient assessment to avoid distractions and to find and prioritize care for all of the patient's injuries and conditions.

Environmental and Personnel Considerations

You've probably already experienced some of the environmental factors that can affect patient assessment and care. Among others, they include scene chaos, violent or dangerous situations, high noise levels, or crowds of bystanders. Extremes of temperature can also complicate your call. A pedestrian struck by a vehicle on a cold winter day is threatened as much by hypothermia as his injuries. In some situations, you may need to perform only critical functions at the scene and then move the patient into the more controlled environment of your ambulance.

Even crowds of responders can be a problem, in some instances. Although having enough help is crucial, it is also important to use personnel wisely (Figure 11-4). A large number of rescuers moving around can be just as distracting as a large number of bystanders. In such situations, some of the rescuers might be staged nearby and brought to the scene when and if necessary. Some may also be assigned to control bystanders.

A large number of rescuers moving around can be just as distracting as a large number of bystanders.

As a rule, assessment is best achieved by one rescuer. A single paramedic can gather information and provide treatment sequentially. In the case of two paramedics, one paramedic can assess the patient while the other provides simultaneous treatment. With multiple responders, however, assessment and history may take place by "committee," which often leads to disorganized management.

ASSESSMENT/MANAGEMENT CHOREOGRAPHY

Although too many people, or multitier responders, may make it hard to acquire a patient history and conduct a secondary assessment, it becomes even more difficult if the responders are all at the same professional level and have no clear direction. It is important to plan for these events so that personnel have designated roles. (See Chapter 3 on incident command.) These roles may be rotated among team members so that no one is left out, but there must be a plan to avoid "freelancing." If there is only one advanced or critical care paramedic, then that person must assume all ALS roles.

In the case of a two-person advanced or critical care paramedic team, an effective preplan involves the roles of team leader and patient care provider, assigned on an alternating basis. Paramedics who work together regularly may develop their own plan, but a universally understood plan allows for other rescuers to participate in a rescue without interrupting the flow. Although the dynamics of field situations may necessitate changes in plans, a general "game plan" can go a long way toward preventing chaos. If field dynamics dictate a change in the preplanned roles, you are still working from a solid base. In setting up a two-person team, keep in mind the following descriptions of team leader and patient care provider roles.

Team Leader

The team leader is usually the person who will accompany the patient through to definitive care. The paramedic charged with this role should establish contact and maintain dialogue with the patient. He obtains the history, performs the secondary assessment, and presents the patient, in both verbal and written reports. During multiple-casualty situations, the team leader acts as the initial EMS commander.

The team leader must maintain overall patient perspective and provide leadership to the team by designating tasks and coordinating transport. Although the team leader must actively participate in critical interventions, it is important that this person not fall into the trap of trying to do everything alone. During advanced care calls, for example, the team leader's tasks might include the

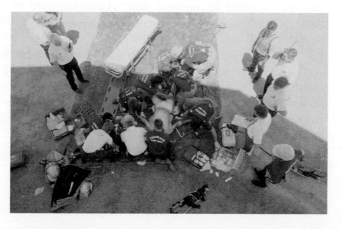

FIGURE 11-4 When multiple responders are on the scene, everyone should have a designated task.

following: reading the ECG, talking on the radio and giving drug orders, controlling the drug box, and keeping notes on drug administrations and effects. Actual treatment, however, would be left to the designated patient care provider.

Patient Care Provider

The patient care provider should ensure "scene cover" (i.e., watching the team leader's back). This person should gather scene information, talk to relatives and bystanders, and obtain vital signs. The patient care provider performs any skills or interventions requested by the team leader, such as attaching monitoring leads, administering oxygen, obtaining venous access, administering medications, and securing transport equipment. In multiple-casualty situations, the patient care provider acts as the triage group leader. During advanced care calls, he administers drugs, monitors tube placement, and oversees other personnel at the scene.

> **Content Review**
>
> ### ROLES OF PATIENT CARE PROVIDER
>
> - Provides scene cover
> - Gathers scene information
> - Talks to relatives/bystanders
> - Obtains vital signs
> - Performs interventions
> - Acts as triage group leader

LAYERED RESPONSE AND MULTIPLE-SERVICE SITUATIONS

You may encounter a variety of emergency response personnel and agencies at the scene of a call. Some EMS systems consist entirely of advanced care ambulances. Other systems use layered response models with mixes of primary care and advanced care staff. In addition, many communities have fire- or police-based emergency medical responder systems. And you may respond to calls where other first-aid or health-care personnel are already on scene: industrial accidents, swimming pools, or nursing and extended care facilities. Other calls may involve specialized responders, such as HAZMAT teams, utility services, or social service personnel.

Paramedics often have the most advanced patient care backgrounds and are responsible for overall patient care. As the team leader, you may be responsible for establishing the roles and delegating tasks regarding patient care. Ensure that you establish and maintain effective communications with the designated leaders of all responding agencies. Take a few moments to establish roles and responsibilities for all services at the scene.

Delegate patient care tasks for the personnel who will work around the patient. Ensure that you are aware of each responder's training and capabilities. Remember that you, as team leader, are ultimately responsible for the care of the patient and the actions of all responders involved in patient care.

THE RIGHT EQUIPMENT

If you do not have the right equipment readily available, you have compromised patient care.

Having the right equipment at the patient's side is essential. As a paramedic, you must be prepared to manage many conditions and injuries or changes in the patient's condition. As already mentioned, assessment and management must usually be done simultaneously. If you do not have the right equipment readily available, then you have compromised patient care and, in fact, the patient may die.

Think of your equipment as items in a backpack. Just like backpacking, you must downsize your equipment to minimum weight and bulk to facilitate rapid movement. At the same time, you need certain essential equipment to ensure survival—in this case, patient survival. The following is a list of the essential equipment for paramedic management of life-threatening conditions. You must bring these items to the side of every patient, regardless of what you initially think you may need:

- Infection Control
  - Infection control supplies (e.g., gloves, eye shields, face masks)

- Airway Control
  - Oral airways
  - Nasal airways
  - Suction (electric or manual)
  - Rigid tonsil-tip and flexible suction catheters
  - Laryngoscope and blades
  - Endotracheal tubes, stylettes, syringes, tape
- Breathing
  - Pocket mask
  - Bag-valve mask
  - Spare masks in various sizes
  - Oxygen tank and regulator
  - Oxygen masks, cannulas, and extension tubing
  - Occlusive dressings
  - Large bore IV catheter for thoracic decompression
- Circulation
  - Dressings
  - Bandages and tape
  - Sphygmomanometer, stethoscope
  - Note pad and pen or pencil
- Disability
  - Rigid collars
  - Flashlight
- Dysrhythmia
  - Cardiac monitor/defibrillator
- Exposure and Protection
  - Scissors
  - Space blankets or something to cover the patient

You may also pack some optional "take-in" equipment, such as drug therapy and venous access supplies. The method by which these supplies are carried may depend on how your system is designed (e.g., paramedic ambulances versus paramedics in nontransporting vehicles). It may also depend on local protocols, flexibility of standing orders, the number of paramedic responders in your area, and the difficulty of accessing patients because of terrain or some other problem.

In most cases, venous access supplies should be carried with the drug box, since venous access is required to administer most medications. The drug box should also contain any medications allowed in the formulary.

GENERAL APPROACH TO THE PATIENT

In addition to having the essential equipment, you need to have the essential demeanour to calm or reassure the patient. You must look and act the part of a professional while exhibiting the compassion and understanding associated with an effective "bedside manner." Although patients may not have the ability to rate your medical performance, they can certainly rate your people skills and service. Be aware of your body language and the messages it sends, either intentionally or unintentionally. Think carefully about what you say and how you say it—this includes your conversations with other members of the team and anyone else at the scene.

Once again, it helps to preplan your general approach to the patient. This will prevent confusion and improve the accuracy of your assessment. One team member should engage in an active, concerned dialogue with the patient. This same person should also demonstrate the listening skills needed to collect information and

Be aware of your body language and the messages it sends, either intentionally or unintentionally.

to convey a caring attitude. Taking notes may prevent asking the same question repeatedly and ensure that you acquire and pass on accurate data.

By approaching the patient with the right equipment and the right attitude, you minimize confusion and stand ready to provide effective emergency care.

The following sections briefly review the steps of the assessment that you will perform systematically on all patients. To review the assessment steps in detail, see Chapter 12.

SCENE ASSESSMENT

The scene assessment has the following components:

- Body substance isolation—Be sure you are wearing disposable gloves and are wearing or have available other protective equipment that may be needed, such as a gown, a mask, and eye protection.
- Scene safety—Observe the scene for any hazards to yourself, other rescuers, bystanders, and the patient. This is as important at a medical scene as at a trauma scene.
- Locate all patients, such as those who may have wandered away from a vehicle collision or additional patients in a household where the patient appears to be suffering from carbon monoxide or other toxic exposure.
- Mechanism of injury or nature of the illness—Determine this as well as possible at this stage of the call and remain observant for additional information as the call progresses.

If you determine that you may need additional equipment or support, now is the time to call for help.

PRIMARY ASSESSMENT

After you assess the scene, you quickly begin the primary assessment for the purpose of detecting and treating immediate life threats. The components of the initial assessment are:

- Formation of a general impression/degree of distress
- Mental status assessment (AVPU)
- Airway assessment
- Breathing assessment
- Circulation assessment
- Determination of the patient's priority for further on-scene care or immediate transport

Depending on your findings during the primary assessment, you might determine that one of the following approaches is appropriate for the patient's priority status.

Resuscitative Approach

Take the resuscitation approach whenever you suspect a life-threatening problem:

- Cardiac or respiratory arrest
- Respiratory distress or failure
- Unstable dysrhythmias
- Status epilepticus (series of generalized motor seizures without an intervening return of consciousness)

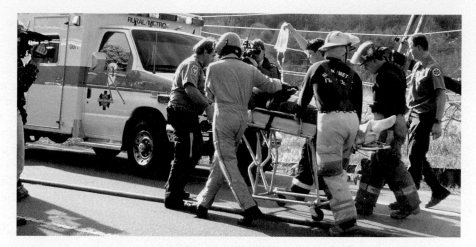

- Coma or altered mental status
- Shock or hypotension
- Major trauma
- Possible C-spine injury

In these cases, you must take immediate resuscitative action (such as CPR and defibrillation and ventilation) or other critical action (such as supplemental oxygen, control of major bleeding, or C-spine immobilization). Additional assessment and care can be performed after resuscitation and the rapid trauma assessment or en route to the hospital.

Contemplative Approach

Use the contemplative approach when immediate intervention is not necessary, such as with stable chest pain or a mild allergic reaction. In such situations, the focused history and secondary assessment, followed by any required interventions, will be performed at the scene, before transport to the hospital.

Immediate Evacuation

In some situations, you will need to immediately evacuate the patient to the ambulance (Figure 11-5). For example, a patient with severe internal bleeding requires life-saving interventions beyond a paramedic's skills. You might also resort to immediate evacuation if the scene is too chaotic for rational assessment or if it is too unsafe or unstable.

In these cases, initiate life-saving interventions, and prepare the patient for immediate transport. For trauma patients, use minimum stabilization. Apply a hard collar, and use an immobilization device, such as a backboard or clamshell, to stabilize the patient's injuries. Continue with assessment and definitive treatments and procedures once you are en route.

FOCUSED HISTORY AND SECONDARY ASSESSMENT

Following the primary assessment, you will perform the focused history and secondary assessment. Based on the patient's chief complaint and the information you have gathered during the primary assessment, you should consider your patient to belong to one of the following four categories:

1. Trauma patient with a significant mechanism of injury or altered mental status

2. Trauma patient with an isolated injury
3. Medical patient who is responsive
4. Medical patient who is unresponsive

For a trauma patient with a significant mechanism of injury or altered mental status or for an unresponsive medical patient, perform a rapid trauma assessment for the trauma patient or rapid medical assessment for the medical patient. For the trauma patient with an isolated injury or for the responsive medical patient, perform a secondary assessment focused on body systems related to the chief complaint.

For a medical patient, gather the history before performing the secondary assessment, unless the patient is unable to provide a history and there are no family members or bystanders who can provide information. For a trauma patient, gather the history after you have performed the secondary assessment. (Of course, elements of the history and the secondary assessment are often obtained simultaneously if partners are working together or as you talk to the responsive patient while assessing him.)

THE ONGOING ASSESSMENT AND THE DETAILED ASSESSMENT

The ongoing assessment must be performed on all patients to monitor and to observe trends in the patient's condition—every 5 minutes if the patient is unstable, every 15 minutes if the patient is stable. Ongoing assessments must be performed until the patient is transferred to the care of hospital personnel. The ongoing assessment includes evaluation of the following:

- Mental status
- Airway, breathing, and circulation (ABCs)
- Transport priorities
- Vital signs
- Focused assessment of any problem areas or conditions
- Effectiveness of interventions
- Management plans

The detailed assessment is similar to but more thorough than the rapid trauma assessment. It is generally performed only on trauma patients and only if time and the patient's condition permit. The purpose is to find any injuries or conditions that may have been missed during earlier assessments. In a critical patient, continuing ongoing assessments are more important than a detailed assessment.

IDENTIFICATION OF LIFE-THREATENING PROBLEMS

At all stages of the assessment, from primary assessment through ongoing assessments, from the scene to the ambulance to arrival at the hospital, you must actively and continuously look for and manage any life-threatening problems.

At all stages of the assessment, you must actively and continuously look for and manage any life-threatening problems.

You need to rapidly determine the chief complaint and to assess the distress in a systematic manner. Obtain baseline vital signs along with the focused secondary assessment, but if partners are working together, one may obtain the baseline vital signs earlier in the assessment. Focus on the relevant portions of the history and the secondary findings. For example, a history of appendicitis would be relevant for a patient complaining of right lower quadrant pain, less relevant for a trauma patient with possible spinal injury.

If you have an educated suspicion of what you are looking for, then you will be able to ask more productive questions. However, you are less likely to find something if you do not suspect it. For this reason, throughout your assessment, keep in mind the mechanism of injury and the nature of the illness (as determined, starting with the primary assessment and the patient's chief complaint). Listen carefully to everything the patient says. With experience, you will develop skill at multitasking—asking questions, listening to answers, and caring for the patient almost simultaneously. However, until you gain that experience, and unless you are actively managing a life-threatening condition, ask questions and just listen. Allow your partner to perform necessary tasks so that you do not miss any important clues.

The ability of a patient to describe symptoms and a paramedic's ability to listen greatly affect the quality and outcome of an assessment. The severity of pain does not always correlate well with the life-threatening potential of a condition. For example, a long splinter jammed under a fingernail will certainly cause pain, but few lives have been lost to such an injury. Conversely, some patients, especially the elderly, suffer myocardial infarctions with only vague symptoms that do not include chest pain. In addition, the location of pain and its source do not always correlate well, especially if it is visceral pain. For example, gallbladder attacks are often characterized by pain that is referred to the shoulder. As a paramedic, you must listen with your ears and then use your knowledge base of various illnesses and diseases to interpret what the patient says.

Basically your role as paramedic is to rapidly and accurately assess the patient and then to treat for the worst case scenario. This is the underlying principle of assessment-based management—your guide for providing effective emergency care.

The underlying principle of assessment-based management is to rapidly and accurately assess the patient and then to treat for the worst case scenario.

PRESENTING THE PATIENT

The ability to communicate effectively is the key to transferring patient information, whether in an out-of-hospital setting or within the hospital itself. Although neither basic nor advanced life support interventions may be required for every patient, a skill that will be used on every single patient is that of effective presentation, whether it is over the radio or telephone, in writing, or in face-to-face transfers at the receiving facility. Despite the frequency with which paramedics present patients, this is often the weakest link in patient care.

ESTABLISHING TRUST AND CREDIBILITY

Effective presentation and communication skills help establish a paramedic's credibility (Figure 11-6). They also inspire the trust and confidence of patients and other medical personnel. If you present your assessment, your findings, and your treatment in a clear, concise manner, you give the impression of a job well done. A poor presentation, conversely, implies poor assessment and poor patient care.

Other health-care providers have little time or interest in listening to rambling, disjointed presentations that cover unimportant details while omitting vital information. Use the SOAP format or some variation of it. Not only does SOAP help you organize your presentation, but most health-care providers also have become accustomed to listening to it and know what to expect. (SOAP stands for *s*ubjective findings, *o*bjective findings, *a*ssessment, and *p*lan. For a detailed description, see Chapter 9.)

The way in which you present the patient has direct implications for the person's care and recovery. Poor presentations compromise patient care. They lead to incomplete or even incorrect medical orders. If you do not communicate a patient's needs or status completely or accurately, a person may be denied some form of treatment based on the information that you have conveyed.

As a paramedic, you will be an extension of the supervisory physician, working under his licence. No doctor is going to issue orders for medications or other

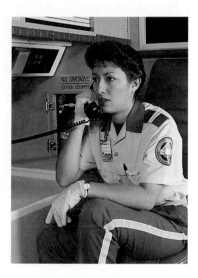

FIGURE 11-6 A clear, concise patient report will enable the hospital staff to prepare for the needs of the patient.

Content Review

SOAP
- Subjective findings
- Objective findings
- Assessment
- Plan

Poor presentations compromise patient care.

patient care based on guesswork. You are the doctor's eyes and ears at the emergency scene, and it is essential that you provide accurate information about both the patient and the emergency situation.

DEVELOPING EFFECTIVE PRESENTATION SKILLS

The most effective oral presentations usually meet these guidelines:

- Last less than one minute
- Are very concise and clear
- Avoid extensive use of medical jargon
- Follow a basic format, usually the SOAP format or some variation
- Include both pertinent findings and pertinent negatives (findings that might be expected, given the patient's complaint or condition, but are absent or denied by the patient)
- Conclude with specific actions, requests, or questions related to the plan

The best way to become proficient at presenting patients is to plan ahead and to practise. Start with an end in mind—know what particular areas of information will be asked for or expected so that you can be ready with that information. As you become more experienced, the flow of information will become second nature to you. Until that time, use a preprinted form to help you organize your thoughts and information and to take notes during the patient workup. Practise presenting both simulated and real patients, perhaps at company or unit drills. Listen to other paramedics as they present patients and learn from them. Adopt their good habits and avoid their bad ones.

An ideal presentation should include the following:

- Patient identification, age, sex, and degree of distress
- If relevant, include supplemental information, such as the patient's weight
- Chief complaint (why a patient called)
- Present illness/injury
  - Pertinent details about the present problem
  - Pertinent negatives
- Past medical history
  - Allergies
  - Medications
  - Pertinent medical history
- Physical signs
  - Vital signs
  - Pertinent positive findings
  - Pertinent negative findings
- Assessment
  - Paramedic impression
- Plan
  - What has been done and the patient's response
  - Orders requested

Remember, the key to developing presentation skills is repetition and an understanding of the format being used. Once you have mastered this, you can transfer the patient with the satisfaction and confidence of a job well done. (For more detail on this topic, review Chapters 8 and 9 on communications and documentation.)

Plan ahead. Know what particular areas of information will be asked for or expected so that you can be ready with that information.

REVIEW OF COMMON COMPLAINTS

To develop as an entry-level practitioner at the paramedic level, it is important to participate in scenario-based reviews of commonly encountered complaints. As mentioned, you might take part in company or unit drills in which you will observe and work with experienced paramedics. You might also participate in laboratory-based simulations.

PRACTICE SESSIONS

The goal of practice sessions is to choreograph the roles and actions of the EMS response team. These sessions will give you the chance to practise assessment and decision making on cases that you are likely to encounter in out-of-hospital situations. They also give you the opportunity to provide intervention based on your assessment and to reinforce the modalities in local and/or regional treatment protocols. Finally, you can practise patient presentation, both verbally and in written form. At all phases, you get the benefit of feedback from the team members and crew with whom you will be working.

LABORATORY-BASED SIMULATIONS

Laboratory-based simulations require you to assess a preprogrammed patient or mannequin. You will make decisions relative to interventions and transport. You will also provide interventions, package the patient (or mannequin), and transport. Ideally, you will work as part of a team and practise the various roles assigned to team members, including that of patient.

SELF-MOTIVATION

The chance to practise does not stop at the classroom or at your unit. While a paramedic student or the new member of a team, take advantage of every opportunity to practise your new skills. Recruit family members or friends—or even a teddy bear—as volunteer patients. What is important is to practise, practise, practise—until you feel comfortable with as many different situations as possible.

SUMMARY

Assessment forms the basis of patient care. To make correct decisions, you must gather information and then evaluate and synthesize it. A variety of factors may affect assessment and the decision-making process itself. Some of these factors include paramedic attitude; uncooperative patients; obvious but distracting injuries; narrow, or tunnel, vision; the environment; patient compliance; and personnel considerations.

It is important to have the right equipment readily available to treat immediately life-threatening conditions. Effective communication and transfer of patient information—whether done face to face, over the telephone or radio, or in writing—is crucial to presenting the patient and ensuring continuation of effective care.

Remember, the best way to develop good assessment skills is to practise until you become comfortable with a wide range of patient complaints.

CHAPTER 12

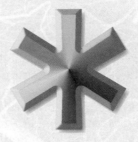

Anatomy and Physiology

Objectives

Part 1: The Cell and the Cellular Environment (begins on p. 466)

After reading Part 1 of this chapter, you should be able to:

1. Describe the structure and function of the normal cell. (pp. 466–470)
2. List types of tissue. (p. 470)
3. Define organs, organ systems, the organism, and system integration. (pp. 470–474)

4. Discuss the cellular environment (fluids and electrolytes), including osmosis and diffusion. (pp. 474–483)
5. Discuss acid-base balance and pH. (pp. 483–486)

Part 2: Body Systems (begins on p. 486)

After reading Part 2 of this chapter, you should be able to:

1. Describe the anatomy and physiology of the integumentary system, including the skin, hair, and nails. (pp. 486–489)

2. Describe the anatomy and physiology of the hematopoietic system, including the components of the blood, and discuss hemostasis, the

Continued

Objectives Continued

hematocrit, and hemoglobin. (pp. 489–500)

3. Describe the anatomy and physiology of the musculoskeletal system, including bones, joints, skeletal organization, and muscular tissue and structure. (pp. 500–522)

4. Describe the anatomy and physiology of the head, face, and neck and their relation to the physiology of the central nervous system. (pp. 532–536)

5. Describe the anatomy and physiology of the spine, including the cervical, thoracic, lumbar, and sacral spine and the coccyx. (pp. 536–542)

6. Describe the anatomy and physiology of the thorax, including its skeletal and muscular structure and the organs and vessels contained within it. (pp. 542–547)

7. Describe the anatomy and physiology of the nervous system, including the neuron, the central nervous system (brain and spine), and the peripheral nervous system (somatic, autonomic, sympathetic, and parasympathetic divisions). (pp. 547–565)

8. Describe the anatomy and physiology of the endocrine system, including the glands and other organs with endocrine activity. (pp. 565–576)

9. Describe the anatomy and physiology of the cardiovascular system, including the heart and the circulatory system. (pp. 576–590)

10. Describe the physiology of perfusion. (pp. 590–596)

11. Describe the anatomy of the respiratory system (upper and lower airway and pediatric airway) and the physiology of the respiratory system (respiration and ventilation and measures of respiratory function). (pp. 596–610)

12. Describe the anatomy and physiology of the abdomen, including its divisions and the organs and vessels contained within it. (pp. 610–613)

13. Describe the anatomy and physiology of the digestive system, including the digestive tract and the accessory organs of digestion, and the spleen. (pp. 613–616)

14. Describe the anatomy and physiology of the urinary system, including the kidneys, ureters, urinary bladder, and urethra. (pp. 616–622)

15. Describe the anatomy and physiology of the female reproductive system, the menstrual cycle, and the pregnant uterus. (pp. 623–629)

16. Describe the anatomy and physiology of the male reproductive system. (pp. 629–630)

INTRODUCTION

An understanding of basic human anatomy and physiology is fundamental to paramedic practice. Part 1 of this chapter presents an overview of the organization of human body systems, including the following:

- The cell
- Tissues
- Organs
- Organ systems
- The organism
- System integration
- Fluids and electrolytes
- Acid-base balance

Part 2 describes the major body systems:

- The integumentary system
- The blood
- The musculoskeletal system
- The head, face, and neck
- The spine and thorax
- The nervous system
- The endocrine system
- The cardiovascular system
- The respiratory system
- The abdomen
- The digestive system and spleen
- The urinary system
- The reproductive system

Part 1: The Cell and the Cellular Environment

THE NORMAL CELL

✱ **cell** the basic structural unit of all plants and animals. Cells are specialized to carry out all the body's basic functions.

The fundamental unit of the human body is the **cell** (Figure 12-1). It contains all necessary components to turn essential nutrients into energy, remove waste products, reproduce, and carry on other essential life functions.

There are two kingdoms of cells: *prokaryotes* and *eukaryotes*. Prokaryotes are the cells of lower plants and animals, such as blue-green algae and bacteria. Their structure is very simple, with an indistinct nucleus that is not encased in a membrane and without any other internal structures. Eukaryotes are the cells of higher plants and animals, such as most algae, fungi, protozoa—and humans.

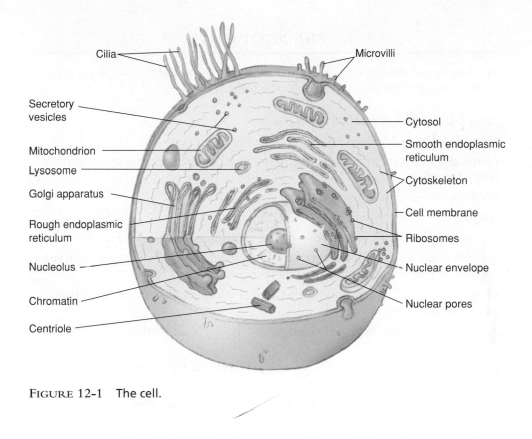

Cilia

Microvilli

Secretory
vesicles

Cytosol

Mitochondrion

Smooth endoplasmic
reticulum

Lysosome

Cytoskeleton

Golgi apparatus

Cell membrane

Rough endoplasmic
reticulum

Ribosomes

Nucleolus

Nuclear envelope

Chromatin

Nuclear pores

Centriole

FIGURE 12-1   The cell.

Eukaryotes are, of course, more complex than prokaryotes. The cell structure discussed on the following pages relates to the eukaryotes.

CELL STRUCTURE

A cell is something like a small, self-sustaining city. Within the cell, specialized structures perform specific functions. In a normal cell, all the structures and functions work together to maintain a normal, balanced environment. Each cell has three main elements: the cell membrane, the cytoplasm, and the organelles.

The Cell Membrane

The **cell membrane** (sometimes called the *plasma membrane*) is the outer covering that encircles and protects the cell.

The membrane is selectively permeable, or **semipermeable,** which means that it allows certain substances to pass from one side to the other but does not allow others to pass. Vital functions of the cell membrane, made possible by its selective permeability, include electrolyte and fluid balance and the transfer of enzymes, hormones, and nutrients into and out of the cell. These functions will be discussed in greater detail later.

Without the cell membrane, the interior contents of a cell would be exposed to the extracellular environment and quickly die. That is why the bacterial cellular membrane is the site targeted by many antibiotic drugs—because destroying the cell membrane kills the cell.

Content Review

MAIN ELEMENTS OF THE CELL

• Cell membrane
• Cytoplasm
• Organelles

✱ **cell membrane** also *plasma membrane;* the outer covering of a cell.

✱ **semipermeable** able to allow some, but not all, substances to pass through. Cell membranes are semipermeable.

THE ROOT CYT

To understand the discussion of cells, take note of the root *cyt*—which means "cell." Words with this root include the following:

cytoplasm—thick fluid that fills a cell.

cytosol—clear liquid portion of the cytoplasm in a cell.

cytoskeleton—structure of protein filaments that supports the internal structure of a cell.

erythrocyte—red blood cell.

leukocyte—white blood cell.

thrombocyte—blood cell responsible for clotting; also called a *platelet*.

lymphocyte—a type of leukocyte, or white blood cell, that attacks foreign substances as part of the body's immune response.

phagocyte—a cell that has the ability to ingest other cells and such substances as bacteria and cell debris.

phagocytosis—ingestion and digestion of bacteria and other substances by phagocytes.

monocyte—white blood cell with a single nucleus; the largest normal blood cell.

granulocyte—white cell with multiple nuclei that has the appearance of a bag of granules.

cytokine—protein produced by a white blood cell that instructs neighbouring cells to respond in a genetically preprogrammed fashion.

cytotoxin—substance that is poisonous to cells.

cytotoxic—poisonous (toxic) to cells.

The Cytoplasm

✱ **cytoplasm** the thick fluid, or *protoplasm*, that fills a cell.

Cytoplasm is the thick, viscous fluid that fills and gives shape to the cell and is also called *protoplasm*. The clear liquid portion of the cytoplasm is called *cytosol*. Substances dissolved in the cytosol are mainly electrolytes, proteins, glucose (sugar), and lipids (fatty substances). Structures of various sizes and functions are dispersed throughout the cytosol.

The Organelles

✱ **organelles** structures that perform specific functions within a cell.

Structures that perform specific functions within the cell are called **organelles.** Six of the most important organelles are the *nucleus, endoplasmic reticulum, Golgi apparatus, mitochondria, lysosomes,* and *peroxisomes.* A brief discussion of a few of their functions provides an idea of the complex activity that takes place within a cell.

✱ **nucleus** the organelle within a cell that contains the DNA, or genetic material; in the cells of higher organisms, the nucleus is surrounded by a membrane.

- *Nucleus.* The **nucleus** contains the genetic material, deoxyribonucleic acid (DNA), and the enzymes necessary for replication of DNA. DNA determines our inherited traits and also plays a critical ongoing role within our bodies. DNA must be constantly copied and transferred to the cells.

- *Endoplasmic reticulum.* The endoplasmic reticulum is a network of small channels that has both rough and smooth portions. Rough endoplasmic reticulum functions in the synthesis (building) of proteins. Smooth endoplasmic reticulum functions in the synthesis of lipids, some of which are used in the formation of cell membranes, and carbohydrates.

- *Golgi apparatus.* The Golgi apparatus is located near the nucleus of most cells. It performs a variety of functions, including synthesis and packaging of such secretions as mucus and enzymes.

- *Mitochondria.* The mitochondria are the energy factories, sometimes called the "powerhouses," of the cells. They convert essential nutrients into energy sources, often in the form of **adenosine triphosphate (ATP)**.

- *Lysosomes.* Lysosomes contain digestive enzymes. Their functions include protection against disease and production of nutrients, breaking down bacteria and organic debris that has been taken into the cells and releasing usable substances, such as sugars and amino acids.

- *Peroxisomes.* Peroxisomes are similar to lysosomes. Especially abundant in the liver, they absorb and neutralize toxins, such as alcohol.

✳ adenosine triphosphate (ATP) a high-energy compound present in all cells, especially muscle cells; when split by enzyme action, it yields energy. Energy is stored in ATP.

A wide variety of other structures and functions exist within the cell. Within the nucleus, for example, there are one or more smaller organelles called *nucleoli* (plural of *nucleolus*). Another component of the nucleus is *chromatin* (tangles of chromosome filaments containing DNA). Additional organelles exist in the cytoplasm (cytosol) outside the nucleus, including the *cytoskeleton* (a structure of protein filaments that supports the internal structure of the cell), *ribosomes* (granular structures that manufacture proteins—some float free, others attach to the surface of the endoplasmic reticulum, which creates the "rough" endoplasmic reticulum), *vesicles* (which play a role in transferring and storing secretions from the rough endoplasmic reticulum and Golgi complex), and *centrioles* (which play a role in cell division). On the surface of some cells are *microvilli* (folds on the cell surface), and, on some cells, whip-like *cilia* and *flagella* (which move fluids across cell surfaces and move cells through the surrounding extracellular fluid).

CELL FUNCTION

All the cells of the human body have the same general structure and contain the same genetic material but—through a process called *differentiation,* or *maturation*—become specialized. Eventually, cells perform specific functions that are different from the functions performed by other cells. There are seven major functions of cells:

- *Movement* is performed by muscle cells. Skeletal muscles move arms and legs. The smooth muscle around blood vessels causes them to dilate or constrict as necessary. Other smooth muscle moves food and wastes through the digestive tract. Cardiac muscle causes the chambers of the heart to contract. (See Muscle Tissue in the next section.)

- *Conductivity* is the function of nerve cells that creates and transmits an electrical impulse in response to a stimulus.

- *Metabolic absorption* is a function of cells of the intestines and kidneys, which take in nutrients that pass through the body.

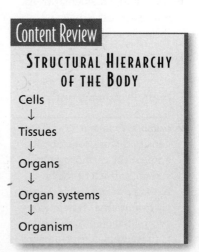

Content Review

STRUCTURAL HIERARCHY OF THE BODY

Cells
↓
Tissues
↓
Organs
↓
Organ systems
↓
Organism

* **tissue** a group of cells that perform a similar function.

* **epithelial tissue** the protective tissue that lines internal and external body tissues. Examples: skin, mucous membranes, the lining of the intestinal tract.

* **muscle tissue** tissue that is capable of contraction when stimulated. There are three types of muscle tissue: *cardiac* (myocardium, or heart muscle), *smooth* (within intestines, surrounding blood vessels), and *skeletal,* or *striated* (allows skeletal movement). Skeletal muscle is mostly under voluntary, or conscious, control; smooth muscle is under involuntary, or unconscious, control; cardiac muscle is capable of spontaneous, or self-excited, contraction.

* **connective tissue** the most abundant body tissue; it provides support, connection, and insulation. Examples: bone, cartilage, fat, blood.

* **nerve tissue** tissue that transmits electrical impulses throughout the body.

* **organ** a group of tissue functioning together. Examples: heart, liver, brain, ovary, eye.

* **organ system** a group of organs that work together. Examples: the cardiovascular system, formed of the heart, blood vessels, and blood; the gastrointestinal system, comprising the mouth, salivary glands, esophagus, stomach, intestines, liver, pancreas, gall bladder, rectum, and anus.

- *Secretion* is performed by glands that produce such substances as hormones, mucus, sweat, and saliva.
- *Excretion* is a function all cells perform as they break down nutrients and expel wastes.
- *Respiration* is the function by which cells take in oxygen, which is used to transform nutrients into energy.
- *Reproduction* is the process by which cells enlarge, divide, and reproduce themselves, replacing dead cells and enabling new tissue growth and healing of wounds. Some cells, such as nerve cells, cannot reproduce—so, for instance, a severed spinal cord cannot repair itself.

TISSUES

Tissue refers to a group of cells that perform a similar function. The following are the four basic types of tissue:

1. **Epithelial tissue** lines internal and external body surfaces and protects the body. In addition, certain types of epithelial tissue perform specialized functions, such as secretion, absorption, diffusion, and filtration. Examples of epithelial tissue are skin, mucous membranes, and the lining of the intestinal tract.

2. **Muscle tissue** has the capability of contraction when stimulated. There are three types of muscle tissue (see Figure 12-42 in the Musculoskeletal System section later in this chapter).
   — *Cardiac muscle* is tissue that is found only within the heart. It has the unique capability of spontaneous contraction without external stimulation.
   — *Smooth muscle* is the muscle found within the intestines and encircling blood vessels. Smooth muscle is generally under the control of the involuntary, or autonomic, component of the nervous system.
   — *Skeletal muscle* is the most abundant muscle type. It allows movement and is mostly under voluntary control.

3. **Connective tissue** is the most abundant tissue in the body. It provides support, connection, and insulation. Examples of connective tissue include bones, cartilage, and fat. Blood is also sometimes classified as connective tissue.

4. **Nerve tissue** is tissue specialized to transmit electrical impulses throughout the body. Examples of nerve tissue include the brain, spinal cord, and peripheral nerves.

ORGANS, ORGAN SYSTEMS, AND THE ORGANISM

A group of tissues functioning together is an **organ.** For example, the pancreas consists of epithelial tissue, connective tissue, and nervous tissue. Together, these tissues perform the essential functions of the pancreas. These functions include production of certain digestive enzymes and regulation of glucose metabolism.

A group of organs that work together is referred to as an **organ system.** The following are important organ systems:

- *Cardiovascular system.* The cardiovascular system consists of the heart, blood vessels, and blood. It transports nutrients and other essential elements to all parts of the body.

- *Respiratory system.* The respiratory system consists of the lungs and associated structures. It provides oxygen to the body, while removing carbon dioxide and other waste products.

- *Gastrointestinal system.* The gastrointestinal system consists of the mouth, salivary glands, esophagus, stomach, intestines, liver, pancreas, gallbladder, rectum, and anus. It takes in complex nutrients and breaks them down into a form that can be readily used by the body. It also aids in the elimination of excess wastes.

- *Genitourinary system.* The genitourinary system consists of the kidneys, ureters, bladder, and urethra. It is important in the elimination of various waste products. It also plays a major role in the regulation of water, electrolytes, blood pressure, and other essential body functions.

- *Reproductive system.* The reproductive system provides for reproduction of the organism. In the female, it consists of the ovaries, fallopian tubes, uterus, and vagina. In the male, it consists of the testes, prostate, seminal vesicles, vas deferens, and penis.

- *Nervous system.* The nervous system consists of the brain, spinal cord, and all peripheral nerves. It controls virtually all bodily functions and is the seat of intellect, awareness, and personality.

- *Endocrine system.* The endocrine system is a control system closely associated with the nervous system. It consists of the pituitary gland, pineal gland, pancreas, testes (male), ovaries (female), adrenal glands, thyroid gland, and parathyroid glands. There is evidence that other organs—such as the heart, kidney, and intestines—have endocrine functions. As noted earlier, the endocrine system exerts its effects through the release of chemical messengers called hormones.

- *Lymphatic system.* The lymphatic system is often considered a part of the cardiovascular system. It consists of the spleen, lymph nodes, lymphatic channels, thoracic duct, and the lymph fluid itself. It is important in fighting disease, in filtration, and in removing waste products of cellular metabolism.

- *Muscular system.* The muscular system is responsible for movement, posture, and heat production. It consists, primarily, of the skeletal muscles.

- *Skeletal system.* The skeletal system consists of the bones, cartilage, and associated connective tissue. It provides for support, protection, and movement. The bone marrow is the site for production of various blood cells, including the red blood cells and certain types of white blood cells.

The sum of all cells, tissues, organs, and organ systems is the **organism.** The failure of any component, from the cellular level to the organ-system level, can result in the development of a serious medical emergency.

✱ **organism** the sum of all the cells, tissues, organs, and organ systems of a living being. Examples: the human organism, a bacterial organism.

The failure of any component of an organism—from the cellular level to the organ system level—can result in a serious medical emergency.

SYSTEM INTEGRATION

The human body is not just a static structure of bones and cavities and tubes. It is a dynamic organization in which cells, tissues, organs, and organ systems perform functions essential to the preservation of the organism. **Homeostasis** is the term for the body's natural tendency to keep the internal environment and metabolism steady and normal. At the cellular level, the body will strive to maintain a very constant environment because cells do not tolerate extreme environmental fluctuations.

A significant amount of energy is needed to maintain the order that is evident in the structures (**anatomy**) and functions (**physiology**) of the organism. Potential energy is stored in the biochemical bonds of cells and tissues in plants and animals, and the kinetic energy necessary to maintain homeostasis is obtained by the breaking of those bonds. Food provides energy substrates, such as sugar, fats, and proteins, which, when broken down, produce the energy for the maintenance of homeostasis. **Metabolism** is the term used to refer to the building up (*anabolism*) and breaking down (*catabolism*) of biochemical substances to produce energy.

The body's cells interact and intercommunicate, rather like a multicellular "social" organism. Communication between the cells consists of electrochemical messages. When something interferes with the normal sending or receiving of these messages, a disease process can begin or advance.

Many intercellular messages are conveyed by substances secreted by various body glands. *Endocrine glands,* sometimes called ductless glands (including the pituitary, thyroid, parathyroid, adrenal glands, the Islets of Langerhans in the pancreas, the testes, and the ovaries), secrete hormones directly into the circulatory system, where they travel to the target organ or tissue. *Exocrine glands* secrete such substances as sweat, saliva, mucus, and digestive enzymes onto the epithelial surfaces of the body (the skin or linings of body cavities and organs) via ducts.

Several types of signalling take place among cells. *Endocrine signalling* (via hormones distributed throughout the body) is one mode of intercellular communication. *Paracrine signalling* (nonendocrine, nonhormonal) involves secretion of chemical mediators by certain cells that act only on nearby cells. In *autocrine signalling,* cells secrete substances that may act on themselves. In *synaptic signalling,* cells secrete specialized chemicals called neurotransmitters, such as norepinephrine, acetylcholine, serotonin, and dopamine, that transmit signals across synapses, the junctions between neurons.

These chemical signals—in the form of hormones and neurotransmitters—are received by various kinds of receptors. Receptors can be nerve endings, sensory organs, or proteins that interact with, and then respond to, the chemical signals and other stimuli. Many of the medications administered by paramedics act on these receptors. *Chemoreceptors* respond to chemical stimuli. Chemoreceptors within the brain respond to increasing levels of carbon dioxide (CO_2) in the cerebrospinal fluid, stimulating respiratory centres in the brainstem to increase the rate and depth of respirations. *Baroreceptors* respond to pressure changes. Baroreceptors in the arch of the aorta and in the carotid sinuses along the carotid artery sense changes in blood pressure, which then cause the cardiac centres in the medulla to alter the heart rate. *Alpha and beta adrenergic receptors* on the surfaces of cells in the bronchi, heart, and blood vessels respond to neurotransmitters and medications, resulting in a variety of cardiovascular and respiratory responses.

As the above examples demonstrate, when normal intercellular communication is interrupted and normal metabolism is disturbed, the body will respond in various ways to compensate and attempt to restore the normal metabolism (i.e., homeostasis).

Each organ system plays a role in maintaining homeostasis. An example is the body's response to the accumulation of cellular carbon dioxide that occurs

---

✳ homeostasis the natural tendency of the body to maintain a steady and normal internal environment.

✳ anatomy the structure of an organism; body structure.

✳ physiology the functions of an organism; the physical and chemical processes of a living thing.

✳ metabolism the total changes that take place during physiological processes.

When something interferes with the electrochemical messages cells send to each other, a disease process can begin or advance.

When normal metabolism is disturbed, the body attempts to restore normal metabolism (i.e., homeostasis).

during exercise. The respiratory system immediately attempts to return the internal environment to its normal state by increasing the respiratory rate and depth to eliminate excess carbon dioxide—which is why runners pant.

The organization of the human body is very complex, with constant interactions occurring within and among the systems to maintain homeostasis. When disease interrupts these interactions, it can cause both local effects (at the specific site of the illness or injury) and systemic effects (throughout the body). When this happens, body cells and systems will respond to restore normal conditions.

To understand how human systems interact, physiologists sometimes view them from an engineering perspective. Various body systems respond to *inputs,* or stressors, that may be sensed by other systems. The system receiving the input responds in some fashion, creating an *output.* The portion of the system creating the output, be it a cell or an organ, is known as the *effector.* For example, consider a large laceration to an extremity with severe blood loss. The drop in blood pressure resulting from the blood loss is sensed by the baroreceptors, which, in turn, cause messages to be sent from the cardiac centre in the medulla to the heart, resulting in an increase in the rate and strength of contractions in an attempt to restore normal blood pressure. By definition, the input would be the drop in pressure sensed by the baroreceptors; the effector would be the heart, which increased its rate in response to signals from the medulla; and the output would be the resultant increase in blood pressure.

This kind of feedback is essential for maintaining stability within a system and homeostasis for the organism. When the output of a system corrects the situation that created the input, it is said to loop, or feed back on the input, and a **negative feedback loop** exists—"negative" because the feedback negates the input caused by the original stressor. To elaborate on the example of the baroreceptors, the output or increase in blood pressure resulting from the increased heart rate feeds back on, or cancels out, the original input (low blood pressure), and the heart (effector) no longer has to maintain an elevated rate. This particular feedback loop is known as the baroreceptor reflex mechanism.

Unfortunately, the grim reality of this model is that blood loss often overwhelms the heart's ability to respond with an increased rate. At that point, the system has lost the ability to compensate, and, as a paramedic, you must intervene by administering fluids and taking other necessary therapeutic measures. When the outputs of effector organs are ineffective in correcting the input condition, *decompensation* is said to have occurred.

In the case of decompensation, the feedback system doesn't or can't restore homeostasis. The opposite problem can also occur when the feedback system goes too far and overcompensates for the original problem. To prevent this, it is important for the body to have some way to stop the output—to restore the heart rate to normal because the inability to control the pulse rate would cause instability in the cardiovascular system and danger to the organism. In fact, the body does have numerous means of controlling or halting output.

Biological systems generally employ negative feedback loops to maintain stability. Positive feedback systems do exist in human physiology. (Positive feedback enhances, rather than negates, the effects of input.) An example would be some short-lived positive feedback loops involved in follicular (egg) development in females. However, these loops work in conjunction with negative feedback loops to maintain stability.

Feedback activity must be orchestrated and synchronized to maintain homeostasis. Two systems work together to maintain homeostasis and to integrate the responses of different systems: the nervous system and the endocrine system. They are functionally and anatomically coupled to allow for this integration. For example, the pituitary gland of the endocrine system is joined with the hypothalamus of the nervous system by a stalk-like structure called the infundibulum. This allows for rapid communication between these two body control systems.

* **negative feedback loop** body mechanisms that work to reverse, or compensate for, a pathophysiological process, (or to reverse any physiological process, whether pathological or nonpathological).

There are important temporal differences in the responses of these two systems. Nervous system response is generally rapid in onset but short lived. An example is the baroreceptor reflex mechanism, mentioned earlier, which is primarily mediated by the nervous system. Conversely, endocrine responses generally take longer—that is, they have a slower onset of action but a longer duration. For example, the pituitary gland secretes antidiuretic hormone (ADH) in response to low blood pressure. ADH acts on the renal (kidney) tubules, causing water to be reabsorbed into the blood instead of being eliminated from the body. This causes an increase in intravascular fluid volume that compensates for the decrease in intravascular volume caused by the blood loss. All these responses are stimulated by pathological alterations or events.

THE CELLULAR ENVIRONMENT: FLUIDS AND ELECTROLYTES

Many pathological conditions, both medical and traumatic, adversely affect the fluid and electrolyte balance of the body. Certain disease processes, such as diabetic ketoacidosis, and heat emergencies are associated with certain electrolyte abnormalities. Severe derangements in fluid and electrolyte status can result in death. For this reason, as a paramedic, you need to have a good understanding of the fluids and electrolytes present in the human body.

WATER

Water is the most abundant substance in the human body. In fact, water accounts for approximately 60 percent of the total body weight (the average for all ages). The total amount of water in the body at any given time is referred to as the **total body water (TBW)**. In an adult weighing 70 kilograms (154 pounds), the amount of total body water would be approximately 42 litres (11 gallons) (Figure 12-2).

Water is distributed into various compartments of the body (Table 12-1). These compartments are separated by cell membranes. The largest compartment is the *intracellular compartment*. This compartment contains the **intracellular fluid (ICF)**, which is all of the fluid found inside body cells. Approximately 75 percent of all body water is found within this compartment. The *extracellular compartment* contains the remaining 25 percent of all body water. It contains the **extracellular fluid (ECF)**, all the fluid found outside the body cells.

There are two divisions within the extracellular compartment. The first contains the **intravascular fluid**—the fluid found outside of cells and within the circulatory system. It is essentially the same as the blood plasma. The remaining compartment contains the **interstitial fluid**—all the fluid found outside the cell membranes, yet not within the circulatory system. For example, minute amounts of fluid are found in the synovial fluid that lubricates the joints, the aqueous humor of the eye, secretions including saliva, gastric juices, bile, and so on.

Total body water and its distribution vary with age and physiological condition. At birth, an infant's TBW is about 75 to 80 percent of its body weight, compared with the 65 percent TBW of the average adult. Infants have a higher TBW for two reasons. First, infants have less fat than adults. (Fat does not absorb water, so the less fat in the body, the more water.) Second, water is essential for the high rates of metabolism that are necessary to promote growth in the infant. The TBW slowly decreases to approximately 70 to 75 percent by age one. Diarrhea is especially worrisome in the infant because it can mean the loss of a significant percentage of TBW. In addition, body systems that compensate for fluid loss are still immature so that infants can rapidly become dangerously dehydrated and subject to electrolyte imbalances. By late childhood, the TBW decreases to 65 to 70 percent.

Some fluid and electrolyte derangements can result in death.

* **total body water (TBW)** the total amount of water in the body at a given time.

* **intracellular fluid (ICF)** the fluid inside the body cells.

* **extracellular fluid (ECF)** the fluid outside the body cells. Extracellular fluid comprises intravascular fluid and interstitial fluid.

* **intravascular fluid** the fluid within the circulatory system; blood plasma.

* **interstitial fluid** the fluid in body tissues that is outside the cells and outside the vascular system.

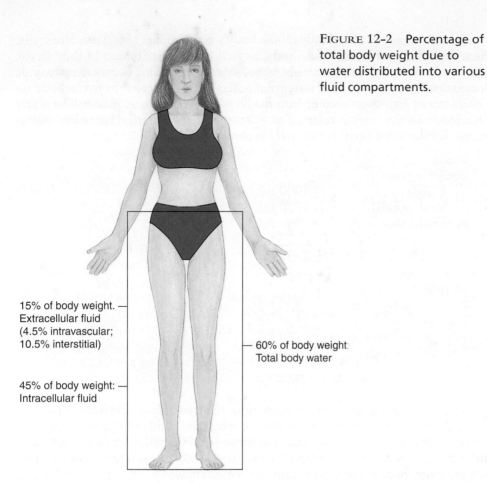

FIGURE 12-2 Percentage of total body weight due to water distributed into various fluid compartments.

15% of body weight. Extracellular fluid (4.5% intravascular; 10.5% interstitial)

60% of body weight: Total body water

45% of body weight: Intracellular fluid

By early adulthood, the TBW of males and females begins to differ. In adult males, TBW constitutes approximately 65 to 70 percent of the body weight, while in adult females the average TBW is 60 to 65 percent. The gender difference is due to hormonal differences that result in the male's greater muscle mass and the female's greater percentage of body fat.

As the human body ages, the loss of muscle mass, increased percentage of fat, and the body's decreasing ability to regulate fluid levels lowers the TBW to around 45 to 55 percent. Due to a decreasing ability to regulate electrolytes and fluid levels, the elderly, like the very young, are at high risk for dehydration and disorders related to electrolyte imbalances.

Hydration

Water is the universal **solvent**. That is, most substances dissolve in water. When they do, various chemical changes take place. For this reason, the water content

✳ **solvent** a substance that dissolves other substances, forming a solution.

Water is the universal solvent. Water is crucial to virtually all of the body's biochemical processes.

Table 12-1	BODY FLUID COMPARTMENTS	
Compartment	Percentage of Total Body Water	Volume in 70 kg Adult
Intracellular fluid	75.0%	31.50 L
Extracellular fluid	25.0%	10.50 L
Interstitial fluid	17.5%	7.35 L
Intravascular fluid	7.5%	3.15 L

of the body is crucial to virtually all the body's biochemical processes. Normally, the total volume of water in the body, as well as the distribution of fluid in the three body compartments, remains relatively constant. This occurs despite wide fluctuations in the amount of water that enters and is excreted from the body on a daily basis. The water coming into the body is referred to as intake. The water excreted from the body is referred to as output. To maintain relative homeostasis, the intake must equal the output, as shown below.

Intake
digestive system:
liquids	1000 mL
food (solids)	1200 mL
metabolic sources:	300 mL
	————
TOTAL:	2500 mL

Output
lungs (water vapour):	400 mL
kidneys (urine):	1500 mL
skin (perspiration):	400 mL
intestines (feces):	200 mL
	————
TOTAL:	2500 mL

Several mechanisms work to maintain a relative balance between input and output. For example, as explained earlier, when the fluid volume drops, the pituitary gland secretes antidiuretic hormone (ADH), which causes the kidney tubules to reabsorb more water into the blood and to excrete less urine. This process helps restore the fluid volume to normal values.

Thirst also regulates fluid intake. The sensation of thirst normally occurs when body fluids decrease, stimulating the person to take in more fluids orally. Conversely, when too many fluids enter the body, the kidneys are activated and more urine is excreted, thus eliminating excess fluid. The body also maintains fluid balance by shifting water from one body space to another.

✱ **dehydration** excessive loss of body fluid.

Content Review

SOME CAUSES OF DEHYDRATION
- Vomiting
- Diarrhea
- Perspiration
- Peritonitis
- Malnutrition
- Burns
- Open wounds

Dehydration Dehydration is an abnormal decrease in the total body water and can result from several factors:

- *Gastrointestinal losses* result from prolonged vomiting, diarrhea, or malabsorption disorders.
- *Increased insensible loss* is loss of water through normal mechanisms that is difficult to detect or measure (e.g., perspiration, water vapour from the lungs, saliva). These can be increased in fever states, during hyperventilation, or with high environmental temperatures.
- *Increased sweating* (also called perspiration or diaphoresis) can result in significant fluid loss. This can occur with many medical conditions or high environmental temperatures.
- *Internal losses* (commonly called "third-space" losses) are losses of fluid into various body fluid compartments. In this situation, fluid is typically lost from the intravascular compartment into the interstitial compartment, effectively taking it out of the circulating volume. This can occur with peritonitis, pancreatitis, or bowel obstruction. It can also occur in poor nutritional states in which there is not enough protein in the vascular system to retain water.
- *Plasma losses* occur from burns, surgical drains and fistulas, and open wounds.

Dehydration rarely involves only the loss of water. More commonly, there is also a loss of electrolytes. At the hospital, fluid replacement will be based on both fluid and electrolyte deficits, once the patient's electrolyte abnormalities are determined through laboratory testing.

Clinically, the dehydrated patient will exhibit dry mucous membranes and poor skin **turgor**. There often is excessive thirst. As it becomes more severe, dehydration will be accompanied by an increased pulse rate, decreased blood pressure, and orthostatic hypotension (increased pulse and decreased blood pressure on rising from a supine position). In infants, the anterior fontanelle may be sunken, and the diaper may be dry or reveal the presence of highly concentrated (dark yellow, strong-smelling) urine. The absence of tears in a crying infant, a capillary refill time greater than two seconds, dry mucosa, and a decrease in urinary output are signs that indicate severe dehydration. The treatment for dehydration is replacement of fluid.

Overhydration **Overhydration** can occur as well. The major sign of overhydration is edema. Patients with heart disease may manifest overhydration much earlier than patients without heart disease. In severe cases of overhydration, overt heart failure may be present. Treatment is directed at removing the excessive fluid.

ELECTROLYTES

Dehydration usually involves loss of both water and electrolytes.

✱ **turgor** normal tension in a cell; the resistance of the skin to deformation. (In a normally hydrated person, the skin, when pinched, will quickly return to its normal formation. In a dehydrated person, the return to normal formation will be slower.)

✱ **overhydration** the presence or retention of an abnormally high amount of body fluid.

HOW TO READ CHEMICAL NOTATION

To describe chemical substances and reactions, scientists use chemical notation, a kind of "shorthand."

Every chemical element has a one- or two-letter abbreviation. Just four elements—hydrogen, oxygen, carbon, and nitrogen—make up more than 99 percent of the body's atoms. These are called the "major elements." Nine "trace elements" account for the remaining less than 1 percent.

Major Element	Symbol	Percent	Trace Element	Symbol
Hydrogen	H	62.0%	Calcium	Ca
Oxygen	O	26.0%	Chlorine	Cl
Carbon	C	10.0%	Iodine	I
Nitrogen	N	1.5%	Iron	Fe
			Magnesium	Mg
			Phosphorus	Ph
			Potassium	K
			Sodium	Na
			Sulphur	S

An *atom* is the smallest particle of an element. A *molecule* is a combination of atoms. The notation for a molecule combines the notations of the included elements. A subscript number after an element indicates the number of atoms of that element. If there is just one atom, there is no number. For example:

NaCl (Sodium chloride, or table salt. A sodium chloride molecule has 1 sodium atom and 1 chlorine atom.)

H_2O (Water. A water molecule has 2 hydrogen atoms and 1 oxygen atom.)

H_2CO_3 (Carbonic acid. A carbonic acid molecule has 2 hydrogen, 1 carbon, and 3 oxygen atoms.)

(continued)

Ions

Each atom is made up of even smaller particles: electrons (that have a negative electrical charge), protons (that have a positive electrical charge), and neutrons (that are uncharged). Protons and neutrons are in the inner core, or nucleus, of the atom, while electrons occupy outer orbits around the nucleus. Sometimes, an atom of an element can lose one or more of its outer electrons or can capture one or more extra electrons from another element.

An *ion* is an atom that has lost one or more negatively charged electrons and now has a positive charge, or an atom that has gained one or more electrons and now has a negative charge. A superscript plus ($^+$) indicates a positively charged cation. A superscript minus ($^-$) indicates a negatively charged anion. For example:

Na^+ (A sodium ion has lost an electron and has a positive charge.)

Ca^{++} (A calcium ion has lost two electrons and has a double positive charge.)

Cl^- (A chloride ion has gained an electron and has a negative charge.)

Electrolytes are substances that form ions when they break down, or dissociate, in water. Remember that the body and its blood are mostly water. The ions formed by dissociation of electrolytes in the body's fluids are a major factor in body metabolism.

Chemical Reactions

Notations for chemical reactions use a plus sign ($+$) to indicate substances that are combined and an arrow ($\rightarrow$) to show the direction of the reaction. The reactants are usually on the left, the product of the reaction on the right.

$$2H + O \rightarrow H_2O$$

(2 hydrogen atoms + 1 oxygen atom → 1 water molecule)

In some circumstances, a reaction may be reversible. That is, separate elements may synthesize (combine), or the synthesized substance may dissociate (break down) into separate components. A two-directional arrow ($\leftrightarrow$) shows that a reaction is reversible and can be read in either direction.

$$CO_2 + H_2O \leftrightarrow H_2CO_3$$

Read as (carbon dioxide + water → carbonic acid) or
(carbonic acid → water + carbon dioxide).

Note that no atoms are gained or lost in a chemical reaction. In the example above, the two oxygen atoms in CO_2 and the single oxygen atom in H_2O combine to equal the three oxygen atoms in H_2CO_3. The hydrogen and carbon atoms are also equal on both sides of the reaction.

Up and down arrows ($\uparrow \downarrow$) are used to indicate an increase or decrease in the substance that follows the arrows. For example:

$\uparrow H^+$ (an increase in hydrogen ions)

$\downarrow CO_2$ (a decrease in carbon dioxide)

The various chemical substances present throughout the body can be classified either as electrolytes or nonelectrolytes. **Electrolytes** are substances that **dissociate** into electrically charged particles when placed into water. The charged particles are referred to as **ions**. Ions with a positive charge are called **cations**, while ions with a negative charge are called **anions**.

An example of this would be the dissociation of the drug sodium bicarbonate when placed in water. Sodium bicarbonate is a neutral salt. When placed in water, it dissociates into two charged particles, as shown below.

$$NaHCO_3 \rightarrow Na^+ + HCO_3^-$$

sodium bicarbonate → sodium cation + bicarbonate anion

neutral salt → cation + anion

Sodium bicarbonate is an example of an electrolyte that is taken into the body as a medication. However, there are many naturally occurring electrolytes present in the body.

The most frequently occurring cations include the following:

- *Sodium* (Na^+). Sodium is the most prevalent cation in the extracellular fluid. It plays a major role in regulating the distribution of water because water is attracted to and moves with sodium. In fact, it is often said that "water follows sodium." Sodium is also important in the transmission of nervous impulses. An abnormal increase in the relative amount of sodium in the body is called *hypernatremia*, while an abnormal decrease is referred to as *hyponatremia*.

- *Potassium* (K^+). Potassium is the most prevalent cation in the intracellular fluid. It is also important in the transmission of electrical impulses. An abnormally high potassium level is called *hyperkalemia*, while an abnormally low potassium level is referred to as *hypokalemia*.

- *Calcium* (Ca^{++}). Calcium has many physiological functions. It plays a major role in muscle contraction as well as nervous impulse transmission. An abnormally increased calcium level is called *hypercalcemia*, while an abnormally decreased calcium level is called *hypocalcemia*.

- *Magnesium* (Mg^{++}). Magnesium is necessary for several biochemical processes that occur in the body and is closely associated with phosphate in many processes. An abnormally increased magnesium level is called *hypermagnesemia*; an abnormally decreased magnesium level is called *hypomagnesemia*.

The most frequently occurring anions include the following:

- *Chloride* (Cl^-). Chloride is an important anion. Its negative charge balances the positive charge associated with the cations. It also plays a major role in fluid balance and renal function. Chloride has a close association with sodium.

- *Bicarbonate* (HCO_3^-). Bicarbonate is the principle **buffer** of the body. This means that it neutralizes the highly acidic hydrogen ion (H^+) and other organic acids. (Buffering will be discussed in more detail later in this chapter.)

- *Phosphate* (HPO_4^-). Phosphate is important in body energy stores. It is closely associated with magnesium in renal function. It also acts as a buffer, primarily in the intracellular space, in much the same manner as bicarbonate.

✱ **electrolyte** a substance that, in water, separates into electrically charged particles.

✱ **dissociate** separate; break down. For example, sodium bicarbonate, when placed in water, dissociates into a sodium cation and a bicarbonate anion.

✱ **ion** a charged particle; an atom or group of atoms whose electrical charge has changed from neutral to positive or negative by losing or gaining one or more electrons. (In an atom's normal, non-ionized state, its positively charged protons and negatively charged electrons balance each other so that the atom's charge is neutral.)

✱ **cation** an ion with a positive charge—so called because it will be attracted to a cathode, or negative pole.

✱ **anion** an ion with a negative charge—so called because it will be attracted to an anode, or positive pole.

✱ **buffer** a substance that tends to preserve or restore a normal acid-base balance by increasing or decreasing the concentration of hydrogen ions.

Many other compounds carry negative charges. Among these are some of the proteins, certain organic acids, and other compounds. Electrolytes are usually measured in *milliequivalents* per litre (mEq/L).

Nonelectrolytes are molecules that do not dissociate into electrically charged particles. These include glucose, urea, proteins, and similar substances.

OSMOSIS AND DIFFUSION

As discussed earlier, the various fluid compartments are separated by cell membranes. These membranes are semipermeable, allowing the passage of certain materials while restricting the passage of others. Compounds with small molecules, such as water (H_2O), pass readily through the membrane; larger compounds, such as proteins, are restricted. This selective movement of fluids results from the presence of pores (openings) in the membrane. Electrolytes do not pass as readily as water through the membrane. This is due not so much to their size as to their electrical charge.

When solutions on opposite sides of a semipermeable membrane are equal in concentration, the relationship is said to be **isotonic.** When the concentration of a given solute (dissolved substance) is greater on one side of the membrane than on the other, it is said to be **hypertonic.** When the concentration is less on one side of the cell membrane, as compared with the other, it is referred to as **hypotonic.** This difference in concentration is known as the **osmotic gradient.**

The natural tendency of the body is to keep the balance of electrolytes and water equal on both sides of the cell membrane. This is an example of homeostasis. If one side of a cell membrane has an increased quantity of a given electrolyte (is hypertonic), there will be a shift of the electrolyte from that side and a shift of water from the other side to restore balance in concentration—the balanced state.

The tendency of molecules to move from an area of higher concentration to an area of lower concentration is referred to as **diffusion** and does not require energy (Figure 12-3). The diffusion of a solute (usually an electrolyte) across a cell

* **isotonic** equal in concentration of solute molecules; solutions may be isotonic to each other.

* **hypertonic** having a greater concentration of solute molecules; one solution may be hypertonic to another.

* **hypotonic** having a lesser concentration of solute molecules; one solution may be hypotonic to another.

* **osmotic gradient** the difference in concentration between solutions on opposite sides of a semipermeable membrane.

* **diffusion** the movement of molecules through a membrane from an area of greater concentration to an area of lesser concentration.

FIGURE 12-3 Diffusion is the movement of a substance from an area of greater concentration to an area of lesser concentration.

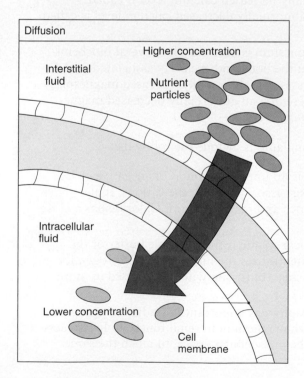

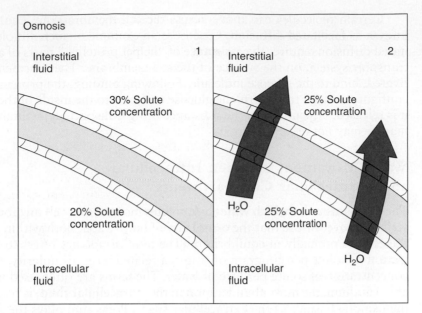

FIGURE 12-4 Osmosis is the movement of water from an area of higher WATER concentration to an area of lesser WATER concentration. Because water is a solvent, it moves from an area of lower SOLUTE concentration to an area of higher SOLUTE concentration.

membrane from the area of higher concentration to the area of lower concentration continues until the natural balance is again attained. This movement from an area of higher concentration to an area of lower concentration is termed a movement *with the osmotic gradient.*

Water also moves across the cell membrane so as to dilute the area of increased electrolyte concentration. The movement of water is more rapid than the movement of electrolytes. This form of diffusion (the passage of any solvent, usually water, through a membrane) is referred to as **osmosis** (Figure 12-4). It occurs in the direction opposite to the direction of solute movement. For example, if a semipermeable membrane separates solutions of water and sodium, and if the concentration of sodium is two times higher on one side of the membrane than on the other, then two things will occur. Sodium will diffuse from the area of higher concentration (the hypertonic side) to the area of lesser concentration (the hypotonic side). Concurrently, water will diffuse in the opposite direction. That is, water will leave the hypotonic side and diffuse across the membrane to the hypertonic side. These actions will continue until the concentration of water and sodium on both sides has equalized.

In addition to diffusion, two other mechanisms—active transport and facilitated diffusion—can transport substances across cell membranes. **Active transport** is the movement of a substance across the cell membrane *against the osmotic gradient* (that is, toward the side that already has more of the substance).

For example, the body requires the cells of the myocardium to be negatively charged on the inside of the cells as compared with the outside. However sodium, with its positive charge, tends to diffuse passively into the cell. This would destroy the negative charge inside the cell. To maintain the desired negative charge, sodium ions are actively pumped out of the cell, while potassium ions are pumped into the cell, by a mechanism known as the sodium-potassium pump. (Sodium and potassium ions are both positive, but more sodium ions are pumped out of the cell than potassium ions are pumped in, creating the desired negative charge inside the cell.)

Active transport is faster than diffusion, but it requires the expenditure of energy, which diffusion does not. Proteins are moved across the cell membrane in a similar fashion.

✳ **osmosis** the passage of a solvent, such as water, through a membrane.

✳ **active transport** movement of a substance through a cell membrane against the osmotic gradient; that is, from an area of lesser concentration to an area of greater concentration, opposite to the normal direction of diffusion.

✱ facilitated diffusion diffusion of a substance, such as glucose, through a cell membrane that requires the assistance of a "helper," or carrier protein.

✱ osmolality the concentration of solute per kilogram of water. *See also* osmolarity.

✱ osmolarity the concentration of solute per litre of water (often used synonymously with *osmolality*).

✱ osmotic pressure the pressure exerted by the concentration of solutes on one side of a membrane that, if hypertonic, tends to "pull" water (cause osmosis) from the other side of the membrane.

✱ oncotic force a form of osmotic pressure exerted by the large protein particles, or colloids, present in blood plasma. In the capillaries, the plasma colloids tend to pull water from the interstitial space across the capillary membrane into the capillary. Oncotic force is also called *colloid osmotic pressure*.

✱ hydrostatic pressure blood pressure or force against vessel walls created by the heart beat. Hydrostatic pressure tends to force water out of the capillaries into the interstitial space.

✱ filtration movement of water out of the plasma across the capillary membrane into the interstitial space.

Certain molecules can move across the cell membrane by another process known as **facilitated diffusion.** Glucose is an example of such a molecule. Facilitated diffusion requires the assistance of "helper proteins," parts of a membrane transport system, on the surface of the cell membrane. These proteins, once activated, bind to the glucose molecule. Following binding, the protein changes its configuration and transports the glucose molecule to the inside of the cell, where it is released. Depending on the substance being transported, facilitated diffusion may or may not require energy.

Water Movement between Intracellular and Extracellular Compartments

The mechanisms by which water and solutes move across cell membranes, as described above, ensure that the **osmolality** of body water, both within and outside the cells, is normally in equilibrium. (The term *osmolality* refers to the concentration of solute per kilogram of water; a related term, **osmolarity,** refers to the concentration of solute per litre of water. The terms are often used interchangeably.) Sodium, the most abundant ion in the extracellular fluid, is responsible for the osmotic balance of the extracellular space. Potassium plays the same role in the intracellular space.

Generally, the osmolality of intracellular fluid does not change very rapidly. However, when there is a change in the osmolality of extracellular fluid, water will move from the intracellular to the extracellular compartment, or vice versa, until osmotic equilibrium is regained.

Water Movement between Intravascular and Interstitial Compartments

Within the extracellular compartment, movement of water between the plasma in the intravascular space and that in the interstitial space is primarily a function of forces at play in the capillary beds.

In general, the movement of water and solutes across a cell membrane is governed by **osmotic pressure.** Osmotic pressure is the pressure exerted by the concentration of solutes on one side of a semipermeable membrane, such as a cell membrane or the thin wall of a capillary. Osmotic pressure can be thought of as a "pull," rather than a "push," because a hypertonic concentration of solutes tends to pull water from the other side of the membrane.

Generally, this is a two-way street as solutes move out of a space while water moves into the space to balance the concentration of solutes on both sides of the membrane. However, there is a somewhat different osmotic mechanism that operates between the plasma inside a capillary and the interstitial space outside the capillary. Blood plasma generates **oncotic force,** which is sometimes called *colloid osmotic pressure*. Plasma proteins are colloids, large particles that do not readily move across the capillary membrane. They tend to remain within the capillary. At the same time, there is very little water in the interstitial space. The small amount of water that does get into the interstitial space is usually taken up by the lymph system. Since there is little water outside the capillary and plasma proteins do not readily move outside the capillary, the forces governing movement of water between the capillary and the interstitial space are almost all on one side, governed by the plasma on the inside of the capillary.

Another force inside the capillaries is **hydrostatic pressure,** which is the blood pressure, or force against the vessel walls, created by contractions of the heart. Hydrostatic pressure does tend to force some water out of the plasma and across the capillary wall into the interstitial space, a process that is called **filtration.** Hydrostatic pressure (a force that favours filtration, pushing water out of the capillary) and oncotic force (a force opposing filtration, pulling water into the capillary) together are responsible for **net filtration,** which is described in *Starling's hypothesis:*

Net filtration = (Forces favouring filtration) − (Forces opposing filtration)

Net filtration in a capillary is normally zero. It works this way: As plasma enters the capillary at the arterial end, hydrostatic pressure forces water to cross the capillary membrane into the interstitial space. This loss of water increases the relative concentration of plasma proteins. By the time the plasma reaches the venous end of the capillary, the oncotic force exerted by the increased concentration of plasma proteins is great enough to pull the water from the interstitial space back into the capillary. The outcome is that water is retained in the intravascular space and does not remain in the interstitial space.

ACID-BASE BALANCE

Acid-base balance is a dynamic relationship that reflects the relative concentration of hydrogen ions (H^+) in the body. Hydrogen ions are acidic and the concentration of these within the body must be maintained within fairly strict limits. Any deviation in the hydrogen ion concentration adversely affects all of the biochemical events that occur in the body. The hydrogen ion concentration is dynamic, changing from second to second.

THE pH SCALE

The total number of hydrogen ions present in the body at any given time is very high. Because of this, the **pH** system of measurement is used. The pH scale is inversely related to hydrogen ion concentration. That is, the greater the hydrogen ion concentration, the lower is the pH. The lower the hydrogen ion concentration, the higher is the pH.

The pH scale is logarithmic, each number representing a value 10 times that of its neighbouring number so that pH 6 represents a hydrogen ion concentration 10 times as great as that represented by pH 7. The following formula represents pH:

$$pH = \log \frac{1}{[H^+]}$$

The pH scale ranges from 1 to 14. A pH of 1 means that only hydrogen ions are present. A pH of 14 means that there are virtually no hydrogen ions present. The pH of water is 7, which is a neutral pH. The pH of the body is normally 7.35 to 7.45 (Table 12-2).

Because hydrogen ions are acidic, a pH below 7.35 is referred to as **acidosis.** A substance that produces negatively charged ions that can neutralize the positively charged hydrogen ions (or other acids) is called an alkali or a base. An excess of alkaline (base) substances or a deficit of acids will produce a pH above 7.45, which is referred to as **alkalosis.** In humans, a variation of only 0.4 of a pH unit in either direction from normal (6.9 or 7.8) can be fatal.

BODILY REGULATION OF ACID-BASE BALANCE

The body is constantly producing hydrogen ions (acids) through metabolism and other biochemical processes. To maintain the acid-base balance, these hydrogen ions must be constantly eliminated from the body. There are three major mechanisms to remove hydrogen ions from the body. The fastest mechanism is often referred to as the *buffer system* or the *bicarbonate buffer system.*

✱ **net filtration** the total loss of water from blood plasma across the capillary membrane into the interstitial space. Normally, hydrostatic pressure forcing water out of the capillary is balanced by oncotic force pulling water into the capillary for a net filtration of zero.

✱ **pH** abbreviation for *potential of hydrogen.* A measure of relative acidity or alkalinity. Since the pH scale is inverse to the concentration of acidic hydrogen ions, the lower the pH, the greater is the acidity; the higher the pH, the greater is the alkalinity. A normal pH range is 7.35 to 7.45.

✱ **acidosis** a high concentration of hydrogen ions; a pH below 7.35.

✱ **alkalosis** a low concentration of hydrogen ions; a pH above 7.45.

Content Review

THREE MECHANISMS OF HYDROGEN ION REMOVAL
• Bicarbonate buffer system
• Respiration
• Kidney function

Table 12-2 — THE pH SCALE AND HYDROGEN ION CONCENTRATIONS

pH		Example	H^+ Concentration*	
Acidic	0	Hydrochloric acid	10^{-0}	(1.0)
	1	Stomach secretions	10^{-1}	(0.1)
	2	Lemon juice	10^{-2}	(0.01)
	3	Cola drinks	10^{-3}	(0.001)
	4	White wine	10^{-4}	(0.0001)
	5	Tomato juice	10^{-5}	(0.00001)
	6	Coffee, urine, saliva	10^{-6}	(0.000001)
Neutral	7	Distilled water	10^{-7}	(0.0000001)
Basic	8	Blood, semen	10^{-8}	(0.00000001)
	9	Bile	10^{-9}	(0.000000001)
	10	Bleach	10^{-10}	(0.0000000001)
	11	Milk of magnesia	10^{-11}	(0.00000000001)
	12	Ammonia water	10^{-12}	(0.000000000001)
	13	Drain opener	10^{-13}	(0.0000000000001)
	14	Lye	10^{-14}	(0.00000000000001)

*Hydrogen ion concentrations are expressed in moles per litre, a quantity based on molecular weight.

The two components of the bicarbonate buffer system are bicarbonate ion (HCO_3^-) and carbonic acid (H_2CO_3). These two compounds are in equilibrium with hydrogen ion (H^+), as follows: In some circumstances, hydrogen ion will combine with bicarbonate ion to produce carbonic acid. In other circumstances, carbonic acid will dissociate into bicarbonate ion and hydrogen ion:

$$H^+ + HCO_3^- \leftrightarrow H_2CO_3$$

hydrogen ion + bicarbonate ion $\leftrightarrow$ carbonic acid

In a healthy individual, for every molecule of carbonic acid, there are 20 molecules of bicarbonate ion. Any change in this 20:1 ratio is immediately corrected without significant change in the total body pH. This occurs in the following manner: An increase in hydrogen ions (acidosis) is corrected as the excess hydrogen ions combine with bicarbonate ions to form carbonic acid. (Thus, an increase in hydrogen ion leads to an increase in carbonic acid—driving the equation above to the right.) Conversely, when there is a deficit in hydrogen ions (alkalosis), carbonic acid will dissociate into bicarbonate ion and hydrogen ion. (Thus, a decrease in hydrogen ion leads to a decrease in carbonic acid—driving the equation above to the left.) (Figure 12-5)

$$\text{Increased Acid: } \uparrow H^+ + HCO_3^- \rightarrow \uparrow H_2CO_3$$
$$\text{Decreased Acid: } \downarrow H^+ + HCO_3^- \rightarrow \downarrow H_2CO_3$$

Carbonic acid is a weak acid that is better tolerated by the body than pure hydrogen ions. However, the body carries this reaction further. Any increase in carbonic acid must also be eliminated.

The elimination of excess carbonic acid takes place as follows: Carbonic acid is unstable and will eventually dissociate into carbon dioxide and water. This

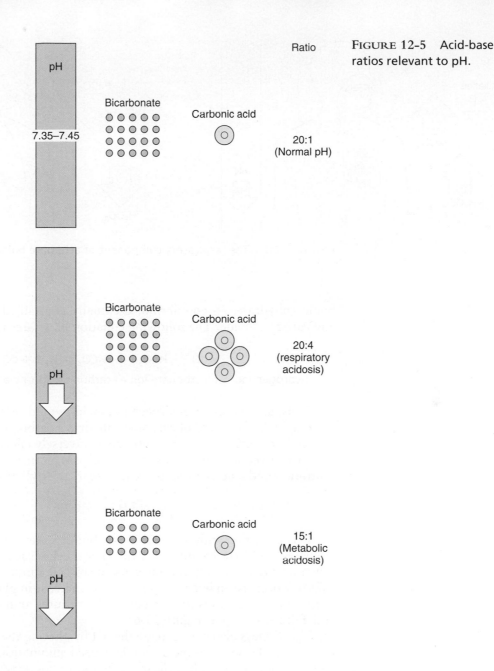

FIGURE 12-5 Acid-base ratios relevant to pH.

normally slow process is speeded up by the blood's erythrocytes, which contain an enzyme called *carbonic anhydrase.* Carbonic anhydrase causes carbonic acid to be converted to carbon dioxide and water very rapidly—so rapidly that carbonic acid exists for only a fraction of a second before it is converted into carbon dioxide and water. Most buffering of acid in the body occurs in the erythrocytes.

The enzyme also works in a reverse fashion, which allows carbon dioxide and water to be quickly converted into carbonic acid. The reaction proceeds in accordance with *LeChetalier's principle.* Given an excess of carbon dioxide on the right side of the equilibrium, a stress is placed on it such that it must shift to the left, which is sometimes referred to as a mass action effect. The net effect of this is the generation of more hydrogen ion, and acidosis. The clinical application of this is that when a patient is said to hypoventilate, that is, retain CO_2, then the accumulation (stress) of increased CO_2 forces the equilibrium to shift to the left, causing what is known as respiratory acidosis. So, with the aid of car-

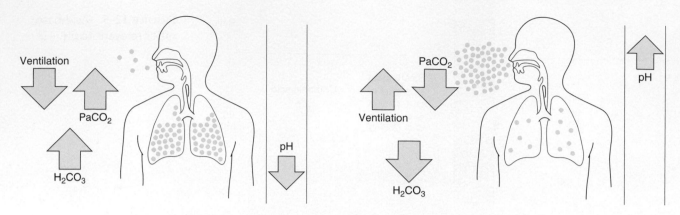

FIGURE 12-6   The respiratory component of acid-base balance.

bonic anhydrase, an equilibrium eventually is attained between hydrogen ion and carbon dioxide. The following equation illustrates this relationship.

$$H^+ + HCO_3^- \leftrightarrow H_2CO_3 \leftrightarrow H_2O + CO_2$$
hydrogen ion + bicarbonate ion $\leftrightarrow$ carbonic acid $\leftrightarrow$ water + carbon dioxide

Thus, an increase in hydrogen ion (acid) would result in an increase in carbonic acid. With the aid of carbonic anhydrase, carbonic acid would quickly dissociate into water and carbon dioxide. Conversely (since the reaction can move in either direction), an increase in CO_2 causes an increase in hydrogen ion concentration and a decrease in pH (increase in acidity), as shown below.

$$\uparrow H^+ \leftrightarrow \uparrow CO_2$$

In conjunction with the bicarbonate buffer system described above, the body regulates acid-base balance by two other mechanisms, respiration and kidney function. Increased respirations cause increased elimination of CO_2, which results in a decrease in hydrogen ions and an increase in pH. Conversely, decreased respirations cause CO_2 to be retained. This causes an increase in hydrogen ions and a decrease in pH (Figure 12-6).

The kidneys also can regulate the pH by altering the concentration of bicarbonate ion (HCO_3^-) in the blood. Increased elimination of HCO_3^- results in a lowered pH. (There is less bicarbonate ion to combine with and eliminate hydrogen ion.) Conversely, retention of HCO_3^- causes an increase in pH. (There is more bicarbonate ion to combine with and eliminate hydrogen ion.) In addition, the kidneys affect the acid-base balance by removing or retaining various chemicals. Normally, the kidneys remove larger metabolic acids, excreting them in the urine, resulting in an increase in pH.

Part 2: Body Systems

THE INTEGUMENTARY SYSTEM

The protective envelope we call the skin is a complex structure. Understanding how it is put together and how it functions will help you appreciate the importance of injuries to it and the value of their proper care.

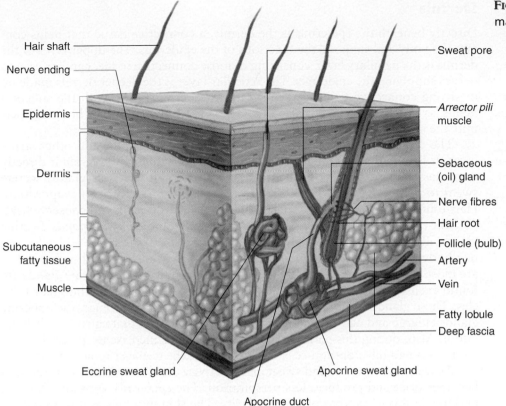

FIGURE 12-7 Layers and major structures of the skin.

Hair shaft

Nerve ending

Epidermis

Dermis

Subcutaneous fatty tissue

Muscle

Sweat pore

Arrector pili muscle

Sebaceous (oil) gland

Nerve fibres

Hair root

Follicle (bulb)

Artery

Vein

Fatty lobule

Deep fascia

Eccrine sweat gland

Apocrine sweat gland

Apocrine duct

THE SKIN

The epidermis, dermis, and subcutaneous tissue layers compose what is commonly known as the skin (Figure 12-7). Each of these layers performs functions essential to helping the body maintain homeostasis, and each plays an important role in the wound repair process.

Epidermis

The outermost skin layer is the **epidermis.** It is generated by a layer of cells just above the dermis (stratum germinativum). These cells divide rapidly, generating a movement of cells upward toward the epidermal surface. As the epidermis contains no vasculature, the further these cells are pushed away from the dermis, the less circulation they receive, and they eventually die. As they die, they flatten and interlock, providing a firm and secure barrier around the body (stratum corneum). The outermost cells are eventually abraded or washed away and then replaced, allowing the epidermis to maintain its thickness. It normally takes two weeks for a cell to move from the dermal border to the surface of the epidermis and another two to four weeks until it is abraded away. This outward movement of cells helps the body resist invasion by bacteria.

A waxy substance called **sebum** lubricates the surface of the epidermis. This lubrication acts much like oil on leather. It keeps the outer layers of the skin flexible, strong, and resistant to penetration by water. The epidermis is also responsible for the pigmentation that protects the skin from the harmful effects of ultraviolet radiation. The thickness of the epidermis varies greatly, depending on the amount of abrasion and pressure it receives. On the soles of the feet, it is very thick and strong, while over the eye, it is microscopic in thickness and very delicate.

Content Review

LAYERS OF THE SKIN
- Epidermis
- Dermis
- Subcutaneous tissue

✱ **epidermis** outermost layer of the skin comprising of dead or dying cells.

✱ **sebum** fatty secretion of the sebaceous gland that helps keep the skin pliable and waterproof.

Dermis

Directly beneath the epidermis is the **dermis**, a connective tissue that helps contain the body and supports the functions of the epidermis. The upper layer of the dermis is the papillary layer, consisting of loose connective tissue, capillaries, and nerves supplying the epidermis. The reticular layer is the deeper dermis made up of strong connective tissue that integrates the dermis firmly with the subcutaneous layer below. This tissue also holds the skin firmly around the body and permits the stretching and flexibility necessary for articulation.

The dermis contains blood vessels, nerve endings, glands, and other structures. It is here that the **sebaceous glands** produce sebum and secrete it directly onto the surface of the skin or into hair follicles. **Sudoriferous glands** secrete sweat to help move heat out of and away from the body through evaporation. Hair follicles produce hair that helps reduce surface abrasion and conserve heat.

The two types of sweat glands are *eccrine glands* and *apocrine glands*. Eccrine glands, also known as merocrine glands, open onto the skin surface and help control body temperature through water excretion. They are widely distributed but are most heavily concentrated in the axilla and genital areas. Apocrine glands are found exclusively in the armpits and genital region, and they open into hair follicles. These glands respond to emotional stress. During adolescence, the apocrine glands enlarge and actively increase the axillary sweating that causes adult body odour. Also, during this period, the sebaceous glands increase their activity, giving the skin an oily appearance. This predisposes the teenager to acne problems.

As we age, sebaceous and sweat gland activity decreases. As a result, the skin becomes drier and produces less perspiration. The epidermis thins and flattens, and the dermis loses some of its vascularity. The skin wrinkles as it loses turgor. In warmer climates, the skin can become thickened, yellowed, and furrowed and take on a weather-beaten appearance. Elderly people develop a variety of spots on the thin skin of the backs of their hands and forearms. Whitish, depigmented marks are known as pseudoscars. Purple spots (purpura) caused by minor capillary bleeding may appear and fade after a few weeks.

In the dermis are several resident body cells responsible for initiating the attack on invading organisms, foreign materials, and damaged cells, and for beginning the repair of damaged tissue. The macrophages and lymphocytes (types of white blood cells) begin the inflammation response by killing invading bodies and triggering a call for other, simliar cells. Mast cells control the microcirculation to tissues and respond to the initial invasion, increasing capillary flow and permeability. Fibroblasts lay down and repair protein strands to strengthen the wound site and begin restoring the skin's integrity.

Subcutaneous Tissue

Subcutaneous tissue is the body layer beneath the dermis. It is rich in fatty or adipose tissue, which helps it absorb the forces of trauma, protecting the tissues and vital organs beneath. Because of its fatty content, heat moves outward through the subcutaneous tissue three times more slowly than through muscles or other layers of the skin; hence it is of great value in conserving body temperature. The body directs blood below the subcutaneous tissue to conserve heat and above it through the dermis when it is necessary to radiate heat.

THE HAIR

Hair is a tactile sensory organ, also playing a role in sexual stimulation and attraction. It covers the entire body, except the palms, soles, and parts of the sex organs. Hair develops from the base of the hair follicle, where it is nourished by

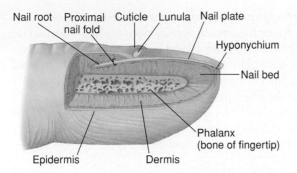

Nail root   Proximal   Cuticle   Lunula   Nail plate
             nail fold

FIGURE 12-8   The nail.

Hyponychium

Nail bed

Phalanx
(bone of fingertip)

Epidermis   Dermis

the papilla, a vast capillary network. An involuntary arrector pili muscle fibre attaches to the base of the hair shaft. When these arrectores pilorum contract, the hair stands erect, and goosebumps appear on the skin.

The two types of hair are vellus and terminal. Vellus hair is short, fine, and lacking pigment (similar to "peach fuzz"). Terminal hair is coarser, thicker, and pigmented. It appears on the eyebrows and scalp, in the armpits and groin of both sexes, and on the faces and bodies of males.

With aging, the hair turns grey from a decrease in pigmentation and its growth declines. A transition from terminal to vellus hair on the scalp causes baldness in both men and women. The opposite occurs in the nares and ears of men, where terminal hair replaces vellus hair. Both genders generally experience a decrease in body hair as they age. Loss of the lateral third of the eyebrow is also normal in the elderly.

THE NAILS

Nails are found at the most distal ends of fingers and toes and are primarily for protection. Nails are strong yet flexible and provide a sharp edge for scratching, scraping, and clawing. They are made up of the nail plate, the nail bed, the proximal nail fold, and the nail root (Figure 12-8). The angle between the proximal nail fold and the nail plate should be less than 180 degrees. Fingernails grow approximately 0.1 mm daily, slightly faster in the summertime. The nail plate lies on a highly vascular nail bed that gives the nail a pink appearance. Nail edges should be smooth and rounded. The nail plates should be smooth, flat, or slightly curved and should feel hard and uniformly thick. As we age, nail growth diminishes because of decreased peripheral circulation. The nails, especially the toenails, become hard, thick, brittle, and yellowish.

THE BLOOD

The **hematopoietic system** consists of blood (both cells and plasma), bone marrow, the liver, the spleen, and the kidneys. The cellular components of blood are formed by the differentiation of a **pluripotent stem cell** in a process termed **hematopoiesis.** In the fetus, hematopoiesis occurs first outside of the bone marrow (*extramedullary hematopoiesis*) in the liver, spleen, lymph nodes, and thymus. By the fourth month, the developing bone marrow begins to produce blood cells (*intramedullary hematopoiesis*). After birth, the bone marrow is the primary site of blood cell production and extramedullary hematopoiesis greatly diminishes, occurring mostly in the liver and spleen. By adulthood, hematopoiesis occurs exclusively in the bone marrow unless a pathological state exists.

In hematopoiesis, the stem cell reproduces to maintain a constant population of cells. Some stem cells then further differentiate into myeloid multipotent stem

✱ **hematopoietic system** body system having to do with the production and development of blood cells, consisting of the bone marrow, liver, spleen, kidneys, and the blood itself.

Content Review

HEMATOPOIETIC SYSTEM COMPONENTS

- Bone marrow
- Liver
- Spleen
- Kidneys
- Blood

✱ **pluripotent stem cell** a cell from which the various types of blood cells can form.

✱ **hematopoiesis** the process through which pluripotent stem cells differentiate into various types of blood cells.

cells that, in turn, differentiate into unipotent progenitors. These unipotent progenitors ultimately mature into basophils, eosinophils, neutrophils, monocytes (types of white blood cells), erythrocytes (red blood cells), and thrombocytes (platelets.) Pluripotent stem cells may also differentiate into common lymphoid stem cells that ultimately mature into lymphocytes (another type of white cell). The kidney, and to a lesser extent the liver, produce **erythropoietin,** the hormone responsible for red blood cell production. The liver also removes toxins from the blood and produces many of the clotting factors and proteins in plasma. The spleen, an important part of the immune system, has cells that scavenge abnormal blood cells and bacteria.

Blood volume normally remains relatively constant at about 6 percent of total body weight. With an average of 80 to 85 millilitres (mL) of blood per kilogram of body weight, a person who weighs 75 kilograms has approximately 6 litres of blood. The body can easily handle up to about one-half litre of lost blood or fluid. An example is routine blood donations where healthy donors tolerate the blood loss without complication.

The major determinants of the blood volume are red cell mass and plasma volume. Red blood cells remain confined to the intravascular compartment. If their destruction remains constant, then only changes in the rate of production can alter the size of the circulating red cell mass. The plasma volume on the other hand can rapidly change due to fluid shifts between the intravascular and extravascular spaces. These fluid shifts help preserve circulating blood volume in the event of acute hemorrhage. Other compensatory mechanisms include vasoconstriction, tachycardia, and increased cardiac contractility to maintain adequate tissue perfusion until significant losses overwhelm these measures. When these compensatory measures fail, the patient enters decompensated shock. Fortunately, young healthy individuals' bodies can compensate for loss of as much as 25 to 30 percent of blood volume.

COMPONENTS OF BLOOD

Blood consists of liquid, or plasma, and of formed elements—red blood cells, white blood cells, and platelets.

Plasma

Plasma is a thick, pale yellow fluid that is 90 to 92 percent water and 6 to 7 percent proteins. Fats, carbohydrates, electrolytes, gases, and certain chemical messengers comprise the remaining 2 to 3 percent. Plasma transports the cellular components of blood and dissolved nutrients throughout the body and, at the same time, transports waste products from cellular metabolism to the liver, kidneys, and lungs, where they can be removed from the body.

Most plasma components can move back and forth across the capillary membranes to the interstitial fluid. However, plasma proteins, such as albumin, are large molecules and have great difficulty diffusing across the membranes. This is fortunate, since they remain in the plasma to help retain water in the capillaries. As noted earlier, this is known as *oncotic force,* or *colloid osmotic pressure.* Plasma proteins perform many other functions, including clotting of blood, dismantling of clots, buffering of the blood's acid-base balance, transporting hormones and regulating their effects, and providing a source of energy.

Electrolytes are also found in the plasma. (As noted earlier, these are chemical substances that dissociate into charged particles in water.) They are essential for nerve conduction, muscle contraction, and water balance. They can easily diffuse across capillary membranes based on their concentration gradients. Carbohydrates

---

✱ **erythropoietin** the hormone responsible for red blood cell production.

Content Review

COMPONENTS OF BLOOD
- Plasma
- Formed elements
  - Red blood cells
  - White blood cells
  - Platelets

✱ **plasma** thick, pale yellow fluid that makes up the liquid part of the blood.

---

in plasma are generally in the form of glucose, the primary energy source for all body tissues. Glucose is especially important to brain cells as they cannot obtain energy from fat metabolism. (Glucose cannot diffuse across most cell membranes without assistance from the hormone insulin.) Plasma also performs a role in gas transport. In addition to being carried by red blood cells, carbon dioxide and oxygen are dissolved and transported in plasma.

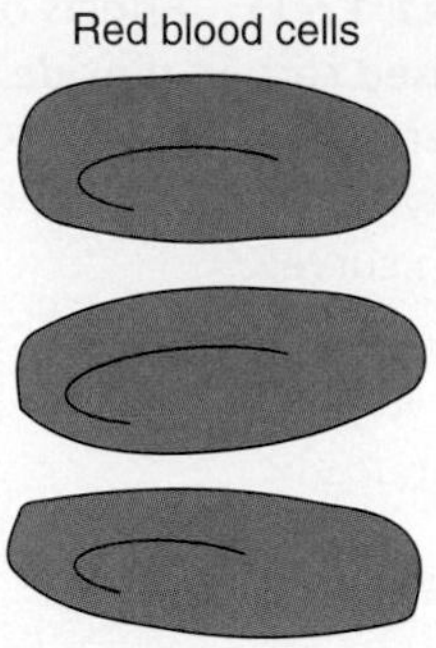

Red Blood Cells

The primary function of blood is to transport oxygen from the lungs to the tissues. At rest, the body consumes about 4 mL of oxygen per kilogram of body weight every minute. Because it stores little oxygen, the body would quickly succumb to anoxia without the continued transport provided by the blood.

The red blood cell (RBC), or **erythrocyte,** is a biconcave disc that does not have a nucleus when mature (Figure 12-9). It contains **hemoglobin** molecules that transport oxygen. Hemoglobin comprises four subunits of *globin,* each bonded to a *heme* (iron containing) molecule. Each globin subunit can bind with one oxygen molecule; thus, each complete hemoglobin molecule can carry up to four oxygen molecules. When all four subunits are carrying an oxygen molecule, the hemoglobin is 100 percent saturated. When fully saturated, each gram of hemoglobin can transport 1.34 mL of oxygen.

Oxygen Transport The effectiveness of oxygen transport depends on many factors. Red blood cell mass (the number of red blood cells present) is obviously a factor in oxygen transport. The greater the number of red blood cells, the greater will be the potential oxygen carrying capacity. The percentage of oxygen bound to hemoglobin increases as the **pO$_2$** increases. This is illustrated in the oxygen-hemoglobin dissociation curve (Figure 12-10). Normal pO$_2$ is approximately 95 mmHg. Based on this, the oxygen-hemoglobin dissociation curve indicates that normal oxygen saturation is about 97 percent. Hemoglobin's affinity for oxygen is also a factor in oxygen transport. Several factors affect oxygen affinity, including pH, **pCO$_2$,** concentration of 2,3-DPG, and temperature.

The lower the pH (that is, the more acidic the blood), the more readily hemoglobin will release oxygen. This shifts the oxygen-hemoglobin dissociation curve to the right. In contrast, alkalosis makes hemoglobin bind to oxygen more tightly. This shifts the oxygen-hemoglobin dissociation curve to the left (Figure 12-11). The pCO$_2$ is directly related to the pH. Thus, in the lungs, as pCO$_2$ decreases with diffusion of CO$_2$ into the alveoli, the quantity of oxygen that binds with the hemoglobin increases. The opposite effect occurs when the

Red blood cells

FIGURE 12-9   Red blood cells.

✳ **erythrocyte** red blood cell.

✳ **hemoglobin** oxygen-bearing molecule in the red blood cells. It is made up of iron-rich red pigment called *heme* and a protein called *globin.*

✳ **pO$_2$** partial pressure of oxygen; (*partial pressure* is the pressure exerted by a given component of a gas containing several components).

✳ **pCO$_2$** partial pressure of carbon dioxide; (*partial pressure* defined—see pO$_2$).

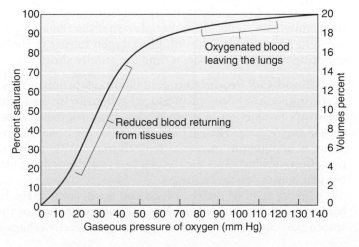

FIGURE 12-10   The oxygen-hemoglobin dissociation curve.

FIGURE 12-11 Effects of pH, increased carbon dioxide, temperature, and 2,3-DPG on the oxygen-hemoglobin dissociation curve.

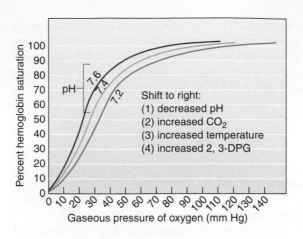

FIGURE 12-11 Effects of pH, increased carbon dioxide, temperature, and 2,3-DPG on the oxygen-hemoglobin dissociation curve.

✱ Bohr effect phenomenon in which a decrease in pCO_2/acidity causes an increase in the quantity of oxygen that binds with the hemoglobin; conversely, an increase in pCO_2/acidity causes the hemoglobin to give up a greater quantity of oxygen.

✱ 2,3-diphosphoglycerate (2,3-DPG) chemical in the red blood cells that affects hemoglobin's affinity for oxygen.

✱ erythropoiesis the process of producing red blood cells.

✱ hemolysis destruction of red blood cells.

✱ sequestration the trapping of red blood cells by an organ, such as the spleen.

blood reaches the tissues. There, waste CO_2 from the tissues diffuses into the blood, causing the hemoglobin to give up more oxygen to the tissues. This is called the **Bohr effect.**

Except for hemoglobin, the most abundant chemical in red blood cells is **2,3-diphosphoglycerate (2,3-DPG).** During prolonged periods of hypoxia, the level of 2,3-DPG increases. This shifts the oxygen-hemoglobin dissociation curve to the right and can increase the pO_2 in the plasma as much as 10 percent more than it otherwise would have been. However, the increased 2,3-DPG makes it more difficult for oxygen to combine with hemoglobin in the lungs. This effect casts doubt on whether 2,3-DPG's effect in hypoxia is as beneficial as was once thought.

An elevation in the body temperature causes a shift to the right of the oxygen-hemoglobin dissociation curve and a decrease in hemoglobin's affinity for blood. Conversely, a fall in body temperature causes hemoglobin to bind oxygen more tightly. During periods of hyperthermia and pyrexia (fever), hemoglobin's decreased affinity for oxygen enhances oxygenation of the peripheral tissues and end organs.

Exercise has several effects on oxygen affinity. First, exercise causes the production and release of carbon dioxide and other acids, especially from the large muscles. It also increases body temperature. Thus, both a decrease in pH and an increase in body temperature will cause hemoglobin to release oxygen more readily. This serves to enhance peripheral tissue oxygenation during strenuous exercise and work.

Importantly, other substances can compete with oxygen for hemoglobin's binding sites. The greater a substance's affinity for the binding sites, the more readily the substance will bind with hemoglobin. The classic example is carbon monoxide (CO). Carbon monoxide has 210 to 250 times oxygen's affinity for hemoglobin and competes for the same binding sites. In carbon monoxide poisoning, when CO binds to one of the hemoglobin molecule's four binding sites, the hemoglobin molecule is altered so that the remaining three oxygen molecules are held more tightly. This inhibits oxygen release in the peripheral tissues, contributing to hypoxia, acidosis, and eventually shock.

Red Blood Cell Production Red blood cell production is termed **erythropoiesis.** Erythropoietin, a hormone produced primarily by the kidney, stimulates the bone marrow's production of erythrocytes. Erythropoietin is secreted when the renal cells sense hypoxia. This, in turn, stimulates the bone marrow to increase RBC production, resulting in increased red cell mass. Although a relatively slow process, this effectively increases the oxygen carrying capacity of blood, thereby increasing oxygen delivery to the tissues.

The life span of the red blood cell is approximately 120 days. Hemorrhage, **hemolysis** (destruction of the RBC), or **sequestration** of the RBCs by the liver or spleen may significantly reduce its life span. Hemorrhage may occur outside the body or be hidden within a body cavity, such as the peritoneum, retroperitoneum, or the gastrointestinal tract. Hemolysis may occur within the circulatory system in sickle cell disease and in rare autoimmune anemias. The spleen and liver contain specialized scavenger cells called macrophages (a type of white blood cell) that can remove damaged or abnormal red blood cells from the circulation.

Laboratory Evaluation of Red Blood Cells and Hemoglobin Red blood cells (RBCs) are quantified or measured and reported in two ways: red blood cell count and hematocrit. The red blood cell count is the total number of RBCs reported in millions per cubic millimetre (mm^3) of blood. Normal values vary with age and sex but, in general, run between 4.2 and 6.0 million/mm^3.

The **hematocrit** is the packed cell volume of red blood cells per unit of blood (Figure 12-12). This measurement is obtained by placing a sample of blood in a centrifuge and spinning it at high speed so that the cellular elements separate from the plasma. The red blood cells are the heaviest blood component, since they carry the iron-containing pigment hemoglobin. They are forced to the bottom of the tube. Above the red blood cells are the white blood cells. On the top of the specimen is the plasma, which consists primarily of water. The RBCs' column height is divided by the blood's total column height (cellular component plus plasma) and reported as a percentage. Normal values range between 40 percent and 52 percent, with females generally running a few percentage points below males.

Another way to determine the status of the red blood cell is to measure the concentration of hemoglobin present. This is typically expressed as the number of grams of hemoglobin present per decilitre of whole blood. The hemoglobin concentration will decrease in two ways. First, when the number of red blood cells present is below normal, the hemoglobin will also be below normal. In some cases, the red blood cell volume can be normal, but the amount of hemoglobin present may be decreased. In emergency medicine, it is commonplace to measure the hemoglobin in addition to the hematocrit (H&H). Both values indicate red blood cell volume and capability. The normal hemoglobin in a man is 12–15 g/dL; for females, it is 10.5–14.0 g/dL.

White Blood Cells

White blood cells, called **leukocytes** or white corpuscles, circulate through the bloodstream and tissues, providing protection from foreign invasion. White blood cells (WBCs) are extremely mobile, travelling through the bloodstream to wherever they are needed to fight infection.

A large population of leukocytes does not move freely within the bloodstream but is attached to the blood vessels' walls. These *marginated* leukocytes may quickly return to the circulating pool in response to stress, corticosteroids, seizures, epinephrine, and exercise. This process is called *demargination*. Marginated leukocytes that attach more firmly to the vascular lining through *adhesion* may then leave the blood vessels by *diapedesis*. This enables the leukocytes to squeeze between the cells lining the blood vessels and to follow chemical signals (**chemotaxis**) to the infection site. There, they may engulf and destroy an invader by **phagocytosis** (Figure 12-13). Others stimulate either chemical or immune responses to fight infection.

Healthy people have 5000 to 9000 white blood cells per microlitre (µL) of blood. An infection can increase that number to more than 16 000. An increase in the white blood cell number is a classic sign of bacterial infection. White blood cells originate in the bone marrow from undifferentiated stem cells. Through a process termed **leukopoiesis,** these stem cells respond to specific growth factors that allow them to differentiate into three mainblasts (immature forms): myeloblasts, monoblasts, and lymphoblasts.

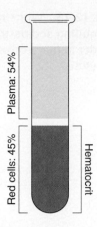

FIGURE 12-12 Hematocrit, including plasma.

✱ **hematocrit** the packed cell volume of red blood cells per unit of blood.

✱ **leukocyte** white blood cell.

✱ **chemotaxis** the movement of white blood cells in response to chemical signals.

✱ **phagocytosis** process in which white blood cells engulf and destroy an invader.

✱ **leukopoiesis** the process through which stem cells differentiate into the white blood cells' immature forms.

Content Review

WHITE BLOOD CELL –BLASTS
- Myeloblasts
- Monoblasts
- Lymphoblasts

FIGURE 12-13 White blood cells engulfing and destroying an invader in the process called phagocytosis.

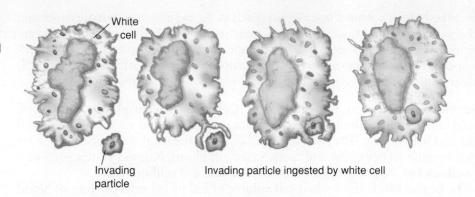

White cell

Invading particle

Invading particle ingested by white cell

White blood cells are categorized as *granulocytes, monocytes,* or *lymphocytes* (Figure 12-14).

Granulocytes Granulocytic white blood cells, so named for the granules they contain, form from stem cells that differentiate in the bone marrow in response to hormonal stimulation. These cells mature through several stages from myeloblast to promyelocyte, myelocyte, metamyelocyte, band form, and mature form (Figure 12-15). Their mature forms are classified by the type of stain they absorb. *Basophils* absorb basic stains and have blue granules. *Eosinophils* absorb acidic stains and contain red granules. *Neutrophils* absorb neither acidic nor basic stains well and contain pale blue and pink granules.

Basophils Basophils are granulocytes that primarily function in allergic reactions. Within their granules, they store all the histamine in the circulating blood. In response to an allergic stimulus, the cells degranulate, releasing histamines that cause vasodilation, bronchoconstriction, rhinorrhea, increased vascular permeability, and increased neutrophil and eosinophil chemotaxis. Basophils also contain heparin, which breaks down blood clots.

Eosinophils Eosinophils are highly specialized members of the granulocytic series. They can inactivate the chemical mediators of acute allergic reactions, thereby modulating the anaphylactic response. They also contain **major basic protein (MBP),** which they release in conjunction with an antibody response shown to fight parasitic infections.

Content Review

WHITE BLOOD CELL CATEGORIES
- Granulocytes
- Monocytes
- Lymphocytes

Content Review

GRANULOCYTE CLASSIFICATIONS
- Basophils
- Eosinophils
- Neutrophils

✱ **major basic protein (MBP)** a larvacidal peptide.

FIGURE 12-14 Types of white blood cells.

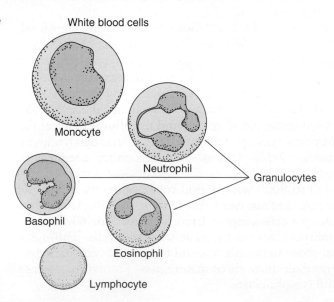

White blood cells

Monocyte

Neutrophil

Basophil

Granulocytes

Eosinophil

Lymphocyte

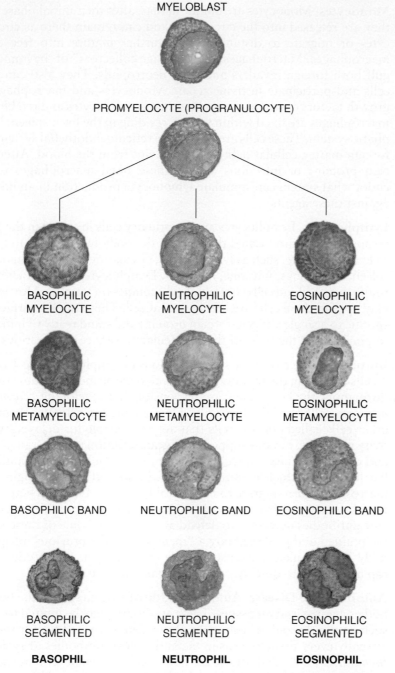

MYELOBLAST

PROMYELOCYTE (PROGRANULOCYTE)

| BASOPHILIC MYELOCYTE | NEUTROPHILIC MYELOCYTE | EOSINOPHILIC MYELOCYTE |

BASOPHILIC METAMYELOCYTE — NEUTROPHILIC METAMYELOCYTE — EOSINOPHILIC METAMYELOCYTE

BASOPHILIC BAND — NEUTROPHILIC BAND — EOSINOPHILIC BAND

BASOPHILIC SEGMENTED — NEUTROPHILIC SEGMENTED — EOSINOPHILIC SEGMENTED

BASOPHIL — **NEUTROPHIL** — **EOSINOPHIL**

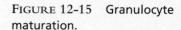

FIGURE 12-15 Granulocyte maturation.

Neutrophils The neutrophils' primary function is to fight infection. They leave the bloodstream by diapedesis and engulf and kill microorganisms that have invaded the body. Once they have phagocytized the microorganism, primary and secondary granules within the neutrophil fuse with the phagosome, and the organism is killed and digested. In severe infections, the total neutrophil count may rise rapidly, with immature (band) forms apparent on the peripheral blood smear under microscopic examination. If the neutrophil count is low (**neutropenia**), the body cannot mount an appropriate response to infection, and the infection may overwhelm the body's defences and kill the individual. Neutropenia may result from primary bone marrow disorders that decrease production, from overwhelming infection, viral syndrome, autoimmune disease, or drugs, and from nutritional deficiencies.

✱ **neutropenia** a low neutrophil count.

Monocytes Monocytes are unique in that, after their initial phase of maturation, they are released into the circulation and can remain there as circulating monocytes or migrate to distant sites to further mature into free or fixed tissue macrophages. Macrophages, the "garbage collectors" of the immune system, engulf both foreign invaders and dead neutrophils. They also can attack tumour cells and participate in tissue repair. Monocytes and macrophages also secrete growth factors to stimulate production of granulocytes and red blood cells. Some macrophages are fixed within tissues, residing in the liver, spleen, lungs, and lymphatic system. These cells are part of the reticuloendothelial system. They remove foreign matter, cellular debris, and proteins from the blood. After engulfing foreign proteins or infectious agents, these fixed macrophages of the reticuloendothelial system can stimulate lymphocyte production in an immune response against these agents.

Lymphocytes Lymphocytes are the primary cells involved in the body's immune response. They are located throughout the body in the circulating blood as well as in other tissues, such as lymph nodes, circulating in lymph fluid, bone marrow, spleen, liver, lungs, intestine, and skin. Lymphocytes are characteristically small, round, white blood cells containing no granules on staining. However similar they may appear, these cells are highly specialized. They contain surface receptor sites specific to a single antigen (foreign protein) and stand ready to initiate the immune response to rid the body of that particular substance or infectious agent.

Immunity The two basic subpopulations of lymphocytes are T cells and B cells. T cells mature in the thymus gland, located in the mediastinum, and then migrate throughout the body. They are responsible for developing *cell-mediated immunity,* also called *cellular immunity.* Once an antigen activates them, they generate other cells called effector cells that are responsible for delayed-type hypersensitivity reactions, tumour suppression, graft rejection (organ transplant rejections), and defence against intracellular organisms. B cells produce antibodies to combat infection, which is termed *humoral immunity.* They originate in the bone marrow and then migrate to peripheral lymphatic tissues. There, they can be exposed to antigens from invading organisms and respond by producing the specific antibodies necessary to defend against them. Some of these B cells' lines are maintained and give the body a "memory" of the previous infection. When the body is subsequently exposed to the same antigen or infection, it generates a rapid response to quickly overwhelm the infection.

Autoimmune Disease Autoimmune disease occurs when the body makes antibodies against its own tissues. These antibodies may be limited to specific organs, such as the thyroid, as occurs in *Hashimoto's thyroiditis.* Or they may involve virtually every tissue type as in the antinuclear antibodies of *systemic lupus erythematosis (SLE)* that attack the body's cell nuclei. Several anemias result from autoimmunity. Mechanisms for the development of autoimmune disease include genetic factors and viral infections.

✱ **autoimmune disease** condition in which the body makes antibodies against its own tissues.

Alterations in Immune Response Several factors can alter the body's immune response. For example, patients who receive an organ transplant must take drugs that inhibit cellular immunity and prevent graft rejection. If they do not, the T cells will recognize the new organ as "not self" and begin the process of attacking it. This is called rejection. Unfortunately, organ-recipient immunosuppressed patients are at risk for infections from many different organisms, including bacteria, viruses, fungi, and protozoa. Human immunodeficiency virus (HIV) effectively destroys cell-mediated immunity by selectively attacking and ultimately killing T cells. This also leaves the patient at risk for opportunistic infections against which the body cannot defend itself, ultimately killing her. Patients who have cancer are often immunocompromised by the disease itself or by chemotherapy agents that also attack the bone marrow. These agents decrease leukocyte production to extremely low levels, leaving the body defenceless against infection. As a paramedic, you must protect your immunosuppressed patients from undue exposure to infection by good handwashing technique, correct IV technique, and proper wound care. If you have an infection, you must take precautions not to transmit it to your patients. If the infection is highly contagious, as in influenza or chicken pox, you may have to work in a non-patient-care setting.

Inflammatory Process The **inflammatory process** is a nonspecific defence mechanism that wards off damage from microorganisms or trauma. It attempts to localize the damage while destroying the source, at the same time facilitating repair of the tissues. Causes of the inflammatory process may be an infectious agent, trauma, chemical, or immunological. After local tissue injury occurs, the damaged tissues release chemical messengers that attract white blood cells (chemotaxis), increase capillary permeability, and cause vasodilation. If bacteria are present, responding neutrophils or macrophages will phagocytize them, and tissue repair begins. The greater capillary permeability and vasodilation allow increased blood flow to the area and enable fluid to leak out of the capillaries. The process of local inflammation results in redness, warmth, swelling, and usually pain. The pain serves as a reminder against overuse, allowing time for rest and repair. Systemic inflammation is an inflammatory reaction, often in response to a bacterial infection. Fever is a common symptom and likely occurs in response to chemical mediators that macrophages release in response to the infectious agent. These chemical mediators act on the brain and lead to stimulation of the sympathetic nervous system, which causes vasoconstriction, heat conservation, and fever. The macrophages also release factors that stimulate the release of leukocytes from the bone marrow, leading to an elevated white blood cell count.

Platelets

Platelets, or **thrombocytes,** are small fragments of large cells called *megakaryocytes*. Like the other blood cells described so far, megakaryocytes come from an undifferentiated stem cell in the bone marrow. The hormone *thrombopoietin* stimulates these stem cells to differentiate through several stages into megakaryocytes, which then mature and break up into platelets, small fragments without nuclei. The normal number of platelets ranges from 150 000 to 450 000 per microlitre of blood. As they function to form a plug at an initial bleeding site and also secrete factors important in clot formation, too few platelets, a condition called *thrombocytopenia,* can lead to bleeding problems and blood loss. Too many platelets, *thrombocytosis,* may cause abnormal clotting, plugs in vessels, and emboli that may travel to the extremities, heart, lungs, or brain. Platelets survive for 7 to 10 days and are removed from circulation by the spleen.

Platelets are activated when they contact injured tissue. This contact stimulates an enzyme within the platelet, causing the surface to become "sticky," which, in turn, leads the platelets to aggregate and form a plug. Platelets also adhere to the damaged tissue to keep the plug in place. As the platelets aggregate, they release chemical messengers that also activate the blood clotting system.

HEMOSTASIS

Hemostasis—from *hemo* (blood) and *stasis* (standing still)—is the term used to describe the combined three mechanisms that work to prevent or control blood loss. These mechanisms include the following:

- Vascular spasms
- Platelet plugs
- Stable fibrin blood clots (coagulation)

Protect your immunosuppressed patients from undue exposure to infection by good handwashing technique, correct IV technique, and proper wound care.

* inflammatory process a nonspecific defence mechanism that wards off damage from microorganisms or trauma.

* thrombocyte blood platelet.

* hemostasis the combined mechanisms that work to prevent or control blood loss.

FIGURE 12-16 Clot
formation.

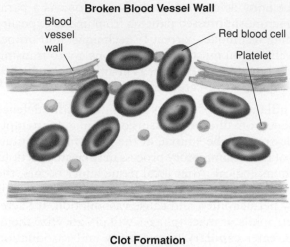

Broken Blood Vessel Wall

Blood vessel wall

Red blood cell

Platelet

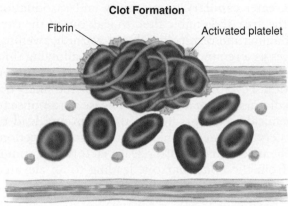

Clot Formation

Fibrin

Activated platelet

When a blood vessel tears, the smooth muscle fibres (tunica media) in the vessel walls contract. This causes vasoconstriction and reduces the size of the tear. Less blood flows through the constricted area, effectively limiting blood loss, and the smaller tear makes it easier for a platelet plug to develop and stop blood loss. At any tear in a blood vessel, platelets aggregate and adhere to collagen, a connective tissue that supports the blood vessels. This forms a platelet plug, which acts much like bubble gum stuck into a hole. The plug is unstable, however, and would permit the vessel to bleed again if not for the formation of a stable fibrin clot. This process, blood coagulation, is initiated, in part, by the platelet plug (Figure 12-16).

Due to the smoothness of the tunica intima, the blood vessels' innermost lining, blood normally flows through the vessels without frictional damage to cells or platelets. Damage to cells or to the vessel lining, however, starts the coagulation cascade. This cascade, or sequence of events, can be activated either by damage to vessels (extrinsic pathway) or by trauma to blood from turbulence (intrinsic pathway). Either results in the cascade's progression to a clot. Most clotting proteins are produced in the liver and circulate in an inactive state. The best known of these are *prothrombin* and *fibrinogen*. The damaged cells send out a chemical message that activates a specific clotting factor. This activates each protein, in turn, until a stable fibrin clot forms. To completely stop the bleeding, the coagulation cascade relies on the platelet plug and the clotting factors to interact. Once the bleeding stops, the inflammatory and healing processes can begin. The coagulation cascade can be summarized thus (Figure 12-17):

1. a. *Intrinsic pathway.* Platelets release substances that lead to the formation of prothrombin activator.

   or

   b. *Extrinsic pathway.* Tissue damage causes platelet aggregation and the formation of prothrombin activator.

2. *Common pathway.* The prothrombin activator, in the presence of calcium, converts prothrombin to thrombin.

3. *Thrombin.* In the presence of calcium, thrombin converts fibrinogen to stable fibrin, which then traps blood cells and more platelets to form a clot.

The development of a clot does not end the coagulation cascade. What the body can do, it usually can undo, given sufficient time. Once a fibrin clot is formed, it releases a chemical called *plasminogen.* Plasminogen is converted to *plasmin* and is then capable of dismantling, or lysing, a clot through the process of **fibrinolysis.** A clot's dismantling generally takes from hours to days. By that time, scarring has begun.

Thrombosis (clot formation), when it occurs in coronary arteries or cerebral vasculature, may lead to heart attack and stroke. To stimulate or speed up fibrinolysis and thus breakdown clots, medical researchers have developed several thrombolytic agents. These agents may help reestablish blood flow to these vital organs, limiting or preventing tissue death and thus helping prevent the patient's disability or death. Thrombolytics are effective only against blockages whose components include a fibrin clot.

Patients who lack certain clotting factors can have bleeding disorders that may complicate their assessment and treatment. Other patients take medications that

✷ **fibrinolysis** the process through which plasmin dismantles a blood clot.

✷ **thrombosis** clot formation, which is extremely dangerous when it occurs in coronary arteries or cerebral vasculature.

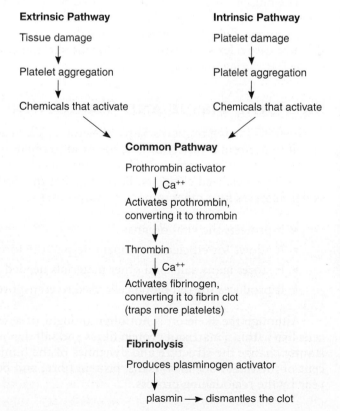

Extrinsic Pathway

Tissue damage
↓
Platelet aggregation
↓
Chemicals that activate

Intrinsic Pathway

Platelet damage
↓
Platelet aggregation
↓
Chemicals that activate

Common Pathway

Prothrombin activator
↓ Ca^{++}
Activates prothrombin, converting it to thrombin
↓
Thrombin
↓ Ca^{++}
Activates fibrinogen, converting it to fibrin clot (traps more platelets)
↓
Fibrinolysis

Produces plasminogen activator
↓
plasmin ⟶ dismantles the clot

FIGURE 12–17   The coagulation cascade.

decrease the effectiveness of platelets or the coagulation cascade. Recall that an enzyme on a platelet membrane makes the membrane sticky. Certain medications, such as aspirin, dipyridamole (Persantine), and ticlopidine (Ticlid), irreversibly alter the enzyme, thus decreasing the platelets' ability to aggregate and initiate the coagulation cascade. Other medications, such as heparin and warfarin (Coumadin), cause changes within the clotting cascade that prevent clot formation. Heparin, in conjunction with antithrombin III (a naturally occurring thrombin inactivator), rapidly inactivates thrombin, which then prevents formation of the fibrin clot. Warfarin (Coumadin) blocks vitamin K activity necessary to generate the activated forms of clotting factors II, VII, IX, and X, effectively interrupting the clotting cascade.

Vitamin K (AquaMEPHYTON) enhances clotting. Certain byproducts of tobacco smoking (especially in females on birth control pills) also enhance clotting. Relative or complete immobility, trauma, polycythemia (high red blood cell count), and cancer may also lead to increased clotting as blood becomes relatively stagnant. This allows platelet activation to begin, which leads to clotting. To counteract the effects of decreased activity, many patients take Aspirin or other antiplatelet inhibitors and wear compressive stockings to facilitate venous drainage from the lower extremities.

THE MUSCULOSKELETAL SYSTEM

The musculoskeletal system is a complex arrangement of levers and fulcrums, powered by biochemical motors, that provides motion and support for the body. It consists of two distinct subsystems, the skeleton and the muscles. The skeleton is the human body's superstructure, while the muscles supply the power of motion to this superstructure, the organs, and the other body components. These subsystems also produce body heat, store essential salts and energy sources, and create the majority of blood cells for transporting oxygen and combating disease.

The musculoskeletal system is covered by the skin and subcutaneous tissue. These elements protect the skeleton and muscles, as well as other body systems, from trauma, fluid loss, infection, and fluctuations in body temperature. The skin also provides some cushioning for the skeletal components, as on the soles of the feet during walking.

SKELETAL TISSUE AND STRUCTURE

As the body's living framework, the skeleton has a structure and design that permits it to perform a variety of functions and to repair itself as needed within limits. The skeleton is a complex, living system of cells, salt deposits, protein fibres, and other specialized elements. Besides giving the body its structural form, the skeleton serves four other important purposes:

- It protects the vital organs.
- It allows for efficient movement despite the forces of gravity.
- It stores many salts and other materials needed for metabolism.
- It produces the red blood cells used to transport oxygen.

Although the skeleton is not often thought of as alive, it is exactly that. Its cells live within a matrix of protein fibres and salt deposits. These living cells constantly change the structure and dynamics of the human frame. In fact, 20 percent of the total bone mass (salts, protein fibre, and bone cells) is replaced each year by the remodelling process.

Content Review

FUNCTIONS OF THE SKELETON

- Gives the body structural form
- Protects vital organs
- Allows for efficient movement
- Stores salts and other materials for metabolism
- Produces red blood cells

Some 20 percent of the total bone mass is replaced each year by the remodelling process.

Bone Structure

The structure of a typical bone consists of numerous aligned cylinders of bone. Minute blood vessels travel lengthwise along the bone through small tubes, called **haversian canals.** These blood vessels are surrounded by layers of salts deposited in collagen fibres. Bone cells called **osteocytes** are trapped within the matrix and maintain the collagen and the calcium, phosphate, carbonate, and other salt crystals. Other bone cells, osteoblasts and osteoclasts, deposit or dissolve these salt deposits as necessary. **Osteoblasts** lay down new bone in areas of stress during growth and during the bone repair cycle. **Osteoclasts** dissolve bone structures that are not carrying the pressures of articulation and support or when the body requires more salts for electrolyte balance. These three types of bone cells maintain a dynamic and efficient structure for supporting and moving the body.

A continuous blood supply brings oxygen and nutrients to the bones and removes carbon dioxide and waste products from them. The blood vessels enter and exit the bone shaft through **perforating canals** and distribute blood to both the bone tissue and the structures located within the medullary canal of the shaft and bone ends. As with any other body tissue, bone tissue becomes ischemic and will eventually die if the blood supply is reduced or cut off. The bone does not show evidence of such degeneration for quite some time, and certainly not during prehospital emergency care. However, the long-term effects of **devascularization** may be devastating.

The long bones, such as those of the forearm (humerus) and thigh (femur), best demonstrate the organization of bone tissue into structural body elements (Figure 12-18). The major areas and tissues of the long bones include the diaphysis, the epiphysis, the metaphysis, the medullary canal, the periosteum, and the articular cartilage.

The Diaphysis The **diaphysis** is the central portion or shaft of the long bone. It consists of a very dense and relatively thin layer of compact bone. Because of its tubular structure, the diaphysis efficiently supports weight and yet is relatively light. Although the design of the bone shaft enables it to carry weight well, lateral forces may cause the shaft to break rather easily.

The Epiphysis Toward the ends of the long bone, its structure changes. The bone's diameter increases dramatically, and the underlying thin, hard, compact bone of the shaft changes to a network of skeletal fibres and strands. This network, called the **epiphysis,** spreads the stresses and pressures of weight bearing over a larger surface. The tissue of the epiphysis in cross-section resembles a rigid bony sponge and is called spongy or **cancellous** bone. Covering this network of fibres is a very thin layer of compact bone supporting the surface that meets and moves against another bone, the **articular surface.**

The Metaphysis The **metaphysis** is an intermediate region between the epiphysis and diaphysis. It is where the diaphysis's hollow tube of compact bone makes the transition to the bone-fibre honeycomb of the epiphysis's cancellous bone. In this region is the **epiphyseal plate,** also called the *growth plate.* During childhood, cartilage is generated here and the plate widens. Osteoblasts from the end of the diaphysis deposit salts within the cartilage's collagen matrix to create new bone tissue. This results in the lengthening of the infant's and then the child's bone. During the growth period, the epiphyseal plate is also weaker than the rest of the bone and associated joints and is thus a frequent site of fractures in pediatric patients.

* **haversian canals** small perforations of the long bones through which the blood vessels and nerves travel into the bone itself.

* **osteocyte** bone-forming cell found in the bone matrix that helps maintain the bone.

* **osteoblast** cell that helps in the creation of new bone during growth and bone repair.

* **osteoclast** bone cell that absorbs and removes excess bone.

* **perforating canals** structures through which blood vessels enter and exit the bone shaft.

* **devascularization** loss of blood vessels from a body part.

* **diaphysis** hollow shaft found in long bones.

* **epiphysis** end of a long bone, including the epiphyseal, or growth plate and supporting structures underlying the joint.

* **cancellous** having a latticework structure, as in the spongy tissue of a bone.

* **articular surface** surface of a bone that moves against another bone.

* **metaphysis** growth zone of a bone, active during the development stages of youth. It is located between the epiphysis and the diaphysis.

* **epiphyseal plate** area of the metaphysis where cartilage is generated during bone growth in childhood; *growth plate.*

FIGURE 12-18 The internal anatomy of a long bone.

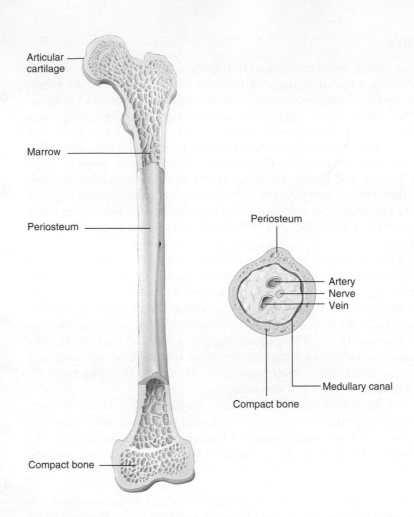

Articular cartilage

Marrow

Periosteum

Periosteum

Artery
Nerve
Vein

Medullary canal

Compact bone

Compact bone

✱ **medullary canal** cavity within a bone that contains the marrow.

✱ **yellow bone marrow** tissue that stores fat in semiliquid form within the internal cavities of a bone.

✱ **red bone marrow** tissue within the internal cavity of a bone responsible for manufacture of erythrocytes and other blood cells.

✱ **periosteum** the tough exterior covering of a bone.

✱ **cartilage** connective tissue providing the articular surfaces of the skeletal system.

Bones are classified according to their general shape.

The Medullary Canal The chamber formed within the hollow diaphysis and the cancellous bone of the epiphysis is called the **medullary canal**. The central medullary canal is filled with **yellow bone marrow** that stores fat in a semiliquid form. The fat is a readily available energy source the body can use quickly and easily. **Red bone marrow** fills the cancellous bone chambers of the larger long bones, the pelvis, and the sternum. It is responsible for the manufacture of erythrocytes and other blood cells.

The Periosteum A tough fibrous membrane called the **periosteum** covers the exterior of the diaphysis. With extensive vasculature and innervation, it transmits sensations of pain when the bone fractures and then initiates the bone repair cycle. Blood vessels and nerves penetrate both the periosteum and compact bone by travelling through the small perforating canals. Tendons intermingle with the collagen fibres of the periosteum and with the collagen fibres of the bony matrix to form strong attachments.

Cartilage A layer of connective tissue called **cartilage** is a continuous collagen extension of the underlying bone and covers a portion of the epiphyseal surface. It is a smooth, strong, and flexible material that functions as the actual surface of articulation between bones. Cartilage is very slippery and somewhat compressible. It permits relatively friction-free joint movement and absorbs some of the shock associated with activity, such as walking.

Bones are classified according to their general shape. Those as described above are considered long bones and include the humerus, radius, ulna, tibia, fibula, metacarpals (hand), metatarsals (foot), and phalanges (fingers and toes). The bones of the wrists and ankles, the carpals and tarsals, are short bones. The bones of the cranium, sternum, ribs, shoulder, and pelvis are classified as flat. Irregularly shaped bones include the bones of the vertebral column and the facial bones. Another special type of bone is the **sesamoid bone,** a bone that grows within tendinous tissue; one example is the kneecap, also called the patella.

Joint Structure

Bones move at, and are held together by, a relatively sophisticated structure called a **joint.**

Types of Joints There are three basic types of joints, which are classified by the amount of movement they permit.

Synarthroses are immovable joints, such as the sutures of the skull or the juncture between jaw and the teeth (which is called a gomphosis). **Amphiarthroses** are joints that allow some very limited movement. Examples include the joints between the vertebrae and between the sacrum and the ilium of the pelvis. **Diarthroses,** or **synovial joints,** permit relatively free movement. Such joints include the elbow, knee, shoulder, and hip.

Diarthroses are divided into three categories of joints based on the movements they allow (Figure 12-19).

- *Monaxial joints*
  - Hinge joints permit bending in a single plane. Examples include the knees, elbows, and fingers.
  - Pivot joints are characterized by the articulation between the atlas (the first cervical vertebrae) and the axis of the spine. They allow the head to rotate through a wide range of motion.

- *Biaxial joints*
  - Condyloid, or gliding, joints provide movement in two directions. They are located at the joints of carpal bones in the wrist and between the clavicle and sternum.
  - Ellipsoidal joints provide a sliding motion in two planes, as between the wrist and the metacarpals.
  - Saddle joints allow for movement in two planes at right angles to each other. Examples are the joints at the bases of the thumbs.

- *Triaxial joints*
  - Ball-and-socket joints permit full motion in a cone of about 180 degrees and allow a limb to rotate. Examples include the hip and shoulder.

These joints permit various types of motion. **Flexion/extension** is the bending motion that reduces/increases the angle between articulating elements. **Adduction/abduction** is the movement of a body part toward/away from the midline. **Rotation** refers to a turning along the axis of a bone or joint. **Circumduction** refers to movement through an arc of a circle.

Ligaments **Ligaments** are bands of connective tissue that hold bones together at joints. They stretch and permit motion at the joint while holding the bone ends firmly in position. The ends of the ligaments attach to the joint ends of each of the associated bones. Ligaments surround the articular region and cross it at many oblique angles. This arrangement ensures that the joint is held together firmly but flexibly enough to permit movement through a designed range of motion.

✴ **sesamoid bone** bone that forms in a tendon.

✴ **joint** area where adjacent bones articulate.

Content Review

TYPES OF JOINTS

- Synarthroses—immovable
- Amphiarthroses—very limited movement
- Diarthroses (synovial joints)—relatively free movement:
  – Monaxial
  – Biaxial
  – Triaxial

✴ **synarthorsis** joint that does not permit movement.

✴ **amphiarthrosis** joint that permits a limited amount of independent motion.

✴ **diarthrosis** a synovial joint.

✴ **synovial joint** joint that permits the greatest degree of independent motion.

✴ **flexion** bending motion that reduces the angle between articulating elements.

✴ **extension** bending motion that increases the angle between articulating elements.

✴ **adduction** movement of a body part toward the midline.

✴ **abduction** movement of a body part away from the midline.

✴ **rotation** a turning along the axis of a bone or joint.

✴ **circumduction** movement at a synovial joint where the distal end of a bone describes a circle but the shaft does not rotate; movement through an arc of a circle.

✴ **ligaments** connective tissue that connects bone to bone and holds joints together.

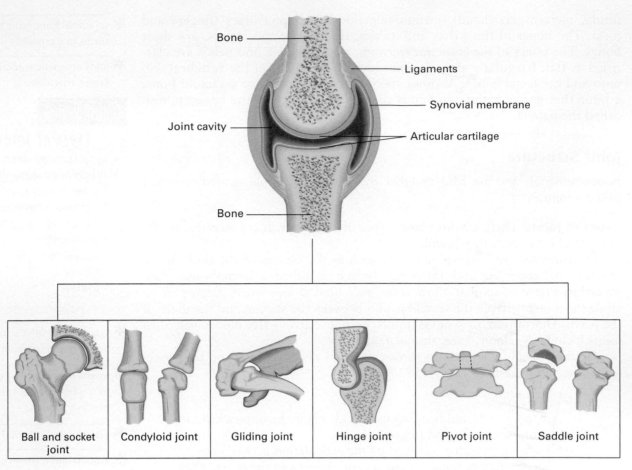

Bone

Ligaments

Synovial membrane

Joint cavity

Articular cartilage

Bone

| Ball and socket joint | Condyloid joint | Gliding joint | Hinge joint | Pivot joint | Saddle joint |

FIGURE 12-19 Types of joints.

* **joint capsule** the ligaments that surround a joint; *synovial capsule.*

* **synovial fluid** substance that lubricates synovial joints.

* **bursae** sacs containing synovial fluid that cushion adjacent structures; singular *bursa.*

* **axial skeleton** bones of the head, thorax, and spine.

Joint Capsule The ligaments surrounding a joint form what is known as the **joint capsule** or *synovial capsule* (Figure 12-20). This chamber holds a small amount of fluid to lubricate the articular surfaces. This oily, viscous substance, known as **synovial fluid,** assists joint motion by reducing friction. Its lubrication reduces friction to about one-fifth that of two pieces of ice sliding together. Small sacs filled with synovial fluid, known as **bursae,** are also located between tendons and ligaments or cartilage in the elbows, knees, and other joints to reduce friction and absorb shock. Synovial fluid flows into and out of the articular cartilage as the joint undergoes pressure and movement. The cartilage acts like a sponge, pushing out fluid as it is compressed and drawing in fluid when it is relaxed. This movement of synovial fluid circulates oxygen, nutrients, and waste products to and from the joint cartilage.

SKELETAL ORGANIZATION

The human skeleton is made up of approximately 206 bones (Figure 12-21). These bones form two major divisions, the axial and the appendicular skeletons.

The **axial skeleton** consists of the bones of the head, thorax, and spine. These bones form the axis of the body, protect the elements of the central nervous system, and make up the thoracic cage, which is the dynamic housing for respiration. The components of the axial skeleton will be discussed under the headings, "The Head, Face, and Neck" and "The Spine and Thorax."

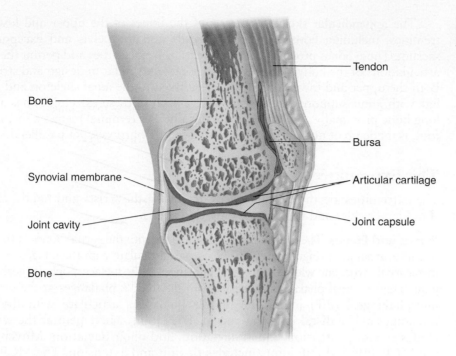

FIGURE 12-20   Structure of a joint.

Tendon

Bone

Bursa

Synovial membrane

Articular cartilage

Joint cavity

Joint capsule

Bone

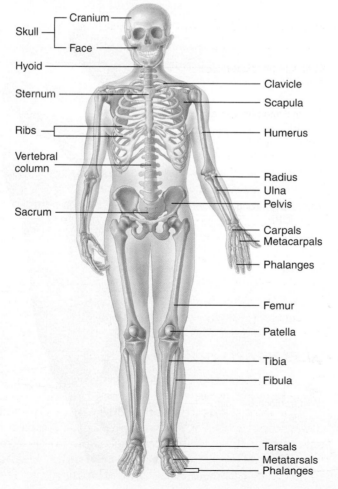

FIGURE 12-21   The human skeleton.

Skull — Cranium

Face

Hyoid

Sternum

Ribs

Vertebral column

Sacrum

Clavicle

Scapula

Humerus

Radius

Ulna

Pelvis

Carpals

Metacarpals

Phalanges

Femur

Patella

Tibia

Fibula

Tarsals

Metatarsals

Phalanges

The Musculoskeletal System   **505**

The **appendicular skeleton** consists of the bones of the upper and lower extremities, including both the shoulder girdle and the pelvis and excepting the sacrum. These bones provide the structure for the extremities and permit the major articulations of the body. Extremity long bones are similar in design and structure. Both the upper and lower extremities are affixed to the axial skeleton and articulate with joints supported by several bones. Each of these extremities has a single long bone proximally and paired bones distally. The terminal member, the hand or foot, is made up of numerous bones with differing purposes, yet parallel designs.

The Extremities

The extremities are the arms and legs, including the wrists and hands, elbows, shoulders, ankles and feet, knees, hips, and pelvis.

Wrists and Hands The radius and ulna articulate with the carpal bones at the wrist, or radiocarpal joint (Figure 12-22). The carpals articulate with the metacarpals. The metacarpals articulate with the proximal phalanges at the metacarpophalangeal (MCP) joint. The proximal phalanges articulate with the middle phalanges at the proximal interphalangeal (PIP) joint. The middle phalanges articulate with the distal phalanges at the distal interphalangeal (DIP) joint. Movement at the wrist includes flexion, extension, radial deviation, and ulnar deviation. Movement at the MCP, PIP, and DIP joints includes flexion and extension. The MCP joints also allow abduction (spreading the fingers out) and adduction (bringing them back together). The major flexor muscles are the flexor carpi radialis and flexor

FIGURE 12-22 Bones and joints of the hand and wrist.

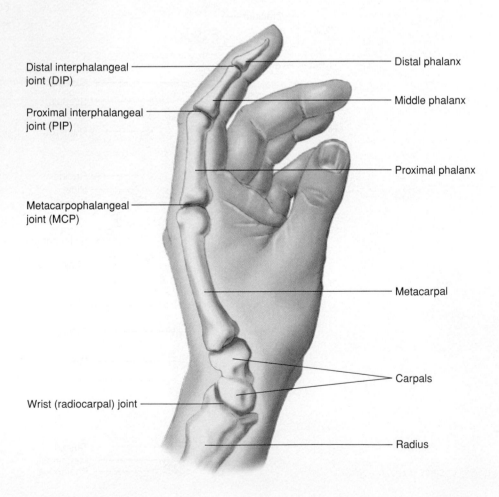

Distal interphalangeal joint (DIP)

Proximal interphalangeal joint (PIP)

Metacarpophalangeal joint (MCP)

Wrist (radiocarpal) joint

Distal phalanx

Middle phalanx

Proximal phalanx

Metacarpal

Carpals

Radius

carpi ulnaris (Figure 12-23). The major extensor muscles are the extensor carpi radialis longus, extensor carpi radialis brevis, and extensor carpi ulnaris.

Elbows The lateral and medial epicondyles (large rounded edges) of the distal humerus, the olecranon process of the proximal ulna, and the proximal radius comprise the elbow joint (Figure 12-24). Between the olecranon process and skin lies a bursa. The ulnar nerve (funny bone) extends through the groove between the olecranon process and the medial epicondyle. The elbow is a hinge joint, allowing flexion and extension. The major flexor muscles are the biceps (Figure 12-25). The

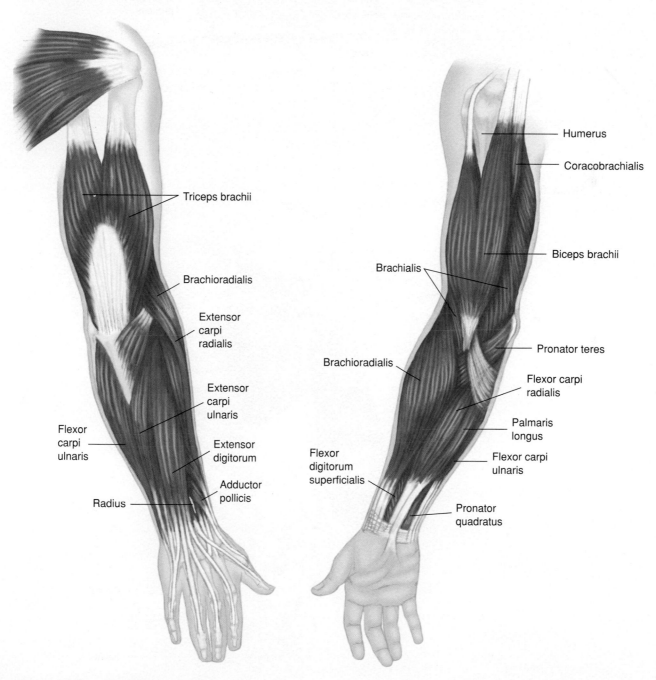

FIGURE 12-23   Muscles of the arm.

FIGURE 12-24 The elbow.

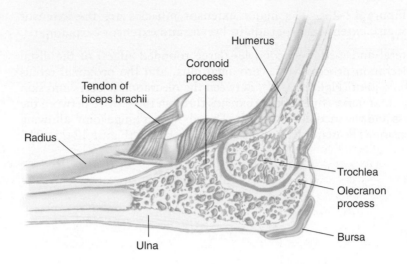

Tendon of
biceps brachii

Coronoid
process

Humerus

Radius

Trochlea

Olecranon
process

Bursa

Ulna

FIGURE 12-25 Elbow flexors.

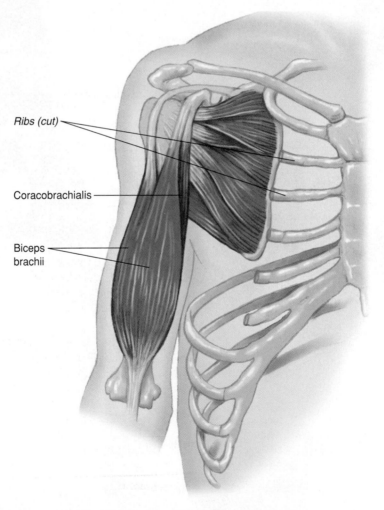

Ribs (cut)

Coracobrachialis

Biceps
brachii

Anterior

major extensor muscles are the triceps (Figure 12-26). Just below the elbow, the relationship of the radius and ulna to the pronator and supinator muscles allows the forearm to supinate (turn palm up) and pronate (turn palm down) (Figure 12-27).

Shoulders The shoulder girdle consists of articulations between the clavicle and the scapula and between the scapula and the head of the humerus (Figure 12-28). The sternoclavicular joint, which joins the clavicle and the manubrium, is the only bony link between the upper extremity and the axial skeleton. Movement at this joint is largely passive and occurs as a result of active movements of the scapula. The distal clavicle articulates with the acromion, or acromion process, of the scapula at the acromioclavicular (AC) joint. The clavicle acts as a strut, keeping the upper limb away from the thorax and permitting a greater range of motion. The AC joint also helps provide stability to the upper limb, reducing the need for muscle energy to keep the shoulder in its proper alignment.

The glenohumeral joint is a ball-and-socket joint that allows flexion, extension, internal and external rotation, abduction, and adduction. It has the greatest range of motion of any joint in the body and as a result is the most frequent site for dislocation. The head of the humerus (ball) fits into the glenoid

FIGURE 12-26   Elbow extensors.

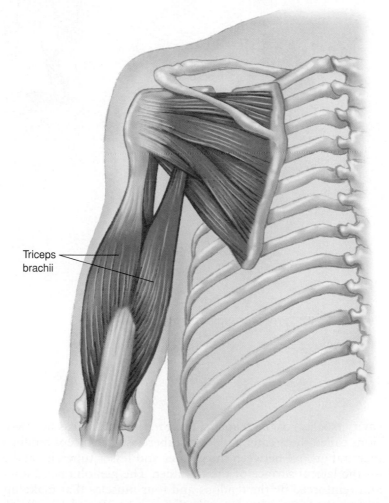

Triceps brachii

Posterior

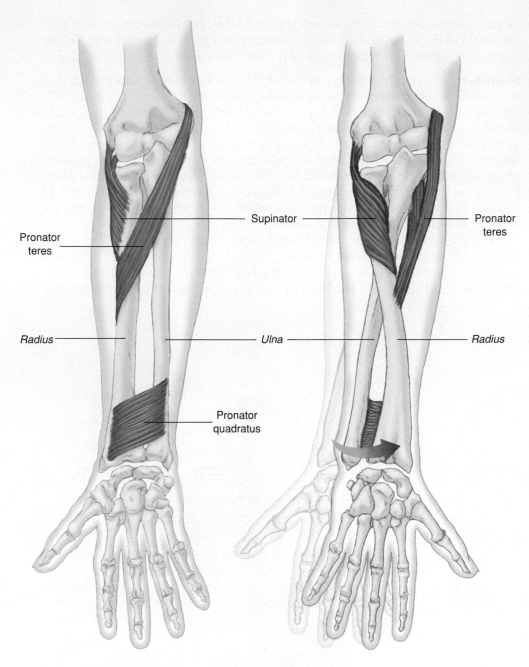

Pronator
teres

Supinator

Pronator
teres

Radius

Ulna

Radius

Pronator
quadratus

FIGURE 12-27   Pronator-supinator muscles.

cavity (socket) of the scapula. The proximal humerus has two rounded protrusions called the greater and lesser tubercles. The biceps tendon runs through the bicipital groove between the greater and lesser tubercles and is easily palpable on the lateral surface of the shoulder. The glenohumeral joint is encapsulated and reinforced by the tendons and four muscles that make up the rotator cuff and by the large deltoid muscle (Figures 12-29 and 12-30). The muscles of the rotator cuff include the supraspinatus, the infraspinatus, the teres minor, and the subscapularis muscles.

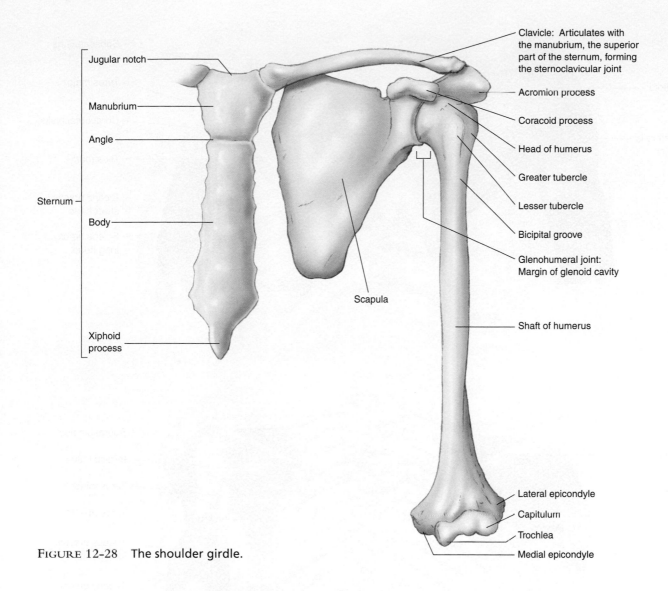

Clavicle: Articulates with the manubrium, the superior part of the sternum, forming the sternoclavicular joint

Jugular notch

Manubrium

Angle

Sternum

Body

Xiphoid process

Acromion process

Coracoid process

Head of humerus

Greater tubercle

Lesser tubercle

Bicipital groove

Glenohumeral joint: Margin of glenoid cavity

Scapula

Shaft of humerus

Lateral epicondyle

Capitulum

Trochlea

Medial epicondyle

FIGURE 12-28   The shoulder girdle.

FIGURE 12-29   Shoulder girdle ligaments.

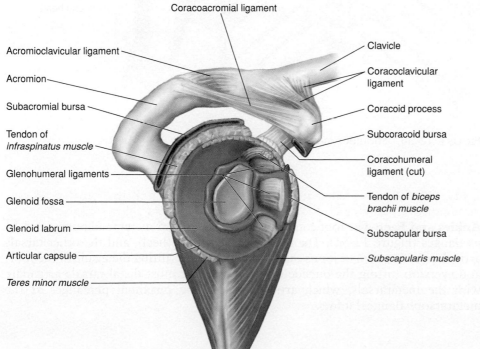

Coracoacromial ligament

Acromioclavicular ligament

Acromion

Subacromial bursa

Tendon of *infraspinatus muscle*

Glenohumeral ligaments

Glenoid fossa

Glenoid labrum

Articular capsule

Teres minor muscle

Clavicle

Coracoclavicular ligament

Coracoid process

Subcoracoid bursa

Coracohumeral ligament (cut)

Tendon of *biceps brachii muscle*

Subscapular bursa

Subscapularis muscle

The Musculoskeletal System   **511**

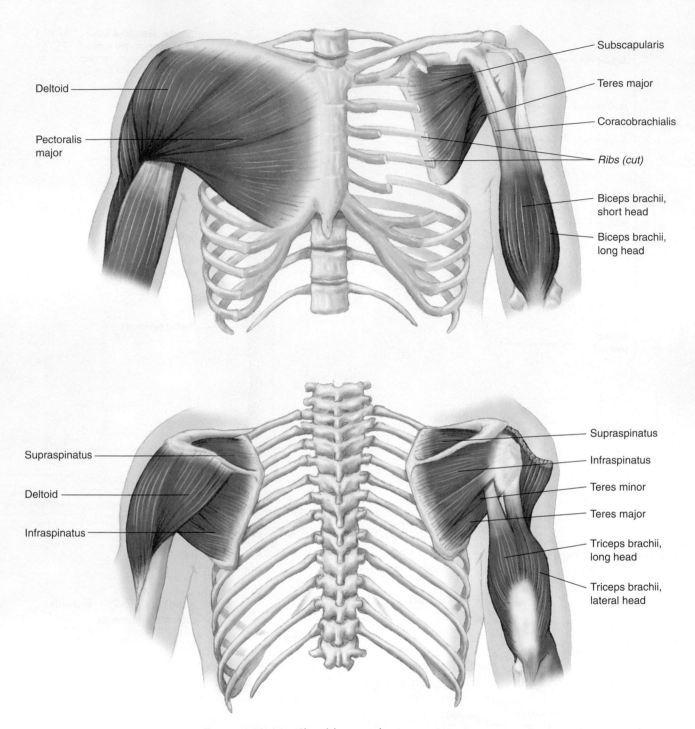

Deltoid

Pectoralis
major

Subscapularis

Teres major

Coracobrachialis

Ribs (cut)

Biceps brachii,
short head

Biceps brachii,
long head

Supraspinatus

Deltoid

Infraspinatus

Supraspinatus

Infraspinatus

Teres minor

Teres major

Triceps brachii,
long head

Triceps brachii,
lateral head

FIGURE 12-30   Shoulder muscles.

Ankles and Feet   The foot comprises 7 tarsal bones, 5 metatarsal bones, and 14
phalanges (Figure 12-31). The talus, the calcaneus (heel), and the other tarsals
articulate in a system of joints that allows inversion (lifting the inside of the foot)
and eversion (lifting the outside of the foot). The most distal tarsals articulate
with the metatarsals, which articulate with the proximal phalanges at the
metatarsophalangeal joints.

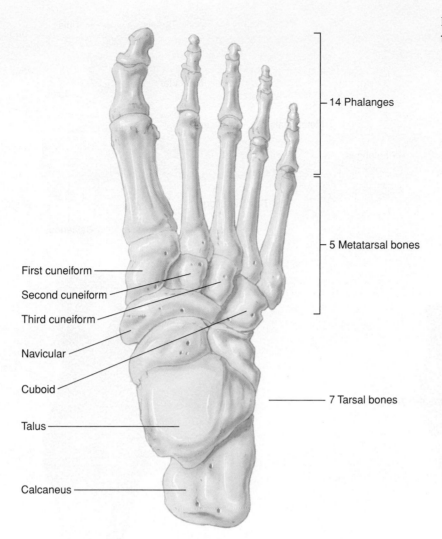

FIGURE 12-31 Bones of the foot.

14 Phalanges

5 Metatarsal bones

First cuneiform

Second cuneiform

Third cuneiform

Navicular

Cuboid

7 Tarsal bones

Talus

Calcaneus

At the ankle joint, the distal tibia (medial malleolus) and the distal fibula (lateral malleolus) articulate with the talus (Figure 12-32). Ligaments stretching from each malleolus to the foot itself hold the ankle joint together. The strong Achilles tendon, which inserts on the calcaneus (heel), also helps maintain the ankle's integrity. Movement in the ankle is limited to dorsiflexion (raising the foot) and plantar flexion (lowering the foot). The major dorsiflexor muscle is the tibialis anterior (Figure 12-33). The major plantar flexor is the gastrocnemius (calf muscle) (Figure 12-34).

Knees The knee joint involves the distal femur, the proximal tibia, and the patella (Figure 12-35). The distal femur and the proximal tibia meet at this joint and are cushioned by the lateral meniscus and the medial meniscus, which form a cartilaginous surface for pain-free movement. The joint capsule contains synovial fluid. Several ligaments surround the knee joint and help maintain its integrity. The medial and lateral collateral ligaments provide side-to-side stability and are easily palpable. The anterior and posterior cruciate ligaments, which give the knee front-to-back stability, lie deep within the joint capsule and are not palpable.

Figure 12-32 The foot and ankle.

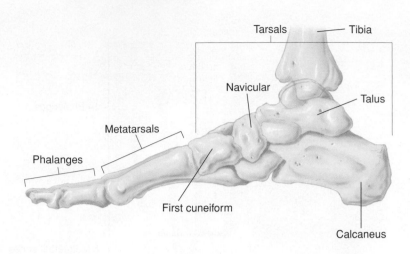

Tarsals — Tibia
Navicular
Talus
Metatarsals
Phalanges
First cuneiform
Calcaneus

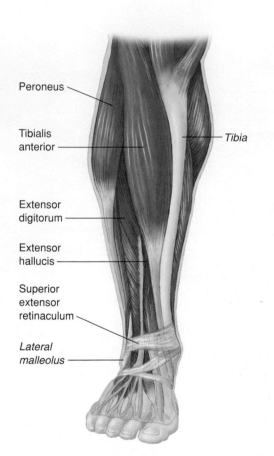

Peroneus
Tibialis anterior
Tibia
Extensor digitorum
Extensor hallucis
Superior extensor retinaculum
Lateral malleolus

Figure 12-33 The dorsiflexors.

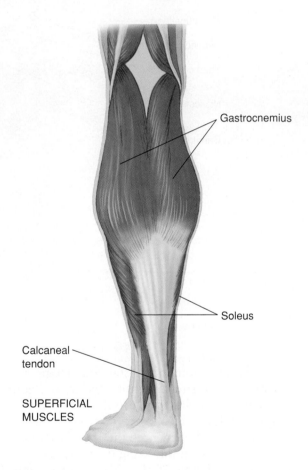

Gastrocnemius
Soleus
Calcaneal tendon
SUPERFICIAL MUSCLES

Figure 12-34 The plantar flexors.

The knee is a modified hinge joint, allowing flexion and extension, with some rotation during flexion. The major flexors are a group of three muscles (biceps femoris, semimembranosus, and semitendinosus) known as the hamstrings (Figure 12-36). The major extensors are a group of four muscles (vastus lateralis, vastus intermedius, vastus medialis, and rectus femoris) known as the quadriceps (Figure 12-37). The femur can rotate on the tibia slightly. The patella lies deep in the middle of the quadriceps tendon, which inserts on the tibial tuberosity below the knee. Concave areas at each side of the patella and below it contain synovial fluid.

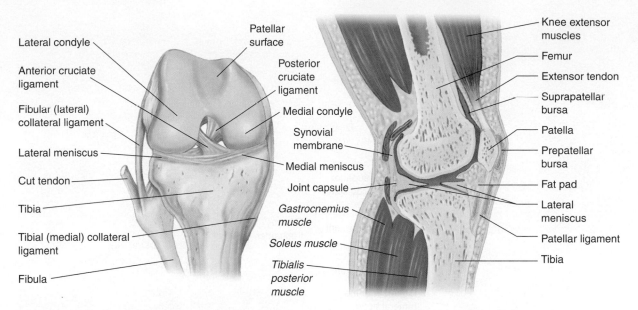

Lateral condyle

Anterior cruciate ligament

Fibular (lateral) collateral ligament

Lateral meniscus

Cut tendon

Tibia

Tibial (medial) collateral ligament

Fibula

Patellar surface

Posterior cruciate ligament

Medial condyle

Synovial membrane

Medial meniscus

Joint capsule

Gastrocnemius muscle

Soleus muscle

Tibialis posterior muscle

Knee extensor muscles

Femur

Extensor tendon

Suprapatellar bursa

Patella

Prepatellar bursa

Fat pad

Lateral meniscus

Patellar ligament

Tibia

FIGURE 12-35 The knee.

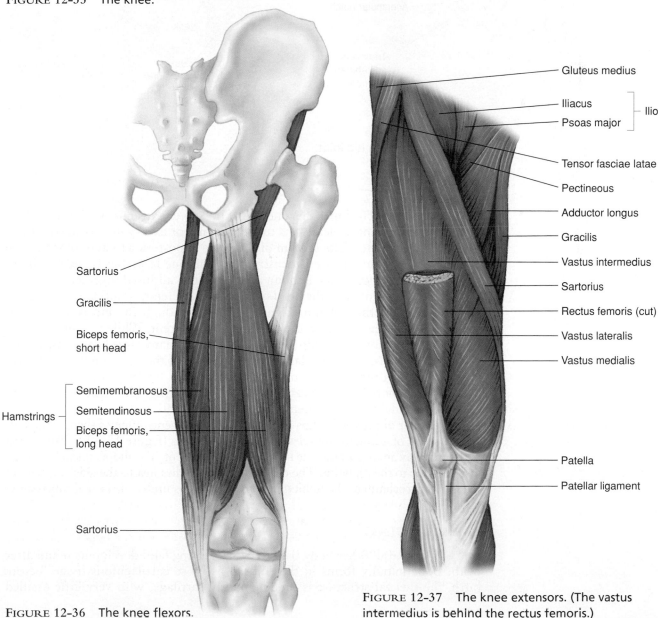

Sartorius

Gracilis

Biceps femoris, short head

Hamstrings

Semimembranosus

Semitendinosus

Biceps femoris, long head

Sartorius

FIGURE 12-36 The knee flexors.

Gluteus medius

Iliacus

Psoas major

Iliopsoas

Tensor fasciae latae

Pectineous

Adductor longus

Gracilis

Vastus intermedius

Sartorius

Rectus femoris (cut)

Vastus lateralis

Vastus medialis

Patella

Patellar ligament

FIGURE 12-37 The knee extensors. (The vastus intermedius is behind the rectus femoris.)

The Musculoskeletal System **515**

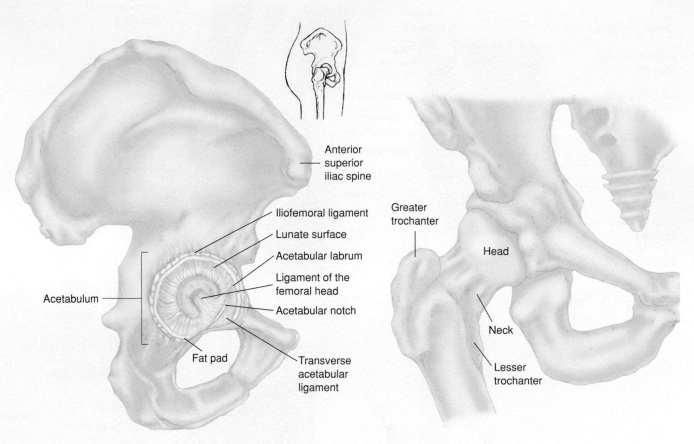

FIGURE 12-38 The hip joint.

Labels in figure: Anterior superior iliac spine; Iliofemoral ligament; Lunate surface; Acetabular labrum; Ligament of the femoral head; Acetabular notch; Acetabulum; Fat pad; Transverse acetabular ligament; Greater trochanter; Head; Neck; Lesser trochanter

Hips and Pelvis The hip is the juncture of the lower extremities with the pelvis. The pelvis is a strong skeletal structure consisting of two symmetrical structures called the inominates. The sacrum of the spine is posterior to and joined to the inominates. Each inominate is constructed from one large flat bone, the ilium, the two irregular bones, the ischium and the pubis, all fused together.

The hip joint involves the head of the proximal femur (ball) and the acetabulum (socket) of the ischium (Figure 12-38). Although the hip is a ball-and-socket joint like the shoulder, the two are very different. While the shoulder has a wide range of motion, the hip joint is restricted by many large ligaments, a bony ridge in the pelvis, and capsular fibres. Hip flexion, the most important movement, occurs via the iliopsoas muscle group (Figure 12-39). Other movements, though much more limited in range than those of the shoulder, include extension, abduction, adduction, and internal and external rotation.

A number of muscle groups control these movements. One of these is the gluteus, a series of adductor muscles and lateral rotators (Figure 12-40). Three bursa in the hip play an important role in pain-free movement. The iliopectineal bursa sits just anterior to the hip joint. The trochanteric bursa lies just to the side and behind the greater trochanter. The ischiogluteal bursa resides under the ischial tuberosity.

BONE AGING

The bones, like all other body tissues, evolve during fetal development and after birth. Bone initially forms in the embryo as loose cartilaginous tissue. Before birth, the skeletal structure is predominantly cartilage, with very little ossified

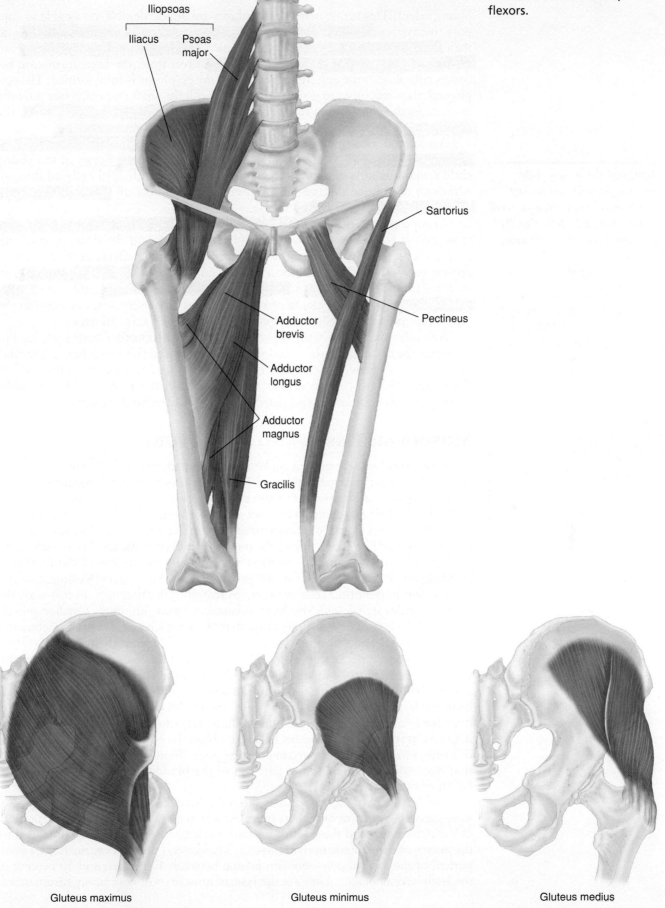

Iliopsoas

Iliacus Psoas major

Sartorius

Adductor brevis

Pectineus

Adductor longus

Adductor magnus

Gracilis

FIGURE 12-39 The hip flexors.

Gluteus maximus

Gluteus minimus

Gluteus medius

FIGURE 12-40 The gluteus muscles.

bone evident. This is one reason that infants are highly flexible yet unable to support themselves. Ossified bone begins to appear along the long bone shafts and then extends to the epiphyseal plates. It also develops within the epiphyses and grows outward to form the articular surfaces. Over time, the bone formation becomes complete to the epiphyseal plate, and the epiphysis is fully formed. The epiphyseal plate continues to generate cartilage, with the shaft and epiphyses growing from it. As the young adult reaches full height and the end of skeletal growth, the epiphyseal plates narrow, become bony, and cease to produce cartilage.

Associated with bone development and aging is the transition from flexible, cartilaginous bone to firm, strong, and fully ossified bone. Bones of the young child remain flexible and do not reach maximum strength until early adulthood. Although each bone matures at a different time, almost all maturation is complete by 18 to 20 years of age.

Around the age of 40, the body begins to lose its ability to maintain the bone structure. It is unable to rebuild the collagen matrix and the deposition of salt crystals is reduced from what it was in earlier years. The effects of these changes appear very slowly. They include a very gradual diminution of bone strength, an increase in bone brittleness, a progressive loss of body height, and some curvature of the spine. The incidence of bone fractures also increases, especially at the high stress points of the lumbar spine and the femur's surgical neck.

Age-related changes in the skeletal system also affect other body systems. For example, the cartilage of the costal-chondral joints and the costal bones (the ribs) becomes less flexible, which leads to shallower, more energy-consuming respirations. Also, the intravertebral discs lose water content and become less flexible, more prone to herniation, and narrower, thus shortening the trunk.

MUSCULAR TISSUE AND STRUCTURE

More than 600 muscle groups make up the muscular system (Figure 12-41). As you might expect, a large number of EMS calls involve injuries to this extensive system. Injuries to it may result from excessive forces indirectly expressed to the muscles and their attachments or from direct trauma, either blunt or penetrating.

There are three types of muscle tissue within the body—cardiac, smooth, and skeletal (Figure 12-42). Of these, the most specialized is the cardiac muscle comprising the myocardium. It contracts rhythmically on its own (automaticity), emitting an electrical impulse in the process (excitability), and passing that impulse along to the other cells of the myocardium (conductivity). In this way, the heart provides its lifelong rhythmic contraction and pumping. Cardiac muscle can also be classified according to its structure, which combines characteristics of both skeletal and smooth muscle and is thus called smooth-striated.

The second muscle type is smooth, or involuntary, muscle, which is not under conscious control but functions at the direction of the autonomic nervous system. These muscles are found in the arterial and venous blood vessels, the bronchioles, the bowel, and many other organs. Smooth muscle contracts to reduce (or relaxes to expand) the lumen (diameter) of the vasculature, airways, or digestive tract. Smooth muscles have the ability to contract over a wide lateral distance, enabling them to accommodate great changes in length, such as those that occur during filling and evacuation of the bladder and contraction and dilation of the arterioles.

The final type of muscle tissue is skeletal (also called striated or voluntary). We have conscious control over these muscles, which are associated with the mobility of the extremities and the body in general. Skeletal muscles are also controlled by the nerves of the somatic nervous system. The skeletal muscles are the largest component of the muscular system, comprising between 40 percent and 50 percent of the body's total weight. They are the type of muscle most commonly traumatized.

Bones of the young child remain flexible and do not reach maximum strength until maturation, which is usually completed by 18 to 20 years of age.

After approximately the age of 40, the body begins to lose the ability to maintain bone structure.

Content Review

TYPES OF MUSCLE
- Cardiac muscle
- Smooth muscle
- Skeletal muscle

FIGURE 12-41
The muscular system (posterior view).

sternocleidomastoid

trapezius

teres minor

teres major

deltoid

triceps

latissimus dorsi

olecranon

lumbodorsal fascia

gluteus maximus

iliotibial band

biceps femoris

semitendinosus

semimembranous

gastrocnemius

soleus

Achilles tendon

FIGURE 12-41 CONTINUED
The muscular system (anterior view).

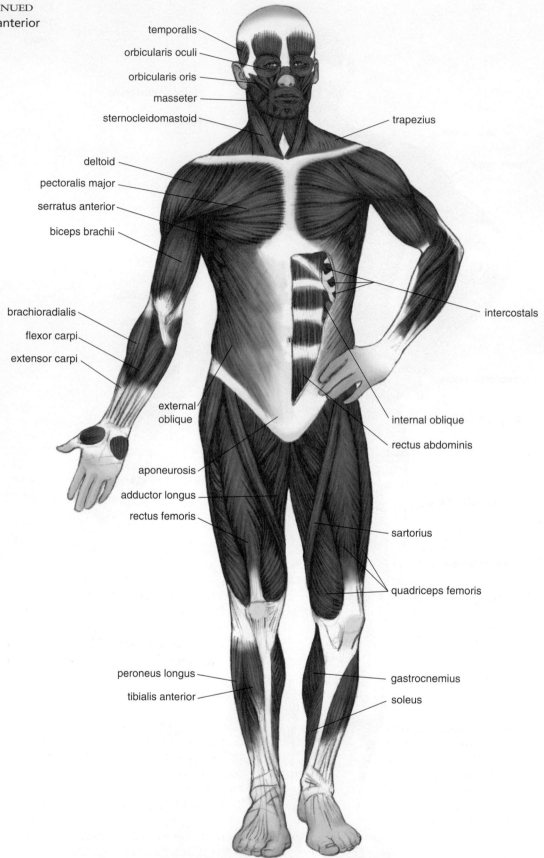

temporalis
orbicularis oculi
orbicularis oris
masseter
sternocleidomastoid
trapezius
deltoid
pectoralis major
serratus anterior
biceps brachii
intercostals
brachioradialis
flexor carpi
extensor carpi
external oblique
internal oblique
rectus abdominis
aponeurosis
adductor longus
rectus femoris
sartorius
quadriceps femoris
peroneus longus
tibialis anterior
gastrocnemius
soleus

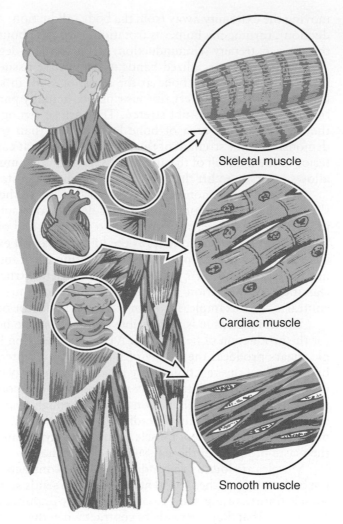

FIGURE 12-42   Three types of muscle.

Skeletal muscle

Cardiac muscle

Smooth muscle

Skeletal muscles lie directly beneath a protective layer of skin and subcutaneous fat. Because of their hunger for oxygen during activity, they have a more than ample supply of blood vessels. Individual muscle cells layer together to form a muscle fibre, many fibres layer together to form a muscle **fasciculus,** and fasciculi layer together to form a muscle body, such as the triceps. A muscle body has a strength of about nine kilograms of lift for each square centimetre of cross-sectional area.

Skeletal muscles attach to the bones at a minimum of two locations. These attachment points are called the origin and the insertion, depending on how the bones move with contraction. The point of attachment that remains stationary as the muscle contracts is the **origin,** while the attachment to the moving bone is the **insertion.**

Muscles usually pair, one on each side of a joint. This configuration is essential because muscles can actively contract, not lengthen. One muscle moves the extremity in one direction by contraction, while the opposing (and relaxed) muscle stretches. The opposing muscle can then, in turn, contract, stretching the first muscle and moving the extremity in the opposite direction. This arrangement, called **opposition,** permits the straightening (extension) and then bending (flexion) of the limbs.

With several muscles attached to a joint with different origins and insertions, the body enjoys a wide variety of motions. In the shoulder, for example, the humerus can travel through several types and ranges of motion. These include

✱ **fasciculus** small bundle of muscle fibres.

✱ **origin** attachment of a muscle to a bone that does not move (or experiences the least movement) when the muscle contracts.

✱ **insertion** attachment of a muscle to a bone that moves when the muscle contracts.

✱ **opposition** pairing of muscles that permits extension and flexion of limbs.

The Musculoskeletal System   **521**

moving the extremity away from the body (abduction) and toward the body (adduction), turning the humerus (rotation) through about 60 degrees, and circling the entire extremity (circumduction) through a 180-degree arc.

Tendons are specialized bands of connective tissue that accomplish the attachment of muscle to bone at the insertion and, in some cases, at the origin (Figure 12-43). These very fibrous ribbons, actually parts of the muscles, are extremely strong and do not stretch. They are so strong that, in some instances, they will break an area of bone loose rather than tear. The Achilles tendon demonstrates the strength of this particular tissue. It can be felt as the band posterior to the malleoli of the ankle. This tendon is the muscle-controlled cord that allows a person to lift the entire body weight when standing on the toes.

The forearm demonstrates the sophistication of the muscle-tendon relationship. As the muscles controlling finger flexion contract, you can feel them tensing in the dorsal forearm. You can also visualize and palpate tendon movement in the distal forearm and wrist as the fingers flex and extend. It is easy to appreciate the damage a deep transverse laceration can cause to the underlying connective tissues and their control of distal skeletal structures. Tendons are often classified by the action they perform when the muscle associated with them contracts—for example, flexor or extensor, abductor or adductor, and so on.

The muscle tissue is responsible not only for the body's movement but also for the production of heat energy. A chemical reaction between oxygen and simple sugars produces the energy of motion. Heat, water, and carbon dioxide are byproducts of this reaction. More than half the energy created by muscle motion is heat that helps maintain body temperature. The body then excretes water in the urine or sweat, expels carbon dioxide through respiration, and dissipates excess heat through the skin via radiation or convection. The body must constantly meet the requirements of muscle tissues for oxygen and nutrients and eliminate the waste products of those tissues, including heat.

Muscles are found in a condition of slight contraction called **tone**. Even while the body is at rest, the central nervous system sends some limited impulses to the muscle fibres causing a few to contract. These impulses give the muscles firmness and ensure that they are ready to contract when the need arises. Muscle tone may be very significant in a well-conditioned athlete or absent (flaccid muscle tone) in someone with peripheral motor nerve disruption.

✱ **tone** state of slight contraction of muscles that gives them firmness and keeps them ready to contract.

FIGURE 12-43 How muscle attaches to bone.

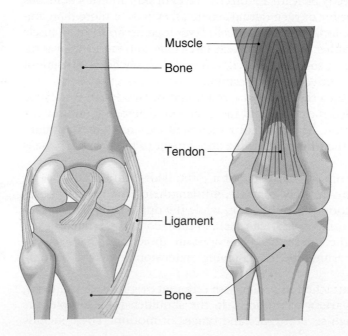

Muscle
Bone
Tendon
Ligament
Bone

THE HEAD, FACE, AND NECK

THE HEAD

The head is made up of three structures that cover the brain: the scalp, the cranium, and the meninges. Each of these structures provides essential protection from the environment and from trauma.

The Scalp

The scalp is a strong and flexible mass of skin, fascia (bands of connective tissue), and muscular tissue that is able to withstand and absorb tremendous kinetic energy. The scalp is also extremely vascular in order to help maintain the brain at the body's core temperature. Scalp hair further insulates the brain from environmental temperatures and, to a lesser degree, from trauma.

The scalp is only loosely attached to the skull and is made up of the overlying skin and a number of thin layers of muscle and connective tissue underneath. Directly beneath the skin and covering the most superior surface of the head is a fibrous connective tissue sheet called the **galea aponeurotica.** Connected anteriorly to it and covering the forehead is a flat sheet of muscle, the frontal muscle. Connected posteriorly and covering the posterior skull surface is the occipitalis muscle. Laterally, the auricularis muscles cover the areas above the ears and between the lateral brow ridge and the occiput. A layer of loose connective tissue beneath these muscles and the galea and just above the periosteum is called the areolar tissue. It contains emissary veins that permit venous blood to flow from the dural sinuses into the venous vessels of the scalp. These emissary veins also exist in the upper reaches of the nasal cavity. These veins become potential routes for infection in scalp wounds or nasal injuries. A helpful way to remember the layers of skin protecting the scalp is the mnemonic SCALP: S—skin; C—connective tissue; A—aponeurotica; L—layer of subaponeurotica (areolar) tissue; P—the periosteum of the skull (the pericranium).

* **galea aponeurotica** connective tissue sheet covering the superior aspect of the cranium.

The Cranium

The bony structure supporting the head and face is the skull. It can be subdivided into two components, the facial bones that form the skeletal base for the face and the vault for the brain, called the **cranium** (Figure 12-44). The cranium actually consists of several bones fused together at pseudo-joints called **sutures.** These bony plates are constructed of two narrow layers of hard compact bone, separated by a layer of cancellous bone. The plates form a strong, light, rigid, and spherical container for the brain. The cranium is, therefore, quite effective in protecting its contents from the direct effects of trauma. This vault, however, provides very little space for internal swelling or hemorrhage. Any expanding lesion within the cranium results in an increase in **intracranial pressure (ICP)**. This reduces cerebral perfusion and can severely damage the delicate brain tissue.

The cranial bones form regions that are helpful in describing the cerebral structures beneath. The anterior or frontal bone begins at the brow ridge and covers the upper and anterior surface of the brain. The parietal bones, one on either side, begin just behind the lateral brow ridge and form the skull above the external portions (pinnae) of the ears. The occipital bone forms the posterior and inferior aspect of the cranium, extending to and forming the foramen magnum. The temporal bones form the lateral cranial surfaces anterior to the ears, while the ethmoid and sphenoid bones, which are very irregular in shape, form the portion of the cranium concealed and protected by the facial bones.

* **cranium** vault-like portion of the skull encasing the brain.

* **sutures** pseudo-joints that join the various bones of the skull to form the cranium.

* **intracranial pressure (ICP)** pressure exerted on the brain by the blood and cerebrospinal fluid.

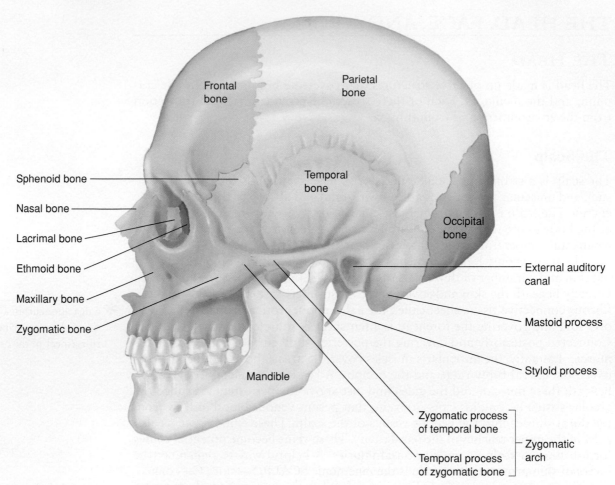

Sphenoid bone

Nasal bone

Lacrimal bone

Ethmoid bone

Maxillary bone

Zygomatic bone

Frontal bone

Parietal bone

Temporal bone

Occipital bone

External auditory canal

Mastoid process

Styloid process

Mandible

Zygomatic process of temporal bone

Temporal process of zygomatic bone

Zygomatic arch

FIGURE 12-44   Bones of the human skull.

The base of the skull consists of portions of the occipital, temporal, sphenoid, and ethmoid bones. This area is important in cases of trauma because the openings, or foramina, for blood vessels, the spinal cord, the auditory canal, and the cranial nerves pass through it. These openings weaken the area, leaving it prone to fracture with serious trauma.

Other anatomical points of interest within the cranium are the cribriform plate and the foramen magnum. The cribriform plate is an irregular portion of the ethmoid bone and a portion of the base of the cranium. It and the remainder of the base of the cranium have rough surfaces against which the brain may abrade, lacerate, or contuse during severe deceleration. The foramen magnum is the largest opening in the skull. It is located at the base of the skull where it meets the spinal column and where the spinal cord exits the cranium.

The Meninges

✱ **meninges** three membranes that surround and protect the brain and spinal cord. They are the dura mater, pia mater, and arachnoid membrane.

✱ **dura mater** tough layer of the meninges firmly attached to the interior of the skull and interior of the spinal column.

The final protective mechanisms for the brain and the spinal cord are the **meninges** (Figure 12-45). They are a group of three tissues between the cranium and the brain and the spinal column and cord. The outermost layer is the **dura mater** (tough mother), a tough connective tissue that provides protection for the central nervous system. The dura mater is actually two layers. The outer layer is the cranium's inner periosteum. The dural layer is made up of tough, continuous connective tissue that extends into the cranial cavity, where it forms partial struc-

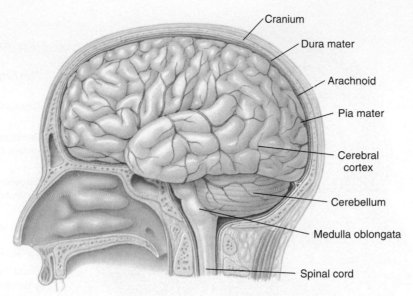

Cranium
Dura mater
Arachnoid
Pia mater
Cerebral cortex
Cerebellum
Medulla oblongata
Spinal cord

FIGURE 12-45 The meninges and skull.

tural divisions (the falx cerebri and the tentorium cerebelli). Above the dura mater lie some of the larger arteries that provide blood flow to the surface of the brain. Between the dural layers lie the dural sinuses, major venous drains for the brain.

The meningeal layer closest to the brain and spinal cord is the **pia mater** (tender mother). It is a delicate tissue, covering all the convolutions of the brain and cord. Although more delicate when compared with the dura mater, the pia mater is still more substantial than brain and spinal cord tissue. The pia mater is a highly vascular tissue with large vessels that supply the superficial areas of the brain.

Separating the two layers of mater is a stratum of connective tissue called the **arachnoid membrane.** It covers the inner dura mater and suspends the brain in the cranial cavity with collagen and elastin fibres. The arachnoid membrane gets its name from its web-like appearance (arachnoid, meaning "spider-like"). Beneath the arachnoid membrane is the subarachnoid space, which is filled with cerebrospinal fluid. This region provides cushioning for the brain when the head is subjected to strong forces of acceleration or deceleration.

✱ **pia mater** inner and most delicate layer of the meninges. It covers the convolutions of the brain and spinal cord.

✱ **arachnoid membrane** middle layer of the meninges.

Cerebrospinal Fluid

Cerebrospinal fluid is a clear, colourless solution of water, proteins, and salts surrounding the central nervous system that absorbs the shock of minor acceleration and deceleration. The brain constantly generates cerebrospinal fluid in the largest two of four spaces (or ventricles) within the substance of the brain. The fluid circulates through the ventricles, then through the subarachnoid space, where it is returned to the venous circulation through the dural sinuses. The cerebrospinal fluid provides buoyancy for the brain and actually floats it in a near-weightless environment within the cranial cavity. This fluid also is a medium through which nutrients and waste products, such as oxygen, proteins, salts, and carbon dioxide, are diffused into and out of the brain tissue.

✱ **cerebrospinal fluid** fluid surrounding and bathing the brain and spinal cord (the elements of the central nervous system).

The Brain

The brain occupies about 80 percent of the interior of the cranium. It is made up of three major structures essential to human function—the cerebrum, cerebellum, and the brainstem.

FIGURE 12-46 The partitions extending into the skull, the falx cerebri and tentorium cerebellum.

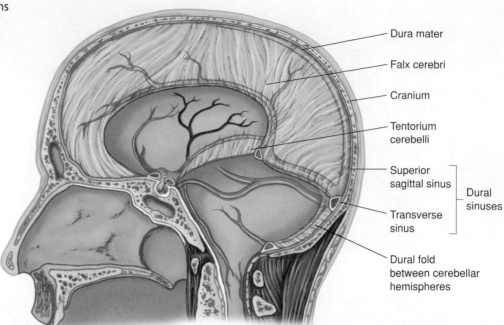

- Dura mater
- Falx cerebri
- Cranium
- Tentorium cerebelli
- Superior sagittal sinus ⎤ Dural sinuses
- Transverse sinus ⎦
- Dural fold between cerebellar hemispheres

✱ **cerebrum** largest part of the brain. It consists of two hemispheres separated by a deep longitudinal fissure. It is the seat of consciousness and the centre of the higher mental functions, such as memory, learning, reasoning, judgment, intelligence, and emotions.

The crossing of nerve impulses from one side of the body to the other takes place just below the medulla oblongata.

The **cerebrum** is the largest element of the nervous system and occupies most of the cranial cavity. It consists of an exterior cortex of grey mater (cell bodies) and is the highest functional portion of the brain. The central portion of the cerebrum is predominantly white matter, mostly communication pathways (axons). The cerebrum is the centre of conscious thought, personality, speech, motor control, and of visual, auditory, and tactile (touch) perception. The cerebrum is regionalized into lobes roughly lying beneath the bones of the cranium (and given the same names). The frontal region is anterior and determines personality. The parietal region, which is superior and posterior, directs motor and sensory activities as well as memory and emotions. The occipital region, which is posterior and inferior, is responsible for sight. Laterally, the temporal regions are the centres for long-term memory, hearing, speech, taste, and smell.

A structure called the falx cerebri divides the cerebrum into right and left hemispheres. A dural partition, the falx cerebri extends into the cranial cavity from the interior and superior surface of the cranium (Figure 12-46). Corresponding to the falx cerebri is a fissure in the cerebrum called the central sulcus. This fissure physically splits the cerebrum into the left and right hemispheres, each of which controls (for the most part) the activities of the opposite side of the body. The crossing of nerve impulses from one side to the other takes place just below the medulla oblongata. The tentorium cerebelli is a similar fibrous sheet within the occipital region, running at right angles to the falx cerebri. It separates the cerebrum from the cerebellum. The brainstem perforates the tentorium through an opening called the tentorium incisura.

The oculomotor nerve (CN-III), which controls pupil size, travels along the tentorium. It is likely to be compressed as intracranial pressure rises or the brain is displaced due to edema, a growing mass, or hemorrhage. This compression causes pupillary disturbances that manifest most commonly on the same side as the problem. If the pressure is great enough, it may affect both sides, and both pupils may dilate and fix.

The left cerebral hemisphere is identified as the dominant hemisphere in most of the population, excepting a few left-handed individuals. It is responsible for mathematical computations (occipital region) and writing (parietal region) and is the centre for language interpretation (occipital region) and speech (frontal region). The right, nondominant cerebral hemisphere processes nonverbal imagery (occipital region).

The **cerebellum** is located directly under the tentorium. It lies posterior and inferior to the cerebrum. The cerebellum "fine tunes" motor control and allows the body to move smoothly from one position to another. Additionally, it is responsible for balance and maintenance of muscle tone.

The **brainstem** is an important central processing centre and the communication junction among the cerebrum, spinal cord, cranial nerves, and cerebellum. It includes the midbrain, the pons, and the medulla oblongata. The **midbrain** makes up the upper portion of the brainstem and consists of the hypothalamus, thalamus, and associated structures. The **hypothalamus** controls much of endocrine function, the vomiting reflex, hunger, thirst, kidney function, body temperature, and emotions. The **thalamus** is the switching centre between the pons and the cerebrum and is a critical element in the **reticular activating system (RAS)**, the system that establishes consciousness. This region also provides the major tracts, or pathways, for the optic and olfactory nerves.

The **pons** acts as the communication interchange between the various components of the central nervous system—the cerebellum, the cerebrum, midbrain, and the spinal cord. It is a bulb-shaped structure directly above the medulla oblongata and appears to be responsible for the sleep component of the reticular activating system.

The last nervous system structure still within the cranial vault is the **medulla oblongata.** It is recognizable as a bulge in the very top of the spinal cord. The medulla contains three important centres—the respiratory centre, the cardiac centre, and the vasomotor centre. The cardiac centre regulates the rate and strength of cardiac contractions. The vasomotor centre controls the distribution of blood and maintains blood pressure. The respiratory centre controls respiratory depth, rate, and rhythm.

To maintain its advanced functioning, the brain has a high metabolic rate. Though the brain accounts for only 2 percent of the body's total weight, it receives about 15 percent of the cardiac output and consumes about 20 percent of the body's oxygen. It requires this circulation whether it is at rest or engaged in activity. Further, this blood supply must be constant because the brain has no stored energy sources. It needs constant supplies of glucose, thiamine (to help metabolize glucose), and oxygen and relies almost solely on aerobic metabolism. If the blood supply stops, unconsciousness follows within 10 seconds, and brain death will ensue within 4 to 6 minutes.

CNS Circulation

Four major arterial vessels provide blood flow to the brain. The first two are the internal carotid arteries. These vessels divide from the common carotid at the carotid sinus and then enter the cranium through its base. The two posterior vessels, the vertebral arteries, ascend along and through the vertebral column. They then enter the base of the skull, where they join and form a singular basilar artery.

The internal carotid and basilar arteries interconnect through the circle of Willis in the base of the brain. This structure is an arterial circle that ensures good circulation to the brain, even if one of the large feeder vessels is obstructed. Various arteries branch out from the circle of Willis and supply the substance of the brain itself.

Venous drainage occurs initially through bridging veins that drain the surface of the cerebrum. They "bridge" with the dural sinuses (large, thin-walled veins). These ultimately drain into the internal jugular veins and then into the superior vena cava.

✱ **cerebellum** portion of the brain located dorsally to the pons and medulla oblongata. It plays an important role in the fine control of voluntary muscular movements.

✱ **brainstem** the part of the brain connecting the cerebral hemispheres with the spinal cord. It comprises the medulla oblongata, the pons, and the midbrain.

✱ **midbrain** portion of the brain connecting the pons and cerebellum with the cerebral hemispheres.

✱ **hypothalamus** portion of the brain important for controlling certain metabolic activities, including the regulation of body temperature.

✱ **thalamus** switching station between the pons and the cerebrum in the brain.

✱ **reticular activating system (RAS)** a series of nervous tissues keeping the human system in a state of consciousness.

✱ **pons** process of tissue responsible for the communication interchange between the cerebellum, the cerebrum, midbrain, and the spinal cord.

✱ **medulla oblongata** lower portion of the brainstem containing the respiratory, cardiac, and vasomotor centres.

Though the brain accounts for only 2 percent of the body's total weight, it consumes about 20 percent of the body's oxygen.

Blood-Brain Barrier

The capillaries of the brain are special in that their walls are thicker and not as permeable as those found elsewhere in the body. They do not permit the interstitial flow of proteins and other materials as freely as do other body capillaries. This ensures that many substances found in the circulatory system, such as some hormones, do not affect the central nervous system cells. Lymphatic circulation is also lacking in the brain and is replaced by the cerebrospinal fluid flow system. This results in a very special and protected environment for central nervous system cells. If blood seeps into the central nervous system tissue, it acts as an irritant, initiating an inflammatory response, resulting in edema.

Cerebral Perfusion Pressure

✳ cerebral perfusion pressure (CPP) the pressure moving blood through the brain.

$$CPP = MAP - ICP$$

✳ autoregulation process that controls blood flow to the brain tissue by causing alterations in the blood pressure.

Cerebral perfusion is exceptionally critical and depends on many factors. Primarily, the pressure within the cranium (intracranial pressure, or ICP) resists blood flow and good perfusion to the central nervous system tissue. Usually, the pressure is less than 10 mmHg and does not significantly impede blood flow as long as the mean arterial blood pressure (MAP is the diastolic blood pressure plus one-third the pulse pressure) is at least 50 mmHg. The pressure moving blood through the cranium is the **cerebral perfusion pressure (CPP).** This is calculated as the mean arterial pressure (MAP) minus the intracranial pressure (ICP). Changes in ICP are met with compensatory changes in blood pressure to ensure adequate cerebral perfusion pressure and cerebral blood flow. This compensating reflex is called **autoregulation.**

Since the cranium is a fixed vault for the structures of the brain, its volume and the pressure within are shared by the occupants. Any expanding mass (tumour), hemorrhage, or edema within the cranium will displace some other occupant, such as the cerebrospinal fluid or blood, since they are the only readily movable media. This displacement maintains the intracranial pressure very effectively, up to a point. When the volumes of cerebrospinal fluid and venous blood are reduced to their limits, however, the intracranial pressure begins to rise. Autoregulation then raises the blood pressure to ensure that there is enough differential (CPP) to provide good cerebral perfusion. However, this increase in blood pressure causes the intracranial pressure to rise still higher and cerebral blood perfusion to diminish even more. As this cycle of increasing intracranial pressure and increasing blood pressure continues, brain injury and death are close at hand.

Cranial Nerves

The cranial nerves are nerve roots originating within the cranium and along the brainstem. They make up 12 distinct pathways that account for some of the more important senses, innervate the facial area, and control significant body functions (see Figure 12-72 in the Nervous System section later in this chapter).

Ascending Reticular Activating System

The ascending reticular activating system is a tract of neurons within the upper brainstem, the pons, and the midbrain that is responsible for the sleep-wake cycle. It is a complex control system that monitors the amount of stimulation the body receives and regulates important bodily functions, such as respiration, heart rate, and peripheral vascular resistance. Injury to the midbrain may result in unconsciousness or coma, while injury to the pons may result in a protracted waking state.

THE FACE

Facial bones make up the anterior and inferior structures of the head and include the zygoma, maxilla, mandible, and nasal bones (Figure 12-47). The **zygoma** is the prominent bone of the cheek. It protects the eyes and the muscles controlling eye and jaw movement. The **maxilla** composes the upper jaw, supports the nasal bone, and provides the lower border of the orbit. The nasal bone is the attachment for the nasal cartilage as it forms the shape of the nose. The last of the facial bones is the **mandible,** or jawbone. It resembles two horizontal "L's," which join anteriorly and hinge underneath the posterior zygomatic arch. Besides forming the beginning of the airway and the alimentary canal, the facial bones form supporting and protective structures for several sense organs, including the tongue (taste), eye (sight), and olfactory nerve (smell).

The facial region, like most other areas of the body, is covered with skin that serves to protect the tissue underneath from trauma and against adverse environmental effects. In the facial region, the skin is very flexible and relatively thin. It also has a very good vascular supply and hemorrhages freely when injured. Beneath the skin is a minimal layer of subcutaneous tissue, and beneath that are the many small muscles that control facial expression and the movements of the mouth, eyes, and eyelids.

Circulation for the facial area is provided by the external carotid artery as it branches into the facial, temporal, and maxillary arteries. The facial artery crosses the mandible, then travels up and along the nasal bone. The maxillary artery runs under the mandible and zygoma, then provides circulation to the cheek area. The temporal artery runs anterior to the ear just posterior to the zygoma. Each major artery has an associated vein paralleling its path.

✱ **zygoma** the cheekbone.

✱ **maxilla** bone of the upper jaw.

✱ **mandible** the jawbone.

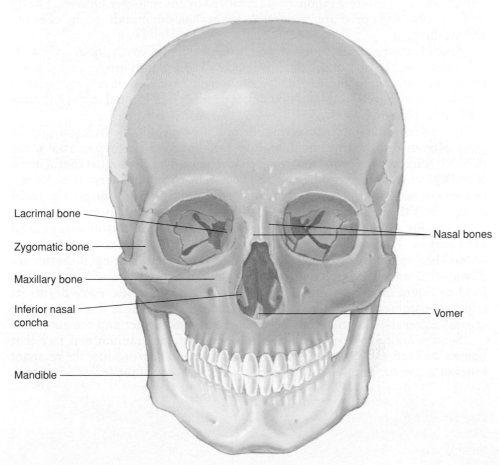

FIGURE 12-47   The facial bones.

The most important cranial nerves traversing this area are the trigeminal (CN-V) and the facial (CN-VII). The trigeminal nerve provides sensation for the face and some motor control over eye movement as well as enables the chewing process. The facial nerve provides motor control to the facial muscles and contributes to the sensation of taste.

The nasal cavity is formed by the juncture of the ethmoid, nasal, and maxillary bones. It is a channel running posteriorly with a bony septum dividing it into left and right chambers and plates protruding medially from the lateral sides. These plates, called turbinates, form support for the vascular mucous membranes that serve to warm, humidify, and collect particulate matter from the incoming air. The lower border of the nasal cavity is formed by the bony hard palate and then, posteriorly, by the more flexible cartilaginous soft palate. The soft palate moves upward to close off the opening of the posterior nasal cavity during swallowing. The nasal bone lies anterior and inferior to the eyes and provides a base for the nasal cartilage. The nasal cartilage defines the shape of the nose and divides the nostrils and their openings, which are called the **nares.**

✱ **nares** the openings of the nostrils.

The oral cavity is formed by the concave shape of the maxillary bone, the palate, and the upper teeth meeting the mandible and the lower teeth. The floor of the chamber consists of musculature and connective tissue that span the mandible and support the tongue. The tongue is a large muscle that occupies much of the oral cavity, provides the taste sensation, and moves food between the teeth during chewing (mastication) and propels the chewed food posteriorly, then inferiorly during swallowing. The tongue connects with the hyoid bone, a free floating U-shaped bone located inferiorly and posteriorly to the mandible. The mandible articulates with the temporal bone at the temporomandibular joint, under the posterior zygoma, and is moved by the masseter muscles. The lip muscles (obicularis oris) are responsible for sealing the mouth during chewing and swallowing.

Special structures are found in and around the oral cavity. Salivary glands provide saliva, the first of the digestive juices. These glands are located just anterior and inferior to the ear, under the tongue, and just inside the inferior mandible. Specialized lymphoid nodules, the tonsils, are located in the posterior wall of the pharynx.

Prominent cranial nerves serving the oral area include the hypoglossal, the glossopharyngeal, the trigeminal, and the facial nerves. The hypoglossal nerve (CN-XII) directs swallowing and tongue movement. The glossopharyngeal nerve (CN-IX) controls saliva production and taste. The trigeminal nerve (CN-V) carries sensations from the facial region and assists in chewing control. The facial nerve (CN-VII) controls the muscles of facial expression and taste.

Posterior and inferior to the oral cavity is a collection of soft tissue called the pharynx. The process of swallowing begins in the pharynx once the bolus of food has been propelled back and down by the tongue. The epiglottis moves downward, while the larynx moves up, sealing the lower airway opening. The food or liquid moves into the esophagus where a peristaltic wave begins its trip to the stomach. This area is of great importance because it maintains the critical segregation of materials between the digestive tract and the airway.

Sinuses are hollow spaces within the bones of the cranium and face that lighten the head, protect the eyes and nasal cavity, and help produce the resonant tones of the voice. They also strengthen this region against the forces of trauma.

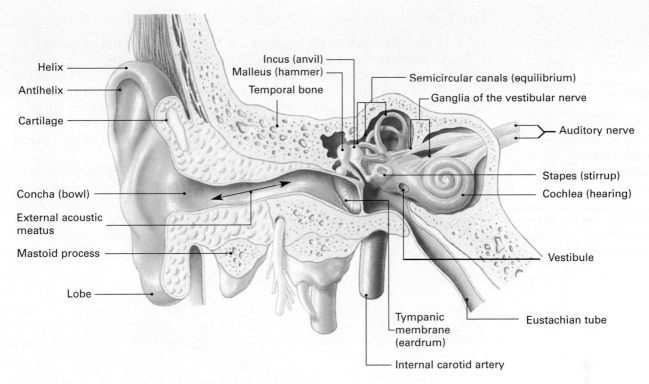

Helix
Antihelix
Cartilage
Concha (bowl)
External acoustic meatus
Mastoid process
Lobe

Incus (anvil)
Malleus (hammer)
Temporal bone

Semicircular canals (equilibrium)
Ganglia of the vestibular nerve
Auditory nerve
Stapes (stirrup)
Cochlea (hearing)
Vestibule
Eustachian tube

Tympanic membrane (eardrum)
Internal carotid artery

FIGURE 12-48   The anatomy of the ear.

The Ear

The outer, visible portion of the ear is termed the **pinna.** It is composed of cartilage and has a poor blood supply. It connects to the external auditory canal, which leads to the eardrum. The external auditory canal contains glands that secrete wax (cerumen) for protection. The ear's important structures are interior and exceptionally well protected from nearly all trauma (Figure 12-48). Only trauma involving great pressure differentials (e.g., blast and diving injuries) or basilar skull fractures are likely to damage this area.

The ear provides the body with two very useful functions, hearing and positional sense. The middle and inner ear contain the structures needed for hearing. Hearing occurs when sound waves cause the tympanic membrane (eardrum) to vibrate. The eardrum transmits the vibrations through three very small bones (the ossicles) to the cochlea, the organ of hearing. These vibrations stimulate the auditory nerve, which, in turn, transmits the signal to the brain.

The **semicircular canals** are responsible for sensing position and motion. They are three hollow, fluid-filled rings set at different angles. When the head moves, fluid in these rings shifts. Small cells with hair-like projections sense the motion and signal the brain to help maintain balance. This positional sense is present even when the eyes are closed. If injury or illness disturbs this area, it transmits excess signals to the brain. Patients then experience a continuous moving sensation known as vertigo.

✱ **pinna** outer, visible portion of the ear.

✱ **semicircular canals** the three rings of the inner ear. They sense the motion of the head and provide positional sense for the body.

The Eye

The eyes provide much of the input we use to interact with our environment. Although they are placed prominently on the face, the eyes are well protected from trauma by a series of facial bones. The frontal bones project above the globe of the eye, while the nasal bones and cartilage protect medially. The bone of the cheek, or zygoma, completes the physical protection both laterally and inferiorly. These bones collectively form the eye socket or **orbit**. The soft tissue of the eyelid and the eyelashes give additional protection to the critical ocular surface.

The eye is a spherical globe, filled with liquid (Figure 12-49). Its major compartment (the posterior chamber) contains a crystal-clear gelatinous fluid called **vitreous humor.** Lining the posterior of the compartment is a light- and colour-sensing tissue known as the **retina.** Images focused on the retina are transmitted to the brain via the optic nerve. The lens separates the posterior and anterior chambers. The lens is responsible for focusing light and images on the retina by

* **orbit** the eye socket.

* **vitreous humor** clear watery fluid filling the posterior chamber of the eye. It is responsible for giving the eye its spherical shape.

* **retina** light- and colour-sensing tissue lining the posterior chamber of the eye.

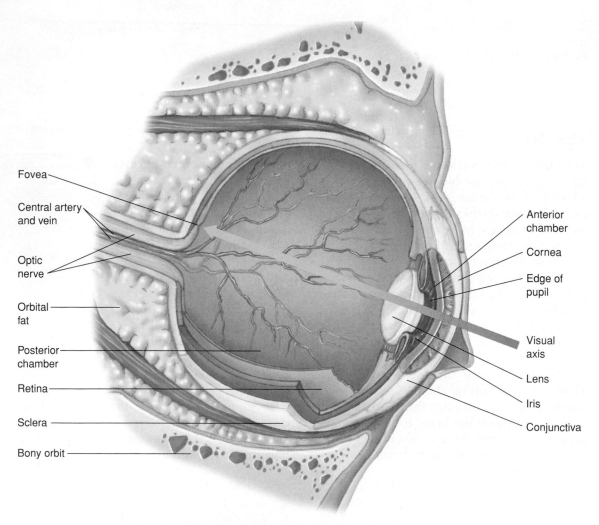

FIGURE 12-49   The anatomy of the eye.

the action of small muscles that change its thickness. A fluid called **aqueous humor**, which is similar to vitreous humor, fills the anterior chamber. The anterior chamber also contains the **iris**, the muscular and coloured portion of the eye that regulates the amount of light reaching the retina. Light enters the eye through the dark opening in the centre of the iris called the **pupil**.

By examining the eye, you can easily identify several of its components, such as the coloured iris and the central black pupil. Bordering the iris is the **sclera**, the white and vascular area that forms the remaining, underlying surface of the exposed eye. The **cornea**, a very thin, clear, and delicate layer, covers both the pupil and the iris. Continuous with the cornea and extending out to the eyelid's interior surface is the **conjunctiva**, another delicate, smooth layer that slides over itself and the cornea when the eye closes or blinks.

The eye is bathed in **lacrimal fluid**, which is produced by almond-shaped lacrimal glands located along the brow ridge just lateral and superior to the eyeball. Lacrimal fluid flows through lacrimal ducts and then over the cornea. Because the cornea does not have blood vessels, the fluid provides crucial lubrication, oxygen, and nutrients. If injury or some other mechanism—for example, a contact lens left in an unconscious patient's eye—prevents this fluid from reaching the cornea, the surface of the eye may be damaged. The lacrimal fluid is drained from the eye into the lacrimal sac, located along the medial orbit, and then empties into the nose.

The last major functional elements of the eye are the muscles that move them and their controlling cranial nerves. These small muscles are attached to the eyeball in the region of the conjunctival fold and are hidden within the eye socket and under the zygomatic arch. The oculomotor (CN-III), trochlear (CN-IV), and abducens (CN-VI) nerves control these muscles, which, in turn, control the eye's motion. The oculomotor nerve controls pupil dilation, conjugate movement (movement of the eyes together), and most of the eye's travel through its normal range of motion. The trochlear nerve moves the eye downward and inward, while the abducens nerve is responsible for eye abduction (outward gaze).

✱ aqueous humor clear fluid filling the anterior chamber of the eye.

✱ iris pigmented portion of the eye. It is the muscular area that constricts or dilates to change the size of the pupil.

✱ pupil dark opening in the centre of the iris through which light enters the eye.

✱ sclera the "white" of the eye.

✱ cornea thin, delicate layer covering the pupil and the iris.

✱ conjunctiva mucous membrane that lines the eyelids.

✱ lacrimal fluid liquid that lubricates the eye.

The Mouth

The lips mark the entrance to the mouth and play a role in the articulation of speech. The mouth houses the tongue, the gums (gingiva), and the teeth (Figure 12-50). The roof of the mouth is formed by the hard palate and the soft palate. The uvula is the peninsular extension of the soft palate that hangs in the back of the mouth. The oral cavity, lined with buccal (cheek/mouth) mucosa, is rich in mucous membranes. The parotid glands, just in front of the ears, and the submandibular glands, just beneath the mandible, secrete digestive enzymes and saliva into the oral cavity (Figure 12-51). The sublingual glands secrete enzymes just beneath the tongue. You can easily palpate these glands under the chin.

The tongue, a large, mobile muscle covered by mucous membranes, has many functions. It helps in chewing by keeping food on the teeth, and it assists in swallowing by moving the food into the oropharynx. It also contains the taste buds and is essential in forming words when we speak.

A highly vascular mucosa lines the gingiva, giving it a pink colour. The teeth are anchored in bony sockets; only their white enamel-covered crowns are visible. An adult normally has 32 permanent teeth, including incisors, canines, premolars, and molars. The pharynx consists of three distinct areas: the nasopharynx (behind the nasal cavity), the oropharynx (back of the throat), and the laryngopharynx (just above the epiglottis). At the back of the throat on either side, the tonsils help separate the oropharynx (food processing) from the nasopharynx (air passage).

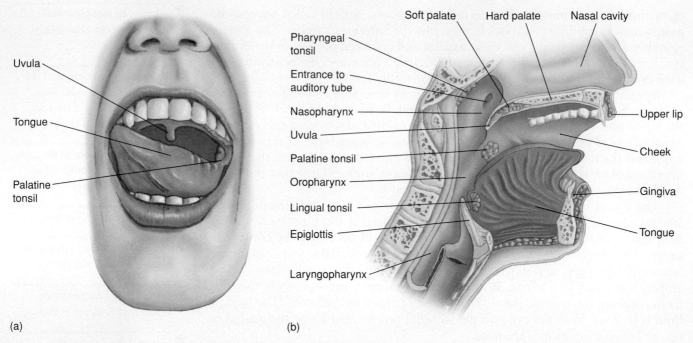

(a)

(b)

FIGURE 12-50 The mouth.

FIGURE 12-51 The salivary glands.

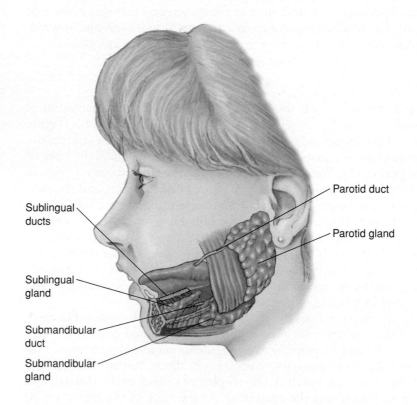

THE NECK

The neck (Figure 12-52) is the region that links the head to the rest of the body. Travelling through this anatomical area are blood for the facial region and brain, air for respiration, food for digestion, and neural communications to sense the body and its environment and to control both the voluntary and involuntary muscles and glands of the body. The neck also contains some of the important muscles used to provide head and shoulder movements as well as the thyroid and parathyroid glands of the endocrine system.

Vasculature of the Neck

The major blood vessels traversing the neck are the carotid arteries and the jugular veins. The carotid arteries arise from the brachiocephalic artery on the right and the aorta on the left. They travel upward and medially along the trachea and split into internal and external carotid arteries at about the level of the larynx's upper border. At this split are the carotid bodies and carotid sinuses, which are responsible for monitoring carbon dioxide and oxygen levels in the blood and blood pressure, respectively. The jugular veins are paired on each side of the neck. The internal jugular vein runs in a sheath with the carotid artery and vagus nerve, while the external jugular vein runs superficially just lateral to the trachea. The jugular veins join the brachiocephalic veins just beneath the clavicles.

Airway Structures

The airway structures of the neck begin with the larynx. It is a prominent hollow cylindrical column made up of the thyroid and cricoid cartilages, atop the trachea.

FIGURE 12-52   The neck.

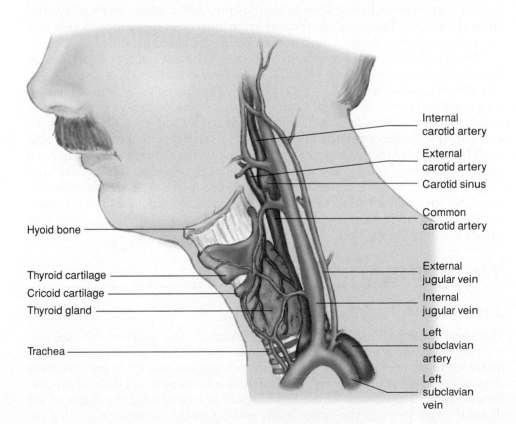

Hyoid bone

Thyroid cartilage
Cricoid cartilage
Thyroid gland

Trachea

Internal carotid artery

External carotid artery

Carotid sinus

Common carotid artery

External jugular vein

Internal jugular vein

Left subclavian artery

Left subclavian vein

The thyroid opening is covered during swallowing by a cartilaginous and soft-tissue flap, the epiglottis. The vocal cords, two folds of connective tissue sitting atop the opening of the larynx, further protect the airway. These cords vibrate with air passage and form sounds; they may also close in spasm to prevent foreign bodies from entering the lower airway. The cricoid cartilage is a circular ring between the thyroid cartilage and the trachea. The trachea is a series of C-shaped cartilages that maintain the tracheal opening. The posterior trachea shares a common border with the anterior surface of the esophagus. The trachea extends inferiorly to just below the sternum, where it bifurcates into the left and right mainstem bronchi at the carina.

Other Structures of the Neck

The cervical portion of the spinal column traverses the neck and provides the skeletal support for both the head and the neck. It is also an attachment point for the ligaments that hold the column together and give it its strength and for the tendons that support and move the head and shoulders.

The cervical spine also contains the spinal cord. The spinal cord is the critical conduit for nervous signals between the brain and the body, and injury to it can be serious, even life threatening. From the spinal cord and at each vertebral junction, the peripheral nerve roots branch out. These structures direct signals to and receive signals from the limbs, internal organs, and sensory structures of the body. (The anatomy of the cervical spine is addressed in detail later in this chapter.)

Other structures within the neck include the esophagus, cranial nerves, thoracic duct, thyroid and parathyroid glands, and brachial plexus. The esophagus is a smooth muscle tube located behind the trachea that carries food and liquid to the stomach. Its anterior border is continuous with the posterior border of the trachea. Some cranial nerves, including the glossopharyngeal (CN-IX) and the vagus (CN-X), traverse the neck. The vagus nerve is essential for many parasympathetic activities including speech, swallowing, and cardiac, respiratory, and visceral function. The glossopharyngeal nerve innervates the carotid bodies and carotid sinuses, monitoring blood oxygen levels and blood pressure.

The **lymphatic system** helps drain fluid from the head and face and assists in fighting infection. A long chain of lymph nodes runs along the side of the neck, behind the ears, and under the chin (Figure 12-53). They are palpable when congested with infectious products. (The lymphatic system is discussed further in the Cardiovascular System section, later in this chapter.) The right and left thoracic ducts deliver lymph to the venous system at the juncture of the jugular and subclavian veins.

The thyroid gland sits over the trachea just below the cricoid cartilage and controls the rate of cellular metabolism as well as the systemic levels of calcium. The brachial plexus is a network of nerves in the lower neck and shoulder responsible for lower arm and hand functions. Lastly, numerous muscles (including the sternocleidomastoid, platysma, and upper trapezius), fascia, and soft tissues are found in the neck.

THE SPINE AND THORAX

THE SPINE

The spine consists of a supporting skeletal structure, the vertebral column, and a central nervous system pathway, the spinal cord. These are important functional elements both for body posture and movement and for communication among the body's many systems. The vertebral column provides skeletal support for and permits movement of the head, assists in maintaining the shape of the thoracic cage, supports the upper body, and forms the posterior aspect of the pelvis. The spinal cord, contained and protected within the vertebral column, is

* **lymphatic system** a network of valveless vessels that drain fluid, called lymph, from the body tissues. Lymph nodes help filter impurities en route to the subclavian vein and thence to the heart.

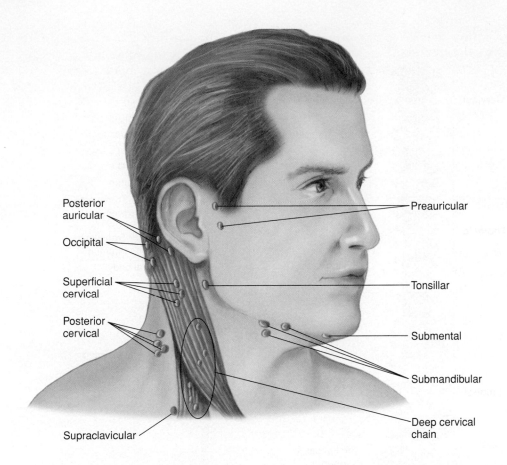

FIGURE 12-53 The lymph nodes of the head and neck.

Posterior auricular

Occipital

Superficial cervical

Posterior cervical

Supraclavicular

Preauricular

Tonsillar

Submental

Submandibular

Deep cervical chain

the main communication conduit of the central nervous system. It is responsible for transmitting messages from the brain to the body organs and tissues and from the sensory nerves in the organs, skin, and other tissues back to the brain.

The Vertebral Column

The vertebral column is a hollow skeletal tube made up of 33 irregular bones, called **vertebrae.** This column attaches to the head, to the bones of the rib cage, and to the pelvis. It provides the central skeletal support structure and a major portion of the axial skeleton. At the same time, the vertebrae provide a protective container for the spinal cord. Several components with differing functions may make up the structure of each individual vertebra.

The major weight-bearing component of a vertebra is the **vertebral body.** It is a cylinder of skeletal tissue made up of cancellous bone surrounded by a layer of hard, compact bone. It lies anterior to the other components of the vertebra.

The size of the vertebral body varies with its location along the spinal column (Figure 12-54). The first two cervical vertebrae (C-1 and C-2) do not have vertebral bodies because of their specialized functions. Below C-1 and C-2, the size of the vertebral bodies increases progressively as you move down the spine because the vertebral column is supporting an increasing portion of the upper body's weight. The lumbar spine has the strongest and largest vertebral bodies due to the weight they bear. Because of the fused nature of the sacrum and coccyx, these regions have no discernable bodies.

A component of the vertebra posterior to the vertebral body is the **spinal canal,** which is the opening, or foramen, that accommodates the spinal cord. This opening is formed by small fused bony structures that are joined together to create a ring. The lateral structures of the ring are called **pedicles,** while the two pos-

* **vertebrae** the 33 bones making up the vertebral column; singular *vertebra.*

* **vertebral body** short column of bone that forms the weight-bearing portion of a vertebra.

* **spinal canal** opening in the vertebrae that accommodates the spinal cord.

* **pedicles** thick, bony struts that connect the vertebral bodies with the spinous and transverse processes and help make up the opening for the spinal canal.

The Spine and Thorax **537**

FIGURE 12-54 Changing dimensions of the vertebral column.

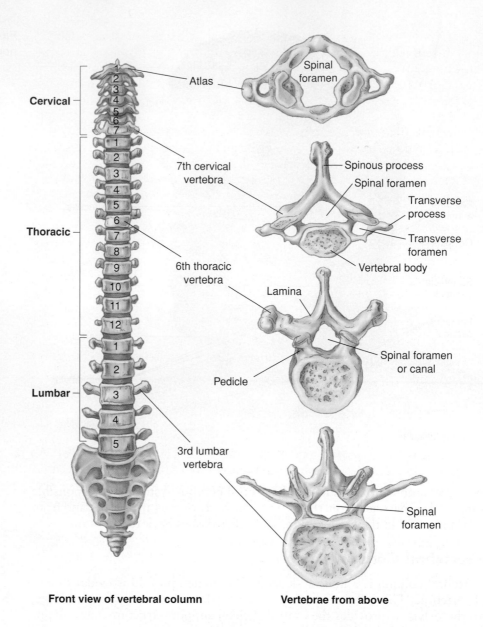

Cervical

Thoracic

Lumbar

Atlas

Spinal foramen

7th cervical vertebra

Spinous process

Spinal foramen

Transverse process

Transverse foramen

Vertebral body

6th thoracic vertebra

Lamina

Pedicle

Spinal foramen or canal

3rd lumbar vertebra

Spinal foramen

Front view of vertebral column   **Vertebrae from above**

✷ laminae posterior bones of a vertebra that help make up the foramen, or opening, of the spinal canal.

✷ transverse process bony outgrowth of the vertebral pedicle that serves as a site for muscle attachment and articulation with the ribs.

✷ spinous process prominence at the posterior part of a vertebra.

✷ intervertebral disc cartilaginous pad between vertebrae that serves as a shock absorber.

terior structures are called **laminae.** The inferior surface of the pedicle contains a notch, called the intervertebral foramen. This notch permits the exit of a peripheral nerve root and spinal vein and the entrance of a spinal artery on each side of the spinal canal and at each vertebral junction.

At the juncture of the pedicle and lamina on each side of a vertebra, there is a bony outgrowth called the **transverse process.** There is also a bony outgrowth where the laminae join, which is called the **spinous process.** The spinous process is the posteriorly and inferiorly oriented bony protrusion that you can feel along the spine.

The spinous and transverse processes are points of attachment for ligaments and tendons. Ligaments hold the vertebrae firmly together and in place while they permit limited motion. The tendons attach muscles to the vertebral column and permit these muscles to move the spine, other bones, and the body. This attachment of muscles and capsule of ligaments protects and strengthens the vertebral column against the forces of trauma.

Between the vertebral bodies are cartilaginous **intervertebral discs.** These discs are formed of a strong yet somewhat flexible outer cover called the annulus fibrosus and a soft and gelatinous inner region called the nucleus pulposus. The intervertebral discs accommodate some motion of the adjacent vertebrae, limit bone wear, and absorb shock along the length of the spinal column. The intervertebral discs make up about 25 percent of the total length of the spinal column, and their degeneration accounts for much of the height loss associated with advancing age.

The elements of the spinal column also have numerous articular surfaces. These surfaces are found on the vertebral bodies, the pedicles, and on the transverse and spinous processes. The articular surfaces enable the spinal column to move around the spinal cord without compressing it, permit articulation with the skull and ribs, and make possible the formation of the rigid, immobile joint of the pelvis.

The vertebral bodies are held firmly together by strong ligaments to ensure that the spinal foramen safely accommodates the spinal cord and that the body has a reasonable range of motion. The anterior longitudinal ligament travels along the anterior surfaces of the vertebral bodies. It provides the major stability of the spinal column and resists hyperextension. The posterior longitudinal ligament travels along the posterior surfaces of the vertebral bodies, within the spinal canal. This ligament helps prevent hyperflexion; when it is disrupted, the result is, frequently, a spinal cord injury. Other ligaments encapsulate the spinous processes (interspinous ligaments) and the transverse processes. These ligaments strengthen and stabilize the column against excessive lateral bending, rotation, and flexion.

Divisions of the Vertebral Column

The vertebral column is divided into five regions: the cervical, the thoracic, the lumbar, the sacral, and the coccygeal (Figure 12-55). Each region is unique in its design and function and has a curve that reverses the curve of the spinal section(s) adjacent to it. The individual vertebrae of the column are identified by the first letter of their region and numbered from superior to inferior. For example, the most inferior of the seven cervical vertebrae is identified as C-7.

Cervical Spine The cervical spine consists of seven cervical vertebrae located between the base of the skull and the shoulders. The cervical spine is the sole skeletal support for the head, which weighs about 7 to 10 kg.

The first two cervical vertebrae have a unique relationship with the head and each other that permits rotation to left and right and nodding of the head. The first cervical vertebra, C-1, is called the atlas (after the Greek god who held up the world) and supports the head. It is securely affixed to the occiput and permits nodding but does not accommodate any twisting or turning motion. It and the next vertebra, C-2, differ from most vertebrae in not having discernible vertebral bodies. Vertebra C-2, called the axis, has a small bony tooth, called the odontoid process or dens, that projects upward. This projection provides a pivotal point around which the atlas and head can rotate from side to side.

The remaining cervical vertebrae permit some rotation as well as flexion, extension, and lateral bending. The range of motion provided by the cervical spine is greater than allowed by any other portion of the spinal column, while the portion of the spinal cord travelling through the region is most critical to life functions. The last cervical vertebra (C-7) is quite noticeable as its spinous process is pronounced and can be felt as the first bony prominence along the spine and just above the shoulders.

Thoracic Spine The thoracic spine consists of 12 thoracic vertebrae. The first rib articulates individually with the first thoracic vertebra at two locations, with the transverse process and with the vertebral body. The next nine ribs articulate with the transverse process and the superior portion of the vertebral body as well

Content Review

DIVISIONS OF THE VERTEBRAL COLUMN
- Cervical spine
- Thoracic spine
- Lumbar spine
- Sacral spine
- Coccygeal spine

The range of motion provided by the cervical spine is the greatest allowed by any region, yet the chord in this region is critical to life functions.

FIGURE 12-55 Divisions of
the veretebral column.

Spinal
Curves

Vertebral
regions

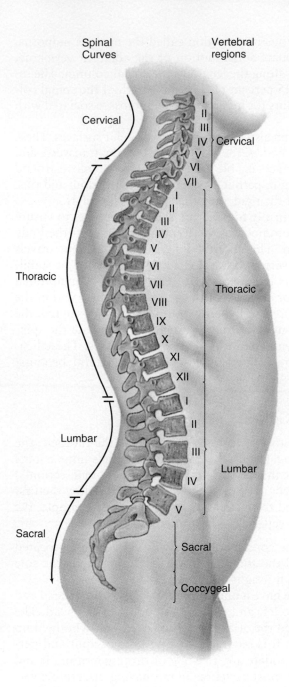

Cervical

Cervical

I
II
III
IV
V
VI
VII

Thoracic

Thoracic

I
II
III
IV
V
VI
VII
VIII
IX
X
XI
XII

Lumbar

Lumbar

I
II
III
IV
V

Sacral

Sacral

Coccygeal

as with the inferior portion of the vertebral body that is adjacent (superior) to it. This system of fixation limits rib movement and increases the strength and rigidity of the thoracic spine. The last two ribs articulate only with the vertebral bodies, which permits greater movement and flexibility.

Because the thoracic spine supports more of the human body than the cervical spine, the thoracic vertebral bodies are larger and stronger. The spinous and transverse processes are also larger and more prominent because they are associated with the musculature holding the upper body erect and with the movement of the thoracic cage during respiration.

Lumbar Spine The five bones of the lumbar spine each carry the weight of the head, neck, and thorax above them. They also bear the forces of bending and lifting above the pelvis. The vertebral bodies are largest in this region of the spinal column, and the intervertebral discs are also the thickest and bear the greatest stress. The lumbar pedicles and lamina are also thick, while the transverse and spinous processes are shorter and stouter than those in the thoracic spine. The spinal foramen is largest in the lumbar region.

Sacral Spine The sacral spine consists of five sacral vertebrae that fuse into the posterior plate of the pelvis. This plate, in conjunction with the two innominate bones of the pelvis, protects the urinary and reproductive organs and attaches the pelvis and lower extremities to the axial skeleton. The articulation with the pelvis occurs at the sacroiliac joint on the lateral surface of the sacrum. This joint is very strong and permits no movement. The upper body balances on the sacrum.

Coccygeal Spine The coccygeal spine is made up of three to five fused vertebrae that represent the residual elements of a tail. They compose the short skeletal end of the vertebral column.

The vertebral column curves through each region of the spine. The cervical and lumbar regions of the spine demonstrate concave curves, while the thoracic and sacral regions represent convex curves. These curves both strengthen the spine and permit a greater range of supported motion.

The Spinal Meninges

The spinal meninges are similar to those covering and protecting the structures within the cranium. They consist of the dura mater, the arachnoid, and the pia mater. The meninges cover the entire spinal cord and the peripheral nerve roots as they leave the spinal column. However, the spinal meninges are not as strongly secured to the spinal column as the meninges are to the cranium. The dura mater is firmly attached to the base of the skull and to a collagen fibre called the coccygeal ligament at the top of the sacrum. These attachments and the dura mater's attachments associated with each pair of peripheral nerve roots help position the cord centrally within the spinal canal yet permit the column to move around the cord (Figure 12-56).

As it does in the brain, cerebrospinal fluid bathes the spinal cord by filling the subarachnoid space. The fluid provides a medium for the exchange of nutri-

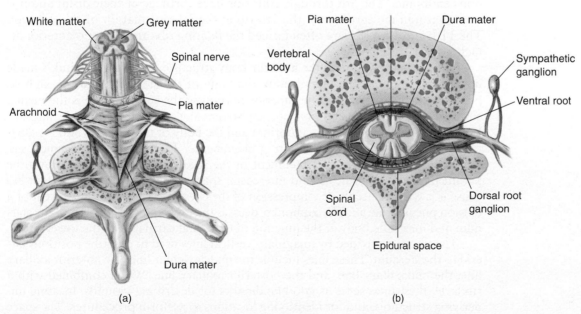

(a)

(b)

FIGURE 12-56 Structural protection of the spinal cord.

ents and waste products and absorbs the shocks of sudden movements. Cerebrospinal fluid is produced in the ventricles of the brain and then circulates through the ventricles and through the arachnoid space of the spinal meninges. The fluid is absorbed by specialized cells (the arachnoid villi) in the lower portion of the lumbar meninges, a region called the spinal cistern.

The distance between the spinal cord and the interior of the vertebral foramen varies in the different spinal regions. The region with the closest tolerance between the cord and the interior surfaces of the spinal foramen is the thoracic spine, where movement of the spinal column is most limited. Although this region is injured only infrequently, just a slight displacement into the vertebral foramen is likely to cause spinal cord injury. The greatest spacing between the cord and the interior of the vertebral column is found in the upper lumbar and upper cervical (C-1 and C-2) regions.

Injuries to the mid- or lower lumbar regions do not endanger the spinal cord because the cord ends at the L-1 level in mature adults. Injury to the lumbar spine can, however, damage the peripheral nerve roots there. The vertebral foramen below L-1 is filled with cerebrospinal fluid and is where the fluid may be most safely removed for diagnostic testing (spinal tap).

THE THORAX

The thoracic cage is the chamber that moves air in and out and where oxygen and carbon dioxide are exchanged to support the body's metabolism. It consists of the thoracic skeleton, diaphragm, and associated musculature. It is also the location of the heart, major blood vessels, and other important structures essential for body function. It contains the trachea, bronchi, and lungs, and the mediastinum. Finally, the dynamics of the chest, respiration, are controlled by a series of centres in the brain and blood vessels.

The Thoracic Skeleton

The thoracic skeleton is defined by 12 pairs of C-shaped ribs, which articulate posteriorly with the thoracic spine and then extend in an anterior and inferior direction (Figure 12-57). The upper seven pairs join the sternum at their cartilaginous endpoints. The 8th through 10th ribs have cartilage at their distal anterior ends that join the cartilage of the 7th rib at the inferior margin of the sternum. The 11th and 12th ribs are often termed the floating ribs and have no anterior attachment.

The sternum completes the anterior bony structure of the thorax and is made up of three sections: the manubrium, the body of the sternum, and the xiphoid process. The manubrium is the superior portion of the sternum and is the medial endpoint of the clavicle and first rib. The sternal angle (also known as the angle of Louis) is the junction of the manubrium and the body of the sternum and is palpable through the skin as an elevation or prominence. This structure has clinical significance as it is the site of attachment of the second rib and quickly allows the paramedic to identify the second intercostal space. This location is important because it is where a needle decompression of the chest is performed in the event of a tension pneumothorax. The xiphoid process is the most inferior portion of the sternum and meets the body at the junction of the costal cartilages of the lower ribs.

The thorax is divided by imaginary vertical lines used to describe positions lateral to the sternum. These lines include the midclavicular line, the anterior axillary line, the midaxillary line, and the posterior axillary line. When combined with a rib level, these lines serve as good landmarks for describing wounds, locating underlying structures, and for identifying locations to perform procedures. The space just inferior to each rib is called an intercostal space and is given the number of the

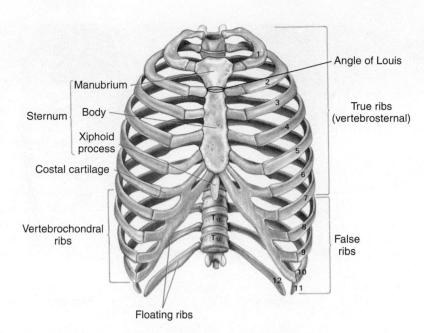

FIGURE 12-57 Skeletal components of the thorax.

Manubrium

Sternum — Body

Xiphoid process

Costal cartilage

Vertebrochondral ribs

Floating ribs

Angle of Louis

True ribs (vertebrosternal)

False ribs

rib above it. For example, the anterior axillary line extends from the anterior margin of the axilla (armpit) inferiorly along the thoracic wall. Its intersection with the fifth intercostal space is generally used in the emergency department to place a thoracostomy tube in patients with pneumothorax or hemothorax. It is not frequently used for prehospital needle decompression because this site is often obscured by the patient's arms or by immobilization devices and blankets.

The thoracic inlet is the superior opening in the thorax. It is narrow in comparison with the thoracic outlet and is defined by the curvature of the first rib, with its posterior attachment at the first thoracic vertebra and ending anteriorly at the manubrium. The thoracic outlet is formed posteriorly by the 12th vertebra, laterally by the curvature of the 12th rib, and extends anteriorly and superiorly along the costal margin to the **xiphisternal joint**.

The Diaphragm

The diaphragm is a muscular, dome-like structure that separates the abdominal cavity from the thoracic cavity. It is affixed to the lower border of the rib cage, while its central and superior margin may extend to the level of the fourth intercostal space anteriorly and the sixth intercostal space posteriorly during maximal expiration. This superior positioning may allow penetrating wounds of the lower half of the thorax to penetrate the diaphragm and enter the abdominal cavity. The aorta, esophagus, and inferior vena cava exit the thoracic cavity through separate openings in this structure. The diaphragm is a major muscle of respiration, contracting to displace the floor of the thoracic cavity downward during inspiration and relaxing and moving upward with expiration.

Associated Musculature

The chest wall musculature along with the shoulder musculature, clavicles, scapula, and humerus provide additional protection to the vital structures within the upper thorax (Figure 12-58). The clavicles articulate laterally with the acromion process of the scapula. The scapula covers the posterior and lateral aspects of the first six ribs and articulates with the humerus to complete the shoulder girdle.

* **xiphisternal joint** union between xiphoid process and body of the sternum.

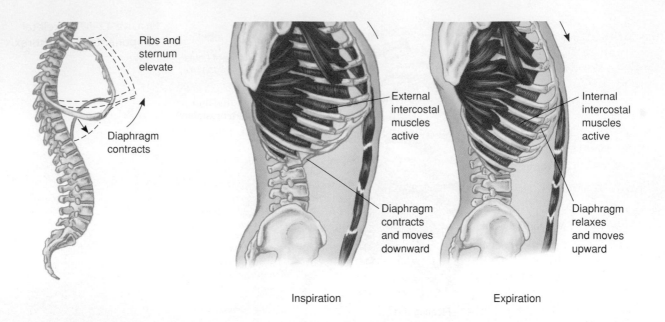

Ribs and sternum elevate

Diaphragm contracts

External intercostal muscles active

Diaphragm contracts and moves downward

Internal intercostal muscles active

Diaphragm relaxes and moves upward

Inspiration

Expiration

FIGURE 12-58   The diaphragm and muscles of the chest change its volume to effect respirations.

Normal inspiration is an active process, while normal expiration is a passive process.

Chest wall muscles between the ribs, called the intercostal muscles, along with the diaphragm and the sternocleidomastoid muscles are the major muscles of respiration. The sternocleidomastoid muscles raise the upper rib and sternum and, with the sternum, the anterior attachments of the next nine ribs. The intercostal muscles contract to further elevate the ribs and increase the anterior-posterior dimension of the thorax. Simultaneously, the diaphragm, which forms the floor of the thorax, contracts and flattens to further increase the volume of the thoracic cavity. As the thoracic volume increases, the pressure within it becomes less than atmospheric. Air rushes in through the tracheobronchial tree and into the alveoli to equalize this pressure gradient, filling the lungs.

As the musculature relaxes, the diaphragm again intrudes upward into the thoracic cavity, the ribs and sternum move inferiorly, and the ribs move closer together in an inferior and posterior direction. This decreases the thoracic volume and increases the intrathoracic pressure. When the pressure within the thorax exceeds that of the surrounding atmosphere, air rushes out. Therefore, exhalation in the resting state is largely a passive activity aided by the elastic recoil of the lungs. Gravity helps facilitate this action with downward displacement of the ribs in either the upright or supine position. This changing of volume to move air in and out is called the bellows effect.

The changing volume and pressure within the thoracic cage also assist with the pumping of blood to and venous return from the systemic circulation. The decreased intrathoracic pressure of inspiration helps move venous blood toward the thorax and heart, while the increased pressure of expiration helps move arterial blood away from the heart and thorax. The changing intrathoracic pressure affects the blood pressure and pulse strength. Normally, the systolic blood pressure and pulse strength fall during inspiration and rise during expiration.

The diaphragm is the primary muscle of respiration. The intercostal muscles are recruited to increase the depth of respiration. As the rate, depth, and work of respiration increase due to exercise or stress from trauma or infection, more accessory muscles of ventilation are recruited. These include the sternocleidomastoid and scalene muscles of the neck for inspiration and the anterior abdominal muscles to aid in forceful exhalation. The rhomboid muscles lift, abduct, and rotate the scapulae to help lift the upper chest with inspiration. The cough reflex, important to keeping the airways clear and alveoli expanded, depends on the addition of the latissimus dorsi muscles located along the posterior and lateral thoracic wall and the erector spinae muscles along the spine to allow for forceful contraction of the thorax.

Trachea, Bronchi, and Lungs

Contained within the thoracic cavity are the tracheobronchial tree and the lungs. The trachea is the hollow and cartilage-supported respiratory pathway through which air moves in and out of the thorax and lungs. It enters through the thoracic inlet and divides into the right and left mainstem bronchi at the carina, located in the upper central thorax. The right and left mainstem bronchi extend for about 3 cm and enter their respective lungs at the **pulmonary hilum.** The pulmonary hilum is also where the pulmonary arteries enter and the pulmonary veins exit the lungs and is the sole point of fixation of the lung in the thoracic cage. The bronchi then further divide into bronchioles, which ultimately terminate in the alveoli. The lungs contain millions of these tiny "grape" shaped alveoli, which are the basic unit of structure and function in the lungs.

    Each lung occupies one side of the thoracic cavity and is divided into lobes. The right lung has three lobes, the upper, middle, and lower. The left lung has two lobes, the upper and lower. The left upper lobe contains the cardiac notch against which the heart rests. The lower section of the left upper lobe (the lingula), projects around the lateral border of the heart and corresponds to the middle lobe of the right lung.

    The lungs are covered by the visceral pleura, a smooth membrane that lines the exterior of the lungs. It folds over on itself at the pulmonary hilum and then lines the inside of the thoracic cavity, becoming the parietal pleura. This dual layer forms a potential space called the pleural space. It contains a small amount of serous (pleural) fluid for lubrication and permits the lungs to expand and contract easily. This dual layer also creates the seal that causes the lungs to expand and contract with the changing volume of the thoracic cavity.

    The trachea, bronchi, and lungs are discussed further in the Respiratory System section later in this chapter.

Mediastinum and Heart

The mediastinum (Figure 12-59) is the central space within the thoracic cavity bounded laterally by the lungs, inferiorly by the diaphragm, and superiorly by the thoracic outlet. The heart is located within and fills most of the mediastinum. (The heart is discussed in detail in the Cardiovascular System section later in this chapter.) Through the mediastinum, the great vessels (see the next section) traverse to and from the heart, and the trachea and esophagus enter the thorax. The esophagus then courses anterior to the aorta before exiting through the diaphragm at the thoracic outlet (esophageal hiatus or foramen).

    The vagus nerve, which provides parasympathetic innervation of thoracic and abdominal viscera, enters the thorax bilaterally through the thoracic inlet and traverses the mediastinum giving branches to the larynx, esophagus, trachea, bronchi, and heart. The vagus nerve then exits the thorax through the esophageal opening in the diaphragm to innervate the abdominal viscera. The phrenic nerve (originating from the third, fourth, and fifth cervical nerve roots) also enters the thorax through the thoracic inlet and traverses the thorax to innervate the diaphragm.

> ✱ **pulmonary hilum** central medial region of the lung where the bronchi and pulmonary vasculature enter the lung.

> *The layers of the pleura and the small volume of fluid between them cause the lungs to move with the thoracic cage.*
>
>

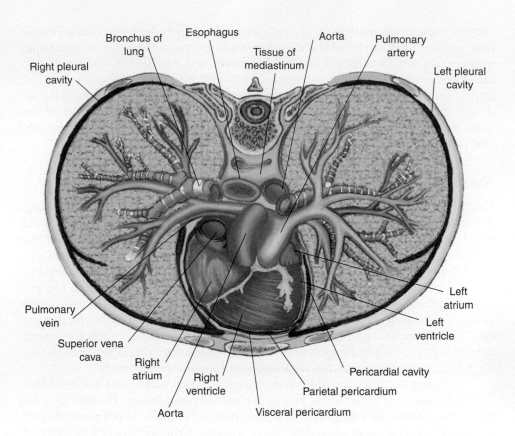

FIGURE 12-59 Structures of the mediastinum and thorax.

Labels on figure: Right pleural cavity · Bronchus of lung · Esophagus · Tissue of mediastinum · Aorta · Pulmonary artery · Left pleural cavity · Pulmonary vein · Superior vena cava · Right atrium · Right ventricle · Aorta · Visceral pericardium · Parietal pericardium · Pericardial cavity · Left ventricle · Left atrium

The thoracic duct (part of the lymphatic system) also traverses the thorax from the thoracic outlet, where it enters through the aortic opening in the diaphragm. It typically crosses the midline from the right side of the aorta in the posterior mediastinum at the level of the fifth thoracic vertebra and then ascends above the level of the left clavicle before arching back downward to empty into the left internal jugular vein. The thoracic duct carries most of the body's lymphatic drainage (all but the right side of the head, neck, thorax, and right upper extremity).

Great Vessels

The **great vessels** are those large arteries and veins that enter and leave the heart and are found in the mediastinum. They are the aorta, the superior and inferior vena cava, the pulmonary arteries, and the pulmonary veins. Injury to these large vascular structures can lead to significant blood loss and death if the condition is not quickly recognized and repaired. The aorta, which is fixed at three positions within the thorax, is not only susceptible to penetrating injury but also to blunt injury by rapid deceleration or shear forces. It is fixed at the annulus where it attaches to the heart, at the **ligamentum arteriosum** near the bifurcation of the pulmonary artery, and at the aortic hiatus where it passes through the diaphragm and enters the abdomen.

Other major vessels that branch from the great vessels in the upper thorax include the subclavian arteries and veins, the common carotid arteries, and the innominate artery (which is the first large branch off the aortic arch dividing into the right common carotid and right subclavian). The internal mammary vessels are inferior branches of the subclavians running along the anterior surface of the pleura, posterior to the costochondral (rib-cartilage) junction. They are often harvested for coronary artery bypass grafts. The intercostal arteries are branches of the thoracic aorta (except for the first two, which arise from branches of the sub-

✱ great vessels the large arteries and veins located in the mediastinum that enter and exit the heart; the aorta, superior and inferior vena cava, pulmonary arteries, and pulmonary veins.

✱ ligamentum arteriosum cord-like remnant of a fetal vessel connecting the pulmonary artery to the aorta at the aortic isthmus.

clavian) that run along the lower margins of the ribs along with the intercostal nerves. Finally, the bronchial arteries (one right and two left) are usually branches of the thoracic aorta that nourish the nonrespiratory tissues of the lung.

Esophagus

The esophagus enters the thorax through the thoracic inlet with and just posterior to the trachea. It continues the length of the mediastinum and exits through the esophageal hiatus of the diaphragm. It is a muscular tube that is contiguous with the posterior wall of the trachea and conducts food and drink from the oral pharynx to the stomach. It moves food and liquid toward the stomach through a rhythmic muscular contraction called peristalsis. During vomiting, peristalsis reverses and propels the emesis up the esophagus.

THE NERVOUS SYSTEM

The nervous system is the body's principal control system. This network of cells, tissues, and organs regulates nearly all bodily functions via electrical impulses transmitted through nerves, all of which are highly susceptible to hypoxia (oxygen deficiency). The endocrine system is closely related to the nervous system. It exerts bodily control via hormones. You will learn more about this system later in this chapter. A third system, the circulatory system, assists in regulatory functions by distributing hormones and other chemical messengers.

The nervous system consists of two main divisions—the central nervous system and the peripheral nervous system. The **central nervous system** consists of the brain and the spinal cord. The **peripheral nervous system** is somewhat more complex. As you look at Figure 12-60, note that the peripheral nervous system is divided into two major subdivisions—the **somatic nervous system,** which governs voluntary functions (those we control consciously), and the **autonomic nervous system** which has two subdivisions—the **sympathetic nervous system** and the **parasympathetic nervous system.** These two subdivisions of the autonomic nervous system work together to carry out involuntary physiological processes, such as regulation of blood pressure, heart rate, and digestion.

You will learn more about these divisions of the nervous system as you continue through the next pages. As you read, it will be helpful if you think of the nervous system as a "living computer." The central nervous system is the central processing unit, and the various divisions of the peripheral nervous system carry on the input and output processes.

FUNDAMENTAL UNIT: THE NEURON

The fundamental unit of the nervous system is the nerve cell, or **neuron.** The neuron includes the *cell body* (soma), containing the nucleus; the *dendrites,* which transmit electrical impulses to the cell body; and the *axons,* which transmit electrical impulses away from the cell body (Figure 12-61).

The transmission of impulses in the nervous system resembles the conduction of electrical impulses through the heart. In its resting state, the neuron is positively charged on the outside and negatively charged on the inside. When electrically stimulated, sodium rapidly surges into the cell and potassium rapidly leaves it so that there is no longer a difference in electrical charge between the inside and the outside. This "depolarization," or loss of the charge difference, is subsequently transmitted down the neuron at an extremely high rate of speed.

The neuron joins with other neurons at junctions called *synapses* (Figure 12-62). The neurons never come into direct contact with each other at these

The nervous system is the body's principal control system.

✴ **central nervous system** the brain and the spinal cord.

✴ **peripheral nervous system** part of the nervous system that extends throughout the body and is composed of the cranial nerves arising from the brain and the peripheral nerves arising from the spinal cord. Its subdivisions are the somatic and the autonomic nervous systems.

✴ **somatic nervous system** part of the nervous system controlling voluntary bodily functions.

✴ **autonomic nervous system** part of the nervous system controlling involuntary bodily functions. It is divided into the sympathetic and the parasympathetic systems.

✴ **sympathetic nervous system** division of the autonomic nervous system that prepares the body for stressful situations. Sympathetic nervous system actions include increased heart rate and dilation of the bronchioles and pupils. Its actions are mediated by the neurotransmitters epinephrine and norepinephrine.

✴ **parasympathetic nervous system** division of the autonomic nervous system that is responsible for controlling vegetative functions. Parasympathetic nervous system actions include decreased heart rate and constriction of the bronchioles and pupils. Its actions are mediated by the neurotransmitter acetylcholine.

✴ **neuron** nerve cell; the fundamental component of the nervous system.

FIGURE 12–60 Overview of
the nervous system.

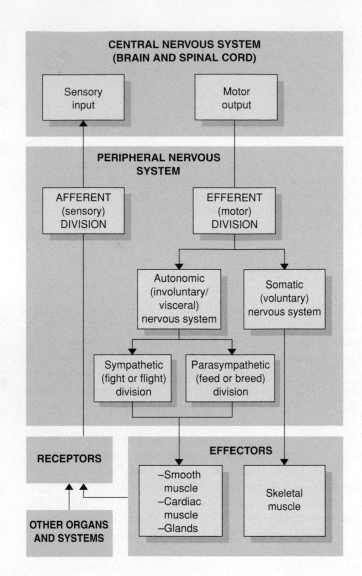

**CENTRAL NERVOUS SYSTEM
(BRAIN AND SPINAL CORD)**

Sensory
input

Motor
output

**PERIPHERAL NERVOUS
SYSTEM**

AFFERENT
(sensory)
DIVISION

EFFERENT
(motor)
DIVISION

Autonomic
(involuntary/
visceral)
nervous system

Somatic
(voluntary)
nervous system

Sympathetic
(fight or flight)
division

Parasympathetic
(feed or breed)
division

RECEPTORS

EFFECTORS

–Smooth
muscle
–Cardiac
muscle
–Glands

Skeletal
muscle

**OTHER ORGANS
AND SYSTEMS**

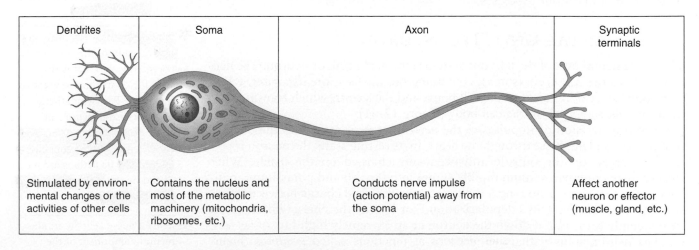

Dendrites	Soma	Axon	Synaptic terminals
Stimulated by environmental changes or the activities of other cells	Contains the nucleus and most of the metabolic machinery (mitochondria, ribosomes, etc.)	Conducts nerve impulse (action potential) away from the soma	Affect another neuron or effector (muscle, gland, etc.)

FIGURE 12–61   Anatomy of a neuron.

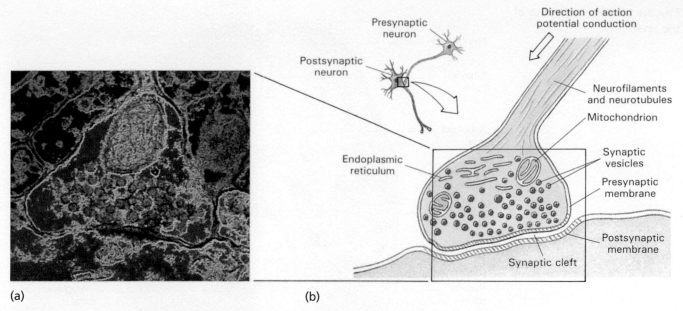

FIGURE 12-62   The synapse: (a) electron micrograph, (b) schematic.

synapses. Instead, on reaching the synapse, the axon causes the release of a chemical **neurotransmitter.** This neurotransmitter, either acetylcholine or norepinephrine, then crosses the gap between the axon of the depolarized neuron and the dendrite of the adjacent neuron. The neurotransmitter stimulates the postsynaptic membrane of the connecting nerve. Acetylcholine is the neurotransmitter of the parasympathetic and voluntary (somatic) nervous systems. Norepinephrine is found in the synaptic terminals of sympathetic nerves. (See the later description of the divisions of the peripheral nervous system.)

THE CENTRAL NERVOUS SYSTEM

Knowledge of the anatomy and physiology of the central nervous system—the brain and the spinal cord—is essential to understanding and treating nervous system emergencies. Note that the basic structures of the central nervous system and some of the related terminology were presented earlier in the chapter under the headings "The Head, Face, and Neck" and "The Spine and Thorax."

Protective Structures

Most of the central nervous system is protected by bony structures. The brain lies within the cranial vault, protected by the skull. Covered by the scalp, the cranium consists of the bones of the head, excluding the facial bones. Bones composing the cranium include two single bones—the frontal and occipital bones—and a series of paired bones—the parietals, temporals, sphenoids, and ethmoids (Figure 12-63; also review Figure 12-44).

The spinal cord is housed inside and is protected by the "spinal canal" formed by the vertebrae of the spinal column (review Figure 12-54).

Protective membranes called the *meninges* cover the entire central nervous system. There are three layers of meninges that pad, or cushion, the brain and spinal cord (Figure 12-64). The durable, outermost layer is referred to as the *dura mater.* The middle layer is a web-like structure known as the *arachnoid membrane.* The innermost layer, directly overlying the central nervous system, is

✱ **neurotransmitter** a substance that is released from the axon terminal of a presynaptic neuron on excitation and that travels across the synaptic cleft to either excite or inhibit the target cell. Examples include acetylcholine, norepinephrine, and dopamine.

Content Review

CENTRAL NERVOUS SYSTEM
• Brain
• Spinal cord

FIGURE 12-63 The bones of the skull.

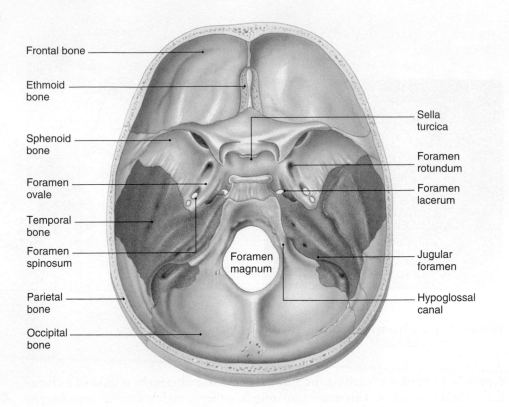

Frontal bone

Ethmoid bone

Sphenoid bone

Foramen ovale

Temporal bone

Foramen spinosum

Parietal bone

Occipital bone

Sella turcica

Foramen rotundum

Foramen lacerum

Foramen magnum

Jugular foramen

Hypoglossal canal

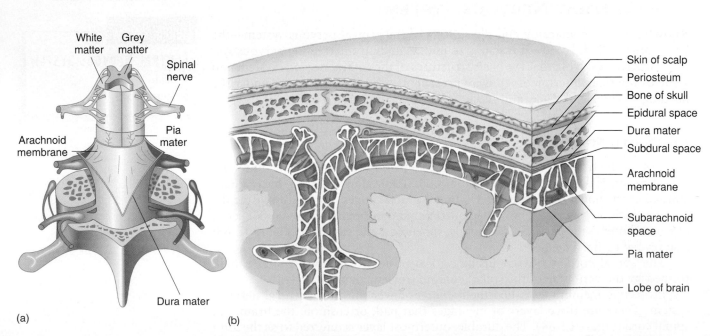

White matter

Grey matter

Spinal nerve

Arachnoid membrane

Pia mater

Dura mater

Skin of scalp

Periosteum

Bone of skull

Epidural space

Dura mater

Subdural space

Arachnoid membrane

Subarachnoid space

Pia mater

Lobe of brain

(a)

(b)

FIGURE 12-64 The meninges: (a) posterior view of the spinal cord showing the meningeal layers; (b) the meninges of the brain.

called the *pia mater*. The space between the pia mater and the arachnoid membrane is referred to as the subarachnoid space, while the space between the dura mater and the arachnoid membrane is called the subdural space. The space outside the dura mater is called the epidural space. Both the brain and the spinal cord are bathed in *cerebrospinal fluid*, a watery, clear fluid that acts as a cushion to protect these organs from physical impact.

The Brain

The brain is the largest part of the central nervous system. The following information provides a general profile of the brain's anatomy and physiology.

Divisions of the Brain Filling the cranial vault, the brain is divided into six major parts: the cerebrum, the diencephalon (which includes the thalamus and hypothalamus), the mesencephalon (midbrain), the pons, the medulla oblongata, and the cerebellum (Figure 12-65).

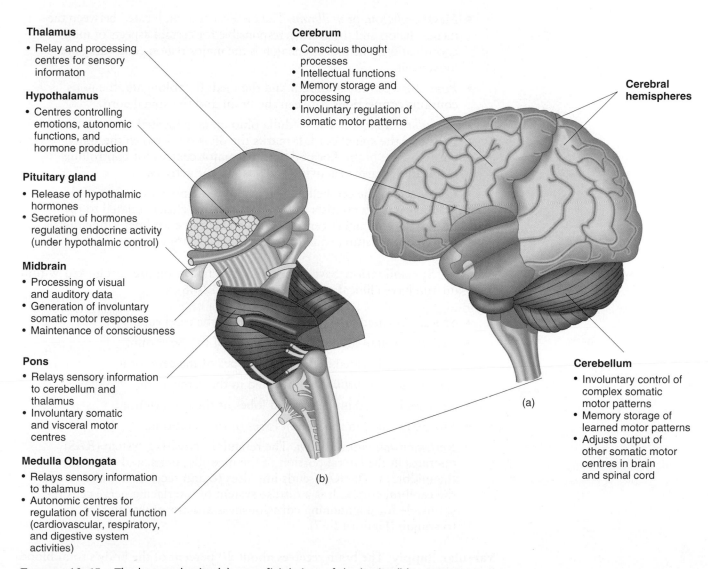

Thalamus
- Relay and processing centres for sensory informaton

Hypothalamus
- Centres controlling emotions, autonomic functions, and hormone production

Pituitary gland
- Release of hypothalmic hormones
- Secretion of hormones regulating endocrine activity (under hypothalmic control)

Midbrain
- Processing of visual and auditory data
- Generation of involuntary somatic motor responses
- Maintenance of consciousness

Pons
- Relays sensory information to cerebellum and thalamus
- Involuntary somatic and visceral motor centres

Medulla Oblongata
- Relays sensory information to thalamus
- Autonomic centres for regulation of visceral function (cardiovascular, respiratory, and digestive system activities)

Cerebrum
- Conscious thought processes
- Intellectual functions
- Memory storage and processing
- Involuntary regulation of somatic motor patterns

Cerebral hemispheres

Cerebellum
- Involuntary control of complex somatic motor patterns
- Memory storage of learned motor patterns
- Adjusts output of other somatic motor centres in brain and spinal cord

(a)

(b)

FIGURE 12-65   The human brain: (a) superficial view of the brain; (b) components of the brainstem.

The cerebrum and diencephalon constitute the *forebrain*.

- *Cerebrum*. The cerebrum is in the anterior and middle area of the cranium. Containing two hemispheres, it is joined by a structure called the *corpus callosum*. The cerebrum governs all sensory and motor actions. It is the seat of intelligence, learning, analysis, memory, and language. The *cerebral cortex* is the outermost layer of the cerebrum.
- *Diencephalon*. Covered by the cerebrum, the diencephalon is sometimes called the *interbrain*. Inside it are the *thalamus, hypothalamus* (which is connected to the pituitary gland), and the *limbic system*. This area is responsible for many involuntary actions, such as temperature regulation, sleep, water balance, stress response, and emotions. It plays a major role in regulating the autonomic nervous system.

The mesencephalon (midbrain), pons, and the medulla oblongata collectively form the *brainstem*. The brainstem and the cerebellum together constitute the *hindbrain*.

- *Mesencephalon*, or *midbrain*. The mesencephalon, located between the diencephalon and the pons, is responsible for certain aspects of motor coordination. The mesencephalon is the major region controlling eye movement.
- *Pons*. Between the midbrain and the medulla oblongata, the pons contains connections between the brain and the spinal cord.
- *Medulla oblongata*. The medulla oblongata is located between the pons and the spinal cord. It marks the division between the spinal cord and the brain. Located here are major centres for controlling respiration, cardiac activity, and vasomotor activity.
- *Cerebellum*. The cerebellum is located in the posterior fossa of the cranial cavity. It consists of two hemispheres closely related to the brainstem and higher centres. The cerebellum coordinates fine motor movement, posture, equilibrium, and muscle tone.

Areas of Specialization Several areas of specialization are recognized within the brain and have clinical application (Figure 12-66).

- *Speech*. Located in the temporal lobe of the cerebrum.
- *Vision*. Located in the occipital cortex of the cerebrum.
- *Personality*. Located in the frontal lobes of the cerebrum.
- *Balance and coordination*. Located in the cerebellum.
- *Sensory*. Located in the parietal lobes of the cerebrum.
- *Motor*. Located in the frontal lobes of the cerebrum.
- *Reticular activating system*. The reticular activating system (RAS) operates in the lateral portion of the medulla, pons, and especially the midbrain. The RAS sends impulses to and receives impulses from the cerebral cortex. It is a diffuse system of interlacing nerve cells responsible for maintaining consciousness and the ability to respond to stimuli (Figure 12-67).

Vascular Supply The brain receives about 20 percent of the body's total blood flow per minute. Blood flow to the brain is provided by two systems. The *carotid system* is anterior, while the *vertebrobasilar system* is posterior. Both join at the

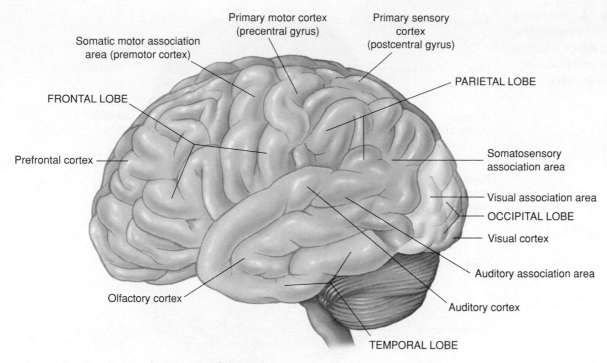

Figure 12-66   External anatomy of the brain.

Circle of Willis before entering the structures of the brain (Figure 12-68). The system is designed so that interruption of any part will not cause significant loss of blood flow to the tissues. Venous drainage of the brain is through the venous sinuses and the internal jugular veins.

Besides blood flow, cerebrospinal fluid bathes the brain and spinal cord. Several chambers within the brain, called ventricles, contain most of the intracranial volume of this fluid.

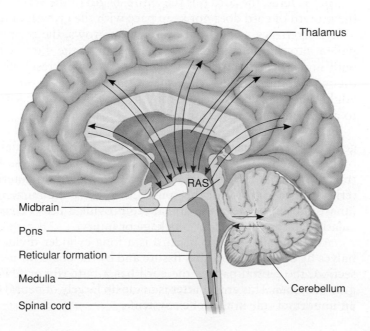

Figure 12-67   The reticular activating system (RAS), which sends and receives messages from various parts of the brain.

FIGURE 12-68 An interior view of the brain showing the Circle of Willis, which is formed by the anterior and posterior communicating arteries.

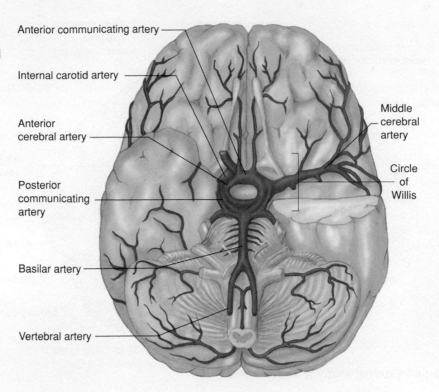

Anterior communicating artery

Internal carotid artery

Anterior cerebral artery

Posterior communicating artery

Basilar artery

Vertebral artery

Middle cerebral artery

Circle of Willis

The Spinal Cord

The **spinal cord** is the central nervous system (CNS) pathway responsible for transmitting sensory input from the body to the brain and for conducting motor impulses from the brain to the body muscles and organs. Through this pathway, the brain monitors and controls most body functions. Additionally, the spinal cord acts as a reflex centre, intercepting sensory signals and initiating short-circuited (reflex) signaling to muscle bodies as needed. If this pathway is compromised, control of the body below the injury is lost.

In the fetus, the cord fills the entire length of the vertebral column. However, the growth of cord does not keep pace with the growth of the vertebral column. This discrepancy means that as a person grows, the peripheral nerve roots are pulled into the spinal foramen. The sheath of the dura below L-2 is thus filled with numerous strands of peripheral nerves. The resulting structure resembles the tail of a horse and is called the cauda equina (Latin for horse's tail). In the adult, the spinal cord extends from the base of the brain (the medulla oblongata) to approximately the L-1 or L-2 level.

Like all central nervous system tissue, the spinal cord constantly needs oxygenated blood. This blood is supplied through paired spinal arteries that branch off the vertebral, cervical, thoracic, and lumbar arteries. These spinal arteries travel through intervertebral foramina, then split into anterior and posterior arteries. On the surface of the spinal cord, there are numerous interconnections (anastomoses) between the arteries to provide a better chance for adequate circulation in case of vascular blockage or injury.

Anatomically, the spinal cord is a long cylinder divided into left and right halves by the **anterior medial fissure** and by the **posterior medial sulcus.** In cross-section, the central part of the cord has a butterfly or "H" shape and appears grey in colour. This **grey matter** is made up largely of neural cell bodies and plays an important role in the reflex system.

✱ **spinal cord** central nervous system pathway responsible for transmitting sensory input from the body to the brain and for conducting motor impulses from the brain to the body muscles and organs.

✱ **anterior medial fissure** deep crease along the ventral surface of the spinal cord that divides the cord into right and left halves.

✱ **posterior medial sulcus** shallow longitudinal groove along the dorsal surface of the spinal cord.

✱ **grey matter** areas in the central nervous system dominated by nerve cell bodies; the central portion of the spinal cord.

The remaining areas, or **white matter,** then form three bundles or columns of myelinated (covered with a protein sheath) nerve fibres on each side of the cord around the grey matter: the anterior white column, the lateral white column, and the posterior white column. This white matter comprises nerve cell pathways called axons. It contains bundles of axons that transmit signals upward to the brain in what are called **ascending tracts** and bundles that transmit signals downward to the body in what are called **descending tracts.** These tracts are paired, one ascending and one descending on each side, and injury may affect either or both.

A thorough discussion of organization and functions of the ascending and descending spinal tracts is beyond the scope of this textbook. However, knowing the functions of some motor and sensory pathways can aid you in recognizing spinal cord injury.

The important ascending (sensory) tracts or fasciculi include the fasciculus gracilis, fasciculus cuneatus, and the spinothalamic tracts. The fasciculus gracilis and fasciculus cuneatus carry sensory impulses of light touch, vibration, and positional sense from the skin, muscles, tendons, and joints to the brain. They are located on the posterior portion of the cord (posterior columns). Their injury causes disruption on the ipsilateral (same side) of the body because the left to right switching occurs at the medulla. The spinothalamic tracts include both lateral and anterior tracts. The anterior pathway conducts pain and temperature, while the lateral pathway conducts touch and pressure sensation. These pathways cross as they enter the cord, and hence injury results in contralateral (opposite side) deficits.

The important descending (motor) spinal nerve tract is the corticospinal tract. It is responsible for voluntary and fine muscle movement on the ipsilateral side of the body. This pathway lies on the posterior and lateral portions of the cord. Two other descending tracts are the reticulospinal and rubrospinal tracts. The reticulospinal tract consists of three sub-tracts, one lateral, one medial, and one anterior. It is thought to be involved in sweating and the muscular activity associated with posturing. The rubrospinal tracts are lateral pathways that affect and control fine motor function of the hands and feet. Injury affects the ipsilateral side of the body with both these pathways.

Spinal Nerves

Spinal nerves are the peripheral nerve roots that branch in pairs from the spinal cord (Figure 12-69). They travel through the intervertebral foramina and have both sensory and motor components. They provide the largest part of the innervation of the skin, muscles, and internal organs.

There are 31 pairs of spinal nerve roots. The first pair exits the spinal column between the skull and the first cervical vertebra. Each of the next 7 pairs exits just below one of the cervical vertebrae and is identified as C-2 through C-8. (Although there are only 7 cervical vertebrae, there are 8 cervical spinal nerves.) There are 12 pairs of thoracic nerves: 5 lumbar, 5 sacral, and 1 coccygeal. Each of these pairs originates just below the vertebra with whose name it is identified. Each spinal nerve pair has two dorsal and two ventral roots. The ventral roots carry motor impulses from the cord to the body, while the dorsal roots carry sensory impulses from the body to the cord. (C-1 and Co [coccygeal]-1 do not have dorsal [sensory] roots.)

The nerve roots often converge in a cluster of nerves called a plexus (Table 12-3). A plexus (or braiding) permits peripheral nerve roots to rejoin and function as a group. The cervical plexus, made up of the first five cervical nerve roots, innervates the neck and produces the phrenic nerve. The phrenic nerve (consisting of peripheral nerve roots C-3 through C-5) is responsible for diaphragm control. The brachial plexus joins the nerves controlling the upper extremity (C-5 through T-1). The lumbar and sacral plexuses control the innervation of the lower extremity.

* **white matter** material that surrounds grey matter in the spinal cord; made up largely of axons.

* **ascending tracts** bundles of axons along the spinal cord that transmit signals from the body to the brain.

* **descending tracts** bundles of axons along the spinal cord that transmit signals from the brain to the body.

* **spinal nerves** 31 pairs of nerves that originate along the spinal cord from anterior and posterior nerve roots.

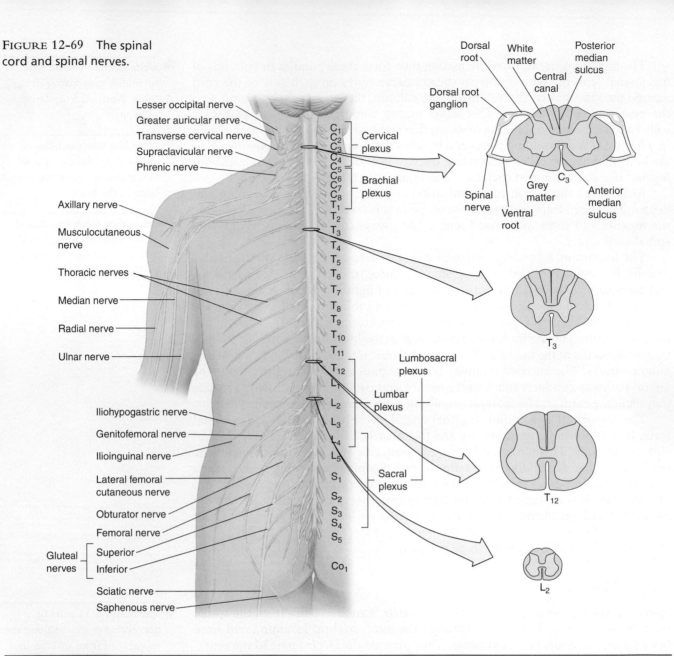

FIGURE 12-69   The spinal cord and spinal nerves.

Table 12-3   SPINAL NERVE PLEXUSES

Plexus	Origin	Nerve	Control	Result of Injury
Cervical	C-1 to C-5	phrenic	diaphragm	respiratory paralysis
Brachial	C-5 to C-8, T-1	axillary	deltoid/skin of shoulder	deltoid muscle paralysis
		radial	triceps/forearm	wristdrop
		median	flexor muscles, forearm, arm	decreased usage
		musculocutaneous	flexor muscles of arm	decreased usage
		ulnar	wrist/hand	claw hand; inability to spread fingers
Lumbar	T-12 to L-4	femoral	lower abdomen, gluteus, thighs	inability to extend leg, flex hip
		obturator	abductor muscles medial thigh	decrease in usage
Sacral	L-4 to S-3	sciatic	lower extremity	decreased usage

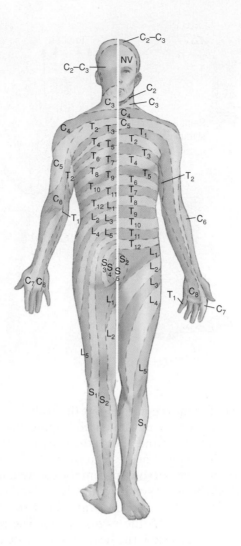

FIGURE 12-70 The dermatomes. Each dermatome corresponds to a spinal nerve.

The sensory components of the spinal nerves innervate specific and discrete areas of the body surface. These areas are called **dermatomes** and are distributed from the occiput of the head to the heel of the foot and buttocks (Figure 12-70). Key locations to recognize for assessment include the collar region (C-3), the little finger (C-7), the nipple line (T-4), the umbilicus (T-10), and the small toe (S-1).

The motor components of the spinal nerve roots also innervate discrete tissues and muscles of the body in regions called **myotomes**. However, as the body grows and matures, some muscles merge and their control is not as specific as it is with the dermatomes. Key myotomes for neurological evaluation include arm extension (C-5), elbow extension (C-7), small finger abduction (T-1), knee extension (L-3), and ankle flexion (S-1). Evaluation of areas controlled by both dermatomes and myotomes can help you identify the spinal cord region associated with an injury.

The spinal cord also performs some primary processing functions, speeding body responses and helping the brain maintain balance and muscle tone. These responses, called reflexes, occur as special neurons in the cord, called interneurons, and intercept sensory signals (Figure 12-71). For example, if you touch a hot stove, the severe pain sends an intense signal to the brain. This strong signal simultaneously triggers an interneuron in the spinal cord to direct a signal to the flexor muscles telling them to contract. The limb withdraws without waiting for the signal sent to the brain to reach it, be processed, and trigger a command to be sent back to the limb. The speed of this reflex action reduces the seriousness of injury. Other reflexes help stabilize the body if it stands in one position for a length of time. As

✳ dermatome topographical region of the body surface innervated by one nerve root.

✳ myotome muscle and tissue of the body innervated by a spinal nerve root.

FIGURE 12-71 The reflex response.

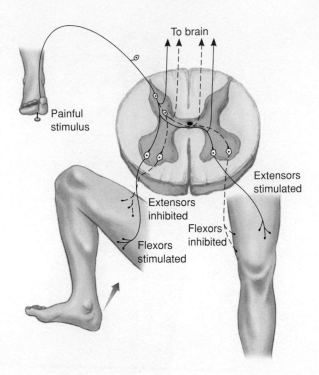

the stretch receptors report the body is moving, the interneurons signal muscles to counteract the movement to help maintain position. This again reduces the body's reaction time and allows the body to stand or maintain a steady position.

The spinal nerves can be further subdivided according to the division of the autonomic nervous system they serve and to their spinal origin. The parasympathetic nervous system controls rest and regenerative functions and consists of the peripheral nerve roots branching from the sacral region and the cranial nerves (predominantly the vagus nerve). The parasympathetic nervous system's major tasks are to slow the heart and increase digestive system activity; the system also plays a role in sexual stimulation. The sympathetic nervous system adjusts the body's metabolic rate to waking activity, provides "fight or flight" functions, and branches from nerves originating in the thoracic and lumbar regions. This system decreases organ and digestive activity through vasoconstriction, constricts the venous blood vessels, and affects the body's metabolic rate through the release of the adrenal hormones norepinephrine and epinephrine. In shock, the sympathetic nervous system causes systemic vasoconstriction to reduce the venous blood volume and increase peripheral vascular resistance. It also increases the heart rate to increase cardiac output in response to dropping preload and blood pressure.

THE PERIPHERAL NERVOUS SYSTEM

Consisting of the cranial and the peripheral nerves, the peripheral nervous system has both voluntary and involuntary components. The 12 pairs of **cranial nerves** originate in the brain and supply nervous control to the head, neck, and certain thoracic and abdominal organs (Figure 12-72). The peripheral nerves, as described previously, originate in the spinal cord and supply nervous control to the periphery.

The four categories of peripheral nerves are as follows:

1. *Somatic Sensory.* These afferent nerves transmit sensations involved in touch, pressure, pain, temperature, and position (proprioception).
2. *Somatic Motor.* These efferent fibres carry impulses to the skeletal (voluntary) muscles.

Content Review

PERIPHERAL NERVOUS SYSTEM
- Voluntary (Somatic)
- Involuntary (Autonomic)
  - Sympathetic
  - Parasympathetic

✳ **cranial nerves** 12 pairs of nerves that extend from the lower surface of the brain.

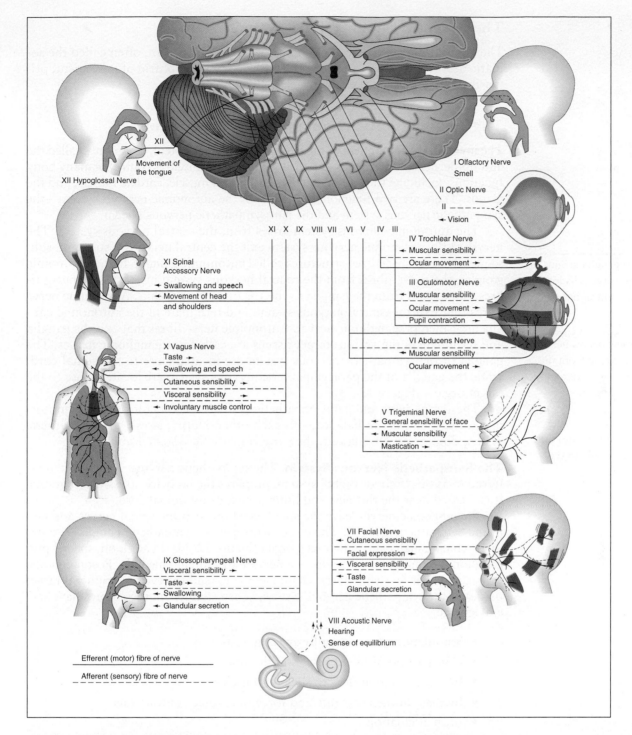

FIGURE 12-72   The cranial nerves.

3. *Visceral (Autonomic) Sensory.* These afferent tracts transmit sensations from the visceral organs. Such sensations as a full bladder or the need to defecate are mediated by visceral sensory fibres.

4. *Visceral (Autonomic) Motor.* These efferent fibres exit the central nervous system and branch to supply nerves to the involuntary cardiac muscle and smooth muscle of the viscera (organs) and to the glands.

The Somatic (Voluntary) Nervous System

The voluntary component of the peripheral nervous system, often called the somatic nervous system, is responsible for the conscious control of movement, primarily controlling the skeletal muscles.

The Autonomic (Involuntary) Nervous System

The involuntary component of the peripheral nervous system, commonly called the autonomic nervous system, is responsible for the unconscious control of many body functions, including those governed by the smooth muscle, cardiac muscle, and the glands. There are two functional divisions of the autonomic nervous system—the sympathetic nervous system and the parasympathetic nervous system.

The autonomic nervous system arises from the central nervous system. The nerves of the autonomic nervous system exit the central nervous system and subsequently enter specialized structures called **autonomic ganglia.** In the autonomic ganglia, the nerve fibres from the central nervous system interact with nerve fibres that extend from the ganglia to the various target organs. Autonomic nerve fibres that exit the central nervous system and terminate in the autonomic ganglia are called **preganglionic nerves.** Autonomic nerve fibres that exit the ganglia and terminate in the various target tissues are called **postganglionic nerves.** The ganglia of the sympathetic nervous system are located close to the spinal cord, while the ganglia of the parasympathetic nervous system are located close to the target organs (Figure 12-73).

The sympathetic and parasympathetic systems are antagonistic. In their normal state, they exist in balance with each other. During stress, the sympathetic system dominates. During rest, the parasympathetic system dominates.

The Sympathetic Nervous System The sympathetic nervous system, often referred to as the "fight or flight" system, prepares the body for stressful situations. It is located near the thoracic and lumbar part of the spinal cord.

Preganglionic nerves leave the spinal cord through the spinal nerves and end in the sympathetic ganglia. There are two types of sympathetic ganglia: sympathetic chain ganglia and collateral ganglia (Figure 12-74). In addition, special preganglionic sympathetic nerve fibres innervate the adrenal medulla. Postganglionic nerves that exit the sympathetic chain ganglia extend to several peripheral target tissues of the sympathetic nervous system. When stimulated, these fibres have several effects.

- Stimulation of secretion by sweat glands
- Constriction of blood vessels in the skin
- Increase in blood flow to skeletal muscles
- Increase in the heart rate and force of cardiac contractions
- Bronchodilation
- Stimulation of energy production

The collateral ganglia are located in the abdominal cavity. Nerves leaving the collateral ganglia innervate many of the organs of the abdomen. Stimulation of these fibres causes several conditions.

- Reduction of blood flow to abdominal organs
- Decreased digestive activity
- Relaxation of smooth muscle in the wall of the urinary bladder
- Release of glucose stores from the liver

✱ **autonomic ganglia** groups of autonomic nerve cells located outside the central nervous system.

✱ **preganglionic nerves** nerve fibres that extend from the central nervous system to the autonomic ganglia.

✱ **postganglionic nerves** nerve fibres that extend from the autonomic ganglia to the target tissues.

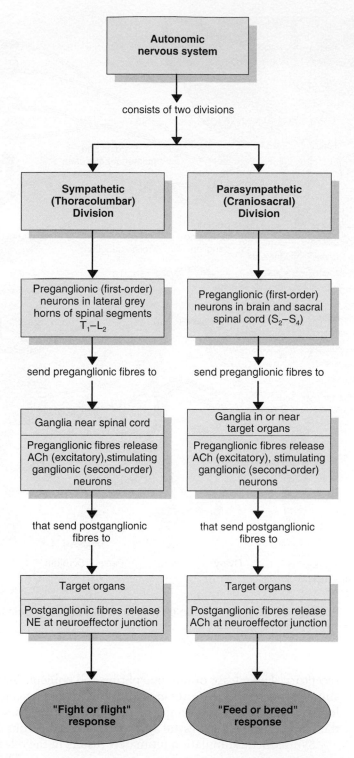

FIGURE 12-73 Components of the autonomic nervous system.

Sympathetic nervous system stimulation also results in direct stimulation of the adrenal medulla, the inner portion of the adrenal gland (Figure 12-75). The adrenal medulla, in turn, releases the hormones norepinephrine (noradrenalin) and epinephrine (adrenalin) into the circulatory system. Approximately 80 percent of the hormones released by the adrenal medulla are epinephrine, while norepinephrine constitutes the remaining 20 percent. Once released, these hormones are carried throughout the body where they cause their intended effects by acting on hormone

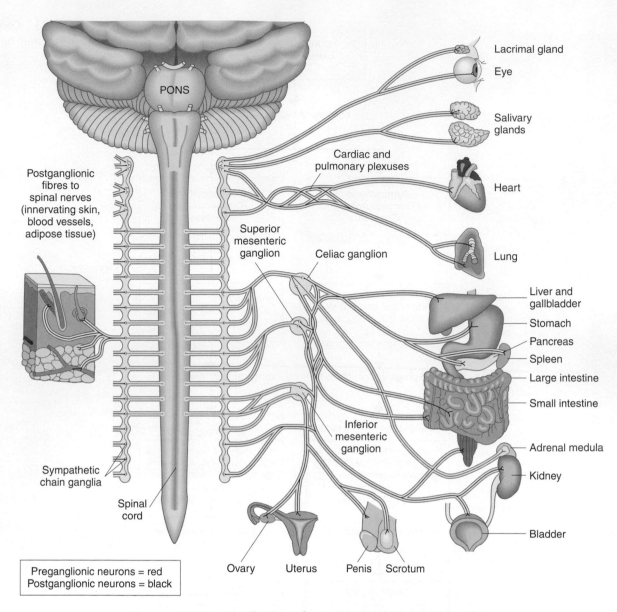

Preganglionic neurons = red
Postganglionic neurons = black

FIGURE 12-74   Distribution of sympathetic postganglionic fibres.

receptors. The release of norepinephrine and epinephrine by the adrenal medulla stimulates tissues that are not innervated by sympathetic nerves. In addition, it prolongs the effects of direct sympathetic stimulation. All these effects serve to prepare the body to deal with stressful and potentially dangerous situations.

Sympathetic stimulation ultimately results in the release of the hormone norepinephrine from postganglionic, presynaptic nerves. The norepinephrine subsequently crosses the synaptic cleft and interacts with adrenergic receptors on the postsynaptic nerves. Shortly thereafter, the norepinephrine is either taken up by the presynaptic neuron for reuse or broken down by enzymes present within the synapse (Figure 12-76). Sympathetic stimulation also results in the release of the hormones epinephrine and norepinephrine from the adrenal medulla. In addition, both epinephrine and norepinephrine interact with specialized adrenergic receptors on the membranes of the target organs. These receptors are located throughout the body. Once stimulated by the appropriate hormone, they cause a response in the organ or organs they control.

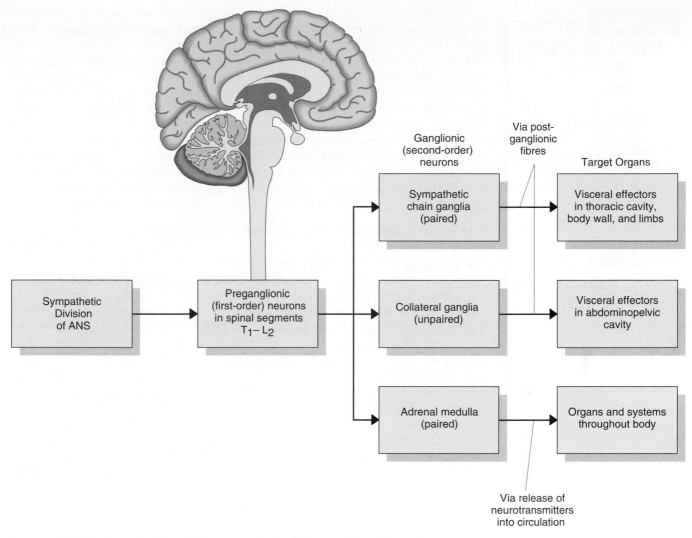

FIGURE 12-75   Organization of the sympathetic division of the autonomic nervous system.

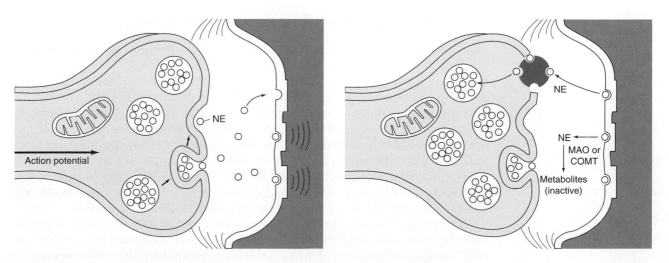

FIGURE 12-76   Physiology of an adrenergic synapse. Norepinephrine is released
from the presynaptic nerve and stimulates receptors on the postsynaptic nerve.
Subsequently, the norepinephrine is either taken up by the presynaptic nerve or
deactivated by enzymes in the synapse.

The two known types of sympathetic receptors are the *adrenergic receptors* and the *dopaminergic receptors*. The adrenergic receptors are generally divided into four types. These four receptors are designated alpha$_1$ (α_1), alpha$_2$ (α_2), beta$_1$ (β_1), and beta$_2$ (β_2). The alpha$_1$ receptors cause peripheral vasoconstriction, mild bronchoconstriction, and stimulation of metabolism. The alpha$_2$ receptors are found on the presynaptic surfaces of sympathetic neuroeffector junctions. Stimulation of alpha$_2$ receptors is inhibitory. These receptors serve to prevent overrelease of norepinephrine in the synapse. When the level of norepinephrine in the synapse gets high enough, the alpha$_2$ receptors are stimulated and norepinephrine release is inhibited. Stimulation of beta$_1$ receptors causes increases in heart rate, cardiac contractile force, and cardiac automaticity and conduction. Stimulation of beta$_2$ receptors causes vasodilation and bronchodilation. Dopaminergic receptors, although not fully understood, evidently cause dilation of the renal, coronary, and cerebral arteries.

The Parasympathetic Nervous System The parasympathetic nervous system, sometimes called the "feed or breed" system, is responsible for controlling vegetative functions, such as normal heart rate and blood pressure.

The parasympathetic nervous system arises from the brain stem and the sacral segments of the spinal cord. The preganglionic neurons of the parasympathetic nervous system are typically much longer than those of the sympathetic nervous system because the ganglia are located close to the target tissues. Parasympathetic nerve fibres that leave the brain stem travel within four of the cranial nerves including the oculomotor nerve (III), the facial nerve (VII), the glossopharyngeal nerve (IX), and the vagus nerve (X). These fibres synapse in the parasympathetic ganglia with short postganglionic fibres that then continue to their target tissues. Postsynaptic fibres innervate much of the body, including the intrinsic eye muscles, the salivary glands, the heart, the lungs, and most of the organs of the abdominal cavity. The sacral segment of the parasympathetic nervous system forms distinct pelvic nerves that innervate ganglia in the kidneys, bladder, sex organs, and the terminal portions of the large intestine (Figure 12-77). Stimulation of the parasympathetic nervous system results in the following conditions:

- Pupillary constriction
- Secretion by digestive glands
- Reduction in heart rate and cardiac contractile force
- Bronchoconstriction
- Increased smooth muscle activity along the digestive tract

These and other functions facilitate the processing of food, energy absorption, relaxation, and reproduction (Figure 12-78).

All preganglionic and postganglionic parasympathetic nerve fibres use acetylcholine as a neurotransmitter. Acetylcholine, when released by presynaptic neurons, crosses the synaptic cleft and activates receptors on the postsynaptic neurons or on the neuroeffector junction. Acetylcholine is also the neurotransmitter for the somatic nervous system and is present in the neuromuscular junction. Acetylcholine is very short lived. Within a fraction of a second after its release, it is deactivated by another chemical called acetylcholinesterase. Acetic acid and choline, which are produced when acetylcholine is deactivated, are taken back up by the presynaptic neuron (Figure 12-79).

The parasympathetic system has two main types of ACh receptors, nicotinic and muscarinic. Knowing these receptors' locations and functions will greatly simplify learning the functions of drugs in this class. Nicotinic$_N$ (neuron) receptors are found in all autonomic ganglia, where acetylcholine serves as the presynaptic neurotransmitter of both the parasympathetic and sympathetic nervous systems. Nicotinic$_M$ (muscle) receptors are found at the neuromuscular junction and initiate muscular contraction as part of the somatic nervous system. Muscarinic receptors

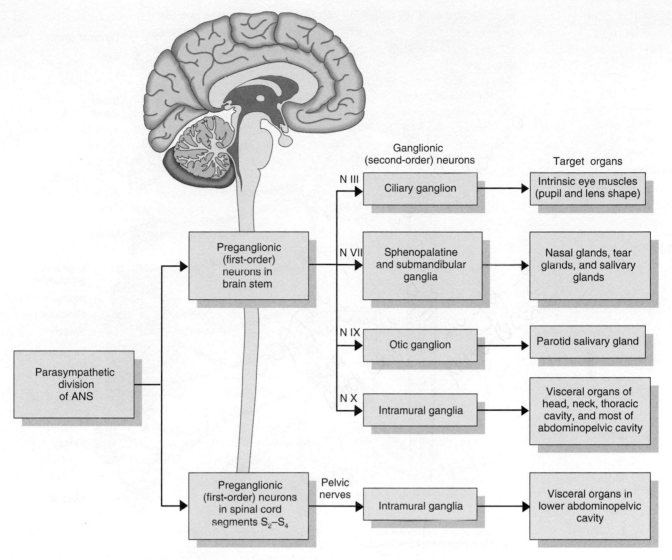

Ganglionic
(second-order) neurons

Target organs

| N III | Ciliary ganglion | Intrinsic eye muscles (pupil and lens shape) |

Preganglionic
(first-order)
neurons in
brain stem

| N VII | Sphenopalatine and submandibular ganglia | Nasal glands, tear glands, and salivary glands |

| N IX | Otic ganglion | Parotid salivary gland |

Parasympathetic
division
of ANS

| N X | Intramural ganglia | Visceral organs of head, neck, thoracic cavity, and most of abdominopelvic cavity |

Preganglionic
(first-order) neurons
in spinal cord
segments S₂–S₄

Pelvic nerves

| Intramural ganglia | Visceral organs in lower abdominopelvic cavity |

FIGURE 12-77   Organization of the parasympathetic division of the autonomic nervous system.

are found in many organs throughout the body and are primarily responsible for promoting the parasympathetic response. Table 12-4 summarizes the locations and actions of the muscarinic receptors.

THE ENDOCRINE SYSTEM

There are eight major glands in the endocrine system: the hypothalamus, pituitary gland, thyroid gland, parathyroid glands, thymus, pancreas, adrenal glands, and gonads. The pineal gland is also an endocrine gland, but much of its function remains unclear. In addition to the endocrine glands, many body tissues have been found to have endocrine function. These include the kidneys, heart, placenta, and parts of the digestive tract.

The endocrine glands are located throughout the body (Figure 12-80). Although Figure 12-80 shows an adult, remember that the thymus is primarily active during childhood, when it plays a role in maturation of the immune system. By adulthood, the thymus is so small that it is not visualized on chest x-rays. The hormones secreted by endocrine glands, their target tissues, and their effects are listed in Table 12-5.

Content Review

ENDOCRINE GLANDS
- Hypothalamus
- Pituitary
- Thyroid
- Parathyroid
- Thymus
- Pancreas
- Adrenals
- Gonads
- Pineal

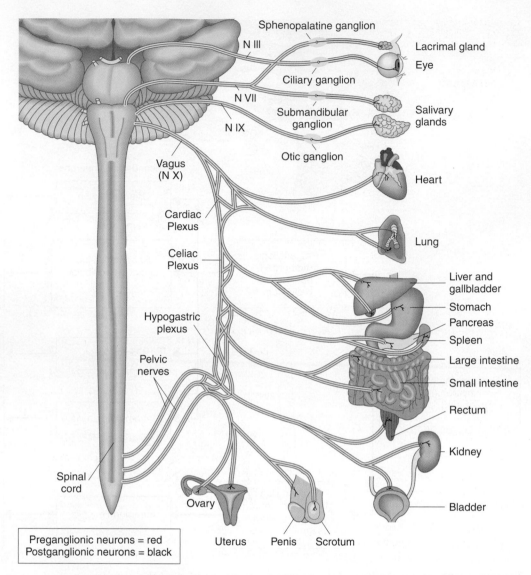

FIGURE 12-78   Distribution of the parasympathetic postganglionic fibres.

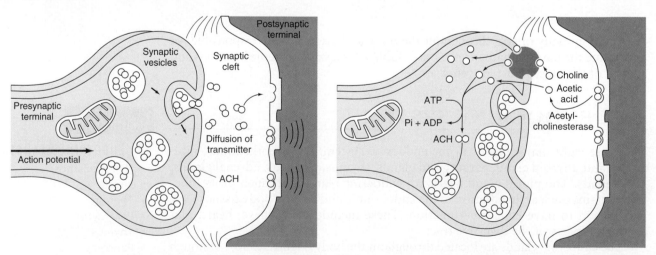

FIGURE 12-79   Physiology of a cholinergic synapse. Acetylcholine is released from the presynaptic nerve and stimulates receptors on the postsynaptic nerve. Subsequently, acetylcholinesterase breaks down the acetylcholine and the presynaptic nerve fibre takes up the products.

Table 12-4 LOCATION AND EFFECT OF MUSCARINIC RECEPTORS

Organ	Functions	Location
Heart	Decreased heart rate	Sinoatrial node
	Decreased conduction rate	Atrioventricular node
Arterioles	Dilation	Coronary
	Dilation	Skin and mucosa
	Dilation	Cerebral
GI tract	Relaxed	Sphincters
	Increased	Motility
	Increased salivation	Salivary glands
	Increased secretion	Exocrine glands
Lungs	Bronchoconstriction	Bronchiole smooth muscle
	Increased mucus production	Bronchial glands
Gallbladder	Contraction	
Urinary bladder	Relaxation	Urinary sphincter
	Contraction	Detrusor muscle
Liver	Glycogen synthesis	
Lacrimal glands	Secretion (increased tearing)	Eye
Eye	Contraction for near vision	Ciliary muscle
	Constriction	Pupil
Penis	Erection	

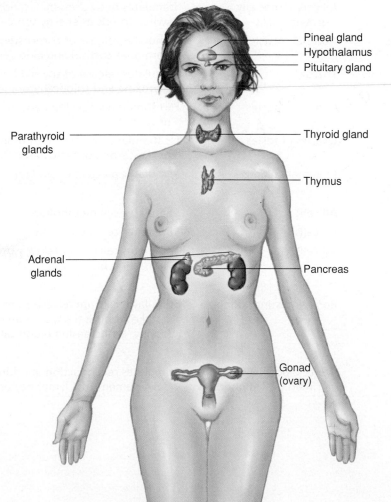

FIGURE 12-80 The major glands of the endocrine system.

Pineal gland
Hypothalamus
Pituitary gland
Parathyroid glands
Thyroid gland
Thymus
Adrenal glands
Pancreas
Gonad (ovary)

Table 12-5   ENDOCRINE SYSTEM: GLANDS, HORMONES, TARGET TISSUES, HORMONE EFFECTS

Gland and Major Hormone(s)	Target Tissues	Major Hormone Effect(s)
Hypothalamus		
Growth hormone-releasing hormone, GHRH	Anterior pituitary	Stimulates release of growth hormone
Growth hormone-inhibiting hormone, GHIH (or somatostatin)	Anterior pituitary	Suppresses release of growth hormone
Corticotropin-releasing hormone, CRH	Anterior pituitary	Stimulates release of adrenocorticotropin
Thyrotropin-releasing hormone, TRH	Anterior pituitary	Stimulates release of thyroid-stimulating hormone
Gonadotropin-releasing hormone, GnRH	Anterior pituitary	Stimulates release of luteinizing hormone and follicle-stimulating hormone
Prolactin-releasing hormone, PRH	Anterior pituitary	Stimulates release of prolactin
Prolactin-inhibiting hormone, PIH	Anterior pituitary	Suppresses release of prolactin
Posterior pituitary gland		
Antidiuretic hormone, ADH	Kidneys	Stimulates increased reabsorption of water into blood volume
Oxytocin	Uterus and breasts of females, kidneys	Stimulates uterine contractions and milk release
Anterior pituitary gland		
Growth hormone, GH	All cells, especially growing cells	Stimulates body growth in childhood; causes switch to fats as energy source
Adrenocorticotropic hormone, ACTH	Adrenal cortexes	Stimulates release of corticosteroidal hormones cortisol and aldosterone
Thyroid-stimulating hormone, TSH	Thyroid	Stimulates release of thyroid hormones thyroxine and triiodothyronine
Follicle-stimulating hormone, FSH	Ovaries or testes	FSH stimulates development of sex cells (ovum or sperm)
Luteinizing hormone, LH	Ovaries or testes	LH stimulates release of hormones (estrogen, progesterone or testosterone)
Prolactin, PRL	Mammary glands	Stimulates production and release of milk
Thyroid gland		
Thyroxine, T_4	All cells	Stimulates cell metabolism
Triiodothyronine, T_3	All cells	Stimulates cell metabolism
Calcitonin	All cells	Stimulates calcium uptake by bones, decreasing blood calcium level
Parathyroid glands		
Parathyroid hormone, PTH	Bone, intestine, kidneys	Stimulates calcium release from bone, calcium uptake from GI tract, calcium reabsorption in kidney, all increasing blood calcium level
Thymus		
Thymosin	White blood cells, primarily T lymphocytes	Stimulates reproduction and functional development of T lymphocytes

Gland and Major Hormone(s)	Target Tissues	Major Hormone Effect(s)
Pancreas		
Glucagon	All cells, particularly in liver, muscle, and fat	Stimulates hepatic glycogenolysis and gluconeogenesis, increasing blood glucose level
Insulin	All cells, particularly in liver, muscle, and fat	Stimulates cellular uptake of glucose, increased rate of synthesis of glycogen, proteins, and fats, decreasing blood glucose level
Somatostatin	Alpha and beta cells in the pancreas	Suppresses secretion of glucagon and insulin within islets of Langerhans
Adrenal medulla		
Epinephrine (or adrenaline)	Muscle, liver, cardiovascular system	Stimulates features of "fight or flight" response to stress
Norepinephrine	Muscle, liver, cardiovascular system	Stimulates vasoconstriction
Adrenal cortex		
Glucocorticoids		
Cortisol	Most cells, particularly white blood cells (cells responsible for inflammatory and immune responses)	Stimulates glucagon-like effects, acts as anti-inflammatory and immunosuppressive agent
Mineralocorticoids		
Aldosterone	Kidneys, blood	Contributes to salt and fluid balance by stimulating kidneys to increase potassium excretion and decrease sodium excretion, increasing blood volume
Androgenic hormones		
Estrogen	Most cells	See effects under Gonads (Ovaries and Testes)
Progesterone	Uterus	
Testosterone	Most cells	
Ovaries		
Estrogen	Most cells, particularly those of female reproductive tract	Stimulates development of secondary sexual characteristics, plays role in maturation of egg before ovulation
Progesterone	Uterus	Stimulates uterine changes necessary for successful pregnancy
Testes		
Testosterone	Most cells, particularly those of male reproductive tract	Stimulates development of secondary sexual characteristics, plays role in development of sperm cells
Pineal gland		
Melatonin	Exact action unknown	Releases melatonin in response to light, may help determine daily, lunar, and reproductive cycles, may affect mood

HYPOTHALAMUS

The *hypothalamus* is located deep within the cerebrum of the brain. Hypothalamic cells act both as nerve cells, or neurons, and as gland cells. The hypothalamus is the junction, or connection, between the central nervous system and the endocrine system. As neurons, many hypothalamic cells receive messages from the autonomic nervous system—peripheral nerves that, among other functions, detect internal conditions, such as blood pressure or blood glucose level, and convey that information to the central nervous system through nerve impulses. Some hypothalamic cells respond by producing nerve impulses that travel to cells in the posterior pituitary gland. Other hypothalamic cells respond as gland cells by producing and releasing hormones into the stalk of tissue that connects the hypothalamus and the anterior pituitary gland.

In response to impulses from the autonomic nervous system, the hypothalamus—and other organs of the endocrine system—can release the hormones that promote homeostasis:

- *Growth hormone-releasing hormone (GHRH)*
- *Growth hormone-inhibiting hormone (GHIH)*
- *Corticotropin-releasing hormone (CRH)*
- *Thyrotropin-releasing hormone (TRH)*
- *Gonadotropin-releasing hormone (GnRH)*
- *Prolactin-releasing hormone (PRH)*
- *Prolactin-inhibiting hormone (PIH)*

As you can see in Table 12-5, most hypothalamic hormones, including thyrotropin-releasing hormone (TRH) and growth hormone-releasing hormone (GHRH), stimulate secretion of pituitary hormones that rouse yet another endocrine gland or body tissue to increased activity. For example, in response to TRH the anterior pituitary releases thyroid stimulating hormone, and thyroid stimulating hormone then acts on the thyroid gland to increase thyroid activity.

The pair of hypothalamic hormones—growth hormone-releasing hormone (GHRH) and growth hormone-inhibiting hormone (GHIH)—demonstrate a major trait of endocrine function: Many hormonal activities are driven not by one hormone but rather by two hormones with opposing effects. GHRH stimulates secretion of growth hormone, and GHIH suppresses secretion of growth hormone. The actual amount of growth hormone secreted by the anterior pituitary depends on the net amount of stimulation (Figure 12-81).

FIGURE 12-81   Regulation by hormone pairs. The net level of stimulation created by the opposing actions of growth hormone-releasing hormone (GHRH) and growth hormone-inhibiting hormone (GHIH) determines the amount of growth hormone (GH) secreted by the anterior pituitary.

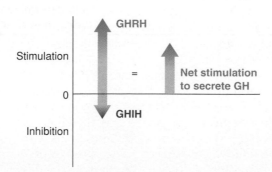

PITUITARY GLAND

The *pituitary gland* is only about the size of a pea. It is divided into posterior and anterior pituitary lobes. These tissues have different embryonic origins and different functional relationships with the hypothalamus. The *posterior pituitary gland* responds to nerve impulses from the hypothalamus, whereas the *anterior pituitary gland* responds to hypothalamic hormones that travel down the stalk that connects the anterior pituitary and hypothalamus. As you look at the target tissues of the anterior pituitary in Table 12-5, you will understand why physiologists once thought of the pituitary gland as the "master gland." Its hormones have a direct impact on endocrine glands throughout the body. The term isn't used much anymore because the dependence of the pituitary on the hypothalamus has been made clear.

As noted above, the pituitary gland has two lobes, the posterior and the anterior.

Posterior Pituitary

The posterior pituitary produces two hormones:

- *Antidiuretic hormone (ADH)*—causes retention of body water
- *Oxytocin*—causes uterine contraction and lactation

Antidiuretic hormone (ADH), also known as vasopressin, causes the kidneys to increase water reabsorption. This retention of water, or antidiuretic effect, results in increased circulating blood volume and decreased urine volume. Increased secretion of ADH is part of the homeostatic mechanism that can counteract losses of blood volume up to about 25 percent. Clinically, you will see increased ADH secretion in early shock states associated with dehydration or hemorrhage. Note that the opposite effect, decreased secretion of ADH, occurs after ingestion of alcohol and when there is a significant rise in circulating blood volume.

Although it is unlikely that a disorder in ADH secretion will present as a medical emergency, you should understand such endocrine dysfunction when patients discuss their medical histories. *Diabetes insipidus,* a disorder marked by large volumes of urine, is caused by inadequate ADH secretion relative to blood volume. The resultant reduction of blood volume, or diuretic effect, appears as excessive urine production. In a 24-hour period, the kidneys normally produce 1 to 1.5 litres of urine. In diabetes insipidus, it is not uncommon for urine output to increase to almost 20 litres per day. You can remember the characteristic urine presentation of diabetes insipidus by remembering that dilute urine has an insipid, or neutral, odour (and taste).

Oxytocin, the natural form of the drug Pitocin, stimulates uterine contraction and lactation in women who have just delivered a baby. Oxytocin actually causes the "letdown" of milk by stimulating contractile cells within the mammary glands. An infant suckling at the breast stimulates receptors in the nipples that causes the release of oxytocin from the posterior pituitary. This, in turn, causes discharge of milk so that the infant can feed. Following delivery, it is recommended that the infant be placed on the breast to suckle, thus stimulating the release of oxytocin. In addition to stimulating milk letdown, the oxytocin stimulates uterine contraction, which can help minimize postpartum bleeding.

In both sexes, oxytocin has a mild antidiuretic effect, which is similar to that of ADH due to their chemical similarity. The relationship between oxytocin and ADH has direct application to emergency medicine. Women in preterm labour are often given an IV fluid bolus in an attempt to suppress uterine contractions without the use of drugs. This works in the following way: The administration of IV fluid bolus causes an increase in circulating blood volume, which is detected by autonomic nerves in the kidneys. An impulse is sent through the hypothalamus to the posterior pituitary, where it causes decreased secretion of ADH. This inhibition of ADH secretion, in turn, triggers decreased secretion of oxytocin, which contributes to the observed increase in urine production and, one hopes, the goal of suppression of preterm labour.

Anterior Pituitary

Because almost all of the anterior pituitary hormones regulate other endocrine glands, disorders directly involving the anterior pituitary are rarely a factor in endocrine emergencies. Table 12-5 lists the six hormones secreted by the anterior pituitary, as well as target tissues and hormone effects. As you can see, five of the six hormones regulate the activity of target glands, while the sixth affects almost all cells:

Five anterior pituitary hormones affect target glands.

1. *Adrenocorticotropic hormone (ACTH)*—targets the adrenal cortexes
2. *Thyroid-stimulating hormone (TSH)*—targets the thyroid
3. *Follicle-stimulating hormone (FSH)*—targets the gonads, or sex organs
4. *Luteinizing hormone (LH)*—also targets the gonads
5. *Prolactin (PRL)*—targets the mammary glands of women

The sixth anterior pituitary hormone has a broader effect.

6. *Growth hormone (GH)*—targets almost all body cells

GH has its most significant effects in children because it is the primary stimulant of skeletal growth. In adults, GH has several physiological effects, but the most significant is metabolic. GH causes adipose cells to release their stored fats into the blood and causes body cells to switch from glucose to fats as the primary energy source. The net effect is that the body uses up fat stores and conserves its sugar stores.

THYROID GLAND

The two lobes of the *thyroid gland* are located in the neck anterior to and just below the cartilage of the larynx, with one lobe on either side of the midline. The two lobes are connected by a small isthmus, or band of tissue, that crosses the trachea at the level of the cricoid cartilage. The thyroid produces three hormones:

1. *Thyroxine (T_4)*—stimulates cell metabolism
2. *Triiodothyronine (T_3)*—stimulates cell metabolism
3. *Calcitonin*—lowers blood calcium levels

The thyroid comprises tiny hollow sacs called follicles, which are filled with a thick fluid called *colloid*. The hormones *thyroxine (T_4)* and *triiodothyronine (T_3)* are produced within the colloid. When stimulated by the pituitary hormone TSH or by environmental conditions, such as cold, the thyroid gland releases these hormones to increase the general rate of cell metabolism.

The thyroid gland also contains perifollicular cells called C cells which produce a different hormone, *calcitonin*. Calcitonin lowers blood calcium levels by increasing uptake of calcium by bones and inhibiting breakdown of bone tissue. Parathyroid hormone has the opposite, or antagonistic, effect on the blood calcium level, which is covered in the following discussion of the parathyroid glands.

Disorders of excessive or deficient production of thyroid hormones T_4 and T_3, are called hyperthyroidism and hypothyroidism, respectively.

PARATHYROID GLANDS

Each *parathyroid gland* is very small, with a maximum diameter of 5 mm and weight of only 35 to 40 mg. Normally, four parathyroid glands are located on the posterior lateral surfaces of the thyroid, one pair above the other. Sometimes, there are more than four parathyroid glands, but only rarely are there fewer. The parathyroid glands secrete:

- *Parathyroid hormone (PTH)*—increases blood calcium levels

PTH increases blood calcium levels through actions on three different target tissues. In bone, the primary target, PTH causes release of calcium into the blood. In the intestines, PTH converts vitamin D into its active form, causing increased absorption of calcium. In the kidneys, PTH causes increased reabsorption of calcium. PTH is the antagonist of calcitonin, and the balance of PTH and calcitonin determines the level of blood calcium. The parathyroid glands rarely cause clinical problems. However, they can be accidentally damaged or removed during surgery, or they may be damaged if the thyroid gland is irradiated. In either case, the loss of parathyroid function may result in hypocalcemia, low blood calcium levels.

THYMUS GLAND

The *thymus* is in the mediastinum just behind the sternum. It is fairly large in children but shrinks into a small remnant of fat and fibrous tissue in adults. Although the thymus is usually considered a lymphatic organ on the basis of its anatomy, its most important function is as an endocrine gland. During childhood, it secretes:

- *Thymosin*—promotes maturation of T lymphocytes

Thymosin is critical to maturation of T lymphocytes, the cells responsible for cell-mediated immunity. The T of T lymphocyte stands for thymus.

PANCREAS

The *pancreas,* located in the upper retroperitoneum behind the stomach and between the duodenum and spleen, comprises both endocrine and exocrine tissues. The exocrine tissues, known as acini, secrete digestive enzymes essential to digestion of fats and proteins into a duct that empties into the small intestine.

The microscopic clusters of endocrine tissue found within the pancreas are known as *islets of Langerhans.* Although there are 1 to 2 million islets interspersed throughout the pancreas, they compose only about 2 percent of its total mass. The three most important types of endocrine cells in the islets of Langerhans are termed *alpha (α), beta (β),* and *delta (δ)* (Figure 12-82). Each type produces and secretes a different hormone. In addition, the islets contain a much smaller number of cells called polypeptide cells. These cells produce pancreatic polypeptide (PP), the function of which is still unclear.

The alpha and beta cells produce two hormones essential for homeostasis of blood glucose:

- *Glucagon*—increases blood glucose
- *Insulin*—decreases blood glucose

FIGURE 12-82 The internal anatomy of the pancreas.

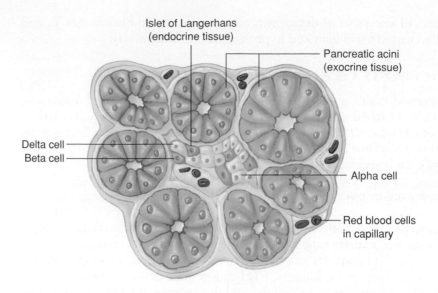

Islet of Langerhans (endocrine tissue)

Pancreatic acini (exocrine tissue)

Delta cell

Beta cell

Alpha cell

Red blood cells in capillary

✱ glycogenolysis the breakdown of glycogen to glucose, primarily by liver cells.

✱ gluconeogenesis conversion of protein and fat to form glucose.

Approximately 25 percent of islet tissue is made up of alpha cells. Alpha cells produce the hormone *glucagon*. When the blood glucose level falls, alpha cells increase secretion of glucagon. Glucagon stimulates the breakdown of glycogen, the complex carbohydrate that is the storage form of glucose, into individual glucose molecules that are released into the blood. This process, called **glycogenolysis,** takes place in more than one tissue, but activity in the liver is by far the most important in raising blood glucose level.

The liver is the largest and heaviest of the internal organs, and so it has many cells that can contain glycogen. In addition, liver cells have the greatest capacity to store glycogen—liver cells can store 5 to 8 percent of their weight as glycogen. Compare this with the capacity of skeletal muscle (1 to 3 percent), another important storage tissue in the body. In addition to stimulating glycogenolysis, the hormone glucagon also stimulates liver breakdown of body proteins and fats with subsequent chemical conversion to glucose. This second process, which produces glucose from nonsugar sources, is called **gluconeogenesis.** Both processes contribute to homeostasis by raising the blood glucose level.

Beta cells make up about 60 percent of islet tissue, and they produce the hormone *insulin*. Insulin is the antagonist of glucagon: Insulin lowers the blood glucose level by increasing the uptake of glucose by body cells. In addition, insulin promotes energy storage in the body by increasing the synthesis of glycogen, protein, and fat. Because the liver removes circulating insulin within 10 to 15 minutes from time of secretion, it must be secreted constantly to sustain an appropriate balance of glucagon and insulin—a balance that results in a steady supply of glucose for immediate use as an energy source and for appropriate energy storage. Loss of functional beta cells leads to increased blood glucose levels as seen in diabetes.

Delta cells, which comprise about 10 percent of islet tissue, produce *somatostatin*. This hormone acts within islets to inhibit secretion of glucagon and insulin. Somatostatin also retards nutrient absorption from the intestines, although its mechanisms of action in the gut are poorly understood. As you look at Table 12-5, note that somatostatin is the same substance as growth hormone-inhibiting hormone (GHIH).

ADRENAL GLANDS

The paired *adrenal glands* are located on the superior surface of the kidneys. Each gland has two distinct anatomical divisions with different functions. The inner portion of the adrenal gland is called the *adrenal medulla,* and its cells behave both as nerve cells and as gland cells. The adrenal medulla is intimately related to the sympathetic component of the autonomic nervous system. When sympathetic nerves carry an impulse into the adrenal medulla, its cells respond by secreting the catecholamine hormones *epinephrine* (or adrenalin) and *norepinephrine* into the bloodstream. The outer portion of the adrenal gland is called the *adrenal cortex,* and it consists of endocrine tissue. The adrenal cortex secretes three classes of steroidal hormones that differ only slightly in chemical structure but have very distinct effects in the body:

1. *Glucocorticoids,* of which *cortisol* is by far the most important, account for 95 percent of adrenocortical hormone production. Like glucagon, they increase the blood glucose level by promoting gluconeogenesis and decreasing glucose utilization as an energy source. If you recall that cortisone is a commonly used medical glucocorticoid, you will realize that this class of hormones also inhibits inflammatory reactions and immune-system responses as well as potentiates the effects of catecholamines. The anterior pituitary hormone that promotes release, ACTH, is secreted in response to stress, trauma, or serious infection.

2. *Mineralocorticoids,* of which *aldosterone* is the most important, contribute to salt and fluid balance in the body by regulating sodium and potassium excretion through the kidneys.

3. *Androgenic* hormones have the same effects as those secreted by gonads, and they will be covered in that discussion.

You may see disorders related to deficient or excessive secretion of adrenal hormones present as medical emergencies.

Gonads

Some differences in the *gonads* are obvious: Ovaries produce eggs, whereas testes produce sperm cells. However, the gonads of both sexes share one vital function: They are the endocrine glands chiefly responsible for the sexual maturation of puberty and any subsequent reproduction.

Ovaries

The *ovaries,* or female gonads, are paired organs about the size of an almond that are located in the pelvis on either side of the uterus. Under the regulation of the anterior pituitary hormones FSH and LH, the ovaries produce:

- *Estrogen*
- *Progesterone*

The hormone *estrogen* promotes the development and maintenance of secondary female sexual characteristics. Estrogen also plays a role in the egg development that precedes ovulation during each menstrual cycle. *Progesterone* is familiarly known as the "hormone of pregnancy" because it is necessary for implantation of the fertilized egg and maintenance of the uterine lining throughout pregnancy. Estrogen also serves to protect the female against heart disease. When estrogen levels fall at menopause, the female's risk of developing heart disease quickly increases to the level of the male's. In addition, the ovaries produce small amounts of *testosterone,* which influences some body changes associated with puberty.

Testes

The male gonads, or *testes*, are located outside of the abdominal cavity in the scrotum. Under the regulation of the anterior pituitary hormones FSH and LH, the testes produce:

- *Testosterone*

The hormone *testosterone* promotes the development and maintenance of secondary male sexual characteristics and plays a role in development of sperm.

PINEAL GLAND

The *pineal gland* is located in the roof of the thalamus in the brain. Its function has remained somewhat elusive. However, it has been shown that the pineal gland releases the hormone *melatonin* in response to changes in light. For example, melatonin production is lowest during daylight hours and highest in the dark of the night. Because of this, the pineal is felt to help determine day-length and lunar cycles and plays a role in controlling the reproductive "biological clock." Melatonin may affect a person's mood. The pineal gland has been implicated in "seasonal affective disorder (SAD)," which is characterized by severe depression during the winter months. Further research will help clarify the role of melatonin.

OTHER ORGANS WITH ENDOCRINE ACTIVITY

We have discussed the principal glands of the endocrine system. Many tissues not considered part of the endocrine system have important endocrine functions. There are organs in other systems that secrete hormones directly into the blood. The placenta can be considered an endocrine gland because of its secretion of *human chorionic gonadotropin (hCG)* throughout gestation. It is the early secretion of hCG that is detected by at-home pregnancy tests. In the digestive tract, gastric and intestinal mucosa produce the hormones *gastrin* and *secretin,* both of which regulate digestive function.

Additionally, there are hormone-producing cells in the atrial walls of the heart. *Atrial natriuretic hormone (ANH)* is secreted by certain atrial cells in response to increased stretching of the atrial walls due to abnormally high blood volume or blood pressure. The hormone ANH is an antagonist to ADH and inhibits secretion of aldosterone, thus contributing to a homeostatic reduction in blood volume by increasing urine production.

The kidneys also have some endocrine function. Certain kidney cells will react to a decrease in blood volume or blood pressure by releasing the enzyme *renin.* Renin acts on *angiotensinogen,* converting it to *angiotensin I.* In the lungs, angiotensin I is converted to *angiotensin II* by *angiotensin-converting enzyme (ACE).* Angiotensin II stimulates the adrenal production of aldosterone, which causes water retention by the kidneys. This leads to increased blood volume and blood pressure. In addition to renin, the kidneys secrete the hormone erythropoietin that stimulates the production of red blood cells by the bone marrow.

THE CARDIOVASCULAR SYSTEM

The cardiovascular system's two major components are the heart and the peripheral blood vessels.

ANATOMY OF THE HEART

The *heart* is a muscular organ, approximately the size of a closed fist. It is in the centre of the chest in the mediastinum, anterior to the spine and posterior to the sternum (Figure 12-83). Approximately two-thirds of the heart's mass is to the left of the midline, with the remainder to the right. The bottom of the heart, or *apex*, is just above the diaphragm, left of the midline. The top of the heart, or *base*, lies at approximately the level of the second rib. The great vessels connect to the heart through the base.

Tissue Layers

The heart consists of three tissue layers: endocardium, myocardium, and pericardium (Figure 12-84). The *endocardium* is the innermost layer. It lines the heart's chambers and is bathed in blood. The *myocardium* is the thick middle layer of the heart. Its cells are unique in that they physically resemble skeletal muscle but have electrical properties similar to smooth muscle. These cells also contain specialized structures that help rapidly conduct electrical impulses from one muscle cell to another, enabling the heart to contract.

The *pericardium* is a protective sac surrounding the heart. It consists of two layers, visceral and parietal. The *visceral pericardium*, also called the *epicardium*, is the inner layer, in contact with the heart muscle itself. The *parietal pericardium* is the outer, fibrous layer. In the pericardial cavity, between these two layers, is about 25 mL of pericardial fluid, a straw-coloured lubricant that reduces friction as the heart beats and changes position. Certain disease processes and injuries can increase the amount of fluid in this sac, compressing the heart and decreasing cardiac output.

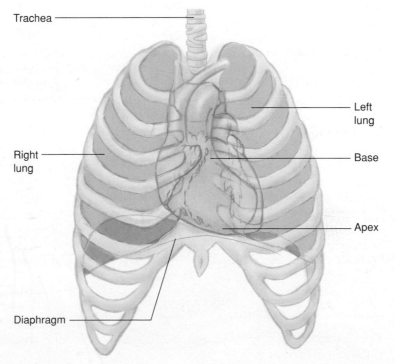

Trachea

Left lung

Right lung

Base

Apex

Diaphragm

FIGURE 12-83   Location of the heart within the chest.

FIGURE 12-84   Layers of
the heart.

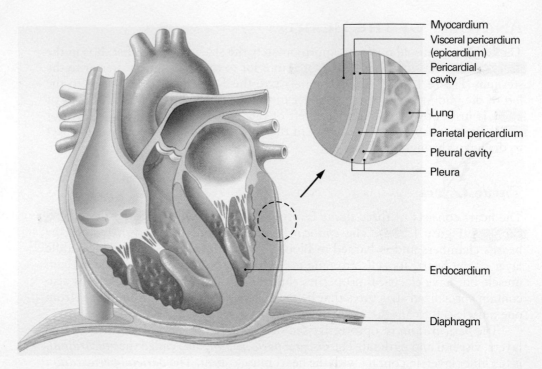

Myocardium
Visceral pericardium
(epicardium)
Pericardial
cavity

Lung
Parietal pericardium
Pleural cavity
Pleura

Endocardium

Diaphragm

Chambers

The heart contains four chambers (Figure 12-85). The *atria*, the two superior chambers, receive incoming blood. The *ventricles*, the two larger, inferior chambers, pump blood out of the heart. The right and left atria are separated by the *interatrial septum*. The ventricles are separated by the *interventricular septum*. Both septa contain fibrous connective tissue as well as contractile muscle. The walls of the atria are much thinner than those of the ventricles and do not contribute significantly to the heart's pumping action.

FIGURE 12-85   The chambers
of the heart.

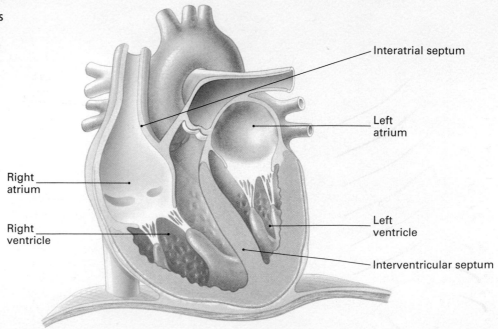

Interatrial septum

Left
atrium

Right
atrium

Left
ventricle

Right
ventricle

Interventricular septum

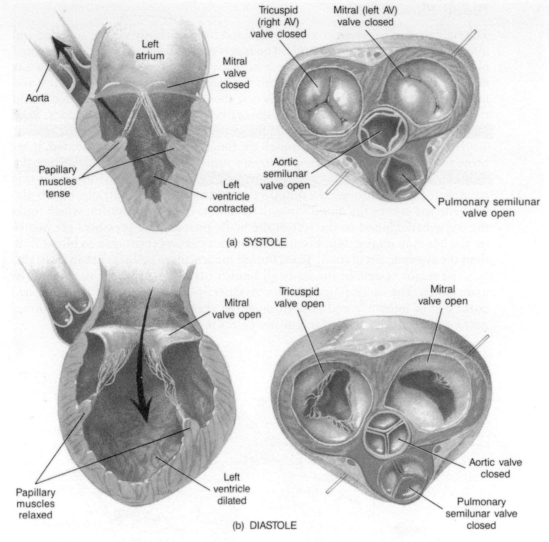

Left atrium

Aorta

Mitral valve closed

Papillary muscles tense

Left ventricle contracted

Tricuspid (right AV) valve closed

Mitral (left AV) valve closed

Aortic semilunar valve open

Pulmonary semilunar valve open

(a) SYSTOLE

Mitral valve open

Tricuspid valve open

Mitral valve open

Papillary muscles relaxed

Left ventricle dilated

Aortic valve closed

Pulmonary semilunar valve closed

(b) DIASTOLE

FIGURE 12-86   The valves of the heart.

Valves

The heart contains two pairs of valves, the *atrioventricular valves* and the *semilunar valves,* made of endocardial and connective tissue (Figure 12-86). The atrioventricular valves control blood flow between the atria and the ventricles. The right atrioventricular valve is called the *tricuspid valve* because it has three leaflets, or cusps. The left atrioventricular valve, called the *mitral valve,* has two leaflets. These valves are connected to specialized *papillary muscles* in the ventricles. When relaxed, these papillary muscles open the valves and allow blood flow between the two chambers. Specialized fibres called *chordae tendoneae* connect the valves' leaflets to the papillary muscles. They prevent the valves from prolapsing into the atria and allowing backflow during ventricular contraction.

The semilunar valves regulate blood flow between the ventricles and the arteries into which they empty. The left semilunar valve, or aortic valve, connects the left ventricle to the aorta. The right semilunar valve, or pulmonic valve, connects the right ventricle to the pulmonary artery. These valves permit one-way movement of blood and prevent backflow.

Blood Flow

The right atrium receives deoxygenated blood from the body via the superior and inferior venae cavae (Figure 12-87). The *superior vena cava* receives deoxygenated blood from the head and upper extremities, the *inferior vena cava* from the areas below the heart. The right atrium pumps this blood through the tricuspid valve and into the right ventricle. The right ventricle then pumps the deoxygenated blood through the pulmonic valve to the *pulmonary artery* and on to the lungs. (The pulmonary artery is the only artery in the body that carries deoxygenated blood.)

After the blood circulates through the lungs and becomes oxygenated, it returns to the left atrium via the *pulmonary veins*. (The pulmonary veins are the only veins in the body that carry oxygenated blood.) The left atrium sends this oxygenated blood through the mitral valve and into the left ventricle. Finally the left ventricle pumps the blood through the aortic valve to the aorta, which feeds the oxygenated blood to the rest of the body. Intracardiac pressures are higher on the left than on the right because the lungs offer less resistance to blood flow than the systemic circulation. Thus, the left myocardium is thicker than the right.

The major vessels of the body all branch off of the aorta, which has three main parts. The *ascending aorta* comes directly from the heart. The *thoracic aorta* curves inferiorly and goes through the chest (or thorax). The *abdominal aorta* goes through the diaphragm and enters the abdomen.

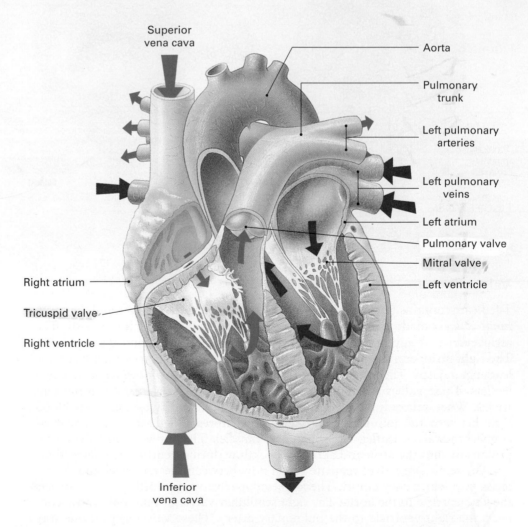

FIGURE 12-87 Blood flow through the heart.

Superior vena cava

Aorta

Pulmonary trunk

Left pulmonary arteries

Left pulmonary veins

Left atrium

Pulmonary valve

Mitral valve

Left ventricle

Right atrium

Tricuspid valve

Right ventricle

Inferior vena cava

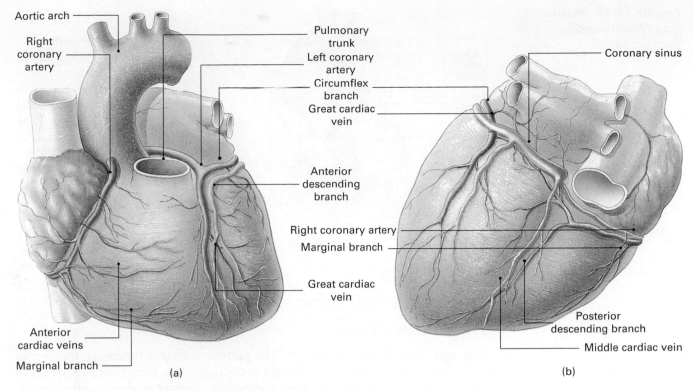

FIGURE 12-88   The coronary circulation: (a) anterior; (b) posterior.

Coronary Circulation

Although the endocardium is bathed in blood, the heart does not receive its nutrients from the blood within its chambers but from the *coronary arteries* (Figure 12-88). The coronary arteries originate in the aorta, just above the leaflets of
the aortic valve. The main coronary arteries lie on the surface of the heart, and
small penetrating arterioles supply the myocardial muscle. The *left coronary artery* supplies the left ventricle, the interventricular septum, part of the right ventricle, and the heart's conduction system. Its two major branches are the *anterior
descending artery* and the *circumflex artery.*

The *right coronary artery* supplies a portion of the right atrium and right ventricle and part of the conduction system. Its two major branches are the *posterior
descending artery* and the *marginal artery.* (Although the blood supply to most
people's hearts follows this pattern, anatomical variants do exist.) The coronary
vessels receive blood during diastole, when the heart relaxes, because the aortic
valve leaflets cover the coronary artery openings (*ostia*) during systole, when the
heart contracts.

Blood drains from the left coronary system via the *anterior great cardiac vein*
and the *lateral marginal veins.* These empty into the *coronary sinus.* The right
coronary artery empties directly into the right atrium via smaller cardiac veins.

Many **anastomoses** (communications between two or more vessels) among
the various branches of the coronary arteries allow *collateral circulation.* Collateral circulation is a protective mechanism that provides an alternative path for
blood flow in case of a blockage somewhere in the system. This is analogous to
a river's developing small tributaries to reach a larger body of water.

✱ **anastomosis** communication
between two or more vessels.

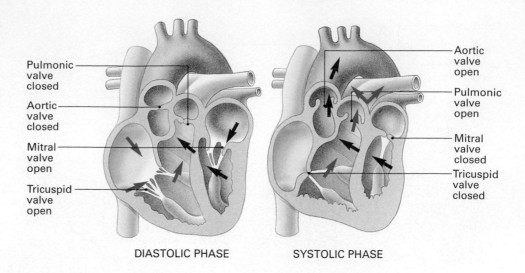

FIGURE 12-89 Relation of blood flow to cardiac contractions.

Pulmonic valve closed
Aortic valve closed
Mitral valve open
Tricuspid valve open

Aortic valve open
Pulmonic valve open
Mitral valve closed
Tricuspid valve closed

DIASTOLIC PHASE   SYSTOLIC PHASE

CARDIAC PHYSIOLOGY

The Cardiac Cycle

Although the heart's right and left sides perform different functions, they act as a unit. The right and left atria contract at the same time, filling both ventricles to their maximum capacities. Both ventricles then contract at the same time, ejecting blood into the pulmonary and systemic circulations. The pressure of the contraction closes the tricuspid and mitral valves and opens the aortic and pulmonic valves at the same time.

The **cardiac cycle** is the sequence of events that occurs between the end of one heart contraction and the end of the next. To evaluate heart sounds and read electrocardiographs, you must thoroughly understand the pumping action of the cardiac cycle (Figure 12-89). Diastole, the first phase of the cardiac cycle, is the relaxation phase. This is when ventricular filling begins. Blood enters the ventricles through the mitral and tricuspid valves. The pulmonic and aortic valves are closed.

During the second phase, systole, the heart contracts. The atria contract first, to finish emptying their blood into the ventricles. Atrial systole is relatively quick and occurs just before ventricular contraction; in healthy hearts, this atrial "kick" boosts cardiac output. The pressure in the ventricles now increases until it exceeds the pressure in the aorta and pulmonary artery. At this point, blood flows out of the ventricles through the pulmonic and aortic valves and into the arteries. The pressure also closes the mitral and tricuspid valves and, if working properly, prevents backflow of blood into the atria. When pressures in the artery exceed the pressures in the ventricles, the valves close, and diastole begins again.

Nervous Control of the Heart

The sympathetic and parasympathetic components of the autonomic nervous system work in direct opposition to one another to regulate the heart. In the heart's normal state the two systems balance. In stressful situations, however, the sympathetic system becomes dominant, while during sleep the parasympathetic system dominates. The sympathetic nervous system innervates the heart through the *cardiac plexus,* a network of nerves at the base of the heart (Figure 12-90).

The sympathetic nerves arise from the thoracic and lumbar regions of the spinal cord, then leave the spinal cord and form the sympathetic chain, which runs along the spinal column. The cardiac plexus arises, in turn, from ganglia in the sympathetic chain and innervates both the atria and ventricles. The chemical

* **cardiac cycle** the period of time from the end of one cardiac contraction to the end of the next.

* **diastole** the period of time when the myocardium is relaxed and cardiac filling and coronary perfusion occur.

* **systole** the period of the cardiac cycle when the myocardium is contracting.

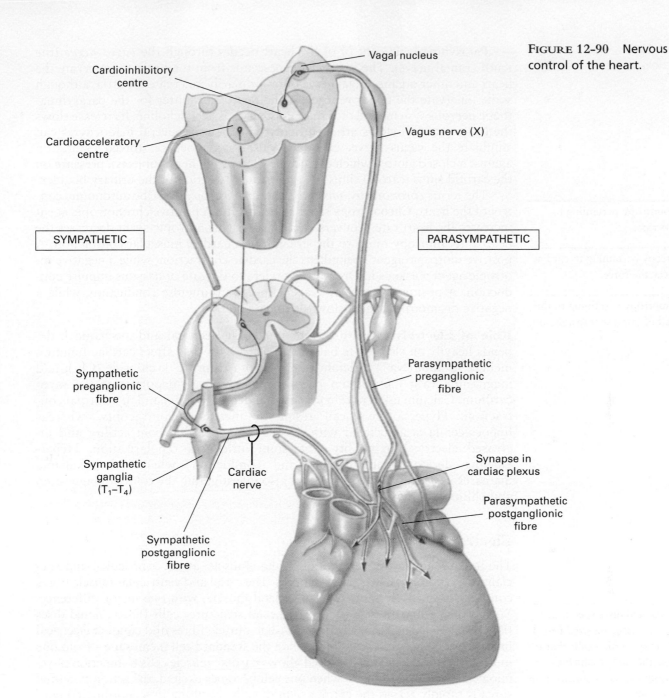

FIGURE 12-90 Nervous control of the heart.

Cardioinhibitory centre

Vagal nucleus

Cardioaccelleratory centre

Vagus nerve (X)

SYMPATHETIC

PARASYMPATHETIC

Sympathetic preganglionic fibre

Parasympathetic preganglionic fibre

Sympathetic ganglia (T_1–T_4)

Cardiac nerve

Synapse in cardiac plexus

Parasympathetic postganglionic fibre

Sympathetic postganglionic fibre

neurotransmitter for the sympathetic nervous system, and thus for the cardiac plexus, is norepinephrine. Its release increases heart rate and cardiac contractile force, primarily through its actions on beta receptors.

As noted earlier, the sympathetic nervous system has two principal types of receptors, alpha and beta. Alpha receptors are located in the peripheral blood vessels and are responsible for vasoconstriction. $Beta_1$ receptors, primarily located in the heart, increase the heart rate and contractility. $Beta_2$ receptors, principally located in the lungs and peripheral blood vessels, cause bronchodilation and peripheral vasodilation. Medications specific to these various receptors cause different physiological effects. For instance, beta blockers slow the heart rate and lower blood pressure by blocking the $beta_1$ receptors, whose job is to increase heart rate and contractility.

Parasympathetic control of the heart occurs through the *vagus nerve* (the tenth cranial nerve). The vagus nerve descends from the brain to innervate the heart and other organs. Vagal nerve fibres primarily innervate the atria, although some innervate the upper ventricles. The neurotransmitter for the parasympathetic nervous system, and thus the vagus nerve, is acetylcholine. Its release slows the heart rate and slows atrioventricular conduction. Several manoeuvres can stimulate the vagus nerve, including Valsalva manoeuvre (forced expiration against a closed glottis, which can occur when lifting heavy objects), pressure on the carotid sinus (carotid sinus massage), and distention of the urinary bladder.

The terms *chronotropy, inotropy,* and *dromotropy* describe autonomic control of the heart. **Chronotropy** refers to heart rate. A positive chronotropic agent increases the heart rate. Conversely, a negative chronotropic agent decreases the heart rate. **Inotropy** refers to the strength of a cardiac muscular contraction. A positive inotropic agent strengthens the cardiac contraction, while a negative inotropic agent weakens it. **Dromotropy** refers to the rate of nervous impulse conduction. A positive dromotropic agent speeds up impulse conduction, while a negative dromotropic agent slows down conduction.

Role of Electrolytes Cardiac function, both electrical and mechanical, depends heavily on electrolyte balances. Electrolytes that affect cardiac function include sodium (Na^+), calcium (Ca^{++}), potassium (K^+), chloride (Cl^-), and magnesium (Mg^{++}). Sodium plays a major role in depolarizing the myocardium. Calcium takes part in myocardial depolarization and myocardial contraction. Hypercalcemia can result in increased contractility, whereas hypocalcemia is associated with decreased myocardial contractility and increased electrical irritability. Potassium influences repolarization. Hyperkalemia decreases automaticity and conduction, whereas hypokalemia increases irritability. New research is also investigating the roles of magnesium and chloride in the cardiac cycle.

Electrophysiology

The heart comprises three types of cardiac muscle: atrial, ventricular, and specialized excitatory and conductive fibres. The atrial and ventricular muscle fibres contract in much the same way as skeletal muscle, with one major difference. Within the cardiac muscle fibres are special structures called **intercalated discs** (Figure 12-91). These discs connect cardiac muscle fibres and conduct electrical impulses quickly—400 times faster than the standard cell membrane—from one muscle fibre to the next. This speed allows cardiac muscle cells to function physiologically as a unit. That is, when one cell becomes excited, the action potential spreads rapidly across the entire group of cells, resulting in a coordinated contraction. This functional unit is a **syncytium**.

The heart has two syncytia—the *atrial syncytium* and the *ventricular syncytium*. The atrial syncytium contracts from superior to inferior so that the atria express blood to the ventricles. The ventricular syncytium, on the other hand, contracts from inferior to superior, expelling blood from the ventricles into the aorta and pulmonary arteries. The syncytia are separated from one another by the fibrous structure that supports the valves and physically separates the atria from the ventricles. The only way an impulse can be conducted from the atria to the ventricles is through the *atrioventricular (AV) bundle.* Cardiac muscle functions according to an "all-or-none" principle. That is, if a single muscle fibre becomes *depolarized,* the action potential will spread through the whole syncytium. Stimulating a single atrial fibre will thus completely depolarize the atria, and stimulating a single ventricular fibre will completely depolarize the ventricles.

❋ chronotropy pertaining to heart rate.

❋ inotropy pertaining to cardiac contractile force.

❋ dromotropy pertaining to the speed of impulse transmission.

❋ intercalated discs specialized bands of tissue inserted between myocardial cells that increase the rate in which the action potential is spread from cell to cell.

❋ syncytium group of cardiac muscle cells that physiologically function as a unit.

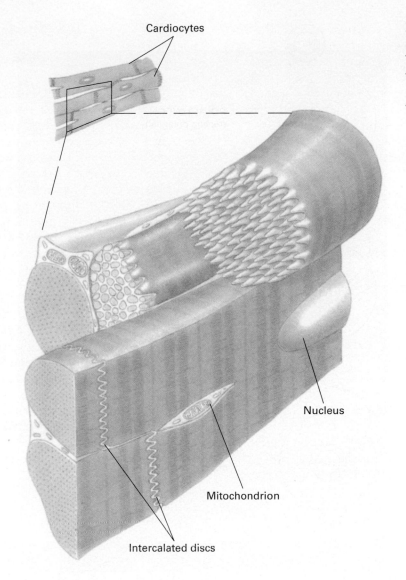

Cardiocytes

Nucleus

Mitochondrion

Intercalated discs

Cardiac Depolarization

Understanding **cardiac depolarization** is essential to interpreting electrocardiograms (ECGs). Normally, an ionic difference exists on the two sides of a cell membrane. The cell's sodium-potassium pump expels sodium (Na^+) from the cell. This leaves more negatively charged anions inside the cell than positively charged cations. Thus, the inside of the cell is more negatively charged than the outside. This difference, called the **resting potential,** can be measured experimentally by placing one probe inside the cell and another outside the cell and determining the difference in millivolts (mV). The resting potential in a myocardial cell is approximately 290 mV (Figure 12-92).

When the myocardial cell is stimulated, the membrane surrounding the cell changes instantaneously to allow sodium ions to rush into the cell, bringing with them their positive charge. This charge is so strong that it gives the inside of the cell a positive charge approximately 120 mV greater than the outside. This influx of sodium and change of membrane polarity is the **action potential.** After the influx of sodium, a slower influx of calcium ions (Ca^{++}) through the calcium channels increases the positive charge inside the cell. Once depolarization occurs in a muscle fibre, it is transmitted throughout the entire syncytium, via the intercalated

* **cardiac depolarization** a reversal of charges at a cell membrane so that the inside of the cell becomes positive in relation to the outside; the opposite of the cell's resting state in which the inside of the cell is negative in relation to the outside.

* **resting potential** the normal electrical state of cardiac cells.

* **action potential** the stimulation of myocardial cells, as evidenced by a change in the membrane electrical charge, that subsequently spreads across the myocardium.

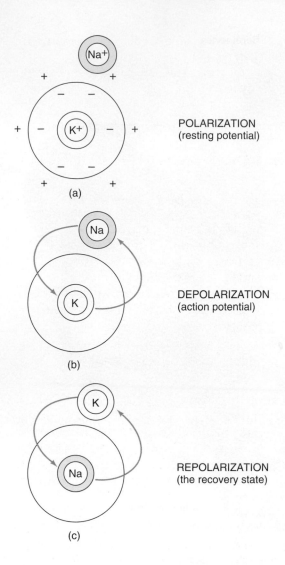

POLARIZATION
(resting potential)

(a)

DEPOLARIZATION
(action potential)

(b)

REPOLARIZATION
(the recovery state)

(c)

discs, until the entire muscle mass is depolarized. Contraction of the muscle follows depolarization.

The cell membrane remains permeable to sodium for only a fraction of a second. Thereafter, sodium influx stops and potassium escapes from inside the cell. This returns the charge inside the cell to normal (negative). In addition, sodium is actively pumped outside the cell, allowing the cell to **repolarize** and return to its normal resting state.

✱ **repolarization** return of a cell to its pre-excitation resting state.

Cardiac Conductive System

The cardiac conductive system stimulates the ventricles to depolarize in the proper direction. As mentioned earlier, the atria contract from superior to inferior and the ventricles from inferior to superior. If the depolarization impulse originated in the atria and spread passively to the ventricles, then the ventricles would depolarize from superior to inferior and would be ineffective. The cardiac conduction system, therefore, must initiate an impulse, spread it through the atria, transmit it quickly to the apex of the heart, and thence stimulate the ventricles to depolarize from inferior to superior. To do this, the conduction system relies on specialized conductive fibres comprising muscle cells that transmit the depolarization potential through the heart much faster than can regular myocardial cells.

To accomplish their task, the cells of the cardiac conductive system have the important properties of excitability, conductivity, automaticity, and contractility.

- **Excitability.** The cells can respond to an electrical stimulus, like all other myocardial cells.
- **Conductivity.** The cells can propagate the electrical impulse from one cell to another.
- **Automaticity.** The individual cells of the conductive system can depolarize without any impulse from an outside source. This property is also called self-excitation. Generally, the cell in the cardiac conductive system with the fastest rate of discharge, or automaticity, becomes the heart's pacemaker. As a rule, the highest cell in the conductive system has the fastest rate of automaticity. Normally, this cell is in the sinoatrial (SA) node, high in the right atrium; however, if one pacemaker cell fails to discharge and depolarize, then the cell with the next fastest rate becomes the pacemaker.
- **Contractility.** Since the cells of the cardiac conductive system are specialized cardiac muscle cells, they retain the ability to contract.

✱ **excitability** ability of the cells to respond to an electrical stimulus.

✱ **conductivity** ability of the cells to propagate the electrical impulse from one cell to another.

✱ **automaticity** pacemaker cells' capability of self-depolarization.

✱ **contractility** ability of muscle cells to contract, or shorten.

Internodal atrial pathways connect the SA node to the AV node (Figure 12-93). These internodal pathways conduct the depolarization impulse to the atrial muscle mass and through the atria to the AV junction. The AV junction (the "gatekeeper") slows the impulse and allows the ventricles time to fill. Then, the impulse passes through the AV junction into the AV node and on to the AV fibres, which conduct the impulse from the atria to the ventricles. In the ventricles, the AV fibres form the *bundle of His*.

The bundle of His subsequently divides into the right and left bundle branches. The *right bundle branch* delivers the impulse to the apex of the right ventricle. From there, the *Purkinje system* spreads it across the myocardium. The *left bundle branch* divides into *anterior and posterior fascicles* that also

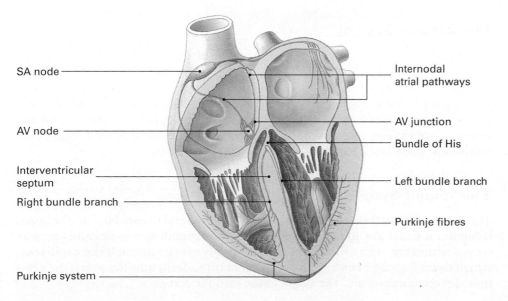

FIGURE 12-93   The cardiac conductive system.

SA node

AV node

Interventricular septum

Right bundle branch

Purkinje system

Internodal atrial pathways

AV junction

Bundle of His

Left bundle branch

Purkinje fibres

ultimately terminate in the Purkinje system. At the same time that the impulse is transmitted to the right ventricle, the Purkinje system spreads it across the mass of the myocardium. Repolarization predominantly occurs in the opposite direction.

Each component of the conductive system has its own intrinsic rate of self-excitation:

SA node = 60–100 beats per minute
AV node = 40–60 beats per minute
Purkinje system = 15–40 beats per minute

ANATOMY OF THE PERIPHERAL CIRCULATION

The peripheral circulation (Figure 12-94) transports oxygenated blood from the heart to the tissues and subsequently transports deoxygenated blood back to the heart. Oxygenated blood leaves the heart via the arterial system, while deoxygenated blood returns via the venous system. (As noted earlier, the exceptions to this rule are the pulmonary artery and the pulmonary veins.)

A capillary wall consists of a single layer of cells. The walls of arteries and veins, however, comprise several layers (Figure 12-95). The arteries' and veins' innermost lining, the *tunica intima,* is a single cell layer thick. The middle layer, the *tunica media,* consists of elastic fibres and muscle. It gives blood vessels their strength and recoil, which results from the difference in pressure inside and outside the vessel. The tunica media is much thicker in arteries than in veins. The outermost lining is the *tunica adventitia,* a fibrous tissue covering. It gives the vessel strength to withstand the pressures generated by the heart's contractions. The cavity inside a vessel is the *lumen.*

The vessels' diameters vary significantly and are directly related to the amount of blood they can transport. The larger the diameter, the greater is the blood flow. In fact, according to **Poiseuille's law** the blood flow through a vessel is directly proportional to the fourth power of the vessel's radius. For example, a vessel with a relative radius of 1 would transport 1 mL per minute of blood at a pressure difference of 100 mmHg. If the vessel's radius were increased to 4, keeping the pressure difference constant, the flow would increase to 256 mL (4^4) per minute.

The Arterial System

The *arterial system,* which carries oxygenated blood from the heart, functions under high pressure. The larger arterial vessels are the *arteries.* The arteries branch into smaller structures called *arterioles,* which control blood flow to various organs by their degree of resistance. The arterioles continue to divide until they become *capillaries,* which are the connection points between the arterial and venous systems. The vascular system and the tissues are able to exchange gases, fluids, and nutrients through the very thin capillary walls.

The Venous System

The *venous system* transports blood from the peripheral tissues back to the heart. It functions under low pressure with the aid of surrounding muscles and one-way valves within the veins. Blood enters the venous system through the capillaries, which drain into the *venules.* The venules, in turn, drain into the *veins,* the veins into the venae cavae, and the venae cavae into the atria.

✳ **Poiseuille's law** a law of physiology stating that blood flow through a vessel is directly proportional to the radius of the vessel to the fourth power.

MAJOR ARTERIES

Internal carotid
External carotid
Common carotid

Subclavian
Innominate

Axillary
Pulmonary

Aorta

Brachial

Radial
Ulnar
Common iliac

Palmar
arches

Digital

Deep femoral
Femoral

Popliteal

Anterior tibial
Peroneal

Posterior tibial

Dorsal pedis

Arcuate

MAJOR VEINS

External jugular
Internal jugular
Innominate
Brachial
Cephalic

Axillary

Basilic   Antecubital

Volar digital

Subclavian
Venae cavae
Splenic artery and vein
Right gastric artery and vein
Hepatic artery and vein

Renal artery and vein
Mesenteric arteries and veins
Common iliac

Great saphenous

Femoral

Popliteal

Peroneal

Posterior tibial

Anterior tibial

Dorsal venous arch

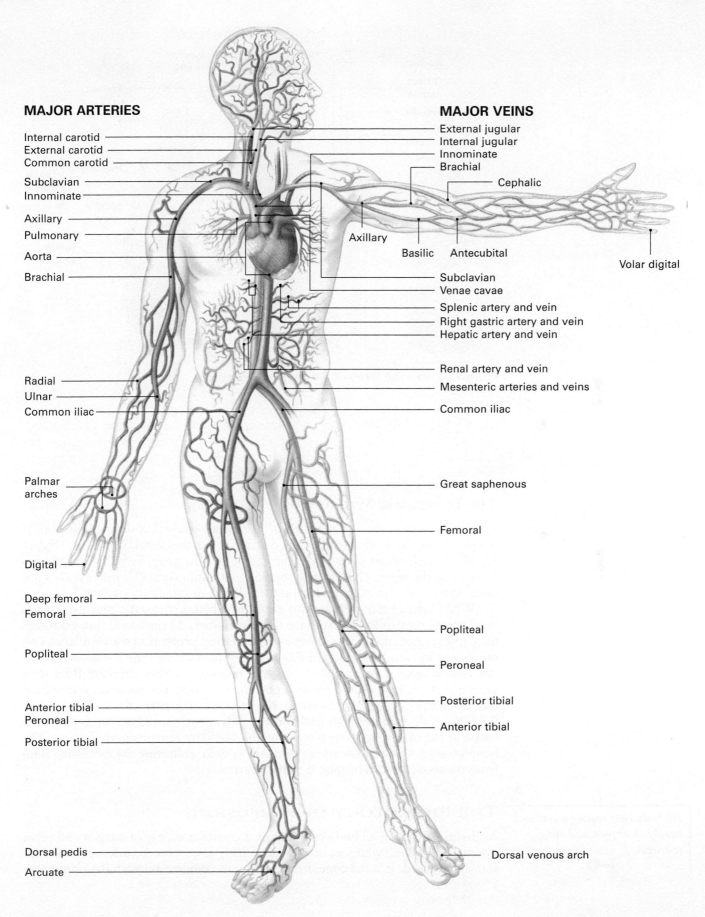

FIGURE 12-94   The circulatory system.

The Cardiovascular System   **589**

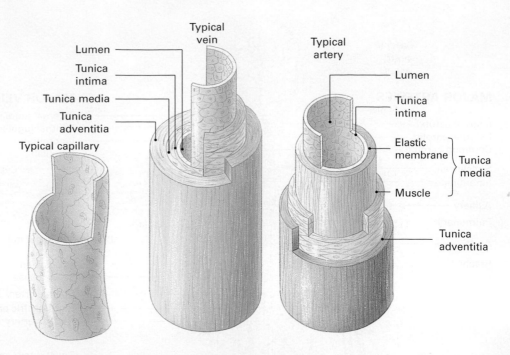

FIGURE 12-95   The layers of the peripheral arteries.

The Lymphatic System

The *lymphatic system* is a network of valveless vessels that drains fluid, called lymph, from the body tissues and delivers it to the subclavian vein (Figure 12-96). Lymph nodes in the neck, the axilla, and the groin help filter impurities en route to the heart. The lymph system plays an important role in the body's immune system. It also plays an important role in our circulatory system.

When arterial blood flows into a capillary bed, hydrostatic pressure pushes fluid across the capillary membrane into the tissues. As the blood flows through the capillary bed, this pressure diminishes. Plasma proteins in the capillaries create an oncotic pressure gradient that draws fluid back into the bloodstream. On the venous side of the capillary bed, the oncotic pressure drawing fluid in is greater than the hydrostatic pressure pushing fluid out. The net effect is that fluid returns to the capillary for its return to the heart. In a perfect system, whatever fluid enters the tissues at one end of the capillary bed should return to the circulation at the other end. In reality, some fluid usually remains in the tissues. The lymph system acts as an auxiliary drainage system, collecting the remaining fluid from the tissues and returning it to the heart.

THE PHYSIOLOGY OF PERFUSION

All body cells require a constant supply of oxygen and other nutrients.

As discussed earlier, all body cells require a constant supply of oxygen and other essential nutrients, while waste products, such as carbon dioxide, must be constantly removed. It is the circulatory system, in conjunction with the respiratory

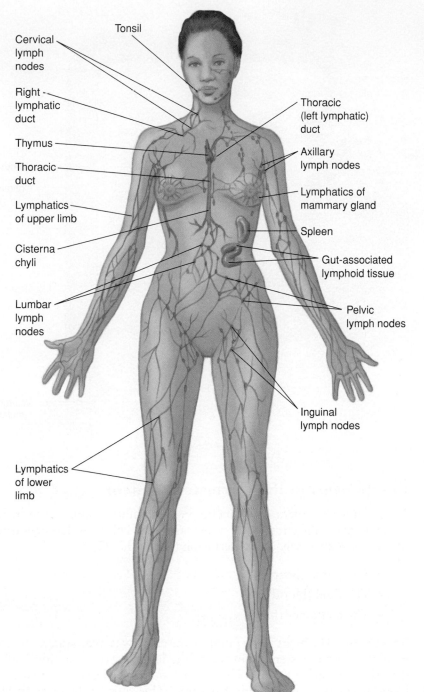

FIGURE 12-96   The lymphatic system.

Tonsil

Cervical lymph nodes

Right lymphatic duct

Thymus

Thoracic duct

Lymphatics of upper limb

Cisterna chyli

Lumbar lymph nodes

Lymphatics of lower limb

Thoracic (left lymphatic) duct

Axillary lymph nodes

Lymphatics of mammary gland

Spleen

Gut-associated lymphoid tissue

Pelvic lymph nodes

Inguinal lymph nodes

✱ **perfusion** the supplying of oxygen and nutrients to the body tissues as a result of the constant passage of blood through the capillaries.

✱ **hypoperfusion** inadequate perfusion of the body tissues, resulting in an inadequate supply of oxygen and nutrients to the body tissues. Also called *shock*.

and gastrointestinal systems, that provides the body's cells with these essential nutrients and removal of wastes. This is accomplished by the passage of blood through the capillaries, the small vessels that interface with body cells, while oxygen and carbon dioxide—nutrients and wastes—are exchanged by movement across the capillary walls and cell membranes. This constant and necessary passage of blood through the body's tissues is called **perfusion.** Inadequate perfusion of body tissues is **hypoperfusion,** which is commonly called *shock.*

FIGURE 12-97 Components of the circulatory system.

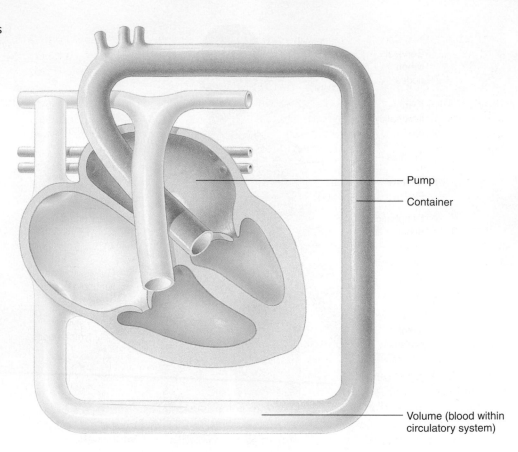

Pump

Container

Volume (blood within circulatory system)

Components of the Circulatory System

Perfusion is dependent on a functioning and intact circulatory system. The three components of the circulatory system are listed below. A derangement in any one of these can adversely affect perfusion (Figure 12-97).

- The pump (heart)
- The fluid (blood)
- The container (blood vessels)

The Pump The heart is the pump of the cardiovascular system. It receives blood from the venous system, pumps it to the lungs for oxygenation and then pumps it to the peripheral tissues. The normal ventricle ejects about two-thirds of the blood it contains at the end of diastole. This ratio is the **ejection fraction.** The amount of blood ejected by the heart in one contraction is referred to as the **stroke volume.** Each time the ventricle pumps blood into the aorta, it generates a pressure wave along the major arteries, which we feel as a pulse. Stroke volume varies between 60 mL and 100 mL, with the average being 70 mL. Three factors affect stroke volume: preload, cardiac contractile force, and afterload.

Preload is the amount of blood delivered to the heart during diastole (when the heart fills with blood between contractions). Preload depends on venous return. The venous system is a capacitance, or storage system. That is, it can be contracted or expanded, to some extent, as needed to meet the physiological demands of the body. When additional oxygenated blood is required, the venous capacitance is reduced, thus increasing the amount of blood delivered to the heart. The greater the preload, the greater is the stroke volume.

✳ **ejection fraction** ratio of blood pumped from the ventricle to the amount remaining at the end of diastole.

✳ **stroke volume** the amount of blood ejected by the heart in one cardiac contraction.

Content Review

FACTORS AFFECTING STROKE VOLUME
- Preload
- Cardiac contractility
- Afterload

✳ **preload** the pressure within the ventricles at the end of diastole, commonly called the *end-diastolic volume.*

Preload also affects **cardiac contractile force**. The greater the volume of preload, the more the ventricles are stretched. The greater the stretch, up to a certain limit, the greater will be the subsequent cardiac contraction. This phenomenon (known as **Starling's law of the heart**) can be illustrated through the example of a rubber band. The more the rubber band is stretched, the greater will be its velocity when released. Myocardial muscle, however, has its limits. If stretched too far, it will not contract properly and will weaken. Think of blowing up a tire. The tension in the walls increases as you put more air in the tire. If you were to put too much air in the tire, the tire would break or bulge from the side. If either of these happened, the tension in the wall would decrease, and if you filled the tire again it would not perform as well as before.

In addition, cardiac contractile force is affected by the circulating hormones called catecholamines (epinephrine and norepinephrine) controlled by the sympathetic nervous system. Catecholamines enhance cardiac contractile force by action on the beta-adrenergic receptors on the surface of the cells.

Finally, stroke volume is affected by afterload. **Afterload** is the resistance against which the ventricle must contract. This resistance must be overcome before ventricular contraction can result in ejection of blood. Afterload is determined by the degree of peripheral vascular resistance, which depends on the amount of vasoconstriction present. (The arterial system can be expanded and contracted to meet the metabolic demands of the body.) An increase in peripheral vascular resistance will decrease stroke volume, and conversely, a decrease in peripheral vascular resistance will allow stroke volume to increase.

The amount of blood pumped by the heart in one minute is referred to as the **cardiac output.** It is a function of stroke volume (millilitres per beat) and heart rate (beats per minute). Cardiac output is usually expressed in millilitres per minute. It can be defined by this equation:

stroke volume (mL/b) × heart rate (bpm) = cardiac output (mL/min)

Since the average stroke volume is 70 mL and the normal heart rate is about 70 beats per minute, the average cardiac output is 4900 millilitres per minute (rounded to 5000 mL/min or 5 L/min).

The foregoing equation illustrates the factors that can affect cardiac output. An increase in stroke volume or an increase in heart rate can increase cardiac output. Conversely, a decrease in stroke volume (in turn, governed by preload, contractile force, and afterload) or a decrease in heart rate can decrease cardiac output.

Blood pressure, the tension exerted by blood against the arterial walls, is dependent on both cardiac output and peripheral vascular resistance.

blood pressure = cardiac output × peripheral vascular resistance

Peripheral vascular resistance is the pressure against which the heart must pump. Since the circulatory system is a closed system, increasing either cardiac output or peripheral vascular resistance will increase blood pressure. Likewise, a decrease in cardiac output or a decrease in peripheral vascular resistance will decrease blood pressure.

The body does its best to keep the blood pressure relatively constant by employing compensatory mechanisms and negative feedback loops to regulate the elements of the above formula. As noted earlier, baroreceptors in the carotid sinuses and in the arch of the aorta closely monitor blood pressure. If blood pressure increases, the baroreceptors send signals to the brain that cause the blood pressure to return to its normal values. This is accomplished by decreasing the heart rate, decreasing the preload, or decreasing peripheral vascular resistance.

The baroreceptors are also stimulated if the blood pressure falls. The heart rate is increased, as is the strength of the cardiac contractions. There is also arteriolar constriction, venous constriction (which results in decreased container size),

* **cardiac contractile force** force of the strength of a contraction of the heart.

* **Starling's law of the heart** law of physiology stating that the more the myocardium is stretched, up to a certain limit, the more forceful the subsequent contraction will be.

* **afterload** the resistance against which the heart must pump.

* **cardiac output** the amount of blood pumped by the heart in one minute.

* **blood pressure** the tension exerted by blood against the arterial walls.

* **peripheral vascular resistance** the resistance of the vessels to the flow of blood: increased when the vessels constrict, decreased when the vessels relax.

and overall increased peripheral vascular resistance. Also, the adrenal medulla (the inner portion of the adrenal gland) is stimulated. This results in the secretion of epinephrine and norepinephrine, which further enhance the response.

The Fluid Blood is the fluid of the cardiovascular system. It is a viscous fluid; that is, it is thicker and more adhesive than water. As a result, blood flows more slowly than water. Blood, which consists of the plasma and the formed elements (red cells, white cells, and platelets), transports oxygen, carbon dioxide, nutrients, hormones, metabolic waste products, and heat.

An adequate amount of blood is required for perfusion. Since the cardiovascular system (the heart and blood vessels) is a closed system, the volume of blood present must be adequate to fill the container, as described below.

The Container Blood vessels (arteries, arterioles, capillaries, venules, and veins) serve as the container of the cardiovascular system. The blood vessels can be thought of as a continuous, closed, and pressurized pipeline by which blood moves throughout the body. Although the heart functions as the pump of the circulatory system, the blood vessels—under the control of the autonomic nervous system—can regulate blood flow to different areas of the body by adjusting their size as well as by selectively rerouting blood through the microcirculation.

Although the arteries and veins, like the heart, are subject to direct stimulation from sympathetic portions of the autonomic nervous system, the microcirculation (comprising the small vessels: the arterioles, capillaries, and venules) is primarily responsive to local tissue needs. The capability of some vessels in the capillary network to adjust their diameter permits the microcirculation to selectively supply undernourished tissue, while temporarily bypassing tissues with no immediate need. Capillaries have a sphincter at the origin of the capillary (between arteriole and capillary), called the *precapillary sphincter*, and another at the end of the capillary (between capillary and venule), called the *postcapillary sphincter*. The precapillary sphincter responds to local tissue conditions, such as acidosis and hypoxia, and opens as more arterial blood is needed. The postcapillary sphincter opens when blood is to be emptied into the venous system.

Blood flow through the vessels is regulated by two factors: peripheral vascular resistance and pressure within the system. Peripheral vascular resistance, as noted earlier, is the resistance to blood flow. Vessels with larger inside diameters offer less resistance, while vessels with smaller inside diameters offer greater resistance. Peripheral vascular resistance is governed by three factors: the length of the vessel, the diameter of the vessel, and blood viscosity.

There is very little resistance to blood flow through the aorta and arteries, but a significant change in peripheral resistance occurs at the arterioles and precapillary sphincters. This is because the inside diameter of the arteriole is much smaller, as compared with those of the aorta and arteries. Additionally, the arteriole has the ability to make a pronounced change in its diameter, as much as fivefold. It tends to do this in response to local tissue needs and autonomic nervous signals.

Contraction of the venous side of the vascular system results in decreased capacitance and increased cardiac preload. The arterial system, on the other hand, provides systemic vascular resistance. An increase in arterial tone increases resistance, which increases blood pressure.

Oxygen Transport

Oxygen is brought into the body via the respiratory system. During inspiration, approximately 500 to 800 mL of atmospheric air is taken in through the upper and lower airways, coming to rest in the alveoli of the lungs.

Surrounding the alveoli are capillaries that are perfused by the pulmonary circulation. The blood that comes into the pulmonary capillaries is oxygen-

The precapillary sphincter responds to local tissue demands, such as acidosis and hypoxia.

depleted blood that was returned from the body to the right atrium of the heart, then pumped by the right ventricle of the heart into the pulmonary arteries and thence into the pulmonary capillaries.

The air in the alveoli contains a concentration of about 13.6 percent oxygen. This is less than the 21-percent concentration of oxygen in atmospheric air because of various factors, including the fact that some air always remains in the alveoli from earlier respirations and oxygen is constantly being absorbed from this air. Nevertheless, alveolar air is far richer in oxygen than blood that enters the pulmonary capillaries.

Another way of stating this is that the *partial pressure of oxygen* present in air in the alveoli of the lungs is greater than the partial pressure of oxygen in the blood within the pulmonary circulation. (In a mix of gases, the portion of the total pressure exerted by each component of the mix is known as the partial pressure of that component.) For this reason, oxygen from the alveoli diffuses across the alveolar-capillary membrane and into the bloodstream—from the area of greater partial pressure to the area of lower partial pressure.

The red blood cells "pick up" this oxygen while passing through the pulmonary capillary bed. Oxygen binds to the hemoglobin molecule of the red blood cells, which serve as the primary carriers of oxygen within the bloodstream. Normally, between 95 percent and 100 percent of the hemoglobin is saturated with oxygen. The oxygen-enriched blood then circulates back to the heart through the venous side of the pulmonary circulation. Passing through the left atrium and into the left ventricle, the oxygen-enriched blood is pumped throughout the body via the systemic circulation.

On reaching capillaries throughout the body, the oxygen-rich blood interfaces with the tissues. The tissues contain cells that are oxygen deficient as a result of normal metabolic activity. Since the partial pressure of oxygen is greater in the bloodstream than in the cells, oxygen will diffuse from the red blood cells across the capillary wall-cell membrane barrier into the cells and tissues.

Overall, the movement and utilization of oxygen in the body is dependent on the following conditions:

- Adequate concentration of inspired oxygen
- Appropriate movement of oxygen across the alveolar/capillary membrane into the arterial bloodstream
- Adequate number of red blood cells to carry the oxygen
- Proper tissue perfusion
- Efficient off-loading of oxygen at the tissue level

The dependence on this set of conditions for oxygen movement and utilization is known as the Fick principle.

Waste Removal

The waste products of cellular metabolism are expelled from the cells and carried away by the blood. Carbon dioxide leaves the bloodstream during the oxygen-carbon dioxide exchange, which occurs through the alveolar/capillary membranes. Carbon dioxide is ultimately eliminated by exhalation from the lungs. Some cellular waste products are expelled into the interstitial fluid and picked up by the lymphatic system. These ultimately flow through the lymph channels into the thoracic duct. The thoracic duct empties the waste products into the venous side of the circulatory system. Other wastes are cleansed from the blood by the kidneys and excreted as urine. Finally, some cellular waste products are emptied into the gastrointestinal system and expelled in the feces.

Content Review

FICK PRINCIPLE
The movement and utilization of oxygen by the body is dependent on:
- Adequate concentration of inspired oxygen
- Appropriate movement of oxygen across the alveolar/capillary membrane into the arterial bloodstream
- Adequate number of red blood cells to carry the oxygen
- Proper tissue perfusion
- Efficient off-loading of oxygen at the tissue level

There is some local control of both tissue perfusion and waste removal. When the amounts of metabolic waste products (such as lactic acid) increase, the tissues subsequently become acidotic. This local acidosis causes nearby precapillary sphincters to relax, thus opening the capillaries and increasing perfusion of the affected tissues. This provides increased capacity for waste elimination and response to local metabolic demands.

THE RESPIRATORY SYSTEM

The respiratory system provides a passage for oxygen, a gas necessary for energy production, to enter the body and for carbon dioxide, a waste product of the body's metabolism, to exit. This gas exchange, called **respiration**, requires a patent, open airway as well as adequate respiratory function. Many pathological processes can inhibit respiration. To understand the interventions that you will use to maintain adequate airway and ventilatory function, you must thoroughly understand the anatomy of the upper and lower airway.

UPPER AIRWAY ANATOMY

The upper airway extends from the mouth and nose to the larynx (Figure 12-98). It includes the nasal cavity, oral cavity, and pharynx. The larynx joins the upper and lower airways.

*** respiration** the exchange of gases between a living organism and its environment.

Content Review

UPPER AIRWAY COMPONENTS
- Nasal cavity
- Oral cavity
- Pharynx

FIGURE 12-98 Anatomy of the upper airway.

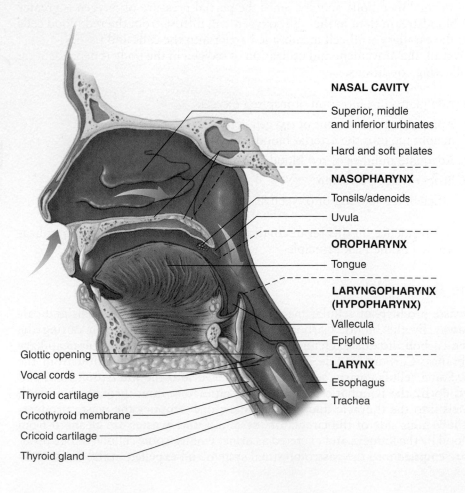

NASAL CAVITY
- Superior, middle and inferior turbinates
- Hard and soft palates

NASOPHARYNX
- Tonsils/adenoids
- Uvula

OROPHARYNX
- Tongue

LARYNGOPHARYNX (HYPOPHARYNX)
- Vallecula
- Epiglottis

LARYNX
- Esophagus
- Trachea

Glottic opening
Vocal cords
Thyroid cartilage
Cricothyroid membrane
Cricoid cartilage
Thyroid gland

The Nasal Cavity

The nasal cavity is the most superior part of the airway. The maxillary, frontal, nasal, ethmoid, and sphenoid bones compose the lateral and superior walls of the nasal cavity. The hard palate forms the floor of the nasal cavity. The cartilaginous and highly vascular **nasal septum** separates the right and left nasal cavities.

Several different structures connect with the nasal cavity. These include the sinuses, the eustachian tubes, and the nasolacrimal ducts. The **sinuses** are air-filled cavities that are lined with a mucous membrane. There are four pairs of sinuses: the ethmoid sinuses, the frontal sinuses, the maxillary sinuses, and the sphenoid sinuses. The sinuses, named for the bone where they are contained, help reduce the overall weight of the head and are thought to assist in heating, purifying, and moistening the inhaled air. The sinuses help trap bacteria entering the nasal cavity. Because of this, they can become infected. Fractures of the upper sinuses (sphenoids) can occasionally cause cerebrospinal fluid (CSF) to leak from the cranial cavity into the nasal cavity. Clinically, this presents with clear fluid draining from the nose (rhinorrhea) and can provide a direct route for the transmission of pathogens to the brain and associated structures.

The **eustachian tubes,** or auditory tubes, connect the ear with the nasal cavity and allow for equalization of pressure on each side of the tympanic membrane. Swallowing can assist in equalizing this pressure. The **nasolacrimal ducts** drain tears and debris from the eyes into the nasal cavity. This can cause the nose to run when someone cries.

Air enters the nasal cavity through the external nares (nostrils). Nasal hairs just inside the external nares initially filter the incoming air. The air then proceeds into the nasal cavity, where it strikes three bony projections, the superior, middle, and inferior turbinates, or conchae. These shell-like structures, which are parallel to the nasal floor, serve as conduits into the sinuses, increase the surface area of the nasal cavity, and cause turbulent airflow. This turbulence helps to filter the air by depositing airborne particles on the **mucous membrane** lining the nasal cavity. Hair-like fibres, called cilia, propel those trapped particles to the back of the pharynx, where they are swallowed.

Because the mucous membrane is covered with **mucus** and has a rich blood supply, it also immediately warms and humidifies the air entering the nose. By the time the air reaches the lower airway, it is at body temperature (37°C), 100 percent humidified, and virtually free of airborne particles. Air proceeds from the nasal cavity through internal nares into the nasopharynx. The tissue of the nasal cavity is extremely delicate and vascular. Because of this, it is susceptible to trauma.

The Oral Cavity

The cheeks, the hard and soft palates, and the tongue form the mouth, or oral cavity. The lips that surround the mouth's opening are fleshy folds of skin. Behind the lips lie the gums and teeth, normally numbering 32 in the adult. Significant force is required to avulse (dislodge) or fracture the teeth. Broken or dislodged teeth can potentially obstruct the airway. The hard palate anteriorly and the soft palate posteriorly form the top of the oral cavity and separate it from the nasal cavity.

The tongue, a large muscle on the bottom of the oral cavity, is the most common airway obstruction. It attaches to the mandible and the hyoid bone through a series of muscles and ligaments. The U-shaped hyoid bone is located just beneath the chin. The hyoid bone is unique. It is the only bone in the axial skeleton that does not articulate with any other bone. Instead, it is suspended by ligaments from the styloid process of the temporal bone and serves to anchor the tongue and larynx, as well as to support the trachea.

***

* nasal septum cartilage that separates the right and left nasal cavities.

* sinus air cavity that conducts fluids from the eustachian tubes and tear ducts to and from the nasopharynx.

* eustachian tube a tube that connects the ear with the nasal cavity.

* nasolacrimal duct narrow tube that carries into the nasal cavity tears and debris that have drained from the eye.

* mucous membranes tissues lining body cavities that communicate with the air; usually contain mucus-secreting cells.

* mucus slippery secretion that lubricates and protects airway surfaces.

The Pharynx

The **pharynx** is a muscular tube that extends vertically from the back of the soft palate to the superior aspect of the esophagus. It allows the air to flow into and out of the respiratory tract and food and liquids to pass into the digestive system. It contains several openings, including the internal nares, the mouth, the larynx, and the esophagus.

The pharynx is divided into three regions: the nasopharynx, the oropharynx, and the laryngopharynx (hypopharynx). The nasopharynx is the uppermost region, extending from the back of the nasal opening to the plane of the soft palate. The oropharynx extends from the plane of the soft palate to the hyoid bone. The adenoids—lymphatic tissue in the mouth and nose—filter bacteria. Either hypertrophy or swelling of the adenoids from infection may make them large enough to obscure your view. The laryngopharynx extends posteriorly from the hyoid bone to the esophagus and anteriorly to the larynx. The laryngopharynx is especially important in airway management.

Because the mouth and pharynx serve dual purposes for respiration and digestion, a number of mechanisms help prevent accidental blockage. To prevent foreign material from entering the trachea and lungs, sensitive nerves activate the body's cough and swallowing mechanisms as well as the **gag reflex.**

Located anteriorly in the hypopharynx is the epiglottis, a leaf-shaped cartilage that prevents food from entering the respiratory tract during swallowing. Just anterior and superior to the epiglottis is the **vallecula,** a fold formed by the base of the tongue and the epiglottis. It is an important landmark for **endotracheal intubation.** A series of ligaments and muscles connects the epiglottis to the hyoid bone and mandible. Immediately behind the hypopharynx are the fourth and fifth cervical vertebral bodies.

The Larynx

The **larynx** is the complex structure that joins the pharynx with the trachea (Figure 12-99). Lying midline in the neck, it is attached to and lies just inferior to the hyoid bone and anterior to the esophagus. It consists of the thyroid and cricoid cartilage (both considered tracheal cartilage), glottic opening, vocal cords, arytenoid cartilage, pyriform fossae, and cricothyroid membrane.

Content Review

REGIONS OF THE PHARYNX
- Nasopharynx
- Oropharynx
- Laryngopharynx

✳ **gag reflex** mechanism that stimulates retching, or striving to vomit, when the soft palate is touched.

✳ **vallecula** depression between the epiglottis and the base of the tongue.

✳ **endotracheal intubation** passing a tube into the trachea to protect and maintain the airway and to permit medication administration and deep suctioning.

✳ **larynx** the complex structure that joins the pharynx with the trachea.

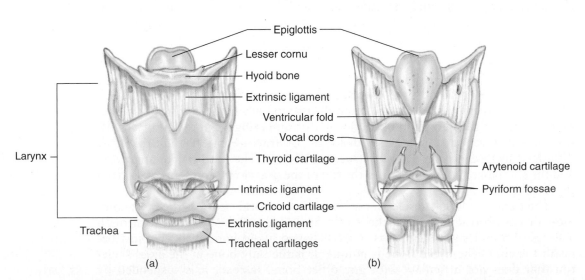

FIGURE 12-99   Internal anatomy of the upper airway.

The main laryngeal cartilage is the shield-shaped thyroid cartilage. Larger in males than in females, the thyroid cartilage forms the anterior prominence called the Adam's apple. The arytenoid cartilage, which forms a pyramid-shaped attachment for the vocal cords posteriorly, is an important landmark for endotracheal intubation. Posteriorly, smooth muscle closes a gap in the thyroid cartilage. Directly behind the Adam's apple, the thyroid cartilage houses the glottic opening, the narrowest part of the adult trachea, which is bordered by the vocal cords. The patency of the glottic opening, or **glottis**, depends heavily on muscle tone. On either side of the glottic opening are the pyriform fossae, recesses that form the lateral borders of the larynx. The thyrohyoid membrane attaches the upper end of the thyroid cartilage to the hyoid bone.

Within the laryngeal cavity lie the true vocal cords, white bands of cartilage that regulate the passage of air through the larynx and produce voice by contraction of the laryngeal muscles. The vocal cords can also close together to prevent foreign bodies from entering the airway. The passage of an endotracheal tube between the vocal cords interferes not only with the creation of sound but also with the protective function of coughing.

Beneath the thyroid cartilage is the cricoid cartilage, which forms the inferior border of the larynx. Often, it is considered the first tracheal ring. Unlike the thyroid and other tracheal cartilages, whose posterior surfaces are open and not fused, the cricoid cartilage forms a complete ring. The esophagus lies behind the cricoid cartilage, and so pressure applied in a posterior direction to the anterior cricoid cartilage occludes the esophagus (**Sellick's manoeuvre**), thus inhibiting vomiting and subsequent **aspiration** during airway management. In children, the cricoid cartilage is the narrowest part of the laryngeal airway. The fibrous **cricothyroid membrane** connects the inferior border of the thyroid cartilage with the superior aspect of the cricoid cartilage. It is the site for surgical airway techniques.

A mucous membrane lines most of the larynx. Rich with nerve endings from the vagus nerve, it is so sensitive that any irritation sparks a cough, or forceful exhalation of a large volume of air. First, air is drawn into the respiratory passageways. Next, the glottic opening shuts tightly, trapping the air within the lungs. Then, the abdominal and thoracic muscles contract, pushing against the diaphragm and increasing intrathoracic pressure. The vocal cords suddenly open, and a burst of air forces foreign particles out of the lungs. The laryngeal mucous membrane is so sensitive that its stimulation by a laryngoscope or endotracheal tube can cause bradycardia (slow pulse rate), hypotension (low blood pressure), and decreased respiratory rate.

Other structures proximate to the larynx and of particular interest when you perform surgical airways are the thyroid gland, carotid arteries, and jugular veins. The thyroid gland is a "bow-tie" shaped endocrine gland located in the neck. It is highly vascular and lies inferior to the cricoid cartilage. It contains two lobes, one on each side of the trachea. These lobes are joined in the middle by the isthmus that extends across the trachea. The carotid arteries run closely along the trachea. Several branches of the carotid arteries cross the trachea. Likewise, the jugular veins lie very close to the trachea. Several branches of the jugular veins, such as the superior thyroid vein, cross the trachea.

LOWER AIRWAY ANATOMY

The lower airway extends from below the larynx to the alveoli (Figure 12-100). This is where the respiratory exchange of oxygen and carbon dioxide occurs. Helpful landmarks are the fourth cervical vertebra at the posterior superior border, and the xiphoid process anterior inferiorly, though the posterior lung extends beyond this inferiorly.

✱ **glottis** lip-like opening between the vocal cords.

✱ **Sellick's manoeuvre** pressure applied in a posterior direction to the anterior cricoid cartilage that occludes the esophagus.

✱ **aspiration** inhaling foreign material, such as vomitus, into the lungs.

✱ **cricothyroid membrane** membrane between the cricoid and thyroid cartilages of the larynx.

Content Review

LOWER AIRWAY COMPONENTS

- Trachea
- Bronchi
- Alveoli
- Lung parenchyma
- Pleura

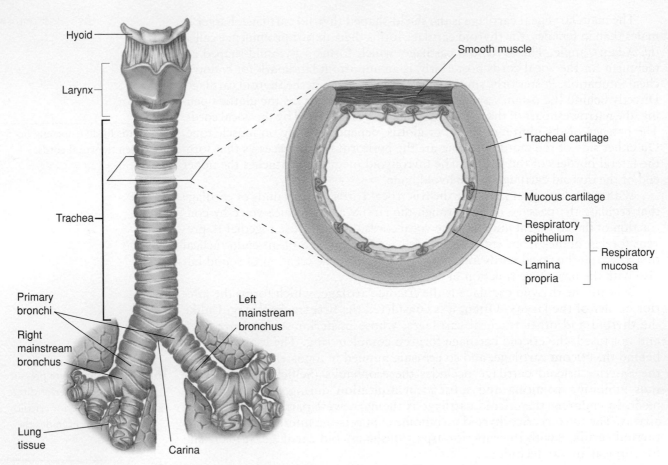

Labels on figure:

Hyoid

Larynx

Trachea

Primary bronchi

Right mainstream bronchus

Lung tissue

Carina

Left mainstream bronchus

Smooth muscle

Tracheal cartilage

Mucous cartilage

Respiratory epithelium

Lamina propria

Respiratory mucosa

FIGURE 12-100   Anatomy of the lower airway.

The Trachea

✱ **trachea** 10- to 12-cm-long tube that connects the larynx to the mainstem bronchi.

As air enters the lower airway from the upper airway, it first enters and then passes through the **trachea.** The trachea is a 10- to 12-centimetre-long tube that connects the larynx to the two mainstem bronchi. It contains cartilaginous, C-shaped, open rings that form a frame to keep it open. The trachea is lined with respiratory epithelium containing cilia and mucus-producing cells. The mucus traps particles that the upper airway did not filter. The cilia then move the trapped particulate matter up into the mouth where it is swallowed or expelled.

The Bronchi

✱ **bronchi** tubes from the trachea into the lungs.

At the carina, the trachea divides, or bifurcates, into the right and left mainstem **bronchi.** The right mainstem bronchus is almost straight, while the left mainstem bronchus angles more acutely to the left. Because of this, the right mainstem is often the site of aspirated foreign bodies. In addition, when an endotracheal tube is inserted too far, it tends to enter the right mainstem bronchus, thus ventilating only the right lung. Mainstem bronchi enter the lung tissue at the hilum, and then divide into the secondary and tertiary bronchi. The secondary and tertiary bronchi ultimately branch into the bronchioles, or small airways.

The bronchioles are encircled with smooth muscle that contains $beta_2$ (β_2) adrenergic receptors. When stimulated, these $beta_2$ receptors relax the bronchial smooth muscle, thus increasing the airway's diameter. This bronchodilation can increase the amount of air transported through the bronchiole. Conversely,

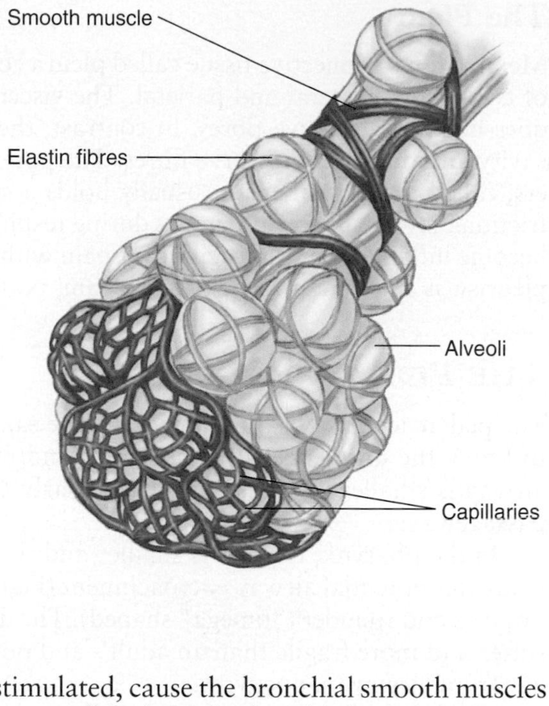

FIGURE 12-101 Anatomy of the alveoli.

Smooth muscle

Elastin fibres

Alveoli

Capillaries

parasympathetic receptors, when stimulated, cause the bronchial smooth muscles to contract, thus reducing the diameter of the bronchiole. This bronchoconstriction can inhibit the movement of air through the bronchiole.

After approximately 22 divisions, the bronchioles turn into the respiratory bronchioles. These structures contain only muscular connective tissue and have a limited capacity for gas exchange. The respiratory bronchioles terminate at the alveoli.

The Alveoli

The respiratory bronchioles divide into the alveolar ducts, which terminate in balloon-like clusters of **alveoli** called alveolar sacs (Figure 12-101). The alveoli contain an alveolar membrane that is only one or two cell layers thick. Because of this, the alveoli compose the key functional unit of the respiratory system. Most oxygen and carbon dioxide gas exchanges take place here, although limited gas exchange may occur in the alveolar ducts and respiratory bronchioles. The alveoli become thinner as they expand. This facilitates diffusion of oxygen and carbon dioxide.

The alveoli's surface area is massive, totalling more than 40 square metres— enough to cover half of a tennis court. These hollow structures resist collapse largely because of the presence of surfactant, a chemical that decreases their surface tension and makes it easier for them to expand. Alveolar collapse (**atelectasis**) can occur if surfactant is insufficient or if the alveoli are not inflated. No gas exchange takes place in atelectatic alveoli.

✱ alveoli microscopic air sacs where most oxygen and carbon dioxide gas exchanges take place.

✱ atelactasis alveolar collapse.

The Lung Parenchyma

The alveoli are the terminal end of the respiratory tree and the functional units of the lungs. As such, they are the core of the lung **parenchyma**. The lung parenchyma is arranged in two pulmonary lobules that form the anatomical division of the lungs. These lobules are further organized into lobes. The right lung has three lobes: the upper lobe, the middle lobe, and the lower lobe. The left lung, which shares thoracic space with the heart, has only two lobes: the upper lobe and the lower lobe.

✱ parenchyma principle or essential parts of an organ.

The Pleura

✱ **pleura** membranous connective tissue covering the lungs.

Membranous connective tissue called **pleura** covers the lungs. The pleura consists of two layers, visceral and parietal. The visceral pleura envelopes the lungs and does not contain nerve fibres. In contrast, the parietal pleura lines the thoracic cavity and does contain nerve fibres. The potential space between these two layers, called the pleural space, usually holds a small amount of fluid that reduces friction between the pleural layers during respiration. Occasionally, the pleura can become inflamed, causing significant pain with respiration. This condition, called pleurisy, is a common cause of chest pain, particularly in cigarette smokers.

THE PEDIATRIC AIRWAY

The pediatric airway is fundamentally the same as an adult's, but you will need to know the differences in relative size and position of some components. The airway is smaller in all aspects, particularly the diameters of the openings and passageways.

In the pharynx, the jaw is smaller and the tongue relatively larger, resulting in greater potential airway encroachment (Figure 12-102). The epiglottis is much floppier and rounder ("omega" shaped). The dental (alveolar) ridge and teeth are softer and more fragile than an adult's and potentially more susceptible to damage from airway manoeuvres.

The larynx lies more superior and anterior in children and is funnel shaped because the cricoid cartilage is undeveloped. Before the age of 10, the cricoid cartilage is the narrowest part of the airway. Most significantly, even a small foreign body or a limited degree of swelling in the pediatric airway can be life threatening. Because of this, young children tend to suffer more problems related to the

FIGURE 12-102 Anatomy of the pediatric airway.

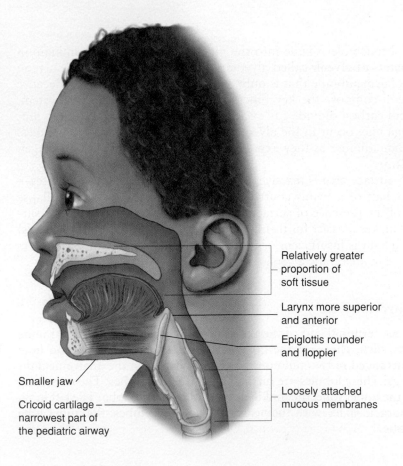

Relatively greater proportion of soft tissue

Larynx more superior and anterior

Epiglottis rounder and floppier

Loosely attached mucous membranes

Smaller jaw

Cricoid cartilage – narrowest part of the pediatric airway

trachea than do older children. A common example is croup (laryngotracheo-bronchitis), a viral infection that causes the soft tissues below the glottis to swell. This can reduce the diameter of the airway, potentially causing serious problems.

The ribs and the cartilage of the pediatric thoracic cage are softer and more pliable. This lack of rigidity lessens the thoracic wall's and accessory muscles' ability to assist lung expansion during inspiration. As a result, infants and children tend to rely more on their diaphragms for breathing. Always pay close attention to these differences when treating pediatric patients, especially those with respiratory complaints.

PHYSIOLOGY OF THE RESPIRATORY SYSTEM

Just as successful airway management requires a firm understanding of airway anatomy, a good outcome for these patients requires a working knowledge of the mechanics of oxygenation and ventilation. Your knowledge of normal respiratory physiology will lay the groundwork for your comprehension of important pathophysiology and will help you determine which actions will ensure optimal patient care.

Respiration and Ventilation

Respiration is the exchange of gases between a living organism and its environment. Pulmonary, or external, respiration occurs in the lungs when the respiratory gases are exchanged between the alveoli and the red blood cells in the pulmonary capillaries through the capillary membranes (Figure 12-103). Cellular, or internal, respiration, on the other hand, occurs in the peripheral capillaries. It is the exchange of the respiratory gases between the red blood cells and the various body tissues. Cellular respiration in the peripheral tissue produces carbon dioxide (CO_2). The blood picks up this waste product in the capillaries and transports it as bicarbonate ions through the venous system to the lungs. Although respiration describes the process of gas exchange in the lungs and peripheral tissues, **ventilation** is the mechanical process that moves air into and out of the lungs. Ventilation is necessary for respiration to occur.

✱ **ventilation** the mechanical process that moves air into and out of the lungs.

The Respiratory Cycle Nothing within the lung parenchyma makes it contract or expand. Pulmonary ventilation, therefore, depends on changes in pressure within the thoracic cavity. These changes occur in a respiratory cycle involving coordinated interaction among the respiratory system, the central nervous system, and the musculoskeletal system.

The thoracic cavity is a closed space, opening to the external environment only through the trachea. The diaphragm separates the thoracic cavity from the abdomen. When the diaphragm contracts, it draws downward, away from the thoracic cavity, thus enlarging it. Likewise, when the muscles between the ribs, or intercostal muscles, contract, they draw the ribcage upward and outward, away from the thoracic cavity, further increasing its volume.

The respiratory cycle begins when the lungs have achieved a normal expiration and the pressure inside the thoracic cavity equals the atmospheric pressure. At this point, respiratory centres in the brain communicate with the diaphragm by way of the phrenic nerve, signalling it to contract and thus initiate the respiratory cycle. As the size of the thorax increases in relation to the volume of air it holds, pressure within the thorax decreases, becoming lower than atmospheric pressure. This negative intrathoracic pressure invites air into the thorax through the airway. Because the visceral and parietal pleura remain in contact with each other under normal circumstances, the highly elastic lungs immediately assume the thoracic cavity's internal contour. These combined factors move air into the lungs (inspiration). At the same time, the alveoli inflate

FIGURE 12-103 Diffusion of gases across an alveolar membrane.

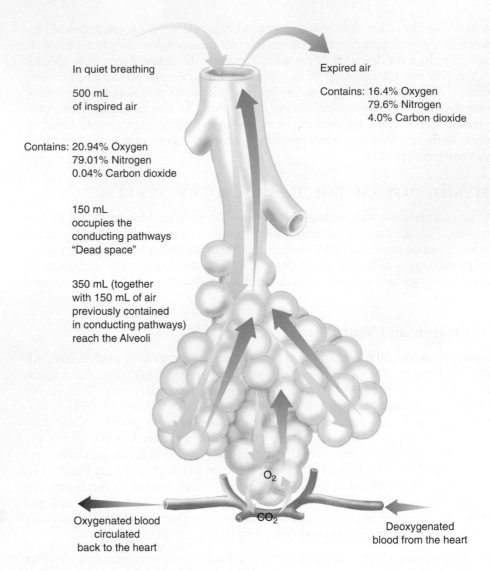

In quiet breathing

500 mL
of inspired air

Contains: 20.94% Oxygen
79.01% Nitrogen
0.04% Carbon dioxide

150 mL
occupies the
conducting pathways
"Dead space"

350 mL (together
with 150 mL of air
previously contained
in conducting pathways)
reach the Alveoli

Expired air

Contains: 16.4% Oxygen
79.6% Nitrogen
4.0% Carbon dioxide

O_2

CO_2

Oxygenated blood
circulated
back to the heart

Deoxygenated
blood from the heart

with the lungs. They become thinner as they expand, allowing oxygen and carbon dioxide to diffuse across their membranes.

When the pressure in the thoracic cavity again reaches that of the atmosphere, the alveoli are maximally inflated. Pulmonary expansion stimulates microscopic stretch receptors in the bronchi and bronchioles. These receptors signal the respiratory centre by way of the vagus nerve to inhibit inspiration, and the air influx stops. This process is primarily protective, as it prevents overinflation of the lungs.

At the end of inspiration, the respiratory muscles now relax, thus decreasing the size of the chest cavity and, in turn, increasing the intrathoracic pressure. The naturally elastic lungs recoil, forcing air out through the airway (expiration) until intrathoracic and atmospheric pressures are equal once again. Normal expiration is a passive process, while inspiration is an active process, using energy. In respiratory inadequacy, when this process fails to provide satisfactory gas exchange, the patient may use accessory respiratory muscles, such as the strap muscles of her neck and her abdominal muscles, to augment her efforts to expand the thoracic cavity.

Pulmonary Circulation Respiration also requires an intact circulatory system. In fact, during each cardiac cycle, the heart pumps as much blood to the lungs as it pumps to the peripheral tissues. In the capillaries, these cells take oxygen from red blood cells coming from the arterial system and give up carbon dioxide to

FIGURE 12-104 Pulmonary circulation.

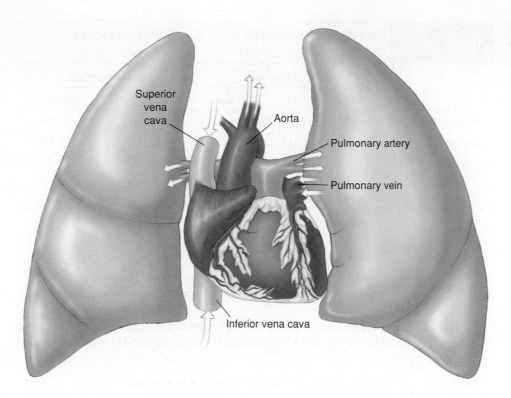

blood returning to the venous system. The venous system carries this deoxygenated blood to the right side of the heart, and the right ventricle pumps it into the pulmonary artery (Figure 12-104).

The pulmonary artery immediately branches into the right and the left pulmonary arteries, each supplying its respective lung. In turn, both branches quickly fan into smaller arteries that end in the pulmonary capillaries. These capillaries are spread over the surfaces of the alveoli, where the red blood cells exchange carbon dioxide for oxygen. The pulmonary capillaries recombine into larger veins, eventually terminating in the pulmonary vein. The pulmonary vein empties the oxygenated blood into the left atrium of the heart. Finally, the heart transports the oxygenated blood through the left ventricle and into the systemic arterial system via the aorta and its tributaries.

The lungs themselves receive little of their blood supply from the pulmonary arteries or veins. Instead, bronchial arteries that branch from the aorta supply most of their blood. Bronchial veins return this blood from the lungs to the superior vena cava.

Measuring Oxygen and Carbon Dioxide Levels

You can determine the amount of oxygen and carbon dioxide in the blood by measuring their partial pressures. **Partial pressure** is the pressure exerted by each component of a gas mixture. In other words, the partial pressure of a gas is its percentage of the mixture's total pressure. The partial pressure of oxygen at normal atmospheric pressure, for example, is the percentage of oxygen in atmospheric air (21 percent) multiplied by the atmospheric pressure at sea level (760 torr, or 2.6 kilograms per square centimetre):

$$0.21 \times 760 \text{ torr} = 159.6 \text{ torr}$$

(Note that torr and mmHg are the same measures of pressure.) Earth's atmosphere consists of four major respiratory gases: nitrogen (N_2), oxygen (O_2), carbon

✱ **partial pressure** the pressure exerted by each component of a gas mixture.

Table 12-6 PARTIAL PRESSURES AND CONCENTRATIONS OF GASES

	Partial Pressure		Concentration	
	Atmospheric	Alveolar	Atmospheric	Alveolar
Nitrogen	597.0 torr	569.0 torr	78.62%	74.9%
Oxygen	159.0 torr	104.0 torr	20.84%	13.7%
Carbon Dioxide	0.3 torr	40.0 torr	0.04%	5.2%
Water	3.7 torr	47.0 torr	0.50%	6.2%
TOTAL	760.0 torr	760.0 torr	100.00%	100.0%

dioxide (CO_2), and water (H_2O). Although nitrogen is metabolically inert, it is needed to inflate gas-filled body cavities, such as the chest. Table 12-6 lists these four respiratory gases' partial pressures and concentrations in the environment and in the alveoli.

Since alveolar partial pressure and arterial partial pressure are essentially the same in the normal lung, normal arterial partial pressures for oxygen and carbon dioxide may be expressed:

Oxygen (PaO_2) = 100 torr (average = 80–100)

Carbon dioxide ($PaCO_2$) = 40 torr (average = 35–45)

* __PA__ alveolar partial pressure.

* __Pa__ arterial partial pressure.

* __diffusion__ movement of a gas from an area of higher concentration to an area of lower concentration.

Alveolar partial pressures are abbreviated __PA__ (PAO_2 and $PACO_2$), while arterial partial pressures are abbreviated __Pa__ (PaO_2 and $PaCO_2$). Because these values are usually the same, however, they typically appear as the shortened notations PO_2 and PCO_2.

__Diffusion__ __Diffusion__ is the movement of a gas from an area of higher concentration to an area of lower concentration, attempting to reach equilibrium. Diffusion transfers gases between the lungs and the blood and between the blood and the peripheral tissues. The rate of diffusion of a gas across the pulmonary membranes depends on the gas's solubility in water. For example, carbon dioxide is 21 times more soluble in water than oxygen and readily crosses the pulmonary capillary membranes. In the peripheral tissues, the gradient (direction of diffusion) for CO_2 is from the tissue, where its concentration is high, to the capillary blood, where its concentration is low.

In the lungs, oxygen dissolves in water at the alveolar membrane and leaves the area of higher concentration, the alveoli, and enters the area of lower concentration, the venous blood in the pulmonary capillaries. Concurrently, carbon dioxide leaves the area of higher concentration, the arterial blood, and enters the area of lower concentration, the alveoli. The blood returns from the pulmonary vein to the heart and then moves into the systemic circulation.

__Oxygen Concentration in the Blood__ Oxygen diffuses into the blood plasma, where most of it combines with hemoglobin and is measured as oxygen saturation (SaO_2). The remainder is dissolved in the blood and is measured as the PaO_2. Hemoglobin approaches 100 percent saturation when the PaO_2 of dissolved oxygen reaches 90 to 100 torr. Each gram of saturated hemoglobin carries 1.34 mL of oxygen. Oxygen saturation is the ratio of the blood's actual oxygen content to its total oxygen-carrying capacity:

Oxygen saturation = O_2 content/O_2 capacity × 100(%)

The hemoglobin molecule carries the vast majority of oxygen in the blood (approximately 97 percent). Very little oxygen dissolves in the plasma. Since partial pressure measurements detect only the amount of oxygen dissolved in the plasma and do not always reflect the total oxygen saturation, they can be misleading. For example, a patient who has suffered carbon monoxide poisoning cannot transport enough oxygen to the peripheral tissues, since carbon monoxide displaces oxygen from the hemoglobin molecule. But an arterial blood gas sample might reveal a normal or high PaO_2. This would indicate that adequate oxygen was reaching the blood. In fact, however, an inadequate amount of hemoglobin would be available to transport the oxygen to the peripheral tissues, resulting in peripheral hypoxia.

Several factors can affect oxygen concentrations in the blood:

- *Decreased hemoglobin concentration* (anemia, hemorrhage)
- *Inadequate alveolar ventilation* due to low inspired-oxygen concentration, respiratory muscle paralysis, and pulmonary conditions, such as emphysema, asthma, or pneumothorax
- *Decreased diffusion across the pulmonary membrane* when diffusion distance increases or the pulmonary membrane changes; for example, when fluid enters the space between the alveolar membrane and the pulmonary capillary membrane, as in pneumonia, chronic obstructive pulmonary disease (COPD), or pulmonary edema (swelling).
- *Ventilation/perfusion mismatch* occurs when a portion of the alveoli collapses, as in atelectasis. Blood travels past these collapsed alveoli without oxygenation (shunting), without carbon dioxide, and without oxygen uptake. This can result from **hypoventilation,** which can occur secondary to pain or inability to inspire (traumatic asphyxia). When the lung collapses, as in **pneumothorax, hemothorax,** or a combination of the two, less surface area is available for gas exchange. Alternatively, a ventilation/perfusion mismatch can occur when blood is prevented from reaching the alveolar capillary membranes but alveolar ventilation remains adequate. This occurs when a blood clot travels to or is formed in the pulmonary arterial system, a condition known as pulmonary thromboembolism.

✳ **hypoventilation** reduction in breathing rate and depth.

✳ **pneumothorax** accumulation of air or gas in the pleural cavity.

✳ **hemothorax** accumulation in the pleural cavity of blood or fluid containing blood.

You can correct oxygen derangements by increasing ventilation, administering supplemental oxygen, using intermittent positive pressure ventilation (IPPV), or administering drugs to correct underlying problems, such as pulmonary edema, asthma, or **pulmonary embolism.** The emergency being treated determines the desired fractional concentration of oxygen (**FiO_2**) to be delivered. It is crucial to remember not to withhold oxygen from any patient whose clinical condition indicates its need.

✳ **pulmonary embolism** blood clot that travels to the pulmonary circulation and hinders oxygenation of the blood.

✳ **FiO_2** concentration of oxygen in inspired air.

Carbon Dioxide Concentration in the Blood The blood transports carbon dioxide mainly in the form of bicarbonate ion (HCO_3^-). It carries approximately 70 percent as bicarbonate and approximately 20 percent combined with hemoglobin. Less than 7 percent is dissolved in the plasma. Several factors influence carbon dioxide's concentration in the blood, including increased CO_2 production and/or decreased CO_2 elimination:

- *Hyperventilation lowers CO_2 levels* and can be the result of an increased respiratory rate or deeper respiration, both of which increase the minute volume. (We will discuss minute volume more completely later.)

- *Increased CO_2 production* can be caused by:
  — Fever
  — Muscle exertion
  — Shivering
  — Metabolic processes resulting in the formation of metabolic acids
- *Decreased CO_2 elimination* (increased CO_2 levels in the blood) resulting from decreased alveolar ventilation is commonly caused by hypoventilation due to
  — Respiratory depression by drugs
  — Airway obstruction
  — Impairment of the respiratory muscles
  — Obstructive diseases, such as asthma and emphysema

* **hypercarbia** excess of carbon dioxide in the blood.

Increased CO_2 levels (**hypercarbia**) are usually treated by increasing the rate and/or volume of ventilation and by correcting the underlying cause.

Regulation of Respiration

* **respiratory rate** the number of times a person breathes in one minute.

Respiratory Rate The number of times a person breathes in one minute, the **respiratory rate,** is unique in that both voluntary and involuntary nervous system mechanisms control it. We do not ordinarily need to make a conscious effort to breathe; our brains automatically regulate this function. However, we can voluntarily override our involuntary respirations until physical and chemical mechanisms signal the nervous system's respiratory centres to provide involuntarily impulses and correct any breathing irregularities.

Nervous Impulses from the Respiratory Centre The main respiratory centre lies in the *medulla oblongata* in the brainstem. Various neurons within the medulla initiate impulses that result in respiration. A rise in the frequency of these impulses increases the respiratory rate. Conversely, a decrease in their frequency decreases the respiratory rate. The medulla is connected to the respiratory muscles primarily via the vagus nerve. This is an involuntary pathway. If the medulla fails to initiate respiration, an additional control centre in the pons, called the *apneustic centre,* assumes respiratory control to ensure the continuation of respirations. A third centre, the *pneumotaxic centre,* also in the pons, controls expiration.

Stretch Receptors During inspiration, the lungs become distended, activating stretch receptors. As the degree of stretch increases, these receptors fire more frequently. The impulses they send to the brainstem inhibit the medullary cells, decreasing the inspiratory stimulus. Thus, the respiratory muscles relax, allowing the elastic lungs to recoil and expel air from the body. As the stretch decreases, the stretch receptors stop firing. This process, called the *Hering-Breuer reflex,* prevents overexpansion of the lungs.

Chemoreceptors Other involuntary respiration controls include central chemical receptors in the medulla and peripheral chemoreceptors in the carotid bodies and in the arch of the aorta. These chemoreceptors are stimulated by decreased PaO_2, increased $PaCO_2$, and decreased pH. (The pH scale expresses the degree of acidity or alkalinity. A lower pH indicates greater acidity; a higher pH indicates greater alkalinity. The chapter on the general principles of pathophysiology discusses pH in greater detail.) Cerebrospinal fluid (CSF) pH is the primary control of respiratory centre stimulation. The CSF pH responds very quickly to changes in arterial PCO_2. Any increase in $PaCO_2$ will decrease CSF pH, which will, in turn, stimulate the central chemoreceptors to increase respiration. Conversely, low $PaCO_2$ levels will raise CSF pH, in turn, decreasing chemoreceptor stimulation and slowing respiratory activity. Because $PaCO_2$ is inversely related to CSF pH, $PaCO_2$ is seen as the normal neuroregulatory control of respirations. Additionally, any increase in the arterial $PaCO_2$ stimulates the peripheral chemoreceptors to signal the brainstem to increase respiration, thus speeding CO_2 elimination from the body.

Hypoxic Drive The body also constantly monitors the PaO_2 and the pH. In fact, **hypoxemia** (decreased partial pressure of oxygen in the blood) is a profound stimulus of respiration in a normal individual. People with chronic respiratory disease, such as emphysema and chronic bronchitis, tend to retain CO_2 and, therefore, have a chronically elevated $PaCO_2$. Chemoreceptors in the periphery eventually become accustomed to this chronic condition, and the central nervous system stops using $PaCO_2$ to regulate respiration. This activates a default mechanism called **hypoxic drive,** which increases respiratory stimulation when PaO_2 falls and inhibits respiratory stimulation when PaO_2 climbs. High-volume oxygen administration to people with this condition can cause respiratory arrest. Because high-flow oxygen can quickly double or even triple the PaO_2, peripheral chemoreceptors stop stimulating the respiratory centres, causing **apnea.** (Although this is a potential threat, it is never appropriate to withhold oxygen from a patient for whom oxygen therapy is indicated; if the respiratory effort becomes inadequate, ventilatory assistance will be necessary.)

Measures of Respiratory Function

The respiratory rate is the number of respiratory cycles per minute, normally 12 to 20 breaths per minute in adults, 18 to 24 in children, and 40 to 60 in infants. Several factors affect respiratory rate:

- Fever—increases rate
- Emotion—increases rate
- Pain—increases rate
- Hypoxia (inadequate tissue oxygenation)—increases rate
- Acidosis—increases rate
- Stimulant drugs—increase rate
- Depressant drugs—decrease rate
- Sleep—decreases rate

Paramedics must fully understand ventilatory mechanics and capacities for the average adult's respiratory system. This knowledge will enable you to adapt your mechanical ventilation techniques to your patient's size, lung compliance, need for hyperventilation, or other individual requirements. It is especially crucial in situations that call for advanced mechanical ventilator skills. Respiratory capacities and measurements with which you must be familiar include:

- *Total Lung Capacity (TLC).* This is the maximum lung capacity—the total amount of air contained in the lung at the end of maximal inspiration. In the average adult male, this volume is approximately 6 litres.
- *Tidal Volume (V_T).* The tidal volume is the average volume of gas inhaled or exhaled in one respiratory cycle. In the adult male, this is approximately 500 mL (5–7 mL/kg).
- *Dead Space Volume (V_D).* The dead space volume is the amount of gas in the tidal volume that remains in air passageways unavailable for gas exchange. It is approximately 150 mL in the adult male. Anatomical dead space includes the trachea and bronchi. Obstructions or diseases, such as chronic obstructive pulmonary disease or atelectasis, can cause physiological dead space.

✳ **hypoxemia** decreased blood oxygen level.

✳ **hypoxic drive** mechanism that increases respiratory stimulation when blood oxygen falls and inhibits respiratory stimulation when blood oxygen climbs.

✳ **apnea** absence of breathing.

✳ **total lung capacity** maximum lung capacity.

✳ **tidal volume** average volume of gas inhaled or exhaled in one respiratory cycle.

- *Alveolar Volume (V_A).* The alveolar volume is the amount of gas in the tidal volume that reaches the alveoli for gas exchange. It is the difference between tidal volume and dead-space volume (approximately 350 mL in the adult male):

$$V_A = V_T - V_D$$

- *Minute Volume (V_{min}).* The minute volume is the amount of gas moved in and out of the respiratory tract in one minute:

$$V_{min} = VT \times \text{respiratory rate}$$

- *Alveolar Minute Volume ($V_{A\text{-}min}$).* The alveolar minute volume is the amount of gas that reaches the alveoli for gas exchange in one minute:

$$V_{A\text{-}min} = (V_T - V_D) \times \text{respiratory rate}$$

or

$$V_{A\text{-}min} = V_A \times \text{respiratory rate}$$

- *Inspiratory Reserve Volume (IRV).* The inspiratory reserve volume is the amount of air that can be maximally inhaled after a normal inspiration.
- *Expiratory Reserve Volume (ERV).* The expiratory reserve volume is the amount of air that can be maximally exhaled after a normal expiration.
- *Residual Volume (RV).* The residual volume is the amount of air remaining in the lungs at the end of maximal expiration.
- *Functional Residual Capacity (FRC).* The functional residual capacity is the volume of gas that remains in the lungs at the end of normal expiration:

$$FRC = ERV + RV$$

- *Forced Expiratory Volume (FEV).* The forced expiratory volume is the amount of air that can be maximally expired after maximum inspiration.

THE ABDOMEN

The abdominal cavity is bound by the diaphragm superiorly; the pelvis inferiorly; the vertebral column, the posterior and inferior ribs, and the back muscles (psoas and paraspinal muscles) posteriorly; the muscles of the flank laterally; and the abdominal muscles anteriorly (Figure 12-105). The cavity is divided into three spaces: the **peritoneal space** (containing those organs or portions of organs covered by the abdominal [peritoneal] lining); the **retroperitoneal space** (containing those organs posterior to the peritoneal lining); and the **pelvic space** (containing the organs within the pelvis). Anatomical landmarks of this area include the centrally located umbilicus (the navel), the xiphoid process (tip of the sternum) at the upper and central abdominal border, the bony ridges of the pelvis (the iliac crests) inferiorly and laterally, and the pubic prominence inferiorly.

The abdomen is divided into four subregions by imaginary vertical and horizontal lines intersecting at the umbilicus (naval) and forming the right and left upper and lower quadrants. The right upper quadrant contains the gallbladder, right kidney, most of the liver, some small bowel, a portion of the ascending and transverse colon, and a small portion of the pancreas. The left upper quadrant

✳ **minute volume** amount of gas inhaled and exhaled in one minute.

✳ **peritoneal space** division of the abdominal cavity containing those organs or portions of organs covered by the peritoneum.

✳ **retroperitoneal space** division of the abdominal cavity containing those organs posterior to the peritoneal lining.

✳ **pelvic space** division of the abdominal cavity containing those organs located within the pelvis.

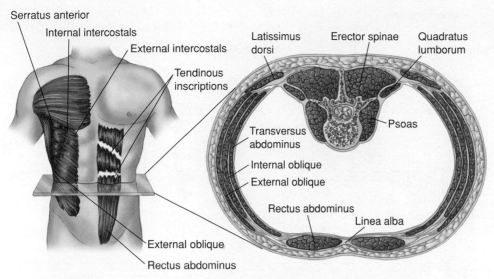

Serratus anterior
Internal intercostals
External intercostals
Tendinous inscriptions
External oblique
Rectus abdominus

Latissimus dorsi
Erector spinae
Quadratus lumborum
Psoas
Transversus abdominus
Internal oblique
External oblique
Rectus abdominus
Linea alba

a. Anterior view of the trunk, showing superficial and deep members of the oblique and rectus groups.

b. Diagrammatic sectional view through the abdominal region.

FIGURE 12-105 Muscles protecting the organs of the abdominal cavity.

contains the stomach, spleen, left kidney, most of the pancreas, and a portion of the liver, small bowel, and transverse and descending colon. The right lower quadrant contains the appendix, and portions of the urinary bladder, small bowel, ascending colon, rectum, and female genitalia. The left lower quadrant contains the sigmoid colon and portions of the urinary bladder, small bowel, descending colon, rectum, and female genitalia.

The major structures within the abdomen include the digestive tract, the accessory organs of digestion, the spleen, the structures and organs of the urinary system, and the female reproductive organs. (The male reproductive organs, or genitalia, are considered to be part of the urinary system. The female reproductive organs are separate from the urinary system and include the reproductive organs within the abdomen as well as the external genitalia.)

ABDOMINAL VASCULATURE

The abdominal contents are supplied with blood via the abdominal aorta, which travels along and to the left of the spinal column. It sends forth many branches to discrete organs and the bowel (Figure 12-106). The abdominal aorta bifurcates at the upper sacral level into two large iliac arteries. These eventually become the femoral arteries as they traverse and then exit the pelvis. The attachment of these arteries to the pelvic structure is quite firm and may result in their tearing if the pelvis is fractured and displaced. The inferior vena cava is located along the spinal column and collects venous blood from the lower extremities and the abdomen, relatively parallel to the arterial system, returning it to the heart. The abdomen also houses a special circulatory system, the portal system. This venous subsystem collects venous blood and the fluid and nutrients absorbed by the bowel and transports them to the liver. The liver detoxifies the fluid, stores excess nutrients, adds nutrients when they are deficient, and then sends the blood/nutrient/fluid mixture into the inferior vena cava, just below the heart. There, it mixes with venous blood and is circulated through the heart and then the rest of the body.

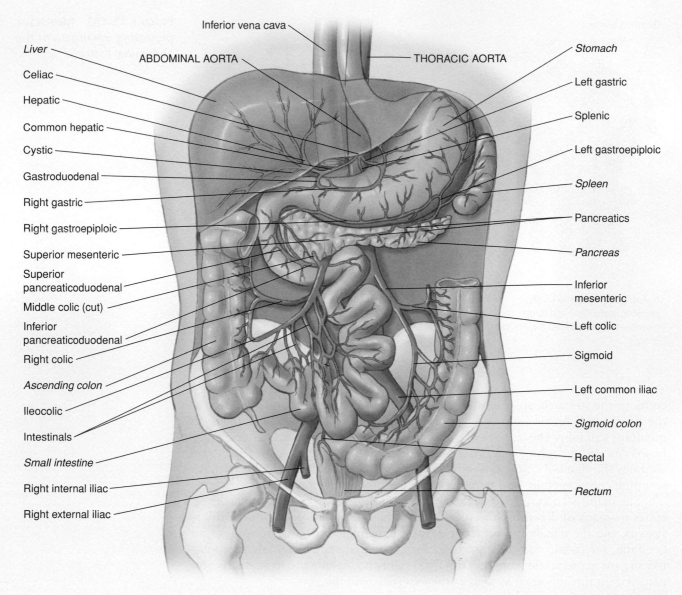

Inferior vena cava

ABDOMINAL AORTA

THORACIC AORTA

Liver

Celiac

Hepatic

Common hepatic

Cystic

Gastroduodenal

Right gastric

Right gastroepiploic

Superior mesenteric

Superior pancreaticoduodenal

Middle colic (cut)

Inferior pancreaticoduodenal

Right colic

Ascending colon

Ileocolic

Intestinals

Small intestine

Right internal iliac

Right external iliac

Stomach

Left gastric

Splenic

Left gastroepiploic

Spleen

Pancreatics

Pancreas

Inferior mesenteric

Left colic

Sigmoid

Left common iliac

Sigmoid colon

Rectal

Rectum

FIGURE 12-106   The abdominal arteries.

THE PERITONEUM

Many of the abdominal organs are covered by a serous membrane called the **peritoneum** (Figure 12-107). This tissue resembles the pleura of the lungs and functions in a similar manner. The parietal peritoneum covers the most of the interior surface of the anterior and lateral abdominal cavity, while the visceral peritoneum covers the individual organs. A small amount of fluid is found between the peritoneal layers and permits free movement of the bowel during digestion.

The digestive tract is restrained and prevented from tangling by a structure called the **mesentery.** The mesentery is a double fold of peritoneum containing blood vessels, lymphatic vessels, nerves, and fatty tissue. It suspends the bowel from the posterior abdominal wall. An additional fold of mesentery, called the omentum, also covers, insulates, and protects the anterior surface of the abdomen. The thickness of the omentum varies with the size and percentage of body fat of the patient. It may be several centimetres thick in the obese patient or very narrow in the thin and muscular patient.

✱ **peritoneum** fine fibrous tissue surrounding the interior of most of the abdominal cavity and covering most of the small bowel and some of the abdominal organs.

✱ **mesentery** double fold of peritoneum that supports the major portion of the small bowel, suspending it from the posterior abdominal wall.

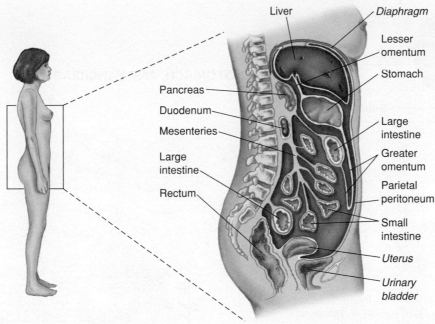

FIGURE 12-107 Reflections of the peritoneum.

Most of the abdominal structures are covered by peritoneum, excepting the kidneys, duodenum, pancreas, urinary bladder, the posterior portions of the ascending and descending colon, and the rectum. Most of the major vascular structures within the abdomen are also retroperitoneal. An organ's relation to the peritoneum becomes important in trauma because irritation of the peritoneum (peritonitis) presents with more apparent signs and symptoms than does hemorrhage or the release of other fluids into the retroperitoneal space.

The abdominal cavity is a dynamic place. The diaphragm moves up and down, displacing the abdominal contents with each breath. With deep expiration, the central portion of the diaphragm moves as far upward as the fourth intercostal space, anteriorly (the nipple line), and the seventh intercostal space (the inferior tips of the scapulae), posteriorly. (The edge of the diaphragm attaches to the border of the rib cage.) During forced and maximal expiration, the diaphragm moves as much as 9 cm inferiorly. This movement displaces the abdominal contents up and down with each breath.

Additionally, the volume of substance within the hollow organs varies—an empty (10 mL) versus a distended (500 mL) bladder or a full (1.5 L) versus an empty stomach. The digestive tract is also suspended from the back of the abdominal cavity and is permitted some movement as it digests food. This dynamic movement becomes an important consideration when anticipating abdominal injury due to blunt or penetrating trauma

THE DIGESTIVE SYSTEM

The digestive system includes the digestive tract and the accessory organs of digestion (Figure 12-108). The digestive tract (also called the *alimentary canal*) is the muscular tube that physically and chemically breaks down and absorbs the fluids and nutrients from the food we eat. The accessory organs of digestion include the liver, gallbladder, and pancreas. These organs prepare and store digestive enzymes and perform other important body functions.

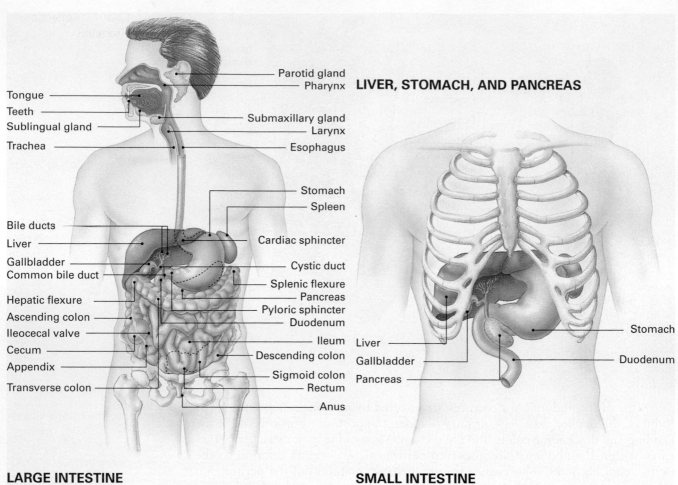

LIVER, STOMACH, AND PANCREAS

Parotid gland
Pharynx
Tongue
Teeth
Sublingual gland
Submaxillary gland
Larynx
Trachea
Esophagus
Stomach
Spleen
Bile ducts
Liver
Cardiac sphincter
Gallbladder
Common bile duct
Cystic duct
Splenic flexure
Hepatic flexure
Pancreas
Ascending colon
Pyloric sphincter
Ileocecal valve
Duodenum
Cecum
Ileum
Appendix
Descending colon
Transverse colon
Sigmoid colon
Rectum
Anus

Liver
Gallbladder
Pancreas
Stomach
Duodenum

LARGE INTESTINE

Esophagus
Diaphragm
Stomach
Duodenum
Hepatic flexure
Ascending colon
Splenic flexure
Ileocecal valve
Transverse colon
Cecum
Descending colon
Appendix
Rectum
Sigmoid colon
Anus

SMALL INTESTINE

Ascending colon
Duodenum
Transverse colon
Jejunum
Cecum
Descending colon
Sigmoid colon
Ileum

FIGURE 12-108   The digestive tract and accessory organs.

THE DIGESTIVE TRACT

The **digestive tract** is a thin, 7.6-metre long, hollow muscular tube responsible for churning the material to be digested, for excreting digestive juices to be mixed with it, and for absorbing nutrients and then water. Abdominal components of the digestive tract consist of the stomach, the small bowel (duodenum, jejunum, and ileum), the large bowel (or colon), the rectum, and the anus. These structures fill the anterior and lateral aspects of the abdominal cavity, except for the area occupied by the liver.

The esophagus enters the abdomen through the hiatus of the diaphragm (just posterior to the xiphoid process) and then deposits its contents into the stomach. The stomach is a J-shaped muscular container that mixes the ingested material with hydrochloric acid and enzymes (both produced in the gastric wall) into a thick fluid called **chyme**. The acid released by the stomach increases the gastric acidity (pH) to between 1.5 and 2.0. This is a very acidic fluid that would damage the stomach and the initial lining of the small bowel if not for the continuous production of a protective mucus. The stomach is highly variable in size, depending on the amount of material it contains. It can distend to hold as much as 1.5 litres of food after a large meal.

Chyme is released in small boluses into the first component of the small bowel, the duodenum. The duodenum is approximately 30 cm in length and is where the digesting material is mixed with bile from the liver (stored in the gallbladder) and pancreatic digestive juices. These agents raise the pH of the chyme (returning it toward neutral) and help release the nutrients it contains.

The digesting food is propelled along the small and large bowels by waves of contraction called **peristalsis**. The muscles of the digestive tract constrict the bowel's lumen behind a mass of food, then progressively constrict the lumen in the direction of desired movement. The resulting rhythmic constriction moves the digesting material through the tract. As chyme enters the next two segments of the small bowel (the jejunum and the ileum), the mixing decreases, and the nutrients, released by the physical and chemical digestion processes, are absorbed, directed to the liver for detoxification, and then released into the circulatory system.

As the food continues its travel through the digestive tract, it arrives at the large bowel. Here, masses of bacteria assist in releasing vitamins and fluid from the digesting food, while the large bowel absorbs most of the remaining fluid content. The water serves to hydrate the body while the digestive juices are reabsorbed and reprocessed to rejoin the digestive process upstream again. The large bowel ascends superiorly along the right side of the abdomen (ascending colon), traverses the abdomen just below the liver and stomach (transverse colon), then descends along the left lateral abdomen (descending colon). It aligns with the rectum through the S-shaped sigmoid colon where the end waste products of the digestive process (feces) await excretion (defecation) through the terminal valve, the anus.

ACCESSORY ORGANS OF DIGESTION

The liver is a vascular structure responsible for detoxifying the blood, removing damaged or aged erythrocytes, and storing glycogen and other important agents for body metabolism. The liver also assists in the osmotic regulation of fluids in the blood and plays a role in the clotting process. Finally, the liver detoxifies materials absorbed by the digestive system and either stores or releases nutrients to ensure that the body's metabolic needs are met. It is located in the right upper quadrant, just below the diaphragm and extends into the medial portion of the left upper quadrant. It is the largest abdominal organ, accounting for 2.5 percent of total body weight. It receives about 25 percent of cardiac output and holds the greatest blood reserve of any body organ. The lower portion of its mass can

* **digestive tract** internal passageway that begins at the mouth and ends at the anus; also called the *alimentary canal.*

* **chyme** semifluid mixture of ingested food and digestive secretions found in the stomach and small intestine.

* **peristalsis** wave-like muscular motion of the esophagus and bowel that moves food through the digestive system.

occasionally be palpated just below the margin of the rib cage. It is suspended in its location by several ligaments, including the ligamentum teres, and connects to the omentum inferiorly. The liver is a solid organ but is rather delicate in nature. It is contained within a fibrous capsule (visceral peritoneum) that serves to retard hemorrhage and helps hold the liver together if injured by blunt trauma. When injured, the liver will regenerate to some degree but will not function as efficiently as before the injury.

The gallbladder is a small hollow organ located behind and beneath the liver. It receives bile (a waste product from the reprocessing of red blood cells) from the liver and stores it until it is needed during digestion of fatty foods. It then constricts and sends bile through the bile duct and into the duodenum. Bile helps the body by emulsifying (breaking apart and suspending) ingested fats that would otherwise remain as clumps during the digestive process.

The other accessory digestive organ is the pancreas. It is responsible for the production of glucagon and insulin, hormones responsible for the regulation of blood glucose levels and the transport of glucose across cell membranes. The pancreas also produces very powerful digestive enzymes that help return the pH of the chyme to normal and break down proteins. These enzymes enter the duodenum through the common bile duct. Like the liver, the pancreas is a solid, though delicate, organ, encapsulated in a serous membrane. It is located in the medial and lower portion of the left upper quadrant and extends into the medial portion of the right upper quadrant. The duodenum wraps around the right pancreatic border. If the cells of the pancreas are damaged, the pancreatic enzymes become active and begin to "self-digest" pancreatic tissue. If these enzymes are released into the retroperitoneal space, they will also damage surrounding tissue.

THE SPLEEN

The spleen is not an accessory organ of digestion but rather a part of the immune system. It is a very vascular organ about the size of the palm of the hand and is located behind the stomach and lateral to the kidney in the left upper quadrant. The spleen performs some immunological functions and also stores a large volume of blood. It is the most fragile abdominal organ, though well protected in its location by the rib cage, spine, and **flank** and back muscles. The spleen, however, can be injured during blunt trauma, especially with impacts affecting the left flank, and when injured, it bleeds heavily.

THE URINARY SYSTEM

The urinary system contains four major structures, the kidneys, ureters, urinary bladder, and urethra (Figure 12-109). First, we will discuss the structures and functions of the urinary system, focusing on the kidneys. Then, we will cover the additional structures of the male genitourinary system.

THE KIDNEYS

The left kidney lies in the upper abdomen behind the spleen, and the right kidney lies behind the liver. These locations correspond to the left and right areas of the small of the back, or the flanks. A healthy **kidney** in a young adult is about the size of a fist and contains about one million **nephrons,** the microscopic structures that produce urine. With aging comes a normal loss of nephrons—10 percent per decade of life after age 40—so you should always be alert to the possibility of compromised kidney function in elderly patients.

* **flanks** the part of the back below the ribs and above the hip bones.

* **kidney** an organ that produces urine and performs other functions related to the urinary system.

* **nephron** a microscopic structure within the kidney that produces urine.

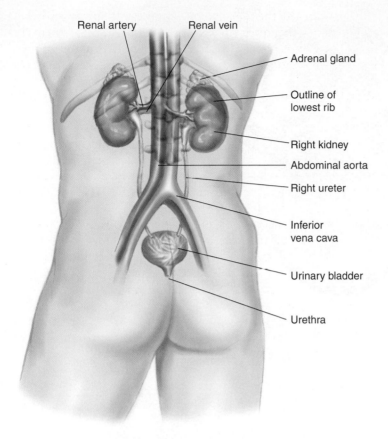

Renal artery   Renal vein

Adrenal gland

Outline of
lowest rib

Right kidney

Abdominal aorta

Right ureter

Inferior
vena cava

Urinary bladder

Urethra

FIGURE 12-109   Anatomy of the urinary system, posterior view.

Gross and Microscopic Anatomy of the Kidney

The renal artery and vein, as well as nerves, lymphatic vessels, and the ureter, pass into the kidney through the notched region called the **hilum.** The tissue of the kidney itself is visibly divided into an outer region, the **cortex,** and an inner region, the **medulla.** Medullary tissue is divided into fan-shaped regions, or **pyramids.** Each pyramid ends in a portion of tissue called the **papilla,** which projects into the hollow space of the **renal pelvis** (Figure 12-110). The spaces of the pelvis come together at the origin of the ureter. Urine forms in the cortical and medullary tissue of the kidney and leaves the kidney through the renal pelvis and ureter.

The functional unit of the kidney, the nephron, forms urine (Figure 12-111). Each nephron consists of a tubule divided into structurally different portions and capillaries that form a complex net of vessels covering the surface of the tubule. Blood that has entered the kidney through the renal artery flows through successively smaller vessels until it reaches a **glomerulus,** a cluster of capillaries surrounded by **Bowman's capsule,** the cup-shaped, hollow structure that is the first part of the nephron. Water and chemical substances enter the tubule through Bowman's capsule. After passage through successive parts of the tubule—the

* **hilum** the notched part of the kidney where the ureter and other structures join kidney tissue.

* **cortex** the outer tissue of an organ, such as the kidney.

* **medulla** the inner tissue of an organ, such as the kidney.

* **pyramids** the visible tissue structures within the medulla of the kidney.

* **papilla** the tip of a pyramid; it juts into the hollow space of the kidney.

* **renal pelvis** the hollow space of the kidney that junctions with a ureter.

* **glomerulus** a tuft of capillaries from which blood is filtered into a nephron.

* **Bowman's capsule** the hollow, cup-shaped first part of the nephron tubule.

FIGURE 12-110 Cross-section
of the kidney.

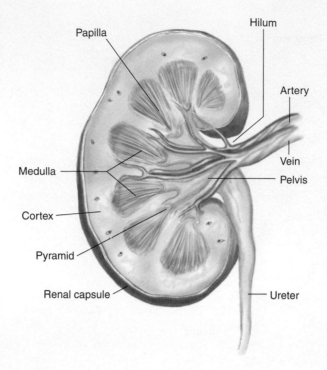

Papilla

Hilum

Artery

Vein

Pelvis

Medulla

Cortex

Pyramid

Renal capsule

Ureter

FIGURE 12-111 Anatomy of
the nephron.

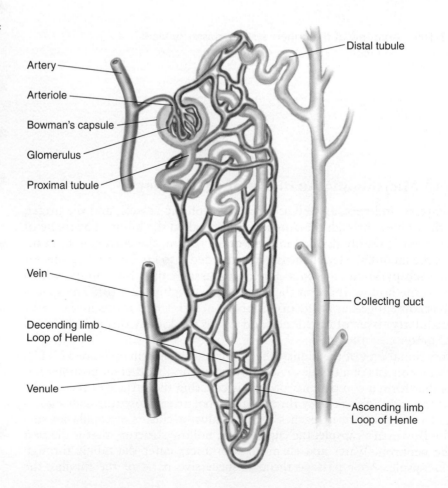

Distal tubule

Artery

Arteriole

Bowman's capsule

Glomerulus

Proximal tubule

Vein

Collecting duct

Decending limb
Loop of Henle

Venule

Ascending limb
Loop of Henle

proximal tubule, descending loop of Henle, ascending loop of Henle, and distal tubule—urine drips into the collecting duct before entering the renal pelvis and ureter.

Kidney Physiology

The physiology of the kidneys is one of the most complex topics in human physiology. Its explanation often requires several book chapters. The following is a brief overview.

Overview of Nephron Physiology Forming and eliminating urine are the basis for two of the kidneys' major functions: (1) maintaining blood volume with proper balance of water, electrolytes, and pH; and (2) retaining key compounds, such as glucose, while excreting wastes, such as urea. A third function, controlling arterial blood pressure, relies both on urine formation and on a second mechanism that does not involve urine production. Last, kidney cells regulate erythrocyte development, but this process does not involve urine formation in any way.

Urine is produced through the interactions among capillary blood flowing over the nephron tubule, the fluid flowing inside the tubule, and the capillary and tubular cells themselves. Three general processes are involved in formation of urine: **glomerular filtration, reabsorption** of substances from the renal tubule into blood, and **secretion** of substances from blood into the renal tubule.

The first step in urine formation is filtration of blood. As blood flows through the capillaries of the glomerulus, water and numerous chemical materials are filtered out of the blood and into Bowman's capsule. Normally, the only blood elements that are not freely filtered into the capsule are blood cells and the plasma proteins, all of which are too large to pass through the pores formed by cell junctions in the capillary walls. Consequently, the fluid formed in the capsule—the **filtrate**—roughly resembles blood plasma, except for the absence of proteins.

The rate at which blood is filtered, the **glomerular filtration rate (GFR)**, averages 180 L/day, the equivalent of 60 complete passages of blood plasma through the glomerular filters. This remarkable efficiency underlies the kidneys' ability to excrete toxic or foreign substances, such as urea or drug metabolites, so quickly that the substances do not accumulate in the blood.

Filtration is a nonselective process based primarily on molecular size (electrical charge is a secondary factor), and it is essential to urine formation. In contrast, reabsorption of substances into the blood and secretion of substances into the renal tubule are highly selective processes. Almost all elements of filtrate are handled independently of the other elements. The processes of reabsorption and secretion are essential to forming urine with the correct composition and volume to compensate for current body conditions, that is, to maintain homeostasis.

Reabsorption and secretion involve intercellular transport, the movement of a molecule across a cell membrane to either enter or exit a cell. Like other intercellular transport processes, they occur in one of three ways: **simple diffusion,** facilitated diffusion, or active transport. Both simple and facilitated diffusion are passive processes: neither requires the cell to spend energy. In simple diffusion, molecules small enough to pass through a cell membrane randomly move into and out of the cell. Because net movement is always from the region of higher concentration to that of lower concentration, simple diffusion leads toward equalization of molecular concentration on both sides of the membrane. Water molecules always move by simple diffusion. **Osmosis** is the process in which water molecules move so that the concentrations of particles dissolved in water (or

* **proximal tubule** the part of the tubule beyond Bowman's capsule.

* **descending loop of Henle** the part of the tubule beyond the proximal tubule.

* **ascending loop of Henle** the part of the tubule beyond the descending loop of Henle.

* **distal tubule** the part of the tubule beyond the ascending loop of Henle.

* **collecting duct** the larger structure beyond the distal tubule into which urine drips.

* **glomerular filtration** the removal from blood of water and other elements, which enter the nephron tubule.

* **reabsorption** the movement of a substance from a nephron tubule back into the blood.

* **secretion** the movement of a substance from the blood into a nephron tubule.

* **filtrate** the fluid produced in Bowman's capsule by filtration of blood.

* **glomerular filtration rate (GFR)** the volume per day at which blood is filtered through capillaries of the glomerulus.

* **simple diffusion** the random motion of molecules from an area of high concentration to an area of lower concentration.

* **osmosis** the diffusion pattern of water in which molecules move to equalize concentrations on both sides of a membrane.

osmolarity) approach equivalence on both sides of a membrane. A solution with a higher concentration than another solution is **hyperosmolar** to the other; a solution with a lower, more dilute concentration is **hypo-osmolar** to the other.

In **facilitated diffusion,** molecules still move from the region of higher concentration to that of lower concentration. However, a molecule-specific carrier in the membrane acts as a tunnel and speeds the molecules' movement through the membrane. The body cells' normal handling of glucose is an example of this process. When insulin binds to a glucose-specific carrier in the cell membrane, glucose can pass into the cell 10 times faster than when insulin is not bound to the carrier.

Active transport is the only process that can produce a net movement of molecules from a region of lower concentration to one of higher concentration. This uphill movement against the concentration gradient is possible because energy is spent to drive the action of the molecule-specific carrier in the membrane. Active transport processes are vital to renal tubular physiology because they allow for the precise balance of reabsorption and secretion that results in independent, homeostatic handling of electrolytes and other substances, such as glucose.

Tubular Handling of Water and Electrolytes Tubular handling of water and electrolytes including sodium (Na^+), potassium (K^+), hydrogen (H^+), and chloride (Cl^-) is the basis for control of blood volume and maintenance of electrolyte balance, including pH. As you recall, Na^+ is the dominant cation in the body's extracellular fluids, including blood, whereas K^+ is the dominant cation in intracellular fluid. Appropriate retention of Na^+ in the body, along with osmotic retention of water, is key to maintaining blood volume. Selective retention of K^+ and H^+, along with anions, such as Cl^-, maintains the balance of blood electrolytes and blood pH.

Filtrate formed in Bowman's capsule enters the proximal tubule (review Figure 12-111). The cells of the proximal tubule have an extensive brush border that maximizes contact between cell membrane and filtrate. They also have high concentrations of molecule-specific carriers in their membranes and maintain a high level of metabolic activity, producing energy that can support active transport. Under normal conditions, about 65 percent of filtered Na^+ and Cl^- is reabsorbed in the proximal tubule, along with osmotic reabsorption of about the same percentage of filtered water. Reabsorption takes place by both passive and active transport processes. Much of the active Na^+ reabsorption is coupled with secretion of H^+ into the tubule; H^+ secretion raises the pH of the arterial-derived blood flowing in capillaries surrounding the tubule. Further handling of H^+ as the filtrate moves through the tubule determines the pH both of the venous blood leaving the kidneys and of the urine excreted from the body.

As filtrate moves through the next part of the nephron, the loop of Henle, its volume and composition change further. Simple diffusion is the dominant process in the first part of the loop. By the time filtrate has moved through the descending limb of the loop, roughly another 20 percent of the filtrate's original water load has been reabsorbed. The cells of the second, ascending limb of the loop of Henle are normally virtually impermeable to water; however, passive and active reabsorption of significant amounts of electrolytes occurs in the same part of the tubule. This reabsorption of electrolytes without reabsorption of water produces a relatively dilute fluid that may exit the collecting duct as dilute urine. Healthy kidneys can produce urine with an osmolarity as low as one-sixth the osmolar concentration of blood plasma, an action termed **diuresis.** A number of hormones alter tubular handling of water and electrolytes (Table 12-7). Some increase the permeability of the distal tubule, collecting duct, or both so that far more water is reabsorbed. **Antidiuresis,** the result of this hormonal activity, can form a very concentrated urine with an osmolarity as high as four times that of plasma.

---

* **hyperosmolar** a solution that has a concentration of the substance greater than that of a second solution.

* **hypo-osmolar** a solution that has a concentration of the substance lower than that of a second solution.

* **facilitated diffusion** a form of molecular diffusion in which a molecule-specific carrier in a cell membrane speeds the molecule's movement from a region of higher concentration to one of lower concentration.

* **active transport** movement of a molecule through a cell membrane from a region of lower concentration to one of higher concentration; movement requires energy consumption within the cell.

* **diuresis** formation and passage of dilute urine, decreasing blood volume.

* **antidiuresis** formation and passage of concentrated urine, preserving blood volume.

Table 12-7 HORMONES THAT AFFECT TUBULAR HANDLING OF WATER AND KEY ELECTROLYTES

Hormone	Target Tissue	Effect(s)
Aldosterone	Distal tubule, collecting duct	Increase in reabsorption of Na^+, Cl^-, and water
		Increase in secretion of K^+
Angiotensin II	Proximal tubule	Increase in reabsorption of Na^+, Cl^-, and water
		Increase in secretion of H^+
Antidiuretic hormone (ADH)	Distal tubule, collecting duct	Increase in reabsorption of water
Atrial natriuretic hormone (ANH)	Distal tubule, collecting duct	Decrease in reabsorption of Na^+ and Cl^-

Note: Aldosterone, ADH, and ANH are discussed in detail in "Endocrinology," Chapter 30; angiotensin II is discussed in "Cardiology," Chapter 28.

Table derived from Arthur C. Guyton and John E. Hall, *Textbook of Medical Physiology*, 9th ed. (Philadelphia: W.B. Saunders Company, 1996).

The ability of healthy kidneys to handle significant swings in water and electrolyte intake is remarkable. Studies have shown that an individual can increase her sodium intake to 10 times the average amount or decrease it to roughly one-tenth the average, and the kidneys will still compensate properly. Blood volume and sodium content will change only modestly from their baseline, normal levels.

Tubular Handling of Glucose and Urea Glucose and urea represent substances that the kidneys handle in opposite fashion. Critical substances, such as glucose, are retained in the body, and wastes, such as urea, are excreted.

Glucose is freely filtered into Bowman's capsule as an element of filtrate. Normally, glucose is completely reabsorbed through an active transport process by the time filtrate leaves the proximal tubule. The body's absolute retention of glucose is usually maintained until the blood glucose level reaches about 10 mmol/L; above that level, glucose begins to be lost in urine. This pattern, in which glucose is completely reabsorbed until a ceiling, or threshold level, of blood glucose is reached, is due to saturation of the active-transport process responsible for reabsorption of glucose. At excessively high blood glucose levels, so much glucose enters the filtrate that the proximal tubule's transport capacity to reabsorb it is insufficient. When this occurs, as in uncontrolled diabetes mellitus type I, the body loses not only glucose but also large amounts of water through **osmotic diuresis.**

Urea, a waste product, is also freely filtered into Bowman's capsule. However, tubular handling of this small molecule is very different from that of glucose. Urea is passively reabsorbed throughout most of the tubule, and about half of the filtered load will remain in urine. Thus, the kidneys' ability to excrete urea efficiently depends on the glomerular filtration rate, or GFR. If blood passes through the glomerular capillaries at an adequate rate, the net result of filtration and passive reabsorption will keep the blood level from rising toward a toxic level. The blood urea nitrogen test, or BUN, directly measures blood concentration of urea and is an indirect indicator of GFR. **Creatinine,** another waste product of metabolism, has larger molecules than urea and is not reabsorbed. Because all of the filtered creatinine will be eliminated in urine, the blood concentration of creatinine is a direct indicator of GFR.

Control of Arterial Blood Pressure The kidneys regulate systemic arterial blood pressure in several ways. Over the long term, they control the body's balance of water and electrolytes, thus maintaining blood volume at a healthy level.

✱ **osmotic diuresis** greatly increased urination and dehydration that results when high levels of glucose cannot be reabsorbed into the blood from the kidney tubules and the osmotic pressure of the glucose in the tubules also prevents water reabsorption.

✱ **creatinine** a waste product caused by metabolism within muscle cells.

BUN and creatinine levels are both important indicators of renal function.

renin an enzyme produced by kidney cells that plays a key role in controlling arterial blood pressure.

In addition, juxtaglomerular cells, specialized cells adjacent to glomerular capillary cells, respond to low blood pressure by releasing an enzyme called **renin.** Within seconds of its release, renin produces significant amounts of the active hormone angiotensin I. As angiotensin I flows through the lungs, angiotensin converting enzyme (ACE) produces angiotensin II, the powerful vasoconstrictor that immediately raises arterial blood pressure. Angiotensin II acts both on kidney tubular cells (see Table 12-7) and on adrenal cells, causing the latter to secrete aldosterone. The renin-angiotensin system has an important role in the maintenance of blood pressure, as noted earlier.

erythropoietin a hormone produced by kidney cells that stimulates maturation of red blood cells.

Control of Erythrocyte Development The kidneys produce 90 percent of the body's **erythropoietin,** a hormone that regulates the rate at which erythrocytes mature in bone marrow. The exact mechanism that produces erythropoietin is unclear. The impact of renal tissue death, however, is clear and profound; the nonkidney sources of erythropoietin can produce only about one-third to one-half the red cell mass (measured as hematocrit) needed by the body.

THE URETERS

ureter a duct that carries urine from kidney to urinary bladder.

Urine drains from the renal pelvis into the **ureter,** the long duct that runs from the kidney to the urinary bladder (review Figure 12-109). Each ureter is about 25 cm long and, like the kidney, is located in the retroperitoneum of the abdomen. A thin muscular layer in the ureters' walls limits their ability to distend in response to internal pressure. The ureters' nerves derive from renal, gonadal, or hypogastric nerve trunks. The microscopic structure of the ureters and the nature of their nerve supply are important in understanding the symptoms caused by kidney stones caught in a ureter.

THE URINARY BLADDER

urinary bladder the muscular organ that stores urine before its elimination from the body.

The **urinary bladder,** the anteriormost organ in the pelvis of both men and women, stores urine. The muscular bladder usually contains at least a small amount of urine, which produces its roughly spherical shape. The bladder neck, through which urine passes during urination, is held in place by ligaments. In women, connective tissue loosely attaches the bladder's posterior wall to the anterior vaginal wall. In men, the bladder's wall bladder is structurally continuous with the prostate gland.

THE URETHRA

urethra the duct that carries urine from the urinary bladder out of the body; in men, it also carries reproductive fluid (semen) to the outside of the body.

The **urethra** is the duct that carries urine from the bladder to the exterior of the body. In women, the urethra is only about 3 to 4 cm long and opens to the external environment via a small orifice just anterior to that of the vagina. In men, the urethra is about 20 cm long and ends at the tip of the penis. The female urethra's shortness is probably one reason the female urinary system is more vulnerable to bacterial infection from environmental (largely skin) sources. Because the male urethra carries both urine and male reproductive fluid, it can be an entry way for sexually transmitted diseases.

THE REPRODUCTIVE SYSTEM

It is important to have an understanding of both the female and the male reproductive systems.

FIGURE 12-112   The vulva.

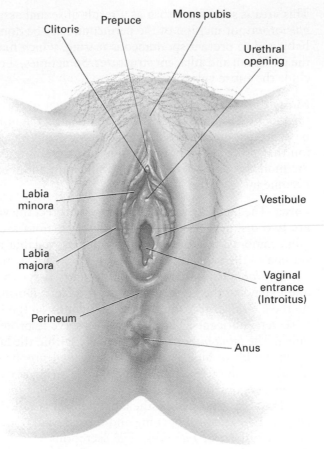

Clitoris Prepuce Mons pubis Urethral opening

Labia minora Vestibule

Labia majora Vaginal entrance (Introitus)

Perineum

Anus

THE FEMALE REPRODUCTIVE SYSTEM

The most important female reproductive organs are internal and are located within the pelvic cavity. These include the ovaries, fallopian tubes, uterus, and vagina, which are essential to reproduction. The external genitalia have accessory functions, in that they protect body openings and play an important role in sexual functioning.

The External Genitalia

The female external genitalia are known collectively as the *vulva*, or *pudendum* (Figure 12-112). These external genitalia consist of highly vascular tissues that protect the entrance to the birth canal. They include the perineum, mons pubis, labia, and clitoris.

   The external genital organs begin to mature and take adult proportions during adolescence. Puberty also marks the appearance of breast buds, pubic hair, and the first period (menarche). The age in which sexual development occurs varies among individuals. As women grow older, ovarian function diminishes, menstrual periods cease, and pubic hair becomes grey and sparse. The labia and clitoris become smaller; the vagina narrows and shortens and its lining (the mucosa) becomes thin, pale, and dry. The ovaries and uterus decrease in size.

Perineum The **perineum** is a roughly diamond-shaped, skin-covered muscular tissue that separates the vagina and the anus. These tissues form a sling-like structure supporting the internal pelvic organs and are able to stretch during childbirth.

✱ **perineum** muscular tissue that separates the vagina and the anus.

This area is sometimes torn as a result of sexual assault or during childbirth. An *episiotomy,* or incision of the perineum, may be done to facilitate delivery of the baby and to prevent spontaneous tearing, which may cause significant injury to the perineum and adjacent structures. Sometimes, the term *perineum* is used to include the entire vulvar area.

Mons Pubis The **mons pubis** is a fatty layer of tissue over the pubic symphysis, the junction of pubic bones. During puberty, the hormone estrogen causes fat to be deposited under the skin, giving it a mound-like shape. This serves as a cushion that protects the pubic symphysis during intercourse. Also, during puberty, the mons becomes covered with pubic hair, and its sebaceous and sweat glands become more active.

＊ mons pubis fatty layer of tissue over the pubic symphysis.

Labia The **labia** are the structures that protect the vagina and the urethra. There are two distinct sets of labia. The labia majora are located laterally, while the labia minora are more medial. Both sets of labia are subject to injury during trauma to the vulvar area, such as occurs with sexual assault.

＊ labia structures that protect the vagina and urethra, including the *labia majora* and the *labia minora.*

The *labia majora* are two folds of fatty tissue that arise from the mons pubis and extend to the perineum, forming a cleft. During puberty, pubic hair grows on the lateral surface, and sebaceous glands on the hairless medial surface begin to secrete lubricants. The labia majora serve to protect the inner structures of the vulva. The *labia minora,* lying medially within the labia majora, are two smaller, thinner folds of highly vascular tissue, well supplied with nerves and sebaceous glands, which secrete lubricating fluid. During sexual arousal, the labia minora become engorged with blood.

The area protected by the labia minora is called the *vestibule.* The vestibule contains the urethral opening and the external opening of the vagina, called the vaginal orifice, or *introitus.* The secretions of two pairs of glands (Skene and Bartholin) lubricate these structures during sexual stimulation. Located within the vestibule is the *hymen.* It is a thin fold of mucous membrane that forms the external border of the vagina, partly closing it.

Clitoris The **clitoris** is highly innervated and richly vascular erectile tissue that lies anterior to the labia minora. This cylindrical structure is a major site of sexual stimulation and orgasm in women. The *prepuce* is a fold of the labia minora that covers the clitoris.

＊ clitoris highly innervated and vascular erectile tissue anterior to the labia minora.

The Internal Genitalia

The internal female reproductive organs are the vagina, the uterus, the fallopian tubes, and the ovaries (Figures 12-113 and 12-114).

Vagina The **vagina** is an elastic canal made up primarily of smooth muscle, 9 to 10 cm in length, that connects the external genitalia to the uterus. It lies between the urethra/bladder and the anus/rectum. Lined with mucous membrane, the vagina extends up and back from the vaginal orifice to the lower end of the uterus (cervix). The vaginal walls are crisscrossed with ridges that allow it to stretch during childbirth, allowing passage of the fetus. The vagina's primary blood supply is the vaginal artery. The pudendal nerve innervates the lower third of the vagina and the external genitalia. The vagina has three functions:

＊ vagina canal that connects the external female genitalia to the uterus.

1. It is the female organ of copulation and receives the penis during sexual intercourse.
2. Often called the birth canal, it forms the final passageway for the infant during childbirth.
3. It provides an outlet for menstrual blood and tissue to leave the body.

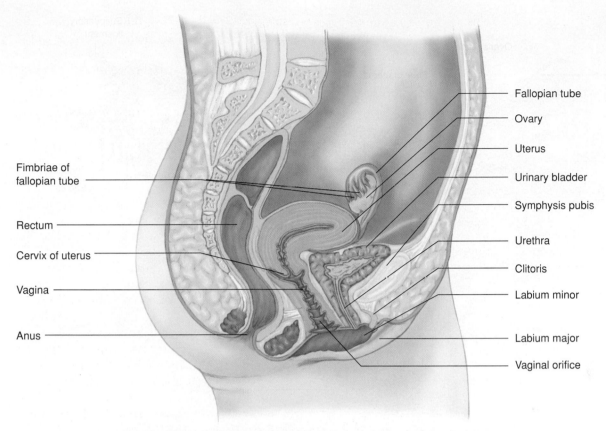

FIGURE 12-113   Cross-sectional anatomy of the female reproductive system.

Uterus The **uterus** is a hollow, thick-walled, muscular, inverted-pear-shaped organ that connects with the vagina. It lies in the centre of the pelvis and is flexed forward between the bladder and rectum above the vagina. Approximately 7.5 cm long and 5 cm wide, the uterus is held loosely in position by ligaments, peritoneal folds, and the pressure of adjacent abdominal structures. The primary function of the uterus is to provide a site for fetal development. During pregnancy, the uterus stretches to a size capable of containing the fetus, placenta, and the associated membranes and amniotic fluid. At term, the gravid uterus measures approximately 40 cm in length. The uterus has an extensive blood supply, primarily from the uterine arteries, which are branches of the internal iliac artery. The autonomic nervous system innervates the uterus. In a nonpregnant state, the uterine cavity is flat and triangular.

The uterus has two major parts: the *body* (or corpus) and the *cervix* (or neck). The upper two-thirds of the uterus form the body and comprise smooth muscle layers. The lower third is the cervix.

The rounded uppermost portion of the body of the uterus is the *fundus*, which lies above the point where the fallopian tubes attach. Measurement of fundal height (distance from the symphysis pubis to the fundus) may be used to estimate gestational age during pregnancy. The fundal height measured in centimetres is generally comparable with the weeks of gestation. For instance, if the fundal height is 30 cm, the gestational age is about 30 weeks. This method of assessing uterine size is most accurate from 22 to 34 weeks.

The body of the uterus has three layers of tissue that make up the uterine wall. The innermost layer or lining is called the **endometrium.** Each month, stimulated by estrogen and progesterone, the endometrium builds up in preparation for the implantation of a fertilized ovum. If fertilization does not occur, the lining degenerates

✱ **uterus** hollow organ in the centre of the abdomen that provides the site for fetal development.

✱ **endometrium** the inner layer of the uterine wall where the fertilized egg implants.

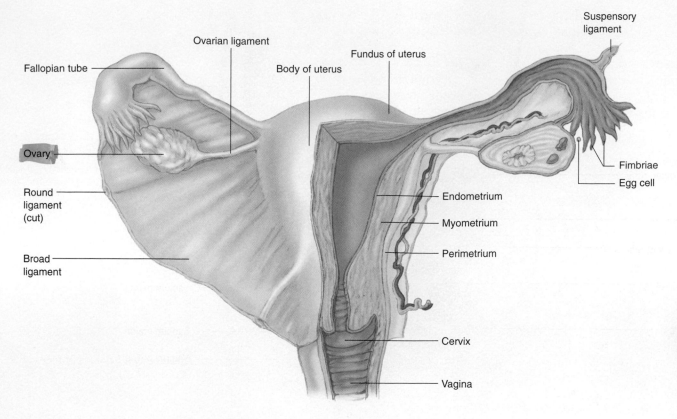

Labels on figure:
Fallopian tube
Ovarian ligament
Body of uterus
Fundus of uterus
Suspensory ligament
Ovary
Round ligament (cut)
Broad ligament
Fimbriae
Egg cell
Endometrium
Myometrium
Perimetrium
Cervix
Vagina

FIGURE 12-114   The uterus, fallopian tubes, and ovaries.

* **myometrium** the thick middle layer of the uterine wall made up of smooth muscle fibres.

* **perimetrium** the serosal peritoneal membrane which forms the outermost layer of the uterine wall.

* **fallopian tubes** thin tubes that extend laterally from the uterus and conduct eggs from the ovaries into the uterine cavity.

and sloughs off. This sloughing of the uterine lining is referred to as the *menses,* or menstrual period.

The thick middle layer of the uterine wall, called the **myometrium** is made up of three distinct layers of smooth muscle fibres. In the outer layer, primarily over the fundus, the fibres run longitudinally, which allows expulsion of the fetus following cervical dilation. The middle (and thicker) layer is made up of figure-eight patterns of interlaced muscle fibres which surround large blood vessels. The contraction of these fibres helps control postdelivery bleeding. The myometrial fibres also contract during menstruation to maximize the sloughing of the endometrium. It has been suggested that menstrual cramps are due to fatigue of the myometrial fibres. The innermost layer of the myometrium comprises circular smooth muscle fibres that form sphincters at the point of fallopian tube attachment and at the internal opening of the cervix.

The outermost layer of the uterine wall is a serous membrane called the **perimetrium** that partially covers the corpus of the uterus. The perimetrium, which is a layer of the visceral peritoneum that lines the abdominal cavity and abdominal organs, does not extend to the cervix. The most significant aspect of this partial coverage is that it allows surgical access to the uterus without the risk of infection that is associated with peritoneal incisions.

The cervix, or neck of the uterus, extends from the narrowest portion of the uterus to connect with the vagina. That distance forms the cervical canal and is only approximately 2.5 cm in length. Elasticity characterizes the cervix. During labour, it dilates to a diameter of approximately 10 cm to allow delivery of the fetus.

Fallopian Tubes The two **fallopian tubes,** also called uterine tubes, are thin flexible tubes that extend laterally from the uterus and curve up and over each ovary on either side. Each tube is approximately 10 cm in length and about 1 cm in diameter (about the size of a pencil lead), except at its ovarian end which is trumpet shaped. Each fallopian tube has two openings, a fimbriated (fringed) end that opens into the abdominal cavity in the area adjacent to the ovaries and a minute opening into the uterus. The function of the tubes is to conduct the egg from the space around the ovaries into the uterine cavity via peristalsis (wave-like muscular contractions). Fertilization usually occurs in the distal third of the fallopian tube.

Ovaries The **ovaries** are the primary female gonads, or sex glands. Almond shaped, the ovaries are situated laterally on either side of the uterus in the upper portion of the pelvic cavity. They have two functions: One function is the secretion of the hormones estrogen and progesterone in response to stimulation from follicle-stimulating hormone (FSH) and luteinizing hormone (LH) secreted from the anterior pituitary gland. The second function of the ovaries is the development and release of eggs (ova) for reproduction.

✳ **ovaries** the primary female sex glands that secrete estrogen and progesterone and produce eggs for reproduction.

The Menstrual Cycle

The female undergoes a monthly hormonal cycle, generally every 28 days, that prepares the uterus to receive a fertilized egg. The onset of the menstrual cycle, that is, the onset of ovulation at puberty, establishes female sexual maturity. This onset, known as **menarche,** usually begins between the ages of 10 and 14. At first, the periods are irregular. Later, they become more regular and predictable. The length of the menstrual cycle may vary from 21 to 32 days. A "normal" menstrual cycle is what is normal for the particular woman. Because of this, it is important to inquire as to the normal length of the patient's menstrual cycle. Regardless of the length of the menstrual cycle, the time from ovulation to menstruation is always 14 days. Any variance in cycle length occurs during the preovulatory phase.

✳ **menarche** the onset of menses, usually occurring between ages 10 and 14.

From puberty to menopause, the female sex hormones (estrogen and progesterone) control the ovarian-menstrual cycle, pregnancy, and lactation. These hormones are not produced at a constant rate, but rather, their production surges and diminishes in a cyclical fashion. The secretion of estrogen and progesterone by the ovaries is controlled by the secretion of FSH and LH.

The Proliferative Phase The first two weeks of the menstrual cycle, known as the proliferative phase, are dominated by estrogen, which causes the uterine lining (endometrium) to thicken and become engorged with blood. In response to a surge of LH at approximately day 14, **ovulation** (release of an egg) takes place.

✳ **ovulation** the release of an egg from the ovary.

At birth, each female's ovary contains some 200 000 ova within immature ovarian follicles known as graafian follicles. This is the female's lifetime supply of ova, which are gradually "used up" through ovulation during her lifetime.

In response to FSH and increased estrogen levels, once during every menstrual cycle, a follicle reaches maturation and ruptures, discharging its egg through the ovary's outer covering into the abdominal cavity. The ruptured follicle, under the influence of LH, develops the corpus luteum, a small yellowish body of cells, which produces progesterone during the second half of the menstrual cycle. If the egg is not fertilized, the corpus luteum will atrophy about three days before the onset of the menstrual phase. If the egg is fertilized, the corpus luteum will produce progesterone until the placenta takes over that function.

The cilia (fine, hair-like structures) on the fimbriated ends of the fallopian tubes draw the egg into the tube and sweep it toward the uterus. If the woman has had sexual intercourse within approximately 24 hours of ovulation, fertilization may take place. If the egg is fertilized, it normally implants in the thickened lining of the uterus, where the fetus subsequently develops. If it is not fertilized, it passes into the uterine cavity and is expelled.

The Secretory Phase The stage of the menstrual cycle immediately surrounding ovulation is referred to as the secretory phase. If the egg is not fertilized, the woman's estrogen level drops sharply while the progesterone level dominates. Uterine vascularity increases during this phase in anticipation of implantation of a fertilized egg.

The Ischemic Phase If fertilization doesn't occur, estrogen and progesterone levels fall. Vascular changes cause the endometrium to become pale and small blood vessels to rupture.

The Menstrual Phase During the menstrual phase, the ischemic endometrium is shed, along with a discharge of blood, mucus, and cellular debris. This is known as **menstruation**. A "normal" menstrual cycle depends on the regular pattern in the individual woman. The first day of the menstrual cycle is the day on which bleeding begins and the menstrual flow usually lasts from three to five days, although this varies from woman to woman. An average blood loss of about 50 mL is common. The absence of a menstrual period in any woman in the childbearing years (generally ages 12 to 55) who is sexually active and whose periods are usually regular should raise the suspicion of pregnancy.

Some women regularly experience marked physical signs and symptoms immediately before the onset of their menstrual period. These are collectively known as **premenstrual syndrome (PMS)**. Although you may hear crude jokes made about PMS, there is no denying the reality of the physical changes that accompany the changing hormonal levels. It is not uncommon for women to report breast tenderness or engorgement, transient weight gain or bloating as a result of fluid retention, excessive fatigue, and/or cravings for specific foods. Women who are prone to migraine headaches may see them increase during the premenstrual period. Other women may have only minimal physical symptoms but are more affected by emotional responses, such as irritability, anxiety, or depression. The severity of PMS varies with each individual and may require treatment focused on relief of symptoms.

Menopause, the cessation of menses, marks the cessation of ovarian function and the cessation of estrogen secretion. Menstrual periods generally continue to occur until a woman is 45 to 55, at which time they begin to decline in frequency and length until they ultimately stop. The end of reproductive life is also known as the "climacteric," which is derived from Greek, meaning "critical time of life." Occasionally, physicians use the term surgical menopause, which means that a woman's periods have stopped because of surgical removal of her uterus, ovaries, or both. The decrease in estrogen levels causes many women to experience hot flashes, night sweats, and mood swings during menopause. It is not uncommon for hormone replacement therapy (oral estrogen, or estrogen and progesterone) to be prescribed for a brief time to help relieve these complaints.

The Pregnant Uterus

The dynamics of pregnancy greatly affect the anatomy of the female abdominal cavity (Figure 12-115). The uterus and its contents grow rapidly from the time of conception until delivery and are well protected during the first trimester (three months) of pregnancy. During the second trimester (12 to 24 weeks), the progressive enlargement of the uterus displaces most of the abdominal contents upward as the growing uterus rises out of the pelvis and its upper border extends above the umbilicus. By 32 weeks and until the end of the pregnancy, the uterus fills the abdominal cavity to the level of the lower rib margin. This enlarging mass in the abdomen also increases the intra-abdominal pressure and displaces the diaphragm upward. This displacement reduces lung capacity at the same time that the physiological changes of pregnancy increase the tidal volume.

✳ **menstruation** sloughing of the uterine lining (endometrium) if a fertilized egg is not implanted. It is controlled by the cyclical release of hormones. Menstruation is also called a *period.*

✳ **premenstrual syndrome (PMS)** a variety of signs and symptoms, such as weight gain, irritability, or specific food cravings associated with the changing hormonal levels that precede menstruation.

✳ **menopause** the cessation of menses and ovarian function resulting from decreased secretion of estrogen.

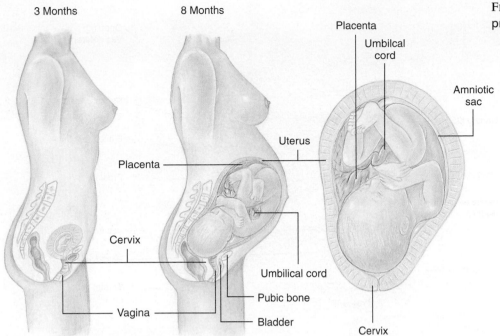

3 Months   8 Months

Placenta
Umbilcal cord
Amniotic sac
Uterus
Placenta
Cervix
Umbilical cord
Pubic bone
Bladder
Vagina
Cervix

FIGURE 12-115 The pregnant uterus.

Pregnancy also affects the maternal physiology by raising the circulatory volume by about 45 percent and, by the third trimester, raising the cardiac rate by about 15 beats per minute and the cardiac output by up to 40 percent. The increase in the vascular volume is accompanied by a less significant increase in the number of erythrocytes. The result is a relative anemia that becomes an important consideration with aggressive fluid resuscitation for the mother in shock. In the last trimester of pregnancy, the uterus is significant in both size and weight and may compress the vena cava, reducing venous return to the heart and inducing a temporary hypotension in the supine patient (supine hypotensive syndrome). Finally, with the developing fetus, there are now two lives to protect when the mother suffers any trauma, especially involving the abdomen.

THE MALE REPRODUCTIVE SYSTEM

As noted earlier, the male reproductive organs are considered to be part of the urinary system (Figure 12-116). Like the female reproductive system, the male reproductive system includes both external and internal genitalia.

The Testes The **testes** are the primary male reproductive organs. They produce both the hormones responsible for sexual maturation and sperm cells, or male sex cells. The testes lie outside of the abdomen in a muscular sac called the scrotum. Normal scrotal temperature is about 2–3°C lower than abdominal temperature, which is critical for development of sperm.

The Epididymis and Vas Deferens Sperm cells pass from the testis into the **epididymis,** a small sac where they are stored. Each testis with its paired epididymis is palpable inside the scrotum. Sperm cells are channelled from the epididymis into the **vas deferens,** a muscular duct that carries them into the pelvis and through the substance of the prostate gland to its opening into the urethra. Sperm cells mix with special fluid before passing into the urethra for ejaculation, or elimination from the body.

The vas deferens passes through an opening in the inguinal ligament known as the *inguinal canal.* The testicular blood supply also runs through this opening, an anatomical weak point that is the site of male hernias.

✳ **testes** primary male reproductive organs that produce hormones responsible for sexual maturation and sperm cells; singular *testis.*

✳ **epididymis** small sac in which sperm cells are stored.

✳ **vas deferens** duct that carries sperm cells to the urethra for ejaculation.

FIGURE 12-116 Anatomy of the male genitourinary system.

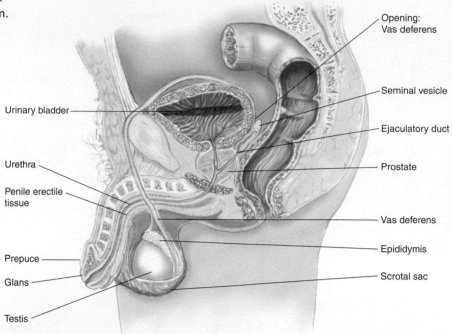

Opening: Vas deferens

Seminal vesicle

Ejaculatory duct

Prostate

Vas deferens

Epididymis

Scrotal sac

Urinary bladder

Urethra

Penile erectile tissue

Prepuce

Glans

Testis

✳ prostate gland gland that surrounds the male urinary bladder neck and is a major source of the fluid that combines with sperm cells to form semen.

✳ penis male organ of copulation.

The Prostate Gland The **prostate gland** surrounds the male urinary bladder neck, and the first part of the urethra runs through its tissue. The prostate gland is a major source of the fluid that combines with sperm to form semen, the ejaculated male reproductive fluid. In emergency care, the prostate is probably most important in its role as part of the urinary system. Because the first part of the urethra passes through the prostate, enlargement of the prostate can narrow or obstruct the urethra and block urine flow.

The Penis The **penis** is the male organ of copulation. Its spongy internal tissues fill with blood to produce penile erection. The skin covering the end of the penis, the *foreskin,* is often surgically removed in infancy through circumcision; the difference in appearance is noticeable.

The male genital organs begin to mature and take adult proportions during adolescence. Puberty also marks a noticeable increase in the size of the testes. As in the female, the actual age in which sexual development occurs will vary widely. As men grow older, the penis decreases in size and the testes hang lower in the scrotum. The pubic hair becomes grey and sparse.

∫UMMARY

An understanding of human anatomy and physiology is basic to paramedic practice. This begins with an understanding of the basic organization of the human body, beginning with the cell and moving on to more complex structures: the tissues, organs, organ systems, and system integration within the organism itself.

Also critical is an understanding of the important body systems including the integumentary system; the blood; the musculoskeletal system; the head, face, and neck; the spine and thorax, the nervous, endocrine, cardiovascular, and respiratory systems; the abdomen, digestive system, and spleen, and the urinary and reproductive systems.

CHAPTER 13

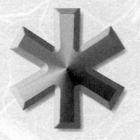

General Principles of Pathophysiology

Objectives

Part 1: How Normal Body Processes Are Altered by Disease and Injury (begins on p. 633)

After reading Part 1 of this chapter, you should be able to:

1. Discuss cellular adaptation, injury, and death. (pp. 633–639)
2. Discuss factors that precipitate disease in the human body. (pp. 639–645)
3. Analyze disease risk. (pp. 646–652)
4. Describe environmental risk factors, combined effects and interaction among risk factors. (pp. 646–652)
5. Discuss familial diseases and associated risk factors. (pp. 646–652)
6. Discuss hypoperfusion. (pp. 652–657)
7. Define cardiogenic, hypovolemic, neurogenic, anaphylactic, and septic shock. (pp. 657–661)
8. Describe multiple organ dysfunction syndrome. (pp. 662–664)

Continued

Part 2: The Body's Defences against Disease and Injury (begins on p. 664)

After reading Part 2 of this chapter, you should be able to:

1. Define the characteristics of the immune response. (pp. 668–670)
2. Discuss induction of the immune system. (pp. 669–670)
3. Describe the inflammation response and its systemic manifestations. (pp. 670–676)
4. Discuss the role of mast cells, the plasma protein system, cellular components, and resolution and repair as part of the inflammation response. (pp. 672–676)

5. Discuss hypersensitivity. (pp. 676–678)
6. Describe deficiencies in immunity and inflammation. (pp. 678–680)
7. Describe homeostasis as a dynamic steady state. (p. 682)
8. Describe neuroendocrine regulation. (pp. 682–685)
9. Discuss the interrelationships among stress, coping, and illness. (pp. 686–687)

INTRODUCTION

As a paramedic, you will assess your patient (noting the patient's complaints, signs, and symptoms) and plan a course of treatment. If you understand basic human physiology (how the body functions normally) and pathophysiology (how the body functions in the presence of disease or injury), you will be far more able to understand the probable causes of common assessment findings and, consequently, far more able to choose effective treatments.

General principles of pathophysiology are presented in this chapter. Before reading this chapter, be familiar with the fundamentals of anatomy and normal physiology as presented in Chapter 12—especially the sections on the cell and cellular environment.

This chapter is divided into two parts:

Part 1: How Normal Body Processes Are Altered by Disease and Injury

Part 2: The Body's Defences against Disease and Injury

Part 1: How Normal Body Processes Are Altered by Disease and Injury

PATHOPHYSIOLOGY

Pathology, from the root *patho* meaning "disease," is the study of disease and its causes. **Pathophysiology** is the study of how diseases alter the normal physiological processes of the human body. The concept of "disease" may include both medical illness and injury.

As a paramedic, you should realize that our understanding of pathophysiology, as a consequence of basic science and clinical outcomes research, is constantly expanding. This expansion has resulted in many changes and improvements in how we care for patients.

One example of this is the assessment and management of shock. From the origin of EMS until the mid-1980s, emergency department and EMS personnel depended on hypotension with tachycardia (low blood pressure with an accelerated pulse rate) as the primary indicators of shock in trauma and medical patients. Basic scientific research has revealed the pathophysiology of shock to be a cellular event, with many compensatory mechanisms occurring before a patient actually presents with hypotension and tachycardia. A patient with this combination of vital signs has already been in shock for an undetermined amount of time without any intervention and will probably not have a good outcome. Clinical research validated what had been deduced from basic scientific research, and the standard of care shifted from using the presence of hypotension and tachycardia to using the mechanism of injury and earlier, more subtle clinical signs and symptoms as the catalysts for responding to shock before it has advanced beyond the stage where it can be effectively reversed.

In this chapter, we will discuss the elements of physiology and pathophysiology: more about the cell (its function and environment), the role of genetics, the interplay and integration of systems to maintain homeostasis, and the impact of system disorders that result in stress, disease, and death. You will confirm, as you read, that an understanding of the cell is critical to an understanding of all these topics.

> * **pathology** the study of disease and its causes.

> * **pathophysiology** the study of how diseases alter normal physiology.

> *Keep in mind that our understanding of pathophysiology, as a consequence of basic science and clinical outcomes research, is constantly expanding. This has resulted in changes and improvements in how we care for patients.*
>
>

> *In shock, many physiological changes occur before the classic signs, hypotension and rapid pulse, become evident. Therefore, you must treat for shock promptly based on the mechanism of injury and early, subtle signs and symptoms, without waiting for the classic signs to appear.*
>
>

HOW CELLS RESPOND TO CHANGE AND INJURY

Keep in mind the concept of homeostasis: the body's tendency to maintain a constantly balanced environment and to correct or compensate for any change that upsets the balance. In this section, we will look at a variety of mechanisms by which cells respond to change and potential or actual injury.

CELLULAR ADAPTATION

Cells, tissues, organs, and even entire organ systems can adapt to both normal and injurious (pathological) conditions. For example, the growth of the uterus during pregnancy is a response to a normal change in condition. Dilation of the left ventricle after a myocardial infarction is an example of response to a pathological condition.

Adaptation to external stressors results in alterations in structure and function at the cellular level. These alterations are classified as atrophy, hypertrophy, hyperplasia, metaplasia, and dysplasia.

> **Content Review**
>
> **CELLULAR ADAPTIONS**
> Atrophy
> Hypertrophy
> Hyperplasia
> Metaplasia
> Dysplasia

Many of these cellular adaptations are successful, at least in the short run, but may also be part of the process of a disease. Therefore, it is sometimes hard to distinguish an adaptive change that is a successful response to a functional demand from one that is pathological in nature.

Atrophy

The size of an individual cell is generally determined by its workload. The cell's size will be sufficient to meet the demands placed on it by the body without wasting energy or vital nutrients. If demands decrease, cell size will also decrease to meet the demands efficiently, using minimal energy and nutrients. The cell will use less oxygen and ATP, due to its decrease in size, and the number of organelles within the cytoplasm will decrease. The process of decreasing size and increasing efficiency is known as **atrophy.**

In addition to a decrease in workload, a variety of other causes of atrophy have been identified. Atrophy may occur as a result of disuse, lack of stimulation, lack of nervous impulses, decreased nutrient supply, ischemia (lack of oxygen), or a decreased vascular (blood) supply.

Atrophy generally affects the cells found in skeletal muscle, the heart, the brain, and the sex organs.

Hypertrophy

When there is an increase in workload, a cell will often respond, in the opposite direction from atrophy, as **hypertrophy.** Hypertrophy is an increase in the size of the cell and its functional mass, including an increase in the number of organelles. The increased functional mass allows the cell to meet the increased demand. Hypertrophy of the myocardium (heart muscle) gradually occurs in response to aerobic exercise. When the heart enlarges as a consequence of a pathological event, such as after an AMI (acute myocardial infarction, or heart attack), the term applied is **dilation.** In a dilated state, the heart muscle cells have increased in size, often with a decrease in the force of contraction.

It is thought that cells that undergo hypertrophy are those that must enlarge in mass because they are unable to increase their numbers through division as in hyperplasia, described below. Hypertrophy most commonly affects cells of the heart and kidneys (enlarged heart, enlarged kidney).

Hyperplasia

Another type of response to an increased workload is **hyperplasia.** Hyperplasia is an increase in the number of cells through cell division. Cell division and duplication also include duplication of the genetic material (DNA) and the nucleus in a process called **mitosis.** Cells capable of undergoing hyperplasia include epithelial, glandular, and epidermal cells. Others, such as skeletal, cardiac, and nerve tissues, cannot divide by mitosis and therefore cannot undergo hyperplasia.

Hyperplasia is very commonly seen along with hypertrophy because the demand placed on cells in a specific area often affects cells and tissues throughout the body, some of which respond through hypertrophy and others through hyperplasia.

Metaplasia

Sometimes, damaged or destroyed cells of one type are replaced by cells of another type in a process called **metaplasia.** Metaplasia often involves replacement of one type of epithelial cell with another type of epithelial cell.

atrophy a decrease in cell size resulting from a decreased workload.

hypertrophy an increase in cell size resulting from an increased workload.

dilation enlargement. In reference to the heart, an abnormal enlargement resulting from pathology.

hyperplasia an increase in number of cells resulting from an increased workload.

mitosis cell division with division of the nucleus; each daughter cell contains the same number of chromosomes as the mother cell. Mitosis is the process by which the body grows.

metaplasia replacement of one type of cell by another type of cell that is not normal for that tissue.

This process can be seen in chronic inflammation or irritation of the respiratory tract from inhalation of irritants, commonly cigarette smoke. The irritants in the smoke will damage and destroy the ciliated columnar epithelial cells of the trachea and larger airways. The response by the body will be to replace these cells with stratified squamous epithelial cells. The squamous epithelium is less likely to be damaged by the carcinogens in the smoke. However, the squamous epithelial cells do not secrete mucus or have cilia, thus causing loss of a vital protective mechanism. In addition, the stratified squamous epithelial cells have a higher tendency to become malignant (cancerous).

Metaplasia is reversible if the causative factor is removed in time. If the person stops smoking before a malignancy (cancer) develops, the body will replace the stratified squamous cells with normal ciliated columnar cells.

Dysplasia

The last adaptive mechanism of cellular response is **dysplasia.** Dysplasia is an abnormal change in cell size, shape, and appearance due to some type of external stressor. (Dysplasia is related to hyperplasia and is often called abnormal or atypical hyperplasia.)

With dysplasia, the external stressor is usually chronic inflammation due to chronic irritation of the tissue. The changes seen result from the irritation and inflammation of the cells. As a result, there is cellular proliferation to protect underlying cells. If the irritant is removed early on, then the cellular changes are often reversible.

Dysplastic cells have a high tendency to cause malignant (cancerous) changes if they are present for an extended period of time. For example, dysplasia of the female cervix potentially leads to cervical cancer.

* **dysplasia** a change in cell size, shape, or appearance caused by an external stressor.

CELLULAR INJURY

In addition to the cellular adaptations just described, there is an enormous variety of cellular responses to injury or insult. In this section, we will discuss the seven most common mechanisms of cellular injury—hypoxia, chemicals, infectious agents, immunological/inflammatory reactions, physical agents, nutritional factors, and genetic factors—and provide examples of the ways cells respond to these types of injury in the effort to restore homeostasis.

> ### Content Review
> ### FORMS OF CELLULAR INJURY
> Hypoxia
> Chemicals
> Infectious agents
> Inflammatory reactions
> Physical agents
> Nutritional factors
> Genetic factors

Hypoxic Injury

The most common cause of cellular injury is **hypoxia,** or oxygen deficiency. Hypoxia can have various causes, usually a deficit in the respiratory or cardiovascular system. Such causes include an inadequate amount of oxygen being taken into the lungs (as from a lack of oxygen in the environment, an occluded airway, or inadequate respiration), a condition that prevents oxygen in the lungs from passing into the bloodstream (as with emphysema), inadequate pumping of blood throughout the body (as in congestive heart failure), or a blockage in the arterial system that prevents oxygenated blood from reaching the cells (as in myocardial infarction or stroke). A blockage or reduction of the delivery of oxygenated blood to the cells is known as **ischemia.**

Ischemia can also result if there is a deficiency of red blood cells to carry the oxygenated hemoglobin, a deficiency of hemoglobin in the blood, or a lack of available binding sites as occurs in patients with carbon monoxide poisoning. As the cell becomes progressively more ischemic, the intracellular metabolism becomes *anaerobic* (without oxygen). With anaerobic metabolism, there is a

* **hypoxia** oxygen deficiency.

* **ischemia** a blockage in the delivery of oxygenated blood to the cells.

marked decrease in cellular ATP production and an increase in the production of harmful acids, primarily lactic acid. The cell and some of its organelles then begin to swell due to increased levels of sodium that result from the breakdown of the sodium-potassium ATP pump. In those cells that use fats as their primary sources of energy, fat may accumulate within the cells, worsening the swelling.

If oxygen is supplied to the cell in time, the injury is reversible. But if oxygen is not supplied, the cell begins to break down, and the cell membrane ruptures, releasing lysosomes and digestive enzymes into the extracellular environment. As a result, the cellular injury has progressed from reversible to irreversible. The result is the cellular and tissue death, called *infarction*.

Chemical Injury

Cellular injury due to chemical products is very common. Deadly chemicals can be found under our sinks, in our walls, in our work environments, and everywhere around us. Harmful chemical agents include heavy metals, such as lead, carbon monoxide, ethanol (alcohol), drugs (misused medicinal drugs as well as street drugs), and insecticides, among others. Some, such as cyanide, cause cell damage and death within minutes. Others, such as common air pollutants, cause injury through prolonged exposure.

Children make up a large percentage of the population affected by chemicals. From accidental ingestion of poisons, such as cleaning products, to ingestion of lead-based paint chips, to ingestion of ethanol products, children lead the way. However, persons of all ages can suffer injury from chemical agents.

Chemicals can damage the body in many ways. Injuries to the cells cause disruption of the cellular membrane resulting in enzymatic reactions, alteration of coagulation, and eventually death of the cell.

Infectious Injury

Infectious, or disease-causing, agents are a common cause of cellular injury. A healthy person harbours many microorganisms (living things so tiny they are invisible to the naked eye) in various body sites. These include bacteria, viruses, fungi, and parasites. The vast majority are harmless, some even useful, to their human hosts. Only a few cause infection or disease. Those that do are known as **pathogens.**

The body has a variety of entry-blocking barriers and mechanisms that ward off most pathogens. The chief barrier is the skin. Mucous secretions trap pathogens and are another important barrier. Normal bacteria, enzymes, gastric acids, and other body substances destroy many pathogens. Coughing, sneezing, vomiting, and elimination of urine and feces also rid the body of pathogens.

When a pathogen does succeed in invading the body, three things can happen: First, it may multiply and spread, overwhelming the body's defences. Second, the body and the pathogen may battle to a draw, producing a chronic infection that is kept in check but is not destroyed by the body. Third, the body's defences, with or without the assistance of medical treatment, may defeat and destroy the pathogen.

The greater the number of body cells invaded or destroyed by a pathogen, the greater the risk of serious or permanent damage to the body. An example would be a localized infection of the hand as compared with widespread peritonitis of the abdominal cavity.

The degree of damage or injury that can be created by a pathogen depends on its numbers, its virulence (or pathogenicity), and the body's ability to contain

Patients suffering a heart attack should be thought of as having myocardial ischemia. Myocardial infarction is irreversible, and we hope to intervene before this occurs.

* **pathogen** a microorganism capable of producing infection or disease.

Content Review

PATHOGENS VS. THE BODY: THREE POSSIBLE OUTCOMES

Pathogen wins.
Pathogen and body battle to a draw.
Body defeats pathogen.

or destroy it. Virulence is dependent on three factors: first, the pathogen's ability to invade and destroy cells; second, its ability to produce toxins; and third, its ability to produce hypersensitivity (allergic) reactions.

Immunological/Inflammatory Injury

Protective responses of the body can cause cell injury and even death. The body's responses to cell injury are inflammation and immune responses in which the body attacks invading foreign substances. Sometimes, an exaggerated immune response called *hypersensitivity* (allergy), or even a life-threatening *anaphylactic* response, may develop. Any immune response, whether mild or severe, not only attacks foreign cells, but also tends to injure healthy body cells in the same area, in particular damaging or interfering with the function of the cell membrane. Once the foreign cells are destroyed, the injured body cells will generally begin to repair themselves.

Immunological responses will be discussed in greater detail later in this chapter.

Injurious Physical Agents

Cellular damage can be caused by physical agents. Extreme variances in temperature, whether hot or cold, can cause injury to the epidermis and underlying tissue, as from a burn or frostbite. Electrical burns, including lightning injuries, cause severe cellular damage. Hyperthermia and hypothermia (exposure to unusually warm or cool environmental temperatures) can also cause cell damage by altering body temperature, breathing patterns, and so on.

Other physical agents that can cause cellular damage include atmospheric pressure changes (for example, in a blast injury or deep-sea-diving injury), exposure to ionizing radiation (x-rays, nuclear radiation), illumination (eyestrain from fluorescent lighting, skin cancers from ultraviolet radiation), noise (hearing impairment), and mechanical stresses (blunt or penetrating trauma, irritation to the skin, repetitive-motion injuries, overexertion back injuries).

Injurious Nutritional Imbalances

Improper nutrition contributes to one of the most widely publicized forms of cellular injury: atherosclerosis caused by the deposition of lipids, cholesterol, and calcium inside arteries. Many nutritionists identify excessive intake of saturated fats and cholesterol as major contributing causes. Others place the blame on excessive carbohydrate (glucose) intake, which triggers increased insulin secretion, which, in turn, stimulates production of cholesterol by the liver. Whatever the underlying causes, the result is a narrowing diameter of the arteries, which decreases the amount of oxygenated blood that reaches target cells, increasing the risk of ischemia to vital organs, such as the heart and brain.

Problems other than atherosclerosis can also be caused or exacerbated by nutritional imbalances. In diabetic patients, an imbalance between insulin levels and carbohydrate intake causes complex, often severe metabolism problems.

Although excessive intake of nutrients may cause such problems as those mentioned above, insufficient intake of nutrients can cause other problems. The cells require proteins, carbohydrates, lipids, vitamins, and minerals for their metabolism and survival. Deficient intake of any of these nutrients can cause cellular damage and illness.

More commonly in less-developed countries, less commonly in North America, malnutrition and starvation lead to cellular injury and such diseases as beriberi, scurvy, and rickets, which are all caused by vitamin deficiencies in the diet.

Atherosclerosis is a disease almost solely limited to developed countries that have drifted away from a balanced agrarian diet.

Table 13-1 RESUSCITATION FLUIDS

Diagnosis	Resuscitation Fluid Used			
	First Choice	**Second Choice**	**Third Choice**	**Fourth Choice**
Hemorrhagic Shock	Whole blood	Packed RBCs	Plasma or plasma substitute	Ringer's Lactate or normal saline
Shock Due to Plasma Loss (Burns)	Plasma	Plasma substitute	Ringer's Lactate or normal saline	—
Dehydration	Ringer's Lactate or normal saline	—	—	—

(resulting from blood loss), where whole blood is the fluid of first choice, packed red blood cells are now more frequently used than whole blood.

Before blood, or blood products, can be administered to a patient, they must be typed and cross-matched to prevent a severe allergic reaction. The exception to this is fresh frozen plasma, which does not require cross-matching. If there is not adequate time for typing and cross-matching, O-negative blood (type O, Rh negative), the universal type, can be administered.

Transfusion Reaction

Blood and blood products are not used in the field. However, on occasion, you may be called on to transport a patient with blood infusing. Because of this, you must be able to recognize the signs and symptoms of a transfusion reaction. Transfusion reactions occur when there is a discrepancy between the blood type of the patient and the type of the blood being transfused. In addition to the ABO and Rh types, there are many minor types that can cause a transfusion reaction. Common signs and symptoms of a transfusion reaction include fever, chills, hives, hypotension, palpitations, tachycardia, flushing of the skin, headaches, loss of consciousness, nausea, vomiting, or shortness of breath.

If a transfusion reaction is suspected, *immediately* stop the transfusion and save the substance being transfused. A rapid IV fluid infusion should be started to prevent renal damage. Quickly assess the patient's mental status. Administer oxygen and contact medical direction. The medical direction physician may request the administration of mannitol (Osmotrol), diphenhydramine (Benadryl), or furosemide (Lasix). These drugs are used to maintain renal function, which is often severely compromised during a transfusion reaction.

In addition to overt reaction, you must always be alert for signs of fluid overload and congestive heart failure secondary to transfusion. This is evidenced by increased dyspnea, pulmonary congestion, edema, and altered mental status. If fluid overload is suspected, stop the infusion and start a crystalloid solution at a TKO (to keep open) rate. Administer oxygen and contact the medical direction physician.

Be alert for signs and symptoms of transfusion reaction. If they occur, immediately stop the transfusion.

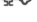

Intravenous Fluids

Intravenous fluids are the most common products used in prehospital care for fluid and electrolyte therapy. Intravenous fluids occur in two general forms—colloids and crystalloids.

Colloids Colloids contain proteins, or other high-molecular-weight molecules, that tend to remain in the intravascular space for an extended period of time. In addition, as described earlier, colloids have oncotic force (colloid osmotic pres-

✱ **colloids** substances, such as proteins or starches, consisting of large molecules or molecule aggregates that disperse evenly within a liquid without forming a true solution.

sure), which means they tend to attract water into the intravascular space from the interstitial space and the intracellular space. Thus, a small amount of a colloid can be administered to a patient with a greater-than-expected increase in intravascular volume. The following are examples of colloids:

- *Plasma protein fraction (Plasmanate)* is a protein-containing colloid. The principal protein present is **albumin,** which is suspended along with other proteins in a saline solvent.
- *Salt-poor albumin* contains only human albumin. Each gram of albumin holds approximately 18 mL of water in the bloodstream.
- *Dextran* is not a protein but a large sugar molecule with osmotic properties similar to albumin. It comes in two molecular weights: 40 000 and 70 000 Daltons. Dextran 40 has 2 to 2.5 times the colloid osmotic pressure of albumin.
- *Hetastarch (Hespan)*, like dextran, is a sugar molecule with osmotic properties similar to protein. It does not appear to share many of dextran's side effects.

✱ **albumin** a protein commonly present in plant and animal tissues. In the blood, albumin works to maintain blood volume and blood pressure and provides colloid osmotic pressure, which prevents plasma loss from the capillaries.

Colloid replacement therapy, at present, does not have a role in prehospital care except under rare circumstances. The colloid products are expensive and have a short shelf life.

Crystalloids Crystalloids are the primary compounds used in prehospital intravenous fluid therapy. There are multiple fluid preparations. It is often helpful to classify them according to their **tonicity** relative to plasma:

✱ **crystalloids** substances capable of crystallization. In solution, unlike colloids, they can diffuse through a membrane, such as a capillary wall.

- *Isotonic solutions* have electrolyte composition similar to the blood plasma. When placed into a normally hydrated patient, they will not cause a significant fluid or electrolyte shift. Examples: normal saline (0.9 percent sodium chloride, also written as 0.9% NaCl), Ringer's Lactate.
- *Hypertonic solutions* have a higher solute concentration than the cells have. These fluids will tend to cause a fluid shift out of the interstitial space and intracellular compartment into the intravascular space when administered to a normally hydrated patient. Later, there will be a diffusion of solute in the opposite direction. Examples: plasmanate, dextran.
- *Hypotonic solutions* have a lower solute concentration than the cells have. When administered to a normally hydrated patient, they will cause a movement of fluid from the intravascular space into the interstitial space and intracellular compartment. Later, solutes will move in an opposite direction. Example: 5 percent dextrose in water (D_5W).

✱ **tonicity** solute concentration or osmotic pressure relative to the blood plasma or body cells.

Intravenous replacement fluids should be chosen based on the needs of the patient and the patient's underlying problem. Choosing fluids is typically guided by laboratory studies obtained in the hospital. However, these studies are not available in the prehospital setting. Hemorrhage occurs so fast that there is usually not time for a significant fluid shift to occur between the intravascular space and interstitial/intracellular spaces. Because of this, isotonic replacement fluids, such as Ringer's Lactate and normal saline, should be used. (See Figure 13-3.)

Certain conditions, such as gastroenteritis (characterized by diarrhea, vomiting, and fever) can cause a patient to lose water more rapidly than the patient loses sodium. These patients will have a deficit in total body water (TBW) due to reduced water intake, excessive water loss, or a combination of both. When

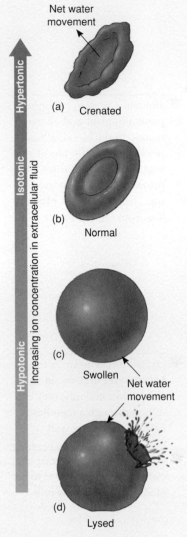

Net water
movement

Hypertonic

(a) Crenated

Isotonic

(b)
Normal

Increasing ion concentration in extracellular fluid

Hypotonic

(c)
Swollen
Net water
movement

(d)
Lysed

FIGURE 13-3   The effects of hypertonic, isotonic, and hypotonic solutions on red blood cells.

The three most commonly used fluids in prehospital care are Ringer's Lactate, normal saline, and D_5W.

Content Review

ACID–BASE DERANGEMENTS
Respiratory acidosis
Respiratory alkalosis
Metabolic acidosis
Metabolic alkalosis

water is lost in this manner, the level of sodium in the serum can increase, resulting in hypernatremia (elevated sodium levels). Patients with hypernatremia primarily need water. Because of this, hypotonic intravenous solutions, such as 0.45 percent sodium chloride (half-normal saline) are often chosen, as they provide the needed water with less sodium. However, it is important to point out that even in cases of hypernatremia, initial fluid replacement therapy should be with an isotonic solution until adequate blood pressure and adequate tissue perfusion have been restored.

Some replacement fluids contain a single element, such as sodium chloride or dextrose, while others contain multiple elements. Solutions such as Ringer's Lactate are designed so that the concentration of electrolytes is very similar to that of the plasma. As a result, these solutions are referred to as balanced salt solutions.

The most commonly used solutions in prehospital care are Ringer's Lactate solution, 0.9 percent sodium chloride (normal saline), and 5 percent dextrose in water (D_5W).

- *Ringer's Lactate* is an isotonic electrolyte solution of sodium chloride, potassium chloride, calcium chloride, and sodium lactate in water.
- *Normal saline* is an electrolyte solution of sodium chloride in water. It is isotonic with the extracellular fluid.
- *D_5W* is a hypotonic glucose solution used to keep a vein open and to supply calories necessary for cell metabolism. Although it will have an initial effect of increasing the circulatory volume, glucose molecules rapidly diffuse across the vascular membrane. Water follows the glucose into the interstitial space, resulting in an increase in interstitial water.

Both Ringer's Lactate solution and normal saline are used for fluid replacement because their administration causes an immediate expansion of the circulatory volume. However, as was noted earlier, due to the movement of electrolytes and water, two-thirds of either of these solutions are lost into the interstitial space within one hour.

ACID–BASE DERANGEMENTS

An increase in hydrogen ions (as occurs, for example, in cardiac arrest) triggers an alteration in acid-base balance. Hydrogen ions immediately combine with bicarbonate ions. This combination results in the formation of carbonic acid, which then dissociates into carbon dioxide and water with the assistance of carbonic anhydrase. Carbon dioxide is eliminated by the lungs, and water is eliminated through the kidneys. Any change in a component of this equation affects the other components. For example:

$$\uparrow H^+ + HCO_3^- \rightarrow \uparrow H_2CO_3 \rightarrow H_2O + \uparrow CO_2$$

Conversely, if the amount of carbon dioxide is increased, the equation is driven in the other direction, resulting in an increase in hydrogen ions (acid).

$$\uparrow CO_2 + H_2O \rightarrow \uparrow H_2CO_3 \rightarrow \uparrow H^+ + HCO_3^-$$

Both types of acid-base derangements, alkalosis and acidosis, can be divided into two categories based on the underlying causes. Changes in the concentration of CO_2 result from changes in respiratory function. Thus, an acidosis caused by retained CO_2 is referred to as *respiratory acidosis*. An alkalosis caused by the excess removal of CO_2 is called *respiratory alkalosis*. However, if acidosis results from the production of metabolic acids, such as lactic acid, then *metabolic acidosis* is said to exist. If an alkalosis is caused by the excess elimination of hydrogen ion, it is termed *metabolic alkalosis*.

Respiratory Acidosis

Respiratory acidosis is caused by the retention of CO_2. This can result from impaired ventilation due to problems occurring either in the lungs or in the respiratory centre of the brain. The CO_2 level is increased and the pH is decreased.

$$\downarrow \text{RESPIRATION} = \uparrow CO_2 + H_2O \rightarrow \uparrow H_2CO_3 \rightarrow \uparrow H^+ + HCO_3^-$$

Treatment is directed at improving ventilation.

✱ **respiratory acidosis** acidity caused by abnormal retention of carbon dioxide resulting from impaired ventilation.

Respiratory Alkalosis

Respiratory alkalosis results from increased respiration and excessive elimination of CO_2. This can occur with anxiety or following ascent to a high altitude. The CO_2 level is decreased and the pH is increased.

$$\uparrow \text{RESPIRATION} = \downarrow CO_2 + H_2O \rightarrow \downarrow H_2CO_3 \rightarrow \downarrow H^+ + HCO_3^-$$

Treatment, if required, consists of increasing the CO_2 level by emotionally supporting the patient and coaching him to reduce his respiratory rate.

✱ **respiratory alkalosis** alkalinity caused by excessive elimination of carbon dioxide resulting from increased respirations.

Metabolic Acidosis

Metabolic acidosis results from the production of metabolic acids, such as lactic acid, which consume bicarbonate ions. In addition, it can result from dehydration (as from diarrhea, vomiting) diabetes, and medication usage. The pH is decreased, and the CO_2 level is normal.

$$\uparrow H^+ + HCO_3^- \rightarrow \uparrow H_2CO_3 \rightarrow H_2O + \uparrow CO_2$$

In addition to treating the underlying cause, treatment includes ventilation, which causes the elimination of CO_2 and, subsequently, hydrogen ion (Figure 13-4). On rare occasions, an IV bolus of sodium bicarbonate ($NaHCO_3$) may be required.

✱ **metabolic acidosis** acidity caused by an increase in acid, often because of increased production of acids during metabolism or from causes such as vomiting, diarrhea, diabetes, or medication.

Metabolic Alkalosis

Metabolic alkalosis occurs much less frequently than metabolic acidosis. It is usually caused by the administration of **diuretics,** loss of chloride ions associated with prolonged vomiting, or the overzealous administration of sodium bicarbonate. The pH is increased and the CO_2 level is normal.

$$\downarrow H^+ + HCO_3^- \rightarrow \downarrow H_2CO_3 \rightarrow H_2O + \downarrow CO_2$$

Treatment consists of correcting the underlying cause.

Usually, both respiratory and metabolic components are present in an acid-base derangement. The type of acid-base derangement present can only be determined by arterial blood gas studies. These, of course, are only available in the hospital setting. Arterial blood gases report the pH, $PaCO_2$, PaO_2, bicarbonate concentration, and oxygen saturation.

✱ **metabolic alkalosis** alkalinity caused by an increase in plasma bicarbonate resulting from causes including diuresis, vomiting, or ingestion of too much sodium bicarbonate.

✱ **diuretic** an agent that increases urine secretion and elimination of body water.

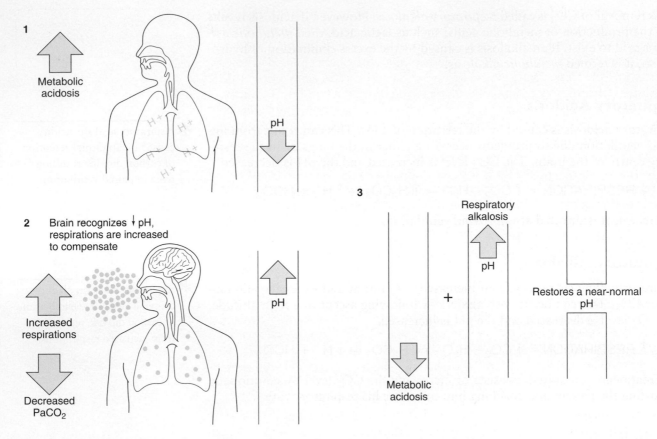

1 Metabolic acidosis

pH

2 Brain recognizes ↓ pH, respirations are increased to compensate

Increased respirations

Decreased PaCO₂

pH

3 Respiratory alkalosis

pH

+

Metabolic acidosis

Restores a near-normal pH

FIGURE 13-4 Compensation for metabolic acidosis begins with an increase in respirations.

GENETICS AND OTHER CAUSES OF DISEASE

When we think of disease, we are likely to think first of infections caused by pathogens, including bacteria, viruses, fungi, and parasites. In recent years, great strides have been made in the medical treatment of infectious diseases, but many diseases result from genetic causes, which have been far more difficult to identify and treat. The picture is additionally complicated by the fact that many diseases result from a combination of genetic and environmental factors (including lifestyle factors) as well as such factors as age and gender.

Even a family history of a particular disease does not necessarily mean that the disease has a purely genetic origin because families also share environmental and lifestyle factors that may cause or contribute to the family disease. Although family history points to the possibility of genetic causes, these cannot be confirmed, much less treated, until scientists are able to make definitive identifications of the defective genes or chromosomes that cause or contribute to particular diseases.

At present, there is increasing progress in identifying and understanding genetic and other noninfectious causes of disease. Many promising advances in gene therapies (the replacement of defective genes with normal genes) and other therapies for diseases have been made.

GENETICS, ENVIRONMENT, LIFESTYLE, AGE, AND GENDER

As noted earlier, our inherited traits are determined by molecules of deoxyribonucleic acid, or DNA, which form structures called genes, which reside on larger structures called chromosomes within the nuclei of all our cells. We inherit our genetic structure from our parents. Every one of a person's somatic cells (all the cells except the sex cells) contains 46 chromosomes. The sex cells, however, contain only 23 chromosomes each. The sex cells contribute these 23 chromosomes to the offspring. Thus, the offspring receives 23 chromosomes from the father and 23 chromosomes from the mother, resulting in a total of 46 chromosomes. Occasionally, one or more of a person's genes or chromosomes is abnormal, and this may cause a congenital disease (one we are born with) or a propensity toward acquiring a disease later in life.

Some diseases are thought to be purely genetic. For example, cystic fibrosis, which affects mainly people of European origin, and sickle cell disease, which affects mainly people of African origin, are known to be caused by disorders of single genes. They affect different populations to a different degree because of the evolutionary history of those populations. A genetic disease may be caused by a single defective gene or by several defective genes or chromosomes. Single-gene causes are, obviously, easier for medical researchers to identify and potentially devise treatments for than are other, more complex genetic causes of disease.

Other diseases are caused by a combination of genetic and environmental factors and are called *multifactorial disorders*. For example, Type II (adult-onset) diabetes has a very high correlation with family history of the disease. However, it is also affected by environmental and lifestyle factors, such as a high-fat or high carbohydrate diet and lack of exercise, which results in obesity, and with age. (There is a higher incidence of Type II diabetes in overweight people, and the disease tends to appear in middle age or later.) Heart disease, which is highly correlated with family history and age, also has a gender/hormonal factor: Women appear to be somewhat protected from heart disease before menopause, when their bodies are still producing estrogen. Following menopause, women quickly "catch up" with men in the development of heart disease. Estrogen replacement therapy used to be readily prescribed following menopause in the belief that it prolonged protection against heart disease. This idea is now being challenged by new studies.

Clinical practitioners and epidemiologists, respectively, study diseases from the point of view of their effects on individuals and from the point of view of their effects on populations as a whole.

- *Effects on Individuals.* Physicians and other clinical practitioners study the effects of diseases on individuals and find it instructive to view the development of diseases as products of the interactions among three factors: *host, agent,* and *environment*. This establishes a framework for determining how one, or a combination of these factors, may precipitate a disease state. Genetic predisposition, gender, and ethnic origin are determinants related to the host. These may interact with a specific agent, in a specific type of environment, to cause illness. The agent may be a bacterium, toxin, gunshot, or other pathophysiological process. The environment may be defined by the local climate, socioeconomic or demographic features, culture, religion, and associated factors. Determination of how the host, agent, and environment interact may yield solutions to curing a disease process. Injury and trauma are now being viewed as "diseases," in the sense of how the interaction of host, agent, and environment may contribute to an understanding of what, until now, have been perceived as social problems.

- *Effects on Populations.* Epidemiologists, who study the effects of diseases on populations, generally report disease data with three basic measures: *incidence, prevalence,* and *mortality. Morbidity,* a term commonly used in discussing disease statistics, can be more precisely

Every human somatic cell contains 46 chromosomes (23 pairs).

Most disease processes are multifactorial in origin.

Content Review

CAUSATIVE ANALYSIS OF DISEASE

Clinical Factors:

Host

Agent

Environment

Epidemiological Factors:

Incidence

Prevalence

Mortality

reported as incidence and prevalence. *Incidence* is the number of new cases of the disease that are reported in a given time, usually one year. *Prevalence* is the proportion of the total population who are affected by the disease at a given time. (Prevalence is higher than incidence, as those who acquire the disease each year are added to those who already have the disease.) *Mortality* is the rate of death from the disease.

Epidemiologists and clinical practitioners are now collaborating to study risk factors, such as the relationship between smoking and lung cancer. Risk factor analysis is both statistical and complex. Although the correlation of smoking to lung cancer is extremely high, not everyone who smokes develops lung cancer and not everyone who develops lung cancer has been a smoker. Risk factor analysis would compare the number of smokers with nonsmokers among lung cancer cases, the pack/year (number of packs per day × number of years) history of the smokers with lung cancer, factors that might have aggravated or mitigated the effects of smoking, and so on.

FAMILY HISTORY AND ASSOCIATED RISK FACTORS

It is important for those who have a family history of a particular disease not to conclude that acquiring the disease is their destiny and there is nothing they can do about it. This is not always true. Most diseases with a genetic component that come on during adulthood also have associated risk factors that can be modified to prevent, delay, or reduce the impact of the disease.

Consider the variety of possible risk factors for disease: People who live in less-developed countries are often at higher risk for disease from microorganisms flourishing in their water supply and disease transmission caused by poor sanitation. Physical conditions commonly seen in larger North American cities as well as rural areas, such as inadequate housing, poor nutrition, and little or no medical attention, potentiate disease transmission. Chemical factors, such as smoke, smog, illicit drug use, occupational chemical exposure, and additives in food, are causative agents for a variety of diseases.

Personal habit is among the most publicized—and controllable—causes of disease in our society. For example, predisposing factors for cardiovascular disease include smoking, alcohol consumption, inactivity, and obesity. Unfortunately, changes in individual lifestyle often occur only after a disease has already manifested itself. As we age, the predisposing factors and causative agents take their toll. The body's ability to defend itself against disease decreases due to the effects of aging on our immunological system and other compensatory mechanisms.

The following is a discussion of some of the most common diseases in which both genetics and other risk factors play a role. You will notice, as you read, that the causation of various diseases varies widely and that although the causes are known for some diseases, the causes of other diseases are still not clearly understood.

Immunological Disorders

A number of immunological disorders, such as rheumatic fever, allergies, and asthma, are more prevalent among those with a family history of the disorder, but they also involve other risk factors.

Rheumatic fever is an inflammatory reaction to an infection but is not an infection itself. There seems to be a hereditary factor, but inadequate nutrition and crowded living conditions are contributing factors.

Allergies often have a family-history factor (and some allergies can be passed from the mother to the fetus during pregnancy). However, allergic reactions are triggered by exposure to allergens and can usually be controlled by avoiding or reducing the presence of allergens as well as with medication.

Asthma sufferers may inherit the propensity for airway narrowing in response to various stimuli, but other triggering factors, including stress, overexertion, exposure to cold air, and stimuli such as pollens, dust mites, cockroach detritus, and smoke, may be identified and, perhaps, controlled.

Cancer

A wide variety of family-history and environmental factors are included among the risk factors for cancer. Some kinds of cancer, such as breast and colorectal cancers, tend to cluster in families and seem to have a combination of genetic and environmental causes. Others, such as lung cancer, are more strongly identified with environmental causes.

For *breast cancer,* the greatest risk factor is age, with the majority occurring after age 60 and the greatest risk after age 75. A history of breast cancer in a first-degree relative (mother, sister, or daughter) increases the risk by two or three times. Some progress has been made in identifying genes for certain breast cancers. Lifestyle factors, such as lack of exercise and obesity, may contribute slightly to the incidence of breast cancer, but these have not been proven.

As with breast cancer, *colorectal cancer* risk factors include age (with the incidence rising after age 40 and peaking between 60 and 75) and family history (incidence in a first-degree relative increases the risk by two or three times). There are gender factors, with rectal cancer being more common in men and colon cancer more common in women. Diet may also be a risk factor, although recent studies have failed to confirm a link between a high-fat, low-fibre diet and colorectal cancer. (However, a high-fat, low-fibre diet has been positively linked to heart disease and other health problems.)

The causes of *lung cancer* are overwhelmingly environmental. Smoking, including inhalation of second-hand smoke, has been identified as the main cause of 90 percent of lung cancers in men and 70 percent of lung cancers in women. Lung cancer can also be caused by inhaling such substances as asbestos, arsenic, and nickel, usually in the workplace.

Endocrine Disorders

The most common endocrine disorder is *diabetes mellitus,* which is a leading cause of blindness, heart disease, kidney failure, and premature death. The causes of diabetes are complex and still not well understood.

There are two major types of diabetes: Type I and Type II. Type I diabetes usually occurs before age 40, sometimes in childhood. Although it is less prevalent than Type II diabetes (accounting for about 20 percent of diabetes cases), it is more severe. In the Type I diabetic, the pancreas produces no or almost no insulin, which is required for the cellular utilization of glucose, the body's chief source of energy. Type I diabetics must take insulin daily. There is some association of Type I diabetes with family history (siblings of Type I diabetics have a 6-percent risk compared with 0.3 percent in the general population), and medical researchers have pinpointed some possible genetic factors. Other causative factors may include autoimmunity disorders and viral infections that invade the pancreas and destroy the insulin-producing cells.

Type II diabetes accounts for about 80 percent of all diabetes cases. It usually occurs after age 40 and the incidence increases with age. It clusters much more strongly in families than does Type I diabetes (siblings have a 10- to 15-percent risk). In contrast to Type I diabetes, in which there is a total lack of insulin, Type II diabetes is associated with a decreased insulin receptor response or a decrease in insulin production. Diet and exercise may also be factors, since the majority of Type II diabetics are obese. Type II diabetes can often be controlled with diet and exercise or with oral medications.

Hematological Disorders

Hereditary coagulation disorders have been studied by geneticists and physicians in great detail. There are many causes of hereditary hematological disorders, such as gene alteration and histocompatibility (tissue interaction) dysfunctions.

Hemophilia is a bleeding disorder that is caused by a genetic clotting factor deficiency. It can be mild, but if severe, it can cause not only serious bruising but bleeding into the joints, which can lead to crippling deformities. A slight bump on the head can cause bleeding within the skull, often resulting in brain damage and death. The heredity is sex-linked (associated with the sex chromosomes), inherited through the mother and affecting male children almost exclusively. There is no cure, but administration of concentrated clotting factors can improve the condition.

Hemochromatosis is another genetic disorder but, this time, caused by a histocompatibility complex dysfunction. It is marked by an excessive absorption and accumulation of iron in the body, causing weight loss, joint pain, abdominal pain, palpitations, and testicular atrophy in males. It is treated by removing blood from the body at intervals.

Not all blood disorders are genetic. Environmental factors, for example, can cause *anemia* (reduction in circulating red blood cells). For example, some antihypertensive medications and other drugs may cause a drug-induced hemolytic (red-blood-cell-destroying) anemia.

Cardiovascular Disorders

The cardiovascular system can be greatly affected by genetic disorders. Disorders such as *prolongation of the QT interval* (a delay between depolarization and repolarization of the ventricles as revealed in an electrocardiogram) and *mitral-valve prolapse* (an upward ballooning of the valve between the left ventricle and atrium that allows blood to regurgitate back into the atrium when the ventricle contracts) tend to cluster in families.

The Heart and Stroke Foundation of Canada lists heredity as a major risk factor for cardiovascular disease. Those with parents who have *coronary artery disease* (deposits on the walls of the coronary arteries that reduce blood flow to the heart muscle) have an approximately fivefold risk of developing the disease. This is why it is important to ask about family history of congenital heart disease (CHD), hypertension, and stroke when assessing patients with possible cardiovascular disease. However, environmental factors, such as a diet high in saturated fats and cholesterol (or a diet high in carbohydrates) and lack of exercise, also play a large role in cardiovascular disease.

Hypertension (high blood pressure) is a major risk factor, not only for cardiac disease but also for stroke and kidney disease. Studies of family history show that approximately 20 to 40 percent of the causation of hypertension is genetic. The remaining causative factors, then, are environmental and may include high sodium ingestion, lack of physical activity, stress, and obesity.

Not all cardiac disorders have a genetic component. For example, *cardiomyopathy* (disease affecting the heart muscle), is thought to occur secondary to other causes, such as infectious disease, toxin exposure, connective tissue disease, or nutritional deficiencies, which may be partially or totally environmental.

Renal Disorders

Renal (kidney) failure is caused by a variety of factors (primarily diabetes) which may eventually require a patient to receive dialysis treatment several times a week. As the location of dialysis treatment shifts from medical centres to homes and community satellite centres, EMS personnel are increasingly being called to deal with the complications of dialysis. These include problems with vascular access devices (shunts, fistulas), localized infection and sepsis, and electrolyte abnormalities (hyperkalemia), which can result in cardiac arrest.

> *As dialysis treatment shifts from medical centres to homes and community centres, EMS personnel are increasingly being called to deal with complications of dialysis.*

Rheumatic Disorders

Gout is a condition that may have both genetic and environmental causes. It is characterized by severe arthritic pain caused by deposit of crystals in the joints, most commonly the great toe. The crystals form as the result of an abnormally high level of uric acid in the blood that may be caused when the kidneys do not excrete enough uric acid or by high production of uric acid. High production of uric acid may be caused by a hereditary metabolic abnormality. Although the underlying cause may be genetic, attacks of gout can be triggered by environmental factors, such as trauma, alcohol consumption, ingestion of certain foods, stress, or other illnesses. Patients with gout also have a tendency to develop *kidney stones*.

Gastrointestinal Disorders

Gastrointestinal disorders have a variety of causes, and the causes of some are not known. *Lactose intolerance,* for example, is usually identified by the inability of the patient to tolerate milk and some other dairy products. The patient lacks lactase, the enzyme that usually breaks down lactose in the digestive tract. This enzyme deficiency may be congenital (inborn) or may develop later on.

Crohn's disease is a chronic inflammation of the wall of the digestive tract that usually affects the small intestine, the large intestine, or both. The cause is not known, but medical researchers have focused on immune system dysfunction, infection, and diet as the major probabilities. A similar disorder is ulcerative colitis, in which the large intestine becomes inflamed and develops ulcers. As with Crohn's disease, the cause is not known, but an overactive immune response is suspected, and heredity seems to play a role.

Peptic ulcers develop when the normal protective structures and mechanisms, such as mucus production, break down and areas in the lining of the stomach or duodenum are inflamed by stomach acid and digestive juices. Environmental factors, bacterial infection (by *Helicobacter pylori*), diet, stress, and alcohol consumption, are thought to play roles in the development of peptic ulcers. Many medications, particularly nonsteroidal anti-inflammatory medications, are associated with ulcer formation.

Cholecystitis is an inflammation of the gallbladder that usually results from blockage by a gallstone. There may be a genetic predisposition for gallstone formation. Gallstones are more prevalent in women. Other risk factors include age, a high-fat diet, and obesity.

Obesity can be defined as being more than 20 percent over the ideal body weight. Obesity has both environmental and familial risk transmission. Research has shown that children whose parents are obese have a much increased chance of developing obesity. Environmental factors such as proper nutrition and exercise may not be modelled or taught by obese parents, but there also seems to be a genetic factor to many cases of obesity. Obesity has been linked to, or defined as a cause for, such diseases as hypertension, heart disease, and vascular diseases.

Neuromuscular Disorders

Diseases of the nervous and muscular systems also have a variety of causes. *Huntington's disease* (which results in uncontrollable jerking and writhing movements) and muscular dystrophy (which results in progressive muscle weakness) are both known to be caused by genetic defects.

Multiple sclerosis (which affects the nerves of the eye, brain, and spinal cord) seems to have some hereditary factor, with clustering among close relatives. Its exact cause is unknown, but it seems to result when the virus-triggered autoimmune response begins to attack the myelin sheath that protects the nerves.

Alzheimer's disease is thought to cause about 50 percent of dementias, or progressive mental deterioration. Its cause is unknown, but it does cluster strongly in families and appears to be either caused or influenced by specific gene abnormalities.

Psychiatric Disorders

Genetic and biological causes of psychiatric disorders are being studied and increasingly understood. An example is *schizophrenia,* which affects about 1 percent of the population worldwide and is more prevalent than Alzheimer's disease, diabetes, or multiple sclerosis. The person with schizophrenia loses contact with reality and suffers from hallucinations, delusions, abnormal thinking, and disrupted social functioning. People who develop schizophrenia are now thought to be "biologically vulnerable" to the disease, but what makes them vulnerable is not fully understood. The cause may be a genetic predisposition or some problem that occurs before, during, or after birth or a viral infection of the brain.

Another common psychiatric disorder is *manic-depressive illness,* also called *bipolar disorder,* in which the person experiences alternating periods of depression and mania or excitement. It can be mild or severe enough to interfere with the patient's ability to work or function socially. Manic-depressive illness affects about twice as many people as does schizophrenia. It is believed to be hereditary, but the exact gene deficit has not yet been discovered.

HYPOPERFUSION

Many disease processes have a genetic cause.

All body cells require a constant supply of oxygen and other nutrients.

* **hypoperfusion** inadequate perfusion of the body tissues, resulting in an inadequate supply of oxygen and nutrients to the body tissues. Also called *shock*.

All body cells require a constant supply of oxygen and other essential nutrients, while waste products, such as carbon dioxide, must be constantly removed. It is the circulatory system, in conjunction with the respiratory and gastrointestinal systems, that provides the body's cells with these essential nutrients and removal of wastes. This is accomplished by the passage of blood through the capillaries, the small vessels that interface with body cells, while oxygen and carbon dioxide, nutrients and wastes are exchanged by movement across the capillary walls and cell membranes. This constant and necessary passage of blood through the body's tissues is called *perfusion.*

There is some local control of both tissue perfusion and waste removal. When the amounts of metabolic waste products (such as lactic acid) increase, the tissues subsequently become acidotic. This local acidosis causes nearby precapillary sphincters to relax, thus opening the capillaries and increasing perfusion of the affected tissues. This provides increased capacity for waste elimination and response to local metabolic demands.

Inadequate perfusion of body tissues is **hypoperfusion,** which is commonly called shock. Shock occurs first at a cellular level. If allowed to progress, the tissues, organs, organ systems, and ultimately the entire organism is affected. Hypoperfusion is a condition that is progressive (that is, it triggers a self-worsening cycle of pathophysiological events) and fatal if not corrected. It can occur for many reasons, such as trauma, fluid loss, myocardial infarction, infection, allergic reaction, spinal cord injury, and other causes.

Although causes differ, all forms of shock have the same underlying pathophysiology at the cellular and tissue levels. As discussed in the next section, shock may be triggered by anything that affects one or more of these components of the cardiovascular system: the pump (the heart), the fluid (the blood), or the container (the blood vessels).

THE PATHOPHYSIOLOGY OF HYPOPERFUSION

Causes of Hypoperfusion

Hypoperfusion (shock) is almost always a result of inadequate cardiac output. A number of factors can decrease effective cardiac output:

- Inadequate pump
  - Inadequate preload
  - Inadequate cardiac contractile strength
  - Inadequate heart rate
  - Excessive afterload
- Inadequate fluid
  - Hypovolemia (abnormally low circulating blood volume)
- Inadequate container
  - Dilated container without change in fluid volume (inadequate systemic vascular resistance)
  - Leak in container

Occasionally, hypoperfusion can develop even when cardiac output is adequate. This can happen when cell metabolism is so excessive that the body cannot increase perfusion enough to meet the cells' metabolic requirements. It can also happen when abnormal circulatory patterns develop so that circulating blood is bypassing critical tissues.

As mentioned earlier, the conditions that lead to hypoperfusion can result from a number of underlying causes, such as infection, trauma and hemorrhage, loss of plasma through burns, severe cardiac dysrhythmia, central nervous system dysfunction, and many others. But the outcome is always the same: inadequate delivery of oxygen and essential nutrients to, and removal of wastes from, all the tissues of the body, especially the critical tissues (brain, heart, kidneys).

Shock at the Cellular Level

Shock is a complex phenomenon. The causes vary. The signs and symptoms vary. At the simplest level, however, shock is inadequate tissue perfusion. Additionally, all types of shock have this in common: The ultimate outcome is impairment of cellular metabolism. Two characteristics of impaired cellular metabolism in any type of shock are impaired oxygen use and impaired glucose use.

Impaired Use of Oxygen One characteristic of any type of shock is that the cells are either not receiving enough oxygen or are unable to use it effectively. This may be caused by hypoperfusion resulting from reduced cardiac function, inadequate blood volume, or vasodilation (pump, fluid, or container problems).

At the simplest level, shock is inadequate tissue perfusion.

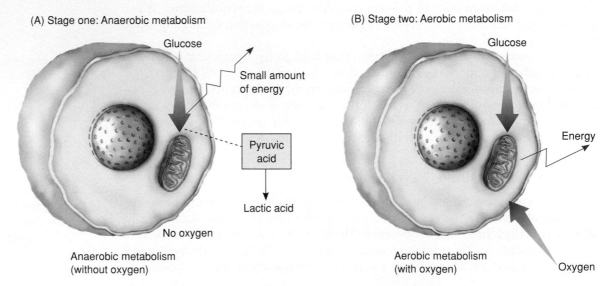

It may result from insufficient red cells to carry the oxygen, from fever that increases cellular oxygen demand, or chemical disruption of cellular metabolism.

When the cells don't receive enough oxygen or cannot use it effectively, they change from **aerobic metabolism** to **anaerobic metabolism**, a far less efficient means of producing energy—as explained below.

The primary energy source for the cells is glucose, taken into the cell with the aid of insulin. Glucose does not provide energy until it is broken down inside the cell. The first stage of glucose breakdown, called glycolysis, is anaerobic (does not require oxygen). Glycolysis produces pyruvic acid but yields very little energy. Thus, by itself, glycolysis is an inefficient utilization of glucose. Therefore, in a normal state of metabolism, a second stage of glucose breakdown is required. During this second stage, which is aerobic (requires oxygen), pyruvic acid is further degraded into carbon dioxide, water, and energy in a process termed the Krebs or citric acid cycle. The energy yield of this second-stage aerobic process is much higher than from the first-stage anaerobic process (Figure 13-5).

During shock, or any condition in which the cells do not receive adequate oxygen or cannot use it effectively, glucose breakdown can only complete the first-stage, anaerobic process of glycolysis and cannot enter into the second-stage, aerobic, citric acid cycle. This causes an accumulation of the end product of glycolysis, pyruvic acid. In these cases, pyruvic acid is quickly degraded to lactic acid. If oxygen is promptly restored to the cells, lactic acid will be reconverted to pyruvic acid. However, if time elapses and the cellular hypoxia is not corrected, lactic acid and other metabolic acids will accumulate. One outcome is that the acidic condition of the blood reduces the ability of hemoglobin in red blood cells to bind with and carry oxygen, which compounds the problem of cellular oxygen deprivation.

The energy that is produced during glucose breakdown is in the form of the chemical adenosine triphosphate (ATP), which is essential to all the metabolic processes in the cells. As just noted, the amount of energy, or ATP, produced during first-stage, anaerobic glycolysis is very small. Without oxygen, when the process of glucose breakdown stops after glycolysis (during which very little energy has been

✳ **aerobic metabolism** the second stage of metabolism, requiring the presence of oxygen, in which the breakdown of glucose (in a process called the Krebs or citric acid cycle) yields a high amount of energy. *Aerobic* means "with oxygen."

✳ **anaerobic metabolism** the first stage of metabolism, which does not require oxygen, in which the breakdown of glucose (in a process called glycolysis) produces pyruvic acid and yields very little energy. *Anaerobic* means "without oxygen."

(A) Stage one: Anaerobic metabolism

Glucose

Small amount of energy

Pyruvic acid

Lactic acid

No oxygen

Anaerobic metabolism (without oxygen)

(B) Stage two: Aerobic metabolism

Glucose

Energy

Oxygen

Aerobic metabolism (with oxygen)

FIGURE 13-5   Glucose breakdown. (A) Stage one, glycolysis, is anaerobic (does not require oxygen). It yields pyruvic acid, with toxic byproducts, such as lactic acid, and very little energy. (B) Stage two is aerobic (requires oxygen). In a process called the Krebs or citric acid cycle, pyruvic acid is degraded into carbon dioxide and water, which produces a much higher yield of energy.

produced), cellular stores of ATP are used up much faster than they can be replaced so that all of the processes of cellular metabolism are gravely impaired.

Because of changes to the internal cell and because blood flow has been slowed by the decreased pumping action and vasodilation, sludging of the blood occurs. This further impedes blood flow. Thus, the normal diffusion of nutrients and wastes in and out of the cells is disrupted, and the balance of the cellular electrolytes is altered. Lysosomes, the organelles that assist in digestion of nutrients, are normally enclosed by a membrane that prevents the digestive enzymes from damaging other cell components. Now, the lysosomes rupture, releasing the lysosomal enzymes into the cell. The sodium-potassium pumping mechanism fails, changing the electrical charge of the cells' internal environment. There is an increase in sodium and water (since water follows sodium) inside the cells, causing cellular edema. The cell membrane then ruptures, allowing lysosomal enzymes and other cellular contents to leak into the interstitial spaces. Cellular death soon follows.

Impaired Use of Glucose The same factors that reduce delivery of oxygen to the cells also reduce delivery of glucose to the cells. In addition, uptake of glucose by the cells may be disrupted by fever, cell damage, or the presence of bacteria, toxins, histamine, or other substances produced or activated by the body's immune and inflammatory responses to disease or injury. Compensatory mechanisms activated by shock may also be responsible for substances that inhibit glucose uptake, including catecholamines and the hormones cortisol and growth hormone.

Glucose that is prevented from entering the cells remains in the blood, resulting in a condition of high serum glucose, or hyperglycemia. Since glucose is the substance from which cells produce energy, the consequences of reduced glucose delivery and uptake are critical.

In the absence of an adequate supply of glucose, certain body cells can create fuel for energy production by converting other substances to glucose. One source is glycogen, the form of glucose that cells store and hold in reserve. Cells convert glycogen to glucose in a process called *glycogenolysis*. However, there is very little stored glycogen in cells other than in the liver, kidneys, and muscles. When glycogen reserves are depleted, which typically occurs in four to eight hours, the cells will then derive energy from the breakdown of fats (*lipolysis*) and from the conversion of noncarbohydrate substrates, such as amino acids from proteins, to glucose (*gluconeogenesis*). The energy costs of glycogenolysis and lipolysis are high and contribute to the failure of cells. But the depletion of proteins in gluconeogenesis will ultimately cause organ failure.

In addition, the anaerobic breakdown of proteins produces ammonia, which is toxic to the cells, and urea, which leads to uric acid, which is also toxic to cells. Finally, when cellular metabolism is impaired, the waste products of metabolism build up in the cells, further impairing cell function and damaging cell membranes.

Impaired use of oxygen and glucose soon leads to cellular death. Cellular death will ultimately lead to tissue death; tissue death will lead to organ failure; and organ failure will lead to death of the individual.

Compensation and Decompensation

Usually, the body is able to compensate for any of the changes described above. However, when the various compensatory mechanisms fail, shock develops and may progress.

Compensation In shock, the fall in cardiac output, detected as a decrease in arterial blood pressure by the baroreceptors, activates several body systems that attempt to reestablish a normal blood pressure—a process known as *compensation*. The sympathetic nervous system stimulates the adrenal gland of the endocrine system to

Cellular death will ultimately lead to tissue death, tissue death to organ failure, and organ failure to death of the individual.

secrete the catecholamines epinephrine and norepinephrine. These chemicals profoundly affect the cardiovascular system, causing an increased heart rate, increased cardiac contractile strength, and arteriolar constriction—all of which serve to elevate the blood pressure.

Another compensatory mechanism, the *renin-angiotensin system,* aids the body in maintaining an adequate blood pressure. When the renin-angiotensin system is activated by a fall in blood pressure, the enzyme *renin* is released from the kidneys into the systemic circulation. Renin acts on a specialized plasma protein called *angiotensin* to produce a substance called *angiotensin I.* Angiotensin I is converted to *angiotensin II* by an enzyme found in the lungs called *angiotensin converting enzyme (ACE).* Angiotensin II is a potent vasoconstrictor. As angiotensin II causes the diameter of the vascular container to decrease, the blood pressure increases. Angiotensin II also stimulates the production of aldosterone, a hormone secreted by the adrenal cortex (outer layer of the adrenal gland) which, in turn, stimulates the kidneys to reabsorb sodium, and, subsequently, water (as noted earlier, "water follows sodium") into peritubular capillaries. The intravascular volume is maintained and elimination of water by the kidneys is reduced.

Another endocrine response by the pituitary gland results in the secretion of antidiuretic hormone (ADH), which also causes the kidneys to reabsorb water, creating an additive effect to that of aldosterone.

The spleen, capable of storing more than 300 mL of blood, can expel up to 200 mL of blood into the venous circulation, consequently increasing blood volume, preload, cardiac output, and blood pressure in response to a sudden drop in blood pressure.

Some passive compensatory responses also occur, with beneficial fluid shifts taking place as a result of simple diffusion. With volume loss, the hydrostatic pressure in capillary beds is reduced, and water from the interstitial spaces diffuses into the capillaries.

All of above-mentioned mechanisms work to compensate for the shock state and may be able to restore normal circulatory volume—if excessive bleeding is managed and the shock state has not progressed too far. In this case, the patient is said to be in **compensated shock.**

Once normal circulatory function and blood pressure are reestablished, the blood pressure will "feed back" on all of the compensatory mechanisms so that all systems can return to normal. In this way, negative feedback loops work to maintain stability by "signalling" the systems to cease the compensatory responses. In this way, stability and homeostasis are maintained.

Decompensation If the conditions causing shock are too serious, or progress too rapidly, compensatory mechanisms may not be able to restore normal function. In those cases, *decompensation* is said to occur, and the patient is in a state of **decompensated shock,** also called **progressive shock.** During decompensated or progressive shock, medical intervention may still be able to correct the condition.

Since all of the "responding" systems have a point at which they can no longer sustain their action (i.e., a limited duration of action), the shock state may progress to a condition where correction, either by the body's own compensatory mechanisms or through medical intervention, is no longer possible. This condition is known as **irreversible shock.**

A critical factor in the downward spiral of decompensation is cardiac depression. The compensatory mechanisms that increase heart rate and contractile strength create a greatly increased demand for oxygen by the myocardium. When arterial blood pressure has fallen sufficiently, however, coronary blood flow is reduced below the level necessary to adequately perfuse the myocardium. The heart is weakened and cardiac output falls even further.

Depression of the vasomotor centre of the brain is another consequence of reduced blood pressure. In early shock, as previously discussed, the sympathetic

Content Review

THE STAGES OF SHOCK
Compensated
Decompensated (progressive)
Irreversible

✱ **compensated shock** early stage of shock during which the body's compensatory mechanisms are able to maintain normal perfusion.

✱ **decompensated shock** advanced stages of shock when the body's compensatory mechanisms are no longer able to maintain normal perfusion; also called **progressive shock.**

✱ **irreversible shock** shock that has progressed so far that no medical intervention can reverse the condition and death is inevitable.

nervous system is stimulated to cause release of catecholamines that support the function of the circulatory system. But when blood pressure falls to a certain point, in the late stages of shock, reduced blood supply to the vasomotor centre results in a slowing, then stoppage, of sympathetic activity.

Metabolic wastes, products of anaerobic metabolism, are released into the slower-flowing blood. The blood in the capillary beds becomes acidic, causing formation of minute blood clots ("sludged" blood), which further slows the flow of blood. And a more generalized, systemic acidosis develops, causing further deterioration of cells and tissues, including the capillary walls.

Capillary cells, like other cells, suffer from lack of oxygen and other nutrients, as well as from the ravages of acidosis. This begins to cause permeability of the capillaries and leakage of fluid into the interstitial spaces. This is another self-perpetuating process, as the decreased circulating volume and anaerobic metabolism cause further cell hypoxia and increased permeability.

Cellular deterioration progresses to tissue deterioration, which progresses to organ failure. (See Multiple Organ Dysfunction Syndrome, later in the chapter.) Medical intervention may save the patient if initiated early enough, but when enough damage has been done to cells, tissues, and organs, no known treatment can help the patient recover. Medical therapies may support function for awhile, but death becomes inevitable.

TYPES OF SHOCK

Shock is usually classified according to the cause. Some newer terminology classifies shock as *cardiogenic* (caused by impaired pumping power of the heart), *hypovolemic* (caused by decreased blood or water volume), *obstructive* (caused by an obstruction that interferes with return of blood to the heart, such as a pulmonary embolism, cardiac tamponade, or tension pneumothorax), and *distributive* (caused by abnormal distribution and return of blood resulting from vasodilation, vasopermeability, or both, as in neurogenic, anaphylactic, or septic shock).

Another more familiar terminology classifies shock as *cardiogenic, hypovolemic, neurogenic, anaphylactic,* and *septic*. The following discussion of types of shock uses these classifications.

Although all types of shock ultimately have the same effects on the body's cells, tissues, and organs, it is important to try to identify the underlying cause because correcting the cause is the most important element in reversing the condition and saving the patient's life. Many of the treatments that you, as a paramedic, will provide for the shock patient will be the same, no matter what the cause or type of shock is, but some differ in important ways. For example, providing IV fluid boluses, which may be appropriate to support circulating volume in the hypovolemic patient, would not be indicated for the patient in cardiogenic shock with pulmonary edema.

Cardiogenic Shock

An inability of the heart to pump enough blood to supply all body parts is referred to as **cardiogenic shock.** Cardiogenic shock is usually the result of severe left ventricular failure secondary to acute myocardial infarction or congestive heart failure. The reduced blood pressure that accompanies this form of shock aggravates the situation by decreasing coronary artery perfusion. With decreased coronary perfusion, the heart muscle becomes even more damaged, thus establishing a vicious cycle that ultimately results in complete pump failure.

During cardiogenic shock, as noted earlier, the activation of compensatory mechanisms can actually worsen the situation. When the peripheral resistance increases in an attempt to maintain blood pressure, the myocardial workload increases. This, in turn, increases the myocardial oxygen demand, further aggravating

The hallmark of decompensated shock is a fall in blood pressure.

Try to identify the underlying cause of shock because correcting the cause is the most important element in reversing the condition and saving the patient's life.

* **cardiogenic shock** shock caused by insufficient cardiac output; the inability of the heart to pump enough blood to perfuse all parts of the body.

myocardial ischemia and infarction. Cardiac output is further depressed and ejection fraction (the percentage of blood in the ventricle that is ejected with each beat) is decreased.

Although the most common cause of cardiogenic shock is severe left ventricular failure, a number of other factors can have the same result. These include chronic progressive heart disease, such as cardiomyopathy, rupture of the papillary heart muscles or interventricular septum, and end-stage valvular disease (mitral stenosis or aortic regurgitation).

Most patients who experience cardiogenic shock will have normal blood volume. However, some patients will be hypovolemic from an excessive use of prescribed diuretics or the severe diaphoresis that accompanies some acute cardiac events. Patients may also experience relative hypovolemia (neurogenic shock) from the vasodilatory (vessel dilation) effects of drugs such as nitroglycerine.

Evaluation and Treatment A major difference between cardiogenic and other types of shock is the presence of pulmonary edema (excess fluid in the lungs), which will probably result in a complaint of difficulty breathing. There may be diminished lung sounds as fluid enters the interstitial spaces of the lungs. As fluid levels rise, wheezes, crackles, or rales may be heard. A productive cough may develop, characterized by white- or pink-tinged foamy sputum. Cyanosis (a dusky blue-grey skin colour) is typical, resulting from the decreased diffusion of oxygen across the alveolar/capillary interface, decreasing oxygen delivery to cells that are already hypoxic because of decreased blood pressure and perfusion. Other signs of shock include altered mentation (resulting from reduced perfusion of the brain) and oliguria (diminished urination resulting from compensatory mechanisms that stimulate reabsorption of water by the kidneys to enhance circulating volume).

Treatment of cardiogenic shock includes the supportive measures that should be provided for shock of any origin: Ensure an open airway, administer oxygen, assist ventilations if necessary (to support oxygenation of myocardial and other body cells), and keep the patient warm (because impaired cellular metabolism is no longer producing enough energy to keep body temperature normal).

In cardiogenic shock, when pulmonary edema is present, elevate the patient's head and shoulders so that gravity can help isolate fluid and create a clear area where oxygen exchange from the alveoli can take place.

A peripheral intravenous line should be established with normal saline at a TKO rate to provide access for medications, but fluid administration should be kept to a minimum to avoid aggravating the edema. (Some patients with chronic heart failure may be on diuretics and suffering dehydration, however, requiring some fluid support.) Since the heart rate may vary from bradycardic (abnormally slow) to tachycardic (abnormally fast), monitoring the heart rate is important. Atropine administration or application of an external pacer may be recommended to manage bradycardia, while extreme tachycardia may be treated by sedation and cardioversion (a type of electric shock) if the patient is awake. Dopamine may be administered to elevate the blood pressure, but it will also increase heart rate. Dobutamine may be administered to increase contractile force with little effect on the heart rate. Follow local protocols.

Hypovolemic Shock

Shock due to a loss of intravascular fluid volume is referred to as **hypovolemic shock.** Possible causes of hypovolemic shock include the following:

- Internal or external hemorrhage (This type of hypovolemic shock is also known as hemorrhagic shock.)
- Traumatic injury
- Long bone or open fractures

Most patients with cardiogenic shock have a normal or increased blood volume.

Provide supportive measures for shock of any origin: Ensure an open airway, administer oxygen, assist ventilations, and keep the patient warm.

✱ **hypovolemic shock** shock caused by a loss of intravascular fluid volume.

- Severe dehydration from vomiting or diarrhea
- Plasma loss from burns
- Excessive sweating
- Diabetic ketoacidosis with resultant **osmotic diuresis**

Hypovolemic shock can also be due to internal third-space loss. Such a condition can occur with bowel obstruction, peritonitis, pancreatitis, or liver failure resulting in ascites (accumulation of fluid within the abdominal cavity).

Evaluation and Treatment The signs of hypovolemic shock are considered the "classic" signs of shock. The mental status becomes altered, progressing from anxiety to lethargy or combativeness to unresponsiveness. The skin becomes pale, cool, and clammy (sweaty). The blood pressure may be normal during compensated shock but then begins to fall. The pulse may be normal in the beginning, then become rapid, finally slowing and disappearing. As the kidneys continue to reabsorb water, urination decreases. Cardiac dysrhythmias may develop in late shock, deteriorating to asystole (absence of heartbeat).

Provide supportive treatment for hypovolemic shock: ensuring airway, oxygen administration, and assisted ventilations if necessary. Control any severe bleeding. Keep the patient warm. If injuries allow, place the patient supine and elevate the legs. An IV bolus of crystalloid solution (such as normal saline or Ringer's Lactate) should be started for fluid replacement.

Neurogenic Shock

Neurogenic shock results from injury to either the brain or the spinal cord, resulting in an interruption of nerve impulses to the arteries. The arteries lose tone and dilate, causing a relative hypovolemia. There has been no loss of fluid, but the container has been enlarged. With this inappropriate vasodilation, a disproportionate amount of blood collects in the capillary bed. This reduces venous return, cardiac output, and arterial blood pressure. Sympathetic nerve impulses to the adrenal glands are lost, which prevents the release of catecholamines and their compensatory effects. With injury high in the cervical spine, there may be interruption of impulses to the peripheral nervous system, causing paralysis and loss of sensation. The respiratory and cardiac centres of the brain may also be affected.

The usual cause of neurogenic shock is central nervous system injury. Neurogenic shock is most commonly due to an injury that has resulted in severe spinal cord injury or total transection of the cord (which may be called *spinal shock*) or injury or deprivation of oxygen or glucose to the medulla of the brain.

Evaluation and Treatment The vasodilation in neurogenic shock causes warm, red skin, and sweat gland malfunction causes dry skin—in contrast to the cool, pale, sweaty skin associated with hypovolemic shock. Because of the lack of compensatory stimulation from catecholamine release, the patient will have a low blood pressure and a slow pulse even in the early stages—again, in contrast to hypovolemic shock.

Treatment for neurogenic shock or spinal shock is similar to treatment for other types of shock and includes support of the airway, oxygenation, ventilation, maintenance of body temperature, and intravenous access. Spinal shock is characterized by hypotension, reflex bradycardia, and warm, dry skin. Because these symptoms signal a likelihood of spinal injury, cervical spine stabilization must be established on first patient contact, and the patient must be immobilized to a backboard as quickly as possible. A thorough search for other causes of shock (e.g., internal hemorrhage) must be made before concluding that a patient's hypotension is due to spinal shock alone. Treatment of spinal shock should include intravenous fluids (especially if there has been blood or fluid loss) and medications that increase

✳ osmotic diuresis greatly increased urination and dehydration due to high levels of glucose that cannot be reabsorbed into the blood from the kidney tubules, causing a loss of water into the urine.

✳ neurogenic shock shock resulting from brain or spinal cord injury that causes an interruption of nerve impulses to the arteries with loss of arterial tone, dilation, and relative hypovolemia.

the blood pressure by increasing peripheral vascular resistance. These include norepinephrine (Levophed) and dopamine (Intropin).

Anaphylactic Shock

When a foreign substance enters the body, the immune system responds to rid the body of the invader. (See the discussion of immunity later in this chapter.) This usually happens with no noticeable effects, and the person is not even aware that an immune response is taking place. Some foreign substances (antigens) provoke an exaggerated immune response (allergic response) that will cause noticeable symptoms, such as a rash (as from contact with poison ivy) or swollen, irritated airway passages (as with hay fever). In rare cases, an allergic response is very severe and life threatening. This kind of severe allergic response is called **anaphylaxis**, or **anaphylactic shock**.

An anaphylactic reaction usually occurs very rapidly. Signs and symptoms most often appear within a minute or less but occasionally may appear an hour or more after exposure. Generally, the faster the reaction develops, the more severe it is likely to be. Death can occur before the patient can get to a hospital, and so prompt intervention is critical. This is a situation when the paramedic at the scene can make the difference between life and death.

Anaphylactic reactions can be triggered by a variety of substances, including foods (especially nuts, eggs, shellfish), venoms, aspirin or nonsteroidal anti-inflammatory drugs (NSAIDS), hormones (animal-derived insulin), preservatives, and others. The most rapid and severe reactions are usually caused by substances injected directly into the circulation, which is one reason that penicillin injections and *Hymenoptera* stings (e.g., from bees, wasps, hornets) are the most common causes of fatal anaphylactic reactions.

Evaluation and Treatment Because the immune responses involved in anaphylaxis can affect different body systems, the signs and symptoms can vary widely:

- Skin
  - Flushing
  - Itching
  - Hives
  - Swelling
  - Cyanosis

- Respiratory system
  - Breathing difficulty
  - Sneezing, coughing
  - Wheezing, stridor
  - Laryngeal edema
  - Laryngospasm

- Cardiovascular system
  - Increased heart rate
  - Decreased blood pressure

- Gastrointestinal system
  - Nausea, vomiting
  - Abdominal cramping
  - Diarrhea

* **anaphylaxis** a life-threatening allergic reaction; also called **anaphylactic shock**.

- Nervous system
  - Altered mental status
  - Dizziness
  - Headache
  - Seizures
  - Tearing

The patient may present with an altered mental status that can progress to unresponsiveness; so, gather a brief history as soon as possible, including previous allergic reactions and any information about what the patient may have ingested or been exposed to that could have caused the present reaction. Be sure the patient is no longer in contact with the allergen; if a stinger is in the skin, scrape it away with a finger nail or scalpel blade.

Since laryngeal edema is often a problem, protecting the patient's airway will be your first concern. Administer oxygen via a nonrebreather mask or, as necessary, by endotracheal intubation. The anaphylactic response causes depletion of circulatory volume by promoting capillary permeability and leaking of fluid into interstitial spaces, and so establish an IV of crystalloid solution (normal saline or Ringer's Lactate) for volume support.

The primary treatment for anaphylaxis is pharmacological. In addition to oxygen, epinephrine is usually administered (if the patient has a history of anaphylaxis, he may be carrying a prescribed spring-loaded epinephrine injector), as are antihistamines (diphenhydramine), corticosteroids (methylprednisolone, hydrocortisone, dexamethasone), and vasopressors (dopamine, norepinephrine, epineprine). Occasionally, an inhaled beta agonist (albuterol) may be required. Follow local protocols.

Septic Shock

Septic shock begins with *septicemia* (also called *sepsis*), an infection that enters the bloodstream and is carried throughout the body. The person may have septicemia for some time before septic shock develops, but eventually toxins released by the invading organism overcome the compensatory mechanisms. Unless it is corrected, septic shock will cause the dysfunction of more than one organ system, resulting in multiple organ dysfunction syndrome (discussed in the next section).

Evaluation and Treatment The signs and symptoms of septic shock are progressive. In the beginning, cardiac output is increased, but toxins causing vasodilation may prevent an increase in blood pressure. The person may seem to be sick but not alarmingly so. By the last stages, toxins have increased permeability of the blood vessels to the point where great amounts of fluid are lost from the vasculature and blood pressure falls drastically.

Signs and symptoms can vary widely as the patient progresses from early to late stages of septic shock. Some patients may have a high fever, but others, especially the elderly or the very young, may have no fever or may even be hypothermic. The skin can be flushed, if fever is present, or very pale and cyanotic in the late stages.

The most susceptible organ system is the respiratory system, and so the patient may present with breathing difficulty and altered lung sounds. The brain may be infected, resulting in altered mental status. Suspicion of septic shock is usually based on a history of recent infection or illness.

Treatment includes administration of high-flow oxygen via a nonrebreather mask or by endotracheal intubation as necessary. An IV of crystalloid solution (normal saline or Ringer's Lactate) should be established, and dopamine may be administered to support the blood pressure. The heart rhythm must be monitored and medications administered to correct any dysrhythmias. Follow local protocols. In the hospital, antibiotic therapy will be initiated.

✱ **septic shock** shock that develops as the result of infection carried by the bloodstream, eventually causing dysfunction of multiple organ systems.

MULTIPLE ORGAN DYSFUNCTION SYNDROME

In the 1970s, a syndrome of multiple organ failure began to be noticed in hospital intensive care units. Medical advances were allowing patients to survive serious illness and trauma—only to die later of complications of the original disease or injury. The syndrome was described in 1975 as *multisystem organ failure*. In 1991, the American College of Chest Physicians and the Society of Critical Care Medicine named it **multiple organ dysfunction syndrome (MODS)**.

MODS is the progressive impairment of two or more organ systems resulting from an uncontrolled inflammatory response to a severe illness or injury. Sepsis and septic shock are the most common causes of MODS, with MODS being the end stage. (The progression from infection to sepsis to septic shock to MODS is known as systemic inflammatory response syndrome, or SIRS).

Actually, MODS can result from any severe disease or injury that triggers a massive systemic inflammatory response—including trauma, burns, surgery, circulatory shock, acute pancreatitis, acute renal failure, and others. Risk factors include age (> 65), malnutrition, and preexisting chronic disease, such as cancer or diabetes. With a mortality rate of 60 to 90 percent, MODS is the major cause of death following sepsis, trauma, and burn injuries.

Pathophysiology of MODS

MODS occurs in two stages. In primary MODS, organ damage results directly from a specific cause, such as ischemia or inadequate perfusion resulting from an episode of shock, trauma, or major surgery. There are stress and inflammatory responses (discussed in detail later in this chapter) to this initial injury, but they may be mild and not readily detectable. However, during this response, neutrophils and macrophages (cells that attack and destroy bacteria, protozoa, foreign cells, and cell debris) as well as mast cells (cells that produce histamine and other components of allergic response) are thought to be "primed" by cytokines (proteins released during an inflammatory or immune response).

The next time there is an insult, such as an additional injury or ischemia or infection—even though the insult may be mild—the primed cells are activated, producing an exaggerated inflammatory response, known as secondary MODS.

Now, the inflammatory response enters a self-perpetuating cycle. As inflammatory mediators are released by the injured organ, they enter the circulation, activating inflammatory responses in organ systems throughout the body. These mediators, especially cytokines, such as tumour necrosis factor (TNF) and interleukin 1 (IL-1), damage the endothelium (cells that line the blood vessels, the heart, and various body cavities). Gram-negative bacteria, if present, release endotoxins that also damage endothelial cells. The injured endothelial cells release factors that aggravate the inflammation and cause vasodilation. The injured epithelium becomes permeable, allowing leakage of fluid into interstitial spaces, and loses much of its anticoagulation function, which allows formation of tiny blood clots (thrombi) in the microvasculature.

The secondary insult also triggers an exaggerated neuroendocrine response. Catecholamine release causes many of the manifestations of MODS, including tachycardia, increased metabolic rates, and increased oxygen consumption. Release of a variety of hormones contributes to the hypermetabolism, and release of endorphins contributes to vasodilation. Additionally, plasma protein systems are activated: specifically, the complement system, the coagulation system, and the kallikrein-kinin system. Plasma proteins are key mediators of the inflammatory response. When activated, each of these systems triggers a cascade of responses, with the overall result of increased vasodilation, vasopermeability, cardiovascular instability, endothelial damage, and clotting abnormalities.

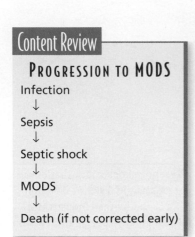

✱ **multiple organ dysfunction syndrome (MODS)** progressive impairment of two or more organ systems resulting from an uncontrolled inflammatory response to a severe illness or injury.

Content Review

PROGRESSION TO MODS

Infection
↓
Sepsis
↓
Septic shock
↓
MODS
↓
Death (if not corrected early)

As a result of the release of the inflammatory mediators and toxins and the plasma protein cascades, a massive immune/inflammatory and coagulation response develops. Vascular changes (vasodilation, increased capillary permeability, selective vasoconstriction, and microvascular thrombi) continue and worsen. Two metabolites that are released have opposing vascular effects: Prostacyclin, also called prostaglandin I_2 (PGI_2) is a vasodilator, while thromboxane A_2 (TXA_2) is a vasoconstrictor. They are released in differing amounts within different organ tissues, contributing to a maldistribution of blood flow to organs and organ systems.

As noted earlier, the release of catecholamines stimulates hypermetabolism within the body cells, which, in turn, creates a greatly increased oxygen demand. Because of lung damage, hypoxemia, and hypoperfusion, a severe oxygen supply/demand imbalance develops. As the cells switch from aerobic to anaerobic metabolism, fuel supplies within the cells (ATP and glucose) are used up faster than they can be replenished. Without adequate ATP, the cells lose their ability to operate the sodium-potassium pump, which is essential to cardiac function. The myocardium is profoundly weakened. Cellular lysosomes begin to break down, releasing lysosomal enzymes that damage the cell membrane and the surrounding cells. Large amounts of lactic acid are released, contributing to acidosis, which further damages the cells. The overall response is similar to that seen in septic and anaphylactic shock, except on a larger scale.

Clinical Presentation of MODS

The cumulative effects of MODS at the cellular and tissue levels begin to cause the breakdown of organ systems: The organs that fail first are not necessarily the organs where the initial insult occurred, and there is a lag time between the initial insult and the onset of organ failure. Dysfunction may develop in the pulmonary, gastrointestinal, hepatic, renal, cardiovascular, hematological, and immune systems. There is decreased cardiac function and myocardial depression, caused by the factors discussed earlier, possibly abetted by release of myocardial depressant factor (MDF) and a decrease in beta-adrenergic receptors in the heart. The smooth muscle of the vascular system fails, with consequent release of capillary sphincters and increased vasodilation.

MODS does not occur in one intense crisis. It will usually develop over two, three, or more weeks. There is no specific therapy for MODS, and the only chance of rescuing the patient from its self-perpetuating spiral toward death is early recognition and initiation of supportive measures. For this reason, it is important to understand how MODS usually presents in the first 24 hours after initial resuscitation.

Although MODS will usually be detected in the hospital, rather than the out-of-hospital setting, there may be occasions when a patient who has not been hospitalized or who has returned home from the hospital is the subject of a call to EMS, or when a patient being transported by EMS from one facility to another is suffering from MODS.

The most common presentation of MODS over time is as follows:

24 Hours after Resuscitation
- Low-grade fever
- Tachycardia (rapid heart rate)
- Dyspnea (breathing difficulty)
- Altered mental status
- General hypermetabolic, hyperdynamic state

Within 24 to 72 Hours
- Pulmonary (lung) failure begins

MODS will usually develop over two, three, or more weeks.

Survival of MODS is dependent on early recognition and supportive care.

Within 7 to 10 Days
- Hepatic (liver) failure begins
- Intestinal failure begins
- Renal (kidney) failure begins

Within 14 to 21 days
- Renal and hepatic failure intensify
- Gastrointestinal collapse
- Immune system collapse

After 21 Days
- Hematological (blood system) failure begins
- Myocardial (heart muscle) failure begins
- Altered mental status resulting from encephalopathy (brain infection)
- Death

Part 2: The Body's Defences against Disease and Injury

As discussed so far in this chapter, the human body is vulnerable to attack by a variety of diseases and foreign invaders as well as to injury. The major focus of Part 2 will be the body's chief defences against disease, invaders, and injury—the immune response and the inflammatory response—and the interactions between the immune and inflammatory responses.

In Part 2, we will also examine hypersensitivity, or allergic and anaphylactic responses, that is, what happens when the immune system overresponds to invasive agents to the extent that the body is actually harming itself. Immune deficiencies will also be discussed, including acquired immune deficiency syndrome, or AIDS.

Finally, we will discuss the interrelationships between stress and disease, including the body's use of the neuroendocrine and immune systems to regulate the stress response. Psychological responses to stress, including various coping mechanisms, are also described.

SELF-DEFENCE MECHANISMS

In Chapter 12, normal body anatomy and physiology were discussed (the normal cell and its environment: fluids and electrolytes, the acid-base balance). In Part 1 of this chapter, we discussed how the body may be attacked or injured (cellular injury, infection, genetic and other causes of disease, hypoperfusion, and multiple organ dysfunction syndrome). In the next sections, we will discuss how the body defends itself from infection and injury.

It is important to keep in mind that the body has powerful ways of defending and healing itself (restoring homeostasis) and that medical intervention is needed only when, on occasion, these natural defence mechanisms are unequal to the task and become overwhelmed.

INFECTIOUS AGENTS

Bacteria

Bacteria are single-cell organisms that consist of internal cytoplasm surrounded by a rigid cell wall. Bacteria are prokaryotic cells that, unlike the eukaryotic cells of the human body, lack an organized nucleus and other intracellular organelles.

✳ **bacteria** (singular *bacterium*) single-cell organisms with a cell membrane and cytoplasm but no organized nucleus. They bind to the cells of a host organism to obtain food and support.

Bacteria can reproduce independently, but they need a host to supply food and other support. Inside the body, they achieve this by binding to host cells.

Bacteria can be cultured and identified readily in most hospital laboratories. Many bacteria are categorized according to their appearance under the microscope after staining with several dyes referred to as *gram stains.* Some bacteria stain blue, while others stain red. Bacteria that stain blue are referred to as *gram-positive* bacteria. They are somewhat similar to each other in their structure. Bacteria that stain red are referred to as *gram-negative* bacteria. They are also somewhat similar to each other in their structure.

Bacteria can cause many of the common infections in medicine, including middle ear infections in children, many cases of tonsillitis, and meningitis. (These kinds of infections can also be caused by viruses, which are discussed in the next section.) Most bacterial infections respond to treatment with drugs called **antibiotics.** Once administered, antibiotics kill or inhibit the growth of invading bacteria. As mentioned earlier, the bacterial cell membrane is the site of action for many antibiotics. Once the cell membrane is broken down, phagocytes (cells that ingest and destroy pathogens and other foreign and abnormal substances) can begin to destroy the bacterium. A variety of antibiotic drugs have been developed with mechanisms of action tailored to different types of bacteria. However, the broad variety of infectious bacteria, and their ability to develop resistance to drugs, makes developing antibiotics to battle them a difficult job.

✱ **antibiotics** substances that destroy or inhibit microorganisms, tiny living bodies invisible to the naked eye. (*Antibiotic* means "destructive to life.")

Some bacteria protect themselves by forming a capsule outside the cell wall that protects the organism from digestion by phagocytes. Some bacteria, such as mycoplasmic bacteria, have no protective capsule but rely on other mechanisms to survive and attack the body. *Mycobacterium tuberculosis,* which has no protective capsule, can actually survive and be transported by phagocytes. Other bacteria simply multiply faster than the body's defence systems can respond. Still others overpower the body's defences by producing enzymes and toxins that attack and injure cells and produce hypersensitivity reactions.

Simple infection is not the only consequence of a bacterial invasion. Many bacteria release poisonous chemicals, or *toxins.* There are two types of toxins produced by bacteria: exotoxins and endotoxins. **Exotoxins** are proteins secreted and released by the bacterial cell during its growth. They travel throughout the body via the blood or lymph, ultimately causing problems. For example, botulism toxin, released by the bacterium *Clostridium botulinum,* blocks the release of cholingeric neurotransmitters at neuromuscular junctions and elsewhere in the autonomic nervous system, causing systemic paralysis. Another example is tetanus, which is caused by the bacterium *Clostridium tetani.* The actual infection by the bacteria is mild and may be limited, for example, to the site of a puncture wound in the foot. Yet, on entering the body, the bacteria release their toxin, *tetanospasmin.* This toxin then travels through the blood to the skeletal muscles, causing the spastic rigidity classically seen in tetanus.

✱ **exotoxins** toxic (poisonous) substances secreted by bacterial cells during their growth.

Endotoxins are complex molecules that are contained in the cell walls of certain gram-negative bacteria. Endotoxins can be released during the destruction of the bacterial cell by phagocytes or even when the bacterial cell is attacked by an antibiotic so that antibiotics cannot control the endotoxic effects of bacteria. When released, endotoxins trigger the inflammatory process and produce fever. In the bloodstream, they can cause widespread clotting within the blood vessels, capillary damage, and hypotension, as well as respiratory distress and fever—a condition known as endotoxin shock. Endotoxins can survive even when the cell that produced them is dead.

✱ **endotoxins** molecules in the walls of certain gram-negative bacteria that are released when the bacterium dies or is destroyed, causing toxic (poisonous) effects on the host body.

Depending on their amount and site of release, the effects of toxins can be local or systemic. When a bacterial organism enters the circulatory system, its released toxins can spread throughout the body. The systemic spread of toxins through the bloodstream is known as **septicemia,** or *sepsis,* and is a grave medical illness.

✱ **septicemia** the systemic spread of toxins through the bloodstream. Also called *sepsis.*

The body encounters the bacterial invasion and release of enzymes and toxins through activation of the immune system. The immune system will mobilize foreign-cell-destroying macrophages (a type of white blood cell) to the site of infection in an attempt to rid the body of the foreign pathogen. As the macrophages attempt to destroy the bacteria, they release substances known as pyrogens. Pyrogens are responsible for causing the increase in temperature known as fever. Pyrogens act on the thermoregulation centre in the hypothalamus to cause the increased body temperature, which is thought to aid in the destruction of pathogens.

Viruses

Most infections are caused by **viruses**. Viruses are much smaller than bacteria and can only be seen with an electron microscope. In addition, they cannot grow without the assistance of another organism. In fact, viruses are referred to as *intracellular parasites,* since they must invade the cells of the organism they infect.

A virus has no organized cellular structure except a protein coat (capsid) surrounding the internal genetic material, deoxyribonucleic acid (DNA) or ribonucleic acid (RNA). With no organized cellular structure or cellular organelles, viruses are incapable of metabolism. Once inside a cell, they take over, using the various cellular enzymes to replicate and produce more viruses, which decreases synthesis of macromolecules vital to the host cell.

Some viruses develop a coating in addition to the capsid, called an envelope. The envelope and the protein capsid allow the virus to resist destruction by the phagocytes of the immune system. However, since viruses cannot reproduce outside a host cell, if the virus does not find a host cell, it will die.

The symptoms of a virus may not be readily apparent because it is hidden within the host cell. After replication is complete, the virus will sometimes destroy the host cell. In other cases, a virus will remain dormant within a cell for months or years. An example is the *varicella zoster virus,* which causes childhood chickenpox and may then remain dormant, only to cause shingles in the adult decades later. Some viruses form a long-term symbiotic relationship with the host cell, resulting in a persistent but unapparent infection.

Viruses do not produce toxins, but they can still cause very serious illnesses. Some viruses are capable of altering the host cell to induce a malignancy (cancer). Others, such as *human immunodeficiency virus (HIV),* which causes AIDS, can proliferate, attacking cells of the immune system and destroying its ability to ward off infections of all types.

Unlike bacteria, viruses are very difficult to treat. Once a virus infects a cell, it can only be killed by destroying the infected cell. Drugs have not yet been developed that can selectively destroy cells infected by viruses while leaving uninfected cells unharmed. This partially explains the dilemma facing researchers trying to find a cure for AIDS. An additional problem is that some viruses mutate (change) frequently, which is why a new flu vaccine must be developed for every flu season. Fortunately, most viral illnesses are mild and fairly self-limiting. (Because viral agents must spread from cell to cell, the immune system is eventually able to "catch" them outside a host cell and destroy them.) Even so, at present, viruses usually cannot be treated with more than symptomatic care.

Other Agents of Infection

Other biological agents that cause human infection include *fungi* (the plural of *fungus*) and parasites.

Fungi, which includes yeast and moulds, are more like plants than animals. Fungi rarely cause human disease, other than minor skin infections, such as athlete's foot and some common vaginal infections. Fungal infections are called *mycoses.* Patients with an impaired immune system, such as HIV patients or patients with organ transplants, suffer fungal infection more commonly than do healthy people. In such patients, the fungi can invade the lungs, blood, and several organs. Treatment of complicated, deep fungal infections has proven difficult, even in the hospital setting.

Parasites range in size from protozoa (single-cell animals not much larger than bacteria) to large intestinal worms. Parasites tend to be more common in the developing nations than in North America. Treatment depends on the organism and the location.

Prions are the most recently recognized classification of infectious agents. Initially thought to be slow-acting viruses, prions differ from viruses in that they are smaller, are made entirely of proteins, and do not have protective capsids.

For more about infectious diseases, see Chapter 37.

THREE LINES OF DEFENCE

There are three chief lines of self-defence against infection and injury. One involves anatomical barriers. The other two—the inflammatory response and the immune response—rely on actions of the leukocytes (white blood cells). Each line of defence can be characterized as external or internal, nonspecific or specific (Table 13-2)—characterizations you may want to keep in mind as you read the following sections and compare the ways these defences protect the body.

Before an infectious agent can attack the body, it has to get past the body's natural anatomical barrier, the epithelium (the skin and the mucous membranes that line the respiratory, gastrointestinal, and genitourinary tracts). The epithelium is more than just a physical barrier; it also provides a chemical defence against infection. The sebaceous glands of the skin secrete fatty and lactic acids, which attack bacteria and fungi. Sweat, tears, and saliva secreted by other glands contain bacteria-attacking enzymes. Various mechanical responses also work to get rid of invading substances. For example, the invader may be coughed or sneezed out of the respiratory tract, flushed out of the urinary tract, or eliminated from the gastrointestinal tract by vomiting or diarrhea.

The anatomical defences are *external* and *nonspecific*. They are considered external because they prevent substances from penetrating the skin or the coverings of internal passageways. They are nonspecific because they defend against all invaders, such as foreign bodies, chemicals, or microorganisms, without targeting any specific type of invader.

If an invading foreign body, chemical, or microorganism penetrates the anatomical barriers and begins to attack internal cells and tissues, two other lines of defence are triggered: the inflammatory response and the immune response. These twin responses of the immune system have contrasting characteristics of speed, specificity, duration (memory), and the plasma systems and cell types that are involved in the response (Table 13-3).

The *inflammatory response*, or *inflammation*, begins within seconds of injury or invasion by a pathogen. As noted earlier, it is nonspecific, attacking any invader by surrounding it with cells and fluids to isolate, destroy, and eliminate it. Inflammation is mediated by multiple plasma protein systems, especially the

> **Content Review**
>
> **THREE LINES OF DEFENCE**
> Anatomical barriers
> Inflammatory response
> Immune response

Table 13-2 THREE LINES OF DEFENCE AGAINST INFECTION AND INJURY

	External	Internal	Nonspecific	Specific
Anatomical Barriers	External		Nonspecific	
Inflammatory Response		Internal	Nonspecific	
Immune Response		Internal		Specific

Table 13-3 — CHARACTERISTICS OF THE INFLAMMATORY AND IMMUNE RESPONSES

	Inflammatory Response	Immune Response
Speed	Fast	Slow
Specificity	Nonspecific	Specific
Duration (Memory)	Transient (no memory)	Long-term (memory)
Involving Which Plasma Systems	Multiple plasma protein systems (complement, coagulation, kinin systems)	One plasma protein system (immunoglobulin)
Involving Which Cell Type	Multiple cell types (granulocytes, monocytes, macrophages)	One blood cell type (lymphocytes)

complement system, the coagulation system, and the kinin system (which will be explained later) and involves a variety of cell types as it attacks the invader.

The *immune response* develops more slowly (one type of response requires a second exposure after priming by the first exposure to the invader). The immune response is specific, in that it will develop a specialized response for each different invader. It is mediated by just one plasma protein system (immunoglobulin) and attacks the invader mainly with a single cell type (lymphocytes, which are one type of leukocyte, or white blood cell).

Inflammation and the immune response interact in many ways. We will discuss the immune response first because understanding the immune response is necessary for understanding some parts of the inflammatory response.

THE IMMUNE RESPONSE

HOW THE IMMUNE RESPONSE WORKS: AN OVERVIEW

Most viruses, bacteria, fungi, and parasites—as well as noninfectious substances, such as pollens, foods, venoms, drugs, and others, that may enter the body—have proteins on their surface called **antigens**. The immune system detects these antigens as being foreign, or "nonself," and responds to produce substances called **antibodies** that combine with antigens to control or destroy them. This is known as the **immune response**. As part of this process, *memory cells* "remember" the antigen and will trigger an even faster and more effective response to destroy the same antigen if it enters the body again. Such long-term protection against specific foreign substances is known as **immunity**.

CHARACTERISTICS OF THE IMMUNE RESPONSE AND IMMUNITY

The immune response and immunity can be classified as natural versus acquired immunity or humoral versus cell-mediated immunity.

Natural versus Acquired Immunity

Natural immunity is not generated by the immune response. It is inborn, part of the genetic makeup of the individual or the species. For example, dogs are naturally immune to measles, and humans are naturally immune to canine distemper. (Some diseases, such as leukemia, however, can affect more than one species.)

Acquired immunity develops as an outcome of the immune response. Acquired immunity can be either active or passive. *Active acquired immunity* is generated by

* **antigen** a marker on the surface of a cell that identifies it as "self" or "nonself."

* **antibody** a substance produced by B lymphocytes in response to the presence of a foreign antigen that will combine with and control or destroy the antigen, thus preventing infection.

* **immune response** the body's reactions that inactivate or eliminate foreign antigens.

* **immunity** a long-term condition of protection against infection or disease.

* **natural immunity** inborn protection against infection or disease.

* **acquired immunity** protection against infection or disease that is (a) developed by the body after exposure to an antigen, or (b) transferred to the person from an outside source.

the immune system after exposure to an antigen. *Passive acquired immunity* is transferred to a person from an outside source. For example, a mother may transfer antibodies to the fetus. Or antibodies may be administered as an immune serum against an invader, such as rabies, tetanus, or snake venom. Active acquired immunity is long lasting. Passive acquired immunity is temporary.

Humoral versus Cell–Mediated Immunity

A special type of leukocyte (white blood cell) is the **lymphocyte**. Lymphocytes (20 to 35 percent of all leukocytes) are responsible for several critical immune functions, including recognizing foreign antigens, producing antibodies, and developing memory.

As lymphocytes mature, they become one of several types, including B lymphocytes and T lymphocytes. **B lymphocytes** do not attack antigens directly. Instead, they produce the antibodies (immunoglobulins) that attack antigens. B lymphocytes also develop memory, and confer long-term immunity to specific antigens. This type of immunity is called **humoral immunity.** (*Humor* refers to the blood and other fluids of the body; *humoral immunity* refers to the long-lasting antibodies and memory cells present in the blood and lymph.)

T lymphocytes do not produce antibodies. Instead, they recognize the presence of a foreign antigen and attack it directly. This type of immunity is called **cell-mediated immunity.**

INDUCTION OF THE IMMUNE RESPONSE

The immune response must be triggered, or induced. The following sections discuss the role of antigens, immunogens, and blood groups.

Antigens and Immunogens

Antigens that can trigger the immune response are called **immunogens.** Not every antigen is an immunogen. That is, not every antigen is capable of triggering the immune response. For example, the immune response is not triggered by antigens present on various helpful bacteria in our bodies.

What makes a molecule an antigen is a chemical structure that is capable of reacting with immune system components, such as antibodies and T lymphocytes. However, having this chemical structure, the ability to *react* once the immune system has been triggered, is not enough to *trigger* the immune system in the first place. To be immunogenic—able to trigger an immune response—an antigen must have additional characteristics.

Characteristics of Antigenic Immunogenicity

- Sufficient foreignness
- Sufficient size
- Sufficient complexity
- Sufficient amounts

Normally, the immune system is not triggered by self-antigens. In fact, the immune system does not just "tolerate" self-antigens; it actively protects them through suppression of the immune system.

Blood Group Antigens

Human leukocyte antigens (HLAs) do not exist on the surface of erythrocytes (red blood cells), but other antigens, known as the blood group antigens, do.

✳ **lymphocyte** a type of leukocyte, or white blood cell, that attacks foreign substances as part of the body's immune response.

✳ **B lymphocytes** white blood cells that, in response to the presence of an antigen, produce antibodies that attack the antigen, develop a memory for the antigen, and confer long-term immunity to the antigen.

✳ **humoral immunity** the long-term immunity to an antigen provided by antibodies produced by B lymphocytes.

✳ **T lymphocytes** white blood cells that do not produce antibodies but, instead, attack antigens directly.

✳ **cell-mediated immunity** the short-term immunity to an antigen provided by T lymphocytes, which directly attack the antigen but do not produce antibodies or memory for the antigen.

✳ **immunogens** antigens that are able to trigger an immune response.

All immunogens are antigens, but not all antigens are immunogens. In other words, only some antigens are capable of triggering an immune response.

There are more than 80 of the red cell antigens that have been grouped into a number of different blood group systems. The two groups that trigger the strongest immune response are the Rh system and the ABO system.

The Rh System The **Rh blood group** is named for the rhesus monkey in which it was first identified. One of several antigens in this group is known as Rh antigen D, or the **Rh factor**. Rh factor is present in about 85 percent of North Americans (Rh positive) but absent in about 15 percent (Rh negative).

Incompatibility between Rh positive and Rh negative blood can cause harmful immune responses. For example, if a patient with Rh negative blood receives a transfusion of Rh positive blood, a primary immune response is triggered. A second transfusion of Rh positive blood may cause a severe transfusion reaction.

Hemolytic disease of the newborn may result from Rh incompatibility between mother and fetus. Problems will usually not occur in a first pregnancy where the mother is Rh negative and the fetus is Rh positive because few fetal erythrocytes cross the placental barrier to the mother. However, a significant number of fetal erythrocytes do enter the mother's bloodstream at birth when the placenta separates from the uterus. These may (depending on several factors) activate a primary immune response and development of Rh antibodies. If the fetus in her next pregnancy is also Rh positive, the mother's Rh antibodies can cross the placenta and destroy the red blood cells of the fetus. This is actually a rare occurrence. Rh incompatibility occurs in only about 10 percent of pregnancies. Since not all such incompatibilities produce Rh antibodies in the mother, only about 5 percent of women ever have babies with hemolytic disease, even after numerous pregnancies.

The ABO System The **ABO blood group** consists of only two antigens, named A and B. Persons with blood type A carry only A antigens on their red blood cells. Those with blood type B carry only B antigens. Those with blood type AB carry both, and those with blood type O carry neither.

An immune response will be activated in a person with type A blood who receives a transfusion of type B blood, which is recognized as nonself. The same will happen when a person with type B blood receives type A blood. People with type O blood are known as *universal donors* because type O blood has no antigens that will trigger an immune response in any other group. Those with type AB blood are known as *universal recipients* because they have both types of antigens and will not produce antibodies in response to any other blood groups.

Mother-fetus ABO incompatibility is more common than Rh incompatibility, occurring in about 20 to 25 percent of pregnancies, but only 10 percent of ABO incompatibilities will result in hemolytic disease of the infant.

INFLAMMATION

INFLAMMATION CONTRASTED WITH THE IMMUNE RESPONSE

Inflammation, also called the *inflammatory response,* is the body's response to cellular injury. It differs from the immune response in many ways. (Review Tables 13-2 and 13-3.) As you read the following sections, keep these points in mind:

- The immune response develops *slowly;* inflammation develops *swiftly.*
- The immune response is *specific* (targets specific antigens); inflammation is *nonspecific* (it attacks all unwanted substances in the same way). In fact, inflammation is sometimes called "the nonspecific immune response."

✳ **Rh blood group** a group of antigens discovered on the red blood cells of rhesus monkeys that is also present to some extent in humans.

✳ **Rh factor** an antigen in the Rh blood group that is also known as antigen D. About 85 percent of North Americans have the Rh factor (are Rh positive), while about 15 percent do not have the Rh factor (are Rh negative). Rh positive and Rh negative blood are incompatible; that is, a person who is Rh negative can experience a severe immune response if Rh positive blood is introduced, as through a transfusion or during childbirth.

✳ **ABO blood group** two antigens known as A and B. A person may have either (type A or type B), both (type AB), or neither (type O). An immune response will be activated whenever a person receives blood containing A or B antigen if this antigen is not already present in his own blood.

✳ **inflammation** the body's response to cellular injury; also called the *inflammatory response.* In contrast to the immune response, inflammation develops swiftly, is nonspecific (attacks all unwanted substances in the same way), and is temporary, leading to healing.

- The immune response is *long lasting* (memory cells will remember an antigen and trigger a swift response on reexposure, even years later); inflammation is *temporary,* lasting only until the immediate threat is conquered—usually only a few days to two weeks.

- The immune response involves *one type of white blood cell* (lymphocytes); inflammation involves *platelets and many types of white cells* (the granulatory cells called neutrophils, basophils, and eosinophils; the monocytes that mature into macrophages).

- The immune response involves *one type of plasma protein* (immunoglobulins, also called antibodies); inflammation involves *several plasma protein systems* (complement, coagulation, and kinin).

However, the immune response and inflammation are interdependent. For example, macrophages that are developed during the inflammatory response must ingest antigens before helper T cells can recognize them and trigger the immune response. Conversely, IgE antibody produced by B cells during an immune response can stimulate mast cells to activate inflammation.

Although inflammation differs from the immune response in many ways, inflammation and the immune response are both considered to be part of the body's immune system.

HOW INFLAMMATION WORKS: AN OVERVIEW

Inflammation is somewhat easier to understand than the immune response because we have all observed it. The immune response is often hidden; your body's immune system may be knocking out an infectious antigen without your ever being aware of it. However, if you cut your finger, you will probably be acutely aware of the inflammatory process. You will actually see the redness and swelling and feel the pain. You may observe the formation of pus. As days go by, you will see the progress of wound healing and, perhaps, scar formation.

This is not to say that inflammation is simple; in its way, it is as complex as the immune response. There are several phases to inflammation. After each phase, healing may take place, and that will be the end of it. If healing doesn't take place, inflammation moves into its next phase. However, healing is the goal of all the phases.

Phases of Inflammation

Phase 1: Acute inflammation → healing
(If healing doesn't take place, moves to phase 2)
Phase 2: Chronic inflammation → healing
(If healing doesn't take place, moves to phase 3)
Phase 3: Granuloma formation
Phase 4: Healing

During each phase, the components of inflammation work together to perform four functions.

The Four Functions of Inflammation (During All Phases)

1. Destroy and remove unwanted substances
2. Wall off the infected and inflamed area
3. Stimulate the immune response
4. Promote healing

Content Review

FOUR FUNCTIONS OF INFLAMMATION
Destroy and remove unwanted substances
Wall off the infected and inflamed area
Stimulate the immune response
Promote healing

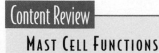
Content Review

MAST CELL FUNCTIONS
Degranulation
Synthesis

FIGURE 13-6 The inflammatory response.

ACUTE INFLAMMATORY RESPONSE

Acute inflammation is triggered by any injury, whether lethal or nonlethal, to the body's cells. As discussed earlier in this chapter, cell injury can result from causes such as hypoxia, chemicals, infectious agents (bacteria, viruses, fungi, parasites), trauma, heat extremes, radiation, nutritional imbalances, genetic factors, and even the injurious effects of the immune and inflammatory responses themselves. When cells are injured, the acute inflammatory response begins within seconds (Figure 13-6).

The basic mechanics are always the same: (1) Blood vessels contract and dilate to move additional blood to the site. Then, (2) vascular permeability increases so that (3) white cells and plasma proteins can move through the capillary walls and into the tissues to begin the tasks of destroying the invader and healing the injury site (Figure 13-7).

MAST CELLS

Mast cells, which resemble bags of granules, are the chief activators of the inflammatory response. They are not blood cells. Instead, they reside in connective tissues just outside the blood vessels.

Mast cells activate the inflammatory response through two functions: *degranulation* and *synthesis* (Figure 13-8).

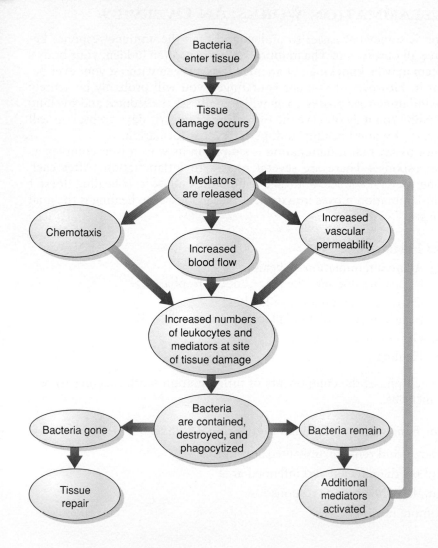

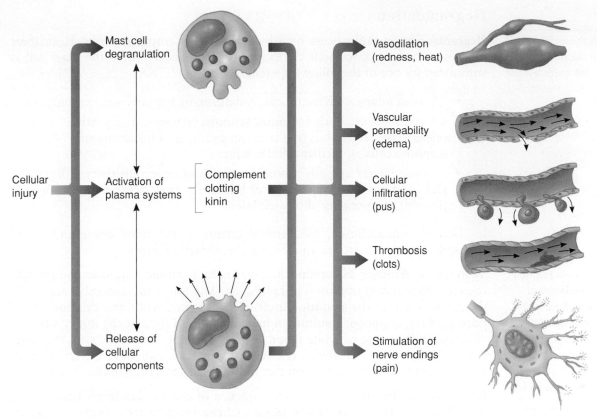

FIGURE 13-7   The acute inflammatory response.

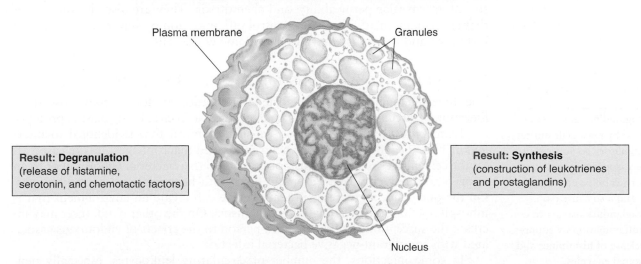

Cause: Mast cell stimulated by:
- Physical injury (e.g., trauma, radiation, temperature extremes)
- Chemical agent (e.g., toxin, venom, enzyme, neutrophil-produced protein)
- Immunological process (e.g., allergic reaction/IgE antibody, activated complement)

Plasma membrane

Granules

Result: Degranulation
(release of histamine, serotonin, and chemotactic factors)

Result: Synthesis
(construction of leukotrienes and prostaglandins)

Nucleus

FIGURE 13-8   Mast cell degranulation and synthesis.

Degranulation

Degranulation is the process by which mast cells empty granules from their interior into the extracellular environment. This occurs when the mast cell is stimulated by one of the following events:

- *Physical injury,* such as trauma, radiation, or temperature extremes
- *Chemical agents,* such as toxins, venoms, enzymes, or a protein released by neutrophils (the latter an example of inflammatory response causing further cellular injury)
- *Immunological and direct processes,* such as hypersensitivity (allergic) reactions involving release of IgE antibody or activation of complement components (discussed later)

During degranulation, biochemical agents in the mast cell granules are released, notably vasoactive amines and chemotactic factors.

Vasoactive Amines Histamine is a vasoactive amine (organic compound) released during degranulation of mast cells. The effect of vasoactive amines is the constriction of the smooth muscle of large vessel walls and dilation of the postcapillary sphincter, resulting in increased blood flow at the injury site.

Basophils (a type of white blood cell) also release histamine, with the same effect. Additionally, **serotonin,** released by platelets, can have effects of both vasoconstriction and vasodilation that may affect blood flow to the affected site.

Chemotactic Factors Another consequence of degranulation of mast cells is the release of various **chemotactic factors.** Chemotactic factors are chemicals that attract white cells to the site of inflammation. This attraction of white cells is called **chemotaxis.**

Synthesis

When stimulated, mast cells synthesize, or construct, two substances that play important roles in inflammation: leukotrienes and prostaglandins.

Leukotrienes, also known as *slow-reacting substances of anaphylaxis (SRS-A),* have actions similar to histamines—vasoconstriction and increased permeability—as well as chemotaxis. However, they are more important in the later stages of inflammation because they promote slower and longer-lasting effects than do histamines. Like leukotrienes, **prostaglandins** cause increased vasoconstruction, vascular permeability, and chemotaxis. They are also the substances that cause pain. In addition, they control inflammation by suppressing release of histamine and lysosomal enzymes from some white cells.

SYSTEMIC RESPONSES OF ACUTE INFLAMMATION

The three chief manifestations of acute inflammation are fever, leukocytosis (proliferation of circulating white cells), and an increase in circulating plasma proteins.

Endogenous pyrogen is a fever-causing chemical that is identical to interleukin 1 (IL-1) and is released by neutrophils and macrophages. It is released after the cell engages in phagocytosis or is exposed to a bacterial endotoxin or to an antigen-antibody complex. Fever can have both beneficial and harmful effects. On the one hand, an increase in temperature can create an environment that is inhospitable to some invading microorganisms. On the other hand, fever may increase the susceptibility of the infected person to the effects of endotoxins associated with some gram-negative bacterial infections.

In some infections, the number of circulating leukocytes, especially neutrophils, increases. Several components of the inflammatory response stimulate production of neutrophils, including a component of the complement system. Phagocytes produce a factor that induces production of granulocytes, including neutrophils, eosinophils, and basophils.

Plasma proteins called *acute phase reactants,* mostly produced in the liver, increase during inflammation. Their synthesis is stimulated by various interleukins. Many of these act to inhibit and control the inflammatory response.

CHRONIC INFLAMMATORY RESPONSES

Defined simply, chronic inflammation is any inflammation that lasts longer than two weeks. It may be caused by a foreign object or substance that persists in the wound, for example, a splinter, glass, or dirt. Or it may accompany a persistent bacterial infection. This can occur because some microorganisms have cell walls with a high lipid or wax content that resist phagocytosis. Other microorganisms can survive inside a macrophage. Still others produce toxins that persist even after the bacterium is dead, continuing to incite inflammatory responses. Inflammation can also be prolonged by the presence of chemicals and other irritants.

During chronic inflammation, large numbers of neutrophils—the phagocytes that were first on the scene during acute inflammation—degranulate and die. Now, the neutrophils are replaced by components that have taken longer to develop, and there is a large infiltration of lymphocytes from the immune response and of macrophages that have matured from monocytes. In addition to attacking foreign invaders, macrophages produce a factor that stimulates **fibroblasts,** cells that secrete collagen, a critical factor in wound healing.

As neutrophils, lymphocytes, and macrophages die, they infiltrate the tissues, sometimes forming a cavity that contains these dead cells, bits of dead tissue, and tissue fluid, a mixture called **pus.** Enzymes present in pus eventually cause it to self-digest, and it is removed through the epithelium or the lymph system.

Occasionally, when macrophages are unable to destroy the foreign invader, a **granuloma** will form to wall off the infection from the rest of the body. The granuloma is formed as large numbers of macrophages, other white cells, and fibroblasts are drawn to the site and surround it. Cells decay within the granuloma, and the released acids and lysosomes break the cellular debris down to basic components and fluid. The fluid eventually diffuses out of the granuloma, leaving a hollow, hard-walled structure buried in the tissues. Some granulomas persist for the life of the individual. Granuloma formation is common in leprosy and tuberculosis, which are caused by mycobacteria, bacteria that resist destruction by phagocytes.

Tissue repair and possible scar formation are the final stages of inflammation and will be discussed in more detail later.

✱ **fibroblasts** cells that secrete collagen, a critical factor in wound healing.

✱ **pus** a liquid mixture of dead cells, bits of dead tissue, and tissue fluid that may accumulate in inflamed tissues.

✱ **granuloma** a tumour or growth that forms when foreign bodies that cannot be destroyed by macrophages are surrounded and walled off.

LOCAL INFLAMMATORY RESPONSES

All the manifestations observed at the local inflammation site result from (1) vascular changes and (2) exudation. Redness and heat result from vascular dilation and increased blood flow to the area. Swelling and pain result from the vascular permeability that permits infiltration of exudate into the tissues.

Exudate has three functions:

1. To dilute toxins released by bacteria and the toxic products of dying cells

2. To bring plasma proteins and leukocytes to the site to attack the invaders

3. To carry away the products of inflammation (e.g., toxins, dead cells, pus)

The composition of exudate varies with the stage of inflammation and the type of injury or infection. Early exudate (serous exudate) is watery with few plasma proteins or leukocytes, as in a blister. In a severe or advanced inflammation, the exudate may be thick and clotted (fibrinous exudate), as in lobar pneumonia. In persistent bacterial infections, the exudate contains pus (purulent, or suppurative, exudate), as with cysts and abscesses. If bleeding is present, the exudate contains blood (hemorrhagic exudate).

The lesions (infected areas or wounds) that result from inflammation vary, depending on the organ affected. In myocardial infarction, cellular death results in the replacement of dead tissue by scar tissue. An infarction of brain tissue may result in liquefactive necrosis, in which the dead cells liquefy and are contained in walled cysts. In the liver, destroyed cells result in the regeneration of liver cells.

Keep in mind that inflammation can only occur in vascularized tissues (tissues to which blood can flow). When perfusion is cut off, as in a gangrenous limb or a limb distal to a tourniquet, inflammation cannot take place—and without inflammation, healing cannot take place.

RESOLUTION AND REPAIR

Healing begins during acute inflammation and may continue for as long as two years. The best outcome is **resolution,** the complete restoration of normal structure and function. This can happen if the damage was minor, there are no complications, and the tissues are capable of *regeneration* through the proliferation of the remaining cells. If resolution is not possible, then **repair** takes place with scarring being the end result. This happens if the wound is large, an abscess or granuloma has formed, or fibrin remains in the damaged tissues.

Both resolution and repair begin in the same way, with the *débridement,* or "cleaning up," of the site. Débridement involves phagocytosis of dead cells and debris and dissolution of fibrin cells (scabs). After débridement, there is a draining away of exudate, toxins, and particles from the site, and vascular dilation and permeability are reversed. At this point, either regeneration and resolution or repair and scar formation will take place. Minor wounds with little tissue loss, like paper cuts, close and heal easily, while more extensive wounds require more complex processes of sealing, filling, and contracting the wound.

VARIANCES IN IMMUNITY AND INFLAMMATION

Sometimes, the immune and inflammatory systems work "too well" and sometimes not well enough. Hypersensitivity reactions are an example of the former and immune deficiency diseases an example of the latter.

HYPERSENSITIVITY

Immune responses are normally protective and helpful. **Hypersensitivity,** however, is an exaggerated and harmful immune response. The word *hypersensitivity* is often used as a synonym for *allergy.* However, *hypersensitivity* is also used as an umbrella term for allergy and two other categories of harmful immune response, which are defined as follows:

Three Types of Hypersensitivity

1. **Allergy**—an exaggerated immune response to an environmental antigen, such as pollen or bee venom

* **resolution** the complete healing of a wound and return of tissues to their normal structure and function; the ending of inflammation with no scar formation.

* **repair** healing of a wound with scar formation.

* **hypersensitivity** an exaggerated and harmful immune response; an umbrella term for allergy, autoimmunity, and isoimmunity.

* **allergy** exaggerated immune response to an environmental antigen.

2. **Autoimmunity**—a disturbance in the body's normal tolerance for self-antigens, as in hyperthyroidism or rheumatic fever

3. **Isoimmunity** (also called *alloimmunity*)—an immune reaction between members of the same species, commonly of one person against the antigens of another person, as in the reaction of a mother to her infant's Rh negative factor or in transplant rejections

The exact cause of such pathological immune responses is not known, but at least three factors seem to be involved: (1) the original insult (exposure to the antigen); (2) the person's genetic makeup, which determines susceptibility to the insult; and (3) an immunological process that boosts the response beyond normal bounds.

Hypersensitivity reactions are classified as **immediate hypersensitivity reactions** or **delayed hypersensitivity reactions,** depending on how long it takes the secondary reaction to appear after reexposure to an antigen. The swiftest immediate hypersensitivity reaction is *anaphylaxis,* a severe allergic response that usually develops within minutes of reexposure. (Review anaphylactic shock earlier in this chapter. Also see Chapter 31, "Allergies and Anaphylaxis.")

Mechanisms of Hypersensitivity

Usually, when a hypersensitivity reaction takes place, inflammation is triggered and results in destruction of healthy tissues. Four mechanisms, or types, of hypersensitivity that cause this destructive reaction have been identified.

Mechanisms of Hypersensitivity Reaction

- Type I—IgE-mediated allergen reactions
- Type II—tissue-specific reactions
- Type III—immune-complex-mediated reactions
- Type IV—cell-mediated reactions

In reality, hypersensitivity reactions are not so easy to categorize. Most involve more than one type of mechanism.

Type I—IgE Reactions IgE is the immunoglobulin most involved in allergic reactions. The first exposure to the allergen (antigen that causes allergic reaction) stimulates B lymphocytes to produce IgE antibodies. These bind to receptors on mast cells in the tissues near blood vessels. On reexposure, the allergen binds to the IgE on the mast cell, which causes degranulation of the mast cell, release of histamine, and triggering of the inflammatory response.

Type II—Tissue-Specific Reactions Most tissues contain tissue-specific antigens, so called because they exist on the cells of only some body tissues. An immune response against one of these will affect only the organs or tissues that present that particular antigen.

Type III—Immune-Complex-Mediated Reactions These result from antigen-antibody complexes, or immune complexes, formed when an antibody meets and binds to a specific antigen. The immune complexes generally circulate for a time before being deposited in vessel walls or other tissues. For this reason, the organs that are affected may have very little connection with where or how the antigen or the immune complex originated.

Type IV—Cell-Mediated Tissue Reactions Types I, II, and III hypersensitivity reactions are mediated by an antibody. Type IV reactions are activated directly

✱ **autoimmunity** an immune response to self-antigens, which the body normally tolerates.

✱ **isoimmunity** an immune response to antigens from another member of the same species, for example, Rh reactions between a mother and her infant or in transplant rejections; also called *alloimmunity.*

✱ **immediate hypersensitivity reaction** a swiftly occurring secondary hypersensitivity reaction (one that occurs after reexposure to an antigen). Immediate hypersensitivity reactions are usually more severe than delayed reactions. The swiftest and most severe such reaction is anaphylaxis.

✱ **delayed hypersensitivity reaction** a hypersensitivity reaction that takes place after the elapse of some time following reexposure to an antigen. Delayed hypersensitivity reactions are usually less severe than immediate reactions.

Content Review

FOUR TYPES OF HYPERSENSITIVITY REACTIONS

Type I—IgE reactions
Type II—Tissue-specific reactions
Type III—Immune-complex-mediated reactions
Type IV—cell-mediated tissue reactions

by T cells and do not involve an antibody. There are two cell-mediated mechanisms. One involves Td cells, which produce lymphokine that activates other cells, such as macrophages. The other involves Tc cells that directly attack and destroy antigen-bearing cells and their toxins.

DEFICIENCIES IN IMMUNITY AND INFLAMMATION

Content Review

TWO TYPES OF IMMUNE DEFICIENCY

Congenital (inborn)
Acquired (after birth)

Immune deficiency disorders result from impaired function of some component of the immune system, including phagocytes, complement, and lymphocytes (T cells and B cells), with lymphocyte dysfunction being the primary cause. Immune deficiency can be congenital (inborn) or acquired (after birth). The most common manifestations of immune deficiency are recurrent infections because the body's ability to ward off invaders has been damaged.

Congenital Immune Deficiencies

Congenital, or primary, immune deficiency develops if the development of lymphocytes in the fetus or embryo is impaired or halted. Different immune-deficiency diseases may develop, depending on whether the T cells, the B cells, or both have been affected.

In the *DiGeorge syndrome,* there is a lack or partial lack of thymus development, resulting in a severe decrease in T cell production and function. *Bruton agammaglobulinemia* is caused by impaired development of B cell precursors, resulting in B cells that cannot produce IgM or IgD antibodies. In *bare lymphocyte syndrome,* lymphocytes and macrophages are unable to produce Class I or Class II HLA, which disrupts the ability of cells to recognize self- or nonself substances, resulting in severe infections that are usually fatal before age five.

Sometimes, there is a defect that depresses the function of just a small portion of the immune system. For example, in *Wiskott-Aldrich syndrome,* IgM antibody production is reduced. *Selective IgA deficiency* is the most common immune deficiency. IgA is the antibody present in mucous membranes. People with IgA deficiency frequently suffer from sinus, lung, and gastrointestinal infections.

Some immune system deficiencies cause a decreased ability to respond to one particular antigen. For example, in *chronic mucocutaneous candidiasis,* the T lymphocytes are unable to resist candida infections.

Acquired Immune Deficiencies

Acquired, or secondary, immune deficiencies develop after birth and do not result from genetic factors. They can be caused by or associated with pregnancy, infections, and diseases, such as diabetes or cirrhosis. The elderly are more prone to acquired immune deficiencies than the young. Among the factors that can severely affect immune function are nutritional deficiencies, medical treatment, trauma, and stress. Of special interest is the fatal acquired immune disorder, AIDS.

Nutritional Deficiencies Critical deficits in calorie or protein ingestion can lead to depression of T cell production and function. Complement activity, neutrophil chemotaxis, and the ability of neutrophils to kill bacteria are also seriously affected by starvation. Zinc deficiencies and vitamin deficiencies can affect both B cell and T cell functions.

Iatrogenic Deficiencies Iatrogenic deficiencies are those that are caused by medical treatment. Some drugs depress blood cell formation in the bone marrow. Others trigger immune responses that destroy granulocytes. Immunosuppressive drugs administered in the treatment for transplants, cancer, or autoimmune diseases suppress B and T cell functions and antibody production. Radiation treatment for cancer exacerbates this effect. Surgery and anesthesia also can suppress B and T cell functions, with severely depressed white cell levels persisting for several weeks after surgery. Surgical removal of the spleen depresses humor response against encapsulated bacteria, depresses IgM levels, and decreases the levels of opsonins.

Deficiencies Caused by Trauma Burn victims are especially susceptible to bacterial infection. Not only has the normal barrier presented by the skin been disrupted, but thermal burns also appear to decrease neutrophil function, complement levels, and other immune functions while increasing immunosuppressive functions, which further depress immune function.

Deficiencies Caused by Stress It has long been suggested that persons undergoing emotional stress (major stresses, such as divorce, but also minor stresses, such as studying for final exams) are more prone to illness. The speculation was that stress has deleterious effects on immune function. Research into the possible mechanisms of stress-induced immune deficiency are just getting underway. (Stress and susceptibility to disease will be discussed later in the chapter.)

AIDS AIDS is an acronym for *acquired immune deficiency syndrome,* which has become the best known acquired immune deficiency disorder. AIDS is a syndrome of disorders that develop from infection with **HIV,** the *human immunodeficiency virus.*

HIV is a retrovirus; that is, it carries its genetic information in RNA rather than DNA molecules. As a retrovirus, HIV infects target cells by binding to receptors on their surfaces, then inserting the HIV RNA into the cell. There, the RNA is converted into DNA and becomes part of the infected cell's genetic material. HIV can remain dormant inside the host cell for years; however, once the cell is activated (and the mechanism by which this occurs is not fully understood), HIV proliferates, kills the host cell, and can then infect other cells. The result is a pervasive breakdown of the immune defences, making the body vulnerable to a wide variety of infections and disorders.

HIV can infect anybody, male or female, homosexual or heterosexual, mostly through the exchange of body fluids during sexual intercourse or through injection. In North America, most cases, to date, have involved homosexual men and intravenous drug users. However, preventive measures (safe sex practices, including use of condoms, and clean-needle programs) have reduced the incidence of HIV/AIDS among homosexual populations and drug users. An increasing proportion of new patients are females who have acquired the infection during heterosexual intercourse. In other parts of the world, HIV/AIDS occurs equally among men and women.

The possibility of acquiring HIV/AIDS by contact with patients or accidental needle sticks fostered something of a panic among health-care workers when AIDS first spread so alarmingly across North America during the 1970s. Universal precautions (body substance isolation practices) have been widely adopted—including the use of disposable gloves, protective eyewear, masks, and gowns, as appropriate, to avoid contact with any body fluids, along with improved techniques for handling needles and other sharps. These measures have proven effective in reducing the fear of HIV/AIDS infection and also in making such infections very rare among health-care workers.

Until recently, the vast majority of those with AIDS died within five years of the development of severe symptoms. This picture has improved somewhat in the developed nations with the initiation of treatments involving multiple chemotherapies (treatment "cocktails") that have shown success in prolonging

✱ **AIDS** *acquired immune deficiency syndrome,* a group of signs, symptoms, and disorders that often develop as a consequence of HIV infection.

✱ **HIV** *human immunodeficiency virus,* a virus that breaks down the immune defences, making the body vulnerable to a variety of infections and disorders.

Universal precautions, including body substance isolation practices, have been effective in relieving fears of HIV/AIDS infection and in making such infections very rare among health-care workers.

life, greatly improving feelings of health and well-being, and suppressing measurable blood levels of HIV.

It is not yet known if such treatments can eradicate HIV and cure AIDS. One fear is that the treatments suppress but do not totally destroy the HIV virus, which "hides" somewhere in the body, waiting to proliferate at some later date. Another fear is that HIV will develop strains that are resistant to the treatments that appear to be successful in the short term. Nevertheless, the success of these treatments has caused the first feelings of optimism since AIDS was identified. Preventive measures have also helped greatly reduce the number of new cases reported in North America. In some parts of the world, however, including Africa and Asia, HIV/AIDS is still spreading at an extremely alarming rate, with seriously inadequate reporting, prevention, and treatment.

Replacement Therapies for Immune Deficiencies

Advances have been made in the treatment of immune deficiencies through the use of replacement therapies, such as those listed below.

Replacement Therapies

- *Gamma globulin therapy*—Gamma globulin is administered to individuals with B cell deficiencies that cause immunoglobulin (antibody) deficiencies.

- *Transplantation and transfusion*—HLA-matched bone marrow is transplanted into patients suffering *severe combined immune deficiencies (SCID),* which is caused by a lack of the stem cells from which T cells and B cells develop. In patients who lack a thymus or have a defective thymus, fetal thymus tissue may be transplanted. Enzyme deficiencies that cause SCID have been treated with transfusions of red blood cells that contain the needed enzyme. Other substances have been transfused into individuals to help restore T cell function and reactivity against certain antigens.

- *Gene therapy*—Therapies involving identification of defective genes that are responsible for immune disorders, and replacement of these defective genes with cloned normal genes, are in the early stages of development and use.

STRESS AND DISEASE

Stress is a word that is used a lot in modern life. You might have a stressful job, feel stressed out by too many demands on your job, or be going through a lot of emotional stress in connection with a personal relationship. In some situations, you may be acutely aware of some of the physiological components of stress, for example, sweaty palms and a pounding heart just before you have to get up and give a speech. If so, you already have a basic understanding of stress that can help you grasp the physiological and medical concepts of stress and how stress is related to disease.

CONCEPTS OF STRESS

Mind and body interact. There is a cause-and-effect relationship between stress and disease.

Today, it is commonly understood that mind and body interact. It was not always so. In fact, the concept that psychological states influence physiological states—and particularly that there is a cause-effect relationship between stress and disease—dates primarily from the work of Hans Selye, an Austrian-born Canadian physician and educator, in the 1940s.

General Adaptation Syndrome

Selye was not studying stress when he made his discovery. Instead, he was trying to identify a new sex hormone. He was injecting ovarian extracts into laboratory rats when he discovered the following triad of physiological effects:

Triad of Stress Effects

- Enlargement of the cortex (outer portion) of the adrenal gland
- Atrophy of the thymus gland and other lymphatic structures
- Development of bleeding ulcers of the stomach and duodenum

Selye soon discovered that this triad of effects was not a response only to the ovarian extracts. The same effects occurred when he subjected the rats to other stimuli, such as cold, surgical injury, and restraint. He concluded that the triad of effects was not specific to any particular stimulus but composed a nonspecific response to any noxious stimulus, or stressor. (**Stress** is generally defined as a state of physical or psychological arousal to a stimulus. Selye originally intended to use the word *stress* for the stimulus, or cause, but through a mistranslation of his work, *stress* came to mean the arousal, or effect. Selye then coined the word **stressor** for the stimulus/cause.)

Because the same responses occurred to a wide array of stimuli, Selye named it the **general adaptation syndrome (GAS).** Later, he identified three stages in the development of GAS:

Stages of GAS

- *Stage I, Alarm*—The sympathetic nervous system is aroused and mobilized in the "fight or flight" response syndrome. Pupils dilate, heart rate increases, and bronchial passages dilate. In addition, blood glucose levels rise, digestion slows, blood pressure rises, and the flow of blood to the skeletal muscles increases. At the same time, the endocrine system is aroused, resulting in secretion by the pituitary and adrenal glands of hormones that enhance the body's readiness to meet the challenge.

- *Stage II, Resistance, or Adaptation*—The person begins to cope with the situation. Sympathetic nervous system responses and circulating hormones return to normal. In most situations, this is the last stage; the stress is resolved. If the stress is very severe or prolonged, however, stress is not resolved, and stage III occurs.

- *Stage III, Exhaustion*—This is the stage sometimes known as "burnout." During this stage, the triad of physiological effects described by Selye occurs. The person can no longer cope with or resolve the stress, and physical illness may ensue.

The stages of GAS begin with **physiological stress,** defined by Selye as a chemical or physical disturbance in the cells or tissue fluid produced by a change, either in the external environment or within the body itself, that requires a response to counteract the disturbance. Selye identified three components of physiological stress: (1) the stressor that initiates the disturbance, (2) the chemical or physical disturbance the stressor produces, and (3) the body's counteracting (adaptational) response.

Psychological Mediators and Specificity

Since Selye defined GAS, others who have studied adaption to stress have refined the concept. For example, more attention has been paid to the psychological

---

* **stress** a state of physical or psychological arousal to stimulus.

* **stressor** the stimulus or cause of stress.

* **general adaptation syndrome (GAS)** a sequence of stress response stages: stage I, alarm; stage II, resistance or adaptation; stage III, exhaustion.

Content Review

GENERAL ADAPTATION SYNDROME (GAS)

Stage I—Alarm
Stage II—Resistance, or adaptation
Stage III—Exhaustion

* **physiological stress** a chemical or physical disturbance in the cells or tissue fluid produced by a change in the external environment or within the body.

mediators of stress. Experiments have shown that there is no direct correlation between stressor and response. People react differently to the same stressor. One person may take in stride the same situation that greatly upsets another person, and the degree of physiological response may be governed more by the psychological, emotional, or social response to the stressor than to the stressor itself. In particular, research has demonstrated pituitary gland and adrenal cortex sensitivity to emotional/psychological/social influences.

Another way in which recent research has diverged from Selye's original hypotheses concerns specificity. Selye postulated that the triad of physiological responses he identified was nonspecific; it was the same for any stressor. It is now thought that although the triad of responses he identified may occur in response to a wide variety of stressors, the total body response to different stressors must be specific, that is, targeted toward correction of the specific disturbance. For example, the body reacts to cold by shivering and to heat through vasodilation and sweating.

Homeostasis as a Dynamic Steady State

An older definition of homeostasis states that the body maintains itself at a "constant" composition. More recently, homeostasis has been described as a **dynamic steady state.** This takes into account the concept of **turnover,** the continual synthesis and breakdown of all body substances (e.g., fats, proteins). Thus, the internal environment of the body is always changing, not constant, but the net effect of all the changes is the dynamic (always changing), yet steady (tending always toward normal balance) state.

Stressors cause a series of reactions that alter the dynamic steady state. Usually, there is a return to normal, which may be rapid or slow. If a disturbance in the dynamic steady state, for example, a high blood glucose level, is prolonged and a causative stressor is no longer present, it is considered a sign of disease.

STRESS RESPONSES

Alteration of the immune system is the ultimate outcome of a stress response that resists quick and successful adaption. The interactions of psychological, neurological, endocrinological, and immunological factors that lead to this outcome are known as **psychoneuroimmunological regulation.**

The **stress response** is initiated by a stressor. The input of the stressor into the central nervous system, as mediated by the person's psychological response, leads to production of corticotropin-releasing factor (CRF) from the hypothalamus, which, in turn, stimulates responses by the sympathetic nervous system and the endocrine system (neuroendocrine regulation), which then affect the immune system. This chain of events is outlined in Figure 13-9 and described in the next sections.

Neuroendocrine Regulation

As mentioned above, when a person encounters a stressor and has a psychological response to the stressor, the sympathetic nervous system is stimulated by *corticotropin-releasing factor (CRF).* In turn, this stimulates the release of catecholamines, cortisol, and other hormones.

Catecholamines Sympathetic nervous system stimulation results in the release of norepinephrine (noradrenalin), and epinephrine (adrenalin), which constitute the category of hormones called *catecholamines.* The nerves of the sympathetic nervous system exit the spine at the thoracic and lumbar levels, and norepineph-

---

✱ dynamic steady state homeostasis; the tendency of the body to maintain a net constant composition, although the components of the body's internal environment are always changing.

✱ turnover the continual synthesis and breakdown of body substances that results in the dynamic steady state.

✱ psychoneuroimmunological regulation the interactions of psychological, neurological, endocrinological, and immunological factors that contribute to alteration of the immune system as an outcome of a stress response that is not quickly resolved.

✱ stress response changes within the body initiated by a stressor.

Content Review

HORMONES PRODUCED IN RESPONSE TO STRESS

Catecholamines
(norepinephrine and
epinephrine)
Cortisol
Beta endorphins
Growth hormone
Prolactin

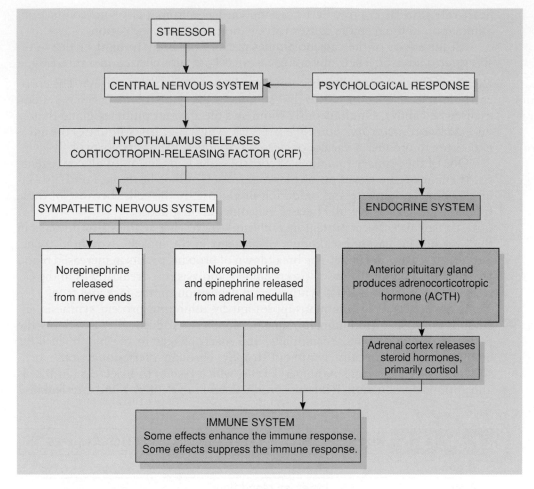

FIGURE 13-9   The stress response: effects on the sympathetic nervous, endocrine, and immune systems.

rine is released into the synaptic spaces (the spaces between the presynaptic ganglia and the postsynaptic nerves).

Additionally, sympathetic nervous system stimulation results in direct stimulation of the adrenal medulla, the inner portion of the adrenal gland. The adrenal medulla, in turn, releases the norepinephrine and epinephrine into the circulatory system. Approximately 80 percent of the hormones released by the adrenal medulla are epinephrine, while norepinephrine constitutes the remaining 20 percent. Once released, these hormones are carried throughout the body, where their effects (preparing the body to deal with stressful situations) act on hormone receptors.

Both epinephrine and norepinephrine interact with specialized adrenergic receptors on the membranes of target organs. These receptors are located throughout the body. Once stimulated by the appropriate hormone, they cause a response in the organ or organs they control.

The adrenergic receptors are generally divided into four types, designated alpha 1 (α_1), alpha 2 (α_2), beta 1 (β_1), and beta 2 (β_2). The α_1 receptors cause peripheral vasoconstriction, mild bronchoconstriction, and stimulation of metabolism. The α_2 receptors are found on the presynaptic surfaces of sympathetic neuroeffector junctions. Stimulation of α_2 receptors is inhibitory. These receptors serve to prevent overrelease of norepinephrine in the synapse. When the level of norepinephrine in the synapse gets high enough, the α_2 receptors are stimulated and norepinephrine release is inhibited. Stimulation of β_1 receptors causes increases in heart rate, cardiac contractile force, and cardiac automaticity and conduction. Stimulation of β_2 receptors causes vasodilation and bronchodilation.

All the effects of the catecholamines prepare the body to fight or flee in response to a stressor. Their physiological effects are summarized in Table 13-4.

Cortisol Cortisol is another hormone produced in response to stress. The corticotropin-releasing factor (CRF) that stimulates the sympathetic nervous system, as discussed above, simultaneously stimulates the anterior pituitary gland to produce *adrenocorticotropic hormone (ACTH)*, which, in turn, stimulates the adrenal cortex to produce a variety of steroid hormones, primarily cortisol.

One of the primary functions of cortisol is the stimulation of gluconeogenesis. It enhances the elevation of blood glucose by other hormones and also inhibits peripheral uptake and oxidation of glucose by the cells. Because of these functions, it has the overall effect of elevating blood glucose.

Cortisol also affects protein metabolism—increasing synthesis of proteins in the liver but increasing breakdown of proteins in the muscle, lymphoid tissue, fatty tissues, skin, and bone. The breakdown of proteins results in increased blood levels of amino acids. Cortisol also promotes lipolysis (fat breakdown) in the extremities and lipogenesis (fat synthesis and deposition) in the face and trunk.

Cortisol acts as an immunosuppressant by inhibiting protein synthesis, including synthesis of immunoglobulins (antibodies). Additionally, it reduces the numbers of lymphocytes, eosinophils, and macrophages in the blood. In large amounts, cortisol can cause lymphoid atrophy. Through a series of actions, cortisol diminishes the actions of helper T cells, which results in a decrease in B cells and antibody production. It inhibits production of interleukin-1 and interleukin-2

✱ **cortisol** a steroid hormone released by the adrenal cortex that regulates the metabolism of fats, carbohydrates, sodium, potassium, and proteins and also has an anti-inflammatory effect.

Table 13-4 PHYSIOLOGICAL EFFECTS OF CATECHOLAMINES

Organ	Effects
Brain	Increased blood flow
	Increased glucose metabolism
Cardiovascular system	Increased contractile force and rate
	Peripheral vasoconstriction
Pulmonary system	Increased ventilation
	Bronchodilation
	Increased oxygen supply
Liver	Increased glucose production
	Increased gluconeogenesis
	Increased glycogenolysis
	Decreased glycogen synthesis
Gastrointestinal and genitourinary tracts	Decreased protein synthesis
Muscle	Increased glycogenolysis
	Increased contraction
	Increased dilation of skeletal muscle vasculature
Skeleton	Decreased glucose uptake and utilization (insulin release decreased)
Adipose (fatty) tissue	Increased lipolysis
	Increased fatty acids and glycerol
Skin	Decreased blood flow
Lymphoid tissue	Increased protein breakdown (shrinkage of lymphoid tissue)

and, consequently, blocks cell-mediated immunity and generation of fever. It inhibits the accumulation of leukocytes at the site of inflammation and inhibits release of substances that are critical in the inflammatory response, including kinins, prostaglandins, and histamine. Cortisol also inhibits fibroblast proliferation during an inflammatory response, which, in turn, causes poor wound healing and increased susceptibility to wound infection.

In the gastrointestinal tract, cortisol increases gastric secretions, occasionally enough to cause ulcer formation. Cortisol also suppresses the release of sex hormones, including testosterone and estradiol.

The immunosuppressive actions of cortisol seem clearly harmful, and yet its production in response to stress indicates that it is beneficial in protecting against stress. Its beneficial effects in stress, however, are not well understood. It has been suggested that its promotion of gluconeogenesis helps ensure an adequate source of glucose as energy for body tissues, especially nerve tissues. Pooled amino acids from protein breakdown may promote protein synthesis in some cells. Its depressive influence on inflammatory responses may play a role in decreasing peripheral blood flow and redirecting blood to critical organs or sites of injury. Suppression of immune function may also help prevent tissue damage that results from prolonged immune responses.

Cortisol—produced in response to stress—has harmful immunosuppressive actions and yet seems to have a little-understood beneficial effect in protecting against stress.

Role of the Immune System

During a stress response, as noted earlier, there is a complex interaction among the nervous and endocrine systems and the immune system. As a consequence, a variety of immune-related disorders are associated with stress.

The specific mechanisms by which stress leads to immune-related disorders is the subject of ongoing research but is not yet well understood. However, research points to the substances that serve as communicators between the cells of the nervous system, the endocrine system, and the immune system—including hormones, neurotransmitters, neuropeptides, and cytokines—as the pathways of cause and effect.

The pathway is not a straight line. The directional arrows of cause and effect move forward, backward, and in circles. Many components of the immune system can be affected by the factors produced by the neuroendocrine system. Conversely, immune system products can affect components of the neuroendocrine system. Here are two examples:

- *Pathway 1: central nervous system to immune system*—The central nervous system *stimulates* the hypothalamus to produce CRF → which *stimulates* the pituitary gland to produce ACTH → which *stimulates* the adrenal gland to secrete cortisol → which *suppresses* the development of macrophages, T cells, B cells, and natural killer (NK) cells, a lymphocyte specially adapted to recognize and kill virally infected cells and malignant cells.

- *Pathway 2: immune system to central nervous system*—During immune system response, macrophages secrete cytokines → which stimulate the hypothalamus to secrete CRF (which begins Pathway 1 again).

The above are only two examples of the many pathways and interactions that take place among the nervous, endocrine, and immune systems.

The suppression of immune system function that is caused by stress-related products of the sympathetic nervous and endocrine systems—especially catecholamines and cortisol—has been linked to a number of immune-mediated diseases, as listed in Table 13-5.

Table 13-5 STRESS- AND IMMUNE-RELATED DISEASES AND CONDITIONS

Target Organ	Diseases and Conditions
Cardiovascular system	Coronary artery disease Hypertension Stroke Dysrhythmias
Muscles	Tension headaches Muscle-related backaches
Connective tissues	Rheumatoid arthritis
Pulmonary system	Asthma Hay fever
Immune system	Immunosuppression or immune deficiency
Gastrointestinal system	Ulcer Irritable bowel syndrome Ulcerative colitis
Genitourinary system	Diuresis Impotence
Skin	Eczema Acne
Endocrine system	Diabetes mellitus
Central nervous system	Fatigue Depression Insomnia

STRESS, COPING, AND ILLNESS INTERRELATIONSHIPS

Research has shown that the ability to cope with stress has significant effects on associated illnesses. Those who cope positively with stress have a reduced chance of becoming ill in the first place and a better chance of getting better or getting better faster if they do become ill. Conversely, those who don't cope as well with stress have a greater chance of becoming ill, prolonging the course of illness, or of not surviving an illness.

Physiological stress is caused by events that directly affect the body, such as a burn, extreme cold, or starvation. *Psychological stress* consists of the unpleasant emotions caused by life events, such as taking exams or getting a divorce. The effects that these stresses will have on the body depend on the individual's ability to cope with them. Some people are "thrown" by events others would perceive as relatively minor, such as a traffic jam or a sprained ankle. Others can take in stride events that others would find very difficult, such as loss of a job or a long-term disability.

The effects of stress, including the degree to which stress causes or affects illness, are moderated by the type, duration, and severity of the stressor in combination with the individual's perception and ability to cope with it. Stressors that are the most likely to have a negative effect on immunity and disease have been characterized as those that are not only undesirable but also are uncontrollable and that overtax the person's ability to cope.

Effective and ineffective coping have been seen to have potentially different effects in healthy persons, symptomatic persons (those who already have some manifestations of disease), and persons who are undergoing medical treatment.

Potential Effects of Stress Based on Effectiveness of Coping

- *In a healthy person:*
  Effective coping → Transient effects, return to normal function
  Ineffective coping → Significant stress effects, illness

- *In a symptomatic person:*
  Effective coping → Little or no effect on symptoms
  Ineffective coping → Exacerbation of symptoms, illness

- *In a person undergoing medical treatment:*
  Effective coping → Person does not perceive the treatment itself as stressful → Treatment is more likely to have a positive effect on symptoms and the course of illness

  Ineffective coping → Person perceives the treatment itself as stressful → Treatment is more likely to have a negative effect on symptoms and the course of illness

Because of the importance of coping ability in the interplay between stress and illness, attention is increasingly being paid to providing counselling and support systems—including family members, friends, and other support networks—to assist persons who are ill or in stressful life situations. There is recognition that supporting the patient's ability to cope is a critical adjunct to medical treatment itself.

SUMMARY

Pathophysiology is the study of how disease and injury alter normal physiology (body processes). The cell is the basic unit of life. Cells exist in an environment of fluids and electrolytes. When something interferes with normal cell function, the normal cell environment, or normal cell intercommunication, disease can begin or advance.

Cells can be injured in a variety of ways, including hypoxia, chemicals, infectious agents, immunological/inflammatory injuries, and others. Diseases can be caused by genetic factors, environmental factors, or a combination of factors (multifactorial diseases).

The body responds to cellular injury in a variety of ways to restore homeostasis, the body's normal dynamic steady state. Cells can adapt through atrophy, hypertrophy, hyperplasia, metaplasia, and dysplasia. Negative feedback mechanisms work to correct, or compensate for, shock—if shock has not progressed too far.

Perfusion of the tissues is necessary to provide essential nutrients to the cells (especially oxygen and glucose) and to remove wastes. Inadequate perfusion, called hypoperfusion or shock, can be caused by a problem in any of the three parts of the cardiovascular system (the heart, the blood vessels, or the blood), sometimes abetted by problems in the respiratory or gastrointestinal system in which the normal intake and transfer of oxygen and glucose may be interrupted. If not corrected, shock continues in a downward spiral toward irreversible shock, possible multiple organ dysfunction syndrome (MODS), and death.

The body's chief means of self-defence is the immune system and the immune and inflammatory responses, which work to attack and destroy infectious agents and other unwanted invaders. Occasionally, the immune response system works "too well," as in hypersensitivity reactions, or not well enough, as in immune deficiency disorders. Stress can also contribute to disease through the interactions of the nervous, endocrine, and immune systems.

CHAPTER 14

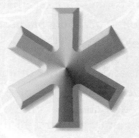

General Principles of Pharmacology

Objectives

Part 1: Basic Pharmacology (begins on p. 690)
After reading Part 1 of this chapter, you should be able to:

1. Describe important historical trends in pharmacology. (p. 690)
2. Differentiate among the chemical, generic (nonproprietary), and trade (proprietary) names of a drug. (pp. 690–691)
3. List the four main sources of drug products. (p. 691)
4. List the authoritative sources for drug information. (pp. 691–692)
5. List legislative acts controlling drug use and abuse in Canada. (pp. 692–694)
6. Differentiate among the schedules of controlled drugs and list examples of substances in each schedule. (p. 693)
7. Discuss standardization of drugs. (p. 694)
8. Discuss the paramedic's responsibilities and scope of management pertinent to the administration of medications. (pp. 694–696)
9. Discuss special considerations in drug treatment with regard to pregnant, pediatric, and geriatric patients. (pp. 696–697)
10. Review the specific anatomy and physiology pertinent to pharmacology. (pp. 698–710)
11. List and describe liquid and solid drug forms. (p. 704)
12. List and describe general properties of drugs. (pp. 705–707)
13. List and differentiate routes of drug administration. (pp. 702–704)
14. Differentiate between enteral and parenteral routes of drug administration. (pp. 703–704)
15. Describe mechanisms of drug action. (pp. 705–707)

Continued

16. List and differentiate the phases of drug activity, including the pharmaceutical, pharmacokinetic, and pharmacodynamic phases. (pp. 698–710)

17. Describe the processes called pharmacokinetics, pharmacodynamics, including theories of drug action, drug-response relationships, factors altering drug responses, predictable drug responses, iatrogenic drug responses, and unpredictable adverse drug responses. (pp. 698–710)

18. Differentiate among drug interactions. (pp. 709–710)

19. Discuss considerations for storing and securing medications. (p. 704)

20. List the components of a drug profile by classification. (p. 692)

Part 2: Drug Classifications (begins on p. 710)

After reading Part 2 of this chapter, you should be able to:

1. Describe how drugs are classified. (pp. 710–711)

2. Review the specific anatomy and physiology pertinent to pharmacology with additional attention to autonomic pharmacology. (pp. 711–760)

3. List and describe common prehospital medications, including indications, contraindications, side effects, routes of administration, and dosages. (pp. 711–760)

4. Given several patient scenarios, identify medications likely to be prescribed and those that are likely part of the prehospital treatment regimen. (pp. 711–760)

5. Given various patient medications, assess the pathophysiology of a patient's condition by identifying classifications of drugs. (pp. 710–760)

INTRODUCTION

The use of herbs and minerals to treat the sick and injured has been documented as long ago as 2000 B.C.E. Ancient Egyptians, Arabs, and Greeks probably passed formulations down through generations by word of mouth for centuries until they were finally recorded in pharmacopeias. By the end of the Renaissance, pharmacology was a distinct and growing discipline, separate from medicine. During the seventeenth and eighteenth centuries, tinctures of opium, coca, and digitalis were available. The related concept of vaccination with biological extracts began in 1796 with Edward Jenner's smallpox inoculations. By the nineteenth century, atropine, chloroform, codeine, ether, and morphine were in use. The discoveries of animal insulin and penicillin in the early twentieth century dramatically changed the treatment of endocrine/metabolic and infectious diseases. Now, at the start of the twenty-first century, recombinant DNA technology has produced human insulin and tissue plasminogen activator (tPA). These drugs have markedly changed the treatment of diabetes and cardiovascular disease.

Presently in Canada, Health Canada is allowing many previously prescription-only drugs to be available over the counter. This is due, in part, to a growing consumer awareness of health care and to consumer marketing by the pharmaceutical industry. The industry is actively seeking drugs that appeal widely to the consumer for treatments and cures. Pharmaceutical research to limit aging or increase the life span is growing rapidly. The federal government also offers incentives to pharmaceutical companies to research drugs for rare diseases. These so-called "orphan drugs" are often expensive to investigate and have a limited sales potential, making them less profitable to develop and manufacture than others.

General principles of pharmacology are presented in this chapter, which is divided into two parts:

Part 1: Basic Pharmacology
Part 2: Drug Classifications

Part 1: Basic Pharmacology

Part 1 concerns the basics of pharmacology. Drug names (including chemical, generic, and brand names) will be explained. The sources of drugs, reference materials for drugs, components of a drug profile, and legal considerations will be described. A major focus of Part 1 will be the safe and effective administration of medications, including the "six rights" (right medication, dose, time, route, patient, and documentation) as well as special considerations in medication administration for pregnant, pediatric, and geriatric patients. Finally, basic concepts of pharmacology, specifically pharmacokinetics and pharmacodynamics, will be examined.

NAMES

Drugs are chemicals used to diagnose, treat, or prevent disease. **Pharmacology** is the study of drugs and their actions on the body. To study and converse about pharmacology, health-care professionals must have a systematic method for naming drugs. The most detailed name for any drug is its chemical description, which states its chemical composition and molecular structure. Ethyl-1-methyl-

4-phenylisonipecotate hydrochloride, for example, is a chemical name. A generic name is usually suggested by the manufacturer. In the case of ethyl-1-methyl-4-phenylisonipecotate hydrochloride, the generic name is meperidine hydrochloride. To foster brand loyalty among its customers, the manufacturer gives the drug a brand name (sometimes called a trade name or proprietary name)—in our example, Demerol. The brand name is a proper name and should be capitalized. Most manufacturers also register the name as a trademark, so the stylized ® or ™ may follow the name, as in Demerol®. Another example is the widely prescribed sedative Valium:

- *Chemical Name:* 7-chloro-1, 3-dihydro-1-methyl-5-phenyl-2H-1, 4-benzodiazepin-2-one
- *Generic Name:* diazepam
- *Brand Name:* Valium®

Content Review

DRUG NAMES

- Chemical name
- Generic name
- Brand name

SOURCES

The four main sources of drugs are plants, animals, minerals, and the laboratory (synthetic). Plants may be the oldest source of medications; primitive people probably used them directly as "herbal" medicines. Indirectly, plant extracts, such as gums and oils, have long been a source of medications. Examples include the purple foxglove, a source of digitalis (a glycoside), and the deadly nightshade, a source of atropine (an alkaloid). Animal extracts are another important source of drugs. For many years the primary sources of insulin for treating diabetes mellitus were the extracts of bovine (cow) and porcine (pig) pancreas. Minerals are inorganic sources of drugs such as calcium chloride and magnesium sulphate. Synthetic drugs are created in the laboratory. They may provide alternative sources of medications for those found in nature, or they may be entirely new medications not found in nature.

REFERENCE MATERIALS

Obtaining information on drugs can be difficult. Using multiple sources of information about drugs is usually a good idea. Every book about drugs, including this one, has a disclaimer regarding doses and current uses, referring the reader to local medical direction for the final word. Using multiple sources and comparing the authors' statements about a drug may lead you to the best available information. EMS providers generally like small, short guides that they can carry in a shirt pocket. These usually include important details about drugs that prehospital providers administer along with a long list of commonly prescribed drugs and their classes. These EMS guides will be useful if you clearly understand the drugs used in your system and have a working knowledge of commonly prescribed drug classes.

Drug inserts, the printed fact sheets that drug manufacturers supply with most medications contain information required by Health Canada. The *Compendium of Pharmaceuticals and Specialties* (CPS), published by the Canadian Pharmacists Association, is a comprehensive guide, with information on product monographs, generic and brand names, product identification photographs, therapeutic classification, and clinical information. Another popular source of information is the American *Physician's Desk Reference*. Most hospitals have extensive resources on medications. Health Canada, through the Therapeutic Products Directorate, maintains an online Drug Product Database. Several smaller, pocket-sized drug references are available, designed for nurses and paramedics.

Content Review

SOURCES OF DRUG INFORMATION

- *Compendium of Pharmaceuticals and Specialties (CPS)*
- *Health Canada Drug Product Database*
- *Physician's Desk Reference*
- *Drug Information*

It is helpful to carry a pharmaceutical reference in paramedic response vehicles.

Recently, drug information databases have become available for handheld computers or personal digital assistants (PDAs).

COMPONENTS OF A DRUG PROFILE

A drug's profile describes its various properties. As a paramedic student, you will become familiar with drug profiles as you study specific medications. A typical drug profile will contain the following information:

- *Names.* These most frequently include the generic and trade names, although the occasional reference will include chemical names.
- *Classification.* This is the broad group to which the drug belongs. Knowing classifications is essential to understanding the properties of drugs.
- *Mechanism of action.* The way in which a drug causes its effects—its pharmacodynamics.
- *Indications.* Conditions that make administration of the drug appropriate (as approved by Health Canada).
- *Pharmacokinetics.* How the drug is absorbed, distributed, and eliminated; typically includes onset and duration of action.
- *Side effects/adverse reactions.* The drug's untoward or undesired effects.
- *Routes of administration.* How the drug is given.
- *Contraindications.* Conditions that make it inappropriate to give the drug. Unlike when the drug is simply not indicated, a contraindication means that a predictable harmful event will occur if the drug is given in this situation.
- *Dosage.* The amount of the drug that should be given.
- *How supplied.* This typically includes the common concentrations of the available preparations; many drugs come in different concentrations.
- *Special considerations.* How the drug may affect pediatric, geriatric, or pregnant patients.

Drug profiles may also include other components, such as its interactions with other drugs or with foods when appropriate.

Know and obey the laws and regulations governing medications and their administration.

Content Review

DRUG LAWS AND REGULATIONS
- Federal law
- Provincial and territorial laws and regulations
- Individual agency regulations

LEGAL

Knowing and obeying the laws and regulations governing medications and their administration will be an important part of your career. These laws and regulations come from three distinct authorities: federal law, provincial and territorial laws and regulations, and individual agency regulations.

Health Canada's Therapeutic Products Directorate regulates pharmaceutical drugs and medical devices. The Food and Drugs Act and Regulations require manufacturers to present scientific evidence of a product's safety, efficacy, and quality before Health Canada will grant market authorization.

The federal government strictly regulates controlled substances because of their high potential for abuse. Since not all drugs cause the same level of physical or psychological dependence, they do not all need to be regulated in the same way (Table 14-1). Most emergency medical services administer only a few controlled substances, usually a narcotic analgesic, such as morphine sulphate, and a benzodiazepine anticonvulsant, such as diazepam.

The majority of the remaining drugs provided by EMS are prescription drugs—those whose use the Therapeutic Products Directorate of Health Canada has designated sufficiently dangerous to require the supervision of a health-care practitioner (physician, dentist, and in some jurisdictions, nurse practitioner or certified physician's assistant). For emergency medical services, this means the physician medical director is in effect prescribing the drugs in advance, based on the assessments and judgments of EMS providers in the field.

Over-the-counter (OTC) medications are generally available in small doses and, when taken as recommended, present a low risk to patients. Of the few OTC drugs that EMS providers administer, acetaminophen and aspirin are probably the most common. Although laws vary across jurisdictions, they require most EMS providers to obtain a physician's order (either written, verbal, or standing) to administer OTC drugs.

Federal drug laws require that certain substances be appropriately secured, distributed, and accounted for. Because of the complexity of this issue and the

Table 14-1 — SCHEDULES OF CONTROLLED DRUGS

Category	Description	Examples
Narcotics Schedule	Stringently restricted drugs: The letter N must appear on all labels and professional advertisements.	**Coca leaf derivatives** • Cocaine **Opiates and opiate derivatives** • Morphine • Codeine • Methadone • Hydromorphone • Meperidine **Other drugs** • Phencyclidine • Cannabis
Schedule F	Prescription drugs: Although not controlled drugs, agents in this category include some with a relatively low abuse potential; the symbol Pr must appear on their labels.	**Anxiolytics** • Benzodiazepines
Schedule G	Controlled drugs: Prescriptions are controlled because of the abuse potential with these drugs.	**Narcotic analgesics** • Nalbuphine • Butorphanol **Stimulants** • Amphetamines **Barbiturates** • Phenobarbital • Amobarbital • Secobarbital
Schedule H	Restricted drugs: These are typically street drugs with no recognized medicinal properties.	**Hallucinogens** • Peyote • LSD • Mescaline
Nonprescription Drug Schedule (Group 3)	These drugs are available only in the pharmacy and are used only on the recommendation of a physician. They have limited access.	**Analgesics** • Low-dose codeine preparations **Other drugs** • Insulin • Nitroglycerine • Muscle relaxants

large variability of drugs used in EMS systems across the country, specific answers to these concerns are not practical here. Consult your local protocols, laws, and most importantly, medical director for guidance in this area.

Province and Territory Provincial and territorial laws vary widely. Some provinces and territories have legislated which medications are appropriate for paramedics to give, while others have left those decisions to local control. Local control varies as well. In some areas, regional EMS authorities set the local standards; in others, the individual medical directors and department directors do. In all cases, however, the physician medical director can delegate to paramedics the authority to administer medications, either by written, verbal, or standing order. You must know the laws of the province and territory in which you practise.

Local In each community, local leaders are responsible for ensuring public safety. Local EMS agencies have the responsibility to create local policies and procedures to ensure the public well-being. An excellent example of a local procedure protecting the patient (and thereby the individual EMS provider and agency) would be a requirement to use a pulse oximeter whenever a patient is sedated or paralyzed. Although this requirement would not have the force of law, it would locally help ensure that local EMS providers do not overlook hypoxia in these patients.

Standards Because some generic drugs affect patients differently from how their brand name counterparts do, standardization of drugs is a necessity. Despite federal standards, drugs sold or distributed by various manufacturers may have biological or therapeutic differences. An **assay** determines the amount and purity of a given chemical in a preparation in the laboratory (in vitro). Although, two generically equivalent preparations may contain the same amount of a given chemical (drug), they may have different therapeutic effects. This relative therapeutic effectiveness of chemically equivalent drugs is their **bioequivalence**. Bioequivalence is determined by a **bioassay**, which attempts to ascertain the drug's availability in a biological model (in vivo). Again, the *Compendium of Pharmaceuticals and Specialities* (USP) is the best standard in Canada.

* **assay** test that determines the amount and purity of a given chemical in a preparation in the laboratory.

* **bioequivalence** relative therapeutic effectiveness of chemically equivalent drugs.

* **bioassay** test to ascertain a drug's availability in a biological model.

PATIENT CARE: THE SAFE AND EFFECTIVE ADMINISTRATION OF MEDICATIONS

Paramedics are responsible for the standard of care for patients in their charge. They are, therefore, personally responsible—legally, morally, and ethically—for the safe and effective administration of medications. The following guidelines will help you meet that responsibility:

- Know the indications, and contraindications, and cautions for all medications you administer.
- Practise proper technique.
- Know how to observe and document drug effects.
- Maintain current knowledge of pharmacology.
- Establish and maintain professional relationships with other health-care providers.
- Understand pharmacokinetics and pharmacodynamics.
- Have current medication references available.
- Take careful drug histories including:
  - Name, strength, and daily dose of prescribed drugs
  - Over-the-counter drugs

- Vitamins
- Herbal medications
- Folk medicine or folk remedies
- Allergies
- Evaluate the compliance, dosage, and adverse reactions.
- Consult with medical direction when appropriate.

SIX RIGHTS OF MEDICATION ADMINISTRATION

No pharmacology chapter would be complete without discussing the six rights of medication administration. They include the right medication, the right dose, the right time, the right route, the right patient, and the right documentation.

Right Medication When following a physician's verbal medication order, repeat the order back to her to confirm that you both intend the same thing for the patient. Inspect the label on the drug at least three times before giving the medication to the patient: first, as you remove the medication from the drug box or cabinet; second, as you draw the medication into the syringe or dole the tablet into a cup; and third, immediately before you administer the medication. Failure to confirm the medication name is one of the most common medication administration errors. If you have any question about a drug, do not administer it without confirmation. Showing the medication container to your partner and asking for confirmation is an easy way to further ensure that you are giving the right drug.

Right Dose To reduce medication errors, many drugs come in unit **dose packaging**. That is, the package contains a single dose for a single patient. Dosages of many emergency drugs, however, are based on patient weight, and so a prefilled syringe may not contain the exact amount a patient needs. You will have to calculate the correct dose. One good practice for identifying potential medication errors is to consider the number of unit dose packages needed for a single dose. If your calculations tell you to open 10 vials for one dose of medication, prudence requires you to check the calculation and dose carefully. The package may contain a unit dose of the wrong medication, or you may have miscalculated.

Right Time Although paramedics usually give medications in urgent and emergent situations, rather than on a schedule, timing can still be very important. Giving nitroglycerine tablets too soon may precipitate hypotension; if epinephrine is not repeated on time during cardiac arrest, it may not help to lower the threshold for defibrillation. Note that some medications should be administered over a specific length of time. Take care to give medications punctually and to document their administration promptly.

Right Route You often will have to choose from among several treatments for a particular problem. In these cases, knowing the principles of pharmacokinetics can help greatly in giving your patient the medication via the right route. For example, you know that administering epinephrine intravenously is more effective than administering it subcutaneously to the patient in anaphylactic shock because her blood is being shunted away from the skin will guide you to the proper administration route.

Right Patient As the paramedic's role in health care expands, you will find yourself caring for more people than just "the patient in the back of the ambulance." You will deal with multiple patients, and the potential for giving medication to the wrong patient will be real. You will have to identify patients by name before administering medications.

Right Documentation The drugs you administer in the field do not stop affecting your patients when those patients enter the hospital. As a result, you must completely document all of your care, especially any drugs you have administered,

Content Review

SIX RIGHTS OF MEDICATION ADMINISTRATION
- Right medication
- Right dose
- Right time
- Right route
- Right patient
- Right documentation

✱ **dose packaging** medication packages contain a single dose for a single patient.

so that long after you have left for your next call, other providers will know what drugs your patient has had.

SPECIAL CONSIDERATIONS

Pregnant Patients Any time you administer drugs to a woman of childbearing years, you must consider the possibility that she is pregnant. Treating pregnant patients clearly means treating two patients. Although emphasis appropriately seems to centre on the mother during care, you must understand that many drugs that affect the mother also affect the fetus. A drug's possible benefits to the mother must clearly outweigh its potential risks to the fetus. For example, some situations, such as cardiac arrest, justify giving the mother medications that may harm the fetus because the drug's possible harm to the fetus is clearly outweighed by the fetus's certain death if the mother dies.

Pregnancy presents two particular pharmacological problems: changes in the mother's anatomy and physiology, and the potential for drugs to harm the fetus. Because the mother is supporting the fetus entirely, her heart rate, cardiac output, and blood volume will increase. This altered maternal physiology can affect the onset and duration of action of many medications. During the first trimester of pregnancy the ingestion of some drugs (**teratogenic drugs**) may potentially deform, injure, or kill the fetus. During the last trimester, drugs administered to the mother may pass through the placenta to the fetus. Some of these drugs will have unwanted effects on the fetus. Others may not be metabolized or excreted, possibly resulting in toxic accumulations. Additionally, a breast-feeding mother's milk may pass some drugs to her infant.

Under some conditions, of course, the health and safety of mother and fetus demand the use of drugs during pregnancy. Examples include pregnancy-induced diabetes, hypertension, and seizure disorders. To help health-care providers determine when drugs are needed during pregnancy, the American Food and Drug Administration (FDA) has developed the classification system shown in Table 14-2, which is also observed in Canada. Always consult medical direction for any questions about drug safety in pregnancy.

Pediatric Patients Several physiological factors affect pharmacokinetics in newborns and young children. These patients' absorption of oral medications is less than an adult's due to various differences in gastric pH, gastric emptying time, and low enzyme levels. A newborn's skin is thinner than is an older patient's and is therefore more permeable to topically administered drugs. This can result in unexpected toxicity. Older children still have less gastric acid than adults do, but their gastric emptying times reach an adult's around the sixth to eighth month of life. Because children up to a year old have diminished plasma protein concentrations, drugs that bind to proteins have higher **free drug availability.** That is, a greater proportion of the drug will be available in the body to cause either desired or undesired effects. Water distribution is different in the neonate as well. Neonates have a much higher proportion of extracellular fluid (nearly 80 percent) than adults (50 to 55 percent). This greater amount of water means a greater volume and, with less than expected protein binding, may require higher drug doses. The premature infant is especially susceptible to drugs penetrating the *blood-brain barrier* because her immature connective tissues form a weaker obstacle.

The newborn's metabolic rates may be much lower than an adult's, but they rise rapidly and by a few years of age may triple an adult's. These metabolic rates then decline steadily until early adolescence, when they reach adult levels. A newborn's low metabolic rates and incompletely developed hepatic system put her at higher risk for toxic interactions. Neonates' metabolic pathways also are different from an adult's, meaning that some drugs will not have the expected effect or may have other, unexpected effects. Finally, the neonatal renal

✱ **teratogenic drug** medication that may deform or kill the fetus.

Children are not "small adults." Drug dosages must consider the various physiological differences.

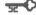

✱ **free drug availability** proportion of a drug available in the body to cause either desired or undesired effects.

Table 14-2	AMERICAN FDA PREGNANCY CATEGORIES
Category	**Description**
A	Adequate studies in pregnant women have not demonstrated a risk to the fetus in the first trimester or later trimesters.
B	Animal studies have not demonstrated a risk to the fetus, *but* there are no adequate studies in pregnant women. OR Adequate studies in pregnant women have not demonstrated a risk to the fetus in the first trimester and there is no risk in the last trimester, *but* animal studies have demonstrated adverse effects.
C	Animal studies have demonstrated adverse effects, *but* there are no adequate studies in pregnant women; however, benefits may be acceptable despite the potential risks. OR No adequate animal studies or adequate studies of pregnant women have been done.
D	Fetal risk has been demonstrated. In certain circumstances, benefits could outweigh the risks.
X	Fetal risk has been demonstrated. This risk outweighs any possible benefit to the mother. Avoid using in pregnant or potentially pregnant patients.

and hepatic systems' immaturity delays elimination of many drugs and their metabolites. Dosing schedules may have to be adjusted to accommodate longer half-lives until these systems mature at about six months to one year of age.

With all these factors, a pediatric patient's drug function can differ radically from an adult's. Pediatric drug dosages must be individualized to minimize the risks of toxicity. Body surface area and weight are the two most common factors in calculating dosages. The Broselow tape gives a good approximation for children of average height/weight ratio. It bases its calculations on the child's height (length), and assumes the child's weight is at the 50th percentile for her height (Figure 14-1). The Broselow tape primarily addresses drugs administered in the critical care setting.

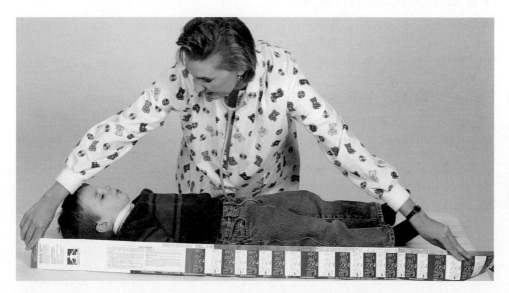

FIGURE 14-1   A Broselow tape is useful for calculating drug dosages for pediatric patients.

Geriatric Patients Significant changes in pharmacokinetics may also occur in patients older than about 60 years. They may absorb oral medications more slowly due to decreased gastrointestinal motility. Decreased plasma protein concentration may alter distribution of drugs in their systems, leaving free drugs that would otherwise have been protein bound. Body fat increases and muscle mass decreases with age; therefore, lipid soluble drugs may have greater deposition, thereby lowering the amount of available drug. Absorption and distribution of intramuscular injections may alter if volumes are inappropriate for the remaining muscle mass. Because the liver primarily handles biotransformation, depressed liver function in an aging patient may delay or prolong drug action. The aging process may also slow elimination by the renal system.

Older patients are also more likely to be on multiple medications or to have multiple underlying disease processes. Various medication interactions can have a severe impact on patients. For example, sildenafil (Viagra) and nitroglycerine given together may cause severe hypotension. Underlying diseases may affect therapeutics in unexpected ways. Congestive heart failure, for instance, may cause congestion of the gastrointestinal tract's vasculature, delaying the absorption of oral medications. The congestive heart failure patient may also have compromised renal function, delaying elimination of drugs.

> *Use caution when administering medications to older patients because they are apt to be on multiple medications.*
>
>

PHARMACOLOGY

Pharmacology is the study of drugs and their interactions with the body. Drugs do not confer any new properties on cells or tissues; they only modify or exploit existing functions. Drugs may be given for their local action (in which case systemic absorption of the drug is discouraged) or for systemic action. Although generally given for a specific effect, drugs tend to have multiple actions at multiple sites, and so they must be thought of in terms of their systemic effects, rather than in terms of an isolated single effect. Pharmacology's two major divisions are pharmacokinetics and pharmacodynamics. You have already learned that **pharmacokinetics** addresses how drugs are transported into and out of the body. **Pharmacodynamics** deals with drugs' effects once they reach the target tissues.

* **pharmacokinetics** how drugs are transported into and out of the body.

* **pharmacodynamics** how a drug interacts with the body to cause its effects.

PHARMACOKINETICS

Strictly defined, pharmacokinetics is the study of the basic processes that determine the duration and intensity of a drug's effect. These four processes are absorption, distribution, biotransformation, and elimination.

Review of Physiology of Transport

Pharmacokinetics is dependent on the body's various physiological mechanisms that move substances across the body's compartments. These mechanisms can be broken down into two broad categories based on their energy requirements and then further classified. A mechanism is referred to as **active transport** if it requires the use of energy to move a substance. This energy is achieved by the breakdown of high-energy chemical bonds found in chemicals such as ATP (adenosine triphosphate). ATP is broken down into ADP (adenosine diphosphate) liberating a considerable amount of biochemical energy. A common example of an active transport mechanism is the sodium-potassium (Na^+-K^+) pump. This is a protein pump that actively moves potassium ions into the cell and sodium ions out of the cell. Because this movement goes *against* the ions' concentration gradients, it must use energy.

> ### Content Review
> #### PHARMACOKINETIC PROCESSES
> * Absorption
> * Distribution
> * Biotransformation
> * Elimination

* **active transport** requires the use of energy to move a substance.

Large molecules, such as glucose and most of the amino acids, do not readily pass through the cell membrane because of their size. These molecules are moved across the cell membrane with the help of special "carrier" proteins found on the surface of the target cells. These large molecules are "carried" across the cell membrane in a special transport process called **carrier-mediated diffusion** or **facilitated diffusion.** Once the molecule to be transported binds with the carrier protein, the configuration of the cell membrane changes, allowing the large molecule to enter the target cell. Insulin, an important hormone secreted by the endocrine pancreas, can increase the rate of carrier-mediated glucose transport from 10- to 20-fold. This is the principal mechanism by which insulin controls glucose use in the body.

Most drugs travel through the body by means of **passive transport,** the movement of a substance without the use of energy. This requires the presence of concentration gradients in a solution. Diffusion and osmosis are forms of passive transport. **Diffusion** involves the movement of solute in the solution, while **osmosis** involves the movement of the solvent (usually water). In diffusion, the solute's molecules or ions move *down* their concentration gradients from an area of higher concentration to an area of lower concentration. Conversely, in osmosis, the solvent's molecules move *up* the concentration gradient from an area of low solute concentration to an area of higher solute concentration. Another way of looking at this is to think of osmosis as simply the diffusion of solvent from an area of high *solvent* concentration to an area of low *solvent* concentration. A final type of passive transport is **filtration.** This is simply the movement of molecules across a membrane down a *pressure* gradient, from an area of high pressure to an area of lower pressure. This pressure typically results from the hydrostatic force of blood pressure.

Absorption

When a drug is administered to a patient, it must find its way to the site of action. If a drug is given orally or injected into any place except the bloodstream, its absorption into the bloodstream is the first step in this process. (Since drugs given intravenously or intra-arterially enter directly into the bloodstream, no absorption needs occur.) Several factors affect a drug's absorption. The body absorbs most drugs faster when they are given intramuscularly than when they are given subcutaneously. This is because muscles are more vascular than subcutaneous tissue. Of course, anything that slows blood flow will delay absorption. Shock and hypothermia are just two examples. Conversely, processes such as fever and hyperthermia increase peripheral blood flow and speed absorption.

Drugs given orally (enterally) must first survive the digestive processes before being absorbed across the mucosa of the gastrointestinal (GI) system. If a drug is not soluble in water, it will have difficulty being absorbed. Time-released medications take advantage of this with an enteric coating that slowly releases the medication. Some drugs have an enteric coating that will not dissolve in the more acidic environment of the stomach but will dissolve in the alkaline environment of the duodenum. This allows a drug that would irritate the stomach or be destroyed by stomach acid to be passed through the stomach into the duodenum and absorbed there. Besides being able to survive stomach acid, a drug must also be somewhat lipid (fat) soluble in order to cross the cells' lipid two-layered (bilayered) membranes. Many drugs **ionize,** or become electrically charged or polar, following administration. Generally speaking, ionized drugs do not absorb across the membranes of cells (lipid bilayers), but fortunately, most drugs do not fully ionize. Instead, they reach an equilibrium between their ionized and nonionized forms, and the nonionized form can be absorbed. A drug's pH also affects the extent to which it ionizes. A drug that is a weak acid will ionize much more substantially in an alkaline environment than in an acidic environment; conversely, an alkaline drug will ionize more readily in an acidic environment than in an alkaline environment. For

* **carrier-mediated diffusion** or **facilitated diffusion** process in which carrier proteins transport large molecules across the cell membrane.

* **passive transport** movement of a substance without the use of energy.

* **diffusion** movement of solute in a solution from an area of higher concentration to an area of lower concentration.

* **osmosis** movement of solvent in a solution from an area of lower solute concentration to an area of higher solute concentration.

* **filtration** movement of molecules across a membrane from an area of higher pressure to an area of lower pressure.

* **ionize** to become electrically charged or polar.

example, Aspirin (an acidic drug) does not dissociate well in the stomach (an acidic environment) and is therefore readily absorbed there.

The nature of the absorbing surface and the blood flow to the administration site also affect drug absorption. The rate of absorption is directly related to the amount of surface area available for absorption. The greater the area, the faster is the absorption. Much of the gastrointestinal system has multiple invaginations, or folds, that increase its surface area. Also, the greater the blood flow is to an area, the faster will be the rate of absorption. Again, the GI tract has a rich vascular system with many capillaries that perfuse its absorbing surfaces, allowing nutrients (and drugs) to diffuse into the bloodstream.

Finally, the drug's concentration affects its absorption. Because drugs diffuse in the body, the higher their concentration, the more rapidly the body will absorb them. This principle is frequently used when giving a "loading dose" of a drug and following it with a "maintenance infusion." The loading dose is typically a larger dose of the same concentration of the drug. On occasion, a more concentrated solution of the drug is used as the loading dose. Regardless, the desired effect is to rapidly raise the amount of the drug in the system to a therapeutic level. This is typically followed by a continuous infusion of the drug at a lower concentration, or slower administration rate, to keep it at the therapeutic level.

Bioavailability is the measure of the amount of a drug that is still active after it reaches its target tissue. This is the bottom line as far as absorption is concerned. The goal of administering a drug is to ensure sufficient bioavailability of the drug at the target tissue in order to produce the desired effect, after considering all the absorption factors.

✱ bioavailability amount of a drug that is still active after it reaches its target tissue.

Distribution

Once a drug has entered the bloodstream, it must be distributed throughout the body. Most drugs will pass easily from the bloodstream, through the interstitial spaces, into the target cells. Some drugs, however, will bind to proteins found in the blood, most commonly albumin, and remain in the body for a prolonged time. They thus have a sustained release from the bloodstream and a prolonged period of action. The therapeutic effects of a drug are primarily due to the unbound portion of the drug in the blood. A drug that is bound to plasma proteins cannot cross membranes and reach the target cells. Thus, only the unbound drug is in equilibrium with the target cells and can cross the cell membranes.

Changing the bloodstream's pH can affect the protein-binding action of a drug. Tricyclic antidepressants (TCAs), for instance, are strongly bound to plasma proteins. Making the blood more alkaline increases protein binding of the TCA molecules. Therefore, in addition to supportive therapy, serious overdoses of TCAs are treated by administering sodium bicarbonate. Sodium bicarbonate makes the blood more alkaline (raises the pH) causing increased binding of the TCA to serum proteins. Cumulatively, this decreases the amount of free drug in the blood, thus decreasing the adverse effects. Sodium bicarbonate administration also facilitates elimination of the drug through the urine.

The presence of other serum protein binding drugs can also affect drug-protein binding. For example, the drug warfarin (Coumadin) is highly protein-bound (99 percent). Its therapeutic effects are due to the 1 percent of the drug that is unbound and circulating in the bloodstream. Aspirin molecules bind to the same binding site on the serum proteins as do warfarin molecules. Thus, when Aspirin is administered to a patient on warfarin, it displaces some of the protein-bound warfarin, increasing the amount of free (unbound) warfarin in the blood. Even if it displaces only 1 percent of the total warfarin, it effectively doubles the available warfarin. This can lead to unwanted side effects, such as hemorrhage.

Albumin is one of the chief proteins in the blood that is available for binding with drugs. When albumin levels are low (hypoalbuminemia), as occurs in malnutrition, drugs that are normally protein bound rise to much greater blood levels than anticipated. For example, consider a patient who has been taking warfarin without difficulty. If she develops hypoalbuminemia, her normal dose of warfarin will result in much more of the drug being available in the body, possibly leading to dangerous bleeding.

Certain organs exclude some drugs from distribution. For example, the tight junctions of the capillary endothelial cells in the central nervous system (CNS) vasculature form a **blood-brain barrier**. These cells are packed together so tightly that only non-protein-bound, highly lipid-soluble drugs can cross into the CNS. The so-called **placental barrier** can likewise prevent drugs from reaching a fetus, although it is not the solid barrier that its name implies. The fetus is exposed to almost every drug that the mother takes. But because any drug must traverse the maternal blood supply and cross the capillary membranes into the placenta (fetal) circulation, delivering drugs to a fetus requires them to be lipid soluble, nonionized and non-protein-bound. This may slow some drugs or reduce their placental transfer to benign levels.

Other drugs are deposited in specific tissues. Fatty tissue, for example, can serve as a drug depot, or reservoir. Because blood flow is lower in fatty areas than in muscular areas, fatty tissue is a relatively stable depot; it can neither absorb nor release a large amount of drug in a short time. Similarly, bones and teeth can accumulate high amounts of drugs that bind to calcium, especially tetracycline antibiotics.

Biotransformation

Like other chemicals that enter the body, drugs are metabolized, or broken down into different chemicals (metabolites). The special name given to the **metabolism** of drugs is **biotransformation**. Biotransformation has one of two effects on most drugs: (1) It can transform the drug into a more or less active metabolite, or (2) it can make the drug more water soluble (or less lipid soluble) to facilitate elimination. Some drugs, such as lidocaine, are totally metabolized before elimination, others only partially, and still others not at all. The body will transform some molecules of most drugs and eliminate others without transformation. Protein-bound drugs are not available for biotransformation. Some so-called **prodrugs** (or parent drugs) are not active when administered, but biotransformation converts them into active metabolites.

Many biotransformation processes occur in the liver. The endoplasmic reticula of hepatocytes (liver cells) contain microsomal enzymes that perform much of the metabolizing. (Smaller quantities of these enzymes are also found in the kidney, lung, and GI tract.) Because the blood supply from the GI tract passes through the liver via the portal vein, all drugs absorbed in the GI tract pass through the liver before moving on through the systemic circulation. The first pass through the liver may partially or completely inactivate many drugs. This **first-pass effect** is why some drugs cannot be given orally but instead must be given intravenously to bypass the GI tract and prevent first-pass hepatic metabolism. It also is why drugs that can be given either orally or intravenously may require a much higher oral dose than IV dose. Because we can observe the extent of first-pass metabolism, we can predict how much to increase a dose of an oral medication to deliver an effective amount of the drug into the general circulation.

The liver's microsomal enzymes react with drugs in two ways: phase-I, or nonsynthetic reactions; and phase-II, or synthetic reactions. *Phase-I reactions* most often **oxidize** the parent drug, although they may reduce it or **hydrolyze** it. These nonsynthetic reactions make the drug more water soluble to ease excretion. A

* **blood-brain barrier** tight junctions of the capillary endothelial cells in the central nervous system vasculature through which only non-protein-bound, highly lipid-soluble drugs can pass.

* **placental barrier** biochemical barrier at the maternal/fetal interface that restricts certain molecules.

* **metabolism** the body's breaking down of chemicals into different chemicals.

* **biotransformation** special name given to the metabolism of drugs.

* **prodrug (parent drug)** medication that is not active when administered but whose biotransformation converts it into active metabolites.

* **first-pass effect** the liver's partial or complete inactivation of a drug before it reaches the systemic circulation.

* **oxidation** the loss of hydrogen atoms or the acceptance of an oxygen atom. This increases the positive charge (or lessens the negative charge) on the molecule.

* **hydrolysis** the breakage of a chemical bond by adding water, or by incorporating a hydroxyl (OH^-) group into one fragment and a hydrogen ion (H^+) into the other.

number of drugs and chemicals increase the activity of, or induce, the microsomal enzyme that causes phase-I reactions. This means that more enzyme is produced and drugs will be metabolized more rapidly. Because the microsomal enzymes are nonspecific, they can be induced by one drug or chemical and then biotransform other drugs or chemicals. *Phase-II reactions,* which are also called conjugation reactions, combine the prodrug or its metabolites with an endogenous (naturally occurring) chemical, usually making the drug more polar and easier to excrete.

Elimination

Whether they are unchanged or metabolized before elimination, most drugs (toxins and metabolites) are excreted in the urine. Some are excreted in the feces or in expired air.

Renal excretion occurs through two major processes: glomerular filtration and tubular secretion. Glomerular filtration is a function of glomerular filtration pressure, which, in turn, results from blood pressure and blood flow through the kidneys. Conditions that affect blood pressure and blood flow can affect renal elimination. Specialized transport systems in the walls of the proximal kidney tubules secrete drugs into the urine. These "pumps" are active transport systems and require energy in the form of adenosine triphosphate (ATP) to function. Some are specialized and transport only specific chemicals, while others can transport a range of similar chemicals. When drugs compete for the same pump, toxicity or other unwanted effects can result; however, combinations of some drugs can take advantage of this specialization to prolong their circulation. For example, probenecid blocks renal tubular pumps and competes for them with many antibiotics, among them penicillin, ampicillin, and oxacillin. Probenecid thus is sometimes given with those antibiotics to increase and prolong their blood levels.

The same factors that affect absorption at any other site also affect reabsorption in the renal tubules. Of particular concern is the urine pH. Lipid soluble and nonionized molecules are readily reabsorbed. Changing the urine pH (usually by administering sodium bicarbonate to make it more alkaline) can affect the reabsorption in the renal tubules. For example, if a drug becomes ionized in a more alkaline environment, then making the urine more alkaline will interfere with reabsorption and cause more of the drug to be excreted. Some drugs and their metabolites can be eliminated in the expired air. This is the basis of the breath test that police use to determine a driver's blood alcohol level. Ethanol is released in the expired air in proportion to its concentration in the bloodstream. Although the liver degrades most ingested ethanol, exhalation releases a measurable quantity. Drugs also can be excreted in the feces. In enterohepatic circulation, if a drug (or its metabolites) is excreted into the intestines from bile, the body may reabsorb the drug and experience a sustained effect. Additionally, drugs may be excreted through sweat, saliva, and breast milk. Excretion through sweat glands is rarely a significant mechanism for elimination. Excretion through mammary glands becomes a concern when nursing mothers take medications.

Drug Routes

The route of a drug's administration clearly has an impact on the drug's absorption and distribution. The route's impact on biotransformation and elimination may not be so clear. The bloodstream will more quickly absorb and distribute water soluble drugs if given in more vascular compartments than if given in less vascular compartments. Oral or nasogastric administration of alkaline drugs may allow the gastric acids to neutralize the drug and prevent its absorption. The liver's first-pass effect may biotransform some orally administered drugs and degrade them almost immediately.

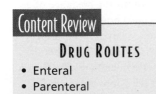

Content Review

DRUG ROUTES
- Enteral
- Parenteral

Enteral Routes **Enteral routes** deliver medications by absorption through the gastrointestinal tract, which goes from the mouth to the stomach and on through the intestines to the rectum. The routes may be oral, orogastric/nasogastric, sublingual, buccal, or rectal.

* *Oral (PO).* The oral route is good for self-administered drugs. Most home medications are administered by this route. The drug must be able to tolerate the acidic gastric environment and be absorbed. Few emergency drugs are administered through this route.
* *Orogastric/nasogastric tube (OG/NG).* This route is generally used for oral medications when the patient already has the tube in place for other reasons.
* *Sublingual (SL).* This is a good route for self-administration and for excellent absorption from the sublingual capillary bed without the problems of gastric acidity or absorption.
* *Buccal.* Absorption through this route between the cheek and gum is similar to sublingual absorption.
* *Rectal (PR).* This route is usually reserved for unconscious or vomiting patients or patients who cannot cooperate with oral or IV administration (small children).

Parenteral Routes Broadly defined, **parenteral** denotes any area outside the gastrointestinal tract; however, additional, specific criteria apply to parenteral drug administration. Parenteral routes typically use needles to inject medications into the circulatory system or tissues. Consequently, some forms of parenteral drug delivery afford the most rapid drug delivery and absorption.

* *Intravenous (IV).* With its rapid onset, this is the preferred route in most emergencies.
* *Endotracheal (ET).* This is an alternative route for *selected* medications in an emergency.
* *Intraosseous (IO).* The intraosseous route delivers drugs to the medullary space of bones. Most often used as an alternative to IV administration in pediatric emergencies, it also has limited use in adults.
* *Umbilical.* Both the umbilical vein and umbilical artery can provide an alternative to IV administration in newborns.
* *Intramuscular (IM).* The intramuscular route allows a slower absorption than does IV administration, as the drug passes into the capillaries.
* *Subcutaneous (SC, SQ, SubQ).* This route is slower than the IM route because the subcutaneous tissue is less vascular than the muscular tissue.
* *Inhalation/Nebulized.* This route, which offers very rapid absorption, is especially useful for delivering drugs whose target tissues are in the lungs.
* *Topical.* Topical administration delivers drugs directly to the skin.
* *Transdermal.* For drugs that can be absorbed through the skin, the transdermal route allows slow, continuous release.
* *Nasal.* Useful for delivering drugs directly to the nasal mucosa, the nasal route has an expanding role in delivering systemically acting drugs.

* **enteral route** delivery of a medication through the gastrointestinal tract.

* **parenteral route** delivery of a medication outside of the gastrointestinal tract, typically using needles to inject medications into the circulatory system or tissues.

Most emergency medications are given intravenously to avoid drug degradation in the liver.

- *Instillation.* Instillation is similar to topical administration but places the drug directly into a wound or an eye.
- *Intradermal.* For allergy testing, intradermal administration delivers a drug or biological agent between the dermal layers.

Drug Forms

Drugs come in many forms. Solid forms, generally given orally, include the following:

- *Pills.* Drugs shaped spherically to be easy to swallow.
- *Powders.* Although they are not as popular as they once were, some powdered drugs are still in use.
- *Tablets.* Powders compressed into a disc-like form.
- *Suppositories.* Drugs mixed with a wax-like base that melts at body temperature, allowing absorption by rectal or vaginal tissue.
- *Capsules.* Gelatin containers filled with powders or tiny pills; the gelatin dissolves, releasing the drug into the gastrointestinal tract.

Liquid drugs are usually solutions of a solid drug dissolved in a solvent. Some can be given parenterally, while others must be given enterally.

- *Solutions.* The most common liquid preparations. They are generally water based; some may be oil based.
- *Tinctures.* Prepared using an alcohol extraction process; some alcohol usually remains in the final drug preparation.
- *Suspensions.* Preparations in which the solid does not dissolve in the solvent; if left alone, the solid portion will precipitate out.
- *Emulsions.* Suspensions with an oily substance in the solvent, even when well mixed, globules of oil separate out of the solution.
- *Spirits.* Solution of a volatile drug in alcohol.
- *Elixirs.* Alcohol and water solvent, often with flavourings added to improve the taste.
- *Syrups.* Sugar, water, and drug solutions.

Some drugs come in a gaseous form. The most common drug supplied this way is oxygen. Paramedics may also find nitrous oxide (N_2O) used as an inhaled analgesic in ambulances and emergency departments.

Drug Storage

Certain guidelines should dictate the manner in which drugs are stored; their properties may be altered by the environment in which they are stored. Although some EMS units are parked in heated stations, others are kept outdoors and exposed to the elements. EMS systems must consider the storage requirements of all drugs and diluents when deciding operational issues, such as vehicle design and posting policies (as occurs in system status management). This rapidly becomes a clinical issue because the actual potency of most medications is altered if they are not stored in proper conditions. Examples of variables to consider when determining the proper method of drug storage include temperature, light, moisture, and shelf-life.

PHARMACODYNAMICS

When we consider a drug's pharmacodynamics, or effects on the body, we are specifically interested in its mechanisms of action and the relationship between its concentration and its effect.

Actions of Drugs

Drugs can act in four different ways. They may bind to a receptor site, change the physical properties of cells, chemically combine with other chemicals, or alter a normal metabolic pathway. Each of these actions involves a physiochemical interaction between the drug and a functionally important molecule in the body.

Drugs That Act by Binding to a Receptor Site Most drugs operate by binding to a **receptor**. Almost all drug receptors are protein molecules on the surfaces of cells. They are part of the body's normal regulatory stimulation/inhibition function and can be stimulated or inhibited by chemicals. Each different receptor's name generally corresponds to the drug that stimulates it. For example, if an opiate stimulates the receptor, then the receptor is an opioid receptor. When multiple drugs stimulate the same receptor, standard practice is to use the generic name.

The force of attraction between a drug and a receptor is called their **affinity**. The greater the affinity, the stronger is the bond. Different drugs may bind to the same type of receptor site, but the strength of their bond may vary. The binding site's shape determines its receptivity to other chemicals, whether they are drugs or endogenous substances. These binding sites are relatively specific—a nonopiate drug generally will not affect an opiate binding site, although occasionally a drug with a similar receptor binding site will unexpectedly cross-react. Receptors can also have subtypes. At least five subtypes of adrenergic receptors, for example, are important to paramedic practice.

A drug's pharmacodynamics also involve its ability to cause the expected response, or **efficacy.** Just as different drugs may have different affinities for a site, they may also have different efficacies; that is, drug A may cause a stronger response than drug B does. Affinity and efficacy are not directly related. Drug A may cause a stronger response than drug B does, even though drug B binds to the receptor site more strongly than drug A does.

When a drug binds with its specific type of receptor, a chemical change occurs that ultimately leads to the drug's effect. In most cases, drugs will either stimulate or inhibit the cell's normal biochemical actions. In fact, a drug cannot impart a new function to a cell. Some drugs may interact with a receptor and directly result in the desired effect. Other drugs, however, may interact with a receptor and cause the release or production of a second compound. This secondary compound, or **second messenger,** includes such compounds as calcium or cyclic adenosine monophosphate (cAMP). Cyclic AMP is the most common second messenger. It has a multitude of effects inside the cell. These secondary messengers are particularly important in the endocrine system, as they principally occur in endocrine glands. Once cAMP is formed inside the cell, it activates still other enzymes, usually in a cascading action. That is, the first enzyme activates another enzyme, which activates a third enzyme, and so forth. This is important in that it amplifies the action so that even a small amount of a drug (or hormone) acting on the cell surface can initiate a powerful, cascading, activating force for the entire cell.

The number of receptors on a target cell usually does not remain constant on a daily basis, or even from minute to minute. This is because the receptor proteins

✱ receptor specialized protein that combines with a drug resulting in a biochemical effect.

✱ affinity force of attraction between a drug and a receptor.

✱ efficacy a drug's ability to cause the expected response.

✱ second messenger chemical that participates in complex cascading reactions that eventually cause a drug's desired effect.

down-regulation binding of a drug or hormone to a target cell receptor that causes the number of receptors to decrease.

up-regulation a drug causes the formation of more receptors than normal.

agonist drug that binds to a receptor and causes it to initiate the expected response.

antagonist drug that binds to a receptor but does not cause it to initiate the expected response.

agonist-antagonist (partial agonist) drug that binds to a receptor and stimulates some of its effects but blocks others.

competitive antagonism one drug binds to a receptor and causes the expected effect while also blocking another drug from triggering the same receptor.

noncompetitive antagonism the binding of an antagonist causes a deformity of the binding site that prevents an agonist from fitting and binding.

irreversible antagonism a competitive antagonist permanently binds with a receptor site.

are often destroyed during the course of their function. At other times, they are either reactivated or remanufactured by the protein-manufacturing mechanism of the cell. Binding of a drug (or hormone) to a target cell receptor causes the number of receptors to decrease. This process is **down-regulation** of the receptors. It results in a decreased responsiveness of the target cell to the drug or hormone as the number of available active receptors decreases. In other cases, but less commonly, a drug (or hormone) can cause the formation of more receptors than normal. This process, **up-regulation,** increases the target tissue's sensitivity to the particular drug or hormone.

Chemicals that stimulate a receptor site generally fall into two broad categories, agonists and antagonists. **Agonists** bind to the receptor and cause it to initiate the expected response. **Antagonists** bind to a site but do not cause the receptor to initiate the expected response. Some drugs, **agonist-antagonists** (also called **partial agonists**), may do both. Nalbuphine (Nubain), for instance, stimulates some of the opioid agonists' analgesic properties but partially blocks others, such as respiratory depression.

Receptor-mediated drug actions work like a lock (the receptor) and key (the agonist). If you put the key in the lock and turn it, the lock will open. An antagonist is like a key that fits into the lock but will not turn and cannot open the lock. Target tissues generally have many receptors, and so to take the analogy another step, imagine that to get maximal effect, a single key (agonist) must move around and open many doors (trigger many biochemical responses). An agonist-antagonist would be a key that unlocks and opens a door but gets stuck in the lock. That is, the drug will cause the expected effect, but that drug will also block another drug from triggering the same receptor. This **competitive antagonism** is considered *surmountable* because a sufficiently large dose of the agonist can overcome the antagonism.

Noncompetitive antagonism can also occur. Continuing the lock, key, and door analogy, imagine the door is barred. This antagonism would be *insurmountable;* no amount of agonist could overcome it. Noncompetitive antagonism occurs because the binding of the antagonist at a different site causes a deformity of the binding site that actually prevents the agonist from fitting and binding. **Irreversible antagonism** may also occur when a competitive antagonist permanently binds with a receptor site. When this occurs, no amount of agonist will stimulate the receptor. For the effects of such an antagonist to wear off, the body must create new receptors.

Two drugs may appear to be antagonists while actually acting independently. This physiological antagonism can occur when one drug's effects counteract another's. Although neither agent chemically affects the other, their net effect is antagonistic. An example of a receptor, agonist, antagonist, and agonist-antagonist can be described using an opiate receptor. These receptors occur naturally in the brain and respond to natural endorphins. Morphine sulphate acts as an agonist. It binds to the opiate receptor and causes the expected response of pain relief. Naloxone (Narcan) acts as an antagonist. It will bind to the opiate receptor but will not initiate the pain relief. It will prevent morphine sulphate from binding to the site and thus effectively blocks the morphine and its response. If the patient is given nalbuphine (Nubain), an agonist-antagonist, it will bind to the opiate receptor and relieve pain, but it is less efficacious than morphine. The nalbuphine blocks morphine from the receptor like an antagonist but stimulates the receptor on its own like an agonist, although to a lesser extent.

Drugs That Act by Changing Physical Properties Some drugs change the physical properties of a part of the body. Drugs that change the osmotic balance across membranes are good examples of this type of drug action. The osmotic diuretic mannitol (Osmotrol), for instance, increases urine output by increasing the blood's osmolarity, or osmotic "pull." This increased osmolarity triggers the normal regulatory systems to decrease water reabsorption in the renal tubules, thereby reducing the total amount of water in the body.

Drugs That Act by Chemically Combining with Other Substances Drugs that participate in chemical reactions that change the chemical nature of their substrates (the chemical or substance on which a drug acts) play a large role in paramedic practice. For example, isopropyl alcohol, which is often used to disinfect skin before percutaneous needle insertion for phlebotomy or IV cannulation, denatures the proteins on the surface of bacterial cells. This ruptures the cells, destroying the bacteria. Antacids are another example. They act by chemically neutralizing the hydrochloric acid in the stomach. Sodium bicarbonate given intravenously chemically neutralizes some of the acids in the bloodstream, effectively making the blood more alkalotic.

Drugs That Act by Altering a Normal Metabolic Pathway Some anticancer and antiviral drugs are chemical analogues of normal metabolic substrates. In a process that has been dubbed a counterfeit incorporation mechanism, these drugs can be incorporated into the products of metabolism of cancer cells. Since these drugs are not really the expected substrate, the anticipated product either will not form or, if formed, will be substantially or completely inactive.

Responses to Drug Administration

When a drug is administered, a response is obviously anticipated. The actual response may be the one desired, or it may be an unintended **side effect**. Most, if not all, drugs have at least some minor side effects. Because our knowledge of pharmacology and physiology has not yet arrived at the point where we can engineer the perfect drug, we must weigh the need for the desired response against the dangers of side effects. In essence, every time we give a medication, we must carefully weigh the risks against the benefits. Although undesirable, side effects are predictable. Iatrogenic responses, however, are not predictable. In general, the term *iatrogenic* refers to a disease or response induced by the actions of a care provider. Derived from the Greek *iatros* (physician) and *gennan* (to produce), it literally means *physician produced*. Negligence is not the only cause of iatrogenic responses. Some common unintended adverse responses to drugs include the following:

* *Allergic reaction.* Also known as hypersensitivity; this effect occurs as the drug is antigenic and activates the immune system, causing effects that are normally more profound than seen in the general population.
* *Idiosyncrasy.* A drug effect that is unique to the individual; it is different from that seen or expected in the population in general.
* *Tolerance.* Decreased response to the same amount of drug after repeated administrations.
* *Cross-tolerance.* Tolerance for a drug that develops after administration of a different drug. Morphine and other opioid agents are common examples. Tolerance for one agent implies tolerance for others as well.
* *Tachyphylaxis.* Rapidly occurring tolerance to a drug that may occur after a single dose. This typically occurs with sympathetic agonists, specifically decongestant and bronchodilation agents.
* *Cumulative effect.* Increased effectiveness when a drug is given in several doses.
* *Drug dependence.* The patient becomes accustomed to the drug's presence in her body and will suffer from withdrawal symptoms on its absence. The dependence may be physiological or psychological.

* **side effect** unintended response to a drug.

Always weigh the need for a drug's desired response against the dangers of its side effects.

- *Drug interaction.* The effects of one drug alter the response to another drug.
- *Drug antagonism.* The effects of one drug block the response to another drug.
- *Summation.* Also known as an additive effect. Two drugs that both have the same effect are given together, analogous to $1+1=2$.
- *Synergism.* Two drugs that both have the same effect are given together and produce a response greater than the sum of their individual responses, analogous to $1+1=3$.
- *Potentiation.* One drug enhances the effect of another. A common example is promethazine (Phenergan) enhancing the effects of morphine.
- *Interference.* The direct biochemical interaction between two drugs; one drug affects the pharmacology of another drug.

Drug–Response Relationship

To have its optimal desired or therapeutic effects, a drug must reach appropriate concentrations at its site of action. The magnitude of the response therefore depends on the dosage and the drug's course through the body over time. Factors that can affect the drug's concentration may be pharmaceutical (the dosage form's disintegration and the drug's dissolution), pharmacokinetic (the drug's absorption, distribution, metabolism, and excretion), or pharmacodynamic (drug-receptor interaction). To predict how the drug will affect different people, a **drug-response relationship** thus correlates different amounts of drug to the resultant clinical response.

Most of the information needed to describe drug-response relationships comes from **plasma-level profiles,** which describe the lengths of onset, duration, and termination of action, as well as the drug's minimum effective concentration and toxic levels. The **onset of action** is the time from administration until a medication reaches its **minimum effective concentration** (the minimum level of drug necessary to cause a given effect). The length of time the amount of drug remains above this level is its **duration of action. Termination of action** is measured from when the drug's level drops below the minimum effective concentration until it is eliminated from the body.

The ratio of a drug's lethal dose for 50 percent of the population (LD_{50}) to its effective dose for 50 percent of the population (ED_{50}) is its **therapeutic index** (TI) or LD_{50}/ED_{50}. The therapeutic index represents the drug's margin of safety. As the range between effective dose and lethal dose decreases, the value of TI decreases; that is, it becomes closer to one. TI values of close to one indicate a very small margin of safety. In other words, the effective dose and lethal dose of a drug whose TI value is close to one are nearly the same. This drug would be very difficult to effectively dose without causing toxicity.

The last component of the drug-response relationship, the **biological half-life,** is the time the body takes to clear one-half of the drug. Although the rates of metabolism and excretion both affect it, a drug's half-life ($t_{1/2}$) is independent of its concentration. For example, if the concentration of a drug were 500 µg/dL after administration and 250 µg/dL in 10 minutes, then its half-life would be 10 minutes. After another 10 minutes, 125 µg/dL would remain.

Factors Altering Drug Response

Different individuals may have different responses to the same drug. Factors that alter the standard drug-response relationship include the following:

✷ **drug-response relationship** correlation of different amounts of a drug to clinical response.

✷ **plasma-level profile** describes the lengths of onset, duration, and termination of action, as well as the drug's minimum effective concentration and toxic levels.

✷ **onset of action** the time from administration until a medication reaches its minimum effective concentration.

✷ **minimum effective concentration** minimum level of a drug needed to cause a given effect.

✷ **duration of action** length of time the amount of drug remains above its minimum effective concentration.

✷ **termination of action** time from when the drug's level drops below its minimum effective concentration until it is eliminated from the body.

✷ **therapeutic index** ratio of a drug's lethal dose for 50 percent of the population to its effective dose for 50 percent of the population.

✷ **biological half-life** time the body takes to clear one-half of a drug.

- *Age.* The liver and kidney functions of infants are not yet fully developed, and so the response to drugs may be altered. Likewise, as we age, the functions of these organs begin to deteriorate. As a result, infants and the elderly are most susceptible to having an altered response to a drug.

- *Body mass.* The more body mass a person has, the more fluid is potentially available to dilute a drug. A given amount of drug will cause a higher concentration in a person with little body mass than in a much larger person. Thus, most drug dosages are stated in terms of body mass.

- *Sex.* Most differences in drug response due to sex result from the relative body masses of men and women. The different distribution and amounts of body fat also affect the amounts of drug available at any given time.

- *Environmental milieu.* Various stimuli in a patient's environment affect her response to a given drug. This is most clearly seen with drugs affecting mood or behaviour. The same dose of an antianxiety medication, such as diazepam (Valium), will have different effects, depending on the patient's mood or surroundings. For example, if the patient were afraid of heights, her usual dose of diazepam would not likely help her remain calm while rappelling from the top of a tall building. Surrounding conditions may also affect the distribution or elimination of a drug. Heat, for example, causes vasodilation and increases perspiration, both of which may alter the rate at which the body distributes and eliminates a drug.

- *Time of administration.* If a patient takes a drug immediately after eating, its absorption will be different from her taking the same drug before breakfast in the morning. Some drugs may cause nausea if taken on an empty stomach and must therefore be taken only after eating.

- *Pathological state.* Several disease states alter the drug-response relationship. Most notable are renal and hepatic dysfunctions, both of which may lead to excess accumulation of a drug in the body. Renal failure is likely to decrease elimination of drugs, while hepatic failure may decrease or inhibit their metabolism, prolonging their duration of action. Acid-base disturbances may alter a drug's solubility or the extent to which it ionizes, thus changing its absorption rate.

- *Genetic factors.* Genetic traits, such as the lack of specific enzymes or lowered basal metabolic rate, alter drug absorption or biotransformation and thus modify the patient's response.

- *Psychological factors.* A patient's mental state can also affect her response to a drug. The best known example of this is the placebo effect. Essentially, if a patient believes that a drug will have a given effect, then she is much more likely to perceive that the effect has occurred.

Drug Interactions

Drug interactions occur whenever two or more drugs are available in the same patient. The interaction can increase, decrease, or have no effect on their combined actions. Any number of variables may cause these drug-drug interactions:

- One drug could alter the rate of intestinal absorption.
- The two drugs could compete for plasma protein binding, resulting in one's accumulation at the other's expense.
- One drug could alter the other's metabolism, thus increasing or decreasing either's bioavailability.
- One drug's action at a receptor site may be antagonistic or synergistic to another's.
- One drug could alter the other's rate of excretion through the kidneys.
- One drug could alter the balance of electrolytes necessary for the other drug's expected result.

In addition to drug-drug interactions, other types of interactions are possible. They include a drug's effects on the rate of absorption of food and nutrients, alteration of enzymes, and food-initiated alteration of drug excretion. Alcohol consumption and smoking may also cause interactions with drugs. Finally, some drugs are incompatible with each other. As an example, catecholamines, such as epinephrine, will precipitate in an alkaline solution, such as sodium bicarbonate.

Part 2: Drug Classifications

Part 2 begins with a discussion of how drugs are classified, that is, how drugs are organized into groups with common characteristics, most often according to the body system affected. The remainder of Part 2 discusses drugs and subgroups of drugs that are included in the following major classifications:

- Drugs used to affect the nervous system
- Drugs used to affect the cardiovascular system
- Drugs used to affect the respiratory system
- Drugs used to affect the gastrointestinal system
- Drugs used to affect the eyes
- Drugs used to affect the ears
- Drugs used to affect the endocrine system
- Drugs used to treat cancer
- Drugs used to treat infectious diseases and inflammation
- Drugs used to affect the skin
- Drugs used to supplement the diet
- Drugs used to treat poisoning and overdoses

CLASSIFYING DRUGS

The enormous amount of material that you must learn about pharmacology can easily become overwhelming. The best way to surmount this challenge is to break the information into manageable groups. Drugs can be classified many ways. You will often find them listed by the body system they affect, by their mechanism of action, or by their indications. Drugs also can be classified by source or by chemical class. Understanding the properties of drug classes (or the model drug of a class) can increase your understanding of drugs and quicken your learning of new drugs.

Grouping medications according to their uses is a very practical way of classifying them. For example, one class of drugs is used to treat heart dysrhythmias, another to treat hypertension. Although the specific dosing regimens and contraindications vary among medications within any class, their general properties are consistent. If you understand those general principles, learning the specific information about individual medications becomes much easier. Thinking in terms of prototypical medications usually helps describe each classification. A **prototype** is a drug that best demonstrates the class's common properties and illustrates its particular characteristics.

In the rest of this chapter, we will look at specific classifications of medications that you as a paramedic will commonly either administer or encounter. Even though you may not frequently administer medications from every classification, knowing how they work remains important. It will help you understand the implications of medications your patients may be taking themselves or getting from another caregiver. An example often cited to demonstrate the importance of understanding the classes of medications, even those that you will rarely administer, is the patient who has taken an overdose of tricyclic antidepressants. Based on your knowledge of this classification, you will know to increase your index of suspicion for hypotension and abnormal cardiac rhythms.

DRUGS USED TO AFFECT THE NERVOUS SYSTEM

The two major divisions of the nervous system are the central nervous system and the peripheral nervous system (Figure 14-2). The *central nervous system* includes the brain and spinal cord; all nerves that originate and terminate within either the brain or the spinal cord are considered central. The *peripheral nervous system* comprises everything else. If a neuron originates within the brain and terminates outside the spinal cord, it is part of the peripheral nervous system, which, in turn, consists of the somatic nervous system and the autonomic nervous system. The

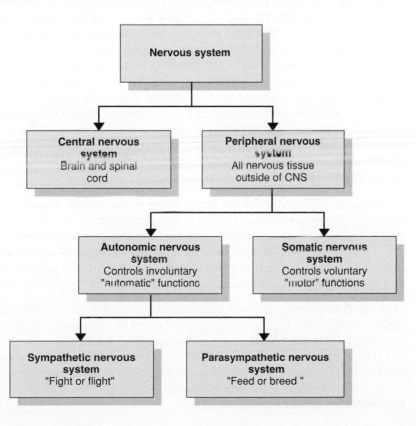

FIGURE 14-2 Functional organization of the autonomic nervous system.

somatic nervous system controls voluntary, or motor, functions. The *autonomic nervous system,* which controls involuntary, or automatic, functions, is further divided into the sympathetic and parasympathetic nervous systems. The two major groupings of medications used to affect the nervous system are those that affect the central nervous system and those that affect the autonomic nervous system.

CENTRAL NERVOUS SYSTEM MEDICATIONS

Many pathological conditions involve the central nervous system (CNS). As a result, a great number of drugs have been developed to affect the CNS, including analgesics, anesthetics, drugs to treat anxiety and insomnia, anticonvulsants, stimulants, psychotherapeutic agents (antidepressants and antimanic agents), and drugs used to treat specific nervous system disorders, such as Parkinson's disease. Obviously, this is a very broad classification with many different types of agents. Having a firm grasp on the basic physiology involved will help you understand the various drugs you encounter.

Analgesics and Antagonists

Analgesics are medications that relieve the sensation of pain. The distinction between **analgesia,** the absence of the sensation of *pain,* and **anesthesia,** the absence of *all* sensation, is important. Where an analgesic decreases the specific sensation of pain, an anesthetic prevents all sensation, often impairing consciousness in the process. A frequently used class of medications, analgesics are available by prescription or over the counter. The two basic subclasses of analgesics are opioid agonists and their derivatives and nonopioid derivatives. Opioid antagonists, which we also discuss in this section, reverse the effects of opioid analgesics; **adjunct medications** enhance the effects of other analgesics.

Opioid Agonists An opioid is chemically similar to opium, which is extracted from the poppy plant and has been used for centuries for its analgesic and hallucinatory effects. Opium and all its derivatives effectively treat pain because of their similarity to natural pain-reducing peptides called *endorphins.* Endorphins and, by extension, opioid drugs, work by decreasing the sensory neurons' ability to propagate pain impulses to the spinal cord and brain.

The prototype opioid drug is morphine. Several of morphine's effects make it useful for clinical practice. At therapeutic doses, morphine causes analgesia, euphoria, sedation, and miosis (pupil constriction). It also decreases cardiac preload and afterload, which makes it useful in treating myocardial infarction and pulmonary edema. At higher doses, it may cause respiratory depression and hypotension. Give morphine with caution to patients at high risk for respiratory failure (COPD and asthma) and hypotension (trauma patients with hypovolemia).

Nonopioid Analgesics Three broad types of nonopioid medications also have analgesic properties, several of which also share antipyretic (fever-fighting) properties. These are such *salicylates* as Aspirin, such *nonsteroidal anti-inflammatory drugs (NSAIDS)* as ibuprofen, and such *para-aminophenol derivates* as acetaminophen. The drugs in each of these classes affect the production of prostaglandins and cyclo-oxygenase, important neurotransmitters involved in the pain response.

Opioid Antagonists Opioid antagonists are useful in reversing the effects of opioid drugs. This typically is necessary to treat respiratory depression. Nalaxone (Narcan) is the prototype opioid antagonist. It competitively binds with opioid receptors but without causing the effects of opioid bonding. It is commonly used to treat overdoses of heroin and other opioid derivatives; however, it has a shorter half-life than most opioid drugs, and so repeated doses may be necessary to prevent its unwanted side effects.

✱ **analgesic** medication that relieves the sensation of pain.

✱ **analgesia** the absence of the sensation of pain.

✱ **anesthesia** the absence of all sensations.

✱ **adjunct medication** agent that enhances the effects of other drugs.

Give morphine with caution to patients at high risk for respiratory failure and hypotension.

Adjunct Medications Adjunct medications are given concurrently with other drugs to enhance their effects. Although they may have only limited or no analgesic properties by themselves, when combined with a true analgesic, they either prolong or intensify its effect. Examples of adjunct medications are benzodiazepines (diazepam [Valium], lorazepam (Ativan), midazolam [Versed]), antihistamines (promethazine [Phenergan]) and caffeine. We will discuss many of these agents in separate sections.

Opioid Agonist–Antagonists An opioid agonist-antagonist displays both agonistic and antagonistic properties. Pentazocine (Talwin) is the prototype for this class. Nalbuphine (Nubain) is commonly used in field care. It is an agonist because, like opioids, it decreases pain response, and it is an antagonist because it has fewer respiratory depressant and addictive side effects. Butorphanol (Stadol) is another common opioid agonist-antagonist.

Anesthetics

Unlike analgesics, an **anesthetic** induces a state of anesthesia, or loss of sensation to touch or pain. Anesthetics are useful during unpleasant procedures, such as surgery or electrical cardioversion. At low levels of anesthesia, patients may have a decreased sensation of pain but remain conscious. **Neuroleptanesthesia,** a type of anesthesia that combines this effect with amnesia, is useful in procedures that require the patient to remain alert and responsive.

> ✱ **anesthetic** medication that induces a loss of sensation to touch or pain.

> ✱ **neuroleptanesthesia** anesthesia that combines decreased sensation of pain with amnesia while the patient remains conscious.

Anesthetics as a group tend to cause respiratory, central nervous system (CNS), and cardiovascular depression. Different agents affect these systems to different degrees and are typically chosen for their ability to produce the desired effect with minimal side effects. Anesthetic agents are rarely used singly; rather, several different agents are typically given together to achieve a balanced anesthetic result. For example, intubating a conscious patient requires her natural gag reflex to be inhibited. Neuromuscular blocking agents, such as succinylcholine, are used to induce paralysis. Because this would be a terribly frightening and potentially painful procedure, antianxiety, amnesic, and analgesic agents are also given to produce the desired anesthetic effect.

Anesthetics are given either by inhalation or injection. The gaseous anesthetics given by inhalation include halothane, enflurane, and nitrous oxide. The first clinically useful anesthetic was ether, a gas. Its discovery marked a new generation in surgical care, but it is very flammable. The modern gaseous anesthetics are much less volatile while still decreasing consciousness and sensation as required. These drugs, by some as yet unidentified mechanism, hyperpolarize neural membranes, making depolarization more difficult. This decreases the firing rates of neural impulses and, therefore, the propagation of action potentials through the nervous system, thus reducing sensation. These effects appear to depend on the gases' solubility. The rate of onset of anesthesia further depends on several additional factors, including cardiac output, inhaled concentration of gas, pulmonary minute volume, and end organ perfusion. Because these gases clear mostly through the lungs, respiratory rate and depth affect the duration of their effect. Although halothane is the prototype of inhaled anesthetics, nitrous oxide is the only medication in this class with which you are likely to have much involvement.

Most anesthetics used outside the operating room are given intravenously. This gives them a considerably faster onset and shorter duration, making them much more useful in emergency care. Paramedics primarily use these agents to assist with intubation in rapid sequence intubation. They include several pharmacological classes including ultra-short acting barbiturates (thiopental [Pentothal] and methohexital [Brevital]), benzodiazepines (diazepam [Valium] and midazolam [Versed]), and opioids (fentanyl [Sublimaze], remifentanil [Ultiva]).

We discuss barbiturates' and benzodiazepines' mechanisms of action in the section on antianxiety and sedative-hypnotics.

Anesthetics are also given locally to block sensation for procedures like suturing and most dentistry. These agents are injected into the skin around the nerves that innervate the area of the procedure. They decrease the nerve's ability to depolarize and propagate the impulse from this area to the brain. Cocaine's first clinical use was as a topical anesthetic of the eye in 1884. The current prototype of this class is lidocaine (Xylocaine). It is frequently mixed with epinephrine. The epinephrine causes local vasoconstriction, decreasing bleeding and systemic absorption of the drug.

Antianxiety and Sedative-Hypnotic Drugs

* **sedation** state of decreased anxiety and inhibitions.

* **hypnosis** instigation of sleep.

Antianxiety and sedative-hypnotic drugs are generally used to decrease anxiety, induce amnesia, and assist sleeping and as part of a balanced approach to anesthesia. **Sedation** refers to a state of decreased anxiety and inhibitions. **Hypnosis** in this context refers to the instigation of sleep. Sleep may be categorized as either rapid eye movement (REM) or non-rapid eye movement (non-REM). REM sleep is characterized by rapid eye movements and lack of motor control. Most dreaming is thought to occur during REM sleep. Insomnia, or difficulty sleeping, typically presents with increased latency (the period of time between lying down and going to sleep) or awakening during sleep.

The two main pharmacological classes within this functional class are benzodiazepines and barbiturates. Alcohol is also in this functional class. Benzodiazepines and barbiturates work in similar ways. Benzodiazepines are frequently prescribed for oral use and are relatively safe and effective for treating general anxiety and insomnia. Barbiturates, which have broader general depressant activities and a higher potential for abuse, are used much less frequently than benzodiazepines. Before the release of benzodiazepines in the 1960s, however, barbiturates were the drug of choice for treating anxiety and insomnia.

Both benzodiazepines and barbiturates hyperpolarize the membrane of central nervous system neurons, which decreases their response to stimuli. Gamma-aminobutyric acid (GABA) is the chief inhibitory neurotransmitter in the central nervous system. GABA receptors are dispersed widely throughout the CNS on proteins that make up chloride ion channels in the cell membrane. When GABA combines with these receptors, the channel "opens," and chloride, which is more prevalent outside the cell, diffuses through the channel. As chloride is an anion, or negative ion, it makes the inside of the cell more negative than the outside. This hyperpolarizes the membrane and makes it more difficult to depolarize. Depolarization therefore requires a larger stimulus to cause the cell to fire. Both benzodiazepines and barbiturates increase the GABA receptor-chloride ion channel complexes' potential for binding with GABA, and both are dose dependent. At low doses, they decrease anxiety and cause sedation. As the dose increases, they induce sleep (hypnosis) and, at higher doses, anesthesia. Because benzodiazepines only increase the effectiveness of GABA, the amount of GABA present limits their effects. This actually makes benzodiazepines much safer than barbiturates, which at high doses can actually mimic GABA's effects and thus can have unlimited effects. Benzodiazepines and barbiturates are also useful in treating convulsions.

Just as opiates have an antagonist in naloxone (Narcan), benzodiazepines have an antagonist in flumazenil (Romazicon). Flumazenil competitively binds with the benzodiazepine receptors in the GABA receptor-chloride ion channel complex without causing the effects of benzodiazepines. This reverses the sedation from benzodiazepines, but it can occasionally have untoward consequences, specifically if a patient depends on benzodiazepines for seizure control, is withdrawing from alcohol, or is taking tricyclic antidepressants. In these cases, the patient may develop seizures following the administration of flumazenil.

Antiseizure or Antiepileptic Drugs

Seizures are a state of hyperactivity of either a section of the brain (partial seizure) or all of the brain (generalized seizure). They may or may not be accompanied by convulsions. Therefore, although the medications in this functional class may be called anticonvulsants, they are more appropriately referred to as antiseizure or antiepileptic drugs. The goal of seizure management is to balance the elimination of the seizures against the side effects of the medications used to treat them. Controlling seizures is a lifelong process for most patients and requires diligent compliance with medication dosing regimens.

Partial (or focal) seizures erupt from a specific focus and are described in terms of alterations in consciousness or behaviour. These may be further divided into simple or complex partial seizures based on the specific area of the brain in which the focus is located. Complex partial seizures are also known as psychomotor seizures and are characterized by repetitive motions.

Generalized seizures involve both hemispheres of the brain and are described in terms of visible motor activity. Grand mal seizures involve periods of muscle rigidity (tonic stage) followed by spasmodic twitching (clonic stage) and then flaccidity and a gradual return to consciousness (postictal stage). Petit mal seizures are also generalized but do not have obvious convulsions. They involve brief losses of consciousness that may occur hundreds of times a day. They are also called absence seizures and are treated differently from other types of seizures. Finally, status epilepticus is a life-threatening condition characterized by uninterrupted grand mal seizures lasting more than 30 minutes or by two or more tonic-clonic seizures without an intervening lucid interval. The preferred therapy for each type of seizure differs.

Seizures are treated through several general mechanisms. The most common is direct action on the sodium and calcium ion channels in the neural membranes. Phenytoin (Dilantin) and carbamazepine (Tegretol) both inhibit the influx of sodium into the cell, thus decreasing the cell's ability to depolarize and propagate seizures. Valproic acid and ethosuximide act similarly, but they interact with calcium channels in the hypothalmus, where absence seizures typically begin. These two drugs are particularly useful because they are specific to hyperactive neurons and therefore have few side effects. Other medications, such as benzodiazepines and barbiturates, interact with the GABA receptor-chloride ion channel complex, as explained in the section on antianxiety and sedative-hypnotic drugs.

Antiseizure medications include several phamacological classes, such as benzodiazepines (diazepam [Valium] and lorazepam (Ativan]), barbiturates (phenobarbitol [Luminal]), hydantoins (phenytoin [Dilantin], fosphenytoin [Ccrcbyx]), succinimides (ethosuximide [Zarontin]), and miscellaneous medications, such as valproic acid (Depakote). Table 14-3 lists the preferred medication for treating each type of seizure.

> *The goal of seizure management is to balance the elimination of the seizures against the side effects of the medications used to treat them.*
>
>

Central Nervous System Stimulants

Stimulating the central nervous system is desirable in certain circumstances, such as fatigue, drowsiness, narcolepsy, obesity, and attention deficit hyperactivity disorder. Broadly, two techniques may accomplish this:

- Increasing the release or effectiveness of excitatory neurotransmitters
- Decreasing the release or effectiveness of inhibitory neurotransmitters

Within the functional class of CNS stimulants are three pharmacological classes, amphetamines, methylphenidates, and methylxanthines.

Table 14-3	ANTISEIZURE MEDICATIONS
Type of Seizure	**Drug of Choice**
Partial Seizures	Phenytoin
	Carbamazepine
Grand Mal	Carbamazepine
	Phenytoin
	Phenobarbitol
Absence	Valproic acid
	Ethosuximide

The amphetamines also include methamphetamine and dextroamphetamine. These drugs all increase the release of excitatory neurotransmitters, including norepinephrine and dopamine. Norepinephrine is the primary cause of these drugs' effects, which include an increased wakefulness and awareness as well as a decreased appetite. Amphetamines' most common uses, therefore, are treating drowsiness and fatigue and suppressing the appetite. Most of amphetamines' side effects result from overstimulation; they include tachycardia and other dysrhythmias, hypertension, convulsions, insomnia, and occasionally psychoses with hallucinations and agitation. Examples of this class include amphetamine sulphate (the prototype) and Dexedrine.

Methylphenidate, marketed as Ritalin, is the most commonly prescribed drug for attention deficit hyperactivity disorder (ADHD). Although it is chemically different from the amphetamines, its pharmacological mechanism of action is similar. Also, like the amphetamines, it has a high abuse potential and is therefore listed as a Schedule II controlled substance. Although treating hyperactivity with a stimulant may seem odd, it is quite effective. Frequently, the cause of inappropriate behaviour in a child with ADHD is an inability to concentrate or focus. Ritalin's stimulant effects increase this ability, and the unwanted behaviour often diminishes.

The methylxanthines include caffeine, aminophylline, and theophylline. Although caffeine, the prototype drug in this class, has few clinical uses, it is frequently ingested in coffee, colas, and chocolates. Theophylline's relaxing effects on bronchial smooth muscle make it helpful in treating asthma. The methylxanthines' mechanism of action is unclear, but it seems to block adenosine receptors. Adenosine is an endogenous neurotransmitter that is used clinically for certain types of tachycardias. Because methylxanthines block the adenosine receptors, larger than normal doses may be needed to achieve the desired result. This class's side effects are similar to the amphetamines', but they have a much lower potential for abuse and are not controlled drugs.

Psychotherapeutic Medications

* **psychotherapeutic medication** drug used to treat mental dysfunction.

Psychotherapeutic medications treat mental dysfunction. Unlike other disease states, we do not thoroughly understand the pathophysiology of mental dysfunction; therefore, we base much of our pharmacological treatment of these conditions on our limited knowledge and on clinical correlation (scientific observation that these medications are indeed effective, even if we do not fully understand their mechanisms). Medications are typically only one tactic in a balanced strategy for treating mental illness. Depending on the specific disorder, physicians will use other treatments, such as psychotherapy and electroconvulsive therapy, in conjunction with pharmaceutical interventions.

Although we do not completely understand these diseases' specific pathologies, they seem to involve the monoamine neurotransmitters in the central nervous system. These neurotransmitters (norepinephrine, dopamine, serotonin) have been implicated in the control and regulation of emotions. Imbalances in these neurotransmitters, especially dopamine, appear to be at least involved in, if not responsible for, most mental disease. Regulating these and other excitatory and inhibitory neurotransmitters forms the basis for psychopharmaceutical therapy. Schizophrenia appears to be related to an increased release of dopamine, and so treatment is aimed at blocking dopamine receptors. Depression seems to be related to inadequate amounts of these neurotransmitters, and so treatment is aimed at increasing their release or duration.

The major diseases treated with psychotherapeutic medications are schizophrenia, depression, and bipolar disorder. *The Diagnostic and Statistical Manual,* fourth edition (*DSM-IV*), published by the American Psychiatric Association, gives schizophrenia's chief characteristics as a lack of contact with reality and disorganized thinking. Its many different manifestations include delusions, hallucinations (auditory more frequently than visual), disorganized and incoherent speech, and grossly disorganized or catatonic behaviour. Schizophrenia is typically treated with antipsychotic medications, frequently in conjunction with medications from other classes, such as antianxiety drugs or antidepressants. **Extrapyramidal symptoms (EPS)**, a common side effect of antipsychotic medications, include muscle tremors and parkinsonism-like effects. As a result, antipsychotic medications are also known as **neuroleptic** (literally, *affecting the nerves*) drugs.

The two chief pharmaceutical classes of antipsychotics and neuroleptics are phenothiazines and butyrophenones. Both have been mainstays of psychiatry since the mid-1950s and are considered traditional antipsychotic drugs. Medications in this group block dopamine, muscarinic acetylcholine, histamine, and $alpha_1$ adrenergic receptors in the central nervous system. These medications' therapeutic effects appear to come from blocking the dopamine receptors; their side effects are fairly well understood to originate in blocking the other receptors. The phenothiazines' and butyrophenones' mechanisms of action are the same; they differ only in potency and pharmacokinetics. The distinction between potency and strength is important. Strength refers to the drug's concentration, while potency is the amount of drug necessary to produce the desired effect. Although the phenothiazines are considered low-potency and the butyrophenones are considered high-potency, they both produce the same effect. The differences in potency and pharmacokinetics determine which class of medication will be prescribed. Chlorpromazine (Thorazine) is the prototype phenothiazine; haloperidol (Haldol) is the prototype of the butyrophenones.

Since the phenothiazines' and the butyrophenones' mechanisms of action are identical, their common side effects are also similar: extrapyramidal symptoms from cholinergic blockade in the basal ganglia of the cerebral hemispheres; orthostatic hypotension from blockage of $alpha_1$ adrenergic receptors; sedation; and sexual dysfunction. Treatment for these side effects typically involves modifying the drug dose. Diphenhydramine (Benadryl), an antihistamine with anticholinergic properties, is indicated for treating acute dystonic reactions (manifestations of EPS), which often present with tongue and neck spasms. Patients with a newly prescribed antipsychotic may experience these effects and contact EMS. Fortunately, treatment with diphenhydramine is effective and rapid. Orthostatic hypotension is treated in the usual fashion described in Chapter 19, Hemorrhage and Shock.

Other medications used to treat psychotic conditions are considered atypical antipsychotics. Although their mechanisms of action are similar to those of the traditional antipsychotics, the atypical antipsychotics block more specific receptors. This specificity allows them to function much like traditional antipsychotics, but without causing the prominent extrapyramidal symptoms. These drugs include clozapine (Clozaril) and risperidone (Risperdal).

Content Review

MAJOR DISEASES TREATED WITH PSYCHOTHERAPEUTIC MEDICATIONS

- Schizophrenia
- Depression
- Bipolar disorder

✱ **extrapyramidal symptoms (EPS)** common side effects of antipsychotic medications that include muscle tremors and parkinsonism-like effects.

✱ **neuroleptic** antipsychotic (literally, *affecting the nerves*).

Content Review

MAJOR CLASSES OF ANTIPSYCHOTIC MEDICATIONS

- Phenothiazines
- Butyrophenones

Be alert for the development of extrapyramidal symptoms any time you administer phenothiazine.

Another functional class of psychotherapeutic medications includes the antidepressants. The *DSM-IV* characterizes major depressive episodes as causing significantly depressed mood, loss of interest in things that normally give the patient pleasure, weight loss or gain, sleeping disturbances, suicide attempts, feelings of hopelessness and helplessness, loss of energy, agitation or withdrawal, and an inability to concentrate. Although the specific pathology of this disease is not yet known, it appears to be related to an insufficiency of monoamine neurotransmitters (norepinephrine and serotonin). Thus, the pharmaceutical interventions for this disease appear to increase the number of neurotransmitters released in the brain. The several ways of doing this include increasing the amount of neurotransmitter produced in the presynaptic terminal, increasing the amount of neurotransmitter released from the presynaptic terminal, and blocking the neurotransmitter's reuptake (reabsorption by the presynaptic terminal). This results in a net increase in the neurotransmitter. The antidepressants comprise three pharmacological classes: tricyclic antidepressants, selective serotonin reuptake inhibitors, and monoamine oxidase inhibitors.

Tricyclic antidepressants (TCAs) are frequently used in treating depression because they are effective, relatively safe, and have few significant side effects when taken in therapeutic dosages. TCAs act by blocking the reuptake of norepinephrine and serotonin, thus extending the duration of their action (Figure 14-3). Unfortunately, they also have anticholinergic properties that cause many side effects, including blurred vision, dry mouth, urinary retention, and tachycardia. Another frequent side effect, orthostatic hypotension, is likely due to the alpha$_1$ adrenergic blockade. This is commonly seen when patients try to stand up too quickly and become dizzy. Additionally, because TCAs can lower the seizure threshold, patients with existing seizure disorders are at risk for convulsions. Unfortunately, when taken in overdose, TCAs can have very significant cardiotoxic effects that make them a favoured means of attempting suicide among depressed patients. These effects include myocardial infarction and dysrhythmias. Partly because of this potential for overdose, TCAs have fallen behind the newer selective serotonin reuptake inhibitors as the drug of choice for depression. Overdoses of these medications also frequently cause marked hypotension. Treatment of TCA overdoses is primarily supportive, with sodium bicarbonate given to increase the excretion of TCAs by alkalanizing the urine. The prototype tricyclic antidepressant, imipramine (Tofranil), was also the first one on the market. Other common examples include amitriptyline (Elavil), desipramine (Norpramin), and nortriptyline (Pamelor).

Selective serotonin reuptake inhibitors (SSRIs) are a recent addition to the antidepressants. The prototype is fluoxetine (Prozac). These drugs' antidepres-

FIGURE 14-3   Effects of TCAs on reuptake of serotonin and norepenephrine.

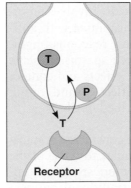

(a) Neurotransmission without TCA

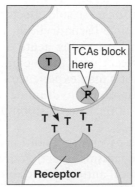

(b) Neurotransmission with TCA

sant effects are comparable with the TCAs', but because the SSRIs selectively block the reuptake of serotonin, they do not affect dopamine or norepinephrine. Nor do they block histaminic or cholinergic receptors, thus avoiding many of the TCAs' side effects. The primary adverse reactions to SSRIs are sexual dysfunction, headache, and nausea. Other selective serotonin reuptake inhibitors include sertraline (Zoloft) and paroxetine (Paxil).

A third pharmacological class of psychotherapeutic medications includes the monoamine oxidase inhibitors (MAOIs). The monoamine neurotransmitters are thought to be insufficient in depression. Monoamine oxidase, an enzyme, metabolizes monoamines into inactive metabolites. MAOIs inhibit monoamine oxidase and block the monoamines' breakdown, thus increasing their availability. Monoamine oxidase is also present in the liver and has a significant role in metabolizing foods that contain tyramine, a substance that increases the release of norepinephrine. The MAOIs' major side effect is hypertensive crisis brought on by the consumption of foods rich in tyramine, such as cheese and red wine. By inhibiting monoamine oxidase, these drugs also decrease the body's ability to inactivate tyramine; they therefore promote the release of norepinephrine, a potent vasopressor. Because of this and other unwanted side effects, MAOIs are not commonly used anymore; rather, they are reserved for treating depression that is refractory to TCAs and SSRIs. The prototype of this class is phenelzine (Nardil).

Patients with bipolar disorder (manic depression) exhibit cyclic swings from mania to depression with periods of normalcy in between. According to the *DSM-IV*, the manic phases of this disease are characterized by hyperactivity, thoughts of grandeur or inflated self-esteem, decreased need for sleep, increased goal-oriented behaviour, increased productivity, flight of ideas (moving from thought to thought with little connection between them), distractibility, and increased risk taking. Lithium is the drug of choice for the management of bipolar disorder. It is frequently given in conjunction with benzodiazepines or antipsychotics. Lithium's mechanism of action is unknown, but it effectively decreases the signs of mania without causing sedation. Adverse reactions include headache, dizziness, fatigue, nausea, and vomiting. Recently, two antiseizure medications—carbamazepine (Tegretol) and valproic acid (Depakote)—have proven successful in treating bipolar disorder.

Drugs Used to Treat Parkinson's Disease

Parkinson's disease is a nervous disorder caused by the destruction of dopamine-releasing neurons in the *substantia nigra,* a part of the basal ganglia, which is a specialized area of the brain involved in controlling fine movements. Dysfunction of parts of the basal ganglia causes the extrapyramidal symptoms (EPS) often seen as a side effect of antipsychotic medications.

Parkinson's disease is characterized by dyskinesia (dysfunctional movements), such as involuntary tremors, unsteady gait, and postural instability. Severe cases also involve bradykinesia (slow movements) and akinesia (the absence of movement). In the later stages, patients frequently present with psychological impairment, including dementia, depression, and impaired memory. Parkinson's is a progressive disease that usually begins in middle age with subtle signs and progresses to a state of incapacitation. Although no treatments can cure Parkinson's or even slow its progression, treating the symptoms can return some function to the patient. The goal in treating these patients is to restore their ability to function without causing unacceptable side effects. Some remarkably effective drugs are available. Unfortunately, they usually are effective for only several years. After that, signs and symptoms return and often are more severe than before treatment began.

Lithium, widely used in the treatment of bipolar disorder, has a very low therapeutic index.

The medications that are effective in treating Parkinson's disease are also effective in treating the extrapyramidal side effects (EPS) of antipsychotics. This is because fine motor control is based, in part, on a balance between inhibitory and excitatory neurotransmitters. In the basal ganglia, dopamine, an inhibitory transmitter, opposes acetylcholine, an excitatory neurotransmitter. Parkinson's disease and the medications that cause EPS both decrease the number of presynaptic terminals that release dopamine in the basal ganglia. This allows the excitatory stimulus of acetylcholine to dominate, ultimately impeding fine motor control.

Pharmacological therapy for Parkinson's disease seeks to restore the balance of dopamine and acetylcholine. This may be done either by increasing the stimulation of dopamine receptors or by decreasing the stimulation of acetylcholine receptors. Drugs can do this either through dopaminergic effects or through anticholinergic effects. Dopaminergic effects increase the release of dopamine from the neuron, directly stimulate the dopamine receptors, or decrease the breakdown of however much dopamine is being released. Anticholinergic effects prevent acetylcholine's effects either by reducing the amount of the neurotransmitter released or by directly blocking the acetylcholine receptors.

Dopamine cannot be given directly to patients with Parkinson's disease because it cannot cross the blood-brain barrier and consequently would be ineffective in treating the disease while still causing many side effects. The drug of choice in treating Parkinson's disease, therefore, is levodopa, an inactive drug that readily crosses the blood-brain barrier. Levodopa is absorbed by the dopamine-releasing neuron terminals, where the enzyme decarboxylase metabolizes it into dopamine, thus increasing the amount of dopamine available for release. Levodopa is very effective and reduces symptoms in the vast majority of patients. As previously mentioned, however, symptoms will return within a period of years as the disease progresses. Levodopa's side effects include nausea, vomiting, and ironically, for unknown reasons, dyskinesias. Because it is converted to dopamine, levodopa may also have cardiovascular effects, including tachycardias and hypertension.

When given alone, levodopa is metabolized primarily outside the brain, where it is ineffective. To prevent this, Sinemet, the most popular anti-Parkinson preparation available, combines levodopa with an inactive ingredient, carbidopa. Although carbidopa by itself produces no effects, it prevents levodopa's conversion into dopamine in the periphery. Because carbidopa does not cross the blood-brain barrier, however, levodopa can still be metabolized in the CNS. This decreases the incidence of cardiovascular side effects and enables lower doses of levodopa to be effective. Sinemet's side effects are essentially those of levodopa by itself. Nausea and vomiting, stimulated from within the CNS, remain problematic.

Another dopaminergic medication, amantadine (Symmetrel), promotes the release of dopamine from those dopamine-releasing neurons that remain unaffected by the disease. It has a rapid onset but generally becomes ineffective in less than a year. Although it can be effective alone, it is usually given in conjunction with Sinemet or levodopa. Several other medications, such as bromocriptine, directly stimulate the dopamine receptors instead of attempting to increase the amount of dopamine released.

One additional dopaminergic approach is to decrease the breakdown of dopamine after it has been released. The enzyme responsible for breaking down such monoamines as norepinephrine, dopamine, and serotonin is monoamine oxidase. (We have previously described monoamine oxidase inhibitors in our discussion of their role in depression.) One monoamine oxidase inhibitor, selegiline (Carbex), is specific for monoamine oxidase type B. This MAO-B enzyme is involved only in the breakdown of dopamine. (MAO-A is responsible for breaking down norepinephrine and serotonin.) By selectively inhibiting the breakdown of dopamine, selegiline increases the amount available for binding with dopamine receptors, thus promoting the dopamine-acetylcholine balance. This selective blockage avoids increased norepinephrine levels that can lead to undesired tachycardia and hypertension.

As opposed to dopaminergic medications, which act on the dopamine side of the dopamine-acetylcholine balance, anticholinergic medications act on the acetylcholine side to block the acetylcholine receptors. The prototype anticholinergic, atropine, was initially used in this context with success, but it also had the typical peripheral anticholinergic side effects of blurred vision, dry mouth, and urinary hesitancy. More recently developed medications affect the CNS more than they do the peripheral nervous system. The prototype centrally acting anticholinergic medication is benztropine (Cogentin). Another example is diphenhydramine (Benadryl), which is more frequently administered for its antihistaminic properties.

AUTONOMIC NERVOUS SYSTEM MEDICATIONS

The **autonomic nervous system** is the part of the nervous system that controls involuntary (automatic) actions. Many medications used in prehospital care directly affect the autonomic nervous system. It is essential that you have a good understanding of this aspect of the nervous system and the ways in which emergency medications affect it.

The two functional divisions of the autonomic nervous system are the sympathetic nervous system and the parasympathetic nervous system. The sympathetic nervous system allows the body to function under stress. It is often referred to as the fight-or-flight aspect of the nervous system. The parasympathetic nervous system primarily controls vegetative functions, such as digestion of food. It is often referred to as the feed-or-breed or the rest-and-repose aspect of the nervous system. The parasympathetic nervous system and the sympathetic nervous system work in constant opposition to control organ responses. For example, the sympathetic nervous system stimulates specific receptors in the heart that increase the heart rate. At the same time, the parasympathetic nervous system stimulates specific receptors that decrease the heart rate. The net result is the resting heart rate. When the body's physiological needs dictate an increased heart rate, the sympathetic stimuli dominate the parasympathetic effects. Conversely, when the body needs to rest (with a decreased heart rate), the parasympathetic stimuli predominate.

Basic Anatomy and Physiology

The autonomic nervous system arises from the central nervous system. The nerves of the autonomic nervous system exit the central nervous system and subsequently enter specialized structures called **autonomic ganglia**. In the autonomic ganglia, the nerve fibres from the central nervous system interact with nerve fibres that extend from the ganglia to the various target organs. Autonomic nerve fibres that exit the central nervous system and terminate in the autonomic ganglia are called **preganglionic nerves**. Autonomic nerve fibres that exit the ganglia and terminate in the various target tissues are called **postganglionic nerves**. The ganglia of the sympathetic nervous system are located close to the spinal cord, while the ganglia of the parasympathetic nervous system are located close to the target organs (Figure 12-73, page 561).

No actual physical connection exists between two nerve cells or between a nerve cell and the organ it innervates. Instead, there is a space, or synapse, between nerve cells. The space between a nerve cell and the target organ is a **neuroeffector junction**. Specialized chemicals called **neurotransmitters** conduct the nervous impulse between nerve cells or between a nerve cell and its target organ.

* **autonomic nervous system** the part of the nervous system that controls involuntary actions.

* **autonomic ganglia** groups of autonomic nerve cells located outside the central nervous system.

* **preganglionic nerves** nerve fibres that extend from the central nervous system to the autonomic ganglia.

* **postganglionic nerves** nerve fibres that extend from the autonomic ganglia to the target tissues.

* **neuroeffector junction** specialized synapse between a nerve cell and the organ or tissue it innervates.

* **neurotransmitter** chemical messenger that conducts a nervous impulse across a synapse.

Neurotransmitters are released from presynaptic neurons and subsequently act on postsynaptic neurons or on the designated target organ. When released by the nerve ending, the neurotransmitter travels across the synapse and activates membrane receptors on the adjoining nerve or target tissue. The neurotransmitter is then either deactivated or taken back up into the presynaptic neuron.

The two neurotransmitters of the autonomic nervous system are acetylcholine and norepinephrine. Acetylcholine is utilized in the preganglionic nerves of the sympathetic nervous system and in both the preganglionic and the postganglionic nerves of the parasympathetic nervous system. Norepinephrine is the postganglionic neurotransmitter of the sympathetic nervous system. Synapses that use acetylcholine as the neurotransmitter are **cholinergic** synapses. Synapses that use norepinephrine as the neurotransmitter are **adrenergic** synapses.

The anatomy and physiology of the autonomic nervous system were discussed in detail in Chapter 12.

Drugs Used to Affect the Parasympathetic Nervous System

The parasympathetic system uses acetylcholine as a neurotransmitter. Acetylcholine (ACL) released by presynaptic neurons activates receptors on the postsynaptic neurons or on the neuroeffector junction.

Receptors that are specialized for acetylcholine are termed cholinergic receptors. Medications that stimulate them are known as cholinergics (**parasympathomimetics**), and those that block them are known as anticholinergics or cholinergic blockers (**parasympatholytics**).

Cholinergics Cholinergic drugs act either directly or indirectly. Direct-acting cholinergics (also called cholinergic esters) simulate the effects of ACh by directly binding with the cholinergic receptors. Drugs in this class generally produce the same effects as cholinergic stimulation, mostly focused on the muscarinic receptors. Their adverse effects are related primarily to decreased heart rate, decreased peripheral vascular resistance resulting in hypotension and excessive salivation, urination, defecation, and sweating. Vomiting and abdominal cramps may also occur. The acronym SLUDGE (**s**alivation, **l**acrimation, **u**rination, **d**efecation, **g**astric motility, **e**mesis) is helpful for remembering these effects.

The prototype direct-acting cholinergic is bethanechol (Urecholine). Its pharmacokinetics make it a good clinical substitute for acetylcholine. It is not broken down by cholinesterase, the enzyme responsible for destroying acetylcholine, and therefore it has a longer duration of action. Most of its effects are on muscarinic receptors in the urinary bladder and gastrointestinal tract. It may be given orally or subcutaneously. Thus, it is used primarily to increase micturition (urination) and peristalsis. Adverse effects are rare but related to its parasympathomimetic effects. Another direct-acting cholinergic medication, pilocarpine, is used as a topical treatment for glaucoma.

Indirect-acting cholinergic drugs affect acetylcholinesterase. By inhibiting its actions in degrading acetylcholine, they prolong the cholinergic response. These drugs affect both muscarinic and nicotinic receptors and therefore have little specificity. Their uses are limited primarily to treating myasthenia gravis, some types of poisoning, and glaucoma as well as for reversing nondepolarizing neuromuscular blockade.

The two basic types of indirect-acting cholinergic drugs are reversible inhibitors and irreversible inhibitors. Both types bind with cholinesterase (ChE), acting as a substitute for ACh. In doing so, they prevent ChE from destroying ACh. The difference between the reversible and irreversible inhibitors is how

* **cholinergic** pertaining to the neurotransmitter acetylcholine.

* **adrenergic** pertaining to the neurotransmitter norepinephrine.

* **parasympathomimetic** drug or other substance that causes effects like those of the parasympathetic nervous system (also called cholinergic).

* **parasympatholytic** drug or other substance that blocks or inhibits the actions of the parasympathetic nervous system (also called anticholinergic).

Content Review

SLUDGE EFFECTS OF CHOLINERGIC MEDICATIONS

- Salivation
- Lacrimation
- Urination
- Defecation
- Gastric motility
- Emesis

long they remain bound with cholinesterase. The reversible inhibitors remain bound with cholinesterase much longer than with acetylcholine but eventually release it. The irreversible inhibitors, too, will eventually release cholinesterase, but they remain bound for so long that, from a practical standpoint, they can be considered irreversible.

Neostigmine (Prostigmin) is the prototype reversible cholinesterase inhibitor. It is used to treat myasthenia gravis, an illness characterized by muscle weakness and progressive fatigue. This illness is an autoimmune disease that destroys the nicotinic$_M$ receptors at the neuromuscular junction. With fewer of these receptors, muscles cannot be stimulated as well and weakness occurs. Neostigmine treats the symptoms of myasthenia gravis by blocking the degradation of ACh, thereby prolonging its effects and increasing motor strength. Its primary side effects are due to the stimulation of muscarinic receptors and include the SLUDGE responses. Fortunately, these responses may be treated effectively with a cholinergic blocker. Neostigmine can also reverse a nondepolarizing neuromuscular blockade. This use is fairly uncommon, however, because such blockades typically are administered only intentionally as part of anesthesia or before intubation.

Physostigmine (Antilirium) is another reversible cholinesterase inhibitor. Its mechanism is similar to neostigmine's, with their primary difference being in their pharmacokinetics. Although neostigmine is poorly absorbed across the cell membrane, physostigmine crosses rapidly and therefore has a shorter onset and may be given in lower doses. Physostigmine's chief use is for reversing overdoses of atropine, an anticholinergic drug that blocks muscarinic receptors.

Irreversible cholinesterase inhibitors have only one clinical function, the treatment of glaucoma, and only one drug, echothiophate (Phospholine Iodide), has been approved for that purpose. Cholinesterase inhibitors, however, are very useful as insecticides (organophosphates), and unfortunately, their mechanism of action is also very attractive for makers of chemical weapons. They are the chief component in nerve gases, such as VX and sarin. They cause extensive stimulation of cholinergic receptors, ultimately resulting in the SLUDGE response. Toxic levels may also affect nicotinic$_M$ receptors, leading to paralysis. Treatment for such toxic exposures involves drugs, such as high doses of atropine or pralidoxime (Protopam, 2-PAM), to block the effects of the accumulating acetylcholine. Pralidoxime can encourage irreversible cholinesterase inhibitors to release cholinesterase.

Anticholinergics Anticholinergic agents oppose the parasympathetic (cholinergic) nervous system. Just as there are multiple types of cholinergic receptors, there are multiple classes of cholinergic receptor antagonists. We will discuss agents that selectively block muscarinic and nicotinic receptors as well as nonselective blockers (ganglionic blockers). A special subclass of nicotinic receptors in neuromuscular blocking drugs.

Muscarinic Cholinergic Antagonists Cholinergic antagonists block the effects of acetylcholine almost exclusively at the muscarinic receptors. They are often called anticholinergics or parasympatholytics. They work by competitively binding with muscarinic receptors without stimulating them. As a result, these receptors cannot bind with acetylcholine.

The prototype anticholinergic drug is atropine, which is widely used to block muscarinic receptors and is commonly administered in the field. Found in the plant *Atropa belladonna,* atropine is one of several drugs classified as belladonna alkaloids (scopolamine is also in this classification). Readily absorbed through both enteral and parenteral routes, it has therapeutic effects at dose-dependent levels at most sites with muscarinic receptors. At low doses, atropine decreases secretion from salivary and bronchial glands as well as from the sympathetically innervated sweat glands. At moderate doses, it increases heart rate and causes mydriasis (dilated pupils) and blurry vision. At higher doses, it decreases gastric

Content Review

TYPES OF PARASYMPATHETIC ACETYLCHOLINE RECEPTORS
- Muscarinic
- Nicotinic
  - Nicotinic$_N$ (neuron)
  - Nicotinic$_M$ (muscle)

Content Review

EFFECTS OF ATROPINE
OVERDOSE

- Hot as hell
- Blind as a bat
- Dry as a bone
- Red as a beet
- Mad as a hatter

motility and stomach acid secretion. Atropine is also useful in reversing overdoses of muscarinic agonists (cholinergics or cholinesterase inhibitors). Its side effects, which are predictable, include dry mouth, blurred vision and photophobia, urinary retention, increased intraocular pressure, tachycardia, constipation, and anhidrosis (decreased sweating), which may cause hyperthermia. A helpful mnemonic for remembering the effects of atropine overdose is "hot as hell, blind as a bat, dry as a bone, red as a beet, mad as a hatter."

Scopolamine is another belladonna anticholinergic. Its actions are similar to atropine's, but unlike atropine, scopolamine causes sedation and antiemesis. Thus, its primary purpose is to prevent motion sickness. It is available as a transdermal patch.

Several synthetic medications mimic the effects of the belladonna alkaloids while minimizing their side effects. Ipratropium bromide (Atrovent), an inhaled anticholinergic, is effective in treating asthma because it relaxes the bronchial smooth muscle and causes bronchodilation. It is frequently administered along with an inhaled beta-adrenergic agonist. Because it is inhaled and has little systemic effect, ipratropium bromide avoids many of atropine's side effects.

Other anticholinergic drugs include dicyclomine (Bentyl) and benztropine (Cogentin).

Nicotinic Cholinergic Antagonists Nicotinic cholinergic antagonists block acetylcholine only at nicotinic sites. They include ganglionic blocking agents that block the nicotinic$_N$ receptors in the autonomic ganglia and neuromuscular blocking agents that block nicotinic$_M$ receptors at the neuromuscular junction.

Ganglionic Blocking Agents Ganglionic blockade is produced by competitive antagonism with acetylcholine at the nicotinic$_N$ receptors in the autonomic ganglia. This can, in effect, turn off the entire autonomic nervous system. The two drugs in this class are trimethaphan (Arfonad) and mecamylamine (Inversine). Both are used to treat hypertension. The adverse effects of ganglionic blockade include signs associated with antimuscarinic drugs like atropine—dry mouth, blurred vision, urinary retention, and tachycardia. Other adverse effects arising from the vasodilation and decreased preload caused by sympathetic blockage include profound hypotension, with orthostatic hypotension even more evident. Trimethaphan is administered primarily for hypertensive crisis when other treatments are ineffective. These agents are almost never used anymore because they are not selective and many superior agents are available.

Neuromuscular blockers affect nicotinic$_M$ receptors.

Neuromuscular Blocking Agents Neuromuscular blockade produces a state of paralysis without affecting consciousness. Imagine how terrifying it would be to be fully conscious and aware but completely paralyzed, unable to move or breathe. Neuromuscular blockade is caused by competitive antagonism of nicotinic$_M$ receptors at the neuromuscular junction. This is useful during surgery as part of anesthesia and during electroconvulsive therapy for depression. These agents are most often used in the field to facilitate intubation.

Neuromuscular blocking agents are either depolarizing or nondepolarizing, depending on their mechanism of action. Most are nondepolarizing; only one depolarizing drug, succinylcholine (Anectine), is commonly used in the clinical setting. Tubocurarine, while not frequently used clinically, is the oldest neuromuscular blocker and the prototype nondepolarizing agent. It produces neuromuscular blockade by binding with the nicotinic$_M$ receptor sites without causing muscle depolarization. Succinylcholine acts in the same manner, but like acetylcholine, it does cause muscle depolarization when it binds with the nicotinic$_M$ receptor. It is useful as a neuromuscular blocker because, in contrast to ACh, which rapidly separates from the receptor, it remains bound, preventing the muscle's repolarization. Several nondepolarizing agents are available; the specific agent chosen depends on its rate of onset and duration of action. Succinylcholine has the shortest onset and duration of action because it has a naturally occurring enzyme, pseudocholinesterase, which degrades it.

Ganglionic-Stimulating Agents Nicotinic$_N$ receptors reside at the ganglia of both the parasympathetic and the sympathetic nervous systems. The alkaloid nicotine stimulates these receptors. Nicotine is found in tobacco and, although it has no therapeutic uses, is of interest for two reasons. Historically, nicotine, along with muscarine, led to a much better understanding of the autonomic nervous system's specific receptors. It is also one of the most abused drugs in the world.

Nicotine may cause a variety of responses, most of which are dose related. At low doses, like those from smoking, nicotine causes excitation at the autonomic ganglia. This affects both the parasympathetic and the sympathetic nervous systems. The parasympathetic response causes increased salivation, peristalsis, and secretion of gastric acid. The sympathetic response causes the release of norepinephrine and epinephrine. These lead to increases in heart rate, myocardial contractility, vasoconstriction, and blood pressure, all of which increase the heart's workload. Sympathetic stimulation also increases awareness and suppresses fatigue and appetite.

Drugs Used to Affect the Sympathetic Nervous System

Medications that stimulate the sympathetic nervous system are **sympathomimetics.** Medications that inhibit the sympathetic nervous system are called **sympatholytics.** Some medications are pure alpha agonists, while others are pure alpha antagonists. Some medications are pure beta agonists, while others are pure beta antagonists. Such medications as epinephrine stimulate both alpha and beta receptors. Other medications, such as the bronchodilators, are termed beta selective, since they act more on beta$_2$ receptors than on beta$_1$ receptors.

The sympathetic nervous system releases norepinephrine from postganglionic end terminals and epinephrine from the adrenal medulla. These neurotransmitters bind with adrenergic receptors. (Epinephrine is also called adrenalin because of its release from the adrenal medulla; hence the term *adren*-ergic). There are two main types of adrenergic receptors, each with two subtypes. These receptors' effects depend primarily on their locations. Table 14-4 describes the chief locations and primary actions of each receptor.

✱ **sympathomimetic** drug or other substance that causes effects like those of the sympathetic nervous system (also called adrenergic).

✱ **sympatholytic** drug or other substance that blocks the actions of the sympathetic nervous system (also call antiadrenergic).

Table 14-4 LOCATION OF ADRENERGIC RECEPTORS AND EFFECTS OF STIMULATION

Receptor	Response to Stimulation	Location
Alpha 1 (α_1)	Constriction	Arterioles
	Constriction	Veins
	Mydriasis	Eye
	Ejaculation	Penis
Alpha 2 (α_2)	Presynaptic terminals inhibition*	
Beta 1 (β_1)	Increased heart rate	Heart
	Increased conductivity	
	Increased automaticity	
	Increased contractility	
	Renin release	Kidney
Beta 2 (β_2)	Bronchodilation	Lungs
	Dilation	Arterioles
	Inhibition of contractions	Uterus
	Tremors	Skeletal muscle
Dopaminergic	Vasodilation (increased blood flow)	Kidney

*Stimulation of α_2 adrenergic receptors inhibits the continued release of norepinephrine from the presynaptic terminal. It is a feedback mechanism that limits the adrenergic response at that synapse. These receptors have no other identified peripheral effects.

The primary clinical purpose for medications that stimulate alpha$_1$ receptors is peripheral vasoconstriction. Constriction of the arterioles increases afterload, while constriction of venules increases preload (decreasing venous capacitance or pooling). Both of these effects increase systolic and diastolic blood pressure and represent the chief therapeutic indication for alpha$_1$ agonists. Stimulation of alpha$_1$ receptors locally may be useful in combination with local anesthetics. The main reason to add the alpha$_1$ agonist in this context is to cause local vasoconstriction so that the systemic absorption of the anesthetic will decrease and its duration will increase. Alpha$_1$ agonists are also useful topically to decrease nasal congestion caused by dilation and engorgement of nasal blood vessels. The primary adverse responses to alpha$_1$ agonist agents are hypertension and local tissue necrosis. If a medication with significant alpha$_1$ properties infiltrates the surrounding tissue or distal body parts, such as fingers, toes, earlobes or nose, inadequate local blood flow due to profound vasoconstriction will likely kill the tissue. Also, alpha$_1$ stimulation may cause reflex bradycardia due to the feedback mechanism that regulates blood pressure. As baroreceptors detect a rise in blood pressure, the heart rate decreases to compensate.

Alpha$_1$ antagonism is indicated almost exclusively for controlling hypertension. By preventing the peripheral vasoconstriction of alpha$_1$ stimulation, these agents decrease blood pressure. They are also useful in treating local tissue necrosis caused by infiltration of alpha$_1$ agonists. Injecting alpha$_1$ antagonists into the area surrounding the infiltration prevents tissue death from excessive vasoconstriction. The effects of pheochromocytoma, a tumour of the adrenal medulla that causes the release of large amounts of catecholamine, may be treated with an alpha$_1$ blocker. The most common adverse effects of alpha$_1$ antagonism are orthostatic hypotension and reflex tachycardia. Just as alpha$_1$ stimulation may increase blood pressure and cause a baroreceptor-mediated bradycardia, the hypotension from alpha$_1$ blockage may lead to reflex tachycardia from the same mechanism. Other side effects include nasal congestion and inhibition of ejaculation. These agents may also increase blood volume. This is ironic, since their primary indication is hypertension. As another feedback mechanism detects hypotension, the kidneys begin to reabsorb sodium and water to increase blood volume. This is typically addressed by use of a diuretic concomitant with the alpha$_1$ antagonist.

Beta$_1$ stimulation increases heart rate, contractility, and conduction. Its primary indications are cardiac arrest and hypotension resulting from inadequate pumping. During cardiac arrest, beta$_1$ activation may stimulate contractions or increase the force of any existing contractions. Even if the heart is only fibrillating, these agents may increase the effectiveness of electrical defibrillation. In cardiogenic shock, when the heart is not pumping with enough force to overcome the afterload created by peripheral vascular resistance, beta$_1$ agonists can adequately increase the contractions' force. The chief adverse effects of beta$_1$ agonists include tachycardia, dysrhythmias, and chest pain from increasing workload.

Beta$_1$ antagonists are among the most frequently prescribed medications. Their most common use is to control blood pressure. By blocking the effects of beta$_1$ stimulation, they decrease heart rate (choronotropy) and contractility (inotropy). These agents are also effective in treating supraventricular tachycardias because they decrease the rate of impulse generation at the SA node (negative chronotropic effects) while also slowing conductivity through the AV node (negative dromotropic effects). Blocking beta$_1$ stimulation also helps treat angina pectoris and reduces the recurrence of myocardial infarction. Its main adverse effects are symptomatic bradycardia, hypotension, and AV block.

Beta$_2$ agonists are used to treat asthma and other conditions with excessive narrowing of the bronchioles. By stimulating beta$_2$ receptors in the lungs, these agents relax the bronchial smooth muscle and cause bronchodilation. Beta$_2$ agonists can also cause uterine smooth muscle relaxation, which may help suppress preterm labour. Their primary adverse effects are muscle tremors and "bleed over" effects on unintended beta$_1$ stimulation, such as tachycardias.

Although beta$_2$ blockade serves no clinically useful purpose, nonselective beta blockers have side effects of beta$_2$ blockade. Chief among these is bronchoconstriction and inhibition of glycogenolysis, the release of stored glycogen by the liver and skeletal muscles. Beta$_2$ stimulation causes glycogenesis. Antagonizing the beta$_2$ receptors can inhibit this release. Although this is not typically a problem for most people, it can be very problematic for diabetics. It not only makes hypoglycemia more likely but also masks one of its common early warning signs, tachycardia.

Adrenergic Agonists Drugs that stimulate the effects of adrenergic receptors work either directly, indirectly, or through a combination of the two. The direct acting agents bind with the receptor and cause the same response as the normal neurotransmitter. In fact, most of the drugs in this category either are synthetically produced versions of the naturally occurring neurotransmitter or are derivatives of those synthetically produced versions. The indirect acting agents stimulate the release of epinephrine from the adrenal medulla and of norepinephrine from the presynaptic terminals. In turn, the epinephrine and norepinephrine stimulate the adrenergic receptors. The mixed actions of direct-indirect acting medications combine these mechanisms.

The most frequently used adrenergic agents are chemically and functionally similar to the endogenous neurotransmitters. These drugs, which are called catecholamines, include norepinephrine, epinephrine, and dopamine. Synthetic catecholamines are also available. They include dobutamine and isoproterenol. Noncatecholamine adrenergic agents, including ephedrine, phenylephrine, and terbutaline, also affect the adrenergic receptors and have useful clinical applications.

Almost all the drugs in this section act on more than one type of receptor. Their specificity varies and is important in determining their uses. Table 14-5 lists their actions on various receptors.

Adrenergic Antagonists Unlike most adrenergic agonists, the majority of available adrenergic antagonists are remarkably selective in which receptor they affect. This selectivity, however, occurs only at therapeutic doses. At higher doses, most agents lose their selectivity and begin affecting other receptors as well.

The two basic subcategories of alpha adrenergic antagonists are noncompetitive long-acting and competitive short-acting. They differ chiefly in the stability of their bond with the receptor. The prototype noncompetitive long-acting alpha antagonist is phenoxybenzamine (Dibenzyline). The prototype competitive

> **Content Review**
>
> **COMMON CATECHOLAMINES**
> * Natural
>   - Epinephrine
>   - Norepinephrine
>   - Dopamine
> * Synthetic
>   - Isoproterenol
>   - Dobutamine

Table 14-5   ADRENERGIC RECEPTOR SPECIFICITY

Medication	Receptor				
	Alpha$_1$	**Alpha$_2$**	**Beta$_1$**	**Beta$_2$**	**Dopaminergic**
Phenylephrine	✔				
Norepinephrine	✔	✔	✔		
Ephedrine	✔	✔	✔	✔	
Epinephrine	✔	✔	✔	✔	
Dobutamine			✔		
Dopamine*			✔		✔
Isoproterenol			✔	✔	
Terbutaline				✔	

*Receptor specificity is dose dependent. The higher the dose, the less dopaminergic effects are seen.

short-acting antagonist is prazosin (Minipress). Prazosin also is the prototype for all alpha adrenergic antagonists. Phentolamine (Regitine) is an important nonselective alpha antagonist because of its effects in reversing tissue necrosis caused by catecholamine infiltration.

Beta adrenergic antagonists are more commonly referred to as beta-blockers. Propranolol (Inderal) is the prototype beta-blocker. It is a nonselective antagonist, which means that it blocks both beta$_1$ and beta$_2$ receptors. It is used to treat tachycardia, hypertension, and angina, all results of beta$_1$ blockade. Because it is nonselective, it also has the side effects of beta$_2$ blockade—bronchoconstriction and inhibited glycogenolysis. Propranolol was the first clinically employed beta-blocker, but its use has declined since the development of more selective beta$_1$ antagonists. The prototype of these cardioselective beta-blockers is metoprolol (Lopressor). At normal doses, metoprolol is selective for only beta$_1$ receptors; therefore, it does not cause propranolol's problematic side effects for asthmatics and diabetics. Atenolol (Tenormin) is another commonly used cardioselective beta-blocker.

Skeletal Muscle Relaxants Skeletal muscle relaxants are used to treat muscle spasm from injury and muscle spasticity from CNS injuries or diseases such as multiple sclerosis. Treatment can involve centrally acting agents or direct acting agents.

The centrally acting muscle relaxants' mechanism is not clear, but it appears to be associated with general sedation. The prototype centrally acting skeletal muscle relaxant is baclofen (Lioresal), which is indicated in the treatment of spasticity. Although baclofen is effective in the treatment of muscle spasticity, it is generally ineffective in muscle spasm. Several drugs are effective in treating muscle spasm, including cyclobenzaprine (Flexeril) and carisoprodol (Soma).

The prototype of the direct acting muscle relaxants is dantrolene (Dantrium). Unlike the centrally acting agents, dantrolene's mechanism is well understood. It decreases the release of calcium from the sarcoplasmic reticulum in response to action potentials propagated from the neuromuscular junction. This calcium is required for the cross-bridge binding of the actin and myosin filaments in the muscle fibres responsible for contraction. Dantrolene is indicated for treating the spasticity associated with multiple sclerosis and cerebral palsy. It is also indicated for treating malignant hyperthermia, which is, on rare occasion, seen with some anesthetics and succinylcholine. This hyperthermia results from muscular contractions. Since dantrolene decreases these contractions, the heat that they generate also decreases. Dantrolene is not effective in treating muscle spasm.

DRUGS USED TO AFFECT THE CARDIOVASCULAR SYSTEM

Cardiovascular drugs have traditionally composed one of the largest parts of the paramedic's pharmacological "tool box." Although this is changing with the expansion of paramedic practice, cardiovascular care (and agents used in that care) remains an important and integral part of a paramedic's knowledge base.

CLASSES OF CARDIOVASCULAR DRUGS

The drugs used to treat cardiovascular disease generally fall into the two broad functional classifications of antidysrhythmics and antihypertensives.

Antidysrhythmics

Antidysrhythmic drugs (Table 14-6) are used to treat and prevent abnormal cardiac rhythms. Used inappropriately, these medications can also cause dysrhythmias or deterioration in existing rhythms.

✱ **antidysrhythmic** drug used to treat and prevent abnormal cardiac rhythms.

Table 14-6 ANTIDYSRHYTHMIC CLASSIFICATIONS AND EXAMPLES

General Action	Class	Prototype	ECG Effects
Sodium Channel Blockers	IA	Quinidine,* procainamide, disopyramide	Widened QRS, prolonged QT
	IB	Lidocaine,* phenytoin, tocainide, mexiletine	Widened QRS, prolonged QT
	IC	Flecainide,* propafenone	Prolonged PR, widened QRS
	I (Misc.)	Moricizine*	Prolonged PR, widened QRS
Beta-Blockers	II	Propranolol,* acebutolol, esmolol	Prolonged PR, bradycardias
Potassium Channel Blockers	III	Bretylium,* amiodarone	Prolonged QT
Calcium Channel Blockers	IV	Verapamil,* diltiazem	Prolonged PR, bradycardias
Miscellaneous		Adenosine, digoxin	Prolonged PR, bradycardias

* prototype

Sodium Channel Blockers (Class I) All the medications in this general class affect the sodium influx in phases 0 and 4 of fast potentials. This slows the propagation of impulses down the specialized conduction system of the atria and ventricles, although it does not affect the SA or AV node.

Class IA drugs include quinidine (Quinidex), procainamide (Pronestyl), and disopyramide (Norpace). In addition to slowing conduction, these drugs also decrease the repolarization rate. This widens the QRS complex and prolongs the QT interval. Quinidine is the prototype for this class, but procainamide is administered more frequently in emergency medicine. Procainamide is indicated in the treatment of atrial fibrillation with rapid ventricular response and ventricular dysrhythmias. Quinidine has a similar mechanism of action, but it also has anticholinergic properties that may induce unintended tachycardias.

Class IB drugs include lidocaine (Xylocaine), phenytoin (Dilantin), tocainide (Tonocard) and mexiletine (Mexitil). Unlike Class IA drugs, Class IB drugs increase the rate of repolarization. They also reduce automaticity in ventricular cells, which makes them effective in treating rhythms originating from ectopic ventricular foci. Lidocaine is the drug of choice for treating ventricular tachycardia and ventricular fibrillation. Although lidocaine was once used prophlactically for patients with myocardial infarction, its use is now limited to life-threatening dysrhythmias. When given in overdose, lidocaine has significant CNS side effects, including tinnitus, confusion, and convulsions.

Class IC drugs include flecainide (Tambocor) and propafenone (Rythmol). They decrease conduction velocity through the atria and ventricles as well as through the bundle of His and the Purkinje network. Like the Class IA drugs, they delay ventricular repolarization. Both of these medications, which are administered orally, are given to prevent recurrence of ventricular dysrhythmias, but both also have prodysrhythmic properties; that is, they are likely to cause dysrhythmias as well as treat them. They also depress myocardial contractility and are therefore reserved for potentially lethal ventricular dysrhythmias that do not respond to any other conventional therapy.

Moricizine (Ethmozine) has additional properties that exclude it from the other Class I subclasses. It blocks sodium influx during fast potential depolarization, thereby decreasing conduction velocity, but it can also depress myocardial contractility. Like the Class IC drugs, it is reserved for the treatment of ventricular dysrhythmias refractory to other conventional therapy.

Content Review

Antidysrhythmics are routinely classified in the Vaughn-Williams and Singh Classification System.

- I: Na^+ channel blockers
  - –1A
  - –1B
  - –1C
- II: Beta-blockers
- III: K^+ channel blockers
- IV: Miscellaneous

Beta-Blockers (Class II) The drugs in this class, propranolol (Inderal), acebutolol (Sectral) and esmolol (Brevibloc) are all beta adrenergic antagonists. Propranolol is nonselective, while acebutolol and esmolol are both selective for the $beta_1$ receptors in the heart. Of the many beta-blockers, these are the only ones approved for the treatment of dysrhythmias. They are indicated in the treatment of tachycardias resulting from excessive sympathetic stimulation. The $beta_1$ receptor in the heart is attached to the calcium channels. Blocking the $beta_1$ receptors thus blocks the calcium channel and prevents the gradual influx of calcium in phase 0 of the slow potential. As a result, the effects of beta-blocker therapy on dysrhythmias are almost identical to those of calcium channel blockers. Propranolol is the prototype Class II drug. Because it is nonselective, it also blocks the effect of $beta_2$ receptors, which leads to many of its side effects.

Potassium Channel Blockers (Class III) Potassium-channel-blocking drugs are also known as antiadrenergic medications because of their complex actions on sympathetic terminals. They include bretylium (Bretylol) and amiodarone (Cordarone); bretylium is the prototype. They act on the potassium channels in the fast potentials. By blocking the efflux of potassium, bretylium prolongs repolarization and the effective refractory period. It is indicated in the treatment of ventricular fibrillation and refractory ventricular tachycardia. It causes an initial release, then an inhibition, of norepinephrine at the sympathetic end terminals. This delayed repolarization prolongs the QT interval; consequently, bretylium's primary and frequent side effect is hypotension.

Calcium Channel Blockers (Class IV) Calcium channel blockers' effect on the heart is almost identical to that of beta-blockers. They decrease SA and AV node automaticity, but most of their usefulness arises from decreasing conductivity through the AV node. They effectively slow the ventricular conduction of atrial fibrillation and flutter, and they can terminate supraventricular tachycardias originating from a reentrant circuit. Verapamil (Isoptin) and diltiazem (Cardizem) are the only two calcium channel blockers that affect the heart. Verapamil is the prototype. Their chief side effect is hypotension and bradycardia.

Miscellaneous Antidysrhythmics Adenosine (Adenocard) and digoxin (Lanoxin) are both effective antidysrhythmics. Magnesium is the drug of choice in *torsade de pointes,* a type of polymorphic ventricular tachycardia. We will briefly discuss each.

Adenosine does not fit any of the previous categories. It is an endogenous nucleoside with a very short half-life (about 10 seconds). It acts on both potassium and calcium channels, increasing potassium efflux and inhibiting calcium influx. This results in a hyperpolarization that effectively slows the conduction of slow potentials, such as those found in the SA and AV nodes. It has little effect on the fast potentials in the ventricles and is not particularly effective on ventricular tachycardias or atrial fibrillation or flutter. Because of its short half-life, its side effects are short lived, but they can be alarming. They include facial flushing, shortness of breath, chest pain, and marked bradycardias. Adenosine must be given as a rapid IV push, as the drug is rapidly metabolized. Doses should be increased in patients taking adenosine blockers, such as aminophylline or caffeine. They should be decreased in patients taking adenosine uptake inhibitors, such as dipyridamole (Persantine) and carbamazepine (Tegretol).

Digoxin (Lanoxin) is a paradoxical drug. Its many effects on the heart make it both an effective antidysrhythmic and a potent prodysrhythmic (generator of dysrhythmias). Although we do not clearly understand its specific actions on the heart's electrical activity, we do understand its effects. Digoxin decreases the intrinsic firing rate in the SA node, whereas it decreases conduction velocity in the AV node. Both of these effects are due to its increasing the strength of the parasympathetic effects on the heart. In the Purkinje fibres and ventricular myocardial cells, it decreases the effective refractory period and increases automaticity, both of which may explain its ability to increase ventricular dysrhythmias. To compound this, by depressing SA node activity, digoxin makes ectopic ventricular beats more likely to assume the pacing activity of the heart. Its side effects include bradycardias, AV blocks, PVCs, ventricular tachycardia, ventricular fibrillation, and atrial fibrillation. Actually, there are few dysrhythmias that digoxin does not produce. In addition, digoxin has a very narrow therapeutic index, meaning that it is difficult to find a patient's effective dose without producing side effects. Digoxin also increases cardiac contractility. It is indicated for atrial fibrillation with rapid ventricular conduction and chronic treatment of congestive heart failure.

Magnesium is the drug of choice in *torsade de pointes*, a polymorphic ventricular tachycardia, and in other ventricular dysrhythmias refractory to other therapy. Its mechanism of action is not known, but it may act on the sodium or potassium channels or on $Na^+K^+ATPase$.

Antihypertensives

Hypertension is a major contributor to coronary artery disease, stroke, and blindness. Fortunately, available drugs can effectively manage blood pressure in the vast majority of patients with limited side effects. Multiple studies have shown conclusively that controlling blood pressure decreases both morbidity and mortality. Blood pressure is equal to cardiac output times the peripheral vascular resistance:

$$blood\ pressure = cardiac\ output \times peripheral\ vascular\ resistance$$

Cardiac output is equal to the heart rate times the stroke volume:

$$cardiac\ output = heart\ rate \times stroke\ volume$$

Antihypertensive agents can manipulate each of these factors. The primary determinant of peripheral vascular resistance is the diameter of peripheral arterioles, which are affected by alpha$_1$ receptors. Heart rate is affected by both muscarinic receptors of the parasympathetic nervous system and beta$_1$ receptors of the sympathetic nervous system; however, hypertension control typically manipulates only beta$_1$ receptors. Stroke volume is affected by contractility and volume. Recall Starling's law, which states that preload and stroke volume are proportionate; that is, as preload increases, stroke volume increases (up to a point); and as preload decreases, stroke volume decreases. Drugs that affect blood volume control hypertension by manipulating preload.

Several pharmacological classes of medications are used to control blood pressure. The major approaches to dealing with hypertension are diuretics, beta-blockers and other antiadrenergic drugs, angiotensin-converting enzyme (ACE) inhibitors, calcium channel blockers, and direct vasodilators. Of these, diuretics and beta-blockers are the most frequently prescribed, and they are effective in many patients. The remaining agents are used when diuretics or beta-blockers are contraindicated or when those approaches are not effective, although ACE inhibitors are gaining increasing popularity. Often, physicians must prescribe multiple drugs to manage hypertension effectively. In these cases, they will pick one drug from two or more classes that complement each other. For example, a physician might prescribe a diuretic with a beta-blocker.

Diuretics Diuretics reduce circulating blood volume by increasing the amount of urine. This reduces preload to the heart, which, in turn, reduces cardiac output. The main categories of diuretics include loop diuretics (high-ceiling diuretics), thiazides, and potassium-sparing diuretics. They all affect the reabsorption of sodium and chloride and create an osmotic gradient that decreases the reabsorption of water. These classes differ according to which area of the nephron

> ### Content Review
> ### PHARMACOLOGICAL CLASSES OF ANTIHYPERTENSIVES
> - Diuretics
> - Beta-blockers and antiadrenergic drugs
> - ACE inhibitors
> - Calcium channel blockers
> - Direct vasodilators

✱ **antihypertensive** drug used to treat hypertension.

✱ **diuretic** drug used to reduce circulating blood volume by increasing the amount of urine.

they affect. In general, the earlier in the nephron the drug works, the more sodium and water will be affected. Almost all electrolytes and other small particles in the blood are filtered through the glomerulus. Most sodium and water (approximately 65 percent) is reabsorbed in the proximal convoluted tubule. Another 20 percent is reabsorbed in the thick portion of the ascending loop of Henle, while only about 1 to 5 percent is recaptured in the distal convoluted tubule and collecting duct. Therefore, a drug that decreases sodium reabsorption in the proximal convoluted tubule will cause the kidneys to excrete more water than will a drug that works on the distal convoluted tubule.

Loop diuretics profoundly affect circulating blood volume. In fact, they decrease blood volume so well that they are typically considered excessive for treating moderate hypertension. They are, however, one of the primary tools in treating left ventricular heart failure (congestive heart failure). Their use for hypertension is typically because other diuretics have failed. Furosemide (Lasix) is the prototype of this class. Furosemide blocks sodium reabsorption in the thick portion of the ascending loop of Henle (hence, the name *loop diuretic*). In doing so, it decreases the pull of water from the tubule and into the capillary bed, thus decreasing fluid volume. Furosemide's main side effects are hyponatremia, hypovolemia, hypokalemia, and dehydration. Because the decrease in volume is most noticeable as decreased preload, orthostatic hypotension is a problem. Reflex tachycardia may also occur as the baroreceptors detect decreased blood pressure and attempt to compensate by increasing the heart rate. This happens in individuals with hypertension because the homeostatic thermostat has been set too high. In other words, the body believes that what is actually hypertension is normal and tries to maintain a higher blood pressure than is healthy. This reflex tachycardia is frequently treated with concurrent administration of a loop diuretic with a beta$_1$ blocker. Hypokalemia is frequently treated by increasing dietary potassium intake (bananas are rich in potassium) or by prescribing potassium supplements. An unexplained side effect of loop diuretics is ototoxicity (tinnitus and deafness). Administering loop diuretics slowly can decrease ototoxicity.

Thiazides have a mechanism similar to loop diuretics. The main difference is that the thiazides' mechanism affects the early part of the distal convoluted tubules and therefore cannot block as much sodium from reabsorption. Thiazides are often the drugs of choice in hypertension treatment because they can decrease fluid volume sufficiently to prevent hypertension but not so much that they promote hypotension. The prototype thiazide is hydrochlorothiazide (HydroDIURIL). This class has essentially the same side effects as loop diuretics. One important distinction is that thiazides depend on the glomerular filtration rate, while loop diuretics do not. Thus, loop diuretics may be preferred for patients with renal disease.

Potassium-sparing diuretics have a slightly different mechanism than do other diuretics. Although they still affect sodium absorption, they do so by inhibiting either the effects of aldosterone on the distal tubules (as does spironolactone) or the specific sodium-potassium exchange mechanism (as does triamterene). Acting so late in the nephritic loop, these agents are not very potent diuretics. In fact, they are rarely used alone but instead are typically administered in conjunction with either a loop diuretic or a thiazide diuretic. They are useful as adjuncts to other diuretics because they not only decrease sodium reabsorption (although in small volumes) but also increase potassium reabsorption. This helps limit the other diuretics' hypokalemic effects. Spironolactone (Aldactone) is the prototype potassium-sparing diuretic.

Although not used in the treatment of hypertension, osmotic diuretics are important because they alter the reabsorption of water in the proximal convoluted tubule. To do this, they use an osmotically large sugar molecule that is freely filtered through the glomerulus and pulls water after it. Mannitol (Osmitrol), the prototype osmotic diuretic, is used to treat increased intracranial and intraocular pressure.

Loop diuretics, particularly furosemide (Lasix), play a major role in the emergency treatment of CHF and acute pulmonary edema.

Adrenergic-Inhibiting Agents Inhibiting the effects of adrenergic stimulation can also control hypertension. Several broad mechanisms accomplish this: beta adrenergic antagonism, centrally acting alpha adrenergic antagonism, adrenergic neuron blockade, $alpha_1$ blockade, and alpha/beta blockade.

Beta Adrenergic Antagonists From Table 14-4 in our earlier discussion of $beta_1$ blockers, you will recall that most $beta_1$ receptors are in the heart but some also exist in the juxtaglomerular cells of the kidney. Selective $beta_1$ blockade is useful in treating hypertension for several reasons. It decreases contractility, thereby directly decreasing cardiac output. It also reduces reflex tachycardia by inhibiting sympathetically induced compensatory increases in heart rate. Finally, it represses renin release from the kidneys, which, in turn, inhibits the vasoconstriction activated by the renin-angiotensin-aldosterone system. The prototype selective $beta_1$ blocker is metropolol (Lopressor); the prototype nonselective beta-blocker is propranolol (Inderal). The section on $beta_1$ blockers discussed these agents' side effects.

Beta-blockers have proven to decrease both short-term and long-term mortality associated with acute MI.

Centrally Acting Adrenergic Inhibitors Centrally acting adrenergic inhibitors reduce hypertension by inhibiting CNS stimulation of adrenergic receptors. In effect, they are CNS $alpha_2$ agonists. Recall that $alpha_2$ receptors are located on the presynaptic end terminals in the sympathetic nervous system. When stimulated, they inhibit the release of norepinephrine to counterbalance sympathetic stimulation. By increasing the stimulation of $alpha_2$ receptors in the section of the CNS responsible for cardiovascular regulation, centrally acting adrenergic inhibitors decrease the sympathetic stimulation of both $alpha_1$ and $beta_2$ receptors. The net effect is to decrease heart rate and contractility by decreasing release of norepinephrine at $beta_1$ receptors and to promote vasodilation by decreasing norepinephrine release at $alpha_1$ receptors at vascular smooth muscle. The prototype drug in this category is clonidine (Catapres). Although it does have some side effects, notably drowsiness and dry mouth, clonidine is a relatively safe and frequently prescribed antihypertensive agent. Methyldopa (Aldomet) is another centrally acting antihypertensive with a mechanism similar to clonidine.

Peripheral Adrenergic Neuron-Blocking Agents Like the centrally acting adrenergic inhibitors, peripheral adrenergic neuron-blocking agents work indirectly to decrease stimulation of adrenergic receptors. They do this by decreasing the amount of norepinephrine released from sympathetic presynaptic terminals. These agents are no longer commonly used.

The prototype of this class is reserpine (Serpalan). Reserpine has two actions that decrease the amount of norepinephrine released. First, it decreases the synthesis of norepinephrine. Second, it exposes norepinephrine in the terminal vesicles to monoamine oxidase, an enzyme that destroys it. This decreases stimulation of $alpha_1$ receptors, resulting in peripheral vasodilation, and of $beta_1$ receptors, resulting in decreased heart rate and contractility. The decreased peripheral vascular resistance and cardiac output, in turn, lower blood pressure.

Reserpine also decreases synthesis of several CNS neurotransmitters (serotonin and other catecholamines). This causes reserpine's primary adverse effect, depression. Reserpine, therefore, is not frequently used as an antihypertensive. Additional side effects include gastrointestinal cramps and increased stomach acid production. Other drugs with similar actions include guanethidine (Ismeline) and guanadrel (Hylorel).

Alpha1 Antagonists This chapter's section on drugs affecting the sympathetic nervous system discusses the $alpha_1$ receptor antagonists in detail. Only their specific action will be repeated here. The prototype selective $alpha_1$ antagonist is prazosin (Minipress). It decreases blood pressure by competitively blocking the $alpha_1$ receptors, thereby inhibiting the sympathetically mediated increases in peripheral vascular resistance. By causing the arterioles to dilate, prazosin directly decreases afterload. By causing the venules to dilate, it promotes venous pooling, which decreases preload. The decreased afterload and preload help to lower blood pressure. Terazosin (Hytrin) is another drug with similar properties.

Combined Alpha/Beta Antagonists Labetalol (Normodyne) and carvedilol (Coreg) competitively bind with both alpha$_1$ and beta$_1$ receptors, increasing their antihypertensive actions. Hypertension is treated by decreasing alpha$_1$-mediated vasoconstriction, which, again, decreases both preload and afterload. Beta$_1$ blockade decreases heart rate, contractility, and renin release from kidneys. By blocking the release of renin, which promotes vasoconstriction, these agents decrease peripheral vascular resistance even further. Labetalol is commonly used to treat hypertensive crisis and is rapidly replacing the use of sublingual nifedipine (Procardia) for this purpose.

Angiotensin-Converting Enzyme (ACE) Inhibitors Agents in this class interrupt the renin-angiotensin-aldosterone system (RAAS) by preventing the conversion of angiotensin I to angiotensin II. Angiotensin II is one of the most potent vasoconstrictors yet discovered. By decreasing the amount of circulating angiotensin II, peripheral vascular resistance can be decreased, which leads to a decrease in blood pressure.

The juxtaglomerular apparatus in the kidneys releases renin in response to decreases in blood volume, sodium concentration, and blood pressure. Renin acts as an enzyme to convert the inactive protein angiotensinogen into angiotensin I. Neither angiotensinogen nor angiotensin I has much pharmaceutical effect, but angiotensin-converting enzyme (ACE) almost immediately converts angiotensin I in the blood into angiotensin II. (ACE is found in the lumen of almost all vessels and is found in the lungs in very high concentrations.) Angiotensin II causes both systemic and local vasoconstriction, with more pronounced effects on arterioles than on venules. It also lessens water loss by decreasing renal filtration secondary to renal vasoconstriction. Finally, angiotensin II also increases the release of aldosterone, a corticosteroid produced in the adrenal cortex. Aldosterone, in turn, increases sodium and water reabsorption in the distal convoluted tubule of the nephrons.

Angiotensin-converting enzyme inhibitors are very effective in treating hypertension and have also shown success in managing heart failure and renal failure. ACE inhibitors block the conversion of angiotensin I to angiotensin II, thereby providing a host of beneficial effects for patients with hypertension. These include a rapid decrease in arteriolar constriction, which lowers peripheral vascular resistance and afterload. Although it does cause some dilation of the venules, this effect is limited. Because of the limited decrease in preload, orthostatic hypotension, common in other antihypertensives, is not a significant concern with ACE inhibitors. These agents also appear to be effective in preventing some of the untoward structural changes in the heart and blood vessels that angiotensin II causes over time.

In addition to their role in the treatment of hypertension, ACE inhibitors play an important role in the treatment of CHF by decreasing afterload.

The prototype ACE inhibitor is captopril (Capoten). Captopril acts like all ACE inhibitors to prevent hypertension. Its main advantage is the absence of side effects common to other antihypertensives. It does not interfere with beta receptors, and so it does not decrease the ability to exercise or respond to hemorrhage. It does not cause potassium loss like many diuretics, and it does not cause depression or drowsiness. Because it has no effect on sexual desire or performance, it is much more attractive to many patients who might not comply with other medications. Other common ACE inhibitors include enalapril (Vasotec) and lisinopril (Zestril). These medications are all taken orally. For intravenous use in hypertensive crisis, enalaprilat (Vasotec I.V.) is available.

The most dangerous side effect of ACE inhibitors is pronounced hypotension after the first dose. This can be minimized by reducing initial doses, and it does not recur. The main adverse effects of continual use are a persistent cough and angioedema.

Angiotensin II Receptor Antagonists This recently developed classification of antihypertensive drugs also acts on the renin-angiotensin-aldosterone system. Angiotensin II receptor antagonists achieve the same effects as the ACE inhibitors without the side effects of cough or angioedema. The prototype of this new class is losartan (Cozaar).

Calcium Channel-Blocking Agents We have already discussed two calcium channel blockers, verapamil and diltiazem, in the section on antidysrhythmics. Another structural subclass of calcium channel blockers is the dihydropyridines. The prototype dihydropyridine is nifedipine (Procardia, Adalat). Nifedipine, as well as the other members of the dihydropyridines, differ from verapamil and diltiazem in that they do not affect the calcium channels of the heart at therapeutic doses. Rather, they act only on the vascular smooth muscle of the arterioles. These agents act by blocking the calcium channels in the arterioles. Calcium, which is required for muscle contraction, is released from sarcoplasmic reticulum on activation by an action potential. When it enters the muscle cell through calcium channels, muscle contraction ensues. Blocking the calcium channels prevents the arterioles' smooth muscle from contracting and therefore dilates these vessels. When this occurs, peripheral vascular resistance decreases and blood pressure falls as a result of lower afterload. Because nifedipine has little effect on veins, it does not cause a corresponding drop in preload and consequently avoids orthostatic hypotension. Although nifedipine does not affect the cardiac electrical conduction system, it is effective in dilating the coronary arteries and arterioles and thereby helps increase coronary perfusion. The primary indications for nifedipine are angina pectoris and chronic treatment of hypertension. Its primary side effects include reflex tachycardia (responding to a baroreceptor to decreased blood pressure), facial flushing, dizziness, headache, and peripheral edema. It has been used commonly for the emergent reduction of blood pressure in the field; however, labetalol is replacing it.

Nifedipine was used extensively for emergent reduction of blood pressure. Now, other agents, such as labetalol, are preferred.

Direct Vasodilators We have already discussed several drugs that cause vasodilation. Two specific classes of vasodilators are those that dilate arterioles and those that dilate both arterioles and veins. All these drugs are used to decrease blood pressure.

Selective dilation of arterioles causes a decrease in peripheral vascular resistance or afterload. This is the resistance that the heart must overcome in order to eject blood. Decreasing peripheral vascular resistance lowers blood pressure, increases cardiac output, and reduces cardiac workload. Conversely, dilating the veins increases capacitance and decreases preload, the amount of blood in the heart before contraction. Starling's law tells us that as preload increases, so do stroke volume and cardiac output (up to a point). By decreasing preload, venodilators decrease both blood pressure and cardiac output.

Hydralizine (Apresoline) is the prototype for the selective arteriole dilators. It is effective in decreasing peripheral vascular resistance and afterload and thus lowering blood pressure. Its primary side effects are reflex tachycardia and increased blood volume. Both occur as a compensatory mechanism to lowered blood pressure, and both have the effect of increasing cardiac workload. As a result, hydralazine is almost always prescribed in conjunction with a beta-blocker and a diuretic. It is frequently used in the treatment of pregnancy-induced hypertension.

Minoxidil (Loniten) is another selective arteriole dilator with properties similar to those of hydralazine. One side effect deserves comment. It produces hypertrichosis (excessive hair growth) in about 80 percent of those taking it. Although this is particularly irritating when it occurs all over a patient's body, it can become a therapeutic effect when the drug is applied as a topical ointment. Minoxidil is marketed in this form as Rogaine to treat hair loss.

Unlike hydralazine, sodium nitroprusside (Nipride) acts on both arterioles and veins. It is the fastest-acting antihypertensive available and is the drug of

Hydralizine (Apresoline) is the preferred antihypertensive for the management of pregnancy-induced hypertension.

choice in hypertensive emergencies. It is very potent and is given via controlled IV infusion. Its effects are almost immediate and end within minutes of drug cessation; therefore, blood pressure must be carefully and continuously monitored during infusion, preferably in the ICU. Sodium nitroprusside has several significant side effects. Obviously, hypotension can be a problem when this medication is not carefully administered. Because cyanide and thyocyanate are byproducts of nitroprusside metabolism, other adverse effects include cyanide poisoning and thyocyanate toxicity.

Ganglionic-Blocking Agents Ganglionic-blocking agents are nicotinic$_N$ antagonists. The prototype is trimethaphan (Arfonad). Since nicotinic$_N$ receptors exist at the ganglia of both the sympathetic and the parasympathetic nervous systems, competitive antagonism of these receptors turns off the entire autonomic nervous system, obviously not a very selective approach. When this happens, the effects on each organ system are determined by the predominant autonomic tone (the division of the ANS that normally has the greater influence on that organ). Because the arteries and veins have predominant sympathetic control, they dilate in response to trimethaphan administration. This reduces both preload and afterload, and blood pressure drops. Trimethaphan also directly affects vascular smooth muscle, causing dilation and the release of histamine, which is also a vasodilator.

Cardiac Glycosides The cardiac glycosides occur naturally in the foxglove plant. The two drugs in the class, digoxin (Lanoxin) and digitoxin (Crystodigin), are chemically related. These drugs are also known as digitalis glycosides. Digoxin is the prototype. One of the 10 most frequently prescribed medications in North America, it is indicated for heart failure and some types of dysrhythmias. Digoxin's mechanism of action is complex. It blocks the effects of Na$^+$K$^+$ATPase, an enzyme responsible for returning ion flow to normal levels after muscle depolarization. By interfering with this sodium-potassium pump, digoxin increases the intracellular levels of sodium. Because sodium is also involved in a reciprocal exchange with calcium, a buildup of intracellular sodium leads to a similar buildup of intracellular calcium. These elevated levels of intracellular calcium increase the strength of muscle contraction and are the basis for digoxin's primary indication. Digoxin reduces the symptoms of congestive heart failure by increasing myocardial contractility and cardiac output. This diminishes the dilation of the heart's chambers frequently seen in left heart failure because it enables the heart to effectively pump blood out of its ventricles, thus decreasing the engorgement typical of this condition. Increasing cardiac output decreases the sympathetic discharge mediated by baroreceptor reflexes, resulting in reduced afterload. Furthermore, digoxin indirectly lessens preload by increasing renal blood flow, which results in higher glomerular filtration and decreased blood volume. Digoxin also has antidysrhythmic effects, which we discuss more thoroughly in the section on antidysrhythmic medications.

Although digoxin effectively treats the symptoms of heart failure, it also is potentially dangerous. Its therapeutic index is very small, and the individual variability is large. This leads to toxicity in some individuals, even though they have normal digoxin levels. Digoxin's chief adverse effects are dysrhythmias. In fact, digoxin frequently induces some of the same dysrhythmias it is used to treat. Other side effects include fatigue, anorexia, nausea and vomiting, and blurred vision with a yellowish haze and halos around dark objects.

Other Vasodilators and Antianginals The drugs discussed in this section have vasodilatory properties that are useful in reducing blood pressure, but they are most commonly used to treat angina. The three basic types of angina pectoris (chest pain) are stable (exertional) angina; unstable angina; and variant, or Prinzmetal's, angina. Stable and unstable angina have the same pathophysiology and differ only by causation: stable angina occurs after exercise as a result of increased myocardial oxygen demand; unstable angina occurs without exertion.

Digitalis (Lanoxin) is still frequently used to increase cardiac output in CHF and to control the rate of ventricular response in atrial fibrillation.

Both result from an imbalance between myocardial supply and demand. A buildup of plaque (atherosclerosis) along the walls of coronary arteries decreases these vessels' diameter and, as a result, the amount of blood flow to the heart. The same imbalance causes Prinzmetal's angina but it results from vasospasm instead of plaque buildup. The medications discussed in this section all either increase oxygen supply or decrease oxygen demand.

In addition to their previously discussed use as antihypertensives and anti-dysrhythmics, calcium channel blockers have a role in the treatment of angina. The three calcium channel blockers most frequently used for this purpose are verapamil (Calan, Isoptin), diltiazem (Cardizem), and nifedipine (Procardia). Recall that calcium is an integral part of both depolarization and muscle contraction. The effects of blocking its entry into the cells are twofold. All these agents directly affect vascular smooth muscle, leading to dilation of the arterioles and, to a lesser degree, of the venules. This arterial dilation decreases peripheral vascular resistance and, as a result, afterload, which, in turn, directly decreases the workload of the heart and myocardial oxygen demand. Verapamil and diltiazem also reduce SA and AV node conductivity, which can decrease reflex tachycardia and dysrhythmias. Nifedipine has relatively few effects on the heart and thus has limited antidysrhythmic properties. The calcium channel blockers are effective in all forms of angina. A primary side effect of these agents is hypotension.

Organic nitrates are potent vasodilators used to treat all forms of angina. First used clinically in 1879, nitroglycerine (Nitrostat) is the oldest of these drugs and is the category's prototype. Other agents include isosorbide (Isordil, Sorbitrate) and amyl nitrite. Nitroglycerine acts on vascular smooth muscle via a complex series of events to decrease intracellular calcium, thus causing vasodilation. Nitroglycerine primarily dilates veins, rather than arterioles. This decreases preload and thus decreases myocardial workload, which is its primary antianginal effect. In Prinzmetal's angina, nitroglycerine reverses coronary artery spasm and increases oxygen supply.

Nitroglycerine is effective in the management of angina pectoris as it decreases cardiac work.

Nitroglycerine is very lipid soluble, which allows it to cross membranes easily. Because of this, it is readily absorbed and can be administered via sublingual, buccal, and transdermal routes. The primary concern with nitroglycerine is orthostatic hypotension, a side effect more common in the presence of right ventricular failure. Other common side effects include headache and reflex tachycardia. Headache is frequently used as an indicator of the effectiveness of nitroglycerine, which rapidly loses its potency when exposed to light. Although orthostatic hypotension is a serious concern with the administration of nitroglycerine, this condition typically responds well to fluid infusions.

Hemostatic Agents

Hemostasis is the stoppage of bleeding. It is a series of events in response to a tear in a blood vessel. Damage to the vessel's intima (innermost layer) exposes the underlying collagen and triggers a release of two naturally occurring substances, adenosine diphosphate (ADP) and thromboxane A_2 (TXA_2). Both ADP and TXA_2 stimulate the aggregation of platelets and vasoconstriction. The vasoconstriction decreases the flow of blood past the tear, thus allowing the newly "sticky" platelets to form a plug that temporarily occludes the bleeding.

Although this plug effectively halts bleeding for the short term, it must be reinforced to continue the stoppage until the tear can be permanently repaired. Stabilizing the plug requires a complex cascade of events involving the activation of naturally occurring factors and ending with the conversion of prothrombin into thrombin. The thrombin then converts fibrinogen into fibrin, a strand-like substance that attaches to the vessel's surface and contracts in a mesh web over the platelet plug to form a blood clot. Several of the factors involved need vitamin K

* **hemostasis** the stoppage of bleeding.

to carry out their functions. A vitamin K deficiency inhibits clotting and makes uncontrolled bleeding more likely. Conversely, limiting the clotting cascade to the immediate area of the vessel injury is important for obvious reasons. The protein antithrombin III is key in this process. Antithrombin III binds with several of the factors needed for clotting, thus inhibiting their ability to coagulate.

Once the vessel has been permanently repaired, the fibrin mesh must be broken down. This process, called fibrinolysis, involves another cascading system that ends with the activation of plasminogen into plasmin, which, in turn, breaks up the clot. Tissue plasminogen activator, a substance in the tissue, activates this last conversion.

Thrombi (blood clots that obstruct vessels or heart cavities) are the primary pathology in several clinical conditions, including myocardial infarction, stroke, and pulmonary embolism. Drugs can effectively treat the causes of these conditions by decreasing platelet aggregation (antiplatelet drugs), interfering with the clotting cascade (anticoagulants) or directly breaking up the thrombus (thrombolytics).

Antiplatelets Antiplatelet drugs decrease the formation of platelet plugs. The prototype antiplatelet drug is aspirin. Aspirin inhibits cyclo-oxygenase, an enzyme needed for the synthesis of thromboxane A_2 (TXA_2). Remember that TXA_2 causes platelets to aggregate and promotes local vasoconstriction. By inhibiting TXA_2, aspirin decreases the formation of platelet plugs and potential thrombi. Aspirin, as well as other antiplatelet and anticoagulant drugs, has no effect on existing thrombi; it only curbs the formation of new thrombi. Aspirin is indicated in the acute treatment of developing myocardial infarction. It is also useful in preventing the recurrence of MI and of ischemic stroke following transient ischemic attacks (TIAs).

One of aspirin's primary side effects is bleeding. Aspirin also may lead to an increase in gastric ulcers, which are a frequent source of gastrointestinal hemorrhage. By both stimulating the development of a potential source of bleeding as well as blocking an important mechanism for stopping that bleeding, aspirin can cause dangerous blood loss. Other antiplatelet drugs include dipyridamole (Persantine), Abciximab (ReoPro), and ticlopidine (Ticlid).

Anticoagulants Anticoagulants interrupt the clotting cascade. The two main types of anticoagulants are parenteral and oral. The prototype parenteral anticoagulant is heparin, a substance derived from the lungs of cattle or the intestines of pigs. Its primary mechanism of action is to enhance antithrombin III's ability to inhibit the clotting cascade. Because heparin is very polar, it is very poorly absorbed and must be given parenterally. Heparin injections and infusions are indicated in treating and preventing deep vein thrombosis, pulmonary embolism, and some forms of stroke. Heparin also is used frequently in conjunction with thrombolytics to treat myocardial infarction. Finally, it is used to keep rubber-capped IV catheters (Hep-Locks) free from clots. As you would expect, bleeding is heparin's primary side effect. Other untoward effects include thrombocytopenia (decreased platelet counts) and allergic reactions. Heparin is measured in units, rather than milligrams. A unit is that amount of heparin necessary to keep 1 mL of sheep plasma from clotting for one hour. Using this measurement is necessary because heparin's potency varies greatly when measured in milligrams.

Protamine sulphate is available as a heparin antagonist. Protamine can reverse the effects of heparin in the presence of dangerous and unintended bleeding by binding with heparin. This prevents heparin from binding with antithrombin III and enhancing its anticlotting abilities.

The prototype oral anticoagulant is warfarin (Coumadin). Warfarin's history serves as a useful reminder of its primary side effect. Warfarin was first developed as a rat poison that killed through uncontrolled bleeding. After noticing that a patient who attempted suicide by ingesting warfarin did not, in fact, die, its clinical use was investigated. Needless to say, this drug's primary side effect is bleeding.

Content Review

DRUGS USED TO TREAT THROMBI

- Antiplatelets
- Anticoagulants
- Thrombolytics

✱ **antiplatelet** drug that decreases the formation of platelet plugs.

✱ **anticoagulant** drug that interrupts the clotting cascade.

Warfarin prevents coagulation by antagonizing the effects of vitamin K, which is needed for the synthesis of multiple factors involved in the clotting cascade. It is prescribed for chronic use to prevent thrombi in high-risk patients, such as those who have hip replacements or artificial heart valves or those who are in atrial fibrillation. Because warfarin easily crosses the placental barrier and has dangerous *teratogenic* (capable of causing malformations) properties, it is contraindicated in pregnant patients. It also interacts adversely with many other medications. Like heparin, warfarin may lead to bleeding. In cases of overdose, you may give vitamin K as an antidote.

Thrombolytics Thrombolytics act directly on thrombi to break them up. The several available thrombolytics share a similar mechanism of action. The prototype drug of this class is streptokinase (Streptase). Other thrombolytics include alteplase (tPA), reteplase (Retavase), and anistreplase (Eminase). These medications all dissolve clots effectively; they differ primarily in their administration and risk of bleeding side effects.

* **thrombolytic** drug that acts directly on thrombi to break them down.

Streptokinase, which is derived from the *Streptococcus* bacterium, is the oldest available thrombolytic. Its mechanism of action is to promote plasminogen's conversion to plasmin. Since plasmin dissolves the fibrin mesh of clots, it can directly treat the cause of most myocardial infarctions and some strokes, as opposed to antiplatelet agents and anticoagulants, which can only prevent potential future thrombi. Streptokinase also breaks down fibrinogen, the precursor to fibrin. Although this action does not serve a clinical purpose (the problematic clot has already been formed), it does play an important role in streptokinase's chief side effect, bleeding. Other side effects include allergic reaction, hypotension, and fever.

Alteplase (Activase) is produced by recombinant DNA technology that is identical to the naturally occurring tissue plasminogen activator (hence its common name, tPA).

The window of opportunity for thrombolytic therapy is limited. Because of this, some EMS systems administer thrombolytics in the prehospital setting. Many have chosen to use reteplase (Retavase) because of its ease of administration (two 10-unit boluses administered 30 minutes apart).

Antihyperlipidemic Agents

Elevated levels of low-density lipoproteins (LDLs) have been clearly indicated as a causative factor in coronary artery disease. Lipoproteins are essentially transport mechanisms for lipids (triglycerides and cholesterol). Because lipids are insoluble in plasma, the body coats them in a plasma-soluble shell in order to transport them to their target destinations. Lipoproteins are categorized as very low-density (VLDL), low-density (LDL), intermediate-density (IDL), and high-density (HDL). Low-density lipoproteins contain most of the cholesterol in the blood and are required for transporting cholesterol from the liver to the peripheral tissues. Conversely, high-density lipoproteins (HDLs) carry cholesterol from the peripheral tissues to the liver, where it is broken down.

HDLs have been described as good cholesterol because they lower blood cholesterol levels and decrease the risk of coronary artery disease (CAD). LDLs are known as bad cholesterol because they increase blood cholesterol levels and the risk of CAD. As blood cholesterol levels increase, fatty plaque is deposited under the arteries' endothelial tissues. Atherosclerosis then develops, and coronary arteries decrease in diameter. Coronary vasoconstriction, in turn, reduces blood flow to the heart and, in times of increased myocardial oxygen demand, may lead to angina. Also, newly deposited plaque is often unstable. Typically, the plaque is under the endothelial tissues, which cap the plaque deposits. As the deposits age, the cap usually becomes fairly stable. In some cases, however, the cap breaks open and exposes the plaque to the blood. When this happens, platelet aggregation and coagulation begin. If the developing clot breaks free of the vessel, it becomes a thrombus and may completely occlude a coronary artery, leading to myocardial infarction.

The goal in lowering LDL levels is to prevent atherosclerosis and subsequent CAD. Although raising HDL levels would help accomplish this, no pharmaceutical means of doing so currently exists. By far, the best way to lower LDL levels remains dietary modification. If this is not sufficient, several classifications of **antihyperlipidemic** medications may be used. The most common are drugs that inhibit hydroxymethylglutaryl coenzyme A (HMG CoA) reductase. The liver must have HMG CoA to synthesize cholesterol. By inhibiting this enzyme, HMG CoA agents lower LDL levels; however, they also increase the number of LDL receptors in the liver, causing a further uptake of LDL.

Five HMG CoA reductase inhibitors are available. Because the names of all five end in *–statin,* these agents are also known as statins. They include lovastatin (Mevacor) and simvastatin (Zocor). Lovastatin is the HMG CoA reductase inhibitors' prototype. Overall, these drugs are well tolerated. Their chief side effects are headache, rash, and flushing. In rare cases, they may cause hepatotoxicity and lead to liver failure.

Bile-acid-binding resins can also reduce LDL levels. Inert substances that have no direct biological activity, these agents pass straight through the GI system without being absorbed and are excreted in feces. They are useful, however, in that they indirectly increase the number of LDL receptors in the liver by binding with bile acids, thus decreasing the bile acids' availability. Because the liver needs cholesterol to synthesize bile acids, it must have more cholesterol to compensate for the decrease in bile acids. The body therefore increases the LDL receptors on the liver. As more LDLs remain in the liver, their levels in the blood drop. Since the body does not absorb bile-acid-binding agents, they have no systemic effects. Their chief untoward effect is constipation. Cholestyramine (Questran) is the prototype.

DRUGS USED TO AFFECT THE RESPIRATORY SYSTEM

Drugs that affect the respiratory system are useful for several purposes. The most obvious is the treatment of asthma, but this class also includes cough suppressants, nasal decongestants, and antihistamines.

ANTIASTHMATIC MEDICATIONS

Asthma is a common disease that decreases pulmonary function and may limit daily activities. It typically presents with shortness of breath, wheezing, and coughing. Its basic pathophysiology has two components: bronchoconstriction and inflammation. Typically, a response to some sort of allergen sets both these processes in motion. Common culprits include pet dander, mould, and dust. In patients with existing asthma, cold air, tobacco smoke, or other pollutants may bring on acute episodes of shortness of breath.

The response to asthma typically begins with an allergen's binding to an antibody on mast cells. This causes the mast cell membrane to rupture and release its contents, including histamine, leukotrienes, and prostaglandins. These cause immediate bronchoconstriction followed by a slower inflammatory response that can lead to mucus plugs and a further decrease in airway size. The inflammation may, in turn, cause a hyperreactivity to stimuli, and allergens that might not normally produce dyspnea may lead to an acute attack.

✳ anithyperlipidemic drug used to treat high blood cholesterol.

Table 14-7 DRUGS USED IN THE TREATMENT OF ASTHMA

Mechanism of Action	Medication
Bronchodilators	
Nonspecific agonists	Epinephrine
	Ephedrine
Beta$_2$-specific agonists	
Inhaled (short-acting)	Salbutamol (Ventolin)
	Metaproterenol (Alupent)
	Terbutaline (Brethine)
	Bitolterol (Tornalate)
Inhaled (long-acting)	Salmeterol (Serevent)
Methylxanthines	Theophylline (Theo-Dur, Slo-Bid)
	Aminophylline
Anticholinergics	Atropine
	Ipratropium (Atrovent)
Anti-inflammatory agents	
Glucocorticoids	
Inhaled	Beclomethasone (Beclovent)
	Flucticasone (Flovent)
	Triamcinolone (Azmacort)
Oral	Prednisone (Deltasone)
Injected	Methylprednisolone (Solu-Medrol)
	Dexamethasone (Decadron)
Leukotriene Antagonists	Zafirlukast (Accolate)
	Zileuton (Zyflo)
Mast-Cell Membrane Stabilizer	Cromolyn (Intal)

Drug treatment of asthma aims to relieve bronchospasm and decrease inflammation. Specific approaches are categorized as beta$_2$ selective sympathomimetics, nonselective sympathomimetics, methylxanthines, anticholinergics, glucocorticoids, and leukotriene antagonists. Cromolyn (Nasalcrom), a frequently used anti-inflammatory agent, does not fit neatly into any of those categories. Table 14-7 summarizes these agents.

Beta$_2$-Specific Agents Drugs that are selective for beta$_2$ receptors are the mainstay in treating asthma-induced shortness of breath. Salbutamol (Ventolin) is the prototype of this class. In general, these agents relax bronchial smooth muscle, which results in bronchodilation and relief from bronchospasm. Agents from this class are first-line therapy for acute shortness of breath and may also be used daily for prophylaxis. Most are administered via metered dose inhaler or nebulizer. Salbutamol and terbutaline may both be taken orally, and terbutaline may be given by injection. These medications' beta$_2$ specificity is not absolute; some patients may experience beta$_1$ effects, such as tachycardia or dysrhythmias. Patients may also experience tremors resulting from the stimulation of beta$_2$ receptors in smooth muscles. Overall, these agents are very safe.

Nonselective Sympathomimetics Medications that stimulate both beta$_1$ and beta$_2$ receptors as well as alpha receptors are rarely used to treat asthma because they have the undesired effects of increased peripheral vascular resistance and increased risks for tachycardias and other dysrhythmias. Nonselective drugs include epinephrine, ephedrine, and isoproterenol. Epinephrine is the only nonselective sympathomimetic in common use today, due to the availability of selective

Drug treatment of asthma aims to relieve bronchospasm and decrease inflammation.

Early pharmacological intervention in asthma is important in order to minimize inflammation.

agents. It may be given subcutaneously for patients who have severe bronchospasm that does not respond to other treatments.

Methylxanthines The methylxanthines are CNS stimulants that have additional bronchodilatory properties. While they were once first-line therapy for asthma, now they are used only when other drugs, such as beta$_2$-specific agents, are ineffective. We do not know the methylxanthines' specific action, but they may block adenosine receptors. The prototype methylxanthine, theophylline, is taken orally. Aminophylline, an IV medication, is rapidly metabolized into theophylline and therefore has identical effects. These agents' chief side effects are nausea, vomiting, insomnia, restlessness, and dysrhythmias. Aminophylline is still used occasionally in the emergency treatment of acute asthma attacks.

Anticholinergics Ipratropium (Atrovent) is an atropine derivative given by nebulizer. Because stimulating the muscarinic receptors in the lungs results in constriction of bronchial smooth muscle, ipratropium, a muscarinic antagonist, causes bronchodilation. Ipratropium is inhaled and, therefore, has no systemic effects. Ipratropium and beta$_2$ agonists, such as salbutamol, act along different pathways, and so their concurrent administration has an additive effect. Ipratropium's most common side effect is dry mouth. It results from the local effects of the drug that remains in the oropharynx after administration.

Glucocorticoids Glucocorticoids have anti-inflammatory properties. They lower the production and release of inflammatory substances, such as histamine, prostaglandins, and leukotrienes, and they reduce mucus and edema secondary to decreasing vascular permeability. These drugs may be inhaled or taken orally, or they may be given intravenously in emergencies. The prototype inhaled glucocorticoid is beclomethasone; the prototype oral glucocorticoid is prednisone. Primarily preventative, they are taken on a regular schedule as opposed to the as-needed administration of the beta$_2$ agonists. An injectable glucocorticoid (methylprednisolone) is available for use secondary to beta$_2$ agonists in emergencies. When inhaled, glucocorticoids cause few side effects. Those are due mostly to direct exposure on the oropharynx, and gargling after taking the drug can decrease them. Likewise, side effects from the intravenous administrations of methylprednisolone in emergencies are not likely. Given orally or intravenously over long periods, however, glucocorticoids may have profound side effects, including adrenal suppression and hyperglycemia.

Another anti-inflammatory agent used to prevent asthma attacks is cromolyn (Intal), an inhaled powder. Although it is not a glucocorticoid, its actions are similar. Although the inhaled glucocorticoids are relatively safe, cromolyn is even safer. In fact, it is the safest of all antiasthma agents. Its only side effects are coughing or wheezing due to local irritation caused by the powder. Cromolyn is often used for preventing asthma in adults and children. It is also a useful prophylaxis before activities known to cause shortness of breath, such as exercise or mowing grass.

✱ leukotriene mediator released from mast cells on contact with allergens.

Leukotriene Antagonists Leukotrienes are mediators released from mast cells on contact with allergens. They contribute powerfully to both inflammation and bronchoconstriction. Consequently, agents that block their effects are useful in treating asthma. Leukotriene antagonists can either block the synthesis of leukotrienes or block their receptors. Zileuton (Zyflo) is the prototype of those that block the synthesis of leukotrienes. Zafirlukast (Accolate) is the prototype of those that block their receptors.

DRUGS USED FOR RHINITIS AND COUGH

Rhinitis (inflammation of the nasal lining) comprises a group of symptoms including nasal congestion, itching, redness, sneezing, and rhinorrhea (runny nose). Either allergic reactions or viral infections, such as the common cold, may cause it. Drugs that treat the symptoms of rhinitis and cold are commonly found in over-the-counter remedies. In addition, nasal decongestants, antihistamines, and cough suppressants are available in prescription medications. Although manufacturers of cold medications often combine several drugs in one product intended to treat multiple symptoms, we will discuss each class separately.

Nasal Decongestants Nasal congestion is caused by dilated and engorged nasal capillaries. Drugs that constrict these capillaries are effective nasal decongestants. The main pharmacological classification in this functional category is alpha$_1$ agonists. Alpha$_1$ agonists may be given either topically or orally. The chief examples of these agents, phenylephrine, pseudoephedrine, and phenylpropanolamine, can be administered either as a mist or in drops. Topical administration reduces systemic effects but has the undesired local effect of rebound congestion, a form of tolerance. Rebound congestion occurs after long-term use (greater than seven consecutive days). As the drug wears off, congestion becomes progressively worse. This effect ends when the patient stops taking the drug; however, the longer the patient has been using the drug, the more unpleasant stopping becomes.

Antihistamines Antihistamines arrest the effects of histamine by blocking its receptors. **Histamine** is an endogenous substance that affects a wide variety of organ systems. It is noted for its role in allergic reaction. In the vasculature, histamine binds with H$_1$ receptors to cause vasodilation and increased capillary permeability. In the lungs, H$_1$ receptors cause bronchoconstriction. In the gut, H$_2$ receptors cause an increase in gastric acid release. Histamine also acts as a neurotransmitter in the central nervous system. Histamine is synthesized and stored in two types of granulocytes: tissue-bound mast cells and plasma-bound basophils. Both types are full of secretory granules, which are vesicles containing inflammatory mediators, such as histamine, leukotrienes, and prostaglandins, among others. When these cells are exposed to allergens, they develop antibodies on their surfaces. On subsequent exposures, the antibodies bind with their specific allergen. The secretory granules then migrate toward the cell's exterior and fuse with the cell membrane. This causes them to release their contents. Although some available medications stabilize this membrane to prevent the release of these substances, the traditional antihistamines work by antagonizing the histamine receptors.

Commonly thought of as a nuisance, histamines are useful in our immune systems. Only when our immune systems overreact do allergies like hay fever or cedar fever send us running for the antihistamines. The typical symptoms of allergic reaction include most of those associated with rhinitis. Severe allergic reactions (anaphylaxis) may cause hypotension. Although histamines play a major role in mild and moderate allergic reactions, their part in anaphylaxis is minimal; therefore, antihistamines are at best only a secondary drug for treating anaphylaxis. (Epinephrine is the drug of choice.)

Just as there are H$_1$ and H$_2$ histamine receptors, there are H$_1$ and H$_2$ histamine receptor antagonists. When most people refer to antihistamines, they are thinking of H$_1$ receptor antagonists. These agents were in popular use long before the discovery of the H$_2$ receptors. (We discuss H$_2$ receptor antagonists in the section on drugs used to treat peptic ulcer disease.) The chief side effect of antihistamines is sedation, which the early antihistamines all caused to some degree. Now, a second generation of antihistamines that do not cause sedation is available.

The first-generation antihistamines comprise several chemical subclasses. Examples include alkylamines (chlorpheniramine [Chlor-Trimeton]), ethanolamines (diphenhydramine [Benadryl], clemastine (Tavist]), and phenothiazines (promethazine [Phenergan]). Although the different classes of agents have the same actions, they differ in the degree of sedation they cause and in their ability to block other, nonhistamine, receptors. Several antihistamines also have significant anticholinergic properties. In fact, some are used specifically for their anticholinergic

Nasal decongestants, when overused, can elevate both the pulse rate and the blood pressure.

✱ **histamine** an endogenous substance that affects a wide variety of organ systems.

* **antitussive** medication that suppresses the stimulus to cough in the central nervous system.

* **expectorant** medication intended to increase the productivity of a cough.

* **mucolytic** medication intended to make mucus more watery.

Content Review

MAIN INDICATIONS FOR GASTROINTESTINAL DRUG THERAPY
- Peptic ulcers
- Constipation
- Diarrhea and emesis
- Indigestion

---

effects, notably promethazine and dimenhydrinate (Gravol), which are used to reduce motion sickness. Other than the sedation that first-generation antihistamines cause, these agents' primary side effects are constipation and the effects of muscarinic blockade, such as dry mouth. Because they can thicken bronchial secretions, antihistamines should not be used in patients with asthma.

The second-generation antihistamines include terfenadine (Seldane), loratadine (Claritin), cetirizine (Zyrtec), and fexofenadine (Allegra). These agents' actions are similar to the first generation's, with the notable exception that they do not cross the blood-brain barrier and therefore do not cause sedation. In addition, their H_1 receptor antagonism is more pronounced, and their anticholinergic actions are greatly diminished. Terfenadine was used widely until the FDA removed it from the market because it had rare but significant side effects of cardiac dysrhythmias in patients with liver dysfunction or who were taking certain medications. Terfenadine's manufacturer is now marketing fexofenadine (Allegra) as a replacement.

Cough Suppressants Coughing is a complex reflex that depends on functions in the CNS, the PNS, and the respiratory muscles. It is a defence mechanism that aids the removal of foreign particles like smoke and dust. A productive cough is one in which these particles are actually being coughed up. In general, treating a productive cough is not appropriate, as it is performing a useful function. An unproductive cough, however, usually results from an irritated oropharynx and can be troublesome. The three classifications of cough suppressants include one that is supported by evidence and two that are not. **Antitussive** medications suppress the stimulus to cough in the central nervous system. This functional class includes two specific pharmacological types: opioids and nonopioids. The two most common opioid antitussives are codeine and hydrocodone. Both inhibit the stimulus for coughing in the brain but also produce varying degrees of euphoria. The doses required for cough suppression are not high enough to cause euphoria, but these drugs still have the potential for abuse. The nonopioid antitussives, in contrast, do not have the potential for abuse. Dextromethoraphan is the leading drug in this class. Although it is almost never given alone, it is the most common antitussive used in over-the-counter combination products for treating cold and flu symptoms. Diphenhydramine (Benadryl) is also used as a nonopioid antitussive, although its mechanism of action is not clear. Finally, the locally acting anesthetic benzonatate (Tessalon) depresses the cough stimulus by directly reducing oropharyngeal irritation. **Expectorants** are intended to increase the productivity of cough, and **mucolytics** make mucus more watery and, therefore, easier to cough up; however, little data support the effectiveness of either of these approaches to cough suppression.

DRUGS USED TO AFFECT THE GASTROINTESTINAL SYSTEM

The main purposes of drug therapy in the gastrointestinal (GI) system are to treat peptic ulcers, constipation, diarrhea, and emesis, and to aid digestion.

DRUGS USED TO TREAT PEPTIC ULCER DISEASE

Peptic ulcer disease (PUD) is characterized by an imbalance between factors in the gastrointestinal system that increase acidity and those that protect against acidity. PUD may manifest as indigestion, heartburn, or more seriously, as perforated ulcers. If the imbalance becomes too severe, parts of the lining of the GI system may be eaten away, exposing the tissue and vasculature underneath to the highly acidic environment of the stomach or duodenum. The GI system's structure fits its function. Many mucus-lined folds surround the GI lumen. The cells of these folds secrete acids needed to help break down foods; they secrete protective mucus that prevents the acid from injuring the underlying tissue; and finally, they secrete bicarbonates, which buffer the effects of acids on the GI system's absorbing surfaces. To absorb the digested nutrients and supply the mucus-producing cells of the lumen wall with oxygen, the entire GI system is very vascular. If the protective lining covering these vessels is removed, hemorrhage may occur.

Several pathological factors oppose the GI system's defences. Contrary to popular belief, the most common cause of peptic ulcer disease is not stress or alcohol but the *Helicobacter pylori* bacterium. *H. pylori* infests the space between the endothelial cells and the mucus lining of the stomach and duodenum. It can remain there for decades, protected against the acid environment by the mucus layer. Although we are still uncertain how this bacterium promotes ulcers, it apparently decreases the body's ability to produce the protective mucus lining. *H. pylori* by itself, however, does not cause ulcers. Many people remain infected for years and years without signs of PUD. Evidently, predisposing and contributing factors combine with *H. pylori* to cause ulceration. Some of these factors include smoking and long-term use of nonsteroidal anti-inflammatory drugs (NSAIDs) like aspirin and acetaminophen.

The approaches to treating PUD include antibiotics and drugs that block or decrease the secretion of gastric acid. Most often, they are used in conjunction with each other. First, and most effective, are antibiotics. When the *H. pylori* infection is eliminated, the signs of PUD resolve, and recurrence is low. Typically, three antibiotics will be utilized to ensure elimination of the bacteria and prevent resistance. Common medications for this purpose include bismuth (Pepto-Bismol), metronidazole (Flagyl), amoxicillin (Amoxil), and tetracycline (Achromycin V).

Drugs that block or decrease the secretion of gastric acid include H_2 receptor antagonists (H_2RAs), proton pump inhibitors, and anticholinergic agents. Mucosal protectants and antacids are also used.

H_2 receptors occur throughout the gut on the membranes of the parietal cells lining the GI lumen. When stimulated with histamine, they increase the action of H^+, K^+ ATPase, an enzyme that exchanges potassium for hydrogen, leading to increased gastric acid secretion. Acetylcholine and prostaglandin receptors appear along with H_2 receptors. Stimulating the ACh receptors (muscarinic receptors) increases gastric acid secretion; stimulating the prostaglandin receptors inhibits it.

H₂ Receptor Antagonists H_2RA agents block the H_2 receptors in the gut. This inhibits gastric acid secretion and helps return the balance between protective and aggressive factors. Four approved H_2RAs are in use: cimetidine (Tagamet), ranitidine (Zantac), famotidine (Pepcid), and nizatidine (Axid Pulvules). Cimetidine is the oldest of these and serves as the prototype. These agents' primary therapeutic use is for ulcers, gastroesophageal reflux, heartburn or acid indigestion, and preventing aspiration pneumonia during anesthesia. Most of these agents have few significant side effects, with the exception of cimetidine, which may lead to decreased libido, impotence, and CNS effects in some patients. Although these agents could technically be called antihistamines, that name, by tradition, is reserved for the H_1 antagonists. The H_2RAs have no effect on the H_1 receptors and are of no value in allergic reaction.

Proton Pump Inhibitors Proton pump inhibitors act directly on the K^+, H^+ ATPase enzyme that secretes gastric acid. Omeprazole (Prilosec) and lansoprazole (Prevacid) are examples. Omeprazole is the prototype. These agents irreversibly block this enzyme, which means that the body must produce new enzyme in order to begin secreting acid again. This gives proton pump inhibitors a long duration of effect. Side effects, occurring in less than 1 percent of patients, are minor and rare. They include diarrhea and headache.

Antacids Antacids are alkalotic compounds used to increase the gastric environment's pH. Most available products are either aluminum, magnesium, calcium, or sodium compounds. They are used in conjunction with other approaches to PUD and are available over the counter for relief of acid indigestion and heartburn.

Anticholinergics Although it might seem that all muscarinic blocking agents would be effective in decreasing gastric acid secretion, most atropine-like drugs produce too many unwanted effects and therefore are not used. The one exception is pirenzepine (Gastrozepine) because of its ability to selectively block the ACh receptors in the gut.

DRUGS USED TO TREAT CONSTIPATION

Laxatives decrease the firmness of stool and increase the water content. Although an uninformed public frequently uses these agents unnecessarily, laxatives are effective in some situations, specifically with patients for whom excessive strain is inappropriate. These patients include those with recent episiotomy, hemorrhoids, colostomies, or cardiovascular disease (for whom excessive straining may decrease heart rate).

Laxatives are traditionally grouped into four categories based on their mechanism of action: bulk-forming, surfactant, stimulant, and osmotic. The bulk-forming agents, such as methylcellulose (Citrucel) and psyllium (Metamucil), produce a response almost identical to normal dietary fibre intake. Fibre is undigestible and unabsorbable; therefore, it remains in the lumen of the GI system and is passed more or less intact in stool. Most water absorption takes place in the colon. Fibre (or bulk-forming laxatives) in the colon absorbs water, leading to a softer, more bulky stool. Fibre can also provide nutrients for bacteria living in the colon. These bacteria feed and provide even more bulk. The enlarged stool stimulates stretch receptors in the colonic wall, which increases peristalsis. Softening the stool also lessens strain on defecation.

The **surfactant** laxatives include docusate sodium (Colace). They decrease surface tension, which increases water absorption into the feces. They also increase water secretion and limit its reabsorption by the intestinal wall.

Stimulant laxatives increase motility. Like the surfactant laxatives, they also increase water secretion and decrease its absorption. The prototype stimulant laxative is phenolphthalein (Ex-Lax, Correctol). Bisacodyl (Bisacolax) is another example.

The osmotic laxatives are poorly absorbed salts that increase the feces' osmotic pull, thereby increasing their water content. Magnesium hydroxide, the active ingredient in Milk of Magnesia, is the prototype of this class.

DRUGS USED TO TREAT DIARRHEA

Diarrhea is the abnormally frequent passage of soft, liquid stool. It is a symptom of an underlying disease, usually a bacterial infection. It may be caused by an increased gastric motility (the stool does not stay in the colon long enough to have much water absorbed), increased water secretion, or decreased water absorption. Although it is a nuisance, diarrhea is often a helpful process because it increases the expulsion of the offending agent. It is usually self-correcting and does not need to be treated. When treatment is necessary, either specific or nonspecific agents may be used. A specific agent directly treats the cause, usually a bacterium. As you would expect, antibiotics are a common specific antidiarrheal medication.

✱ **antacid** alkalotic compound used to increase the gastric environment's pH.

✱ **laxative** medication used to decrease stool's firmness and increase its water content.

Content Review

CATEGORIES OF LAXATIVES
- Bulk-forming
- Stimulant
- Osmotic
- Surfactant

✱ **surfactant** substance that decreases surface tension.

DRUGS USED TO TREAT EMESIS

Emesis is a complex process that involves different parts of the brain as well as receptors and muscles in the stomach and inner ear. The two involved parts of the brain include the vomiting centre in the medulla and the chemoreceptor trigger zone (CTZ). The vomiting centre stimulates vomiting directly, while the CTZ does so indirectly.

The vomiting centre is stimulated by H₁ and ACh receptors in the pathway between itself and the inner ear, by sensory input from the eyes and nose (unpleasant or disturbing sights and smells), and by other parts of the brain in response to anxiety or fear. The CTZ stimulates the vomiting centre in response to stimuli from serotonin receptors in the stomach and bloodborne substances, such as opioids and ipecac.

Stimulating emesis is rarely desired, but it can be useful in treating certain types of overdoses or poisonings. Ipecac is the drug of choice when stimulating emesis is indicated. It stimulates the CTZ, which, in turn, stimulates the vomiting centre.

Antiemetics Unlike causing emesis, preventing emesis is frequently desirable. **Antiemetics** are indicated in conjunction with chemotherapy, which may cause violent nausea and vomiting. Antiemetics are also indicated in the prophylactic treatment of motion sickness.

Multiple transmitters are involved in the vomiting reflex. They include serotonin, dopamine, acetylcholine, and histamine. Drugs that interfere with any of these transmitters can decrease or prevent nausea and vomiting. This functional class includes several pharmacological subclasses: serotonin antagonists, dopamine antagonists, anticholinergics, and cannabinoids.

Serotonin Antagonists The prototype serotonin antagonist is ondansetron (Zofran). It blocks the serotonin receptors in the CTZ, the stomach, and the small intestines. It is very effective in the treatment of nausea and vomiting associated with chemotherapy, and unlike the dopamine antagonists, it does not cause extrapyramidal effects like dystonia and ataxia. Its most common side effects are headache and diarrhea.

Dopamine Antagonists Both phenothiazines and butyrophenones effectively block dopamine receptors in the CTZ. (This chapter's section on psychotherapeutic medications discusses both these medications at length.) The phenothiazines include prochlorperazine (Compazine) and promethazine (Phenergan), while the butyrophenones include haloperidol (Haldol) and droperidol (Inapsine). Agents from both classes cause side effects of extrapyramidal effects and sedation. Another dopamine antagonist, metoclopramide (Reglan) is neither a phenothiazine nor a butyrophenone. It is unique in that it blocks both serotonin and dopamine receptors in the CTZ.

Cannabinoids The cannabinoids are derivatives of tetrahydrocannabinol (THC) and are effective antiemetics used to treat chemotherapy-induced nausea and vomiting. The two available agents are dronabinol (Marinol) and nabilone (Cesamet). Because both agents are essentially the same as THC (the active ingredient in marijuana), their side effects include euphoria similar to that of marijuana. Although those effects may be desirable for some, they may be intensely unpleasant for others.

DRUGS USED TO AID DIGESTION

Several drugs are available to aid the digestion of carbohydrates and fats. These agents are similar to endogenous digestive enzymes released into the duodenum

Ipecac is the drug of choice when stimulating emesis is indicated.

✱ **antiemetic** medication used to prevent vomiting.

Many of the antiemetics used in emergency care can cause extrapyramidal symptoms. Always be alert for these.

in response to vagal stimulation. Occasionally, supplemental enzymes are necessary for patients whose vagal stimulus has been surgically severed or whose duodenum has been bypassed. Two of these drugs are pancreatin (Entozyme) and pancrelipase (Viokase). Their chief side effects are nausea, vomiting, and abdominal cramping.

DRUGS USED TO AFFECT THE EYES

Ophthalmic drugs are used to treat conditions involving the eyes, primarily glaucoma and trauma. In addition, some ophthalmic agents are used in diagnosing and examining the eyes.

Glaucoma is a degenerative disease that affects the optic nerve. Its causative factors are not clear; however, correlations are known between it and several risk factors, including intraocular pressure, race (its rate is three times higher among black people than among white people), and age. The medications used to treat glaucoma are all aimed at reducing intraocular pressure (IOP). Beta-blockers and cholinergics are the most common. Beta blockade decreases IOP by an unknown mechanism. Timolol (Timoptic) and betaxolol (Betoptic) are examples of this class. Pilocarpine (Isopto Carpine) is the prototype cholinergic drug for treating glaucoma. It stimulates muscarinic receptors in the eye to cause miosis (pupil constriction) and ciliary muscle contraction, which indirectly lowers IOP. Drugs from these classes are given topically. Beta-blockers have few side effects, while pilocarpine causes blurred vision and local irritation.

Some diagnostic procedures call for causing mydriasis (pupil dilation) and cycloplegia (paralysis of the ciliary muscles used to focus vision). The two pharmacological approaches to doing this involve anticholinergics or adrenergic agonists. In this functional class, atropine solutions, such as Atropisol, and scopolamine solutions, such as Isopto Hyoscine, are typical anticholinergics; phenylephrine solution (AK-Dilate) is the class's principal adrenergic agonist. This chapter's sections on anticholinergics and adrenergic agonists discuss these pharmacological classes in more detail.

Tetracaine (Pontocaine) is a local anesthetic of the ester class. (It is related to cocaine, another ester, but not to lidocaine, an amide.) It is used to decrease pain and sensation in the eye from trauma or during ophthalmic procedures.

If tetracaine is administered in the field, remind the patient not to rub her eyes, as she can worsen the injury.

DRUGS USED TO AFFECT THE EARS

Most drugs used to treat conditions involving the ear are aimed at eliminating underlying bacterial or fungal infections or at breaking up impacted ear wax. Chloramphenicol (Chloromycetin Otic) and gentamicin sulphate otic solution (Garamycin) are common antibiotics; carbamide peroxide (Auro Ear Drops) and carbamide peroxide and glycerin (Ear Wax Removal System) are both used to treat ear wax. Finally, several drugs are available to treat swimmer's ear, an inflammation/irritation of the external ear. They include isopropyl alcohol (Auro-Dri Ear Drops) and boric acid and isopropyl alcohol (Aurocaine 2).

Some drugs that are used for other purposes have ototoxic (harmful to the organs or nerves that produce hearing or balance) properties if taken in overdose or administered too quickly. The most common ototoxic symptom is tinnitus, or ringing in the ears. Drugs with ototoxic properties include Aspirin and other NSAIDs, some antibiotics (including erythromycin and vancomycin), and the diuretic furosemide (Lasix).

DRUGS USED TO AFFECT
THE ENDOCRINE SYSTEM

The endocrine system and nervous system together are chiefly responsible for the regulatory activities that maintain homeostasis. The nervous system, with its direct connections between nerves and organs, may be thought of as a "wired" system, while the endocrine system, which releases hormones directly into the bloodstream, may be thought of as "wireless." The endocrine system comprises the following glands: pituitary (anterior and posterior lobes), pineal, thyroid, parathyroid, thymus, adrenal, pancreas, ovaries, and testes. Of these, the pituitary is commonly referred to as the master gland because of its role in controlling the other endocrine glands. (The hypothalmus, in turn, controls many of the pituitary's functions.) Once in the bloodstream, the hormones from these glands circulate widely throughout the body. To be effective, however, they must bind with very specific receptors. This discussion will focus on the pharmacological actions of drugs that affect the various endocrine glands.

DRUGS AFFECTING THE PITUITARY GLAND

The pituitary gland has a posterior and an anterior lobe. Anterior pituitary-like drugs are used to treat abnormal growth: dwarfism, acromegaly, and gigantism. The two posterior pituitary hormones are oxytocin and antidiuretic hormone. Oxytocin is discussed in the section on drugs affecting labour and delivery. Antidiuretic hormone (ADH) promotes water retention. ADH analogues are used to treat diabetes insipidus and nocturnal enuresis (bedwetting). At higher doses, ADH can cause vasoconstriction and increased blood pressure; hence its other name, vasopressin. Vasopressin (Pitressin), desmopressin (Stimate), and lypressin (Diapid) are all available to reverse ADH deficiency.

DRUGS AFFECTING THE PARATHYROID
AND THYROID GLANDS

The parathyroid glands are primarily responsible for regulating calcium levels. Hypoparathyroidism leads to decreased levels of calcium and vitamin D. Treatment, therefore, is through calcium and vitamin D supplements. Hyperparathyroidism leads to high levels of calcium. Because it usually results from tumours, the treatment of choice is surgical removal of all or part of the parathyroid glands.

The thyroid gland produces thyroid hormones, which play a vital role in regulating growth, maturation, and metabolism. Hypothyroidism can occur in children or adults. When it develops in children, it is known as cretinism and manifests itself as dwarfism and mental retardation with characteristic features. Because most growth and maturation in adults is complete, adult onset of hypothyroidism appears as decreased metabolic rate, weight gain, fatigue, and bradycardia. In some cases, myxedema (facial puffiness) may be present. Treatment is aimed at thyroid hormone replacement. The prototype drug, levothyroxine (Synthroid), is also the most commonly used. A synthetic analogue of T_4 (thyroxine), one of the thyroid hormones, levothyroxine generally has no significant side effects when taken in therapeutic doses. Overdose may lead to thyrotoxicosis or thyroid storm. Thyrotoxicosis is a condition in which hyperthyroidism causes an increase in thyroid hormones. Thyroid storm is a severe form of thyrotoxicosis in which the manifestations of the disease increase to life-threatening proportions. Thyroid storm is characterized by tachycardic dysrhythmias, angina, hypertension, and hyperthermia.

Goitres are enlargements of the thyroid gland. They are typically caused by insufficient dietary iodine. In the developed countries, goitre is much rarer than in the less-developed countries and is most commonly caused by Hashimoto's disease, a chronic autoimmune disease. Treatment of goitres is aimed at supplementing the inadequate iodine.

Hyperthyroidism is caused by excessive release of thyroid hormones, typically as a result of tumours. The most common cause of hyperthyroidism in Canada is Grave's disease. It presents with tachycardia, hypertension, hyperthermia, nervousness, insomnia, increased metabolic rate, and weight loss. In severe cases, exophthalmos (protrusion of the eyeballs) may occur. Treatment is typically surgical removal of all or part of the thyroid gland. Radioactive iodine (^{131}I) may also be given for radiation therapy. Propylthiouracil (PTU) may be given alone or as adjunct therapy to surgery or radiation in treating hyperthyroidism.

DRUGS AFFECTING THE ADRENAL CORTEX

The adrenal cortex synthesizes and secretes three classes of hormones: glucocorticoids, mineralocorticoids, and androgens. The glucocorticoids and mineralocorticoids are referred to collectively as corticosteroids, adrenocortiocoids, or corticoids. As their name implies, glucocorticoids increase the production of glucose by enhancing carbohydrate metabolism, promoting gluconeogenesis, and reducing peripheral glucose utilization. The most important glucocorticoid is cortisol. The mineralocorticoids regulate salt and water balance. The primary mineralocorticoid is aldosterone. The androgens are important hormones in regulating sexual maturation and development.

Two diseases typify the disorders associated with the adrenal cortex: Cushing's disease and Addison's disease. Cushing's disease is characterized by hypersecretion of adrenocorticotropic hormone, an anterior pituitary tropic hormone that increases the synthesis of corticoids, leading to excessive glucocorticoid secretion. Common signs and symptoms include hyperglycemia, obesity, hypertension, and electrolyte imbalances. Addison's disease is characterized by hyposecretion of corticoids as a result of damage to the adrenal gland. Common signs and symptoms include hypoglycemia, emaciation, hypotension, hyperkalemia, and hyponatremia.

Treatment of Cushing's disease is typically surgical. Symptomatic pharmacological intervention with an antihypertensive (potassium-sparing diuretics, such as spironolactone [Aldactone], or ACE inhibitors, such as captopril [Capoten]), may be necessary. Drugs that may inhibit the synthesis of corticosteroids (antiadrenals) may also be used as an adjunct to surgery or radiation. In high doses, the antifungal agent ketoconazole (Nizoral) is an effective temporary antiadrenal drug. At such doses, however, it may cause liver dysfunction.

Treatment of Addison's disease is aimed at replacement therapy. Cortisone (Cortistan) and hydrocortisone (SoluCortef) are the drugs of choice. Occasionally, a specific mineralocorticoid is necessary. Fludrocortisone (Florinef Acetate) is the only mineralocorticoid available.

DRUGS AFFECTING THE PANCREAS

Diabetes mellitus is the most important disease involving the pancreas. Diabetes mellitus (as opposed to diabetes insipidus, which involves inadequate ADH secretion) involves inappropriate carbohydrate metabolism. Traditionally, the term diabetes used alone refers to diabetes mellitus, of which the two main types are, logically, Type I and Type II. Type I diabetes is also known as insulin-dependent diabetes mellitus, or IDDM. It results from an inadequate release of insulin from the beta cells of the pancreatic islets. Patients with Type I diabetes rely on insulin replacement therapy to survive. Because IDDM typically manifests itself at an early age (usually before 30 years) it was commonly called juvenile onset diabetes. Most diabetics have Type II diabetes, which is also referred to as non-insulin-dependent diabetes mellitus (NIDDM) and used to be called adult-onset diabetes. It results from a decreased responsiveness to insulin and a lack of synchronization between insulin release and blood glucose levels. Type II diabetes typically begins later in life (after 40 years) and almost always occurs in obese patients. Because they have functioning beta cells that release insulin, Type II diabetics usually do not depend on insulin replacement. Gestational diabetes, a third type, occurs transitionally during pregnancy. Gestational diabetes is a form of stress-induced diabetes in which the mother cannot effectively manage her blood glucose levels during pregnancy without medical intervention. Gestational diabetes resolves itself within hours to days of delivery.

The two main substances involved with regulating blood glucose are insulin and glucagon. Both are secreted from the pancreas and both are used to manage diabetes. Secreted from the beta cells of the pancreatic islets of Langerhans in response to increased blood glucose levels, **insulin** increases cellular transport of glucose, potassium, and amino acids. It also converts glucose into glycogen for storage in the liver and in skeletal muscle. Finally, insulin promotes cell growth and division.

Glucagon, too, is secreted from the pancreatic islets, but by alpha cells rather than by the insulin-producing beta cells. Glucagon's actions are the direct opposite of insulin's; it increases both glycogenolysis (glycogen breakdown into glucose) and gluconeogenesis (the synthesis of glucose from glycerol and amino acids). So, while insulin decreases blood glucose levels, glucagon increases them.

Patients with either Type I or Type II diabetes may experience both hyperglycemia and hypoglycemia. Although hyperglycemia more often results from the disease, hypoglycemia is a common side effect of treatment. The main intervention for patients with IDDM is insulin-replacement therapy. Several insulin preparations are available. The most effective therapy for patients with NIDDM is usually weight loss through diet modification and exercise. When this is not effective, oral hypoglycemic agents and, occasionally, insulin are used. Finally, glucagon and diazoxide (both can be considered hyperglycemic agents) are occasionally used for treating emergency hypoglycemia.

Insulin Preparations Insulin comes from one of three sources. Initially, it came from either beef or pork intestines. Now, recombinant DNA technology has made human insulin available (that is, insulin synthesized with a human RNA template, not harvested directly from humans). Insulin preparations differ primarily in their onset and duration of action and in their incidence of allergic reaction. Insulin preparations may be short acting, intermediate acting, or long acting, depending on their onset and duration of action. (Table 14-8 lists insulin preparations.)

Insulin is also classified as natural (regular) or modified. As their name suggests, the natural insulins are used as they occur in nature. The other insulin preparations have been modified to increase their duration of action and thus decrease the frequency of their administration. All insulin preparations are given subcutaneously, with the exception of regular insulin, which may also be given intravenously. Insulin is not available as an oral medication because the digestive enzymes would rapidly render it inactive, therefore, IDDM patients must take multiple injections every day of their lives. This may discourage compliance in some patients.

The modified insulin preparations include NPH (neutral protamine Hagedorn) insulin, which is regular insulin attached to a large protein designed to delay absorption, and the lente series, which is attached to zinc. Two preparations of lente insulin are available by themselves, lente and ultralente. A third, semilente insulin, is available only in a combination product with other insulins.

Insulin preparations are used for lifelong replacement therapy in IDDM and for emergency treatment of hyperglycemia and hyperkalemia in nondiabetics.

✱ **insulin** substance that decreases blood glucose level.

✱ **glucagon** substance that increases blood glucose level.

Always consider glucagon in the hyperglycemic patient when an IV cannot be started.

Diabetic ketoacidosis (DKA) is best treated by a continuous insulin infusion accompanied by frequent checks of the blood glucose levels.

Table 14-8 INSULIN PREPARATIONS

Classification	Trade Name	Source
Rapid-Acting		
Lispro Insulin	Humalog	Human
Regular Insulin	Humulin R	Human
	Novolin R	Human
	Velosulin BR	Human
	Regular Iletin I	Beef/Pork
	Regular Iletin II	Pork
Intermediate Acting		
NPH Insulin	NPH Iletin I	Beef/Pork
	Pork NPH Iletin II	Pork
	Humulin N	Human
	Novolin N	Human
Lente	Lente Iletin I	Beef/Pork
	Lente Iletin II (Pork)	Pork
	Humulin L	Human
	Novolin L	Human
Long-Acting		
Ultralente	Humulin U	Human
	Ultralente	
Combination Products		
NPH/Regular 70%/30%	Humulin 70/30	Human
	Novolin 70/30	Human
NPH/Regular 50%/50%	Humulin 50/50	Human

(Recall that insulin also increases potassium uptake by cells and is therefore useful in lowering potassium levels). These preparations' primary side effect is unintended hypoglycemia. Because beta$_2$ adrenergic blockers can hide the effects of hypoglycemia, patients may not recognize this condition's signs until they cannot care for themselves. Also, beta-blockers decrease the release of glucagon, so these patients' hypoglycemia may be even worse. Insulin preparations derived from beef or pork, as well as the lentes, may lead to allergic reactions. The natural human insulin preparations do not have this effect.

Oral Hypoglycemic Agents Oral hypoglycemic agents are used to stimulate insulin secretion from the pancreas in patients with NIDDM. These agents are ineffective in people with Type I diabetes, since those patients cannot secrete insulin. This functional class comprises four pharmacological classes: sulphonylureas, biguanides, alpha-glucosidase inhibitors, and thiazolidinediones. The sulphonylureas were the first class of oral hypoglycemics available and, as such, are also known as first-generation or second-generation oral hypoglycemics, depending on when they were released. Drugs in this class include tolbutamide (Orinase), chlorpropamide (Diabinese), glipizide (Glucotrol), and glyburide (Micronase). They work by increasing insulin secretion from the pancreas and may also increase tissue response to insulin. Their major side effect is hypoglycemia.

The only agent in the biguanide class is metformin (Glucophage). It decreases glucose synthesis and increases glucose uptake. It does not stimulate the release of insulin from the pancreas and therefore does not cause hypoglycemia. Its primary side effects are nausea, vomiting, and decreased appetite.

Alpha-glucosidase inhibitors include acarbose (Precose) and miglitol (Glyset). They work by delaying carbohydrate metabolism, which moderates the increase in blood glucose that occurs after meals. These agents' primary side effects are flatulence, cramps, diarrhea, and abdominal distention resulting from colonic bacteria feeding on the increased number of carbohydrates remaining in fecal matter.

Thiazolidinediones are a new class of oral hypoglycemic agents unrelated to the others. The only drug in this class is troglitazone (Rezulin). It works by promoting tissue response to insulin and thus making the available insulin more effective. Troglitazone has no major side effects.

Hyperglycemic Agents Two hyperglycemic agents, glucagon and diazoxide (Proglycem), act to increase blood glucose levels. Glucagon is indicated for the emergency treatment of patients with hypoglycemia. It will frequently be given intramuscularly to hypoglycemic patients in whom an IV line is unobtainable. Occasional side effects are nausea and vomiting and, rarely, allergic reactions. Diazoxide (Proglycem) inhibits insulin release and is typically used only for patients with hyperinsulin secretion resulting from pancreatic tumours; it is more commonly used for hypertension. It is not indicated for treating diabetes-induced hypoglycemia.

$D_{50}W$ (50 percent dextrose in water) is a sugar solution given intravenously for acute hypoglycemia. Its primary side effect is local tissue necrosis if infiltration occurs.

Dilute $D_{50}W$ to $D_{25}W$ for administration to pediatric patients.

DRUGS AFFECTING THE FEMALE REPRODUCTIVE SYSTEM

The main groups of drugs affecting the female reproductive system are estrogens, progestins, oral contraceptives, drugs affecting uterine contraction, and those used to treat infertility.

Estrogens and Progestins Estrogens are produced in females by the ovaries and the ovarian follicles, and in pregnancy by the placenta. Outside pregnancy, the ovaries are the principal source of estrogens. The principal ovarian estrogen is estradiol, of which there are many commercial preparations. The principal indication for estrogen is replacement therapy in postmenopausal women. After menopause, estrogen levels drop significantly and have been indicated as a major increased risk factor for osteoporosis and coronary artery disease. Hormone replacement therapy with estrogen was believed to reverse these risk factors and increase life expectancy; however, it is not without its own risks. There is much debate about the increased chances of breast cancer, heart attack, and stroke associated with hormone replacement therapy. Unfortunately, the data on this issue are conflicting, and no conclusive answers are currently possible. Side effects include nausea, fluid retention, and breast tenderness. The nausea usually diminishes after several months of therapy. Estrogen is also administered in cases of delayed puberty in girls as a result of hypogonadism.

The progestins' principal noncontraceptive use is to counteract the untoward effects of estrogen on the endometrium in hormone replacement therapy for postmenopausal women. They are also used to treat amenorrhea, endometriosis, and dysfunctional uterine bleeding.

Oral Contraceptives Oral contraception is an effective means of preventing pregnancy. All oral contraceptives' primary mechanism of action is the prevention of ovulation, which makes the endometrium less favourable for implantation and promotes the development of a thick mucus plug that blocks access to sperm through the cervix. These contraceptives are either a combination of estrogen and progestin or, in the case of "mini-pills," progestin only. They may also be classified based on their administration cycle as monophasic, biphasic, or triphasic. These classes differ in how they alter the dose of estrogen or progestin throughout the menstrual cycle. Many different preparations are available, although they all work in similar fashion. In general, these drugs are well tolerated and have few side effects. The oral contraceptives' chief side effects are unintended pregnancy (in less than 3 percent of users), thromboembolism (this risk is much lower with the newer low-estrogen-dose preparations), hypertension, and abnormal uterine bleeding. They are in wide use and are one of the most widely prescribed drug classes. They are the second-most popular means of birth control after surgical sterilization (male and female combined).

Uterine Stimulants and Relaxants Drugs that increase uterine contraction (uterine stimulants) are oxytocics (oxytocin means rapid birth). Drugs that relax the uterus or inhibit uterine contraction are tocolytics.

The primary indications for administration of an oxytocic are to induce labour and to treat severe postpartum hemorrhage. Oxytocin is available commercially as Pitocin and Syntocinon. The uterus becomes increasingly sensitive to oxytocin throughout gestation, progressing from relatively insensitive before pregnancy to very sensitive around the time of labour. Oxytocin's chief side effect, water retention, is rarely significant and only so if large volumes of fluid have been administered without careful ongoing assessment. Ergonovine (Ergotrate), a derivative of a rye fungus, is a powerful uterine stimulant. It increases both the force and duration of contraction. Because of this increased duration, ergonovine is only used in the treatment of postpartum hemorrhage.

The tocolytics relax uterine smooth muscle by stimulating the beta$_2$ receptors in the uterus. The two beta$_2$ agonists commonly used for this purpose are terbutaline (Brethine) and ritodrine (Yutopar). Terbutaline's primary use is to treat asthma, but it is commonly used to delay labour even though it is not currently approved for that purpose. Both agents decrease both the force and frequency of contraction. Their chief side effects are the same as those of the other beta$_2$ agonists used to treat asthma: tremors and tachycardia. Occasionally, hyperglycemia may result from glycogenolysis in the liver.

Infertility Agents A number of conditions may cause infertility, which is the inability to become pregnant, and medications can treat only some of them. Most infertility drugs are developed for women and promote maturation of ovarian follicles. Clomiphene (Clomid), urofollitropin (Metrodin), and menotropins (Pergonal) are all within this class, although they each act by a different mechanism. These agents' side effects include ovarian enlargement or cysts, abdominal pain, and menstrual irregularities.

DRUGS AFFECTING THE MALE REPRODUCTIVE SYSTEM

Drugs that affect the male reproductive system include those that treat testosterone deficiency and benign prostatic hyperplasia. Testosterone replacement therapy may be indicated in testosterone deficiency caused by cryptorchidism (failure of one or both of the testes to descend during puberty), orchitis (testicular inflammation), or orchidectomy (testicular removal). It is also used in delayed puberty. Preparations include testosterone enanthate, methyltestosterone (Metandren), and fluoxymesterone (Halotestin).

Benign prostatic hyperplasia is an enlarged prostate. This is a common but problematic age-related disease. By the age of 70, close to 75 percent of men will have symptoms severe enough to seek therapy. These symptoms may include urinary hesitancy and retention. Treatment has traditionally been surgery, but several drugs are available, including finasteride (Proscar), which interferes with the production of an enzyme involved in prostate growth. Side effects may include rash, breast tenderness, headache, impotence, and decreased libido.

DRUGS AFFECTING SEXUAL BEHAVIOUR

For centuries, cultures have searched for drugs that would increase libido and sexual potency. Ironically, the reverse has most commonly been found. The largest category of drugs affecting sexual behaviour do so as a side effect of their intended purpose. Many drug classifications decrease libido in both sexes and inhibit erection and ejaculation. Examples include antihypertensives (beta-blockers, centrally acting alpha antagonists, and diuretics) and antianxiety/antipsychotic medications (benzodiazepines, phenothiazines, MAO inhibitors, and tricyclic antidepressants).

Many drugs are purported to increase libido. The most notable of these is cantharis (Spanish fly). Despite common belief, no evidence indicates that cantharis actually increases sexual appetite. Indeed, it can produce some very dangerous side effects. Hallucinogens, such as LSD and marijuana, as well as alcohol, are also commonly believed to heighten sexuality. Any such effect from these agents is likely an indirect result of decreased inhibitions or anxiety. These drugs all have very different effects, depending on each individual's unique physiology, expectations before use, and surrounding circumstances. They have no proven direct physiological effect on sexual gratification.

Levodopa (L-dopa), an anti-Parkinson's drug, has demonstrated increased libido and improved erectile ability as a side effect of treatment. Whether this results directly from increased autonomic stimulation or indirectly from improved self-esteem achieved in therapy, any improvement seems to be only temporary. Finally, sildenafil (Viagra) was approved in 1998 for pharmacological therapy in patients with erectile dysfunction. Sildenafil acts by relaxing vascular smooth muscle, which increases blood flow to the corpus cavernosum, the sponge-like tissue on the sides of the penis responsible for erection. This drug is unique in that it has no effect in the absence of sexual stimulation. Other drugs used to treat impotence have caused prolonged and painful erections (priapism). The chief side effect of sildenafil is seen when it is used in combination with nitrates. The combined effect of relaxing vascular smooth muscle may lead to a dangerously decreased preload, which may lower blood pressure and lead to myocardial infarction. Prehospital personnel should be aware of this important interaction. If you are called on to treat a patient with chest pain who has taken sildenafil recently, do not give him nitroglycerine or any other nitrate.

If you treat a patient with chest pain who has taken sildenafil recently, do not give him nitroglycerine or any other nitrate.

DRUGS USED TO TREAT CANCER

Drugs used to treat cancer are called antineoplastic agents. A detailed discussion of the many different antineoplastic agents is beyond the scope of this text; however, this section will briefly overview their main classes and prototype drugs.

 antineoplastic agent drug used to treat cancer.

Cancer involves the modification of cellular DNA leading to an abnormal growth of tissues. Of the many known types of cancer, only a few are successfully treated with chemotherapy. In fact, most cancers are best treated by surgical removal of the tumour. Unfortunately, many of the more lethal cancers do not involve a compact growth; rather, they affect the formed elements of the blood, especially leukocytes. Treating these widely dispersed cancers with surgery is not possible, as there is nothing for the surgeon to remove.

Chemotherapy is not nearly as safe or devoid of side effects as antibiotic therapy; however, scientists have yet to identify any unique characteristics of cancer cells that would allow them to develop drugs specific to those cells. Because cancer is the abnormal growth of normal cells, drugs that kill cancerous cells therefore also kill noncancerous cells. Chemotherapy is thus largely a balancing act aimed at maximizing the kill rate of cancer cells while minimizing the death of normal tissue. The one characteristic that most cancer cells share is rapid cell division and replication. Consequently, most antineoplastic agents have their greatest effect on cancer cells during miosis and on young, small cancers that are undergoing rapid growth.

The agents used to kill cancer cells are grouped according to their mechanism of action. Antimetabolite drugs mimic some of the enzymes and proteins needed for DNA replication but do not have the same effects; therefore, they prevent cells from reproducing. Their prototype is fluorouracil (Adrucil). Alkylating agents that interfere with DNA splitting include cyclophosphamide (Cytoxan) and mechlorethamine (Mustargen). Mitotic inhibitors also interfere with cell division; they include vinblastine (Velban) and vincristine (Oncovin).

Chemotherapy's primary side effects include nausea, vomiting, and other gastrointestinal disturbances, as well as hair loss and weakness. Almost all anti-neoplastic agents cause severe side effects and are given in conjunction with antiemetics.

DRUGS USED TO TREAT INFECTIOUS DISEASES AND INFLAMMATION

Infectious diseases are typically caused by bacteria, viruses, or fungi and may be treated with antimicrobial drugs developed to fight those particular invaders. We will discuss each broad class.

Antibiotics An **antibiotic** agent may either kill the offending bacteria (bacteri-cidal agents) or so decrease the bacteria's growth that the patient's immune system can effectively fight the infection (bacteriostatic agents). In general, all these agents share one of several mechanisms. Drugs in the penicillin and cephalosporin classes, as well as vancomycin (Vancocin), are bactericidal and act by inhibiting cell wall synthesis. Unlike animal cells, bacteria have hypertonic cell cytoplasm and depend on the rigid and relatively impermeable cell wall to maintain integrity. When cell wall synthesis is inhibited, osmotic pressure pulls water into the cell, and the cell ruptures, killing the bacteria. The macrolide, aminoglycoside, and tetracycline antibiotics inhibit protein synthesis, preventing the bacterial cell from replicating and thus spreading infection. These agents are usually bacteriostatic but can be bactericidal at high doses. Typical side effects from antibiotics include gastrointestinal dysfunction, which commonly results from a decrease in the nat-ural gastrointestinal bacteria that inhabit the colon.

Antifungal and Antiviral Agents Fungi are parasitic microorganisms that cannot synthesize their own food. Fungal infections (mycoses) may be treated with several drugs. The azole antifungals inhibit fungal growth. Their prototype is ketoconazole (Nizoral). Drugs used to treat viruses work by a variety of mechanisms and include acyclovir (Zovirax) and zidovudine (Retrovir), which is commonly known as AZT. Protease inhibitors are one of the more promising classes of drugs for treating viruses like HIV. Indinavir (Crixivan) is the prototype of this class.

Other Antimicrobial and Antiparasitic Agents Although most diseases treated with the medications discussed in this section are uncommon in the developed countries, they are leading causes of death in the less-developed countries. These diseases include malaria, tuberculosis, leprosy, amebiasis, and helminthiasis. Tuberculosis is increasingly appearing in Canada in patients with compromised immune systems.

Malaria is a parasitic infection common in the tropics. It is transmitted by certain types of mosquitoes or, less commonly, by blood transfusion. Drugs used to treat malaria are called schizonticides. They include chloroquine (Aralen), mefloquine (Lariam), and quinine. Treatment is aimed at either preventing

* **antibiotic** agent that kills or decreases the growth of bacteria.

infestation (prophylactic treatment for individuals travelling to high risk areas) or killing the parasites in infected patients.

Tuberculosis is caused by bacteria that are transmitted through airborne droplets from the coughing and sneezing of infected patients. The bacteria can grow only in well-oxygenated areas. Because of the route of infection and the need for oxygen, most patients with tuberculosis have infestations in the lungs. Once in the lungs, the bacteria are typically "walled off," or enclosed in tubercules, and become dormant and noninfective. If the patient's immune system is compromised, the bacteria may become active again and begin to cause symptoms. Drugs commonly used to treat tuberculosis include isoniazid (Nydrazid, INH) and rifampin (Rifadin).

Amebiasis is a parasitic infection of the intestines common in tropical areas. Transmission most frequently occurs via the oral-fecal route from eating poorly cooked food contaminated by cooks who inadequately wash their hands. Drugs used to treat amebiasis include paromomycin (Humatin) and metronidazole (Flagyl).

Helminthiasis is caused by parasitic worms (helminths), including flatworms and roundworms. These worms usually invade the host's intestinal tract and attach themselves to the lumen wall with hooks or suckers. They cause symptoms by depriving the host of nutrients (especially in children); by obstructing the intestinal lumen, which leads to bowel obstruction; and by producing toxins. Treatment is aimed at either killing the organism outright or destroying its ability to latch onto the intestinal wall so that it passes with the patient's feces. These drugs include mebendazole (Vermox) and niclosamide (Niclocide).

Leprosy, also known as Hansen's disease, is caused by bacteria. It leads to characteristic lesions, footdrop (plantar flexion), and plantar ulceration. Drugs used to treat it include dapsone (DDS, Avlosulfon), and clofazimine (Lamprene).

Nonsteroidal Anti-Inflammatory Drugs NSAIDs (nonsteroidal anti-inflammatory drugs) are commonly used as analgesics and antipyretics (fever reducers). Many are available over the counter, including acetaminophen and ibuprofen. As a group, these agents interfere with the production of prostaglandins, thereby interrupting the inflammatory process. NSAIDs are indicated for the relief of pain, fever, and inflammation associated with common headache, arthritis, dysmenorrhea, and orthopedic injuries. They are also commonly prescribed to relieve pain following trauma and surgery. Other NSAIDs include ketorolac (Toradol), piroxicam (Feldene), and naproxen (Naprosyn).

Uricosuric Drugs Uricosuric drugs are used to treat and prevent acute episodes of gout. Gout is an inflammatory disease caused by an altered metabolism of uric acid and marked by hyperuricemia (high levels of uric acid in the blood). It may present with acute episodes characterized by pain and swelling of joints. Left untreated, gout may lead to crystal deposits in various parts of the body that can cause kidney stones, nephritis, and atherosclerosis. Drugs used to treat gout include colchicine and allopurinol (Zyloprim).

Serums, Vaccines, and Other Immunizing Agents The human body has a complex series of systems that help prevent disease. The most important of these are the anatomical barriers, such as the skin and mucous membranes, that block the entrance of **pathogens** (disease causing organisms including viruses and bacteria). If pathogens get past these protective barriers, our immune system comes into play. This system consists of the spleen, lymph nodes, thymus, leukocytes, and proteins called antibodies in plasma. The ability to respond to pathogens is called **immunity.**

Immunity may be acquired passively or actively. It is passively acquired when antibodies pass directly into a person, either through artificial routes, such

✱ **pathogen** disease-causing organism.

✱ **immunity** the body's ability to respond to the presence of a pathogen.

as injection, or through natural routes, such as the placenta or breast milk. Immunity may also be actively acquired in response to the presence of a pathogen.

Actively acquired immunity occurs when T lymphocytes (a type of leukocyte that becomes specialized in the thymus gland) comes in contact with a new pathogen. The body produces an infinite variety of T-cell configurations. When the pathogen comes into contact with a T cell that is specific to it, that T cell begins to rapidly reproduce. Some of these cells become involved in the immune response to the pathogen, while others act as "memory" cells. The cells involved in the immune response either directly attack the pathogen (cell-mediated immunity) or activate the complement system, a complex cascade of events that leads to the immune response. The memory cells remain in the body in higher numbers so that the next time this specific pathogen enters the body, a much faster response is possible. At the same time, B cells (lymphocytes that differentiate or become more specialized in the body, as opposed to the thymus) that are specific for the invading pathogen begin to produce antibodies for that antigen. This process is called humoral immunity or antibody immunity. When an antibody contacts its specific antigen, it forms a complex that triggers the complement system, leading to the immune response.

Serums and vaccines may augment the immune system. A **serum** is a solution containing whole antibodies for a specific pathogen. The antibodies give the recipient temporary, passive immunity. A **vaccine** contains a modified pathogen that does not actually cause disease but still stimulates the development of antibodies specific to it. These pathogens may be either dead or attenuated (having a decreased disease-causing ability).

The best age for vaccination against disease is within the first two years of life, as the immune system is fairly immature.

Immune Suppressing and Enhancing Agents Available drugs can either suppress the immune system (immunosuppressants) or enhance it (immunomodulators). Suppressing the immune system is indicated to prevent the rejection of transplanted organs and grafted skin. Azathioprine (Imuran) is a commonly used immunosuppressant that acts by decreasing cell-mediated reactions and suppressing antibody production.

Immunomodulating agents enhance the natural immune reaction in immunosuppressed patients, such as those with HIV. Zidovudine (Retrovir), commonly known as AZT, and several protease inhibitors, such as ritonavir (Norvir) and saquinavir (Invirase), are examples of these agents.

DRUGS USED TO AFFECT THE SKIN

Dermatological drugs are used to treat skin irritations. They are common over-the-counter medications. The many different general preparations include baths, soaps, solutions, cleansers, emollients (Lubriderm, Vaseline), skin protectants (Benzoin), wet dressings or soaks (Domeboro Powder), and rubs and liniments (Ben-Gay, Icy Hot). Prophylactic agents, such as sunscreens, are also available to help prevent skin disease and irritation.

DRUGS USED TO SUPPLEMENT THE DIET

Many disease processes affect the production, distribution, and utilization of essential dietary nutrients. Additionally, the body's intricate balance of fluid (including specific amounts of electrolytes) is a vital component in maintaining homeostasis. Dietary supplements can help maintain needed levels of these essential nutrients and fluids.

* **serum** solution containing whole antibodies for a specific pathogen.

* **vaccine** solution containing a modified pathogen that does not actually cause disease but still stimulates the development of antibodies specific to it.

VITAMINS AND MINERALS

Vitamins are organic compounds necessary for many different physiological processes, including metabolism, growth, development, and tissue repair. The body absorbs most vitamins through the gastrointestinal tract following dietary ingestion. Vitamins must be obtained from the diet, as the body cannot manufacture them. In the developed countries, healthy adults usually receive adequate amounts of vitamins and do not need supplements. Vitamin supplements may, however, be indicated for special populations, including pregnant and nursing women, patients with absorption disorders, the chronically ill, surgery patients, alcoholics, and the malnourished. Additionally, people on a strict vegetarian diet may need supplemental vitamins. Vitamins are either fat soluble or water soluble. The liver stores the fat-soluble vitamins (A, D, E, and K), and so the patient will become deficient only after long periods of inadequate vitamin intake. Vitamin D is unique in that the skin produces it with exposure to sunlight. The water-soluble vitamins (C and those in the B complex), must be routinely ingested, as the body does not store them. After short periods of deprivation, patients may begin to experience vitamin deficiency. The B complex vitamins are grouped only because they occur together in foods; otherwise they share no significant characteristics. The individual B vitamins are named for the order in which they were discovered (B_1, B_2, B_3, and so forth). These vitamins also have specific names. For example, B_1 is also known as thiamine, a vitamin that plays a key role in carbohydrate metabolism. Table 14-9 details selected vitamins. Iron is an essential mineral necessary for oxygen transport and several metabolic processes. Iron supplements are the most common mineral supplement. They are indicated for iron deficiency.

FLUIDS AND ELECTROLYTES

Water composes approximately 60 percent of a person's total body weight. The specific composition and amounts of this fluid are vital to a patient's well-being. The specific amounts of electrolytes, such as calcium, potassium, sodium,

Table 14-9 VITAMIN SOURCES AND DEFICIENCIES

Vitamin	Problems Resulting from Deficiency	Source
Fat Soluble		
A	Night blindness, skin lesions	Butter, yellow fruit, green leafy vegetables, milk
D	Bone and muscle pain, weakness, softening of bones	Fish, fortified milk, exposure to sunlight
E	Hyporeflexia, ataxia, anemia	Nuts, green leafy vegetables, wheat
K	Increased bleeding	Liver, green leafy vegetables
Water Soluble		
B_1 (thiamine)	Peripheral neuritis, depression, anorexia, poor memory	Whole grain, beef, pork, peas, beans, nuts
B_2 (riboflavin)	Sore throat, stomatitis, painful or swollen tongue, anemia	Milk, eggs, cheese, green leafy vegetables
B_3 (niacin)	Skin eruptions, diarrhea, enteritis, headache, dizziness, insomnia	Meat, eggs, milk
B_6 (pyridoxine)	Skin lesions, seizures, peripheral neuritis	Liver, meats, eggs, vegetables
B_9 (folic acid)	Megaloblastic anemia	Liver, fresh green vegetables, yeast
B_{12} (cyanocobalamin)	Irreversible nervous system damage, pernicious anemia	Fish, egg yolk, milk
C	Scurvy	Citrus fruits, tomatoes, strawberries

and chlorine, are similarly important. This book's chapter on pathophysiology reviews the physiology of fluids and electrolytes and discusses acid-base balance. The indications and contraindications for administering fluids and electrolytes, as well as these medications' interactions, are covered in Chapter 15 on medication administration and Chapter 19 on hemorrhage and shock.

DRUGS USED TO TREAT POISONING AND OVERDOSES

The treatment for poisoning and overdose depends greatly on the substance involved. In general, therapy aims at eliminating the substance by emptying the gastric contents, by increasing gastric motility in order to decrease the time available for absorption, by alkalinizing the urine with sodium bicarbonate (for tricyclic antidepressant and salicylate overdose), or by filtering the substance from the blood with dialysis. When gastric emptying is indicated, syrup of ipecac is the drug of choice; otherwise, activated charcoal may be used as a gastric absorbent.

Actual antidotes are few; however, some medications are effective in treating certain overdoses or poisonings. General mechanisms for antidote action include receptor site antagonism, blocking enzyme actions involved with metabolism of the substance, and chelation (binding the substance with a stable compound, such as iron, so that it becomes inactive). Specific antidotes include acetylcysteine (Mucomyst) for acetaminophen overdose and deferoxamine for iron chelation. Organophosphates are a common ingredient in insecticides and herbicides as well as chemical weapons. They are aggressive acetylcholinesterase (AChE) inhibitors that prevent the breakdown of acetylcholine, leading to overstimulation of the parasympathetic nervous system as well as neuromuscular junctions. Signs and symptoms of this overstimulation may be remembered by the acronym SLUDGE (salivation, lacrimation, urination, defecation, gastric motility, and emesis). Other signs include bradycardia, hypotension, bronchospasm, muscle fasciculations, miosis (pupil constriction), and respiratory arrest. The antidotes for organophosphate poisoning are atropine and pralidoxamine (2-PAM, Protopam). Atropine antagonizes ACh, while pralidoxamine breaks the organophosphate-acetylcholinesterase bond, freeing AChE to break down the excess ACh.

SUMMARY

Pharmacology is a cornerstone of paramedic practice. Paramedics must have a solid understanding of its foundations (legal issues, terminology, drug forms, and routes), pharmacokinetics, and pharmacodynamics if they are to practise their profession safely. Additionally, paramedics must understand not only the medications they personally administer but also the medications that their patients are taking on an ongoing basis. Although you are not likely to remember everything in this chapter after your first reading, with diligent study and practice, you can master this information. This chapter has barely broken the surface of pharmacology. To continue your education, you should take the time to understand the mechanisms and interactions of the medications your patients are taking. If you do not already know them (you will not, in the majority of cases, as you begin your career), look them up. Many very useful drug references are available today. Most are small and can be easily carried by you on your unit or in your station.

Finally, pharmacology is a dynamic field with new discoveries being made every day. If you take your responsibilities as a paramedic seriously and remain current on the latest changes in this field, you can be sure that you can give your patients the care they deserve.

CHAPTER 15

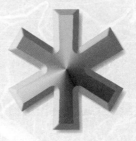

Medication Administration

Objectives

Part 1: Principles and Routes of Medication Administration (begins on p. 763)

After reading Part 1 of this chapter, you should be able to:

1. Review the specific anatomy and physiology pertinent to medication administration. (pp. 766–796)
2. Describe the indications, equipment needed, technique used, precautions, and general principles for the following:
   a. inhalation routes of medication administration. (pp. 770–773)
   b. parenteral routes of medication administration. (pp. 780–796)
   c. percutaneous routes of medication administration. (pp. 766–770)
   d. enteral routes of medication administration, including gastric tube administration and rectal administration. (pp. 773–780)
3. Describe the indications, contraindications, side effects, dosages, and routes of administration for medica-

tions commonly administered by paramedics. (pp. 766–796)
4. Discuss legal aspects affecting medication administration. (pp. 763–764, 766)
5. Discuss the "six rights" of drug administration and correlate them with the principles of medication administration. (p. 763)
6. Differentiate among the percutaneous routes of medication administration. (pp. 766–770)
7. Discuss medical asepsis and the differences between clean and sterile techniques. (pp. 764–765)
8. Describe uses of antiseptics and disinfectants. (pp. 764–765)
9. Describe the use of body substance isolation (BSI) procedures when administering a medication. (p. 764)

Continued

10. Describe disposal of contaminated items and sharps. (p. 765)
11. Synthesize a pharmacological management plan, including medication administration. (pp. 763–796)

Part 2: Intravenous Access, Blood Sampling, and Intraosseous Infusion (begins on p. 796)

After reading Part 2 of this chapter, you should be able to:

1. Review the specific anatomy and physiology pertinent to medication administration. (pp. 796–835)
2. Describe the indications, equipment needed, technique used, precautions, and general principles for the following:

   a. peripheral venous or external jugular cannulation. (pp. 797–824)
   b. intraosseous needle placement and infusion. (pp. 828–835)
   c. obtaining a blood sample. (pp. 824–828)

Part 3: Medical Mathematics (begins on p. 835)

After reading Part 3 of this chapter, you should be able to:

1. Review mathematical equivalents. (pp. 835–838)
2. Differentiate temperature readings between the centigrade and Fahrenheit scales. (p. 837)
3. Discuss formulas as a basis for performing drug calculations. (pp. 838–843)
4. Describe how to perform mathematical conversions from the household system to the metric system. (pp. 836–837)

INTRODUCTION

✱ **medications/drugs** foreign substances placed into the human body.

Medications, or **drugs,** are foreign substances placed into the human body. They serve a variety of purposes, such as controlling specific diseases like hypertension or helping the body fight diseases like cancer and infection.

Medication administration will be an important part of the medical care you provide as a paramedic. You may have to use medications to correct or prevent many life-threatening situations. You may also use drugs to stabilize or comfort a patient in distress. In addition to your knowledge of particular medications and their properties from the previous chapter on pharmacology, you must also be thoroughly skilled in drug administration. Specific drugs require specific routes and administration techniques. Their effectiveness depends directly on their correct route of delivery. Incorrect or sloppy drug administration can have tremendous legal implications for the paramedic. More importantly, it equates to poor care that can harm or even kill the patient.

This chapter discusses the routes and techniques you will use to correctly deliver your patient's medications. It is divided into three parts:

Part 1: Principles and Routes of Medication Administration
Part 2: Intravenous Access, Blood Sampling, and Intraosseous Infusion
Part 3: Medical Mathematics

Part 1: Principles and Routes of Medication Administration

As a paramedic, you are responsible for ensuring that all emergency drugs are in place and ready for immediate use. Therefore, you must know your local drug distribution system. You will have to know where to obtain and replace each drug as it expires or is used up, as another patient may require it at any time. You also will have to thoroughly document the administration and restocking of narcotics, as many local, provincial and territorial, and federal agencies mandate such record keeping.

Always be certain that you correctly give all drugs in the right dose. Medication errors may prove disastrous in terms of patient care and legal responsibility. Your knowledge of drug indications, contraindications, side effects, dosages, and routes of administration is crucial to effective patient care.

You can attain effective pharmacological therapy and eliminate medication errors by following the six "rights" of drug administration:

- *Right person*
- *Right drug*
- *Right dose*
- *Right time*
- *Right route*
- *Right documentation*

Your knowledge of drug indications, dosages, and routes of administration is of paramount importance.

In the field, you will be responsible for the safe and appropriate delivery of medications. If you ever doubt the use or dosage of a medication, contact medical direction immediately. You must repeat back, or echo, all drug orders issued by direct medical command. For example, if medical direction ordered you to administer 25 mg of diphenhydramine (Benadryl), you would echo, "Medic 101 copies the medication order for 25 mg of diphenhydramine to be administered slow IV push." By echoing, you confirm your reception and understanding of the order. If medical direction has issued an inappropriate medication or dosage, echoing may bring it to light and elicit an immediate correction. If you still find the order questionable after echoing, tactfully request clarification or ask about the intent.

Pharmacological therapy permits you to function as an extension of the physician. No room exists for medication errors; once a drug is given, it is difficult, if not impossible, to retrieve. In addition, withholding a needed medication can have catastrophic consequences. Concentration and knowledge are the keys to this component of paramedical care.

If you ever doubt the use or dosage of a medication, contact medical direction immediately.

MEDICAL DIRECTION

Paramedics do not practise autonomously. You will operate under the licence of a medical director who is responsible for all your actions. This responsibility extends to the administration of medications.

Your medical director or medical advisory committee determines which medications you will use and the routes by which you will deliver them. Some medications can be administered via offline medical direction (protocols or written standing orders). You may need specific authorization for others after consulting online or direct medical direction. You must strictly abide by all of your medical director's guidelines.

> *You can ill afford to waste valuable time looking up procedures and directives for the critical patient who requires immediate drug therapy.*
>
>

Knowing all drug administration protocols is essential, especially which drugs to administer under standing orders and which to deliver only after getting authorization from medical direction. You can ill afford to waste valuable time looking up procedures and directives for the critical patient who requires immediate drug therapy. Furthermore, because inappropriate drug delivery can have serious consequences, you may face severe legal ramifications even if your patient suffers no harm.

BODY SUBSTANCE ISOLATION

* **body substance isolation** (BSI) measures to decrease your risk of exposure to blood and body fluids.

* **personal protective equipment** (PPE) generally includes gloves, goggles, and mask.

Establishing routes for drug delivery presents the constant potential for exposure to blood and other body fluids. Always take appropriate **body substance isolation** (BSI) measures, and wear appropriate **personal protective equipment** (PPE) to decrease your risk of exposure. The type of BSI you use will vary according to the delivery route and your patient's condition. At a minimum, you should wear gloves. Optimally, you will also wear goggles and a mask. Remarkably, the simplest form of BSI is often the most neglected: handwashing. Washing your hands before and after patient contact is one of the most effective ways to decrease your exposure to infectious material. Chapter 1 includes a thorough discussion of BSI measures.

MEDICAL ASEPSIS

* **asepsis** a condition free of pathogens.

Medical **asepsis** (*a-*, without; *sepsis,* infection) describes a medical environment free of pathogens. Many paramedical procedures, especially those related to drug administration, place the patient at increased risk for infection. The external environment is full of microorganisms, many of them pathogenic. Such techniques as intravenous access or endotracheal intubation can allow pathogens to enter the patient's body, where they may cause **local** or **systemic** complications.

* **local** limited to one area of the body.

* **systemic** throughout the body.

STERILIZATION

* **sterile** free of all forms of life.

* **medically clean** careful handling to prevent contamination.

The most aseptic environment is a sterile one. A **sterile** environment is free of all forms of life. Generally, environments are sterilized with extensive heat or chemicals. A sterile environment is difficult to attain in the prehospital setting. Consequently, you must practise medically clean techniques to minimize your patient's risk of infection. **Medically clean** techniques involve the careful handling of sterile equipment to prevent contamination. For example, much of the equipment used for drug administration is packaged sterilely. Once you open the package, you must use a medically clean technique to keep the equipment clean and uncontaminated until you use it. If you drop a piece of equipment on a dirty surface, you should discard it and obtain a new piece. Other medically clean techniques, including handwashing, glove changing, and discarding equipment in opened packages, help prevent equipment and patient contamination. Remember, too, that many patients have lowered immunity levels or carry infectious diseases. Thus, keeping the ambulance and equipment clean is another essential medically clean procedure.

DISINFECTANTS AND ANTISEPTICS

* **disinfectant** cleansing agent that is toxic to living tissue.

When administering medications, you must use disinfectants and antiseptics to ensure local cleanliness. Do not confuse disinfectants and antiseptics; the distinction is important. **Disinfectants** are toxic to living tissue. You will therefore use them only on nonliving surfaces or objects, such as the inside of an ambulance or laryngoscope blades after use. Never use disinfectants on living tissue. **Antiseptics** are not toxic to living tissue. They destroy or inhibit pathogenic microorganisms already on living surfaces and are generally used to cleanse the local area before needle puncture. Common antiseptics include alcohol and iodine preparations used either alone or together. Frequently, antiseptics are diluted disinfectants.

* **antiseptic** cleansing agent that is not toxic to living tissue.

DISPOSAL OF CONTAMINATED EQUIPMENT AND SHARPS

Blood and body fluid can harbour infectious material that endangers the health-care provider, family, bystanders, or the patient himself. Many times, the patient is infected with pathogenic organisms long before signs and symptoms appear. Therefore, you must treat all blood and body fluids as potentially infectious.

Treat all blood and body fluids as potentially infectious.

Drug administration commonly involves needles in direct contact with the patient's blood and body fluid. Once used, a needle presents a significant risk. Inadvertent needle sticks, the most common accident in health care as a whole, can transmit diseases between the patient and paramedic. Properly handling needles and other sharps before and after patient use can prevent many of these accidental needle sticks. To minimize or eliminate the risk of an accidental needle stick, take these precautions:

- *Minimize the tasks you perform in a moving ambulance.* Use needles as sparingly as possible in the back of a moving ambulance. When appropriate, perform all interventions involving needles on the scene. While en route, it may be occasionally necessary to have the driver pull the ambulance to the side of the road and stop briefly. Most paramedics become quite proficient at completing these procedures in a moving ambulance.

- *Immediately dispose of used sharps in a sharps container.* A **sharps container** is a rigid, puncture-resistant container clearly marked as biohazardous. You can deposit whole needles and prefilled syringes in it, thus eliminating the need for bending or cutting. Some sharps containers have adapters that permit the easy removal of needles from blood-draw equipment and syringes. You should also dispose of such items as used ampules in the sharps container. Avoid dropping sharps onto the floor for later disposal. In the heat of the moment, you may forget the sharp or mentally misplace it.

- *Recap needles only as a last resort.* If you absolutely must recap a needle, never use two hands to do so. Place the cap on a stationary surface and then place the point of the sharp into the cap using one hand. Although the one-hand method is still hazardous, it at least reduces the chance for an accidental needle stick.

By law, every medical organization must have a biological hazard exposure plan. Be familiar with yours. If you are exposed to blood or other body substances, follow the plan, and immediately notify the appropriate resources. Remember that prevention is the best medicine.

Content Review

NEEDLE-HANDLING PRECAUTIONS

Minimize tasks in a moving ambulance.
Properly dispose of all sharps.
Recap needles only as a last resort.

* **sharps container** rigid, puncture resistant container clearly marked as a biohazard.

MEDICATION ADMINISTRATION AND DOCUMENTATION

When administering medications, proper and thorough documentation is extremely important. You must record all information concerning the patient and the medication including the following:

- Indication for drug administration
- Dosage and route delivered
- Patient response to the medication—both positive and negative

You must also document the patient's condition and vital signs before medication administration as well as after. In addition to communicating all information to those to whom you transfer care, you must record it on a copy of the patient care report.

In emergent and nonemergent situations alike, you will administer a variety of medications through a variety of delivery routes. The routes of drug administration fall into four basic categories: percutaneous, pulmonary, enteral, and parenteral. Technically, drug deliveries through the rectum and pulmonary system are **topical** applications; however, accepted practice classifies these routes separately. Which route you use will depend on the drug you are administering and your patient's status.

PERCUTANEOUS DRUG ADMINISTRATION

Percutaneous medications are applied to and absorbed through the skin or mucous membranes. They are easy to administer and bypass the digestive tract, making their absorption more predictable.

TRANSDERMAL ADMINISTRATION

Medications given by the **transdermal** (*trans-,* across; *dermal,* skin) route promote slow, steady absorption. Nitroglycerine, hormones, and analgesics are commonly administered transdermally. Transdermal delivery can also produce localized effects, as with anti-inflammatories and other bacteriostatic and softening agents. Applying medication locally avoids passing larger quantities of the medication through the entire body, where it is not needed. Transdermal medications include lotions, ointments, creams, foams, wet dressings, adhesive-backed applications, and suppositories.

To administer a transdermal medication, use the following technique:

1. Use appropriate BSI.
2. Confirm the indication, medication, dose, route, and expiration date.
3. Use gloves to avoid contaminating the medication and inadvertently getting it on your skin.
4. Clean and dry your patient's skin at the administration site.
5. Apply medication to the site as specified by the manufacturer. Avoid overdosing or underdosing when using lotion, ointment, cream, or foam.
6. Leave the medication in place for the required time. Monitor the patient for desirable or adverse effects.

You may need to place a dressing over the medication to protect the site and quantity of drug. Carefully follow all recommendations. Administration may

---

Content Review

ROUTES OF DRUG ADMINISTRATION

Percutaneous
Pulmonary
Enteral
Parenteral

---

* **topical medications** material applied to and absorbed through the skin or mucous membranes.

Content Review

PERCUTANEOUS ROUTES

Transdermal
Mucous membrane

---

* **transdermal** absorbed through the skin.

vary subtly, depending on the form of medication and the specific manufacturer's instructions.

Several factors can affect how quickly the skin absorbs transdermal medications. Thin skin, overdose, or penetrating solvents can increase the absorption rate. Conversely, thick skin, scar tissue, or peripheral vascular disease can decrease the rate. If these factors are present, consider alternative sites or dosage adjustments.

MUCOUS MEMBRANES

The mucous membranes absorb medications at a moderate to rapid rate. Similar to transdermal administration, drug delivery through the mucous membranes avoids the digestive tract and complications associated with that route. You can deliver drugs through the mucous membranes at several sites. However, specific drugs are made for specific sites and generally are not interchangeable.

Sublingual

Sublingual drugs are absorbed through the mucous membranes beneath the tongue (*sub-*, below; *lingual*, tongue). The sublingual region is extremely vascular and permits rapid absorption with systemic delivery. These medications are generally dissolvable tablets or sprays. One commonly administered sublingual medication is nitroglycerine.

To administer a medication via the sublingual route, follow these steps:

1. Use appropriate BSI.
2. Confirm the indication, medication, dose, route, and expiration date.
3. Have your patient lift his tongue toward the top and back of his oral cavity.
4. Place the pill or direct the spray between the underside of the tongue and the floor of the oral cavity. Have your patient relax his tongue and mouth. If administering a pill, instruct the patient to let the pill dissolve and not to swallow.
5. Monitor the patient for desirable or adverse effects.

Buccal

The **buccal** region lies in the oral cavity between the cheek and gums. Buccal medications are generally tablets. Hormonal and enzyme preparations are typically given buccally.

To administer a medication buccally, follow these steps:

1. Use appropriate BSI.
2. Confirm the indication, medication, dose, buccal route, and expiration date.
3. Place the medication between the patient's cheek and gum. Instruct the patient to allow the pill or other preparation to dissolve. Ensure that the patient does not swallow the medication.
4. Monitor the patient for desirable or adverse effects.

Content Review

MUCOUS MEMBRANE MEDICATION SITES

Tongue
Cheek
Eye
Nose
Ear

* **sublingual** beneath the tongue.

* **buccal** between the cheek and gums.

Ocular

ocular medication drug administered through the mucous membranes of the eye.

Ocular medications are topical medications that are administered through the mucous membranes of the eye. These are typically local medications for alleviating eye pain, treating infection, decreasing intraocular pressure, or lubricating the eyelid. Medications delivered by way of the eye are labelled for ophthalmic use and packaged as drops or ointments.

If medication is to be administered only to one eye, be sure to medicate the correct eye. The following abbreviations designate right, left, or both eyes:

o.d. right eye *(oculus dexter)*

o.s. left eye *(oculus sinister)*

o.u. both right and left eyes *(oculus uterque)*

To administer a medication via eye drops, use the following technique (Figure 15-1):

1. Use appropriate BSI.
2. Confirm the indication, medication, dose, route, and expiration date.
3. Have your patient lie supine or lay his head back and look toward the ceiling.
4. Pull the lower eyelid downward to expose the conjunctival sac. Never touch the eye.
5. Use a medicine dropper to place the prescribed dosage on the conjunctival sac. Never administer medications directly on the eye unless specifically instructed.
6. Instruct the patient to hold his eye(s) shut for 1–2 minutes.

Ocular medications may also be packaged as ointments. To apply an ointment, follow the same procedure as above, but carefully squeeze the ointment onto the conjunctival sac. If you administer too much medication, carefully blot away the excess drops or ointment with sterile gauze. The ointment will melt as it warms to body temperature and will spread smoothly across the surface of the eye.

FIGURE 15-1 Eye drop administration. Use a medicine dropper to place the prescribed dosage on the conjunctival sac.

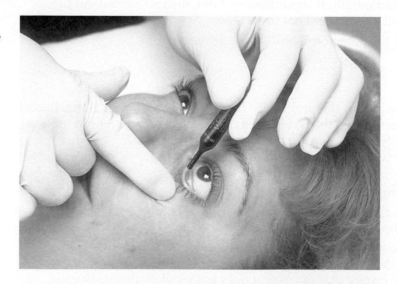

Nasal

The mucous membranes of the nose are another port for topical medication delivery. Given through the nares (nostrils), these **nasal medications** are usually drops or sprays intended for local effect. They commonly treat nasal congestion, hemorrhage, and infection.

✷ **nasal medication** drug administered through the mucous membranes of the nose.

To administer a medication via the nose, use the following technique (Figure 15-2):

1. Use appropriate BSI.
2. Confirm the indication, medication, dose, route, and expiration date.
3. Have the patient blow his nose and tilt his head backward.
4. Use a medicine dropper or squeezable nebulizer to administer the medication into the appropriate nare(s) according to the manufacturer's instructions.
5. Hold the nare(s) shut or tilt the head forward to distribute the medication.
6. Monitor the patient for desirable and undesirable effects.

Aural

Some medications are delivered to the mucous membranes of the ear and ear canal through drops or medicated gauze. These drugs primarily treat local infections and ear pain. Use the following technique to administer medicated drops (Figure 15-3):

1. Use appropriate BSI.
2. Confirm the indication, medication, dose, route, and expiration date.
3. Determine the correct ear for administration.
4. Have the patient lie in the lateral recumbent position with the affected ear upward.
5. Manually open the ear canal: for adult patients, pull the ear up and back; for pediatric patients, pull it down and back.
6. Administer the appropriate dose of medication with a medicine dropper.
7. Have the patient continue to lie with his ear up for 10 minutes.
8. Monitor the patient for desirable and undesirable effects.

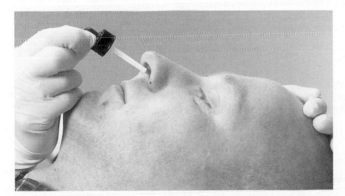

FIGURE 15-2 Nasal medication administration.

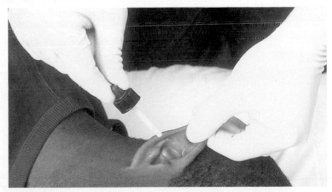

FIGURE 15-3 Aural medication administration. Manually open the ear canal, and administer the appropriate dose.

Using medicated gauze or cotton is generally reserved for the hospital setting. If your local protocols permit you to administer these medications, follow the procedure outlined above, gently inserting the gauze into the ear instead of instilling medicated drops. Avoid tightly packing the ear canal.

PULMONARY DRUG ADMINISTRATION

Special medications can be administered into the pulmonary system via **inhalation** or **injection**. Generally gases, fine mists, or liquids, these drugs include those that promote bronchodilation for respiratory emergencies. Other inhaled drugs are mucolytics, antibiotics, and topical steroids. Inhalation can also be used for humidification and pulmonary decongestion.

NEBULIZER

Typically, drugs administered by inhalation are delivered with the aid of a small volume nebulizer. A **nebulizer** uses pressurized oxygen to disperse a liquid into a fine aerosol spray or mist. Inhalation carries the aerosol into the lungs. Figure 15-4 illustrates a typical nebulizer. The specific design depends on the manufacturer, but they all work on the same principle and typically have the same parts:

- Mouthpiece
- Medication reservoir
- Oxygen port
- Relief valve
- Oxygen tubing
- Oxygen source

To administer a drug with a nebulizer, follow these steps:

1. Use appropriate BSI. Note that paramedics should consider wearing a mask when giving patients nebulized medications.
2. Confirm the indication, medication, dose, route, and expiration date.
3. Put the medication in the medication reservoir. If the medication is not diluted, combine it with 3–5 mL sterile saline solution. This will allow adequate aerosolization. Screw the reservoir in place.

Content Review

PULMONARY MEDICATION MECHANISMS
Nebulizer
Metered dose inhaler
Endotracheal tube

✱ **inhalation** drawing of medication into the lungs along with air during breathing.

✱ **injection** placement of medication in or under the skin with a needle and syringe.

✱ **nebulizer** inhalation aid that disperses liquid into aerosol spray or mist.

FIGURE 15-4   Small volume nebulizer.

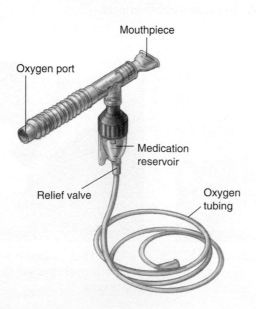

Mouthpiece
Oxygen port
Medication reservoir
Relief valve
Oxygen tubing

4. Assemble the nebulizer.

5. Attach oxygen tubing to the oxygen port and oxygen source.

6. Set the oxygen source regulator for 5–8 litres per minute.
   Note: Never set the oxygen pressure outside of this range.
   Less than 5 L/min will not create enough pressure to aerosolize
   the medication. More than 8 L/min will create too much pressure
   and destroy the oxygen tubing or nebulizer at its weakest point.
   Furthermore, because of pressure restrictions, do not attach the
   nebulizer to an oxygen humidifier.

7. Place the nebulizer in the patient's mouth. Instruct him to exhale
   and then seal his lips around the mouthpiece. Now, have him hold
   the nebulizer and slowly inhale as deeply as possible. On maximum inhalation, instruct the patient to hold in the medication for
   one to two seconds before exhaling. This permits maximum deposition and absorption. Continue this process until the medication
   is completely gone. Typically, this takes 3–5 minutes.

Nebulizers also come preattached to an oxygen facemask in both pediatric and
adult sizes (Figure 15-5). Use nebulization facemasks for pediatric or adult
patients who cannot hold the nebulizer. Nebulizers for those who require long-
term therapy may be powered by a battery or other energy source.

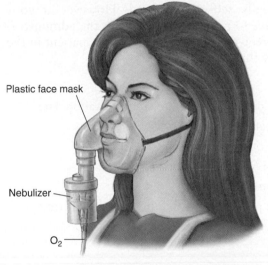

(a) Nebulizer with attached face mask

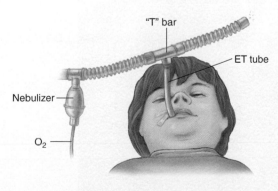

(b) Nebulizer with endotracheal tube

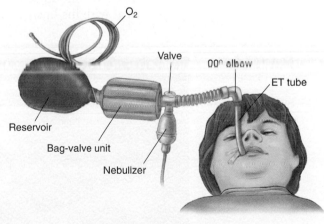

(c) Nebulizer with bag-valve unit

FIGURE 15-5 Nebulizer with attached face mask, endotracheal tube, and bag-valve mask.

For a nebulizer to be effective, the patient must have an adequate tidal volume and respiratory rate. If the tidal volume is shallow or respiratory rate low, the medication will not move from the nebulizer into the lungs. For patients with a poor tidal or respiratory rate who cannot pull the medication into their lungs, you can connect nebulizers to a bag-valve mask or endotracheal tube.

METERED DOSE INHALER

* metered dose inhaler handheld device that produces a medicated spray for inhalation.

Inhaled medications are also delivered through **metered dose inhalers** (MDI). These small, handheld devices produce a medicated spray for inhalation. Patients with conditions like asthma or COPD use metered dose inhalers to deliver a specific, or metered, dose of medication. A metered dose inhaler consists of two parts, a medication canister and a plastic shell and mouthpiece (Figure 15–6). Some metered dose inhalers come equipped with a spacer. The spacer is a cylindrical canister between the inhaler and the mouthpiece. Prior to self-administration, the patient will depress the inhaler sending a measured dose of drug into the spacer. The patient will then breathe in and out of the spacer through the mouthpiece, thus inhaling the drug into the lungs. This system is particularly useful for patients who have a hard time operating and inhaling the metered dose inhaler. This is common in the elderly and in young children. The spacer, when used in conjunction with a metered dose inhaler, is very effective. The MIDI and spacer may be used when dealing with the possibility of the spread of disease, such as SARS.

Metered dose inhalers are usually self-administered. However, if your patient is incapacitated, you may have to physically assist with the administration or educate the patient or his caregivers in its use. To assist a patient in the use of a metered dose inhaler, follow this technique:

1. Use appropriate BSI.
2. Confirm the indication, medication, dose, route, and expiration date.
3. Insert the medication canister into the plastic shell.
4. Remove the cap from the mouthpiece.
5. If required, gently shake the MDI for 2–5 seconds.
6. Instruct the patient to maximally exhale.
7. Place the mouthpiece in the patient's mouth, and have him form a seal with his lips.

FIGURE 15-6 Metered dose inhaler.

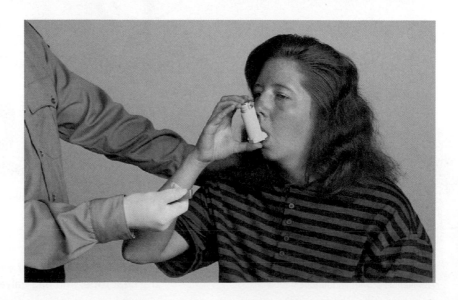

8. As the patient inhales, press the canister's top downward to release the medication.

9. Have the patient hold his breath for several seconds.

10. Remove the inhaler from the patient's mouth and instruct him to breathe slowly.

11. If a second dose is necessary, wait according to the manufacturer's instructions. Repeat.

12. In an acute respiratory emergency involving a patient with a metered dose inhaler, always use a nebulizer instead of the MDI. Although the metered dose inhaler delivers a small amount of medication, the nebulizer delivers larger quantities of medication mixed with water and oxygen.

Nebulizers and metered dose inhalers offer several advantages. In respiratory emergencies, less medication is needed because it reaches its exact site of action. The lower dosage is less likely to promote side effects, and if the patient has an adverse reaction, implementing or discontinuing drug delivery is easy. Furthermore, because the patient can hold the nebulizer, he will benefit from feeling more in control of his overall therapy. Most importantly, if your patient is hypoxic, you can administer inhaled medications with supplemental oxygen.

The nebulizer and metered dose inhaler also have disadvantages. Moving the aerosolized medication into the lungs depends on adequate ventilation. For the patient with a poor tidal and minute volume, nebulized medications are ineffective, as the drug cannot reach its site of action. In these cases, you should use the nebulizer in conjunction with a bag-valve mask or endotracheal tube. Additionally, the patient must exhibit an adequate level of consciousness and manual dexterity to hold the nebulizer and follow instructions correctly.

ENDOTRACHEAL TUBE

When you have not yet established an IV, you can administer certain medications, such as lidocaine (Xylocaine), epinephrine, atropine, and naloxone (Narcan), through an endotracheal tube. Delivering liquid medications into the lungs permits rapid absorption through the pulmonary capillaries. In fact, some authorities believe pulmonary absorption is as fast as intravenous absorption.

When using an endotracheal tube, you must increase conventional IV dosages 2–2.5 times. You also should dilute the medication in normal saline to create 10 mL of solution and then quickly inject it down the endotracheal tube. Several ventilations must follow to aerosolize the medication and enhance its absorption. Ideally, you can pass a commercially manufactured catheter through the endotracheal tube and inject the medication through it. If cardiopulmonary resuscitation (CPR) is underway, stop compressions while you administer the medication, and ventilate for aerosolization.

ENTERAL DRUG ADMINISTRATION

Enteral drug administration is the delivery of any medication that is absorbed through the gastrointestinal tract. The gastrointestinal tract, or alimentary canal, travels from the mouth to the stomach and on through the intestines to the rectum (Figure 15-7). You can administer enteral medications orally, through a gastric tube, or rectally.

Several advantages make the gastrointestinal tract the most common route for medication delivery. Aside from sheer convenience, it is the least expensive route,

Content Review

ENDOTRACHEAL MEDICATIONS
- Lidocaine
- Epinephrine
- Atropine
- Naloxone

* **enteral drug administration** the delivery of any medication that is absorbed through the gastrointestinal tract.

and its use requires little equipment and minimal training. In some instances, after you have delivered a drug, you may be able to retrieve it by inducing vomiting, by removing it from the rectum, or simply by having the patient spit it out.

Conversely, enteral drug administration poses several disadvantages. Physical activity, emotions, or food can significantly alter the gastrointestinal tract's chemical and physical environment, making absorption unreliable. In addition, as all blood from the stomach and small intestine must pass through the hepatic circulatory system (portal circulation), the liver's condition can reduce the medication's effectiveness. A dysfunctional liver can significantly alter drug distribution and, in extreme cases, metabolize therapeutic medications into inert or harmful substances. Furthermore, a patient resistant to or *noncompliant* in taking medications makes administration via the enteral route very difficult.

ORAL ADMINISTRATION

✱ oral drug administration the delivery of any medication that is taken by mouth and swallowed into the lower gastrointestinal tract.

Oral drug administration denotes any medication taken by mouth (oral) and swallowed into the gastrointestinal (GI) tract. From the GI tract, the medication is absorbed and distributed throughout the body. When administering a medication by the oral route, you must be sure that the patient has an adequate level of consciousness to support his airway. Administering an oral medication to a pa-

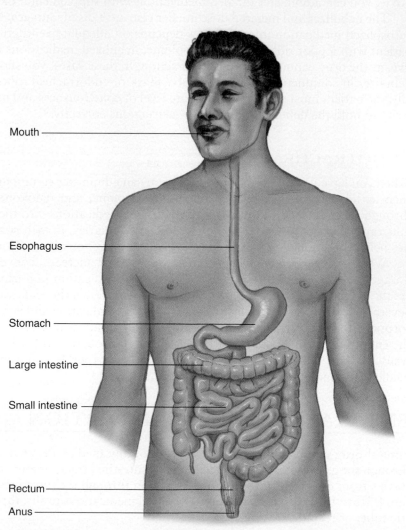

Mouth ——————————

Esophagus ——————————

Stomach ——————————

Large intestine ——————————

Small intestine ——————————

Rectum ——————————

Anus ——————————

FIGURE 15-7   Gastrointestinal tract.

tient who cannot support his airway may result in an airway occlusion or aspiration into the lungs. If aspiration into the lungs occurs, aspiration pneumonia and its deadly consequences may occur.

Medications for oral delivery come in a variety of forms, either solid or liquid.

- *Capsules*. Capsules contain liquid, dry, or beaded medication in a soluble casing. For maximum effectiveness, the patient must swallow them whole.
- *Tablets*. Tablets comprise medicated powder compressed into a small, solid disc. Typically, tablets may be scored to permit breaking in halves or quarters when lesser dosages are required.
- *Pills*. Pills, comprising medicated powder compressed into a small disc, are the same as tablets. In the past, the term *pill* was used to denote a solid medication taken by mouth. Over time, tablet has become the accepted term.
- *Enteric-coated/time-release capsules and tablets*. These forms of medication release the drug gradually as layers of the capsule or tablet slowly erode. Time-release capsules or tablets must be swallowed whole.
- *Elixirs*. Elixirs are liquid medications combined with alcohol or placed in a sweetened fluid.
- *Emulsions*. Emulsions are medications combined with a fat or an oil emulsifier.
- *Lozenges*. Lozenges are solid forms of medication that slowly dissolve in the mouth, thus permitting gradual swallowing.
- *Suspensions*. A suspension is a liquid that contains small particles of solid medication.
- *Syrups*. A syrup is a concentrated solution of sugar in water or another liquid to which a medication is added.

Equipment for Oral Administration

Administering oral medications is simple and easy. The basic equipment that you may need depends on the medication and the patient's status:

- *Soufflé cup*. A soufflé cup is a paper or plastic cup. Placing a solid medication in a soufflé cup makes it easy to see and minimizes contact with the provider's hands.
- *Medicine cup*. A medicine cup is a plastic or glass cup with volumetric measurements on the side. It facilitates giving specific amounts of liquid medication. When you pour medication into the cup, the liquid does not form a flat surface but clings to the sides at a higher level, forming a *meniscus*. To compensate for the meniscus, measure the medication toward the centre, at its lowest level.
- *Medicine dropper*. A medicine dropper has markings for measuring liquid volumes. You will use it for special medications and to administer medications to children or patients who cannot tolerate other forms of oral medication.
- *Teaspoon*. You will use these accurately sized measuring spoons to administer liquid medications. A teaspoon normally holds 5 mL of fluid; however, the volume of household teaspoons varies significantly. To ensure accurate medication administration, use a measured teaspoon or syringe.

Never use household teaspoons to measure medications, as teaspoons vary significantly in volume.

3. Confirm proper tube placement. Disconnect the tube from the drainage or suction unit or clamping device. Clamp the tube from the drainage or suction unit to avoid gastric contents spilling from either device. Attach a cone-tipped syringe to the proximal end of the gastric tube. Gently inject air while auscultating over the stomach. Following this, withdraw the plunger while observing for the presence of gastric fluid or contents, which indicates appropriate placement. Leave the tube disconnected from the drainage or suction unit.

4. Irrigate the gastric tube. To irrigate the gastric tube, draw up 50–100 mL of normal saline into a cone-tipped syringe. Insert the syringe into the open end of the gastric tube. With the syringe tip pointed at the floor, gently inject the saline into the tube. If the saline encounters resistance, look for such problems as tube kinking. Also, have the patient lie on his left side, and reattempt injection. If the saline still meets resistance, reattach the tube to the drainage or suction unit, and contact medical direction for further directives.

5. Prepare the medication(s) for delivery. Crush tablets or empty capsules into 30 mL of warm water. Ensure that all particles are small so that they will not occlude the tube. You may administer liquid medications without further preparation.

6. Draw the medication into a 30–50 mL cone-tipped syringe, and place the tip into open gastric tube. Gently administer the medication into the gastric tube. Forceful application may create considerable distention and patient discomfort.

7. Draw 50–100 mL of warm normal saline into a cone-tipped syringe, and attach it to the open end of the gastric tube. Gently inject the saline. This facilitates the medication's passage into the stomach and rinses the tube, ensuring that the patient receives the entire dose. Repeated administrations may be necessary.

8. Clamp off the distal tube. Use a commercially manufactured device or hemostat to clamp shut the distal portion of the gastric tube for approximately 30 minutes after you administer the medication. Do not reattach to the drainage or suction unit to prevent the medication's inadvertent removal from the stomach.

If you must refill the syringe in order to administer the full dosage of medication, do not allow the syringe to empty completely before you detach it from the gastric tube. This prevents drawing air into the syringe and then introducing it into the stomach, which causes discomfort.

RECTAL ADMINISTRATION

The rectum's extreme vascularity promotes rapid drug absorption. Additionally, because medications given rectally do not pass through the liver, they are not subject to **hepatic alteration;** thus, their absorption is more predictable.

In the emergency setting, you may give certain drugs rectally if you cannot establish an intravenous line or use the oral route. These include diazepam (Valium) for protracted seizures or Aspirin for cardiac or neurological emergencies. In the nonacute setting, you may administer sedatives, antiemetics, or other specially prepared medications rectally.

Rectal administration may prove advantageous with the unconscious or pediatric patient or when administering drugs with an objectionable taste or odour. Unfortunately, drug absorption may be erratic if gross fecal matter exists. In addition, some drugs may cause considerable anal or rectal irritation.

✱ hepatic alteration change in a medication's chemical composition that occurs in the liver.

Rectal medications come in a variety of forms. In the emergency setting, they are typically liquid, thus permitting easy administration and rapid absorption. To administer a rectal medication in the emergent setting follow this technique:

1. Use appropriate BSI.
2. Confirm the indication, medication, dose, route, and expiration date.
3. Draw the correct quantity of medication into a syringe.
4. Place the hub of a 14-gauge Teflon catheter (removed from the angiocatheter) on the end of a needleless syringe (Figure 15-8).
5. Insert the Teflon catheter into the patient's rectum and inject the medication. Try to keep the medication in the lower part of the rectum. Administration higher in the rectum may result in the medication's being absorbed by veins that deliver drug to the portal circulation.
6. Withdraw the catheter and hold the patient's buttocks together, thus permitting retention and absorption.

An alternative technique utilizes a small endotracheal tube instead of the Teflon angiocatheter. Remove the 15/22 mm BVM adapter and connect a syringe to the proximal end of the tube (Figure 15-9). Lubricate the tube and insert it into the rectum. Inject the medication, remove the tube, and hold the patient's buttocks together.

In the nonemergent setting, suppositories or enemas are common methods for rectal administration. Because your responsibilities as a paramedic may include nonemergent clinical settings, you should master these techniques. Additionally, the rectal route may prove beneficial for a pediatric patient who resists oral administration or for whom IV access proves impractical.

Suppositories are medications packaged in a soft, pliable form. Generally refrigerated until they are used, they begin to melt at body temperature in the rectum. Some are lubricated to ease insertion. Suppositories can be lubricated by running a small amount of lukewarm tap water over the suppository before insertion. To administer a suppository, manually insert it into the rectum. Hold the patient's buttocks shut for 5–10 minutes to allow for retention and absorption.

An **enema** is typically a liquid **bolus** of medication that is injected into the rectum. Medications given via this route are typically referred to as small-volume enemas. They are typically prepackaged in a squeezable container with a rectal tip (Figure 15-10).

✳ **suppository** medication packaged in a soft, pliable form, for insertion into the rectum.

✳ **enema** a liquid bolus of medication that is injected into the rectum.

✳ **bolus** concentrated mass of medication.

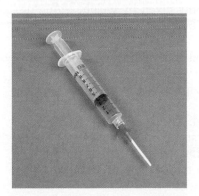

FIGURE 15-8 Catheter placement on needleless syringe.

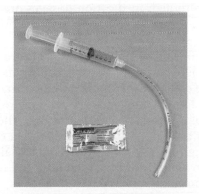

FIGURE 15-9 Syringe attached to endotracheal tube.

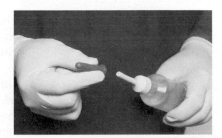

FIGURE 15-10 Prepackaged enema container.

To administer a medicated small-volume enema, use the following technique:

1. Apply appropriate BSI.
2. Confirm the indication, medication, dose, route, and expiration date.
3. Confirm the need for administration via a small-volume enema.
4. Place the patient on his left side. Flex his right leg to expose the anus.
5. Insert the prelubricated rectal tip into the anus, and advance 7.5–10 mm.
6. Gently squeeze the medicated solution of the bottle into the rectum and colon.
7. Hold the patient's buttocks together to enhance absorption into the rectal and intestinal tissue.

Only those medications with specific guidelines for rectal administration should be delivered through this route. Do not administer rectal medications in the presence of diarrhea, rectal bleeding, hemorrhoids, or any other situation involving severe anal irritation.

PARENTERAL DRUG ADMINISTRATION

Parenteral denotes any drug administration outside the gastrointestinal tract. Broadly, this encompasses pulmonary and some topical forms of medication delivery; however, additional, specific criteria apply to parenteral administration. Typically, the parenteral route involves the use of needles as medications are injected into the circulatory system or tissues. Consequently, some forms of parenteral drug delivery afford the most rapid drug delivery and absorption.

SYRINGES AND NEEDLES

Frequently, giving medications via the parenteral route requires a syringe and hypodermic needle.

Syringe

A **syringe** is a plastic tube with which liquid medications can be drawn up, stored, and injected. Syringes range in size from 1 mL to 100 mL and greater. Remember that although medication dosages are generally given by weight (g/mg/µg), syringes represent volume. Therefore, you must be prepared to mathematically convert these measurements.

A syringe's two major components are a barrel and a plunger (Figure 15-11). The tube-like barrel, or body, functions as a reservoir for medication. Markings on its side calibrate its overall volume. Smaller syringes are calibrated in 0.10 mL intervals, larger syringes in 1.0 mL intervals.

The plunger is a device that fits into the barrel. At one end it has a handle for pulling or pushing. At the opposite end, a rubber stopper fits snugly into the barrel. Pulling on the plunger draws material into the barrel; pushing on it expels material from the barrel. The rubber end forms a tight seal from which the fluid medication cannot escape.

The junction of the fluid and rubber stopper measures the total volume of liquid in the syringe. The barrel's maximum volume should correspond closely to the volume of medication needed. For example, to administer 2 mL of medication, a 3-mL syringe would prove most appropriate.

Do not administer rectal medications in the presence of diarrhea, rectal bleeding, hemorrhoids, or any other situation involving severe anal irritation.

* **parenteral** drug administration outside the gastrointestinal tract.

* **syringe** plastic tube with which liquid medications can be drawn up, stored, and injected.

An adapter at the syringe's distal end is compatible with the hub of an IV catheter or, as many cases will require, a hypodermic needle.

Hypodermic Needle

The **hypodermic needle** is a hollow metal tube used with the syringe to administer medications. It is sharp enough to easily puncture tissues, blood vessels, or IV medication ports.

The hypodermic needle's primary components include a hilt and shaft. The hilt is a threaded plastic tube that screws securely onto the syringe's distal adapter. The shaft is a thin metal tube through which medications can flow from the syringe into the delivery site. A bevel at the shaft's distal end accounts for its sharpness (Figure 15-12).

Hypodermic needles come in a variety of gauges and lengths. A needle's **gauge** describes its diameter. Generally, hypodermic needle gauges range from 18 to 27. The gauge and actual diameter are inversely related: the higher the gauge, the smaller is the diameter. Thus, a 25-gauge needle's diameter is smaller than an 18-gauge needle's. Conversely, a 20-gauge needle's diameter is larger than a 22-gauge needle's. Hypodermic needle lengths generally range from 1 cm to 3.5 cm. The package label lists the size of the syringe and the gauge and length of the hypodermic needle.

Because syringes and hypodermic needles frequently involve invasive procedures, they are packaged sterile. Never use either a syringe or a hypodermic needle from a package that has been opened or tampered with. Used hypodermic needles are sharp and present a biohazard. Dispose of them immediately after you complete any task involving their use.

MEDICATION PACKAGING

All medications delivered by the parenteral route are liquids. They are packaged in a variety of containers with which you must be familiar, as obtaining medication from each type requires a different procedure. The kinds of parenteral drug containers include the following:

- Glass ampules
- Single and multidose vials
- Nonconstituted drug vials
- Prefilled syringes
- Intravenous medication fluids

You must also be thoroughly familiar with the information included on the labels of all medication containers:

* **hypodermic needle** hollow metal tube used with the syringe to administer medications.

* **gauge** the size of a needle's diameter.

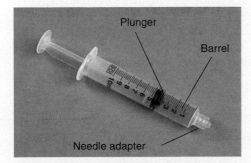

FIGURE 15-11   Syringe.

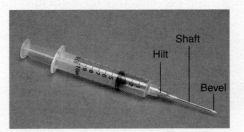

FIGURE 15-12   Hypodermic needle.

- *Name of medication.* The label lists both the generic and trade names of the medication. Always ensure that you have selected the right medication.
- *Expiration date.* All medications have an expiration date after which they cannot be used. Never use an expired medication.
- *Total dose and concentration.* The total dose of drug is the total weight (g/mg/μg) of medication in the container. The concentration represents the weight of the drug per volume of fluid. For example, if 10 mg of a drug were packaged in 10 mL of fluid, the total dose would be 10 mg, and the concentration would be 10 mg/10 mL or 1 mg/mL. Beware—identical drugs can be packaged in different dosages and concentrations, and different drugs can be packaged in similar containers.

These labels are printed directly on the vial, ampule, prefilled syringe, or IV medication bag. Always use them to confirm the correct medication.

Glass Ampules

An **ampule,** or amp, is a breakable glass vessel containing liquid medication. It has a cone shaped top, thin neck, and circular tubular base for storing the medication (Figure 15-13). The thin neck is a vulnerable point where you intentionally break the ampule to retrieve its contents. Ampules usually range in volume from 1 to 5 mL. The least expensive form of drug packaging, they contain single doses of medication.

To obtain medication from a glass ampule, you will need a syringe and needle. Use the following technique (Procedure 15-2):

1. Apply appropriate BSI.
2. Confirm the indication, medication, dose, route, and expiration date.
3. Confirm the ampule label (medication name, dose, and expiration).
4. Hold the ampule upright and tap its top to dislodge any trapped solution. Discard the top in the sharps container.
5. Place gauze around the thin neck and snap it off with your thumb.
6. Place the tip of the hypodermic needle inside the ampule and withdraw the medication into the syringe.
7. Reconfirm the indication, drug, dose, and route of administration.
8. Administer the medication appropriately via the indicated route.
9. Properly dispose of the needle, syringe, and broken glass ampule.

Single and Multidose Vials

Vials are plastic or glass containers with self-sealing rubber tops (Figure 15-14). Vials may contain single or multiple doses of medication; the self-sealing rubber top prevents leakage from punctures and permits multiple access with a syringe and hypodermic needle. The medication inside the vial is packaged in a vacuum.

To obtain medication from a vial, follow these steps (Procedure 15-3):

1. Apply appropriate BSI.
2. Confirm the indication, medication, dose, route, and expiration date.
3. Confirm the vial label (name, dose, and expiration).
4. Determine the volume of medication to be administered.

Always use the label printed directly on the container to confirm the correct medication.

✴ ampule breakable glass vessel containing liquid medication.

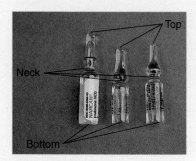

FIGURE 15-13   Ampules.

✴ vial plastic or glass container with a self-sealing rubber top.

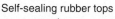
Self-sealing rubber tops

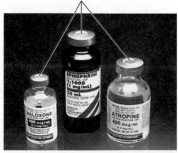

FIGURE 15-14   Vials.

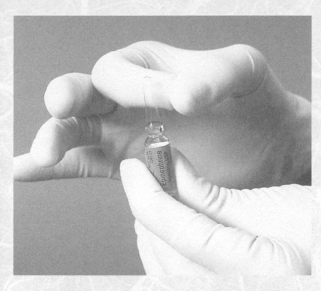

15-2a   Hold the ampule upright and tap its top to dislodge any trapped solution.

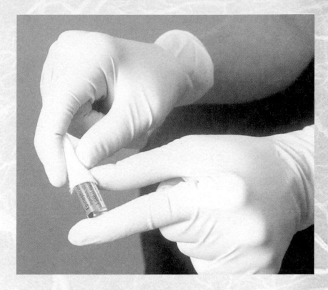

15-2b   Place gauze around the thin neck . . .

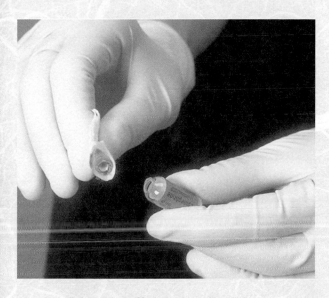

15-2c   and snap it off with your thumb.

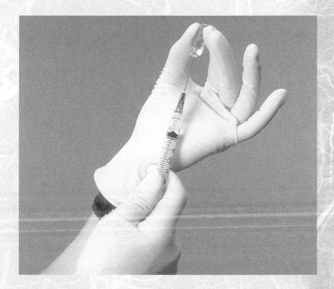

15-2d   Draw up the medication.

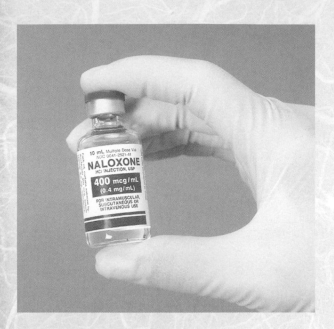

15-3a   Confirm the vial label.

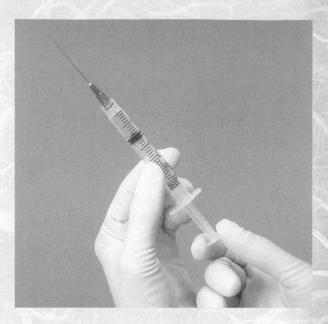

15-3b   Prepare the syringe and hypodermic needle.

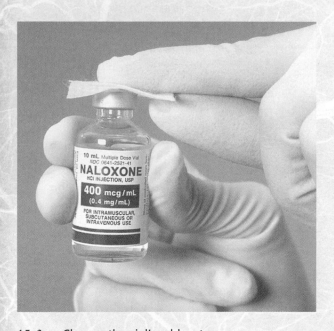

15-3c   Cleanse the vial's rubber top.

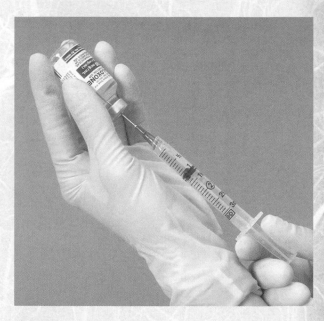

15-3d   Insert the hypodermic needle into the rubber top and draw the air from the syringe into the vial.

5. Prepare the syringe and hypodermic needle. Because the vial is vacuum packed, you will have to replace the volume of medication removed with air in order to maintain equilibrium in the vial. Withdraw the plunger, to draw a volume of air into the syringe equal to the volume of medication to be administered. This technique permits easy medication retrieval from the vial.

6. Cleanse the vial's rubber top with an antiseptic alcohol preparation.

7. Insert the hypodermic needle into the rubber top and draw the air from the syringe into the vial. Then, withdraw the appropriate volume of medication.

8. Reconfirm the indication, drug, dose, and route of administration.

9. Administer appropriately via the indicated route.

10. Properly dispose of the needle, syringe, and vial.

Nonconstituted Drug Vial

The **nonconstituted drug vial**, extends the viability and storage time of drugs that have a short shelf life or are unstable in liquid form. The nonconstituted drug vial actually consists of two vials, one containing a powdered medication and one containing a liquid mixing solution (Figure 15-15). To prepare the drug you must mix it, or reconstitute it, by withdrawing the liquid solution from its vial and placing it in the powdered medication's vial. In a **Mix-o-Vial** system, the two vials are joined and you must squeeze them together to break the seal and mix.

   To prepare a medication from a nonconstituted drug vial, use the following technique (Procedure 15-4):

1. Apply appropriate BSI.
2. Confirm the indication, medication, dose, route, and expiration date.
3. Confirm the vial's label (name, dose, expiration date).
4. Remove all solution from the vial containing the mixing solution, using the same procedure as you would to withdraw medication from a single or multidose vial.
5. With an alcohol preparation, cleanse the top of the vial containing the powdered drug and inject the mixing solution.
6. Gently agitate or shake the vial to ensure complete mixture.
7. Determine the volume of newly constituted medication to be administered.
8. Prepare the syringe and hypodermic needle. Because the vial is vacuum packed, you will have to replace the volume of medication removed with air in order to retain equilibrium in the vial. By withdrawing the plunger, place into the syringe a volume of air equal to the volume of medication that will be removed. This technique permits easy medication retrieval from the vial.
9. Cleanse the medication vial's rubber top with an antiseptic alcohol preparation.
10. Insert the hypodermic needle into the rubber top and withdraw the appropriate volume of medication.
11. Reconfirm the indication, drug, dose, and route of administration.
12. Administer appropriately via the indicated route.
13. Monitor the patient for the desired effects.
14. Properly dispose of the needle and syringe.

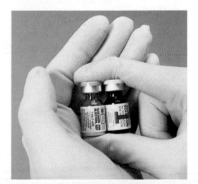

FIGURE 15-15 The nonconstituted drug vial actually consists of two vials, one containing a powdered medication and one containing a liquid mixing solution.

Preparing Medication from a Nonconstituted Drug Vial

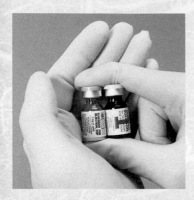

15-4a Nonconsituted drugs come in separate vials. Confirm the labels.

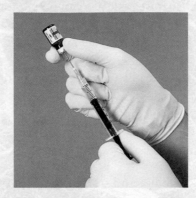

15-4b Remove all solution from the vial containing the mixing solution.

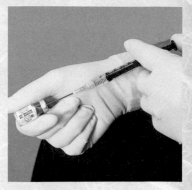

15-4c Cleanse the top of the vial containing the powdered drug and inject the solution.

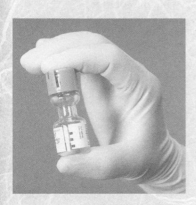

15-4d Agitate or shake the vial to ensure complete mixture.

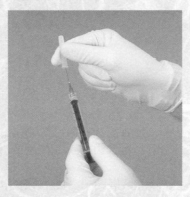

15-4e Prepare a new syringe and hypodermic needle.

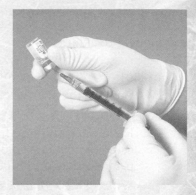

15-4f Withdraw the appropriate volume of medication.

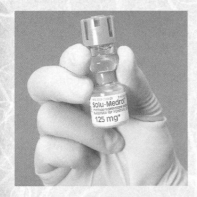

15-4g In the Mix-o-Vial system, the vials are joined at the neck. Confirm the labels.

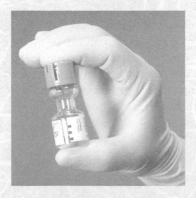

15-4h Squeeze the vials together to break the seal. Agitate or shake to mix completely.

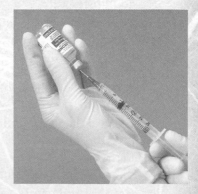

15-4i Withdraw the appropriate volume of medication.

In some instances you may have to place multiple medications into one syringe for a single delivery. For example, meperidine (Demerol) and promethazine (Phenergan) may be delivered in this manner. Meperidine, an analgesic, can cause nausea and vomiting when administered. To decrease the incidence of nausea and vomiting, you can simultaneously administer promethazine, an antiemetic. To perform this task, draw all medications in the appropriate order according to the procedures discussed. Always anticipate total volume and select an appropriate syringe size. To avoid complications, you must always be aware of drug incompatibilities.

Prefilled or Preloaded Syringes

Prefilled or **preloaded syringes** are packaged in tamper-proof containers with the medication already in the syringe. Because the syringe is prefilled, you do not need to draw the medication from another source. Generally, prefilled syringes contain standard dosages, thus decreasing the chance of dosage error.

The prefilled syringe consists of two parts, a syringe and a tube prefilled with liquid medication. The plastic syringe is similar to those described earlier; however, it does not have a plunger. Rather, you screw the prefilled tube into the syringe barrel and secure it (Figure 15-16). Pushing the container into the syringe barrel expels the medication through the attached hypodermic needle.

Follow these steps to administer a medication from a prefilled syringe:

1. Apply appropriate BSI.
2. Confirm the indication, medication, dose, route, and expiration date.
3. Confirm the prefilled syringe label (name, dose, and expiration date).
4. Assemble the prefilled syringe. Remove the pop-off caps and screw together.
5. Reconfirm the indication, drug, dose, and route of administration.
6. Administer appropriately via the indicated route.
7. Properly dispose of the needle and syringe.

Intravenous Medication Solutions

Medicated solutions are another form of parenteral medication. They are packaged in an IV bag and administered as an IV **infusion**. IV medication solutions may be premixed or you may have to mix them. The section on intravenous drug infusions later in this chapter discusses the actual preparation and administration of an infusion.

PARENTERAL ROUTES

Parenterally administered drugs can be absorbed locally or systemically. Additionally, depending on the route of administration, their absorption rate may be

* **prefilled/preloaded syringe** syringe packaged in a tamper-proof container with the medication already in the barrel.

* **medicated solution** parenteral medication packaged in an IV bag and administered as an IV infusion.

* **infusion** liquid medication delivered through a vein.

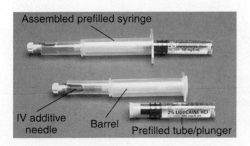

FIGURE 15-16   Prefilled syringes.

Content Review

PARENTERAL ROUTES
Intradermal injection
Subcutaneous injection
Intramuscular injection
Intravenous access
Intraosseous infusion

slow, sustained, or rapid. Parenteral delivery bypasses the digestive tract, thus making the drug's absorption, action, and onset more predictable. Because parenteral routes use hypodermic needles that contact body fluids, the risk of disease transmission is ever present.

Parenteral drug delivery employs the following routes:

- Intradermal injection
- Subcutaneous injection
- Intramuscular injection
- Intravenous access
- Intraosseous infusion

Specific medications require specific routes of parenteral delivery; therefore, you must be competent with every route. In this section, we will discuss the specialized equipment, medications, and routes for intradermal, subcutaneous, and intramuscular injections. Because of their complexity, we will discuss intravenous access and intraosseous infusions separately in the following sections.

Whether you are administering a parenteral injection or an IV bolus or infusion, you should explain the entire procedure to the patient to help alleviate his anxiety. Finally, remember that hypoperfusion (hypovolemia or peripheral vascular disease, for instance) may significantly reduce parenteral absorption.

Intradermal Injection

 intradermal within the dermal layer of the skin.

Using a syringe and hypodermic needle, **intradermal injections** deposit medication into the dermal layer of the skin (*intra-*, within; *derma*, skin). The amount of medication placed in the dermal layer is quite small, typically less than 1 mL (Figure 15-17).

Capillaries in the dermis afford a very slow rate of absorption, with little or no systemic distribution. Rather, the bulk of medication remains localized in the area of administration. Intradermal delivery proves useful for allergy testing and tuberculin skin testing and for administering local anesthetics during suturing, wound débridement, and IV establishment.

Capillaries in the dermis afford a very slow rate of absorption, with little or no systemic distribution.

The forearm and upper back are preferred sites for intradermal injections. They have little hair and are highly visible. Additionally, you should look for sites free of superficial blood vessels, which increase the chance for systemic absorption.

To administer an intradermal injection, you will need the following equipment:

- BSI protection (personal protective equipment)
- Alcohol or betadine antiseptic preparations
- Packaged medication

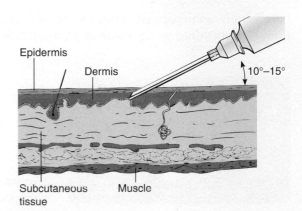

FIGURE 15-17 Intradermal injection.

- Tuberculin syringe (1 mL)
- 25- to 27-gauge needle, 1–2.5 cm long
- Sterile gauze and adhesive bandage

To administer an intradermal injection, follow these steps:

1. Apply appropriate BSI.
2. Confirm the indication, medication, dose, route, and expiration date.
3. Assemble and prepare the needed equipment.
4. Apply BSI and confirm the drug, indication, dosage, and need for intradermal injection.
5. Draw up medication as appropriate.
6. Prepare the site with alcohol or betadine. The intended site must be cleansed of pathogens, thereby decreasing the likelihood of infection. Generally, you will use alcohol or betadine antiseptics. To appropriately cleanse the site, start at the site itself and work outward with an expanding circular motion. This motion will push pathogens away from the intended site of puncture.
7. Pull the patient's skin taut with your nondominant hand.
8. Insert the needle, bevel up, just under the skin, at a 10- to 15-degree angle.
9. Slowly inject the medication, look for a small bump, or wheal, to form as medication is deposited and collects in the intradermal tissue.
10. Remove the needle and dispose of it in the sharps container.
11. Place the adhesive bandage over the site; use the gauze for hemorrhage control if needed.

Do not rub or massage the injection site. This promotes systemic absorption and nullifies the advantage of localized effect.

Subcutaneous Injection

Subcutaneous injections place medication into the subcutaneous tissue (*sub-*, below; *cutaneous*, skin). The subcutaneous layer consists of loose connective tissue between the skin and muscle (Figure 15-18). The subcutaneous tissue has few blood vessels and thus promotes slow, sustained absorption, which prolongs a drug's effect on the body. Like intradermal injections, no more than 1 mL of medication is administered subcutaneously. Administering more than 1 mL of medication can cause irritation and, possibly, an abscess.

 subcutaneous (see subcutaneous tissue) the layer of loose connective tissue between the skin and muscle.

The subcutaneous tissue has few blood vessels and thus promotes slow, sustained absorption, which prolongs a drug's effect on the body.

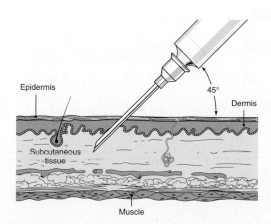

FIGURE 15-18 Subcutaneous injection.

Administer subcutaneous injections where you can easily pinch the skin on the upper arms, thighs, or occasionally, the abdomen (Figure 15-19). Easily pinched skin contains more subcutaneous tissue and readily separates from the muscle. All sites should be free of superficial blood vessels, nerves, and tendons. Additionally, avoid areas with tattoos or bruising.

To perform a subcutaneous injection, you will need the following equipment:

- BSI protection (personal protective equipment)
- Alcohol or betadine antiseptic preparations
- Packaged medication
- Syringe (1–3 mL)
- 24- to 26-gauge hypodermic needle, 1–2.5 cm long
- Sterile gauze and adhesive bandage

To administer a subcutaneous injection, use the following technique (Procedure 15-5):

1. Apply appropriate BSI.
2. Confirm the indication, medication, dose, route, and expiration date.
3. Assemble and prepare the equipment.
4. Draw up the medication as appropriate.
5. Prepare the site with alcohol or betadine as described for an intradermal injection.
6. Gently pinch a 2-cm fold of skin.
7. Insert the needle just into skin at a 45-degree angle with the bevel up.
8. Pull the plunger back to aspirate tissue fluid.
9. If blood appears, the hypodermic needle is in a blood vessel and absorption will be too rapid. Start the procedure over with a new syringe.

FIGURE 15-19 Subcutaneous injection sites (injection sites shown in red).

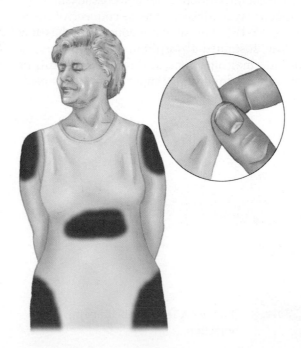

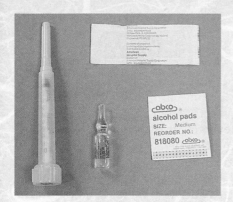

15-5a   Prepare the equipment.

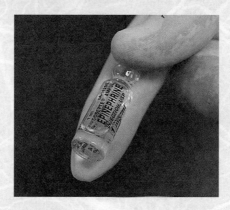

15-5b   Check the medication.

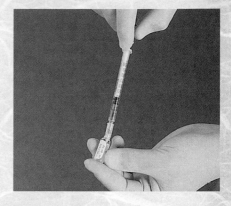

15-5c   Draw up the medication.

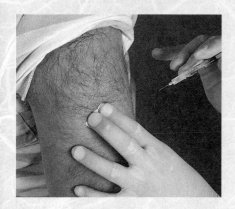

15-5d   Prep the site.

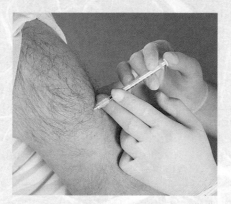

15-5e   Insert the needle at a 45-degree angle.

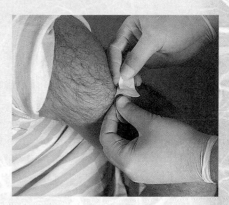

15-5f   Remove the needle and cover the puncture site.

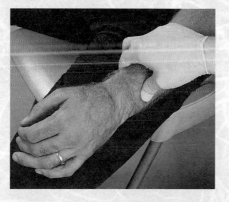

15-5g   Monitor the patient.

10. If no blood appears, proceed to step 11.

11. Slowly inject the medication.

12. Remove the needle and dispose of it in a sharps container.

13. Place an adhesive bandage over the site; use the gauze for hemorrhage control if needed.

14. Monitor the patient.

After you give the injection, gently rubbing or massaging the site will help initiate systemic absorption.

Some authorities recommend using an air plug in the syringe. This is approximately 0.1 mL of air that follows the injection and pushes the medication further into the subcutaneous tissue, thus preventing leakage or medication loss. To place an air plug in the syringe, aspirate approximately 0.1 mL of air into the barrel after you have drawn up the medication. Pointing the needle downward and perpendicular to the ground, tap the syringe with your finger to dislodge the air pocket. It will float to the top of the plunger, and from there it will follow the medication into the subcutaneous tissue.

You can also deliver a subcutaneous injection into the sublingual region, or fleshy tissue below the tongue. To administer a subcutaneous injection, place the hypodermic needle of a small, medication-filled syringe into the sublingual tissue and then inject the medication as appropriate. Epinephrine in severe cases of asthma or anaphylaxis can be administered in this manner.

Intramuscular Injection

Intramuscular injections deposit medication into muscle (*intra-*, within; *muscular,* muscle). Muscle is extremely vascular and permits systemic delivery at a moderate absorption rate. Drug absorption through muscle is also relatively predictable. To reach the muscle, a needle must penetrate the dermal and subcutaneous tissue (Figure 15-20).

Several sites are used for intramuscular injections (Figure 15-21). Depending on the site, varying quantities of medication can be delivered. These sites and their correlating volumes of medication include the following:

- *Deltoid.* The deltoid muscle is three to four finger breadths below the acromial process (the bony bump on the shoulder). It is highly vascular and permits easy access. You can deliver up to 2 mL into this muscle.

- *Dorsal Gluteal.* The dorsal gluteal muscle, or buttock, is a common administration point for intramuscular injections. Injections here can deliver 5 mL of medication or more. They cause little

 intramuscular within the muscle.

Content Review

INTRAMUSCULAR INJECTION SITES

Deltoid
Dorsal gluteal
Vastus lateralis
Rectus femoris

Muscle is extremely vascular and permits systemic delivery at a moderate absorption rate.

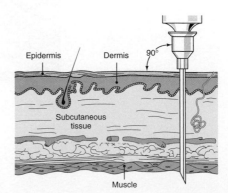

FIGURE 15-20 Intramuscular injection.

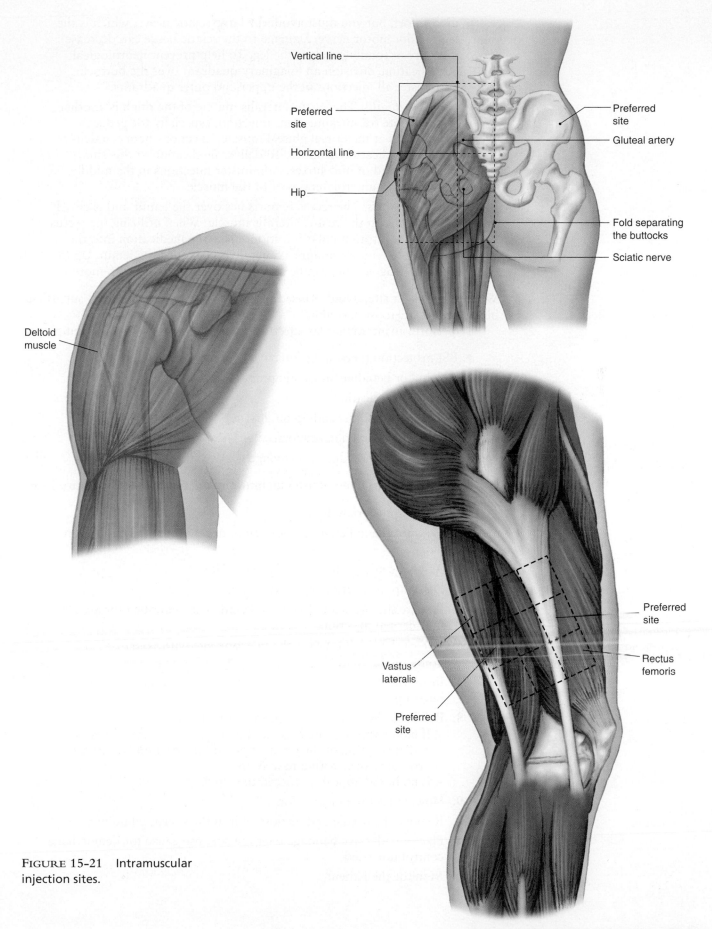

Vertical line

Preferred site

Horizontal line

Hip

Preferred site

Gluteal artery

Fold separating the buttocks

Sciatic nerve

Deltoid muscle

Vastus lateralis

Preferred site

Preferred site

Rectus femoris

FIGURE 15–21   Intramuscular injection sites.

discomfort, but you must avoid the large sciatic nerve, which is the leg's major motor nerve. Damage to the sciatic nerve can decrease mobility or totally paralyze the leg. To help prevent neurological complication, envision an imaginary quadrant over the buttock; administer all injections in the upper and outer quadrants.

- *Vastus Lateralis.* The vastus lateralis muscle of the thigh is another common site for intramuscular injection, especially for pediatric patients. As at the dorsal gluteal muscle, injections here can deliver 5 mL of medication or more. To deliver medication at this site, imagine a grid of nine boxes. Administer injections in the middle, outer box, or anterolateral part of the muscle.

- *Rectus Femoris.* The rectus femoris lies over the femur and is closely associated with the vastus lateralis muscle. When utilizing the rectus femoris for intramuscular injection, place the medication into the centre of the muscle at approximately midshaft of the femur. Up to 5 mL of drug volume can be administered into the rectus femoris.

When choosing a site, avoid bruised or scarred areas. Areas free of superficial blood vessels are most desirable.

To perform an intramuscular injection, you will need the following equipment:

- BSI protection (personal protective equipment)
- Alcohol or betadine antiseptic preparation
- Packaged medication
- Syringe (1–5 mL depending on dosage)
- 21- to 23-gauge hypodermic needle, 1–2.5 cm long
- Sterile gauze and adhesive bandage

Follow these steps to administer an intramuscular injection (Procedure 15-6):

1. Apply appropriate BSI.
2. Confirm the indication, medication, dose, route, and expiration date.
3. Assemble and prepare the needed equipment.
4. Draw up medication as appropriate.
5. Prepare the site with alcohol or betadine as described for an intradermal injection.
6. Stretch the skin taut over the injection site with your nondominant hand.
7. Insert the needle just into skin at a 90-degree angle with the bevel up.
8. Pull back the plunger to aspirate tissue fluid.
   - If blood appears, the hypodermic needle is in a blood vessel, and absorption of the medication will be too rapid. Start the procedure over with a new syringe.
   - If no blood appears, proceed to step 9.
9. Slowly inject the medication.
10. Remove the needle and dispose of it in the sharps container.
11. Place an adhesive bandage over the site; use gauze for hemorrhage control if needed.
12. Monitor the patient.

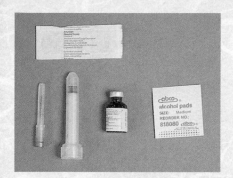

15-6a   Prepare the equipment.

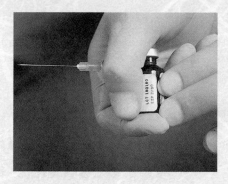

15-6b   Check the medication.

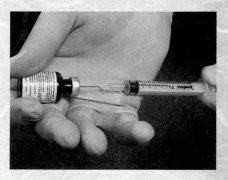

15-6c   Draw up the medication.

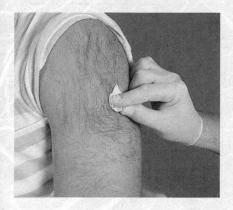

15-6d   Prepare the site.

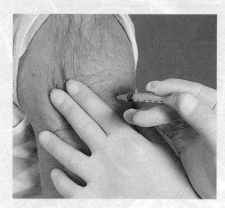

15-6e   Insert the needle at a 90-degree angle.

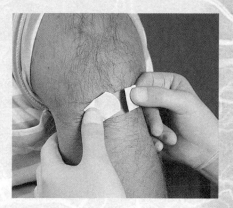

15-6f   Remove the needle and cover the puncture site.

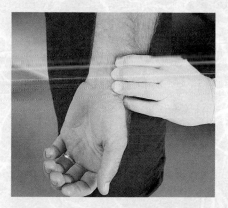

15-6g   Monitor the patient.

After administration, gently rubbing or massaging the site helps to initiate systemic absorption. Do not massage the site, however, if you have administered heparin or another anticoagulant. Again, some authorities recommend a 0.1-mL air plug as described under subcutaneous injection.

Intravenous and Intraosseous Routes

Two important parenteral drug administration routes—intravenous access and intraosseous infusion—are discussed in detail in Part 2.

Part 2: Intravenous Access, Blood Sampling, and Intraosseous Infusion

Objectives

In this part, we will discuss intravenous access, including types of venous access and the variety of equipment required, where and how to establish intravenous access, flow rates, and possible complications. We will also detail intravenous administration of medications (bolus and infusion). Venous blood sampling techniques will also be covered.

Additionally, this part of the chapter provides information on intraosseous medication administration, including techniques, possible complications, and contraindications. Intraosseous administration is a route most often used in pediatric patients under five years of age.

INTRAVENOUS ACCESS

✱ **intravenous access (cannulation)** surgical puncture of a vein to deliver medication or withdraw blood.

Intravenous (IV) access (*intra-*, within; *venous*, vein) or **cannulation,** is a routine paramedic procedure. Circulating blood transports chemicals, proteins, and fluids throughout the body. Venous circulation can likewise deliver medications and fluids into the body and provides an invaluable tool for treating the sick and injured.

The following situations indicate intravenous access:

- Fluid and blood replacement
- Drug administration
- Obtaining venous blood specimens for laboratory analysis

Since veins are easier to locate and penetrate, venous access is preferable to arterial access. Additionally, venous circulation pressure is lower than arterial and presents fewer hemorrhage control complications.

TYPES OF INTRAVENOUS ACCESS

Medical care providers use two types of intravenous access, peripheral and central. As a paramedic, you will most often perform peripheral intravenous access. Central venous access is rarely, if ever, performed in the prehospital setting.

Peripheral Venous Access

Although challenging, **peripheral venous access** is relatively easy to master. As its name implies, it uses peripheral veins. Common sites include the arms and legs and, when necessary, the neck. Figure 15-22 illustrates the specific veins commonly accessed on the hand, forearm, and leg.

As some patients' veins may not be readily visible, you must know venous topography. In these cases, you will have to locate veins based on anatomical layout and palpation. Exhaust all possibilities on the arms before trying to locate the veins of the legs. Leg veins are more difficult to access and present complications more frequently. For neonates and infants, you may access veins in the scalp. Chapter 42 on pediatrics explains that technique.

When establishing a peripheral IV, start at the distal end of the extremity and work proximally. Once you have attempted cannulation, the disruption in blood flow hinders using veins distal to that site. However, the purpose of access also determines site selection. For example, rapid fluid administration requires larger veins like the antecubital fossa, as opposed to the smaller veins of the hand. The external jugular vein is considered a peripheral vein and can be accessed when other peripheral sites are not available.

The major advantage of peripheral venous access is that it is relatively simple to perform because visualizing and accessing the veins is usually easy. Additionally, you can access peripheral veins while simultaneously doing other life-sustaining procedures, such as CPR or endotracheal intubation. Conversely, peripheral veins collapse in hypovolemia, circulatory failure, or hypothermia, thus becoming difficult to locate and access. Furthermore, the peripheral veins of geriatric patients, pediatric patients, or those with peripheral vascular disease may be fragile and difficult to cannulate. Finally, peripheral veins may roll and elude IV placement.

* **peripheral venous access** surgical puncture of a vein in the arm, leg, or neck.

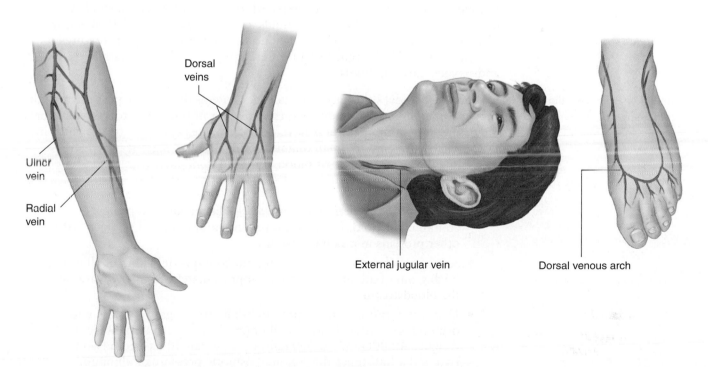

FIGURE 15-22 Peripheral IV access sites: veins of the arm, hand, neck, and foot.

Central Venous Access

* central venous access surgical puncture of the internal jugular, subclavian, or femoral vein.

Central venous access utilizes veins located deep within the body. These include the internal jugular, subclavian, and femoral veins. They are larger than peripheral veins and will not collapse in shock. Central IV lines are placed near the heart for long-term use. Typically, they are used when medical conditions require repeated access for medication and fluid delivery. They also are used for transvenous pacing or for monitoring central venous pressure.

* peripherally inserted central catheter (PICC) line threaded into the central circulation via a peripheral site.

A special type of central line is the peripherally inserted central catheter, or PICC, line. PICC lines are smaller than those routinely used for central access and are threaded into the central circulation via a peripheral site. PICC lines are most often used in infants and children requiring long-term care.

Central venous access is typically restricted to the hospital setting because of its invasive nature and high risk of complications, such as arterial puncture, pneumothorax, and air embolism. Central veins cannot be accessed during procedures like CPR, and they often require a chest x-ray for placement confirmation. You may nonetheless encounter a central line during interfacility transports or in a chronically ill homebound patient. Protocols in some EMS systems allow paramedics to access existing central lines during emergency care. Still other systems allow their paramedics to place certain central lines. Always follow local protocols regarding central line access and insertion. For more information about central venous access, consult a text on advanced venipuncture techniques.

EQUIPMENT AND SUPPLIES FOR VENOUS ACCESS

To establish intravenous access, you will need the following specialized equipment and supplies.

Intravenous Fluids

* intravenous fluid chemically prepared solution tailored to the body's specific needs.

Intravenous fluids are chemically prepared solutions tailored to the body's specific needs. They replace the body's lost fluids and aid the delivery of IV medications. They also can keep a vein patent when no fluid or drug therapy is required.

Intravenous fluids come in four different forms: colloids, crystalloids, blood, and oxygen-carrying fluids.

* colloid intravenous solutions containing large proteins that cannot pass through capillary membranes.

Colloids Colloidal solutions contain large proteins that cannot pass through the capillary membrane. Consequently, they remain in the circulatory system for a long time. In addition, colloids have osmotic properties that attract water into the circulatory system. A small quantity of colloid can significantly increase intravascular volume (volume of blood and fluid contained within the blood vessels). Common colloids include the following:

- *Plasma protein fraction (plasmanate)*. Plasmanate is a protein-containing colloid. Its principal protein, albumin, is suspended with other proteins in a saline solvent.
- *Salt-poor albumin*. Salt-poor albumin contains only human albumin. Each gram of albumin will retain approximately 18 mL of water in the bloodstream.
- *Dextran*. Dextran is not a protein but a large sugar molecule with osmotic properties similar to albumin's. It comes in two molecular weights: 40 000 and 70 000 daltons. Dextran 40 has from two to two-and-a-half times the colloidal osmotic pressure of albumin. Anaphylactic reaction is a possible side effect.

- *Hetastarch (Hespan).* Like Dextran, hetastarch is a sugar molecule with osmotic properties similar to protein's. Hetastarch does not appear to share Dextran's side effects.

Although colloids help maintain vascular volume, using them in the field is not practical. Their high cost, short shelf life, and specific storage requirements suit them better to the hospital setting. However, the paramedic who works in an emergency department, in an aeromedical service, or at a mass-casualty incident may have to administer colloidal solutions.

Crystalloids Crystalloids are the primary prehospital IV solution. Crystalloids contain electrolytes and water but lack colloids' larger proteins and larger molecules. The many preparations of crystalloid solutions are classified by their tonicity (number of particles per unit volume) relative to that of body plasma:

- *Isotonic Solutions.* **Isotonic** solutions have a tonicity equal to blood plasma's. In a normally hydrated patient, they will not cause a significant fluid or electrolyte shift.
- *Hypertonic Solutions.* **Hypertonic** solutions have a higher solute concentration than do the cells. When administered to the normally hydrated patient, they cause fluid to shift out of the intracellular compartment and into the extracellular compartment. Later, the solutes will diffuse in the opposite direction.
- *Hypotonic Solutions.* **Hypotonic** solutions have a lower solute concentration than do the cells. When administered to a normally hydrated patient, they cause fluid to move from the extracellular compartment and into the intracellular compartment. Later, the solutes will move in the opposite direction.

The particular type of IV solution you select depends on your patient's needs. The three most commonly used IV fluids in prehospital care are as follows:

- *Ringer's Lactate.* Ringer's Lactate solution is an isotonic electrolyte solution. It contains sodium chloride, potassium chloride, calcium chloride, and sodium lactate in water.
- *Normal saline solution.* Normal saline is an isotonic electrolyte solution containing 0.90 percent sodium chloride in water.
- *Five-percent dextrose in water* (D_5W). D_5W is a hypotonic glucose solution used to keep a vein patent and to supply calories needed for cellular metabolism. Although D_5W initially increases circulatory volume, glucose molecules rapidly diffuse across the vascular membrane and increase the free water.

Both Ringer's Lactate and normal saline solution are used for fluid replacement because of their immediate ability to expand the circulating volume. However, due to the movement of electrolytes and water, two-thirds of either solution will be lost to the extravascular space within one hour. Crystalloids, such as normal saline mixed with D_5W or half-strength normal saline (0.45 percent), are combinations or modifications of the above solutions.

Occasionally, you will have to warm or cool the IV fluid. A hypothermic patient may benefit from having a crystalloid warmed before and during fluid administration. Warm fluids assist in elevating the patient's core temperature. Conversely, cool fluids may benefit the patient with an increased core temperature.

* **crystalloid** intravenous solutions that contain electrolytes but lack the larger proteins associated with colloids.

Content Review

CRYSTALLOID CLASSES
Isotonic
Hypertonic
Hypotonic

* **isotonic** state in which solutions on opposite sides of a semipermeable membrane are in equal concentration.

* **hypertonic** state in which a solution has a higher solute concentration on one side of a semipermeable membrane than on the other side.

* **hypotonic** state in which a solution has a lower solute concentration on one side of a semipermeable membrane than on the other side.

You can cool or warm fluids by storing them in a special temperature-controlled compartment or by using the heater or air conditioner in the ambulance, helicopter, or mobile intensive care unit. Commercial fluid heaters are available. Their use is detailed later in this chapter. Some fluids, such as blood and some colloids, require constant storage in a cool environment.

Blood The most desirable fluid for replacement is whole blood. Unlike colloids and crystalloids, the hemoglobin in blood carries oxygen. Blood, however, is a precious commodity and must be conserved so that it can be of benefit to the most people. Its use in the field is generally limited to aeromedical services or mass-casualty incidents. O-negative blood's universal compatibility makes it ideal for administration in the field. Chapter 35 on hematology discusses blood in detail.

Oxygen-Carrying Solutions In development are fluids that can carry oxygen and offload it for cellular use. These fluids, which remain experimental at present, show promise for treating hypovolemia in the field.

Packaging of Intravenous Fluids Most intravenous fluids and blood are packaged in soft plastic or vinyl bags of various sizes (50, 100, 250, 500, 1000, 2000, and 3000 mL) (Figure 15-23). Some contain medication that is incompatible with plastic or vinyl and must be packaged in glass bottles.

The IV-fluid container provides important information:

- *Label.* A label on every IV bottle or bag lists the fluid type and expiration date. Like any other medication, intravenous solutions have a shelf life; do not use them after their expiration date. Discard any fluid that appears cloudy, discoloured, or laced with particulate. Additionally, avoid using any fluid when the sealed packaging has been opened or tampered with.
- *Medication Administration Port.* A medication port on IV-solution bags or bottles permits you to inject medication into the fluid for infusion.
- *Administration Set Port.* The administration set port is where you place the spike from the IV administration tubing.

Administration Tubing

Intravenous **administration tubing** connects the solution bag to the IV **cannula** that is inserted into the patient's vein. Administration tubing is made of very flexible clear plastic. You must select from several types of administration tubing according to your patient's need. All tubing is packaged in a sterile container. If the container is opened or appears damaged, select another administration set. Any pathogens on the tubing will enter the patient, possibly causing long-term complications.

Microdrip and Macrodrip Tubing Microdrip administration tubing delivers relatively small amounts of fluid to the patient. It is more appropriate when you need to restrict the overall fluid volume a patient will receive. **Macrodrip** administration tubing delivers relatively large amounts of fluid. It is more appropriate when volume replacement is necessary, as in shock, fluid replacement, or hypotension.

To effectively deliver intravenous fluids, you must be thoroughly familiar with the microdrip and macrodrip administration sets, their components, and their subtle differences (Figure 15-24).

- *Spike.* The **spike** is a sharp-pointed plastic device that you insert into the administration set port on the IV solution bag. A plastic sheath covering the spike keeps it sterile. When the sheath is removed, you

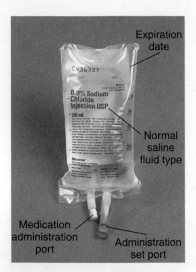

Expiration date

Normal saline fluid type

Medication administration port

Administration set port

FIGURE 15-23 IV solution containers.

Do not use any IV fluids after their expiration date; any fluids that appear cloudy, discoloured, or laced with particulate; or any fluid whose sealed packaging has been opened or tampered with.

✱ **administration tubing** flexible, clear plastic tubing that connects the solution bag to the IV cannula.

✱ **cannula** hollow needle used to puncture a vein.

✱ **microdrip tubing** administration tubing that delivers a relatively small amount of fluid.

✱ **macrodrip tubing** administration tubing that delivers a relatively large amount of fluid.

✱ **spike** sharp-pointed device inserted into the IV solution bag's administration set port.

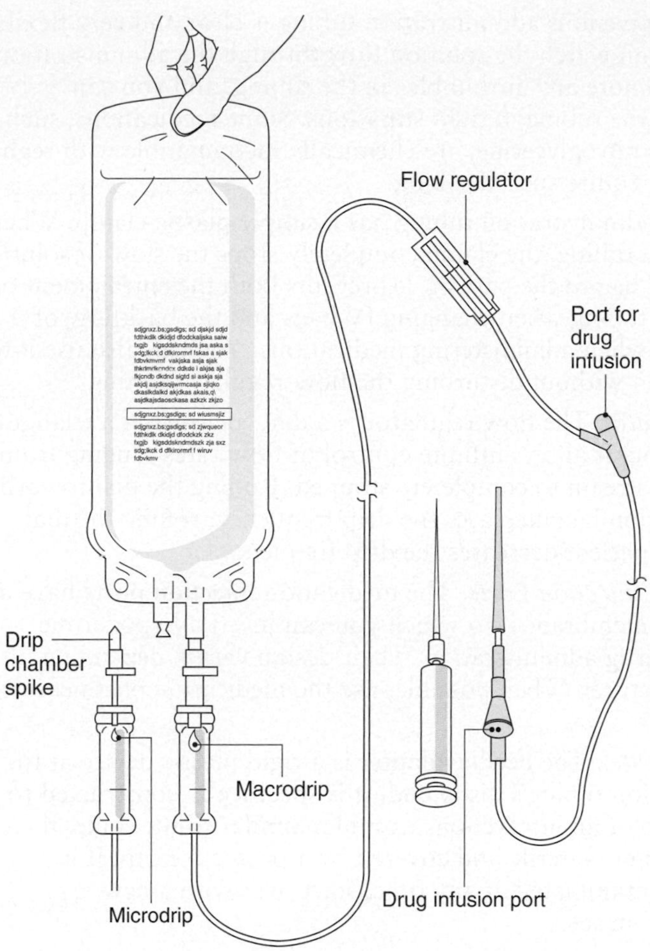

FIGURE 15-24 Macrodrip and microdrip administration sets.

must use a medically clean technique to avoid contaminating the spike. If the spike becomes contaminated, discard the administration set, and start over with new tubing.

- *Drip Chamber.* The **drip chamber** is a clear plastic chamber that allows you to view the **drip rate.** The drip chamber is squeezable; when compressed, it collects fluid from the IV solution bag and acts as a reservoir for administration. For optimal fluid delivery, the drip chamber should be about one-third full; a line on the chamber marks the correct fluid level.

- *Drop Former.* Inside the drip chamber is a **drop former.** In microdrip administration tubing, the drop former is a hollow metal stylet. In macrodrip tubing, it is a large circular opening at the top of the drip chamber. The drop former regulates each drop's size. The narrow metal stylet in the microdrip tubing creates smaller drops; the wider opening in the macrodrip tubing creates larger drops. In either case, the drop former's precise calibration allows you to calculate fluid volumes by counting drops, or **gtts:**

  - Microdrip   60 gtts = 1 mL
  - Macrodrip   10 gtts = 1 mL

Depending on the manufacturer, macrodrip sets may equate 15 or 20 gtts to 1 mL. You must know drops per millilitre to calculate flow rates or medicated infusion dosages.

✱ drip chamber clear plastic chamber that allows visualization of the drip rate.

✱ drip rate pace at which the fluid moves from the bag into the patient.

✱ drop former device that regulates the size of drops.

✱ gtts drops (Latin *guttae,* drops [*gutta,* drop]).

- *Tubing.* Intravenous administration tubing is clear and very flexible. Thus, you can watch the solution flow through the administration set, you can note any air bubbles in the tubing, and you can manipulate the tubing in tight situations. Some medications, such as intravenous nitroglycerine, are chemically incompatible with regular tubing and require special tubing.

- *Clamp.* IV administration tubing has a simple plastic clamp. When slid over the tubing, the clamp completely stops the flow of solution from the IV bag to the patient. It prevents both the entrainment of air into the tubing when changing IV bags and the backflow of medication when administering medications. You can also use it to stop infusion without disturbing the flow-regulator setting.

- *Flow Regulator.* The flow regulator is a dial enclosed in a triangular plastic casing. It allows infinite control of flow rates ranging from a continuous stream to completely stopped. Rolling the dial toward the IV solution bag increases the drip frequency; rolling the dial toward the patient decreases the drip frequency.

- *Medication Injection Ports.* The **medication injection ports** have a self-sealing membrane into which you can insert a hypodermic needle for drug administration. Their design varies, depending on the manufacturer. When possible, use the medication port nearest the patient.

- *Needle Adapter.* The **needle adapter** is a rigid plastic device at the administration tubing's distal end. It is specifically constructed to fit into the hub of an intravenous cannula. Similar to the spike, the needle adapter is sterile and covered by a protective cap. If it becomes contaminated at any time, start over with a new administration set.

IV Extension Tubing **Extension tubing** is IV tubing used to extend the original macrodrip or microdrip setup. Its packaging clearly marks it as such. Like administration sets, extension tubing is sterile and must be handled accordingly.

Extension tubing also permits the paramedic to change the original administration tubing or the IV solution bag with little difficulty. For example, if you have to switch from a macrodrip set to a microdrip set, you can close the clamp on the extension and detach the primary tubing. Once you have flushed the new tubing with fluid, you place the needle adapter into the receiving port on the extension tubing and release the clamp. You can now resume fluid therapy without risking complications or having to painfully reinitiate a second IV line.

Electromechanical Pump Tubing Mechanical infusion devices may require specially manufactured pump tubing. Typically, pump tubing has special components that attach directly to the pump. Additionally, bladders and relief points permit you to void possible air bubbles. Many specific models of electromechanical infusion pumps require specific pump tubing. When using a mechanical infusion pump, be sure to have the appropriate tubing on hand.

Measured Volume Administration Set The **measured volume administration set** can deliver specific volumes of fluid with or without medication. It is especially advantageous for pediatrics, renal failure, or other patients who cannot tolerate fluid overload.

The measured volume administration set consists of either micro- or macrodrip tubing, with the addition of a large **burette chamber** marked in 1-mL increments. The burette chamber holds between 120 mL and 150 mL of fluid. Its components include the following:

✳ **medication injection port** self-sealing membrane into which a hypodermic needle is inserted for drug administration.

✳ **needle adapter** rigid plastic device specifically constructed to fit into the hub of an intravenous cannula.

✳ **extension tubing** IV tubing used to extend a macrodrip or microdrip setup.

✳ **measured volume administration set** IV setup that delivers specific volumes of fluid.

✳ **burette chamber** calibrated chamber of Berutrol IV administration tubing that enables precise measurement and delivery of fluids and medicated solutions.

- Flanged spike
- Clamp
- Airway handle
- Medication injection port
- Burette chamber
- Float valve
- Drip chamber
- Flow regulator
- Medication injection port
- Needle adapter

When opened, the airway handle on top of the burette chamber permits air to be displaced or replaced as fluid enters or exits the chamber. If a medication must be mixed in a specific amount of IV solution, you can add it through the medication administration port after correctly filling the chamber.

Blood Tubing Administering whole blood or blood components requires **blood tubing,** which contains a filter that prevents clots and other debris from entering the patient. Without exception, all blood must be filtered. Blood that is stored or delivered over an extended period is prone to form fibrin clots or to accumulate other debris. If these clots or debris enter the circulatory system, they can travel in the form of an embolus.

Many aeromedical and facility-based paramedics administer blood and must be familiar with blood tubing. Although most ambulances do not carry blood, paramedics may initiate normal saline with blood tubing in anticipation that whole blood or blood products will be required immediately in the emergency department.

Blood tubing comes in two configurations, straight and Y. Y tubing has two administration ports, one for blood and one for IV normal saline solution. Typically, blood is administered with normal saline. Fluids like Ringer's Lactate increase the potential for blood coagulation. The two-port design permits immediate access to normal saline if the blood supply is exhausted or must be shut down, as for a transfusion reaction. When you use Y blood tubing, establish a traditional IV by connecting a bag of normal saline to the tubing. Attach the blood to the second port when needed, while maintaining strict medical asepsis. Using the flow regulator, discontinue the normal saline while opening the clamp regulating the flow of blood. Straight blood tubing has only one reservoir. Therefore, only blood is attached to the tubing. A medication administration port close to the needle adapter allows you to piggyback a secondary line of normal saline into the tubing.

Miscellaneous Administration Sets Some tubing now has a manual dial that can set drops per minute or specific flow rates. Some manufacturers have created a single drip chamber that can create either microdrips or macrodrips.

Intravenous Cannulas

The intravenous cannula permits actual puncture and access into a patient's vein. The distal portion of the administration tubing connects to the IV cannula. The three basic types of IV cannulas are:

- Over-the-needle catheter
- Hollow-needle catheter
- Plastic catheter inserted through a hollow needle

over-the-needle catheter/ angiocatheter semiflexible catheter enclosing a sharp metal stylet.

Over-the-Needle Catheter Often called an **angiocatheter,** the semiflexible **over-the-needle catheter** encloses a sharp metal stylet (needle) (Figure 15-25).

- *Metal stylet (needle).* The metal stylet punctures the skin and blood vessel. Blood flows through the hollow stylet to the flashback chamber.
- *Flashback chamber.* Blood in the clear plastic flashback chamber confirms placement of the stylet in the vein.
- *Teflon catheter.* The Teflon catheter slides over the metal stylet into a successfully punctured vein.
- *Hub.* Located on the back of the Teflon catheter, the hub receives the needle adapter of the administration tubing once removed from the metal stylet.

For peripheral venous access, the over-the-needle catheter is preferred, since it is easy to place and anchor and permits freer movement of the patient.

hollow-needle catheter stylet that does not have a Teflon tube but is itself inserted into the vein and secured there.

Hollow-Needle Catheter For pediatric or other patients with tiny, delicate veins, use **hollow-needle catheters** (Figure 15-26). These catheters do not have a Teflon tube; rather, the metal stylet itself is inserted into the vein and secured there. Because the sharp metal stylet can easily damage the vein, you must insert it very carefully. Some hollow-needle catheters have wings for guidance and securing into a vein. These hollow-needle catheters are referred to as winged catheters or butterfly catheters.

catheter inserted through the needle (intracatheter) Teflon catheter inserted through a large metal stylet.

Catheter Inserted through the Needle The **catheter inserted through the needle** is also called an **intracatheter.** It consists of a Teflon catheter inserted through a large metal stylet (Figure 15-27). Used in the hospital setting to implement central lines, its proper placement requires great skill, as discussed previously.

The size of an intravenous cannula is expressed as its gauge. The *larger* the gauge, the *smaller* is the diameter of the stylet and catheter. For example, a 22-gauge cannula is smaller than a 14-gauge cannula. The larger-diameter, 14-gauge catheter allows greater flow rates than the smaller-diameter 22-gauge cannula. When establishing venous access, choose the cannula size most appropriate for the patient condition. Typical uses for the various sizes of cannulas are as follows:

- *22-gauge:* Small gauges are used for *fragile* veins, such as those of the elderly or children.
- *20-gauge:* Moderate gauges are used for the average adult who does not need fluid replacement.
- *18-gauge, 16-gauge, or 14-gauge:* Larger gauge cannulas are used to increase volume or to administer viscous medications, such as dextrose. Blood can be administered only through a cannula that is 16 gauge or larger.

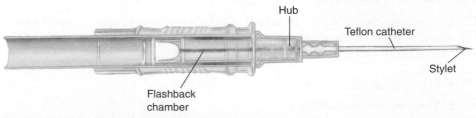

FIGURE 15-25   Over-the-needle catheter.

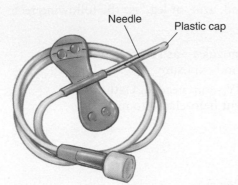

Needle   Plastic cap

FIGURE 15-26   Hollow-needle catheter.

The largest gauge cannula that will fit into a vein is not always appropriate. A cardiac patient with large veins should not receive a 14-gauge cannula for medication administration, just as a multisystems trauma patient with good veins should not receive a 22-gauge cannula for fluid administration. Remember that intravenous access is painful and causes discomfort not only to those receiving it but also to family members watching a loved one in distress.

Miscellaneous Equipment

The **venous constricting band** is a flat rubber band applied proximal to the intended puncture site. It impedes venous return, thereby engorging veins and making them easier to see. This helps you select the best site and makes venipuncture easier. Never restrict arterial blood flow with the constricting band, and never leave it in place longer than two minutes.

Intravenous access is an invasive procedure; therefore, you must use medically clean techniques, including antiseptic preparations, to prevent infection. Applying alcohol and betadine before and after venipuncture decreases the chance of infection.

Once you have established an IV, you must secure it to avoid losing the access. Medical tape and an adhesive bandage are inexpensive and easy to apply. You can also apply clear membranes over the site. Commercial devices manufactured specifically for this task are also available. Have gauze on hand for hemorrhage control if IV cannulation is unsuccessful or if blood leaks from around the site.

Obtaining a venous blood specimen at the time of venipuncture will save the patient from being stuck with a needle again later. This chapter's section on venous blood sampling discusses this technique in detail.

INTRAVENOUS ACCESS IN THE HAND, ARM, AND LEG

As a paramedic, you will most often establish peripheral IVs in the hand, arm, or leg. The veins in these places are relatively easy to locate and accessing them causes the patient less pain. In addition, the likelihood of complications is less with these veins than with the external jugular vein (discussed later) or central IV initiation. Therefore, the veins of the hand, arm, and leg are the primary sites for IV initiation.

Intravenous access is painful and causes discomfort not only to those receiving it but also to family members watching a loved one in distress.

✱ **venous constricting band** flat rubber band used to impede venous return and make veins easier to see.

Never leave the constricting band in place more than two minutes.

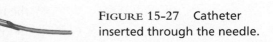

FIGURE 15-27   Catheter inserted through the needle.

To establish a peripheral IV in the hand, arm, or leg, use the following technique (Procedure 15-7):

1. Use the proper BSI—gloves and goggles—as IV access is invasive and presents the potential for blood exposure.

2. Confirm indication and type of IV setup needed. Gather and arrange all supplies and equipment beforehand to make the process easy and accessible:
   - IV fluid
   - Administration set
   - Intravenous cannula
   - Tape or commercial securing device
   - Venous blood drawing equipment
   - Venous constricting band
   - Antiseptic swab (betadine/alcohol)

   When appropriate, explain the entire process to the patient.

3. Prepare all needed equipment. Examine the IV fluid for clarity and expiration date. Ensure the roller clamp is closed. Insert the administration tubing spike in the IV solution bag's administration set port. Squeeze fluid from the IV fluid container into the drip chamber until it reaches the fill line. Open the clamp or flow regulator to flush the solution through the administration tubing and expel trapped air bubbles. Shut down the flow regulator and replace the cap over the needle adapter. Remember that the IV administration set is sterile; if any contamination occurs, you must replace the set with a new one.

4. Select the venipuncture site. Acceptable sites have clearly visible veins and are free of bruising or scarring. Straight veins are easier to cannulate than are crooked ones.

5. Place the constricting band proximal to the intended site of puncture. Tighten it enough to impede venous blood flow without restricting arterial blood passage. Never leave the constricting band in place more than two minutes, as intrinsic changes will occur in the slowed venous blood.

6. Cleanse the venipuncture site. You must cleanse the intended site of pathogens to decrease the likelihood of infection. Alcohol and betadine are the most commonly used antiseptics. Start at the site itself and work outward in an expanding circle. This pushes pathogens away from the puncture site.

7. Insert the intravenous cannula into the vein. With your nondominant hand, pull all local skin taut to stabilize the vein and prevent it from rolling. With the distal bevel of the metal stylet up, insert the cannula into the vein at a 10- to 30-degree angle. Continue until you feel the cannula "pop" into the vein or see blood in the flashback chamber. The metal stylet is now in the vein; however, the Teflon catheter is not. To place the catheter into the vein, lower the angle of the needle and carefully advance the cannula approximately 0.5 cm further. (If you are using a butterfly cannula, it has no Teflon catheter, and you must carefully advance the needle itself.)

8. Holding the metal stylet stationary, slide the Teflon catheter over the needle into the vein. Place a finger over the vein at the catheter tip, and tamponade (press gently downward to occlude the vein), thus preventing blood from flowing from the catheter and air from entraining into the circulatory system. Carefully remove the

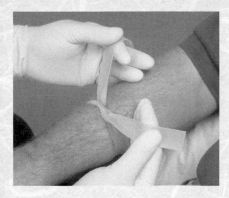

15-7a   Place the constricting band.

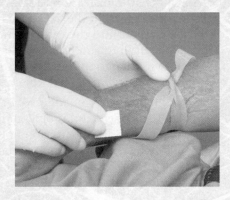

15-7b   Cleanse the venipuncture site.

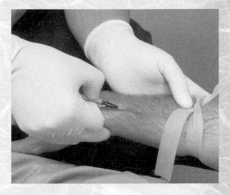

15-7c   Insert the intravenous cannula into the vein.

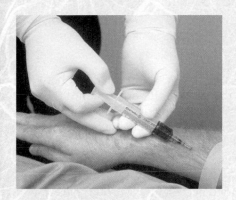

15-7d   Withdraw any blood samples needed.

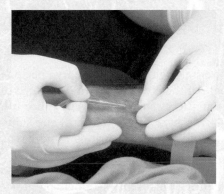

15-7e   Connect the IV tubing.

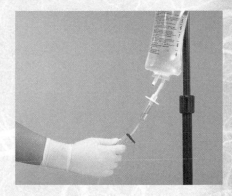

15-7f   Turn on the IV and check the flow.

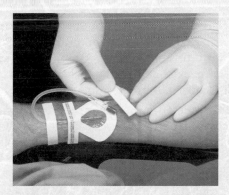

15-7g   Secure the site.

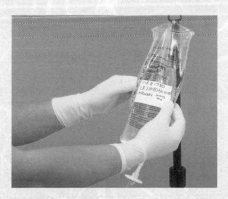

15-7h   Label the intravenous solution bag.

metal stylet and promptly dispose of it in the sharps container. Remove the venous constricting band.

9. Obtain venous blood samples as discussed in the section on venous blood sampling.

10. Attach the administration tubing to the cannula. Remove the protective cap from the needle adapter and tightly secure the needle adapter into the cannula hub. Open the flow regulator and allow the fluid to run freely for several seconds. Adjust the flow rate. Do not let go of the cannula and administration tubing until you have secured them as explained in step 10.

11. Cover the site with an adhesive bandage or other commercial device. Loop the distal tubing and secure with tape. This makes the medication administration port more accessible and attaches the device to the patient more securely. Continue by taping the administration tubing to the patient, proximal to the venipuncture site.

12. Label the intravenous solution bag with the following information:
    - Date and time initiated
    - Person initiating the intravenous access

13. Continually monitor the patient and flow rate.

INTRAVENOUS ACCESS IN THE EXTERNAL JUGULAR VEIN

The external jugular vein is a large peripheral blood vessel in the neck, between the angle of the jaw and the middle third of the clavicle. It connects into the central circulation's subclavian vein. Since it lies so close to the central circulation, cannulation here offers many of the same benefits afforded by central venous access. Fluids and medications rapidly reach the core of the body from this site.

Consider accessing the external jugular vein only after you have exhausted other means of peripheral access or when a patient requires immediate fluid administration. This is an extremely painful site to access, and so you typically will reserve its use for patients with a decreased or total loss of consciousness.

Cannulating the external jugular vein requires essentially the same equipment as other forms of peripheral IV access, plus a 10-mL syringe. You will not need a constricting band. To access the external jugular, use the following technique (Procedure 15-8):

1. Use the appropriate BSI. Prepare all equipment as for peripheral IV access in an arm, hand, or leg. In addition, fill the 10-mL syringe with 3 to 5 mL of sterile saline. Attach the distal part of the syringe to the flashback chamber of a large bore, over-the-needle catheter. Use the proper BSI protection.

2. Place the patient supine or in the Trendelenburg position. This position will increase blood flow to the chest and neck, thus distending the vein and making it easier to see. In addition, the supine-Trendelenburg position decreases the chance of air entering the circulatory system during cannulation.

3. Turn the patient's head to the side opposite of access. This manoeuvre makes the site easier to see and reach; do not perform it if the patient has traumatic head or neck injuries.

Consider accessing the external jugular only after you have exhausted other means of peripheral access or when a patient requires immediate fluid administration.

Peripheral Intravenous Access in an External Jugular Vein

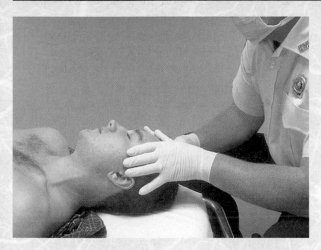

15-8a   Place the patient supine or in the Trendelen-burg position.

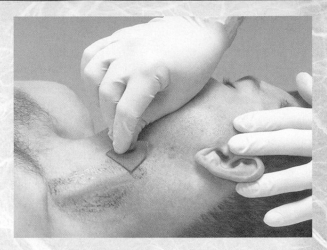

15-8b   Turn the patient's head to the side opposite of access and cleanse the site.

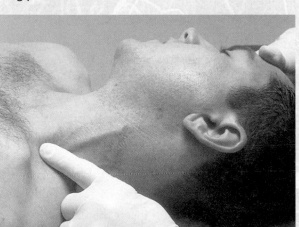

15-8c   Occlude venous return by placing a finger on the external jugular vein just above the clavicle.

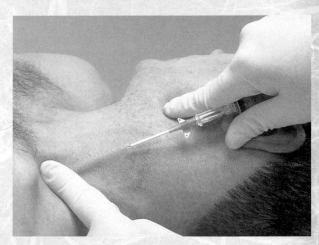

15-8d   Point the catheter at the medial third of the clavicle and insert it, bevel up, at a 10- to 30 degree angle.

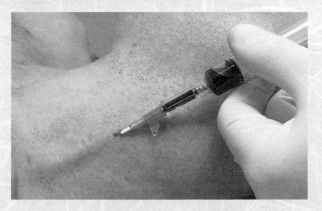

15-8e   Enter the external jugular vein while with-drawing on the plunger of the attached syringe.

4. Cleanse the site with antiseptics. Start at the site of intended puncture and work outward 2 to 5 cm in ever-increasing circles.

5. Occlude venous return by placing a finger on the external jugular vein just above the clavicle. This should distend the vein, again allowing greater visualization and ease of puncture. Never apply a venous constricting band around the patient's neck.

6. Position the intravenous cannula parallel with the vein, midway between the angle of the jaw clavicle. Point the catheter at the medial third of the clavicle and insert it, bevel up, at a 10- to 30-degree angle.

7. Enter the external jugular vein while withdrawing on the plunger of the attached syringe. You will see blood in the syringe or feel a pop as the cannula enters the vein. Once inside the vein, advance the entire angiocatheter another 0.5 cm so the tip of the Teflon catheter lies within the lumen of the vein. Then, slide the Teflon catheter into the vein and remove the metal stylet as previously described. Immediately dispose of the metal stylet.

8. Obtain venous blood samples as discussed in the section on venous blood sampling.

9. Attach the administration tubing to the IV catheter. Allow the intravenous solution to run freely for several seconds. Set the flow rate and secure as appropriate.

10. Monitor the patient for complications.

Although using the external jugular vein has advantages, it also has distinct drawbacks. You may inadvertently puncture the airway or damage the nearby arterial vessels. Additionally, this is a painful entry site for the conscious patient. To minimize risks, perform the procedure very carefully.

INTRAVENOUS ACCESS WITH A MEASURED VOLUME ADMINISTRATION SET

When using a measured volume administration set, follow this procedure (Procedure 15-9):

1. Prepare the tubing by closing all clamps, and insert the flanged spike into the IV solution bag's spike port.

2. Open the airway handle. Open the uppermost clamp and fill the burette chamber with approximately 20 mL of fluid. Squeeze the drip chamber until the fluid reaches the fill line. Open the bottom flow regulator to purge air through the tubing. When all air is purged, close the bottom flow regulator.

3. Continue to fill the burette chamber with the designated amount of solution.

4. Close the uppermost clamp and open the flow regulator until you reach the desired drip rate. Leave the airway handle open so that air replaces the displaced fluid.

To refill the burette chamber, open the uppermost clamp until you have delivered the desired volume; then repeat step 4.

You can also use measured volume administration sets for continuous fluid administration. Fill the burette chamber with at least 30 mL of solution and close the airway handle. Leave the uppermost clamp open and adjust the rate with the lower flow regulator.

Intravenous Access with a Measured Volume Administration Set

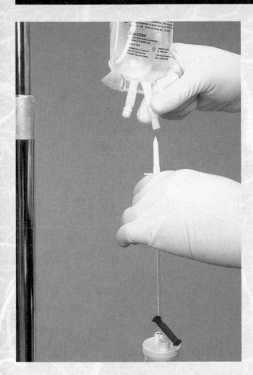

15-9a   Spike the solution bag.

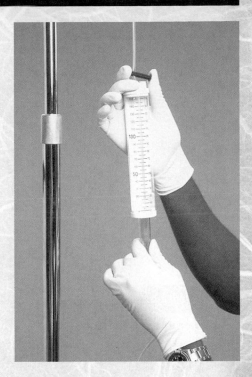

15-9b   Open the uppermost clamp and fill the burette chamber with the desired volume of fluid.

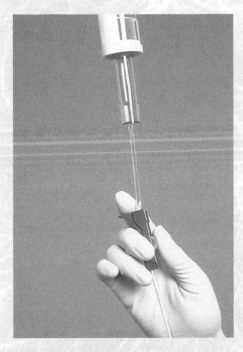

15-9c   Close the uppermost clamp and open the flow regulator.

INTRAVENOUS ACCESS WITH BLOOD TUBING

To establish an IV with blood tubing, use the following procedure:

1. Prepare the tubing by closing all clamps, and insert the flanged spike into the spike port of the blood and/or normal saline solution (Y-configured tubing).

2. Squeeze the drip chamber until it is one-third full and blood covers the filter. Repeat for the normal saline if you are using Y tubing.

3. If you are using straight tubing, piggyback a secondary line of normal saline into the blood tubing, unless you plan to piggyback the straight blood tubing into a large-bore primary line.

4. Flush all tubing with normal saline and blood as appropriate.

5. Attach blood tubing to the intravenous cannula or into a previously established IV line.

6. Ensure patency by infusing a small amount of normal saline. Shut down when you have confirmed patency.

7. Open the clamp(s) and flow regulator(s) that allow blood to move from the bag to the patient. Adjust the flow rate accordingly.

8. When blood therapy is complete or must be discontinued, shut down the flow regulator from the blood supply and open the regulator(s) for the normal saline solution.

FACTORS AFFECTING INTRAVENOUS FLOW RATES

If an IV does not flow properly, check for the following problems and correct them as appropriate.

- *Constricting band.* Has the venous constricting band been removed? This is probably the most common mistake both in and out of the hospital. Additionally, ensure that the patient is not wearing restrictive clothing that interferes with venous blood flow.

- *Edema at the puncture site.* Swelling at the IV site indicates fluid collection caused by infiltration. This **extravasation** occurs if you accidentally puncture the vein more than once, thus allowing IV solution and blood to escape from the second puncture and accumulate in the surrounding tissue. An infiltrated IV site is not usable.

- *Cannula abutting the vein wall or valve.* If the distal tip of the cannula butts against a wall or valve, carefully reposition it. You may have to untape and retape the cannula once you have achieved an adequate flow rate. Additionally, you may need to use an arm board to keep the patient's extremity straight, as flexion may kink the vein at the site and impede the solution's flow.

- *Administration set control valves.* Ensure that the flow regulator is open. Be sure to check the flow regulator and clamps of both the primary and any secondary or extension tubing.

- *IV bag height.* When you move the patient, you may raise the cannulation site above the IV solution bag. This interrupts the solution's gravitational flow from the bag into the patient.

✱ **extravasation** leakage of fluid or medication from the blood vessel that is commonly found with infiltration.

- *Completely filled drip chamber.* Is the drip chamber completely filled? You can easily correct this by inverting the bag and squeezing the fluid from the drip chamber back into the bag.
- *Catheter patency.* A blood clot at the end of the Teflon catheter or needle may obstruct the flow of solution from the IV solution bag into the body. If the flow slows, increase the IV drip rate to keep the catheter or needle clear. If the flow stops completely, cleanse the medication administration port closest to the IV entry site with alcohol preparations and insert a syringe and hypodermic needle. Gently aspirate back on the syringe until the blood clot is pulled into the syringe. Never flush an IV that has stopped running because of a clot. Flushing will force the clot into the circulatory system and can cause occlusions in the heart or lungs.

If flow remains inadequate after you have eliminated all of these possible causes, lower the IV bag below the insertion site. If blood flows into the IV administration tubing, the site is patent and the problem lies elsewhere. If the problem persists, remove the IV and reestablish it on another extremity, using all new equipment. If you do not observe blood return, the site is inoperable.

COMPLICATIONS OF PERIPHERAL INTRAVENOUS ACCESS

Even though it is a routine procedure, intravenous access is not trouble free. It can cause a number of complications.

Pain Pain at the puncture site occurs during needle penetration or with extravasation. To minimize pain, use a smaller gauge catheter or use a 1percent lidocaine solution (without epinephrine) to anesthetize the overlying skin before insertion.

Local Infection Local infection occurs if you do not properly cleanse the site and thus introduce pathogens through the puncture. This complication does not become apparent until after the IV has been established for several hours.

Pyrogenic Reaction Pyrogens (foreign proteins capable of producing fever) in the administration tubing or IV solution can cause a pyrogenic reaction. The abrupt onset of fever (37.8°C–41.2°C), chills, backache, headache, nausea, and vomiting characterize these reactions. Cardiovascular collapse may also result.

Typically, a pyrogenic reaction will occur within 30–60 minutes after you initiate an IV. If you suspect a pyrogenic reaction, immediately terminate the IV and reestablish access in the opposite side with new equipment and fluid.

Typically, pyrogenic reactions occur secondary to the use of intravenous solutions that have been contaminated with a microorganism or other foreign matter. Pyrogenic reactions underscore the need to discard any fluid that is cloudy or any equipment that has been opened.

Allergic Reaction A patient receiving IV therapy may develop an allergic reaction. Most often, allergic reactions accompany the administration of blood or colloidal (protein-containing) solutions. In addition, some patients may react to the latex in some types of IV administration tubing.

The sudden onset of hives (urticaria), itching (pruritis), localized or systemic edema, or shortness of breath may signify an allergic reaction. If you suspect an allergic reaction, stop the IV infusion and remove the IV catheter. Treat the patient as discussed in Chapter 31 on allergies and anaphylaxis.

Content Review

IV ACCESS COMPLICATIONS
Pain
Local infection
Pyrogenic reaction
Allergic reaction
Catheter shear
Inadvertent arterial
  puncture
Circulatory overload
Thrombophlebitis
Thrombus formation
Air embolism
Necrosis
Anticoagulants

✳ **pyrogen** foreign protein capable of producing fever.

Catheter Shear A catheter shear can occur if you pull the Teflon catheter through or over the needle after you have advanced it into the vein. The soft plastic catheter will easily snag on the metal stylet's sharp point and shear off, thus forming a plastic **embolus**. Therefore, never draw the Teflon catheter back over the metal stylet after you have advanced it.

Inadvertent Arterial Puncture Because arteries may lie close to veins, accidental arterial puncture may occur. Arterial blood is bright red and characteristically spurts with each contraction of the heart. When an arterial puncture occurs, immediately remove the catheter and apply direct pressure to the site for at least five minutes. Do not release the pressure until the hemorrhage has stopped.

* **embolus** foreign particle in the blood.

Circulatory Overload Circulatory overload occurs if you administer too much fluid for the patient's condition. You must monitor flow rates carefully, especially for patients with medical conditions, such as kidney failure or heart failure, who are intolerant of excessive fluid. Continually examine the patient for signs of circulatory overload (rales, tachypnea, dyspnea, and jugular venous distention, as discussed in Chapter 6 on physical assessment techniques). If you encounter circulatory overload, adjust the flow rate.

* **circulatory overload** an excess in intravascular fluid volume.

Thrombophlebitis Thrombophlebitis, or inflammation of the vein, is particularly common in long-term intravenous therapy. Redness and edema at the puncture site are typical signs of thrombophlebitis. This complication may also present as pain along the course of the vein, sometimes accompanied by inflammation and tenderness. Typically, thrombophlebitis does not occur until several hours after IV initiation. When you suspect thrombophlebitis, terminate the IV, and apply a warm compress to the site.

* **thrombophlebitis** inflammation of the vein.

Thrombus Formation A thrombus, or blood clot, can form if IV access injures the vessel wall. A thrombus may form around the catheter and occlude the movement of fluid between the IV and the blood vessel. If you suspect a thrombus, you may try to aspirate the clot (see page 813), or discontinue the block IV and restart the IV using new equipment. Do not attempt to dislodge the clot with a fluid bolus, as this may create an embolus that causes neurological or pulmonary complications.

* **thrombus** blood clot.

Air Embolism Air embolism occurs when air enters the vein. Air embolus is most likely to occur during central venous access or when administration tubing has not been properly flushed. Failure to tamponade larger veins during cannulation may allow air into the vein.

* **air embolism** air in the vein.

Necrosis Necrosis, or the sloughing off of dead tissue, occurs later in IV therapy as medication has extravasated into the interstitial space.

* **necrosis** the sloughing off of dead tissue.

Anticoagulants Anticoagulant drugs, such as aspirin, Coumadin, or heparin, increase the chance of bleeding and impede hemorrhage control during IV establishment. They drastically increase the complications of hematoma or infiltration.

* **anticoagulant** drug that inhibits blood clotting.

CHANGING AN IV BAG OR BOTTLE

You may sometimes have to change an IV bag or bottle. This generally occurs when only 50 mL of solution remain and you must continue therapy after those 50 mL are depleted. Changing the solution bag or bottle is a sterile process. If the equipment becomes contaminated, you should dispose of it.

To change the IV solution bag or bottle, use the following technique:

1. Prepare the new IV solution bag or bottle by removing the protective cover from the IV tubing port.

2. Occlude the flow of solution from the depleted bag or bottle by moving the roller clamp on the IV administration tubing.

3. Remove the spike from the depleted IV bag or bottle. Be careful not to drop or contaminate the spike in any way.

4. Insert the spike into the new IV bag or bottle. Ensure that the drip chamber is filled appropriately.

5. Open the roller clamp to the appropriate flow rate.

If air becomes entrained within the administration tubing during this process, cleanse the medication administration port below the trapped air and insert a hypodermic needle and syringe. Pull the plunger back to aspirate the trapped air into the syringe. After you have removed the air, adjust the IV flow rate as needed.

INTRAVENOUS DRUG ADMINISTRATION

Medications can be delivered through an existing IV line. As the IV line is seated directly into a vein, the blood rapidly absorbs these medications and distributes them throughout the body. Intravenous administration avoids many of the barriers to drug absorption in other routes. For example, drugs given via the gastrointestinal tract face enzymes and other chemicals that may deactivate, exacerbate, or in some other way alter the medication being administered. Likewise, local tissues can absorb drugs administered via the subcutaneous or intramuscular routes, thus preventing the total dosage from reaching the bloodstream for delivery. The two methods for administering drugs through an IV line are intravenous bolus and intravenous infusion.

Intravenous Bolus

An intravenous bolus involves injecting the circulatory system with a concentrated dose of drug through the medication administration port of an established IV. This procedure requires the following equipment:

- BSI protection (personal protective equipment)
- Alcohol antiseptic preparation
- Packaged medication
- Syringe (size depends on the volume of drug you will administer)
- 18- to 20-gauge hypodermic needle, 2.5 to 3.5 cm long
- Existing intravenous line with medication port

To administer an intravenous medication bolus, use the following technique (Procedure 15-10):

1. Use appropriate BSI.

2. Confirm the indication, medication, dose, route, and expiration date.

3. Ensure that the primary IV line is patent.

4. Draw up the medication or prepare a prefilled syringe as appropriate.

5. Cleanse the medication port nearest the IV site with an alcohol antiseptic preparation.

6. Insert a hypodermic needle through the port membrane.

7. Pinch the IV line above the medication port. This prevents the medication from travelling toward the fluids bag, forcing it instead toward the patient.

8. Inject the medication as appropriate.

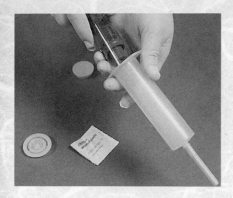

15-10a   Prepare the equipment.

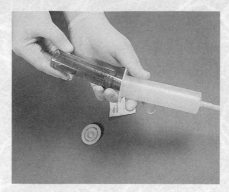

15-10b   Prepare the medication.

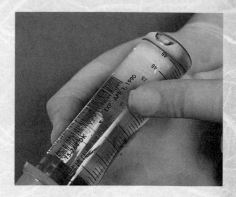

15-10c   Check the label.

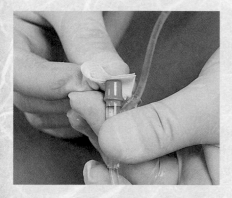

15-10d   Select and clean an administration port.

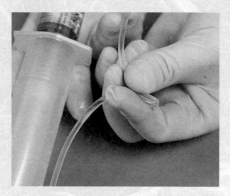

15-10e   Pinch the line.

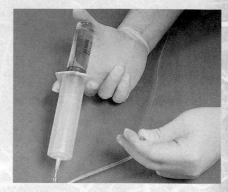

15-10f   Administer the medication.

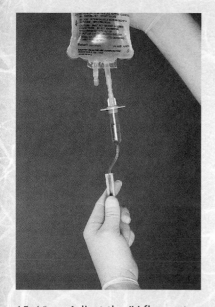

15-10g   Adjust the IV flow rate.

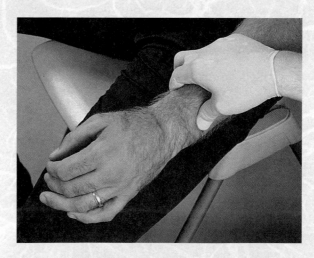

15-10h   Monitor the patient.

9. Remove the hypodermic needle and syringe and release the tubing.

10. Open the flow regulator to allow a 20-mL fluid flush. The fluid will push the medication into the patient's circulatory system. Set the flow rate back to its original rate.

11. Dispose of the hypodermic needle and syringe as appropriate. Monitor the patient for desired or undesired effects.

Intravenous Drug Infusion

Many cardiac drugs and antibiotics are given as intravenous infusions (IV piggybacks). Intravenous drug infusions deliver a steady, continual dose of medication through an existing IV line. You may give them either as an initial dosage or to maintain drug levels after delivering an initial bolus.

Piggybacking IV infusions through an existing intravenous line gives you greater control over medication delivery and allows you easily to discontinue the infusion when therapy is complete or must be stopped. Never administer intravenous infusions as a primary IV line.

IV infusions are contained in bags or bottles of intravenous solution. If the IV infusion is premixed, read the label on the bag for the following information:

Never administer intravenous infusions as a primary IV line.

- Name of medication
- Total dosage in weight mixed in bag
- Concentration (weight per single mL)
- Expiration date

If the infusion is not premixed, make a label listing this information and attach it to the bag (Figure 15-28). Additionally, note the date and time you mixed the infusion, and initial it.

Use the following technique to administer a medication as an IV infusion (Procedure 15-11):

1. Use appropriate BSI.
2. Confirm the indication, medication, dose, route, and expiration date.
3. Establish a primary IV line and ensure patency.

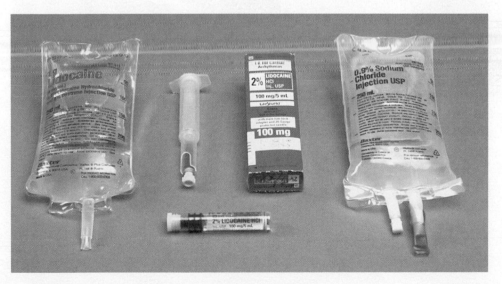

FIGURE 15-28 If an IV solution is not premixed, you will have to mix and label it yourself.

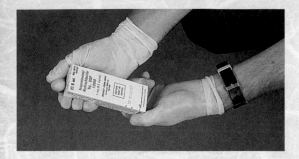

15-11a   Select the drug.

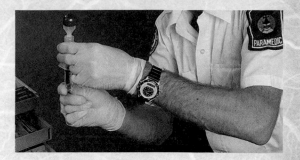

15-11b   Draw up the drug.

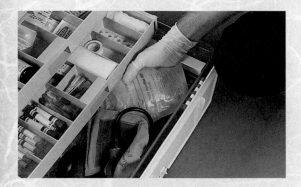

15-11c   Select IV fluid for dilution.

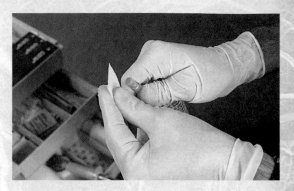

15-11d   Clean the medication addition port.

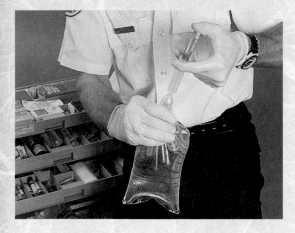

15-11e   Inject the drug into the fluid.

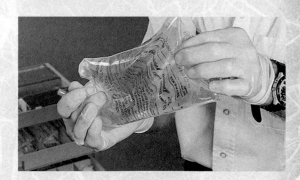

15-11f   Mix the solution.

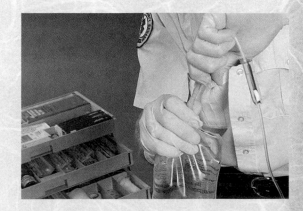

15-11g   Insert an administration set and
connect to the main IV line with the needle.

4. Prepare the infusion bag or bottle. (If the infusion is premixed, continue to step 5.)
   a. Draw up the appropriate quantity of medication from its source with a syringe.
   b. Cleanse the IV bag or bottle's medication port with an alcohol antiseptic wipe.
   c. Insert the hypodermic needle into the medication port and inject the medication.
   d. Gently agitate the bag or bottle to mix its contents.
   e. Label the bag or bottle.

5. Connect administration tubing to the medication bag or bottle and fill the drip chamber to the fluid line. Most infusions require microdrip tubing. If you use a mechanical infusion pump, you may need to use special tubing.

6. Place the hypodermic needle on the administration tubing's needle adapter and flush the tubing with solution. (The needle adapter typically accepts a 20-gauge needle.)

7. Cleanse the medication administration port on the primary line with alcohol and insert the secondary line's hypodermic needle. Secure the hypodermic needle and the secondary administration line with tape or another securing device.

8. Reconfirm the indication, drug, dose, and route of administration.

9. Shut down the primary line so that no fluid will flow from the primary solution bag.

10. Adjust the secondary line to the desired drip rate. If you are using a mechanical infusion pump, set it accordingly.

11. Properly dispose of the needle and syringe.

When the infusion is complete, shut down the secondary line with the flow regulator or a clamp. Open the primary line and adjust it to the indicated drip rate. Remove the hypodermic needle from the medication administration port and properly dispose of all contents. If required by your local protocols, retain the medication bag to verify administration and for quality assurance.

You can also use measured volume administration tubing to administer medicated infusions. First, fill the burette chamber of a measured volume administration device with a specific volume of fluid. Then, you can inject the drug through the medication injection site on top of the burette chamber. You must adjust the flow rate to deliver the precise amount of medication required. In addition, you can mix the medication within the IV bag or bottle as previously described and use the measured volume administration tubing solely for administering the infusion, rather than for mixing it.

Heparin Lock and Saline Lock

When a patient requires occasional IV medication drips or boluses but does not need continuous fluid, heparin locks are used. A **heparin lock** is a peripheral IV port that does not use a bag of fluid. Like a typical IV start, it places an IV cannula into a peripheral vein; however, instead of IV administration tubing, it has attached short tubing with a clamp and a distal medication port (Figure 15-29). A heparin lock decreases the risk of accidental fluid overload and electrolyte derangement. You also may withdraw blood samples from the lock if it is in a suitable vein. For short-term use, saline locks may be used. Sterile saline is injected following the drug. Saline remains in the lock to keep it open. For long-term use, a heparin lock is preferred.

✱ **heparin lock** peripheral IV port that does not use a bag of fluid.

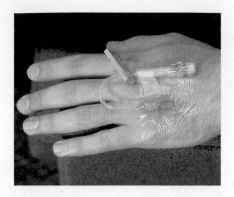

FIGURE 15-29   Heparin lock.

Although it functions the same as a saline lock, a heparin lock is filled with a low concentration solution of heparin, which aids in keeping any blood that gets into the device from clotting. Typically, a drug will be administered through the heparin lock. This is followed by a saline flush to ensure that no drug remains in the lock or hub. Then, the lock and hub are filled with a heparin solution. This aids in keeping the IV site open for a long time.

Initiating a heparin lock requires the following equipment:

- BSI (personal protective equipment)
- IV cannula
- Heparin lock
- Syringe with 3 mL to 5 mL heparin injection device
- Tape or commercial securing device
- Venous blood-drawing equipment
- Venous constricting band
- Antiseptic swab (betadine/alcohol)

To place a heparin lock, follow these steps:

1. Use appropriate BSI.
2. Select the venipuncture site.
3. Place the constricting band proximal to the puncture site.
4. Cleanse the venipuncture site with alcohol or betadine antiseptics.
5. Insert the intravenous cannula into the vein.
6. Slide the Teflon catheter into the vein.
7. Carefully remove the metal stylet and promptly dispose of it into the sharps container. Remove the venous constricting band.
8. Obtain venous blood samples, as explained under Venous Blood Sampling.
9. Attach the heparin lock tubing to the angiocatheter hub.
10. Cleanse the medication port and inject 3 mL to 5 mL of heparin into the lock. Easy flow of the fluid without edema at the puncture site indicates patency. If you encounter resistance or if edema forms, restart the procedure with new equipment.
11. Cover the site with an adhesive bandage or other commercial device. Secure the tubing to the patient.

To administer an IV medication bolus through a heparin lock, assemble the following equipment and supplies:

- BSI protection (personal protective equipment)
- Alcohol antiseptic preparation
- Packaged medication
- Syringe (the size depends on the volume being administered)
- 18- to 20-gauge hypodermic needle 2.5 to 3.5 cm long

After you have gathered all equipment and supplies, use the following technique to administer an IV medication bolus with a heparin lock:

1. Use appropriate BSI.
2. Confirm the indication, medication, dose, route, and expiration date.
3. Draw up the medication, or prepare a prefilled syringe as appropriate.
4. Cleanse the medication port nearest the IV site with alcohol antiseptic preparation.
5. Ensure that the plastic clamp is open.
6. Insert the hypodermic needle through the port membrane.
7. Inject the medication as appropriate.
8. Remove the hypodermic needle and dispose of it in the sharps container.
9. Follow the medication administration with a 10- to 20-mL saline flush from another syringe.
10. Refill the lock with heparin.
11. Properly dispose of the hypodermic needle and syringe. Monitor the patient for desired or undesired effects.

If fluid administration becomes necessary, you can unscrew the medication port and insert IV administration tubing. Periodically flush with sterile saline or heparin to prevent clot formation and occlusion at the Teflon catheter's distal end.

Venous Access Device

A **venous access device** is a surgically implanted port that permits repeated access to the central venous circulation. Implanted just under the skin, venous access devices are constructed of a plastic or stainless steel injection port and flexible catheter. The injection port, which lies just beneath the skin, contains a self-sealing septum that allows repeated penetration and access into the venous circulation. The self-sealing septum is connected to a flexible catheter that is placed within the lumen of a central vein, most often the superior vena cava.

Typically, patients with venous access devices have chronic illnesses that require repeated intravenous access for medication administration, long-term intravenous therapy, or blood sampling. Generally, venous access devices are placed on the anterior chest near the third or fourth rib lateral to the sternum. A venous access device is apparent as a raised circle just beneath the skin.

Use of an indwelling central venous access device requires special training. Delivering a medication through the venous access device requires a special needle specific for the venous access device in question. A common needle, the **Huber needle,** has an opening on the side of its shaft instead of at the tip. When placed into the injection port, this configuration allows easy administration of medication into the venous access device. Never access a venous access device unless you

* **venous access device** surgically implanted port that permits repeated access to central venous circulation.

* **Huber needle** needle that has an opening on the side of the shaft instead of the tip.

have the specific needle unique for the particular device. Always ask the patient, family, or nursing staff about the type of venous access device. Often, they will have a supply of needles for the device.

To administer fluids, medication, or blood through a venous access device, you must first prepare the site using the following technique:

1. Use appropriate BSI.
2. Fill a 10-mL syringe with approximately 7 mL of normal saline.
3. Place a 21- or 22-gauge Huber needle (or other specialized needle) on the end of the syringe.
4. Cleanse the skin over the injection port with povidone-iodine or alcohol preparations.
5. Stabilize the site with one hand while inserting the Huber needle at a 90-degree angle. Gently advance it until it meets resistance. This signals that the needle has contacted the floor of the injection port.
6. Pull back on the plunger and observe for blood return. The presence of blood confirms placement.
7. Slowly inject the normal saline to ensure patency.

To administer the medication by intravenous bolus, use the following technique:

1. Use appropriate BSI.
2. Confirm the indication, medication, dose, route, and expiration date.
3. Prepare the medication, fluid, or blood for administration.
4. Attach a 21- or 22-gauge Huber needle (or other specialized needle) to the end of the syringe.
5. Cleanse the skin over the injection port with povidone-iodine or alcohol preparations.
6. Insert the needle into the injection port at a 90-degree angle until the needle cannot be further advanced. Pull back on the plunger of the syringe and observe for the return of blood. The presence of blood confirms proper placement.
7. Inject the medication as appropriate.
8. Remove and dispose of the syringe appropriately.
9. With another syringe and attached specialized needle, administer a bolus of heparinized saline to clear the catheter of any blood clots or other obstruction.

If the venous access device is not patent or access proves difficult, contact medical direction for further directives.

To administer IV fluids, use the following technique:

1. Use appropriate BSI.
2. Prepare a primary IV line. Be sure to prime or flush the air from the administration tubing.
3. Attach a 21- or 22-gauge Huber needle (or other specialized needle) to the primary IV administration tubing. Insert a 10-mL syringe and hypodermic needle filled with 7 mL of normal saline solution into the tubing medication delivery port nearest the venous access device.
4. Cleanse the skin over the injection port with povidone-iodine or alcohol preparations.

5. Insert the needle into the injection port at a 90-degree angle until it encounters resistance.

6. Pinch the administration tubing above the medication administration port and pull back on the syringe plunger. Observe for the return of blood. The presence of blood confirms proper placement.

7. Gently inject the 7 mL of normal saline solution.

8. Set the primary line to the appropriate flow rate.

If administering a secondary medicated infusion, continue as follows:

1. Prepare a secondary line containing the fluid, blood, or medicated solution for infusion.

2. Attach a hypodermic needle to the needle adapter of the secondary line. Insert the secondary line into a medication administration port on the primary tubing.

3. Shut down the primary line and infuse the medicated solution as appropriate. Look for ease of administration as a sign of patency.

4. When infusion is complete, administer a bolus of heparinized saline to clear the catheter of any blood clots or other obstruction.

Using a venous access device is a very sterile procedure. You must take care to clean the site before delivering medications. Other complications of using a venous access device include infection, thrombus formation, and dislodgment of the catheter tip from the vein.

Electromechanical Infusion Devices

Electromechanical infusion devices permit the precise delivery of fluid and/or medications through electronic regulation. Anytime that intravenous infusion occurs, electromechanical infusion pumps provide optimal delivery. Infusion devices are classified as either infusion controllers or infusion pumps.

Infusion Controllers Infusion controllers are gravity-flow devices that regulate the fluid's passage through the pump. Because infusion controllers do not use positive pressure, they will not force fluids into the **extravascular** space if you infiltrate the vein.

Infusion Pumps Infusion pumps deliver fluids and medications under positive pressure (Figure 15-30). This pressure can cause complications like hematoma or extravasation if you infiltrate the vein. Some infusion pumps contain a pressure monitor and will warn you if they encounter the increased resistance that occurs with infiltration.

Syringe-type infusion pumps are gaining popularity for medical transport. Syringe pumps deliver their medications from a medical syringe without a hypodermic needle instead of from IV solution bags, fluids, or liquid medications (Figure 15-31). You place the syringe containing the medications in the pump, which uses computerized mechanics to gradually depress the plunger at the correct rate. These compact pumps prove advantageous during transport.

Manufacturers make many different electromechanical infusion pumps. Depending on the maker, pump compatibility may require specialized administration tubing. With some computerized pumps, you can enter the basic information and then the pump will perform all medical calculations internally and automatically set the drip rate. Most infusion pumps contain internal monitoring devices that

* **infusion controller** gravity-flow device that regulates fluid's passage through an electromechanical pump.

* **extravascular** outside the vein.

* **infusion pump** device that delivers fluids and medications under positive pressure.

FIGURE 15-30   Infusion pump.

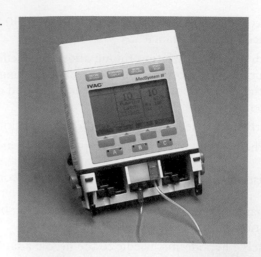

FIGURE 15-31   Syringe-type
infusion pump.

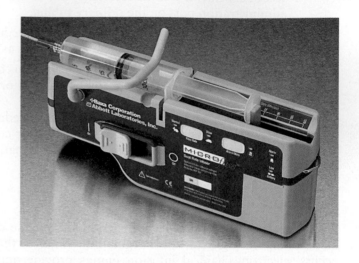

sound an alarm for problems such as infiltration, occlusion, or fluid source depletion. Electronic devices are prone to malfunction, and so you must be prepared to perform all calculations and set the drip rate manually.

VENOUS BLOOD SAMPLING

The laboratory analysis of blood can provide valuable information about the sick or injured patient. The concentrations of electrolytes, gases, hormones, or other chemicals in blood can often shed light on the underlying causes of vague complaints, such as dizziness or generalized weakness. Additionally, blood evaluation can confirm suspected conditions. For example, elevated cardiac enzymes in a patient's blood can confirm a suspected myocardial infarction.

In the field, you often will be the first to assess and treat an ill or injured patient. Many of your interventions can alter the blood's composition and erase important information. If you obtain venous blood samples before performing those interventions, they will enable the physician to evaluate the patient's original status. However, many ambulance services have discontinued or decreased emphasis on obtaining a prehospital venous blood sample.

Venous blood is commonly obtained via venipuncture. Thus, paramedics, who routinely initiate intravenous access, can simultaneously obtain blood samples. Doing so saves considerable hospital time and avoids multiple needle sticks.

You should obtain venous blood in the following situations:

- During peripheral access
- Before drug administration
- When drug administration may be needed

Never stop to draw blood if it will delay critical measures, such as drug administration in cardiac arrest or transport in a multisystems trauma.

Never stop to draw blood if it will delay critical measures.

Equipment for Drawing Blood

You will need the following equipment to obtain venous blood:

Blood tubes Blood tubes are made of glass and have colour-coded, self-sealing rubber tops. Blood tube sizes for adults generally range from 5 to 7 mL; for pediatrics, from 2 mL to 3 mL (Figure 15-32). They are vacuum packed, and some contain a chemical anticoagulant. The different-coloured tops correspond to specific anticoagulants. A label on every blood tube identifies the type of additive and its expiration date. Do not use a blood tube after its expiration date, as both the anticoagulant and the vacuum lose their effectiveness.

Using blood tubes in their correct order is essential. If you do not follow the proper sequence, the various anticoagulants will cause cross-contamination, skewing the results and rendering the blood useless. Table 15-1 lists anticoagulants, the order in which you should use them, and the colours of their tops.

Miscellaneous Equipment Depending on the technique you use to obtain venous blood, you will also need syringes, hypodermic needles, and commercially manufactured plastic sleeves called vacutainers.

* blood tube glass container with colour-coded, self-sealing rubber top.

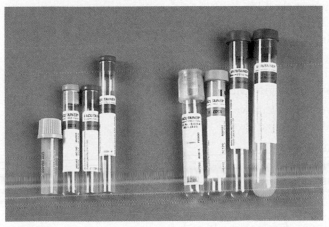

FIGURE 15-32 Blood tubes.

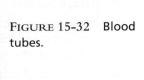

Table 15-1	BLOOD TUBE SEQUENCE	
	Anticoagulant	Colour of Top
1.	none	red
2.	citrate	blue
3.	heparin	green
4.	EDTA	purple
5.	fluoride	grey

Obtaining Venous Blood

Obtaining venous blood is a simple process; however, if the blood is to remain usable, you must pay strict attention to detail. You can obtain blood either from an angiocath or directly from the vein. Which technique you use will depend on the situation. In either case, venous blood samples are best obtained from sturdy veins, such as the cephalic, basilic, or median. Smaller veins, such as those on the back of the hand, are more likely to collapse during retrieval, making the procedure difficult to complete.

Obtaining Venous Blood from an IV Angiocath The most convenient way to obtain venous blood is through an angiocath at the time of peripheral vascular access. In addition to blood tubes, you will need a tube holder (Figure 15-33). The tube holder is commonly referred to as a **vacutainer.** A special adapter called a leur lock fits into the tube holder. The **leur lock** has a rubber-covered needle used to puncture the self-sealing top of the blood tube. The remaining portion of the leur lock protrudes from the tube holder and fits snugly into the hub of the angiocath.

To obtain blood directly from the angiocath, use the following procedure:

1. Use appropriate BSI.
2. Assemble and prepare all equipment. Inspect the blood tubes for expiration or damage and insert the leur lock into the vacutainer.
    Note: Never place blood tubes into the assembled vacutainer and leur lock until you are ready to draw blood. This will destroy the vacuum and render the blood tube useless.
3. Establish IV access with the angiocatheter. Do not connect IV administration tubing.
4. Attach the end of the leur adapter to the hub of the cannula.
5. In correct order, insert the blood tubes so that the rubber-covered needle punctures the self-sealing rubber top. Blood should be pulled into the blood tube.
6. Fill all blood tubes completely, as the amount of anticoagulant is proportional to the tube's volume. Gently agitate the tubes to mix the anticoagulant evenly with the blood.
7. Tamponade the vein and remove the vacutainer and leur lock. Attach the IV and ensure patency.
8. Properly dispose of all sharps.
9. Label all blood tubes with the following information:
    * Patient's first and last name
    * Patient's age and gender
    * Date and time drawn
    * Name of the person drawing the blood

* **vacutainer** device that holds blood tubes.

* **leur lock** adapter with a rubber-covered needle used to puncture a blood tube's self-sealing top.

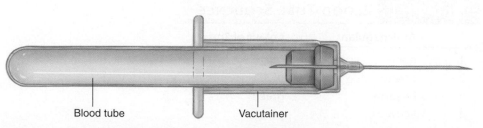

Blood tube   Vacutainer

FIGURE 15-33   Vacutainer with leur sampling needle.

If commercial equipment is not available, use a 20-mL syringe (Figure 15-34). Attach the syringe's needle adapter to the angiocath hub and gently pull back the plunger. Blood will fill the syringe. When the syringe is full, remove it from the angiocath and place the IV line into the angiocath. Carefully attach a hypodermic needle to the syringe to puncture the tops of the blood tubes. In the appropriate order, place the collected blood into the blood tubes and gently agitate. When finished, properly dispose of all sharps and label the blood tubes.

Obtaining Blood Directly from a Vein When IV access is difficult or unobtainable, you may draw blood directly from the vein with a hypodermic needle. This technique is useful for routine sampling that will not require further IV access. To draw blood directly from a vein, you will need the same equipment as for obtaining blood from an angiocath. Instead of a leur lock, however, you will use a **leur sampling needle** (Figure 15-35). A leur sampling needle is similar to the leur lock, but instead of an angiocath adapter, it has a long, exposed needle. The leur sampling needle screws into the vacutainer, and you insert the exposed needle directly into the vein. You will also need a constricting band and antiseptic wipes.

To obtain blood directly from a vein, use the following procedure:

✳ **leur sampling needle** long, exposed needle that screws into the vacutainer and is inserted directly into the vein.

1. Use appropriate BSI.
2. Assemble and prepare all equipment. Inspect the blood tubes for expiration or damage, and insert the leur lock into the vacutainer.
3. Apply the constricting band and select an appropriate puncture site.
4. Cleanse the site with alcohol or betadine.
5. Insert the end of the leur sampling needle into the vein and remove the constricting band.
6. In the correct order, insert each blood tube so that the rubber-covered needle punctures the self-sealing rubber top. Blood should be pulled into the tube.
7. Gently agitate the tube to evenly mix the anticoagulant with the blood. Completely fill all blood tubes, as the anticoagulant is proportional to the volume of the tube.

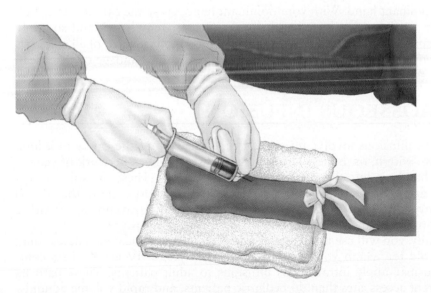
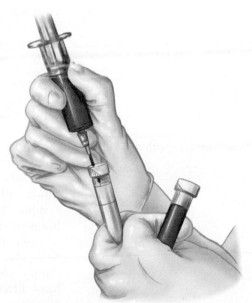

FIGURE 15-34   Obtaining a blood sample with a 20-mL syringe.

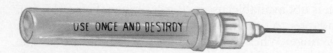

FIGURE 15-35   Leur sampling needle.

8. Place sterile gauze over the site and remove the sampling needle. Properly dispose of all sharps.

9. Cover the puncture site with gauze and tape, or an adhesive bandage.

10. Label all blood tubes with the following information:
    • Patient's first and last name
    • Patient's age and sex
    • Date and time drawn
    • Person drawing the blood

Again, if commercial equipment is not available, you may use a 20-mL syringe. When using a syringe, attach an 18-gauge hypodermic needle to the end of the syringe and insert it into the vein. Gently pull back the plunger to fill the syringe with blood. When the syringe is full, remove the syringe and dress the puncture site. In the appropriate order, inject the collected blood into the blood tubes and gently agitate. When you have finished, properly dispose of all sharps and label the blood tubes.

Complications from drawing blood include damage to the vein wall, inadvertant removal of the IV angiocath and hemoconcentration and hemolysis of the blood sample. **Hemoconcentration** occurs when the constricting band is left in place too long, elevating the numbers of red and white blood cells in the sample. **Hemolysis** is the destruction of red blood cells. When red blood cells are destroyed, they release hemoglobin and potassium, thus rendering the blood unusable. Causes of hemolysis include vigorously shaking the blood tubes after they are filled, using too small a needle for retrieval, or too forcefully aspirating blood into or out of a syringe.

✷ hemoconcentration elevated numbers of red and white blood cells.

✷ hemolysis the destruction of red blood cells.

REMOVING A PERIPHERAL IV

Remove any IV that will not flow or has served its purpose. ⚷

You should remove any IV that will not flow or has served its purpose. To do so, completely occlude the tubing with the flow regulator or clamp. Remove all tape or other securing devices from the tubing and patient. Place a sterile gauze pad over the puncture site. Apply pressure to the gauze with the fingers or thumb of your nondominant hand. With your dominant hand, grasp the cannula at its hub and swiftly remove it, pulling straight back. The site may bleed, and so apply direct pressure with the gauze for five minutes. Immediately dispose of all materials in the appropriate biohazard container. Apply an adhesive bandage or tape clean gauze over the site to protect against infection.

INTRAOSSEOUS INFUSION

✷ intraosseous within the bone.

Intraosseous infusions involve inserting a rigid needle into the cavity of a long bone (*intra-*, within; *os*, bone). The bone marrow contains a network of venous sinusoids that drain into the nutrient and emissary veins. These sinusoids accept fluids and drugs during intraosseous infusion and transport them to the venous system. Any solution or drug that can be administered intravenously, as either bolus or infusion, can be administered by the intraosseous route.

Generally, you will use intraosseous infusions for the critical patient less than five years old for whom you cannot establish peripheral IV access. Less commonly, you may apply intraosseous infusions to adult patients. These patients have different access sites than do pediatric patients, and rapid volume administration is not nearly as effective. Situations that might require an intraosseous route include shock, status epilepticus, trauma, and cardiac arrest, and critical pediatric patients for whom rapid IV access cannot be obtained. Initiate intraosseous lines only after 90 seconds or three unsuccessful attempts to establish peripheral IV access, or according to local protocol.

Initiate intraosseous lines only after 90 seconds or three unsuccessful attempts to establish peripheral IV access.

ACCESS SITE

The bone most commonly used for intraosseous access is the tibia. Pediatric access uses the proximal tibia. Adult or geriatric access uses the distal tibia. To properly locate appropriate sites and avoid complications, you must understand the anatomy and physiology of the tibia (Figure 15-36). The tibia is a long bone that transfers weight from the femur to the foot. In conjunction with the fibula, it facilitates walking. Its three main sections are the diaphysis, which comprises

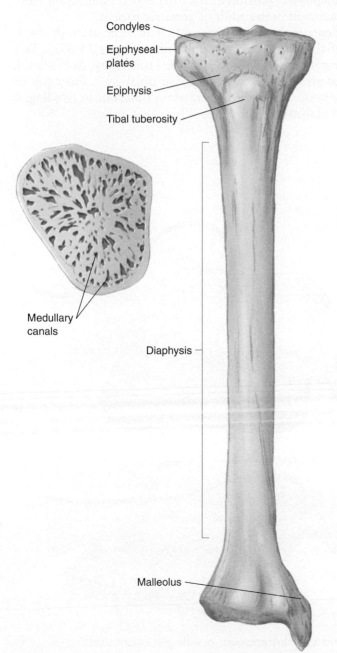

Condyles

Epiphyseal plates

Epiphysis

Tibal tuberosity

Medullary canals

Diaphysis

Malleolus

FIGURE 15-36   Tibia.

the middle, and the two epiphyses, one at either end. Epiphyseal discs, or growth plates, between the diaphysis and the epiphyses, allow the tibia to grow and develop and are present in children. Damage to these discs during intraosseous access can cause long-term growth complications or abnormalities.

Within the diaphysis, the medullary canal holds the vascular bone marrow. When placed correctly, the distal part of the intraosseous needle will lie in the medullary canal. On either side of the proximal tibia are the medial and lateral condyles. You can identify the proximal epiphysis by palpating the condyles.

Between the condyles, on the top of the anterior tibial crest, is a palpable bump called the tibial tuberosity. The tibial tuberosity lies at the level of the epipheseal growth plate, for which it provides an excellent reference. Consequently, the tibial tuberosity is extremely important in locating the appropriate pediatric intraosseous access site.

At the distal end of the tibia lie the lateral malleolus and the medial malleolus. They mark the distal epiphyseal portion of the tibia and are important landmarks for intraosseous placement in the adult or geriatric patient.

For the pediatric patient (under five years old), you will establish intraosseous access on the medial aspect of the proximal tibia (Figure 15-37a). This site is from two to three finger-breadths below the tibial tuberosity. At this level, place the needle on the flat area medial to the anterior tibial crest. For adult or geriatric patients, place the needle at the distal part of the tibia, one to two finger-breadths above the medial malleolus (Figure 15-37b).

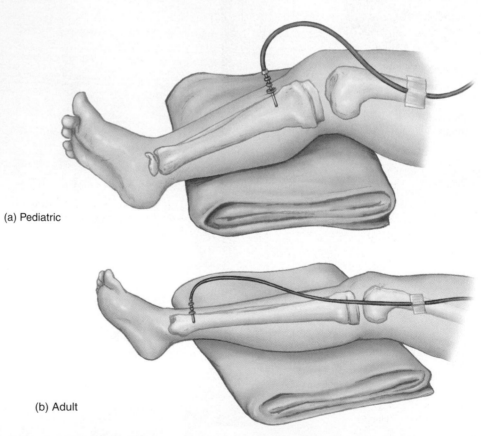

(a) Pediatric

(b) Adult

FIGURE 15-37   Pediatric and adult intraosseous needle placement sites.

EQUIPMENT FOR INTRAOSSEOUS ACCESS

Intraosseous placement requires a specially designed needle and a 10-mL syringe. Manufactured specifically for intraosseous access, an intraosseous needle is a 14- to 18-gauge hollow cannula with a sharp metal **trocar** inside (Figure 15-38). The trocar gives strength for puncture and prevents occlusion during insertion. On placement, the trocar is removed. The intraosseous needle has a plastic handle for insertion and an adjustable plastic disc to stabilize the needle once it is in place. You will attach a 10-mL syringe with 3 to 5 mL of sterile saline to the intraosseous needle. The syringe and saline are used similarly to IV access of the external jugular vein. A large-bore spinal needle with a trocar in place is an acceptable substitute for an intraosseous needle.

* **trocar** a sharp, pointed instrument.

Other equipment for intraosseous placement is similar to that for a peripheral intravenous access line (fluid, administration tubing, tape, antiseptics, and gauze). However, you will not use a constricting band or traditional cannula. Depending on the specific intraosseous needle, you may need an adapter to connect the administration tubing and the needle.

PLACING AN INTRAOSSEOUS INFUSION

To place an intraosseous line, use the following technique (Procedure 15-12):

1. Use appropriate BSI.
2. Determine the indication for intraosseous access.
3. Assemble and check all equipment.
4. Position the patient. Rotate the leg toward the outside to expose the medial, proximal aspect of the tibia.
5. Locate the access site. Palpate the tibia, and use all landmarks.
   - *Pediatric.* Locate the tibial tuberosity. Move from one to two finger-breadths below the tibial tuberosity and find the flat expanse medial to the anterior tibial crest.
   - *Adult or geriatric.* Find the medial malleolus. Move from one to two finger-breadths above the medial malleolus and locate the flat expanse medial to the anterior tibial crest.
6. Cleanse the site with alcohol or betadine. Start at the puncture site and work outward in an expanding circular motion.
7. Perform the puncture. Holding the needle perpendicular to the puncture site, insert it with a twisting motion until you feel a decrease in resistance or a "pop." When this occurs, the needle is in the medullary canal. Do not advance it any further. Generally, you will need to insert the needle only 2 to 4 mm for entry.

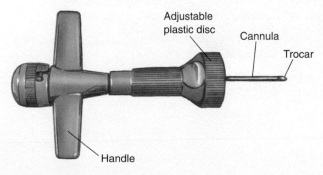

FIGURE 15-38   Intraosseous needle.

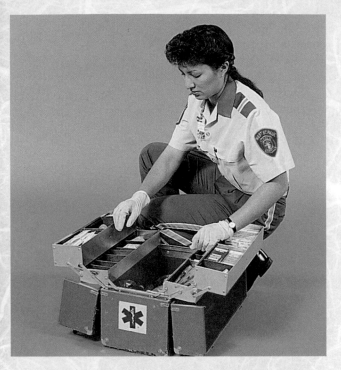

15-12a   Select the medication and prepare the equipment.

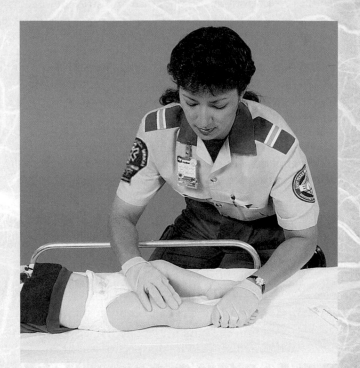

15-12b   Palpate the puncture site and prep with an antiseptic solution.

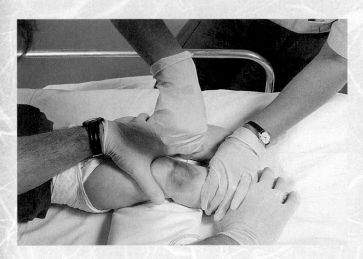

15-12c   Make the puncture.

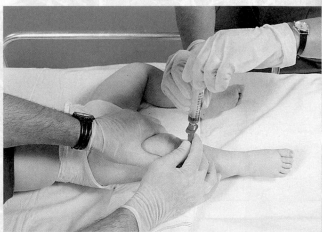

15-12d   Aspirate to confirm proper placement.

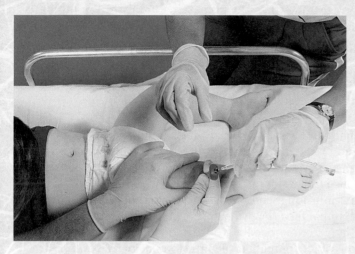

15-12e Connect the IV fluid tubing.

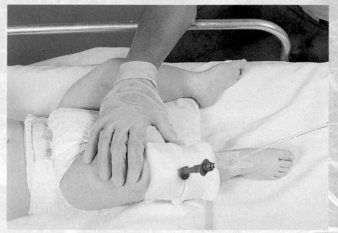

15-12f Secure the needle appropriately.

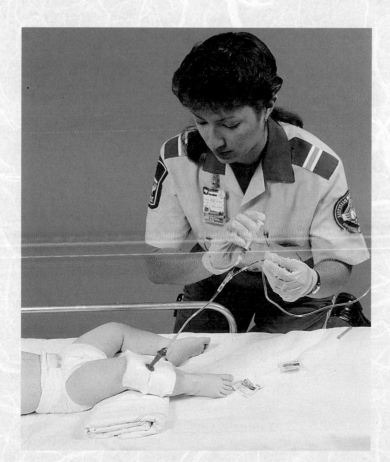

15-12g Administer the medication. Monitor the patient for effects.

8. Remove the trocar and attach the saline-filled syringe. Slowly pull back the plunger to attempt aspiration into the syringe. Easy aspiration of bone marrow and blood confirms correct medullary placement.

9. Once you have confirmed placement, rotate the plastic disc toward the skin to secure the needle.

10. Remove the syringe and attach the prepared administration tubing and solution. Set the appropriate flow rate.

11. Secure the needle as if securing an impaled object by surrounding it with bulky dressings and taping them securely in place. Commercial devices are available.

12. Periodically flush the needle to keep it patent.

Any solution or drug that can be administered by IV bolus or continuous infusion can also be delivered by the intraosseous route. Use the medicinal administration port on the primary administration tubing with the techniques as described under Intravenous Drug Administration.

When an intraosseous infusion is complete, shut down the secondary line with the flow regulator or a clamp. Open the primary line and adjust it to the indicated drip rate. Remove the hypodermic needle from the medication administration port and properly dispose of all contents if the infusion has been exhausted.

INTRAOSSEOUS ACCESS COMPLICATIONS AND PRECAUTIONS

Intraosseous access poses serious potential complications similiar to those of peripheral access: local infection, thrombophlebitis, air embolism, circulatory overload, and allergic reactions, as well as the following:

- *Fracture.* Too large a needle or too forceful an insertion can fracture the tibia, particulary in very young children.

- *Infiltration.* Infiltration occurs when IV solution collects in the local tissues instead of in the intramedullary canal. Infiltration may occur if you run fluids through an incorrectly placed needle or if a fracture has occurred. An infusion that does not run freely or the formation of an edema at the puncture site indicates infiltration. If infiltration occurs, immediately discontinue infusion and restart on the other leg.

- *Growth plate damage.* An improperly located puncture may damage the growth plate and result in long-term growth complications.

- *Complete insertion.* To avoid complete puncture (needle passing through both sides of the tibia), stop advancing the needle once you feel the pop. If complete puncture occurs, remove the needle with a reverse twisting motion and start again on the other leg. Apply direct pressure and a sterile dressing over the site(s) for at least five minutes.

- *Pulmonary embolism.* If bone, fat, or marrow particles make their way into the circulatory system, pulmonary embolism may result. Use proper technique and watch for signs associated with pulmonary embolism (sudden onset of chest pain or shortness of breath).

CONTRAINDICATIONS TO INTRAOSSEOUS PLACEMENT

Do not attempt intraosseous placement in the following situations:

- Fracture to the tibia or femur on the side of access
- Osteogenesis imperfecta—a congenital disease causing fragile bones
- Osteoporosis
- Establishment of a peripheral IV line

You must continually refresh your intraosseous access skills so that you can perform this technique properly when needed.

Part 3: Medical Mathematics

Proper drug administration requires basic mathematical proficiency. Because drug dosages are not always standardized, you may have to calculate amounts according to your patient's age, weight, or other medically related criteria. To properly prepare and administer medications, you must understand roman numerals and be proficient in multiplication, division, fractions, decimal fractions, proportions, and percentages. If you are deficient in one or more of these areas, refer to any text on basic and intermediate math.

METRIC SYSTEM

The metric system's three fundamental units are grams, metres, and litres. Prefixes denote values greater or less than the basic unit. Table 15-2 lists metric prefixes.

The most commonly used prefixes in pharmacology are *kilo-, centi-, milli-,* and *micro-.* The prefix *milli-* (m) refers to 1/1000. Thus, a *millilitre* equals 1/1000 of a litre. Similarly, a milligram is 1/1000 of a gram. The prefix *micro-* expresses 1/1 000 000. A *microgram* is 1/1 000 000 of a gram.

CONVERSION BETWEEN PREFIXES

If you know the prefixes and their numeric equivalents, you can easily convert measurements to smaller or larger units. To convert a measurement to a smaller unit, multiply the original measurement by the numerical equivalent of the smaller measurement's prefix.

Content Review

FUNDAMENTAL METRIC UNITS

Grams—mass
Metres—distance
Litres—volume

Table 15-2	METRIC PREFIXES	
Prefix	**Multiplier**	**Symbol**
kilo	1000	k
hecto	100	h
deka	10	D
deci	1/10 or 0.1	d
centi	1/100 or 0.01	c
milli	1/1000 or 0.001	m
micro	1/1 000 000 or 0.000001	μ

Example 1: Convert 3 grams to milligrams.

Milligrams (1/1000) are smaller than grams; therefore, multiply 3 by 1000:

$$3 \text{ (grams)} \times 1000 \text{ (milli)} = 3000$$

$$3 \text{ grams (g)} = 3000 \text{ milligrams}$$

Example 2: Convert 2.67 litres to millilitres.

Millilitres (1/1000) are smaller than a litre; therefore, multiply 2.67 by 1000:

$$2.67 \text{ litres} \times 1000 \text{ (milli)} = 2670$$

$$2.67 \text{ litres (L)} = 2670 \text{ millilitres (mL)}$$

To convert a measurement to a larger unit, divide the original measurement by the numerical equivalent of the smaller measurement's prefix.

Example 3: Convert 1600 micrograms to grams.

A microgram is 1/1 000 000 the size of a gram; therefore, divide 1600 by 1 000 000:

$$1600/1 \ 000 \ 000 = 0.0016 \text{ grams}$$

$$1600 \text{ micrograms (µg)} = 0.0016 \text{ grams (g)}$$

When converting a measurement to or from a prefix that is not the fundamental unit, first convert the *existing* measurement to the *fundamental* measurement. Then, convert the fundamental measurement to the desired unit.

Example 4: Convert 5.6 milligrams to micrograms.

First, convert the 5.6 milligrams to grams:

$$5.6 \text{ milligrams}/1000 = 0.0056 \text{ grams}$$

$$5.6 \text{ milligrams (mg)} = 0.0056 \text{ grams (g)}$$

Now, convert 0.0056 grams to micrograms as previously described:

$$0.0056 \text{ (grams)} \times 1 \ 000 \ 000 = 5600 \text{ micrograms}$$

$$5.6 \text{ milligrams (mg)} = 5600 \text{ micrograms (µg)}$$

For the beginner, this technique avoids confusion. The more experienced provider will be able to make a direct conversion from milligrams to micrograms.

HOUSEHOLD AND APOTHECARY SYSTEMS OF MEASURE

In the past, pharmacology traditionally used the household and apothecary systems to measure drug dosages. Gradually, the metric system has replaced those systems, but you may occasionally encounter their remnants. Table 15-3 gives the metric equivalents of the household and apothecary units you will most likely encounter.

Table 15-3 METRIC EQUIVALENTS

Household	Apothecary	Metric
1 gallon	4 quarts	3.785 litres
1 quart	1 quart	0.946 litres
16 ounces	approximately 1 pint	473 millilitres
1 cup	approximately ½ pint	approximately 250 millilitres
1 tablespoon		approximately 16 millilitres
1 teaspoon		approximately 4–5 millilitres

WEIGHT CONVERSION

Some medications' dosages are calculated according to kilograms of body weight. To convert pounds to kilograms use the following formula:

$$\text{kilograms} = \text{pounds}/2.2$$

Example 5: How many kilograms does a 182 lb. person weigh?

$$\text{kilograms} = 182 \text{ lb.}/2.2$$

$$\text{kilograms} = 82.7$$

$$182 \text{ pounds (lb.)} = 82.7 \text{ kilograms (kg)}$$

TEMPERATURE

The international thermometric scale measures temperature in degrees Celsius. Although degrees Celsius is often cited interchangeably with degrees centigrade, the two scales are slightly different. For practical purposes, however, you can think of them both as dividing the interval between the freezing and boiling points of water into 100 equal parts, with 0 degree being the freezing point and 100 degrees being the boiling point. The household measurement system, however, divides the interval between the freezing and boiling points of water into 180 equal parts, with 32 degrees being the freezing point and 212 degrees being the boiling point. When taking a body temperature, use the following formulas to convert between degrees Fahrenheit and degrees Celsius:

$$°F = (°C \times 1.8) + 32$$
$$°C = (°F - 32) \div 1.8$$

Example 6: Convert 98.2°F to °C

$$°C = (98.2 - 32) \div 1.8$$

$$°C = 66.2 \div 1.8$$

$$°C = 36.8$$

$$36.8°C = 98.2°F$$

Example 7: Convert 28.4°C to °F

$$°F = (28.4 \times 1.8) + 32$$

$$°F = 51.12 + 32$$

$$°F = 83.1$$

$$83.1°F = 28.4°C$$

✱ **unit** predetermined amount of medication or fluid.

Converting between the different prefixes and between different systems of measurement is crucial in calculating drug dosages. You should continually practise all conversions, not only during your formal education but also throughout your career in the emergency medical services.

UNITS

Some medications are measured in **units.** Penicillin, heparin, and insulin are administered in units. Units do not convert among the metric, household, and apothecary systems.

MEDICAL CALCULATIONS

Frequently, you will have to apply basic mathematical principles to calculate specific quantities before administering medications and fluids. In prehospital care, the following forms of medications often require calculation:

- Oral medications
- Liquid parenteral medications
- Intravenous fluid administration
- Intravenous medication infusions

✱ **stock solution** standard concentration of routinely used medications.

Most medications are provided in **stock solution.** Therefore, you must calculate the exact amount of medication to remove from the stock for administration. To calculate basic drug dosage, you will need three facts:

- Desired dose
- Dosage on hand
- Volume on hand

✱ **desired dose** specific quantity of medication needed.

Desired Dose The **desired dose** is the specific quantity of medication needed. Most dosages are expressed as a weight (grams, milligrams, or micrograms). Dosages may be standard or calculated according to body weight or age.

✱ **concentration** weight per volume.

✱ **dosage on hand** the amount of drug available in a solution.

✱ **volume on hand** the available amount of solution containing a medication.

Dosage and Volume on Hand All liquid medications are packaged as concentrations. **Concentration** refers to weight per volume. A liquid medication's concentration is the drug's weight (grams, milligrams, or micrograms) per volume of liquid (mL) in which it is dissolved. For example, 50 percent dextrose (D_{50}) is packaged as a concentration of 25 grams (weight) dextrose in 50 mL (volume) of water. From the concentration, you can determine the **dosage on hand** (weight) and the **volume on hand.** For 50 percent dextrose, the dosage on hand is 25 grams and the volume on hand is 50 mL. Concentrations are identified on all drug packaging and labels.

Because you cannot see the desired dose dissolved in liquid, you must convert its weight to volume, a readily visible measurement, using the following formula:

$$\text{volume to be administered} = \frac{\text{volume on hand} \times \text{desired dose}}{\text{dosage on hand}}$$

To use this formula, you must express all weight and volume measurements with the same metric prefix. For example, if the desired dose is expressed in *milli*grams, the dosage on hand must also be expressed in *milli*grams, volume on hand in *milli*litres.

CALCULATING DOSAGES FOR ORAL MEDICATIONS

The following example illustrates how to calculate the volume of a specific drug dosage:

> **Example 1:** A physician orders you to administer 90 mg of acetaminophen to a pediatric patient. The liquid acetaminophen is packaged as a concentration of 500 mg in 8 mL of solution. How much of the medication will you administer?

Because you cannot see the 90 mg of acetaminophen, you must convert this weight to a volume. To do so you need these facts:

$$\text{desired dose} = 90 \text{ mg}$$
$$\text{dosage on hand} = 500 \text{ mg}$$
$$\text{volume on hand} = 8 \text{ mL}$$

Use the formula to calculate the dosage's volume:

$$\text{volume to be administered} = \frac{\text{volume on hand (8 mL)} \times \text{desired dose (90 mg)}}{\text{dosage on hand (500 mg)}}$$

$$\text{volume to be administered} = (8 \times 90)/500$$
$$\text{volume to be administered} = 720/500$$
$$\text{volume to be administered} = 1.44 \text{ mL}$$

Administer 1.44 mL of solution to deliver 90 mg of acetaminophen.

Another way to calculate drug dosages is the ratio (fraction) and proportion method. A ratio (fraction) illustrates a relationship between two numbers. A proportion is the comparison of two numerically equivalent ratios. Using the variable x, the above problem can be stated this way:

$$8 \text{ mL}/500 \text{ mg} = x \text{ mL}/90 \text{ mg}$$

To solve the problem, cross-multiply the numerals:

$$\frac{8}{500} = \frac{x}{90}$$
$$720 = 500x$$
$$\frac{720}{500} = x$$
$$1.44 = x$$
$$x = 1.44 \text{ mL}$$

> **Math Summary 1**
>
> $$x \text{ mL} = \frac{8 \text{ mL} \times 90 \text{ mg}}{500 \text{ mg}}$$
> $$x \text{ mL} = \frac{720}{500}$$
> $$x \text{ mL} = 1.44$$

> **Math Summary 2**
>
> $$\frac{8 \text{ mL}}{500 \text{ mg}} = \frac{x \text{ mL}}{90 \text{ mg}}$$
> $$x \text{ mL} = \frac{720}{500}$$
> $$x = 1.44 \text{ mL}$$

CONVERTING PREFIXES

The following example shows how to calculate the volume to be administered when the desired dose, the dosage on hand, and the volume on hand are not all expressed in metric units with the same prefix.

> **Example 2:** A physician orders you to give 250 mg of a drug via IV bolus. The multidose vial contains 2 grams of the drug in 10 mL of solution. How much of the medication should you administer?

Because the desired dose is expressed as *milli*grams, the dosage on hand must be converted from grams to milligrams. In the metric system, 2 grams equal 2000 milligrams. You now know:

$$\text{desired dose} = 250 \text{ mg}$$
$$\text{dosage on hand} = 2000 \text{ mg}$$
$$\text{volume on hand} = 10 \text{ mL}$$

Math Summary 3

$$x \text{ mL} = \frac{10 \text{ mL} \times 250 \text{ mg}}{2000 \text{ mg}}$$

$$x \text{ mL} = \frac{2500}{2000}$$

$$x \text{ mL} = 1.25$$

Now you can use the formula to calculate the volume to be administered:

$$\text{volume to be administered} = \frac{\text{volume on hand (10 mL)} \times \text{desired dose (250 mg)}}{\text{dosage on hand (2000 mg)}}$$

volume to be administered = (10 × 250)/2000

volume to be administered = 2500/2000

volume to be administered = 1.25 mL

Administer 1.25 mL of solution to deliver 250 mg medication.

You can also solve this problem using the ratio proportion as follows:

$$\frac{10 \text{ mL}}{2000 \text{ mg}} = \frac{x \text{ mL}}{250 \text{ mg}}$$

$$2500 = 2000x$$

$$2500/2000 = x$$

$$1.25 = x$$

$$x = 1.25 \text{ mL}$$

Math Summary 4

$$\frac{10 \text{ mL}}{2000 \text{ mg}} = \frac{x \text{ mL}}{250 \text{ mg}}$$

$$x \text{ mL} = \frac{2500}{2000}$$

$$x = 1.25 \text{ mL}$$

Tablets also come in stock doses. If the dosage of one tablet or pill is more than needed, divide the tablet or pill to make the correct dose. Do not divide enteric or time-release capsules.

CALCULATING DOSAGES FOR PARENTERAL MEDICATIONS

You can use the same formula to calculate specific doses and volume for parenteral medication delivery.

Example 3: A physician wants you to administer 5 mg of medication subcutaneously. The ampule contains 10 mg of the drug in 2 mL of solvent. How much medication should you use?

desired dose = 5 mg

dosage on hand = 10 mg

volume on hand = 2 mL

$$\text{volume to be administered} = \frac{\text{volume on hand (2 mL)} \times \text{desired dose (5 mg)}}{\text{dosage on hand (10 mg)}}$$

volume to be administered = (2 × 5)/10

volume to be administered = 10/10

volume to be administered = 1 mL

Administer 1 mL of solution to deliver 5 mg of the medication.

Using the ratio and proportion method, the problem is solved as follows:

Math Summary 5

$$\frac{2 \text{ mL}}{10 \text{ mg}} = \frac{x \text{ mL}}{5 \text{ mg}}$$

$$x \text{ mL} = \frac{10}{10}$$

$$x = 1 \text{ mL}$$

$$\frac{2 \text{ mL}}{10 \text{ mg}} = \frac{x \text{ mL}}{5 \text{ mg}}$$

$$10 = 10x$$

$$10/10 = x$$

$$1 = x$$

$$x = 1 \text{ mL}$$

CALCULATING WEIGHT-DEPENDENT DOSAGES

Occasionally, you will have to calculate the desired dose according to the patient's weight.

> **Example 4:** You must administer 1.5 mg/kg of lidocaine via IV bolus to a patient in stable ventricular tachycardia. The concentration of lidocaine is 100 mg in a prefilled syringe containing 10 mL of solution. The patient weighs 158 lbs.

Start by converting the patient's weight to kilograms:

$$\text{Kilograms} = \text{pounds}/2.2$$

$$\text{Kilograms} = 158 \text{ lb.}/2.2$$

$$\text{Kilograms} = 71.82$$

The patient weighs approximately 72 kg.

Calculate the desired dose:

$$1.5 \text{ mg} \times 72 \text{ kg} = 108 \text{ mg}$$

You now know these three facts:

$$\text{desired dose} = 108 \text{ mg}$$

$$\text{dosage on hand} = 100 \text{ mg}$$

$$\text{volume on hand} = 10 \text{ mL}$$

Use the same formula as before to calculate the volume to be administered:

$$\text{volume to be administered} = \frac{\text{volume on hand (10 mL)} \times \text{desired dose (108 mg)}}{\text{dosage on hand (100 mg)}}$$

$$\text{volume to be administered} = (10 \times 108)/100$$

$$\text{volume to be administered} = 1080/100$$

$$\text{volume to be administered} = 10.8 \text{ mL}$$

Administer 10.8 mL of solution to deliver 108 mg of lidocaine.

After you have calculated the desired dose, you can solve this problem using the ratio and proportion method as previously illustrated.

Math Summary 6

$$x \text{ mL} = \frac{10 \text{ mL} \times 108 \text{ mg}}{100 \text{ mg}}$$

$$x \text{ mL} = \frac{1080}{100}$$

$$x = 10.8 \text{ mL}$$

CALCULATING INFUSION RATES

To deliver fluid or medication through an IV infusion, you must calculate the correct infusion rate in drops per minute. To do so, you must know the administration tubing's drip factor, as well as the volume on hand, desired dose, and dosage on hand.

Medicated Infusions

To calculate the correct IV infusion rate, use the following formula:

$$\text{drops/minute} = \frac{\text{volume on hand} \times \text{drip factor} \times \text{desired dose}}{\text{dosage on hand}}$$

Math Summary 7

$$\frac{10 \text{ mL}}{100 \text{ mg}} = \frac{x \text{ mL}}{108 \text{ mg}}$$

$$x \text{ mL} = \frac{1080}{100}$$

$$x = 10.8 \text{ mL}$$

Example 5: A physician wants you to administer 2 mg/min of lidocaine to a patient. To prepare the infusion, you mix 2 grams of lidocaine in an IV bag containing 500 mL of 5 percent dextrose in water (D_5W). You will use a microdrip administration set (60 gtts/mL). Calculate the infusion rate.

$$\text{desired dose} = 2 \text{ mg}$$
$$\text{dosage on hand} = 2000 \text{ mg (2 grams)}$$
$$\text{volume on hand} = 500 \text{ mL}$$
$$\text{drip factor} = 60 \text{ gtts/mL}$$

$$\text{drops/minute} = \frac{\text{volume on hand (500 mL)} \times \text{drip factor (60 gtts/mL)} \times \text{desired dose (2 mg)}}{\text{dosage on hand (2000 mg)}}$$

$$\text{drops/minute} = (500 \times 60 \times 2)/2000$$
$$\text{drops/minute} = 60\ 000/2000$$
$$\text{drops/minute} = 30$$

Run the infusion at 30 drops/minute to infuse 2 mg lidocaine per minute.

Fluid Volume over Time

Fluids with or without medications may require administration over a specific period. To deliver the fluid correctly, you must calculate volume/time. This calculation, requires the following information:

- Volume to be administered
- Drip factor of the administration set (gtts/mL)
- Total time of infusion (minutes)

✱ infusion rate speed at which a medication is delivered intravenously.

To calculate the **infusion rate,** use this formula:

$$\text{drops/minute} = \frac{\text{volume to be administered (drip factor)}}{\text{time in minutes}}$$

Example 6: A physician tells you to administer 500 mL of normal saline solution to a patient over one hour (60 minutes). The administration tubing is a macrodrip set with a drip factor of 10 gtts/mL. At what drip rate would you run this infusion?

$$\text{volume to be administered} = 500 \text{ mL}$$
$$\text{administration set drip factor (gtts/mL)} = 10 \text{ gtts/mL}$$
$$\text{total time of infusion (minutes)} = 60 \text{ minutes}$$

Calculate the infusion rate:

$$\text{drops/minute} = \frac{(500 \text{ mL})(10 \text{ gtts/mL})}{60 \text{ minutes}}$$

$$\text{drops/minute} = (500 \times 10)/60$$
$$\text{drops/minute} = 5000/60$$
$$\text{drops/minute} = 83.3$$

Set the flow rate at approximately 83 drops per minute to infuse 500 mL of normal saline in almost exactly 60 minutes.

You can use the same formula to determine how long it will take to use all the fluid in a container.

Example 7: You are transporting a patient with an IV antibiotic. The infusion rate is 45 gtts/minute and the administration tubing is a microdrip set (60 gtts/mL); 150 millilitres remain in the 500 millilitre bag of D_5W. How long until the antibiotic will infuse fully?

Use the same formula as in Example 6; however, in this instance you will find time in minutes.

$$45 \text{ drops/minute} = \frac{(150 \text{ mL})(60 \text{ gtts/mL})}{\text{time}}$$
$$45 = (150 \times 60)/\text{time}$$
$$45 = 9000/\text{time}$$
$$\text{time} = 9000/45$$
$$\text{time} = 200$$
$$45 \text{ drops/minute} = 200 \text{ minutes}$$

The antibiotic will infuse fully in 200 minutes, or 3 hours and 20 minutes.

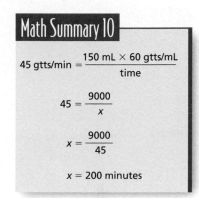

Math Summary 10

$$45 \text{ gtts/min} = \frac{150 \text{ mL} \times 60 \text{ gtts/mL}}{\text{time}}$$
$$45 = \frac{9000}{x}$$
$$x = \frac{9000}{45}$$
$$x = 200 \text{ minutes}$$

Calculating Dosages and Infusion Rates for Infants and Children

Infants and children cannot tolerate under- or overdoses of medication and fluids. When you administer infusions to pediatric patients, you must calculate exact flow rates. Because infants and children differ drastically from adults in size and internal development, their dosages often depend on weight. Most weight-dependent dosages express the patient's weight in kilograms, and so you must make the appropriate conversion from pounds as discussed earlier. Occasionally, you may encounter a medication that is based on body surface area (BSA). Chemotherapeutic agents for children are often based on body surface area. Although you will not initiate such drugs, you may encounter them on critical care transports either by ground or air. Many aids for calculating pediatric drug doses and infusion rates are available, including charts, forms, and length-based resuscitation tapes. Although these devices are helpful, you should not rely on them exclusively. They are no substitute for knowledge.

SUMMARY

Drug administration is a fundamental skill used in the treatment of the sick and the injured. For medications to be effective, they must be *safely* delivered into the body by the *appropriate* route. Many different routes for drug delivery are available to the paramedic; however, specific drugs require specific routes for administration.

It is your responsibility to be familiar with all routes of drug delivery and the techniques for establishing and utilizing them. You will use some routes of medication administration infrequently, and they will quickly fade from memory. Nonetheless, someone's well-being may depend on your ability to utilize such a route in an emergency. Therefore, periodic review of all routes used in medication administration is highly recommended. In addition, you must accurately calculate many drug dosages. Dosage errors and inappropriate medication administration harm patient care and cast serious doubt on your ability.

Appendix A

PCP AND ACP COMPETENCIES

The following table correlates the Paramedic Association of Canada's *National Occupational Competency Profiles for Paramedic Practitioners* with text content. Please refer to the legend below to understand the degree of competency required as a primary care paramedic (PCP) or an advanced care paramedic (ACP).

N The competency is not applicable to the practitioner.

X The practitioner should have a basic awareness of the subject matter of the competency.

A The practitioner must have demonstrated an academic understanding of the competency.

S The practitioner must have demonstrated the competency in a simulated setting (including practical scenarios, skill stations). In Competency Areas 4 and 5, skills must be demonstrated on a human subject where legally and ethically acceptable.

C The practitioner must have demonstrated the competency in a clinical setting with a patient.

P The practitioner must have demonstrated the competency in a field preceptorship with a patient.

AREA 1 PROFESSIONAL RESPONSIBILITIES

Specific Competency	PCP	ACP	Reference Chapter(s)
General Competency 1.1 Function as a professional			
Maintain patient dignity	P	P	**1, 41, 43, 45, 46**
Reflect professionalism through use of appropriate language	P	P	**1, 4, 5**
Dress appropriately and maintain personal hygiene	P	P	**1, 4, 5**
Maintain appropriate personal interaction with patients	A	A	**1, 4**
Maintain patient confidentiality	P	P	**2**
Participate in quality assurance and enhancement programs	A	A	**1, 16**
Utilize community support agencies as appropriate	A	A	**1**
Promote awareness of emergency medical system and profession	P	P	**1**
Participate in professional association	A	A	**1**
Behave ethically	P	P	**1, 2**
Function as patient advocate	P	P	**1, 2**
General Competency 1.2 Participate in continuing education			
Develop personal plan for continuing professional development	A	A	**1**
Self-evaluate and set goals for improvement, as related to professional practice	A	A	**1**
Interpret evidence in medical literature and assess relevance to practice	A	A	**1, Appendix B**

General Competency 1.3 Possess an understanding of the medicolegal aspects of the profession

Comply with scope of practice	P	P	**1, 2, 10, 11**
Recognize "patient rights" and the implications on the role of the provider	A	A	**1, 2**
Include all pertinent and required information on ambulance call report forms	P	P	**1, 2, 6, 9**

General Competency 1.4 Recognize and comply with relevant provincial and federal legislation

Function within relevant legislation, policies, and procedures	A	A	**1, 2, 3, 8**

General Competency 1.5 Function effectively in a team environment

Work collaboratively with a partner	P	P	**1, 11**
Accept and deliver constructive feedback	P	P	**1**
Work collaboratively with other emergency response agencies	P	P	**1, 3, 16**
Work collaboratively with other members of the health care team	P	P	**1, 3, 16**

General Competency 1.6 Make decisions effectively

Exhibit reasonable and prudent judgement	P	P	**10, 11**
Practise effective problem-solving	P	P	**10, 11**
Delegate tasks appropriately	P	P	**11**

AREA 2 COMMUNICATION

Specific Competency	PCP	ACP	Reference Chapter(s)

General Competency 2.1 Practise effective oral communication skills

Deliver an organized, accurate, and relevant report utilizing telecommunication devices	P	P	**8**
Deliver an organized, accurate, and relevant verbal report	P	P	**8, 11**
Deliver an organized, accurate, and relevant patient history	P	P	**8, 11**
Provide information to patient about their situation and how they will be treated	P	P	**4, 42**
Interact effectively with the patient, relatives, and bystanders who are in stressful situations	P	P	**5, 38, 41, 42, 43**
Speak in language appropriate to the listener	P	P	**4, 5, 42**
Use appropriate terminology	P	P	**5, 8, 9**

General Competency 2.2 Practise effective written communication skills

Record organized, accurate, and relevant patient information	P	P	**2, 9**
Prepare professional correspondence	P	P	**8, 9**

General Competency 2.3 Practise effective non-verbal communication skills

Exhibit effective non-verbal behaviour	S	S	**4**
Practise active listening techniques	P	P	**4, 5, 6**
Establish trust and rapport with patients and colleagues	P	P	**4, 5, 6**
Recognize and react appropriately to non-verbal behaviours	P	P	**3, 4, 38**

General Competency 2.4 Practise effective interpersonal relations

Treat others with respect	P	P	**1, 4, 5, 38, 42, 43**
Exhibit empathy and compassion while providing care	P	P	**1, 4, 5, 22, 43**
Recognize and react appropriately to individuals and groups manifesting coping mechanisms	P	P	**1, 42**
Act in a confident manner	P	P	**1, 4, 5, 10**

	PCP	ACP	
Act assertively as required	P	P	**1, 4**
Manage and provide support to patients, bystanders, and relatives manifesting emotional reactions	P	P	**1, 5, 42**
Exhibit diplomacy, tact, and discretion	P	P	**1, 5**
Exhibit conflict resolution skills	S	S	**1, 4**

AREA 3 HEALTH AND SAFETY

Specific Competency	PCP	ACP	Reference Chapter(s)

General Competency 3.1 Maintain good physical and mental health

Maintain balance in personal lifestyle	A	A	1
Develop and maintain an appropriate support system	A	A	1
Manage personal stress	A	A	1
Practise effective strategies to improve physical and mental health related to shift work	A	A	1
Exhibit physical strength and fitness consistent with the requirements of professional practice	A	A	1

General Competency 3.2 Practise safe lifting and moving techniques

Practise safe biomechanics	P	P	**1**
Transfer patient from various positions using applicable equipment and/or techniques	P	P	**24, 1**
Transfer patient using emergency evacuation techniques	S	S	**3, 24, 1**
Secure patient to applicable equipment	P	P	**3, 24, 1**
Lift patient and stretcher in and out of ambulance with partner	P	P	**1**

General Competency 3.3 Create and maintain a safe work environment

Assess scene for safety	P	P	**1, 3, 7**
Address potential occupational hazards	P	P	**1, 3, 7**
Conduct basic extrication	S	S	**3**
Exhibit defusing and self-protection behaviours appropriate for use with patients and bystanders	S	S	**1, 4, 5, 23, 38**
Conduct procedures and operations consistent with Workplace Hazardous Materials Information System (WHMIS) and hazardous materials management requirements	A	A	**3**
Practise infection control techniques	P	P	**1, 7, 19, 37**
Clean and disinfect equipment	P	P	**1, 7, 37**
Clean and disinfect an emergency vehicle	P	P	**1, 3, 37**

AREA 4 ASSESSMENT AND DIAGNOSTICS

Specific Competency	PCP	ACP	Reference Chapter(s)

General Competency 4.1 Conduct triage

Rapidly assess a scene based on the principles of a triage system	S	S	3
Assume different roles in a mass casualty incident	A	A	3
Manage a mass casualty incident	A	A	3

General Competency 4.2 Obtain patient history

Obtain a list of patient's allergies	P	P	**5, 7**
Obtain a list of patient's medications	P	P	**5, 7**
Obtain chief complaint and/or incident history from patient, family members, and/or bystanders	P	P	**5, 7**

Obtain information regarding patient's past medical history	P	P	5, 7
Obtain information about patient's last oral intake	P	P	5, 7
Obtain information regarding incident through accurate and complete scene assessment	P	P	5

General Competency 4.3 Conduct complete physical assessment demonstrating appropriate use of inspection, palpation, percussion, and auscultation, and interpret findings

Conduct primary patient assessment and interpret findings	P	P	7, 10, 11
Conduct secondary patient assessment and interpret findings	P	P	5, 6, 7, 10, 11
Conduct cardiovascular system assessment and interpret findings	P	P	5, 6, 7, 12, 13, 28, 41, 42, 43
Conduct neurological system assessment and interpret findings	P	P	5, 6, 7, 13, 23, 24, 29, 37, 42, 43, 45, 46
Conduct respiratory system assessment and interpret findings	P	P	5, 6, 7, 12, 25, 27, 27a, 42, 43
Conduct obstetrical assessment and interpret findings	S	C	5, 26, 40, 41
Conduct gastrointestinal system assessment and interpret findings	S	P	5, 6, 7, 26, 32, 43
Conduct genitourinary system assessment and interpret findings	S	P	5, 6, 7, 13, 26, 33, 39, 43
Conduct integumentary system assessment and interpret findings	S	S	5, 6, 7, 20, 21, 31, 37, 42, 43
Conduct musculoskeletal assessment and interpret findings	P	P	5, 6, 7, 20, 22, 24, 42, 43
Conduct assessment of the immune system and interpret findings	P	P	13, 31, 43
Conduct assessment of the endocrine system and interpret findings	P	P	5, 13, 30, 43
Conduct assessment of the ears, eyes, nose, and throat and interpret findings	S	S	5, 6, 23, 42
Conduct multisystem assessment and interpret findings	P	P	7, 13, 19, 20, 31, 34, 35, 36, 37, 44
Conduct neonatal assessment and interpret findings	S	C	41
Conduct psychiatric assessment and interpret findings	S	S	5, 38, 43

General Competency 4.4 Assess vital signs

Assess pulse	P	P	6, 7, 41, 42
Assess respiration	P	P	6, 7, 41, 42
Conduct non-invasive temperature monitoring	C	C	6, 42
Measure blood pressure by auscultation	P	P	6, 42
Measure blood pressure by palpation	P	P	6
Measure blood pressure with non-invasive blood pressure monitor	C	C	6, 42
Assess skin condition	P	P	6, 7, 41, 42
Assess pupils	P	P	6, 7, 41, 42
Assess level of mentation	P	P	4, 6, 7, 23, 29, 41, 42

General Competency 4.5 Utilize diagnostic tests

Conduct oximetry testing and interpret findings	C	C	6, 27, 27a, 29
Conduct end-tidal carbon dioxide monitoring and interpret findings	N	C	6, 27, 27a, 29
Conduct glucometric testing and interpret findings	P	P	6
Conduct peripheral venipuncture	N	X	15
Obtain arterial blood samples via radial artery puncture	N	X	Glossary
Conduct invasive core temperature monitoring and interpret findings	N	X	Glossary
Conduct pulmonary artery catheter monitoring and interpret findings	N	X	Glossary
Conduct central venous pressure monitoring and interpret findings	N	X	Glossary
Conduct arterial line monitoring and interpret findings	N	X	Glossary
Interpret laboratory and radiological data	X	A	Glossary
Conduct 3-lead electrocardiogram (ECG) and interpret findings	S	P	6, 7, 28
Obtain 12-lead electrocardiogram and interpret findings	X	A	6, 7, 28

AREA 5 THERAPEUTICS

Specific Competency	PCP	ACP	Reference Chapter(s)
General Competency 5.1 Maintain patency of upper airway and trachea			
Use manual manoeuvres and positioning to maintain airway patency	C	C	27a, 42
Suction oropharynx	S	C	23, 27a, 42
Suction beyond oropharynx	A	C	27a
Utilize oropharyngeal airway	S	C	23, 27a, 41, 42
Utilize nasopharyngeal airway	S	S	23, 27a, 42
Utilize airway devices not requiring visualization of vocal cords and not introduced endotracheally	A	S	27a
Utilize airway devices not requiring visualization of vocal cords and introduced endotracheally	A	S	10, 20, 27a
Utilize airway devices requiring visualization of vocal cords and introduced endotracheally	A	C	27a, 41, 42
Remove airway foreign bodies (AFB)	S	S	7, 27, 42
Remove foreign body by direct techniques	X	S	7, 27, 27a, 42
Conduct percutaneous cricothyroidotomy	X	S	20, 23, 27a, 42
Conduct surgical cricothyroidotomy	N	A	20, 23, 27a, 42
General Competency 5.2 Prepare oxygen delivery devices			
Recognize indications for oxygen administration	A	A	27a, 42
Take appropriate safety precautions	A	A	46
Ensure adequacy of oxygen supply	A	A	27a
Recognize different types of oxygen delivery systems	A	A	27a, 46
General Competency 5.3 Deliver oxygen and administer manual ventilation			
Administer oxygen using nasal cannula	C	C	27a, 42
Administer oxygen using low concentration mask	C	C	27a
Administer oxygen using controlled concentration mask	X	X	27a
Administer oxygen using high concentration mask	C	C	27a, 42
Administer oxygen using pocket mask	S	S	27a
Provide oxgenation and ventilation using bag-valve-mask	C	C	27, 27a, 7, 42, 46
Recognize indications for mechanical ventilation	A	A	27, 27a
Prepare mechanical ventilation equipment	A	A	27a, 46
Provide mechanical ventilation	N	C	27a, 46
General Competency 5.5 Implement measures to maintain hemodynamic stability			
Conduct cardiopulmonary resuscitation (CPR)	S	S	28, 41, 42
Control external hemorrhage through the use of direct pressure and patient positioning	S	S	19, 23
Maintain peripheral intravenous (IV) access devices and infusions of crystalloid solutions without additives	C	P	15, 19, 42
Conduct peripheral intravenous cannulation	A	P	15
Conduct intraosseous needle insertion	X	S	15, 42
Utilize direct pressure infusion devices and intravenous infusions	A	S	19
Administer volume expanders (colloid and non-crystalloid)	X	S	13, 15, 19
Administer blood and/or blood products	X	A	13, 15, 35
Conduct automated external defibrillation	S	S	28
Conduct manual defibrillation	X	S	28
Conduct cardioversion	X	S	28
Conduct transcutaneous pacing	X	S	28
Maintain transvenous pacing	N	A	Glossary
Maintain intra-aortic balloon pumps	N	X	Glossary
Provide routine care for patient with urinary catheter	S	C	46

Provide routine care for patient with ostomy drainage system	A	S	46
Provide routine care for patient with non-catheter urinary drainage system	A	A	46
Monitor chest tubes	X	X	Glossary
Conduct needle thoracostomy	X	S	25, Glossary
Conduct oral and nasal gastric tube insertion	X	S	41, 42, 46
Conduct urinary catheterization	X	A	46, Glossary

General Competency 5.6 Provide basic care for soft tissue injuries

Treat soft tissue injuries	P	P	19, 20
Treat burn	S	S	21, 42, 43
Treat eye injury	S	S	23
Treat penetration wound	S	S	18 20 25 42
Treat local cold injury	S	S	36

General Competency 5.7 Immobilize actual and suspected fractures

Immobilize suspected fractures involving appendicular skeleton	S	S	17, 22, 42, 43
Immobilize suspected fractures involving axial skeleton	P	P	17, 22, 24, 42

General Competency 5.8 Administer medications

Recognize principles of pharmacology as applied to the medications listed in Appendix 5 of the profiles	A	A	14, 22, 23, 27a, 24, 28, 30, 31, 41, 42, Drug cards
Follow safe process for responsible medication administration	S	P	14, 15
Administer medication via subcutaneous route	S	C	14, 15
Administer medication via intramuscular route	S	C	14, 15
Administer medication via intravenous route	X	P	14, 15, 42
Administer medication via intraosseous route	X	S	14, 15, 42
Administer medication via endotracheal route	X	S	14, 15
Administer medication via sublingual route	S	C	14, 15
Administer medication via topical route	X	S	14, 15
Administer medication via oral route	S	C	14, 15
Administer medication via rectal route	X	A	14, 15
Administer medication via inhalation	S	C	14, 15

AREA 6 INTEGRATION

Specific Competency	PCP	ACP	Reference Chapter(s)

General Competency 6.1 Utilize differential diagnosis skills, decision-making skills, and psychomotor skills in providing care to patients

Provide care to patient experiencing illness or injury primarily involving cardiovascular system	P	P	17, 18, 25, 42, 43
Provide care to patient experiencing illness or injury primarily involving neurological system	P	P	17, 18, 19, 29, 42, 43
Provide care to patient experiencing illness or injury primarily involving respiratory system	P	P	17, 18, 20, 21, 25, 27, 27a, 42, 43, 46
Provide care to patient experiencing illness or injury primarily involving genitourinary/reproductive systems	S	S	33, 39, 43
Provide care to patient experiencing illness or injury primarily involving gastrointestinal system	P	P	7, 18, 20, 26, 32, 42, 43
Provide care to patient experiencing illness or injury primarily involving integumentary system	P	P	17, 18, 20, 42, 43
Provide care to patient experiencing illness or injury primarily involving musculoskeletal system	P	P	17, 18, 20, 22, 24, 42, 43
Provide care to patient experiencing illness or injury primarily	S	S	31, 42

involving immune system

Provide care to patient experiencing illness or injury primarily involving endocrine system	S	S	30, 40, 42, 43
Provide care to patient experiencing illness or injury primarily involving the eyes, ears, nose, or throat	S	S	18, 19, 20, 42
Provide care to patient experiencing illness or injury due to poisoning or overdose	S	P	34, 42, 43
Provide care to patient experiencing non-urgent medical problem	P	P	11, 46
Provide care to patient experiencing terminal illness	S	S	29, 45, 46
Provide care to patient experiencing illness or injury due to extremes of temperature or adverse environments	S	S	36, 41, 43
Provide care to patient based on understanding of common physiological, anatomical, incident- and patient-specific field trauma criteria that determine appropriate decisions for triage, transport, and destination	P	P	7, 16
Provide care for patient experiencing psychiatric crisis	S	P	43, 38
Provide care for patient in labour	S	C	40

General Competency 6.2 Provide care to meet the needs of unique patient groups

Provide care for neonatal patient	S	C	40, 41
Provide care for pediatric patient	C	C	6, 23, 26, 27a, 42, 44
Provide care for geriatric patient	C	C	38, 44
Provide care for physically-challenged patient	S	S	42, 45
Provide care for mentally-challenged patient	S	S	45

General Competency 6.3 Conduct ongoing assessments and provide care

Conduct ongoing assessments based on patient presentation and interpret findings	P	P	11, 7, 10
Re-direct priorities based on assessment findings	P	P	7, 10, 11

AREA 7 TRANSPORTATION

Specific Competency	PCP	ACP	Reference Chapter(s)

General Competency 7.1 Prepare ambulance for service

Conduct vehicle maintenance and safety check	P	P	3
Recognize conditions requiring removal of vehicle from service	A	A	3
Utilize all vehicle equipment and vehicle devices within ambulance	S	S	3

General Competency 7.2 Drive ambulance or similar type vehicle

Utilize defensive driving techniques	A	A	1, 3
Utilize safe emergency driving techniques	A	A	1, 3
Drive in a manner that ensures patient comfort and a safe environment for all passengers	A	A	1, 3

General Competency 7.3 Transfer patient to air ambulance

Create safe landing zone for rotary-wing aircraft	A	A	3
Safely approach stationary rotary-wing aircraft	A	A	3
Safely approach stationary fixed-wing aircraft	A	A	3

General Competency 7.4 Transport patient in air ambulance

Prepare patient for air medical transport	A	A	3
Recognize the stressors of flight on patient, crew, and equipment, and the implications for patient care	A	A	3, 16

Appendix B

PREHOSPITAL RESEARCH

Antishock trousers are good. Antishock trousers are bad. Intravenous fluids are good. Intravenous fluids are bad. EMS providers hear these and other similar statements all the time. It can be quite confusing. Furthermore, newspapers and the television news pick up stories from articles in medical journals and report them to the public. How much of these reports can a paramedic believe? Do they apply to all EMS systems? Should they be the basis for changes in prehospital practice?

Research is an increasingly important part of EMS. Many of our ideas about patient care are the result of tradition and have never been evaluated from a scientific standpoint. This is true not just of EMS but also of medicine in general and emergency medicine in particular. Only in the last few years has anyone paid significant attention to laying the foundation for research-proven quality care in EMS.

This appendix will describe three aspects of research as it applies to EMS. First, it will introduce you to the subject of how to interpret research. This will help you understand what to look for in a piece of published research, such as whether to believe the conclusions of the paper and how to apply the research to your EMS system. Second, this appendix will describe what you need to know if you participate in a research project. More and more EMS systems are participating in the research needed to determine how best to care for our patients and to justify what we do. Third, this appendix will list a number of ways you can learn more about research and how it is interpreted.

UNDERSTANDING RESEARCH

HOW A FIELD ADVANCES

Every area of medicine is rapidly changing. EMS is no exception. One of the ways in which a discipline advances is by common sense. No one has to do a research study to conclude that placing heavy sandbags on the sides of an immobilized patient's head can lead to harm if the patient and backboard must be turned on their sides. In this case, using something sturdy and lightweight makes a great deal more sense. Similarly, it is obvious that glass IV bottles are much more likely to break in a moving ambulance than are plastic IV bags. In these cases, common sense guides us in making important decisions.

However, common sense has its limits. In the early years, common sense led us to believe that we could raise the blood pressure of a shock patient by inflating antishock trousers. In fact, it was taught that antishock trousers would potentially autotransfuse two or three units of blood from the lower extremities to the torso. These ideas seemed sound and were based on experiences the military had with gravity suits. It was assumed that the same physiological effects would occur in a shock patient when the trousers were applied. Various researchers began to question the effectiveness of the antishock trousers. First, several studies were conducted that addressed the physiological effects of the trousers. Much to the surprise of many, it was found that the trousers had very little impact on blood pressure in shock patients. Furthermore, it was found that the antishock trousers autotransfused only a very small amount of blood, if any.

Other researchers looked at a much more important and key issue. Do antishock trousers improve patient survival? The research found that the antishock trousers had no beneficial effect on patient survival. In fact, some patients actually did worse when the trousers were applied compared with those who did not have them applied. Because of this research, antishock trousers are no longer routinely used in the prehospital management of hemorrhagic shock.

Several years ago, it was also considered common sense to place a soft cervical collar around the neck of a patient with a suspected cervical-spine injury. That belief is no longer considered valid. Today, common sense tells us that a rigid cervical collar, applied in conjunction with spinal immobilization, does a better job of preventing spine injuries from becoming spinal-cord injuries. It remains to be seen whether this belief will be verified by scientific evidence or if someone will find a better approach.

Sometimes, we have to rely on something a little more substantive than common sense, even when we do not have the hard data to make a definitive statement. In this case, we may try to get a consensus of experts in the field. For example, to develop a course curriculum, a group of team leaders, each responsible for a particular section of the curriculum, would discuss the general direction and approach the curriculum should take. Each team leader would then discuss more specific information with a group of writing experts (authors) and medical content experts (physicians). Because EMS is such a young field, there may frequently be a lack of clear evidence to support certain subjects and interventions. Using this approach, experts would discuss and come to agreement on what should and should not be included in the curriculum.

This approach is used often in medicine when there is conflicting and missing information or when there have been many changes in a short time. The American Heart Association (AHA), for example, periodically uses this approach in updating its guidelines for basic and advanced cardiac life support. The AHA has recently augmented its consensus approach with a set of evidence-based guidelines. These guidelines call on participants in the process to evaluate the strength of available evidence by evaluating the nature of the evidence supporting it. The results of a well-conducted study that has a powerful methodology and many study subjects would receive more weight than a case report (a description of what happened to one or a few patients in an emergency department, for example).

Scientific studies are another way of improving the care our patients receive. To many people, this is the best way to advance a field because it allows practitioners to see exactly how an idea was tested. When done well, a piece of research can have a significant impact on many people's lives. EMS has only recently begun to lay this foundation and establish credibility for itself. In recent years, some of the areas that have received attention from EMS researchers include defibrillation, spine immobilization, aeromedical transport (helicopters), triaging of patients to trauma centres, intravenous fluids, endotracheal intubation by primary care paramedics, time saved by use of lights and sirens, and the value of certain advanced life support interventions.

TYPES OF STUDIES

There are four types of scientific studies that you are likely to encounter: descriptive, case-control, cohort, and intervention studies. Each type of study has its strengths and weaknesses.

Descriptive Studies

In a *descriptive study*, researchers do not attempt to change anything or discover the effects of any intervention. Instead, they carefully evaluate a particular subject according to carefully spelled out criteria. This yields a report that describes the current state of affairs in a particular area. For example, an EMS agency may wish to learn how many defibrillators to purchase and where to place them. To accomplish this, they review their call reports for the last three years to determine how many cardiac arrests the service had and where those arrests occurred. The results give the organization the information it needs in order to station enough defibrillators in the right places. This will increase the likelihood that a defibrillator will be nearby when a patient goes into cardiac arrest.

Descriptive studies are relatively inexpensive and simple to conduct because they usually involve reviewing a database or conducting a survey. They are limited, though, in their scope and applicability because they typically look only at a single system, which may be very different from other systems, and because like a snapshot it shows conditions at only one particular point in time. A *cross-sectional study*, for example, might look at divorce rates among emergency workers. If the rate were found to be high (or low), we would have the answer to the question we asked. However, we would be left with a lot more questions this study would not be able to answer, such as: Is the divorce rate different because of the work these people do? Or is the rate different because of the kind of person drawn to emergency work?

Because they are very weak in their ability to draw conclusions about cause and effect, descriptive studies are not very useful for investigating hypotheses. Instead, they are better suited for laying the foundation for research in a particular area and for suggesting research questions for the future.

Case-Control Studies

A *case-control study* is an example of *retrospective research*, which looks backward in time. By finding patients who have a particular disease or condition and comparing them with people who do not have the disease or condition, a case-control study can allow investigators to determine which factors place someone at risk for developing the disease. An example of this was a landmark study on the effects of cigarette smoking published in 1950. The investigators looked at the health history, including smoking history, of more than 700 patients hospitalized for lung cancer and compared this with the same information obtained from a large number of patients hospitalized for other conditions. They found that patients with lung cancer were significantly more likely to have smoked than were those without lung cancer.[1]

One of the criticisms of case-control studies is a phenomenon called *recall bias*. If you ask someone with lung cancer how long and how much he has smoked, he may, either consciously or unconsciously, give inaccurate answers, depending on whether he believes smoking caused his condition and which answers he believes the investigator wants. He also may not want to admit he was unable to quit smoking and so may be less than completely truthful. Alternatively, he may want to exaggerate the role smoking played in causing his condition so that others will not imitate him. The person without lung cancer is presumably less likely to be subject to these feelings but may still be subject to recall bias. Even the most carefully conducted study can fall victim to this kind of distortion, and so it is important that researchers take it into consideration and do everything they can to minimize it.

Cohort Studies

Like case-control studies, *cohort studies* look at certain characteristics of study subjects (potential risk factors) and the development of disease. In this case, though, we

---

[1]Doll, R. and A.B. Hill. Smoking and carcinoma of the lung; Preliminary report. *British Medical Journal* 2:739, 1950.

do not know yet whether the study subjects have the disease we are studying. Instead, we record which potential risk factors patients have or were exposed to and monitor them to see which ones develop the disease being studied. This is an example of *prospective research*, where the condition being studied has not yet appeared.

This can be quite time consuming, since many conditions take years to develop. Over a long time, study subjects may also move away from the investigators or in other ways be lost to follow-up. This can make such a study quite expensive. Probably one of the best known examples of this type of study is the Framingham Heart Study.[2]

In the early 1950s, investigators began studying more than 5000 middle-aged adults without cardiovascular disease in the Framingham, Massachusetts, area. These people have been monitored and periodically examined for heart disease. Since the researchers did not (and could not) know at the beginning of the study which patients with which risk factors would develop heart disease, this study has given scientists very strong evidence about the roles of cigarette smoking, cholesterol, and high blood pressure in the development of heart disease.

Intervention Studies

In case-control studies, investigators look at patients who have a disease and determine risk factors for development of the disease. In cohort studies, patients are selected on the basis of whether or not they have been exposed to risk factors and monitored for the development of disease. In *experimental* or *intervention studies*, the situation is quite different. In these studies, the investigators determine whether or not a subject is exposed (or treated) instead of depending on nature to determine this. This kind of study, when designed and conducted properly, yields extremely strong evidence about the effects of certain interventions. For this reason, it is often considered the gold standard in research methodology.

The investigators begin, just as they do with case-control and cohort studies, by deciding on a study hypothesis. This consists of an idea that they can test in an objective manner. For instance, a number of years ago, clinicians in King County, Washington, wanted to test the hypothesis that EMTs with automated external defibrillators (AEDs) could increase survival from cardiac arrest just as well as EMTs with manual defibrillators.[3] They trained EMTs to use both machines, set up protocols for their use, decided exactly what data they were going to record, and planned how they were going to be able to tell whether their hypothesis was correct (through selection of the proper statistical tests). They did this very carefully and planned how to conduct the study so that irrelevant factors were eliminated or minimized.

Since the researchers wanted to find out whether EMTs could operate AEDs, they used just one brand of AED. This eliminated one potential source of confounding. A variable that is not being studied, but which may have an effect on the result, is called a *confounding variable* or *nuisance variable*. In this case, the researchers made sure that no one could say increased (or decreased) survival could be attributed to one brand of AED over another since only one AED was being used.

Whenever possible, researchers performing clinical trials attempt to *randomize* the intervention so that there is less chance of interference from a confounding variable. For example, a number of EMTs in King County had been us-

---

[2]Dawber, T.R. *The Framingham Study: The Epidemiology of Atherosclerotic Disease.* Cambridge, MA: Harvard University Press, 1980.

[3]Cummins, R.O., M.S. Eisenberg, P.E. Litwin, et al. Automatic external defibrillators used by emergency medical technicians. *Journal of the American Medical Association* 257:1605–1610, 1987.

ing manual defibrillators for several years and preferred using them. If they had a choice as to which defibrillator they could use, they might select the manual defibrillator for patients with short down times and the automated defibrillators for long or unknown down times. The researchers took this into account by telling the EMTs to use one of the machines for 75 days and then the other for the next 75 days. Although this is not randomization in the strictest sense of the word, this alternation design, or *alternative time sampling*, is an acceptable means of preventing this type of confounding. Another example is the use of one intervention on even days and another on odd days.

As can be seen in this case, it is not always practical, or even possible, to use truly random sampling. In such cases, *systematic sampling* may be a reasonable alternative. This might include, for example, using the study intervention every second or third day. Although systematic sampling is subject to bias, it is better than *convenience sampling*. Convenience sampling, as the name implies, occurs at the convenience of the investigator, which, for example, might be only when that person is working. If the investigator is a paramedic with some seniority who gets some choice over when and where he works, this could lead to significant bias in subject selection.

All clinical trials compare one group that receives an intervention (the *study group*) against at least one other group that does not receive the intervention being studied (the *control group*). In many studies, the control group receives a placebo, something that resembles the intervention but has no physical effect on the study subject. In drug trials, for instance, a placebo is sometimes a sugar pill. In the case of an AED study, it would have been unethical to deny defibrillation to cardiac-arrest patients in the control group, since there was clear evidence that manual defibrillation was saving some lives. So, the researchers used manual defibrillators as their control.

Something else researchers attempt to incorporate into their study designs whenever possible is *blinding*. This refers to whether or not someone knows which is being used, a placebo or an active agent. In an *unblinded* study, everyone involved (the patient, researcher, statistician, and so on) knows when the intervention is and is not being used. *Single blinding* occurs when the patient does not know what he is receiving, but the researcher does. *Double blinding* means that neither the patient nor the researcher knows what the patient is receiving. *Triple blinding* is a less commonly used term that refers to the situation where the patient, the researcher, and the statistician (or principal investigator, who may be functioning in that capacity) do not know whether a patient is receiving the intervention or a placebo.

In the case of a drug study, it can be very important to blind the study subjects and the investigators because of the possibility of *observation bias*. This occurs when, either consciously or unconsciously, someone (either the subject or the investigator) reports an effect because they believe there should be one. This is called the *placebo effect*. Study subjects who receive placebos often report feeling better, even though they did not receive any medication. This effect can occur in as many as a quarter of study subjects and may persist for years afterward. A similar type of bias, known as the *Hawthorne effect*, occurs when outcomes improve during a study just because those participating in the study are aware that experimental attempts are being made to bring about improvement.

In a study where the outcome being studied is as objective as death or survival, there is little or no need for blinding. If, however, a subjective outcome like quality of life after cardiac arrest was being studied, there would be a lot more potential for observation bias. In this case, it would be important to make sure that the investigators determining the quality of life do not know which intervention a patient receives, if at all possible.

Another way in which the King County researchers demonstrated good study design was the way they planned their data collection and statistical analysis. Even with randomization, study subjects may differ from the control subjects in important ways. It thus becomes important for researchers to evaluate the two groups for differences that may confound the results. In this case, they looked at a number of variables, including age, sex, whether or not the arrest was witnessed, initial ECG rhythm, and response times. They found that the two groups were significantly different in a few ways, but they were able to use some sophisticated statistical methods to determine that in this case those differences did not affect patient outcome.

One of the other things they did was to calculate the sample size they would need to detect a difference in survival rates. They calculated that in order to have an 80 percent chance of detecting a difference in survival of more than 15 percent (if a difference truly existed), they would need to have at least 150 patients in each group. This allowed them to plan approximately how long the study would take. The figure of 80 percent is sometimes referred to as the "power of the study" and is directly related to how willing the investigators are to avoid making an error in their conclusions.

There are two types of *statistical error* that researchers can make. A Type I, or alpha, error is accepting a hypothesis when it is false. A Type II, or beta, error is rejecting a hypothesis when it is true. The Type I error rate is set at 0.05 or 5 percent in most research. A commonly accepted Type II error rate is 20 percent or 0.2. The power of a study is equal to 1 – beta. Since many studies set beta at 0.2, the power is 1 – 2 = 0.8 or 80 percent to detect a difference at the magnitude specified by the investigators if a difference truly exists. The Type I and Type II error rates have an inverse relationship; that is, the lower the Type I error rate the investigator wishes to have, the higher is the Type II error rate the investigator will have to tolerate, all other factors being equal. The reverse is also true.

The Type I error rate, or alpha, receives a great deal of attention in published research. Most investigators set alpha at 0.05. This means the researchers will say there is a difference and consider the study to have statistically significant results only if there is a 5 percent chance or less of getting the results they obtained. Another way of looking at a Type I error rate, or alpha, of 0.05 is that there is only a 5 percent chance of rejecting the study hypothesis when it is false, assuming the hypothesis is true.

A good practice many studies follow is to report not just the acceptable alpha of 0.05 but also the actual probability of getting the results obtained in the study. You may see this written as "$P < .01$." This means the chance of finding such a difference in the study groups is less than 1 percent, assuming the hypothesis is true.

Some people have misinterpreted P values in two ways. First, they conclude that because the P value is so small, the hypothesis is absolutely proven beyond a shadow of a doubt. This is not true. No study can definitively prove its hypothesis. All a study can do is assign certain probabilities to the conclusions. All studies also make certain assumptions, such as the type of data to be collected, accuracy of the data, and whether or not samples were selected randomly and independently. If these assumptions are violated, the study's conclusions are suspect.

Second, some people conclude that because there is *statistical* significance (because the P value is so small), there must be *clinical* significance. This is not the case. The researcher determines whether or not there is statistical significance by deciding how much Type I error is acceptable. The researcher and the reader must then determine if there is clinical significance by evaluating the effect of this difference on patient care.

For example, suppose a new drug for hypertension is studied. The investigators find statistically significant differences between the blood pressures in the treated and untreated subjects with $P \ll .01$ (P much less than 1 percent). In other words, if there was no difference between the drug and the control, these results would occur much less than 1 percent of the time. On looking at the data, the reader finds that the experimental drug lowers diastolic blood pressure 0.1 mmHg. Is this a clinically significant difference? Not likely. To see a change that is significant enough to affect patient outcome, the difference would have to be greater.

The Type II error rate, or beta, receives much less attention in most published research. This oversight is unfortunate because, in some cases, investigators fail to get a large enough sample size and so are unable to find a difference even though it exists. A good way to reduce both error rates is to increase the sample size. This solution can lead to some other problems though.

With greater sample size come the difficulties of more data collection, longer times required to conduct the study, and increased expense. Additionally, it may become easier to find differences that are irrelevant. This occurs because a larger sample allows smaller differences to be detected.

Another problem that can arise in clinical trials is violation of protocol. Despite the planning and precautions of the investigators in the King County study, there were some instances in which EMTs used the manual defibrillator when they were supposed to use the AED. In their analysis of the data, they evaluated these cases as a separate group and also with the AED group to which they should have belonged. This is called *intention to treat* analysis and is an appropriate way to manage protocol violations. This approach does increase the difficulty of finding a difference, but this is usually safer than the opposite approach of including these cases in the other treatment group. In this case, when the investigators analyzed the data, they found that the violations did not have an effect on the overall outcome.

In the end, the King County study found that there was no significant difference in survival between the group treated with the manual defibrillator and the group treated with the AED. Since AEDs are less expensive, require less training to operate, are extremely consistent in performance, and can be used in areas where there are fewer cardiac arrests, the investigators concluded that AEDs can make early defibrillation possible for more patients and should be encouraged. This is an example of a study that, because it showed there was no statistically significant difference between two treatments, had great clinical significance.

Table B-1 summarizes the advantages and disadvantages of different types of studies.

COMMON STATISTICAL TESTS

A number of computer programs, including commonly used spreadsheets, are available to calculate statistical tests for researchers and others. This section will briefly describe, in layperson's terms, a few of the more common tests you will find in reading research papers.

Descriptive Statistics

Descriptive statistics describe the nature of a sample. The most common descriptive statistic you will encounter is the *mean*, or average. It is computed by adding the values and dividing by the number of values involved. This gives a look at the average or typical value of a group of numbers in many cases. The mean is especially well suited when the data are what statisticians call "normally distributed." This means that if you graphed the data, they would form a shape similar to a bell curve described by a particular statistical equation. Height of individuals is an example of a normally distributed variable. Most people have a height close to the average, with a few very short and a few very tall people at each end of the graph.

Table B-1   ADVANTAGES AND DISADVANTAGES OF DIFFERENT TYPES OF STUDIES

Study Type	Advantages	Disadvantages
Descriptive	Inexpensive Relatively easy to conduct Can be done in relatively short time	Not good for testing hypotheses Very system specific
Case-Control	Good for testing hypotheses regarding uncommon or rare conditions Lays groundwork for cohort and intervention studies	Subject to recall bias
Cohort	Can provide very strong evidence for effects of risk factors	Not good for uncommon or rare conditions Can be very time consuming Expensive
Intervention	Provides strongest kind of evidence research can produce Can minimize bias through randomization and blinding	Expensive Need to protect study subjects may prolong time needed to conduct a study Study conditions may not be similar to real-life conditions

When the data are not normally distributed, the *median* is a better way of finding a typical value. To compute the median, put the values into numerical order and find the middle value. This is the median, also known as the "fiftieth percentile." For example, if you have seven exam scores, to find the median, you put the scores in order and find the fourth highest (or fourth lowest, since it is the same).

Here is an example of how the median can be more useful than the mean in some situations: In many jurisdictions, the number of emergency calls received by EMS agencies is not normally distributed. There are frequently a few very busy services in urban areas, a good number of moderately busy services, and a larger number of services in rural areas that receive a much smaller number of calls. If you were to compute the mean, or average, it would be skewed by the very busy services, even though there are only a few of them, because they receive such a high number of calls. The median would better reflect the number of calls received by a typical service.

The mean and the median only tell one part of the story. They are called *measures of central tendency* because they indicate the centre of the group in one way or another. A different, but very important quality to know about a group is how spread out it is, or how dispersed the data are.

There are two closely related measures of this that you are likely to see. The first is called the *variance*. To get it, we take each value and subtract the mean from it. We cannot take the average of these numbers and get anything useful because the negative numbers will cancel out the positive numbers and we will get zero. To overcome this, we multiply each number by itself (square it) and add up the squared numbers. We then divide this sum by the number of values we started with (for reasons statisticians can describe, when we are working with samples, we usually divide by one less than the number of values). This is the variance.

To get the *standard deviation* (SD), the other common measure of dispersion, we take the square root of the variance. See Figure B-1 for two examples of variance and standard deviation. The standard deviation gives us valuable information about the data. If two groups of data have the same mean but the second has a standard deviation much larger than the first, the data in the second group are much more spread out than the data in the first group. The SD is also used in many statistical formulas.

Another way we can describe data is to give the *mode*. This is simply the most common value in a set of data. If you graph the data, with the data value on the horizontal axis and the frequency of occurrence on the vertical axis (also known as a frequency distribution), the mode is the value associated with the highest point on the graph.

Inferential Statistics

As noted earlier, the mean, median, variance, and standard deviation are examples of *descriptive statistics*. They describe the nature of a sample of data taken from a *population*, a group we are interested in.

Descriptive statistics are related to, but quite different from, *inferential statistics*. Here, instead of describing the sample, we want to draw inferences about the population the sample came from. In this case, we say we are estimating *parameters* of the population. For example, if the sample is of sufficient size and we make certain assumptions about the population and how the sample was selected, we can estimate the mean value of the population from which we drew our sample. Polling organizations commonly use these techniques in reporting results of their surveys. We must keep in mind, however, the phenomenon of *sampling error*. This is the difference between the value obtained from the sample and the value obtained from the population stemming solely from the fact that only a sample of the population was included.

When researchers find that something occurs with a certain frequency, they usually report this proportion as a percentage. For example, survival from cardiac arrest caused by ventricular fibrillation (VF) may be 20 percent in a particular study. But since the study looked at a sample of patients in VF, this proportion is only an estimate and may, in reality, be higher or lower. Investigators can calculate how much variability exists in this percentage based on the number of observations, the actual data, and how reliable they want the estimate to be.

The variability (not the same as the variance) can then be added and subtracted to the original proportion to give what is called a *confidence interval*. For example, suppose the investigators calculated the variability in the example above with 95 percent confidence and found it was 6 percent. Then, we would have a 95 percent confidence interval of 20 percent plus or minus 6 percent. This means that, assuming the hypothesis is true, we can be 95 percent confident that the actual rate of survival under the conditions studied was between 14 percent and 26 percent.

Confidence intervals are very important in interpreting the value of the research results. If the confidence interval for a proportion like the one above include zero, then there would be a real possibility that there is no actual difference between the study group outcome and the control group outcome. We would conclude that the results are not statistically significant and that there is insufficient reason to believe there is a difference between the two groups.

Quantitative and Qualitative Statistics

There are many tests for finding differences between groups. Statisticians frequently classify them into qualitative and quantitative tests. *Qualitative statistics* usually deal with data that are nonnumerical in nature (e.g., female, male) or that are nonnumerical in nature and have been assigned a number indicating ranking or ordering of importance or severity (stage I, II, and III of certain cancers, for example). These are sometimes called *nominal* and *ordinal data*. Finding the mean of such data may be impossible or absurd, since they are categorical in nature. *Quantitative statistics*, conversely, are numerical in nature, such as temperature measured in degrees on a thermometer or height of an individual measured in centimetres. They are sometimes referred to as continuous data.

Examples of Variance and Standard Deviation

To see how the variance and standard deviation can give valuable information about data, consider this example: Two different paramedic classes take the same midterm exam. The classes are the same size (seven students each) and have the same mean (or average) score, 85 percent. If we did not look any further, we might think the two classes performed the same on the exam. By looking at the variance and standard deviation, though, we can see that they are actually quite different.

Class 1

	Score	Mean	Score − Mean	(Score − Mean)^2
	78	85	−7	49
	81	85	−4	16
	82	85	−3	9
	84	85	−1	1
	87	85	2	4
	89	85	4	16
	94	85	9	81
Sum	595		0	176

Recall that to get the variance we must find the mean, then find the difference between the scores and the mean, square these differences, add them up, and divide by one less than the number of scores. The mean is included in the second column to make it easier to calculate the difference between each score and the mean. The variance is then 176/6 = 29.3. The standard deviation is the square root of 29.3, which is 5.4.

Class 2

	Score	Mean	Score − Mean	(Score − Mean)^2
	82	85	−3	9
	83	85	−2	4
	84	85	−1	1
	85	85	0	0
	86	85	1	1
	87	85	2	4
	88	85	3	9
Sum	595		0	28

Again, to get the variance, we sum the squared differences in the last column and divide by one less than the number of scores: 28/6 = 4.7. The standard deviation is the square root of 4.7, or 2.2, less than half the standard deviation of the first class.

This implies that the scores in the first class are much more spread out than the scores in the second class. When we graph the scores, we can see that this is true:

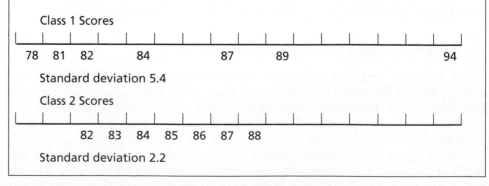

FIGURE B-1   Examples of variance and standard deviation.

Other Types of Data

Commonly used tests you may see in research include *t test*, the *analysis of variance (ANOVA)* and the *chi square test*. Which test is used depends to a great extent on the kind of data involved and the kinds of differences the investigators are looking for. We will not describe these tests here, but the interested reader can consult some of the sources listed at the end of this appendix.

Another test you may see is the *odds ratio*. This is used in case-control studies and consists of the odds of having a risk factor, if the condition is present, divided by the odds of having the risk factor, if the condition is not present. Simply put, the odds ratio describes how strong the association is between a risk factor and the condition it is associated with. The larger the risk factor, the stronger is the association. When you see an odds ratio, look for the confidence interval. Since an odds ratio of 1 indicates that there is no risk associated with the risk factor, if the confidence interval includes 1, there is no statistically significant risk.

For example, suppose investigators surveyed advanced care paramedic students regarding how much education they had received before enrolling in their course. They wanted to test the hypothesis that having at least a university degree is associated with passing the ACP certification exam. After the course is over, they perform the proper calculations and determine that the odds ratio is 1.6. This means a student who passes is 1.6 times as likely to have at least a university degree compared with someone who does not pass the exam. The 95 percent confidence interval, though, is 0.8–2.4.

This means we are 95 percent confident the true odds ratio lies between 0.8 and 2.4. Since the interval includes 1 (keep in mind an odds ratio of 1 means there is no association), we cannot be 95 percent confident that there really is an association, and so we conclude there is no statistically significant relationship between having at least a university degree and passing the ACP exam in this group. However, if the 95 percent confidence interval had been 1.2–2.0, and interval that does not include 1, we would have concluded with 95 percent confidence that there is a statistically significant relationship and that a person who passes the ACP exam is between 1.2 and 2 times as likely to have at least a university degree.

Many other statistical tests are used for different kinds of studies and different kinds of data. The references section at the end of this appendix lists several sources where you can learn more about them.

FORMAT OF A RESEARCH PAPER

When authors submit their findings to a journal, they structure their results in a standardized fashion that allows others to quickly understand what the researchers did and what they found (Table B-2). The first thing to appear after the title and names of the authors is the *abstract*. This is a brief paragraph that summarizes the need for the study, the research methods used, and the results encountered. Many people use the abstract to determine whether or not the paper is one of interest to them and therefore worth reading.

Table B-2	OUTLINE OF RESEARCH PAPER FORMAT
	Abstract
	Introduction
	Methods
	Results
	Discussion
	Summary

The *introduction* is the first section of the paper itself. This is a brief description of pertinent previously published papers on the subject of the investigation. It should describe why the study was undertaken and what the purpose of the study was or what hypothesis the authors wanted to test.

Next comes the *methods* section. This describes exactly how the authors conducted the study, including what population they wished to study, how subjects were selected (and excluded), and what intervention was performed, if any. There should be enough information for interested readers to repeat the experiment should they so desire. The authors should also describe how they determined the sample size, how much statistical power there was to detect a difference, which statistical tests they used to analyze the data, and what level of significance they chose for their statistical tests.

The *results* come next. Here, the researchers provide their data (or a summary of the data), frequently with tables, charts, and graphs to help make sense of the information they gathered. This section presents the data but does not elaborate on it.

The *discussion* section is where the authors interpret their findings and describe the significance of them. There is usually a description of how this new information fits into the field of study and whether it supports or refutes previous research. There should also be a discussion of the limitations of the study, frequently followed by a call for further research to answer the questions raised by the study.

The *summary*, or conclusion, is a very brief (no more than a few sentences) recap of the main findings of the study.

HOW A RESEARCH PAPER IS PUBLISHED

Once the authors of a study have drafted their paper, they submit it to a scientific journal for publication. Each journal has its own particular rules, but all peer-reviewed journals follow the same general procedure. After receiving the paper, the editor sends it to one or more members of a review board, people who have significant expertise either in the field covered by the journal or a related area, such as statistics or research methodology. The reviewers read the paper and evaluate it for its adherence to standards of research methods, its pertinence to the field, and the potential value it has for practitioners. The reviewers send their comments to the editor, who then decides whether to publish it, send it back for revisions, or reject it. A copy editor may go over it for grammar, spelling, and syntax at some point in the process. Many papers submitted by researchers are not published and some journals have reputations for being very selective.

A note here about the term *abstract:* In the prior section, we mentioned that the first part of a research paper is a brief summary paragraph called the abstract. The term *abstract* more commonly describes a brief form of a longer scientific research paper that is often published before the full research paper. The abstract may be presented at national peer meetings and responses to the abstract may form the basis for adjustments to the full research paper that is subsequently published. Abstracts are also published and cited in peer review journals.

The peer-review process has recently begun to receive greater attention than it has in the past. This has been the result, ironically enough, of several studies looking at the quality of published papers. A surprisingly large number of papers, when evaluated objectively for adherence to principles of research methodology, have been shown to be deficient. This has led at least one journal, *Annals of Emergency Medicine*, to review and revamp its review procedures.[4] Reviewers now get train-

---

[4]Waeckerle, J.J., and M.L. Callaham. Medical journals and the science of peer reviewing: Raising the standard. *Annals of Emergency Medicine* July, 28: 75, 1996.

ing in what to look for and how to evaluate papers, and closer attention will be paid to how statistics are used. This may be the beginning of a trend that should improve the quality of the research that is conducted and published.

WHAT TO LOOK FOR WHEN REVIEWING A STUDY

Questions to ask when reviewing a study include the following (Table B-3):

- *Was the research peer reviewed?* This is no guarantee of quality, but it at least indicates that experts have reviewed the study and found it to have some merit. Keep in mind that some journals will deliberately publish papers they know to be of lower quality than usual in order to stir up debate about an important subject.

- *Was there a clear hypothesis or study purpose?* The paper should have a clear description of exactly what the investigators were evaluating and what their study hypothesis was. When a hypothesis is not clearly spelled out, it is very easy for the investigators to draw unjustified conclusions.

- *Was the study approved by an institutional review board (IRB), and was it conducted ethically?* An IRB is a group of people, usually at a hospital or university, who review study proposals to ensure that patients are protected when they participate in research as study subjects.

- *Was the study type appropriate?* Not every investigation lends itself to the format of the randomized controlled clinical trial. It may be necessary, for ethical or financial reasons, to use another format. Evaluate whether the questions the investigator asked were well suited for the type of study they conducted.

- *What population were the researchers studying?* Is the population similar to the one you see?

- *What inclusion and exclusion criteria did the researchers use?* If the investigators excluded the patients most likely to have a condition or patients very similar to the ones you see, the study may have very little to tell you.

- *How did the investigators draw their samples?* Did they use true random sampling? systematic sampling? alternative time sampling? convenience sampling?

- *How many groups were patients divided into, and were patients assigned to control and study groups properly?* The effects of bias and confounding must be taken into account for the study to yield worthwhile results. In particular, ask yourself:
  — For case-control and cohort studies, were selection bias and recall bias taken into account?
  — For randomized controlled studies, were randomization and blind assignment maintained?

- *Were the control and study groups the proper size?* Did the investigators describe the sample size necessary to produce sufficient power to avoid a type II error? What was the power of the study?

- *Were the effects of confounding variables taken into account?* Did the investigators describe potential confounders and how they prevented them from interfering with the study?

Table B-3 QUESTIONS TO ASK WHEN REVIEWING A STUDY

- Was the research peer reviewed?
- Was there a clear hypothesis or study purpose?
- Was the study approved by an institutional review board (IRB), and was it conducted ethically?
- Was the study type appropriate?
- What population were the researchers studying?
- What inclusion and exclusion criteria did the researchers use?
- How did the investigators draw their sample?
- How many groups were patients divided into, and were patients assigned to control and study groups properly?
- Were the control and study groups the proper size?
- Were the effects of confounding variables taken into account?
- What kind of data did the investigators collect, and did they analyze the data with the proper statistical tests?
- Were the results reported properly (e.g., 95 percent confidence interval)?
- How likely is it that the study results would occur by chance alone?
- Are the author's conclusions logical and based on the data?

- *What kind of data did the investigators collect, and did they analyze the data with the proper statistical tests?* There are many tests available, and more than one may be appropriate for the conditions at hand. You may need to consult a statistician or researcher to determine whether or not the investigators used the right tests on the data. Did the investigators clearly determine before data collection took place which tests they were going to use? When the data fail to provide statistically significant results, it is very tempting to perform more tests until one shows significant results. This kind of retrospective testing is called *data snooping* or *data dredging*. If one continues to perform statistical tests, eventually one will be significant just by chance alone. This inappropriate use of statistics is to be avoided.

- *Were the results reported properly?* When a paper includes a proportion or an odds ratio, is there also a 95 percent confidence interval?

- *How likely is it that the study results would occur by chance alone?* Remember that a P value reflects only the odds of seeing the results of a particular piece of research if the study hypothesis is true. A small P value may be very impressive, but it does not prove the study hypothesis. Keep in mind also the difference between association and causation. For example, it would be easy to show that the number of drownings increases with sales of ice cream. An inattentive reader might conclude that the sale of more ice cream causes more drownings to occur. In reality, this is an example of association, not causation. Ice cream sales go up when the weather gets warmer, which is also when more people go swimming and drown. This is also an example of confounding.

- *Are the author's conclusions logical and based on the data?* Occasionally, a journal publishes a paper that goes against everything you know. It can then be difficult to determine whether you need to change your approach to a particular problem or consider the paper an aberration. After all, by chance alone, some studies will show statistically significant results that are the result of chance or coincidence. Sometimes, the prudent course is to see if anyone else can replicate the experiment before changing your practice. This is a good example of how you should be very cautious in changing your practice based on just one study. If the conclusion is a real one and not spurious, someone else should be able to come up with it, too.

And one more consideration that is very important in EMS research:

- *How "good" was the EMS system in which the study was done?* This factor can have a profound effect of the validity of a study. As an extreme example, how valid would the results of a study of the impact of AED use be if the time from arrest to emergency responder arrival was 15 minutes? In this scenario, there would likely be no survivors, no matter what intervention was used!

APPLYING STUDY RESULTS TO YOUR PRACTICE

Once you have evaluated a study, you are in a better position to determine whether or not it should change your practice. Before you do so, though, you need to consider several factors. Rarely do clinicians make significant changes on the basis of one study. Since no study can definitively prove a hypothesis, the reader must look at other studies and his own experience in order to construct an informed opinion. If every other study published on a particular topic comes to very different conclusions from those of the study at hand, the reader has to wonder whether the study was poorly designed, subject to bias of some sort, affected by unknown confounding variables, or just the result of chance. One must evaluate the field and its knowledge base in order to make an informed decision about how to interpret a piece of research.

The clinical significance is another important piece of the puzzle to consider. A P value with lots of zeros (e.g., $P < .0001$) may be very impressive, but not very pertinent. Distinguish between the statistical significance and the clinical significance of the study. Was the difference found in the study large enough to make a real difference to patients?

When investigators conduct their experiments, they have the luxury of selecting patients who meet their criteria and excluding patients who do not. In the real world, things are not quite so tidy. Before we can apply the results of a piece of research to a particular patient, we must be sure the patient is similar enough to the study group to benefit from the intervention.

Finally, EMS providers do not function in a vacuum. Before implementing any significant changes in your practice, speak to the management of your organization and especially to your medical director. You are responsible not only to your patients but also to your bosses and your medical director. Including them in decision making of this nature is essential and will pay off in better patient care overall.

PARTICIPATING IN RESEARCH

Many EMS systems are not content to watch other people advance their field. They have decided to conduct research themselves. They have found that by executing well-designed studies, they can not only improve care in their coverage areas but also improve prehospital care throughout the nation, sharpen the skills of their providers, and rekindle their providers' interest by doing something new and potentially groundbreaking.

Before you participate in such a study, there are certain things you should do and find out (Table B-4). The first step usually is to ask a question. This should involve something of practical importance. Determining the value of a particular intervention (end-tidal CO_2 monitoring, for example) is clearly going to have more impact on EMS than finding out whether ambulances carry 24 four-by-four gauze pads or 48 four-by-four gauze pads.

Once you have focused on the issue and determined exactly what you wish to discover, you can go to the next step. This is where you generate your hypothesis, a statement of exactly what you are going to test. The *null hypothesis* is usually a statement that there is no difference between the groups you are sampling from. The *research* or *alternative hypothesis* is a statement that there is a difference between the groups. This is often, though not always, what you would like to show.

Once you know what you are evaluating, you need to define the *population* you will be studying, or the group you draw your subjects from and to which you plan to generalize your results.

Closely associated with this step is determining the limitations of your study. This might include limited ability to generalize your results because of the patient-selection methods you used, even though you had little or no choice in the methods available to you. Similarly, the population you draw from might be significantly different from other populations.

For example, if you wanted to test for improved survival in hypotensive trauma patients, some of whom received antishock trouser treatment and some of whom did not, you would need to describe your EMS and trauma care system very carefully. You might have a primarily urban population with predominantly penetrating trauma, short transport time to level 1 trauma centres, and experienced paramedics. Your results would have limited applicability to a rural population with predominantly blunt trauma, long transport times to small community hospitals, and less experienced emergency medical responders and primary care paramedics.

The best studies limit themselves to a single question or hypothesis. This is desirable because it allows you to focus better on the question at hand. The downside is that you may not find out everything you wanted to. This is usually considered an acceptable tradeoff. No single study can answer every question.

The next step in conducting a study is usually to get approval from an institutional review board (IRB), sometimes known as the Ethics Review Committee. This allows you to get an outside evaluation of your study methodology and reduces considerably the chance you will be accused of conducting an unethical study. One of the items the IRB will undoubtedly be interested in is the issue of informed consent (consent given by the patient based on full disclosure of information regarding the nature, risks, and benefits of the procedure or study).

Several reports in the media over the last few years have described unethical studies in which subjects were not given the opportunity to give or refuse consent because they were not informed of the risks and benefits of participating in the study. In some cases, subjects actually died because they did not receive standard treatment available at the time of the study. These stories have prompted an

---

Table B-4	THINGS TO FIND OUT BEFORE YOU PARTICIPATE IN A STUDY

- Determine the question.
- Prepare your hypothesis (null hypothesis and research hypothesis).
- Decide what you want to measure and how you will do it.
- Identify the limitations of your study.
- Get the approval of the proper authorities.
- Determine how you will get informed consent from study subjects.
- Gather data, perhaps after conducting pilot trials.
- Analyze the data.
- Determine what you will do with your results (publish, present at a conference, follow up with more studies).

understandable reluctance on the part of many individuals to participate in research. The government even came out with standards for government-funded research that describe stringent requirements for informed consent.

A good *principal investigator* (PI), the person who oversees the study, will be familiar with these requirements and will be able to guide you through them. The PI should also gain the approval of other appropriate agencies, including the medical director and the head of the service involved.

After you have determined how to gain informed consent, you need to gather your data. Sometimes, a pilot trial is undertaken first so you can find unforeseen obstacles to data gathering. Seemingly trivial matters can become very important (such as whether or not EMS providers have to fill out any more forms). A good PI will meet with the EMS providers who are administering the study intervention and collecting the data. The PI should make sure they know how long the study is expected to last. This allows them to make plans and perhaps reschedule certain future activities they had anticipated. The providers collecting data need to know the name of the principal investigator and how to contact him. This is usually, though not always, a physician. Many EMS physicians who conduct field research will recruit a field provider to coordinate and assist with data collection.

Other things to tell those who will be participating are the inclusion and exclusion criteria for enrolling patients in the study, the effect of the study on patient care in general, and the risks and potential benefits to patients in the study. Once everyone understands these factors, you will be prepared to go forward with the study.

After you have collected the data and reached your predetermined sample size, it is time to analyze the data. Use the tests you described in your description of the methods for your study. Be very careful about performing additional tests, especially if your results do not show what you hoped or expected. Data snooping is a dangerous activity. If you perform enough statistical tests, you will eventually find one or more that give you "significant" results. Unfortunately, these results may very well be a product of chance, rather than your intervention. When multiple statistical tests are planned for the same set of data, statisticians adjust for this with multiple-testing procedures to avoid such false results. Similarly, post hoc analysis of subgroups that were not defined before the study can also be dangerous. This can be a good way of generating hypotheses for future studies, but it is not a good basis for drawing conclusions now.

Once you have finished your data analysis, you must decide what to do with your results. If you feel your study addresses a pertinent, timely issue, and you think your methods were well thought out and your study was carefully conducted, you should seriously consider submitting it to a peer-reviewed journal. This is the best way to get such information out to the EMS community.

Alternatively, you may decide to present your findings at a conference. This usually involves summarizing your methods and results either orally or in the form of a poster, or both. This is less time-consuming than writing up a paper for publication but can still get the word out about your results and stimulate others to investigate the same phenomenon.

Do not feel that a "negative" study is worthless. If your study shows no difference in outcome between groups that did and did not receive an intervention, you may have reached important conclusions about the value, or lack of value, of an intervention.

A common result of a well-constructed study is more questions. This frequently stimulates the investigator and others to perform further studies. Once you get involved with researching the answers to questions, you may find yourself a little more skeptical about accepted, untested treatments and more interested in finding out what really works.

LEARNING MORE ABOUT RESEARCH

There are many ways you can learn more about interpreting and conducting research. In 1994, Ferno-Washington of Wilmington, Ohio, published a manual by James Menegazzi called *Research: The Who, What, Why, When, and How*. It is an excellent introduction to this topic and includes the proceedings of the 1992 Winter Assembly of the National Association of EMS Physicians on Research in Prehospital Care Systems.

A number of peer-reviewed medical journals publish articles regarding prehospital care. Three that publish many such articles are *Prehospital Emergency Care*, *Annals of Emergency Medicine*, and *Academic Emergency Medicine*. Sometimes, the *New England Journal of Medicine* and the *Journal of the American Medical Association* also publish articles of an EMS nature. All of these journals should be available at the library of your local hospital or medical school.

The Prehospital Care Research Forum promotes EMS research, and it sponsors an annual supplement to the *Journal of Emergency Medical Services*. This supplement gives selected abstracts from recent EMS studies. The Forum also sponsors oral and poster presentations at the annual *EMS Today* conference.

For the advanced reader who is not afraid of a challenge, there is *Emergency Medical Abstracts*. This is a monthly collection of forty abstracts of articles pertaining to emergency medicine. Only a few of the articles are directly related to EMS, but for the interested reader, the real prize is the audiotape that comes with the abstracts. On the tape, two emergency physicians discuss the abstracts for that month in an educational and often humorous fashion. The frequent criticisms of the methodologies used in the articles can enlighten even the most experienced clinician.

An excellent book for those interested in learning about research methodology is *Studying a Study and Testing a Test: How to Read the Medical Literature* by Richard Riegelman and Robert Hirsch. It includes a great deal more information about many of the topics discussed above.

Probably the most humorous book you will ever see about statistics is *PDQ Statistics* by Geoffrey Norman and David Streiner. This book does not go into detail about how to figure out statistics but instead concentrates on describing these tests in lay terms so that the reader can gain a fuller understanding of what statisticians do.

Finally, talk to others who have an interest in research. Emergency physicians are an especially good source of information about what is new and how to interpret it. EMS is performed by teams and learning how to do it better is often best done in teams, too.

More information on the sources mentioned above can be found in the following:

Brown, L.H., Criss, E.A., and Prasad, N.H. *An Introduction to EMS Research*. Toronto: Brady/Prentice Hall Health, 2002.

Emergency Medical Abstracts, Center for Medical Education, P.O. Box 600, Creamery, Pennsylvania 19430. Phone 1-800-458-4779.

Menegazzi, J. *Research: The Who, What, Why, When, and How*. Wilmington, Ohio: Ferno-Washington, 1994.

Norman, G.R., and D.L. Streiner. *PDQ Statistics*. Hamilton: B.C. Decker Inc., 1996.

Riegelman, R.K., and R.P. Hirsch. *Studying a Study and Testing a Test: How to Read the Medical Literature*, Third Edition. Little, Brown and Company, 1996.

Appendix C

EMERGENCY DRUGS

INTRODUCTION

The following pages describe the drugs commonly used by paramedics. Each medication is listed in either the *Compendium of Pharmaceuticals and Specialties* (CPS) or Health Canada's Drug Product Database. The description identifies the name and class of the drug, includes a brief description, and specifies its indications, contraindications, precautions, common dosages, and routes of administration.

Be sure that your instructor identifies which drugs are used in your EMS system and which need to be modified to indicate your EMS system's specific indications, contraindications, precautions, doses, and methods of administration.

Begin to familiarize yourself with all the information contained on the card when you are presented with the drug name. Reviewing just a few pages each week and then reviewing them as your course progresses will help you commit to memory the essential information about each drug.

Name/Class:	**ACETAMINOPHEN (Tylenol, Anacin-3)/Analgesic, Antipyretic**
Description:	Acetaminophen is a clinically proven analgesic/antipyretic with little effect on platelet function.
Indications:	For mild to moderate pain and fever when Aspirin is otherwise not tolerated.
Contraindications:	Hypersensitivity, children under 3 years.
Precautions:	Patients with hepatic disease; children under 12 years with arthritic conditions; alcoholism; malnutrition; and thrombocytopenia.
Dosage/Route:	325 to 650 mg PO/4 to 6 hours. 650 mg PR/4 to 6 hours.

Name/Class:	**ACTIVATED CHARCOAL (Actidose)/Adsorbent**
Description:	Activated charcoal is a specially prepared charcoal that will adsorb and bind toxins from the gastrointestinal tract.
Indications:	Acute ingested poisoning.
Contraindications:	An airway that cannot be controlled; ingestion of cyanide, mineral acids, caustic alkalis, organic solvents, iron, ethanol, methanol.
Precautions:	Administer only after emesis or in those cases where emesis is contraindicated.
Dosage/Route:	1 g/kg mixed with at least 180 to 250 mL of water, then PO or via an NG tube.

Name/Class:	**ADENOSINE (Adenocard)/Antidysrhythmic**
Description:	Adenosine is a naturally occurring agent that can "chemically cardiovert" PSVT to a normal sinus rhythm. It has a half-life of 10 seconds and does not cause hypotension.
Indications:	Narrow, complex paroxysmal supraventricular tachycardia refractory to vagal manoeuvres.
Contraindications:	Hypersensitivity, 2nd- and 3rd-degree heart block, sinus node disease, or asthma.
Precautions:	It may cause transient dysrhythmias. COPD.
Dosage/Route:	6 mg rapidly (over 1 to 2 s) IV, then flush the line rapidly with 20 mL saline. If ineffective, 12 mg in 1 to 2 min, may be repeated. Ped.: 0.1 mg/kg (over 1 to 2 s) IV followed by rapid 20 mL saline flush, then 0.2 mg/kg in 1 to 2 min to max 12 mg.

Name/Class:	**ALTEPLASE RECOMBINANT (tPA))/Thrombolytic**
Description:	Recombinant DNA-derived form of human tPA promotes thrombolysis by forming plasmin. Plasmin, in turn, degrades fibrin and fibrinogen and, ultimately, the clot.
Indications:	To thrombolyse in acute myocardial infarction, acute ischemic stroke, and pulmonary embolism.
Contraindications:	Active internal bleeding, suspected aortic dissection, traumatic CPR, recent hemorrhagic stroke (6 mo), intracranial or intraspinal surgery or trauma (2 mo), pregnancy, uncontrolled hypertension, or hypersensitivity to thrombolytics.
Precautions:	Recent major surgery, cerebral vascular disease, recent GI or GU bleeding, recent trauma, hypertension, patients over 75 years, current oral anticoagulants, or hemorrhagic ophthalmic conditions.
Dosage/Route:	MI and stroke: 15 mg IV, then 0.75 mg/kg (up to 50 mg) over 30 min, then 0.5 mg/kg (up to 35 mg) over 60 min. Pulmonary embolism: 100 mg IV infusion over 2 hours.

Name/Class:	**AMINOPHYLLINE (Aminophylline, Somophyllin)/Methylxanthine Bronchodilator**
Description:	Aminophylline is a methylxanthine that prolongs bronchodilation and decreased mucus production and has mild cardiac and CNS stimulating effects.
Indications:	Bronchospasm in asthma and COPD refractory to sympathomimetics and other bronchodilators and in CHF.
Contraindications:	Hypersensitivity to methylxanthines or uncontrolled cardiac dysrhythmias.
Precautions:	Cardiovascular disease, hypertension, or taking theophylline, hepatic impairment, diabetes, hyperthyroidism, young children, glaucoma, peptic ulcers, acute influenza or influenza immunization, and the elderly. Watch for PVCs or tachycardia. May cause hypotension.
Dosage/Route:	250 to 500 mg IV over 20 to 30 min. Ped.: 6 mg/kg over 20 to 30 min. Max 12 mg/kg/day.

Name/Class:	**AMIODARONE (Cordarone)/Antidysrhythmic**
Description:	Amiodarone is an antidysrhythmic that prolongs the duration of the action potential and refractory period and relaxes smooth muscles, reducing peripheral vascular resistance and increasing coronary blood flow.
Indications:	Life-threatening ventricular and supraventricular dysrythmias, frequently atrial fibrillation. Cardiac arrest.
Contraindications:	Hypersensitivity, cardiogenic shock, severe sinus bradycardia, or advanced heart block.
Precautions:	Hepatic impairment, pregnancy, nursing mothers, children.
Dosage/Route:	150 to 300 mg IV over 10 min, then 1 mg/min over next 6 hours. Ped.: 5 mg/kg IV/IO, then 15 mg/kg/day. In cardiac arrest: 300 mg IV. May repeat once at 150 mg after 3 to 5 min.

Name/Class:	**AMRINONE (Inocor)/Cardiac Inotrope**
Description:	Amrinone enhances myocardial contractility, increasing output, and reduces systemic vascular resistance.
Indications:	To increase cardiac output in CHF or children in septic shock or myocardial dysfunction.
Contraindications:	Hypersensitivity to amrinone or bisulphites.
Precautions:	CHF immediately after MI (may cause ischemia).
Dosage/Route:	CHF: 0.75 mg/kg IV over 2 to 3 min, then drip at 5 to 15 µg/kg/min titrated to hemodynamic response (may repeat bolus at 30 min).
	Septic shock or myocardial dysfunction in peds.: 0.75 to 1 mg/kg IV over 5 min, repeated up to 2 times to 3 mg/kg, then drip of 5 to 10 µg/min IV.

Name/Class:	**AMYL NITRITE (Amyl Nitrite)/Vasodilator**
Description:	Amyl nitrite is a short-acting vasodilator similar to nitroglycerine. Binds with hemoglobin to help biodegrade cyanide.
Indications:	Acute cyanide poisoning.
Contraindications:	None for acute cyanide poisoning.
Precautions:	None.
Dosage/Route:	0.3 mL ampule/min (crushed) until sodium nitrate infusion is ready. Ped.: same as adult.

Name/Class:	**ANISTREPLASE (APSAC) (Eminase)/Thrombolytic**
Description:	Anistreplase causes thrombolysis by converting plasminogen into plasmin, which then dissolves the fibrin and fibrinogen of the clot.
Indications:	To reduce infarct size in acute MI.
Contraindications:	Active internal bleeding, suspected aortic dissection, traumatic CPR, recent hemorrhagic stroke, intracranial or intraspinal surgery or trauma, tumours, pregnancy, hypertension, hypersensitivity to anistreplase or streptokinase.
Precautions:	Recent major surgery, cerebral vascular disease, recent GI or GU bleeding, recent trauma, hypertension, patients over 75 years, current oral anticoagulants, or hemorrhagic ophthalmic conditions.
Dosage/Route:	30 units IV over 2 to 5 min.

Name/Class:	**ASPIRIN (Acetylsalicylic Acid) (Alka-Seltzer, Bayer, Empirin, St. Joseph Children's)/Analgesic, Antipyretic, Platelet Inhibitor, Anti-inflammatory**
Description:	Aspirin inhibits agents that cause the production of inflammation, pain, and fever. It relieves mild to moderate pain by acting on the peripheral nervous system, lowers body temperature in fever, and powerfully inhibits platelet aggregation.
Indications:	Chest pain suggestive of an MI.
Contraindications:	Hypersensitivity to salicylates, active ulcer disease, asthma.
Precautions:	Allergies to other NSAIDs, bleeding disorders, children or teenagers with varicella or influenza-like symptoms.
Dosage/Route:	160 to 325 mg PO (chewable).

Name/Class:	**ATENOLOL (Tenormin, Apo-Atenolel)/Antidysrhythmic, Antihypertensive**
Description:	Atenolol is a selective beta-blocker that reduces the rate and force of cardiac contraction and lowers cardiac output and blood pressure.
Indications:	Non-Q-wave MI and unstable angina.
Contraindications:	Sinus bradycardia, 2nd- or 3rd-degree heart block, CHF, cardiogenic failure or shock.
Precautions:	Asthma, COPD, or CHF controlled by digitalis and diuretics.
Dosage/Route:	5 mg slow IV (over 5 min), if tolerated, then after 10 min repeat. Ped.: 0.8 to 1.5 mg/kg/day PO (max 2 mg/kg/day).

Name/Class:	**ATRACURIUM (Tracrium)/Nondepolarizing Neuromuscular Blocker**
Description:	Atracurium is a synthetic skeletal muscle relaxant that produces a short-duration neuromuscular blockade.
Indications:	To produce skeletal muscle relaxation to facilitate endotracheal intubation and IPPV.
Contraindications:	Myasthenia gravis.
Precautions:	Asthma, anaphylaxis, cardiovascular or neuromuscular disease, electrolyte or acid-base imbalance, dehydration, or pulmonary impairment.
Dosage/Route:	0.4 to 0.5 mg/kg IV. Ped.: < 2 Y.O. 0.3 to 0.4 mg/kg, otherwise same as adult.

Name/Class:	**ATROPINE/Parasympatholytic**
Description:	Atropine blocks the parasympathetic nervous system, specifically the vagal effects on heart rate. It does not increase contractility but may increase myocardial oxygen demand. Decreases airway secretions.
Indications:	Hemodynamically significant bradycardia, bradyasystolic arrest, and organophosphate poisoning.
Contraindications:	None in the emergency setting.
Precautions:	AMI, glaucoma.
Dosage/Route:	Symptomatic bradycardia: 0.5 to 1 mg IV/2 mg ET. Repeat 3 to 5 min to 0.04 mg/kg. Ped.: 0.02 mg/kg IV, 0.04 mg/kg ET, may repeat in 5 min up to 1 mg. Asystole: 1 mg IV or 2 mg ET, may repeat 3 to 5 min up to 0.04 mg/kg. Organophosphate poisoning: 2 to 5 mg IV/IM/IO/10 to 15 min. Ped.: 0.05 mg/kg IV/IM/IO/10 to 15 min.

Name/Class: **BRETYLIUM (Bretylol) (Bretylate)/Antidysrhythmic**

Description: Bretylium causes a release of norepinephrine, depresses ventricular fibrillation, and reduces ectopy. Bretylium also suppresses ventricular tachydysrhythmias with reentry mechanisms.

Indications: Ventricular fibrillation and ventricular tachycardia.

Contraindications: None in the presence of life-threatening dysrhythmias.

Precautions: Digitalized patients, digitalis-induced dysrhythmias, fixed cardiac output, angina, or renal impairment. May induce postural hypotension.

Dosage/Route: 5 mg/kg IV, then 10 mg/kg/15 to 30 min, to a max 30 mg/kg. Following conversion: 1 to 2 mg/min drip. Ped.: 5 mg/kg IV, repeat 10 mg/kg in 15 to 30 min.

Name/Class: **BUMETANIDE (Bumex)/Loop Diuretic**

Description: Bumetanide is related to furosemide, though it has a faster rate of onset, a greater diuretic potency (40 times), shorter duration, and produces only mild hypotension.

Indications: To promote diuresis in CHF and pulmonary edema.

Contraindications: Hypersensitivity to bumetanide and other sulphonamides.

Precautions: Pregnancy (use only for life-threatening conditions).

Dosage/Route: 0.5 to 1 mg IM/IV over 1 to 2 min, repeat in 2 to 3 hours as needed.

Name/Class: **BUTORPHANOL (Stadol)/Synthetic Narcotic Analgesic**

Description: Butorphanol is a centrally acting synthetic narcotic analgesic about 5 times more potent than morphine. A schedule IV narcotic.

Indications: Moderate to severe pain.

Contraindications: Hypersensitivity, head injury, or undiagnosed abdominal pain.

Precautions: May cause withdrawal in narcotic-dependent patients.

Dosage/Route: 1 mg IV or 3 to 4 mg IM/3 to 4 hours.

Name/Class:	**CALCIUM CHLORIDE (Calcium Chloride)/Electrolyte**
Description:	Calcium chloride increases myocardial contractile force and increases ventricular automaticity.
Indications:	Hyperkalemia, hypocalcemia, hypermagnesemia, and calcium channel blocker toxicity.
Contraindications:	Ventricular fibrillation, hypercalcemia, and possible digitalis toxicity.
Precautions:	It may precipitate toxicity in patients taking digoxin. Ensure the IV line is in a large vein and flushed before using and after calcium.
Dosage/Route:	2 to 4 mg/kg IV (10% solution)/10 min, as needed. Ped.: 20 mg/kg IV (10% solution) repeat at 10 min as needed.

Name/Class:	**CALCIUM GLUCONATE (Kalcinate)/Electrolyte**
Description:	Calcium gluconate increases myocardial contractile force and increases ventricular automaticity. It is more potent than calcium chloride.
Indications:	Hyperkalemia, hypermagnesemia, and calcium channel blocker toxicity.
Contraindications:	Ventricular fibrillation.
Precautions:	It may precipitate toxicity in patients taking digitalis, with renal or cardiac insufficiency, and immobilized patients.
Dosage/Route:	5 to 8 mL of 10% solution, repeated as necessary at 10 min intervals.

Name/Class:	**CAPOTEN (captopril tablets)/Angiotensin-Converting Enzyme (ACE) Inhibitor**
Description:	Lowers blood pressure by specific inhibition of the angiotensin-converting enzyme. Potent vasodilator.
Indications:	Hypertension, congestive heart failure.
Contraindications:	Pregnancy, children.
Precautions:	Impaired renal function, solitary kidney, patients on immunosupressants.
Dosage/Route:	6.25 to 25 mg PO t.i.d.

Name/Class:	**CHLORDIAZEPOXIDE (Librium)/Sedative, Hypnotic**
Description:	Chlordiazepoxide is a benzodiazepine derivative that produces mild sedation and anticonvulsant, skeletal muscle relaxant, and prolonged hypnotic effects.
Indications:	Severe anxiety and tension, acute alcohol withdrawal symptoms (delirium tremeris).
Contraindications:	Hypersensitivity to benzodiazepines, pregnant and nursing mothers, children under 6.
Precautions:	Primary depressive disorders or psychoses, acute alcohol intoxication.
Dosage/Route:	50 to 100 mg IV/IM.

Name/Class:	**CHLORPROMAZINE (Largactil)/Tranquilizer, Antipsychotic**
Description:	Chlorpromazine is a phenothiazine derivative used to manage psychotic episodes by providing strong sedation and moderate extrapyramidal symptoms. Produces reduced initiative, interest, and affect.
Indications:	Acute psychotic episode, intractable hiccups, nausea/vomiting.
Contraindications:	Hypersensitivity to phenothiazines, coma, sedative overdose, acute alcohol withdrawal, and children under 6 months.
Precautions:	Agitated states with depression; seizure disorders; respiratory infection or COPD; glaucoma; diabetes; hypertension; peptic ulcer; prostatic hypertrophy; breast cancer; thyroid, cardiovascular, and hepatic impairment; and patients exposed to extreme heat or organophosphates.
Dosage/Route:	25 to 50 mg IM. Ped.: 0.5 mg/kg IM or 1 mg/kg PR.

Name/Class:	**DEXAMETHASONE (Decadron)/Steroid**
Description:	Dexamethasone is a long-acting synthetic adrenocorticoid with intense anti-inflammatory activity. It prevents the accumulation of inflammation generating cells at the sites of infection or injury.
Indications:	Anaphylaxis, asthma, COPD, spinal cord edema.
Contraindications:	No absolute contraindications in the emergency setting. Relative contraindications: systemic fungal infections, acute infections, tuberculosis, varicella, vaccinia, or live virus vaccinations.
Precautions:	Herpes simplex, keratitis, myasthenia gravis, hepatic or renal impairment, diabetes, CHF, seizures, psychic disorders, hypothyroidism, and GI ulceration.
Dosage/Route:	4 to 24 mg IV/IM. Ped.: 0.5 to 1 mg/kg.

Name/Class:	**DEXTROSE 50% IN WATER (D$_{50}$W)/Carbohydrate**
Description:	Dextrose is a simple sugar that the body can rapidly metabolize to create energy.
Indications:	Hypoglycemia.
Contraindications:	None in hypoglycemia.
Precautions:	Increased ICP. Determine blood glucose level before administration. Ensure good venous access.
Dosage/Route:	25 g D$_{50}$W (50 mL) IV. Ped.: 2 mL/kg of a 25% solution IV.

Name/Class:	**DIAZEPAM (Valium)/Antianxiety, Hypnotic, Anticonvulsant, Sedative**
Description:	Diazepam is a benzodiazepine sedative and skeletal muscle relaxant that reduces tremors, induces amnesia, and reduces the incidence and recurrence of seizures. It relaxes muscle spasms in orthopedic injuries and produces amnesia for painful procedures (cardioversion).
Indications:	Major motor seizures, status epilepticus, premedication before cardioversion, muscle tremors due to injury, and acute anxiety.
Contraindications:	Hypersensitivity to the drug, shock, coma, acute alcoholism, depressed vital signs, obstetrical patients, neonates.
Precautions:	Psychoses, depression, myasthenia gravis, hepatic or renal impairment, addiction, elderly or very ill patients, or COPD. Due to a short half-life of the drug, seizure activity may recur.
Dosage/Route:	Seizures: 5 to 10 mg IV/IM. Ped.: 0.5 to 2 mg IV/IM. Acute anxiety: 2 to 5 mg IV/IM. Ped.: 0.5 to 2 mg IM. Premedication: 5 to 15 mg IV. Ped.: 0.2 to 0.5 mg/kg IV.

Name/Class:	**DIAZOXIDE (Hyperstat)/Antihypertensive**
Description:	Diazoxide is a rapid-acting thiazide nondiuretic hypotensive and hyperglycemia agent that reduces BP and peripheral vascular resistance.
Indications:	Rapidly decreases BP in hypertensive crisis.
Contraindications:	Hypersensitivity to thiazides, cerebral bleeding, eclampsia, significant coronary artery disease.
Precautions:	Diabetes, impaired cerebral or cardiac circulation, renal impairment, corticosteroid or progesterone therapy, gout, or uremia.
Dosage/Route:	1 to 3 mg/kg IV up to 150 mg, repeated/5 to 15 min, as needed. Ped.: same as adult.

Name/Class:	**DIGOXIN (Digoxin, Lanoxin, Novodigoxin)/Cardiac Glycoside**
Description:	Digoxin is a rapid-acting cardiac glycoside used in the treatment of CHF and rapid atrial dysrhythmias. It increases the force and velocity of myocardial contraction and cardiac output. It also decreases conduction through the AV node, thus decreasing heart rate.
Indications:	Increase cardiac output in CHF and to stabilize supraventricular tachydysrhythmias.
Contraindications:	Hypersensitivity, ventricular fibrillation, or ventricular tachycardia except due to CHF.
Precautions:	Reduce dosage if digitoxin taken within 2 weeks. Toxicity potentiated by an MI and with hypokalemia, hypocalcemia, advanced heart disease, incomplete heart block, cor pulmonale, hyperthyroidism, respiratory impairment, children, elderly or debilitated patients, and hypomagnesemia.
Dosage/Route:	0.25 to 0.5 mg slowly IV. Ped.: 10 to 50 µg/kg IV.

Name/Class:	**DIGOXIN IMMUNE FAB (Digibind)/Antidote**
Description:	Digoxin immune FAB comprises fragments of antibodies specific for digoxin (and effective for digitoxin) and prevents the drug from binding to receptor sites.
Indications:	Life-threatening digoxin or digitoxin toxicity.
Contraindications:	Hypersensitivity to sheep products and renal or cardiac failure.
Precautions:	Patients with prior sheep or bovine antibody fragments, renal impairment, and allergies.
Dosage/Route:	Dose dependent on patient digoxin or digitoxin levels.

Name/Class:	**DILTIAZEM (Cardizem, Apo-Diltiaz)/Calcium Channel Blocker**
Description:	Diltiazem is a slow calcium channel blocker similar to verapamil. It dilates coronary and peripheral arteries and arterioles, thus increasing circulation to the heart and reducing peripheral vascular resistance.
Indications:	Supraventricular tachydysrhythmias (atrial fibrillation, atrial flutter, and PSVT refractory to adenosine) and to increase coronary artery perfusion in angina.
Contraindications:	Hypersensitivity, sick sinus syndrome, 2nd- or 3rd-degree heart block, systolic BP < 90, diastolic BP < 60, wide-complex tachycardia and WPW.
Precautions:	CHF (especially with beta-blockers), conduction abnormalities, renal or hepatic impairment, the elderly, and nursing mothers.
Dosage/Route:	0.25 mg/kg IV over 2 min, may repeat as needed with 0.35 mg/kg followed by a drip of 5 to 10 mg/h not to exceed 15 mg/h over 24 hours.

Name/Class:	**DIMENHYDRINATE (Gravol)/Antihistamine**
Description:	Dimenhydrinate is related to diphenhydramine though it is most frequently used for the prevention and treatment of motion sickness and vertigo, rather than any antihistamine properties.
Indications:	To relieve nausea/vomiting associated with motion sickness and narcotic use.
Contraindications:	None in the emergency setting.
Precautions:	Seizure disorders and asthma.
Dosage/Route:	12.5 to 25 mg IV; 50 mg IM/4 hours as needed. Ped.: 1.25 mg/kg/4 hours up to 300 mg/day.

Name/Class:	**DIMERCAPROL (BAL in Oil)/Antidote**
Description:	Dimercaprol is a dithiol compound that combines with the ions of various heavy metals to form nontoxic compounds that can be excreted.
Indications:	Antidote for acute arsenic, mercury, lead, and gold poisoning.
Contraindications:	Hepatic and severe renal impairment and poisonings due to cadmium, iron, selenium, and uranium.
Precautions:	Hypertensive patients.
Dosage/Route:	Gold and arsenic: 2.5 to 3 mg/kg IM. Ped.: same as adult. Mercury: 5 mg/kg IM. Ped.: same as adult. Lead: 4 mg/kg IM. Ped.: same as adult.

Name/Class:	**DIPHENHYDRAMINE (Benadryl)/Antihistamine**
Description:	Diphenhydramine blocks histamine release, thereby reducing bronchoconstriction, vasodilation, and edema.
Indications:	Anaphylaxis, allergic reactions, and dystonic reactions.
Contraindications:	Asthma and other lower respiratory diseases.
Precautions:	May induce hypotension, headache, palpitations, tachycardia, sedation, drowsiness, or disturbed coordination.
Dosage/Route:	25 to 50 mg IV/IM.

Name/Class:	**DOBUTAMINE (Dobutrex)/Sympathomimetic**
Description:	Dobutamine is a synthetic catecholamine and beta agent that increases the strength of cardiac contraction without appreciably increasing rate.
Indications:	To increase cardiac output in congestive heart failure/cardiogenic shock.
Contraindications:	Hypersensitivity to sympathomimetic amines, ventricular tachycardia, and hypovolemia without fluid resuscitation.
Precautions:	Atrial fibrillation or preexisting hypertension.
Dosage/Route:	2 to 20 µg/kg/min IV. Ped.: same as adult.

Name/Class:	**DOPAMINE (Revimine, Intropin)/Sympathomimetic**
Description:	Dopamine is a naturally occurring catecholamine that increases cardiac output without appreciably increasing myocardial oxygen consumption. It maintains renal and mesenteric blood flow while inducing vasoconstriction and increasing systolic blood pressure.
Indications:	Nonhypovolemic hypotension (70 to 100 mmHg) and cardiogenic shock.
Contraindications:	Hypovolemic hypotension without aggressive fluid resuscitation, tachydysrhythmias, ventricular fibrillation, and pheochromocytoma.
Precautions:	Occlusive vascular disease, cold injury, arterial embolism. Ensure adequate fluid resuscitation of the hypovolemic patient.
Dosage/Route:	2 to 5 µg/kg/min up to 20 µg/kg/min, titrated to effect. Ped.: same as adult.

Name/Class:	**DROPERIDOL (Inapsine)/Antiemetic**
Description:	Droperidol is related to haloperidol and antagonizes the emetic properties of morphine-like analgesics. It may also produce hypotension and mild sedation.
Indications:	Nausea and vomiting (second line), to produce a tranquilizing effect, and in some cases as an antipsychotic.
Contraindications:	Intolerance.
Precautions:	Elderly; debilitated; hypotension; hepatic, renal, or cardiac impairment; and Parkinson's disease.
Dosage/Route:	2.5 to 10 mg IV. Ped.: 0.088 to 0.165 mg/kg IV.

Name/Class:	**ENOXAPARIN (Lovenox)/Anticoagulant**
Description:	Enoxaparin is a heparin derivative that prevents the conversion of fibrinogen to fibrin.
Indications:	To inhibit clot formation in unstable angina and non-Q-wave myocardial infarction.
Contraindications:	Hypersensitivity to the drug, pork products or heparin, major active bleeding, or thrombocytopenia.
Precautions:	None.
Dosage/Route:	Unstable angina and non-Q wave MI: 1 mg/kg SC. Pulmonary embolism: 0.5 mg/kg IV.

Name/Class:	**EPINEPHRINE (Adrenalin)/Sympathomimetic**
Description:	Epinephrine is a naturally occurring catecholamine that increases heart rate, cardiac contractile force, myocardial electrical activity, systemic vascular resistance, and systolic blood pressure, and decreases overall airway resistance and automaticity. It also, through bronchial artery constriction, may reduce pulmonary congestion and increase tidal volume and vital capacity.
Indications:	To restore rhythm in cardiac arrest and severe allergic reactions.
Contraindications:	Hypersensitivity to sympathomimetic amines, narrow-angle glaucoma; hemorrhagic, traumatic, or cardiac shock; coronary insufficiency; dysrhythmias; organic brain or heart disease; or during labour.
Precautions:	Elderly, debilitated patients, hypertension, hyperthyroidism, Parkinson's disease, diabetes, tuberculosis, asthma, emphysema, and in children under 6 years.
Dosage/Route:	Arrest: 1 mg of 1:10 000 IV/3 to 5 min (ET: 2 to 2.5 mg 1:1000). Ped.: 0.01 mg/kg 1:10 000 IV/IO (ET: 0.1 mg/kg 1:1000). All subsequent doses 0.1 mg/kg IV/IO. Allergic reactions: 0.3 to 0.5 mg of 1:1000 SC/5 to 15 min as needed or 0.5 to 1 mg of 1:10 000 IV if SC dose ineffective or severe reaction. Ped.: 0.01 mg/kg of 1:1000 SC/10 to 15 min or 0.01 mg/kg of 1:10 000 IV if SC dose ineffective or severe.

Name/Class:	**ESMOLOL (Brevibloc)/Beta-Blocker**
Description:	Esmolol is an ultra-short-acting cardio-selective beta-blocker that inhibits the actions of the catecholamines.
Indications:	Supraventricular tachycardias with rapid ventricular responses.
Contraindications:	Cardiac failure, 2nd- and 3rd-degree block, sinus bradycardia, and cardiogenic shock.
Precautions:	Allergies or bronchial asthma, emphysema, CHF, diabetes, and renal impairment.
Dosage/Route:	500 µg/kg/min IV for 1 min, loading dose, then 50 µg/kg/min for 4 min. If unsuccessful, repeat loading dose every 4 min and increase maintenance dose by 50 µg/kg to 200 µg/kg/min.

Name/Class:	**ETOMIDATE (Amidate)/Hypnotic**
Description:	Etomidate is an ultra-short-acting nonbarbiturate hypnotic with no analgesic effects and limited cardiovascular and respiratory effects.
Indications:	Induce sedation for rapid sequence intubation.
Contraindications:	Hypersensitivity.
Precautions:	Marked hypotension, severe asthma, or severe cardiovascular disease.
Dosage/Route:	0.1 to 0.3 mg/kg IV over 15 to 30 sec. Ped.: children > 10 years, same as for adults.

Name/Class:	**FENTANYL (Sublimaze)/Narcotic Analgesic**
Description:	Fentanyl is a potent synthetic narcotic analgesic similar to morphine and meperidine but with a more rapid and less-prolonged action.
Indications:	Induce sedation for endotracheal intubation.
Contraindications:	MAO inhibitors within 14 days, myasthenia gravis.
Precautions:	Increased intracranial pressure, elderly, debilitated, COPD, respiratory problems, hepatic and renal insufficiency.
Dosage/Route:	25 to 100 µg slow IV (2 to 3 min). Ped.: 2 µg/kg slow IV/IM.

Name/Class:	**FLECAINIDE (Tambocor)/Antidysrhythmic**
Description:	Flecainide is a local anesthetic and antidysrhythmic that slows myocardial conduction and effectively suppresses PVCs and a variety of atrial and ventricular dysrhythmias.
Indications:	Atrial flutter, atrial fibrillation, AV reentrant tachycardia, or SVT associated with Wolff-Parkinson-White syndrome.
Contraindications:	Hypersensitivity, 2nd- or 3rd-degree heart block, right bundle branch block with left hemiblock, cardiogenic shock, or significant hepatic impairment.
Precautions:	CHF, sick sinus syndrome, or renal impairment.
Dosage/Route:	100 mg PO/12 h or 2 mg/kg IV at 10 mg/min. Ped.: 1 to 3 mg/kg/day PO in 3 equal doses (max 8 mg/kg/day).

Name/Class:	**FLUMAZENIL (Anexete, Romazicon)/Benzodiazepine Antagonist**
Description:	Flumazenil is a benzodiazepine antagonist used to reverse the sedative, recall, and psychomotor effects of diazepam, midazolam, and the other benzodiazepines.
Indications:	Respiratory depression secondary to the benzodiazepines.
Contraindications:	Hypersensitivity to flumazenil or benzodiazepines; those patients who take flumazenil for status epilepticus or seizures; seizure-prone patients during labour and delivery; tricyclic antidepressant overdose.
Precautions:	Hepatic impairment, elderly, pregnancy, nursing mothers, head injury, alcohol and drug dependency, and physical dependence on benzodiazepines.
Dosage/Route:	0.2 mg IV over 30 s/min, up to 1 mg.

Name/Class:	**FOSPHENYTOIN (Cerebyx)/Anticonvulsant**
Description:	Fosphenytoin is a drug that, once administered, is converted to phenytoin and causes the anticonvulsant properties associated with that drug.
Indications:	Seizure control and status epilepticus.
Contraindications:	Hypersensitivity, seizures due to hypoglycemia, sinus bradycardia, heart block, Stokes-Adams syndrome, late pregnancy, and lactating mothers.
Precautions:	Hepatic or renal impairment, alcoholism, hypotension, bradycardia, heart block, severe CAD, diabetes, hyperglycemia, or respiratory depression.
Dosage/Route:	15 to 20 mg PE/kg IV given at 100 to 150 mg PE/min (PE = phenytoin equivalent).

Name/Class:	**FUROSEMIDE (Lasix)/Diuretic**
Description:	Furosemide is a rapid-acting, potent diuretic and antihypertensive that inhibits sodium reabsorption by the kidney. Its vasodilating effects reduce venous return and cardiac workload.
Indications:	Congestive heart failure and pulmonary edema.
Contraindications:	Hypersensitivity to furosemide or the sulphonamides, fluid and electrolyte depletion states, heptic coma, pregnancy (except in life-threatening circumstances).
Precautions:	Infants, elderly, hepatic impairment, nephrotic syndrome, cardiogenic shock associated with acute MI, gout, or patients receiving digitalis or potassium-depleting steroids.
Dosage/Route:	40 to 120 mg slow IV. Ped.: 1 mg/kg slow IV.

Name/Class:	**GLUCAGON (GlucaGen)/Hormone, Antihypoglycemic**
Description:	Glucagon is a protein secreted by pancreatic cells that causes a breakdown of stored glycogen into glucose and inhibits the synthesis of glycogen from glucose.
Indications:	Hypoglycemia without IV access and to reverse beta-blocker overdose.
Contraindications:	Hypersensitivity to glucagon or protein compounds.
Precautions:	Cardiovascular or renal impairment. Effective only if there are sufficient stores of glycogen in the liver.
Dosage/Route:	Hypoglycemia: 1 mg IM/SC repeat 5 to 20 min. Ped.: < 10 kg: 0.1 mg/kg IM/SC/IV. Ped: > 10 kg: 1 mg IM/SC/IV. Beta-blocker overdose: 50 to 150 mg/kg IV over 1 min. Ped.: 50 to 150 mg/kg IV over 1 min.

Name/Class:	**HALOPERIDOL (Haldol)/Antipsychotic**
Description:	Haloperidol is believed to block dopamine receptors in the brain associated with mood and behaviour, is a potent antiemetic, and impairs temperature regulation.
Indications:	Acute psychotic episodes.
Contraindications:	Parkinson's disease, seizure disorders, coma, alcohol depression, CNS depression, and thyrotoxicosis, and with other sedatives.
Precautions:	Elderly, debilitated patients, urinary retention, glaucoma, severe cardiovascular disease, or anticonvulsant, anticoagulant, or lithium therapy.
Dosage/Route:	2 to 5 mg IM. Ped.: Children > 3; 0.015 to 0.15 mg/kg/day PO in two or three divided doses.

Name/Class:	**HEPARIN (Heparin)/Anticoagulant**
Description:	Heparin is a rapid-onset anticoagulant, enhancing the effects of antithrombin III and blocking the conversion of prothrombin to thrombin and fibrinogen to fibrin.
Indications:	To prevent thrombus formation in acute MI.
Contraindications:	Hypersensitivity; active bleeding or bleeding tendencies; recent eye, brain, or spinal surgery; shock.
Precautions:	Alcoholism, elderly, allergies, indwelling catheters, elderly, menstruation, pregnancy, or cerebral embolism.
Dosage/Route:	5000 units IV, then 20 000 to 40 000 over 24 hours.

Name/Class:	**HYDRALAZINE (Apresoline)/Antihypertensive**
Description:	Hydralazine reduces blood pressure by arterial vasodilation, increasing cardiac output and renal and cerebral blood flow.
Indications:	Hypertensive crisis and preeclampsia.
Contraindications:	Hypersensitivity, coronary artery or mitral valve disease, AMI, tachydysrhythmias.
Precautions:	CVA, renal impairment, and MAO inhibitor use.
Dosage/Route:	20 to 40 mg IV/IM repeated in 4 to 6 hours. Ped.: 0.1 to 0.5 mg/kg/day IV/IM.

Name/Class:	**HYDROCORTISONE (Solu-Cortef)/Steroid**
Description:	Hydrocortisone is a short-acting synthetic steroid that inhibits histamine formation, storage, and release from mast cells, reducing allergic response.
Indications:	Inflammation during allergic reactions, severe anaphylaxis, asthma, and COPD.
Contraindications:	Hypersensitivity to glucocorticoids.
Precautions:	Limited precautions in acute care.
Dosage/Route:	40 to 250 mg IV/IM. Ped.: 4 to 8 mg/kg/day IV/IM.

Name/Class:	**HYDROXYZINE (Vistaril)/Antihistamine**
Description:	Hydroxyzine is an antihistamine with depressive, sedative, antiemetic, and bronchodilator properties.
Indications:	Acute anxiety, nausea/vomiting.
Contraindications:	Hypersensitivity.
Precautions:	Elderly.
Dosage/Route:	Anxiety: 50 to 100 mg deep IM. Ped.: 1 mg/kg deep IM. Nausea/vomiting: 25 to 50 mg deep IM. Ped.: 1 mg/kg deep IM.

Name/Class:	**IBUPROFEN (Advil, Motrin, Nuprin, Excedrin IB)/Nonsteroidal Anti-inflammatory Drug (NSAID)**
Description:	Ibuprofen is the prototype NSAID with significant analgesic and antipyretic properties. It also inhibits platelet aggregation and increases bleeding time.
Indications:	Reduce fever and relieve minor to moderate pain.
Contraindications:	Sensitivity to Aspirin or other NSAIDs, active peptic ulcer, and bleeding abnormalities.
Precautions:	Hypertension, GI ulceration, hepatic or renal impairment, cardiac decompensation.
Dosage/Route:	200 to 400 mg PO/4 to 6 hours up to 1200 mg/day. Ped.: 5 to 10 mg/kg PO/4 to 6 hours up to 40 mg/kg/day.

Name/Class:	**IBUTILIDE (Corvert)/Antidysrhythmic**
Description:	Ibutilide is a short-acting antidysrhythmic that may convert atrial flutter and fibrillation or may assist with electrical cardioversion.
Indications:	Recent onset atrial flutter and fibrillation.
Contraindications:	Hypersensitivity, hypokalemia, or hypomagnesemia.
Precautions:	CHF, low ejection fraction, recent MI, prolonged QT intervals, hepatic impairment, cardiovascular disorder other than atrial dysrhythmias, or drugs that prolong the QT interval, lactation.
Dosage/Route:	1 mg over 10 min IV. Patients < 60 kg, 0.01 mg/kg IV, may repeat in 10 min as needed.

Name/Class:	**INSULIN (Regular Insulin, Humulin)/Hormone**
Description:	Insulin is a naturally occurring protein that promotes the uptake of glucose by the cells.
Indications:	Hyperglycemia and diabetic coma.
Contraindications:	Hypersensitivity and hypoglycemia.
Precautions:	None.
Dosage/Route:	5 to 10 units IV/IM/SC. Ped.: 2 to 4 units IV/IM/SC.

Name/Class:	**IPECAC SYRUP/Emetic**
Description:	Ipecac syrup is a gastric irritant and acts on the emetic centres of the medulla to induce vomiting. Emesis usually occurs within 5 to 10 minutes.
Indications:	Poisoning and overdose.
Contraindications:	Reduced level of consciousness, corrosive ingestion, petroleum distillate ingestion, alkali ingestion, or antiemetic ingestion (especially phenothiazine).
Precautions:	Monitor the airway and have suction ready. Administer activated charcoal only after emesis. Caution with heart disease patients.
Dosage/Route:	30 mL PO, followed by 1 to 2 glasses of water, repeat in 20 min as needed. Ped.: 15 mL PO followed by 1 to 2 glasses of water, repeat in 20 min as needed.

Name/Class:	**IPRATROPIUM (Atrovent)/Anticholinergic**
Description:	Ipratropium is a bronchodilator used in the treatment of respiratory emergencies that causes bronchial dilation and dries respiratory tract secretions by blocking acetylcholine receptors.
Indications:	Bronchospasm associated with asthma, COPD, and inhaled irritants.
Contraindications:	Hypersensitivity to atropine or its derivatives, or as a primary treatment for acute bronchospasm.
Precautions:	Elderly, cardiovascular disease, or hypertension.
Dosage/Route:	500 µg in 2.5 to 3 mL NS via nebulizer or 2 sprays from a metered dose inhaler. Ped.: 125 to 250 µg in 2.5 to 3 mL NS via nebulizer, or 1 to 2 sprays from a metered dose inhaler.

Name/Class:	**ISOETHARINE (Bronkosol)/Sympathomimetic Bronchodilator**
Description:	Isoetharine is a synthetic sympathomimetic with rapid onset and prolonged duration that relaxes the bronchial smooth muscles, decreasing airway resistance and helping clear secretions.
Indications:	Bronchospasm in asthma and COPD.
Contraindications:	Hypersensitivity to or use of sympathomimetic amines, preexisting tachydysrhythmias, allergy to sodium bisulphite agents.
Precautions:	Elderly, hypertension, acute coronary artery disease, CHF, hyperthyroidism, diabetes, tuberculosis, or seizures.
Dosage/Route:	1 to 2 sprays via metered dose inhaler, 0.5 mL in 2 to 3 mL saline via nebulizer. Ped.: 0.01 mL/kg of 1% solution (max 0.5 mL) diluted in 2 to 3 mL saline by nebulizer.

Name/Class:	**ISOPROTERENOL (Isuprel)/Sympathomimetic**
Description:	Isoproterenol is a synthetic sympathomimetic that results in increased cardiac output by increasing the strength of cardiac contraction and somewhat increasing rate. It also reduces peripheral vascular resistance and venous return.
Indications:	Bradycardia refractory to atropine when pacing is not available and for severe status asthmaticus.
Contraindications:	Cardiogenic shock.
Precautions:	Tachydysrhythmias and those associated with digitalis and acute myocardial infarction.
Dosage/Route:	Bradycardia: 2 to 10 µg/min titrated to cardiac rate. Ped.: 0.1 µg/kg/min titrated to cardiac rate. Status asthmaticus: 1 to 2 sprays, metered dose inhaler. Ped.: same as adult.

Name/Class:	**KETOROLAC (Toradol)/Nonsteroidal Anti-inflammatory Drug (NSAID)**
Description:	Ketorolac is an injectable NSAID that exhibits analgesic, anti-inflammatory, and antipyretic properties without sedative effects.
Indications:	Mild or moderate pain.
Contraindications:	Hypersensitivity to ketorolac, Aspirin, or other NSAIDs, and asthma.
Precautions:	Peptic ulcers, renal or hepatic impairment, or elderly.
Dosage/Route:	30 mg IV/IM (15 mg > 65 Y.O. or weighs < 50 kg)

Name/Class:	**LABETALOL (Trandate, Normodyne)/Beta-Blocker**
Description:	Labetalol is a beta-blocker with some alpha-blocker characteristics. It induces vasodilation, reduces peripheral vascular resistance, and lowers blood pressure.
Indications:	Acute hypertensive crisis.
Contraindications:	Asthma, CHF, 2nd- and 3rd-degree heart block, severe bradycardia, or cardiogenic shock.
Precautions:	COPD, heart failure, hepatic impairment, diabetes, peripheral vascular disease.
Dosage/Route:	20 mg slow IV, then 40 to 80 mg/10 min as needed, up to 300 mg OR a continuous drip 2 mg/min up to 300 mg.

Name/Class:	**LIDOCAINE (Xylocord, Xylocaine)/Antiarrhythmic**
Description:	Lidocaine is an antidysrhythmic that suppresses automaticity and raises stimulation threshold of the ventricles. It also causes sedation, anticonvulsant, and analgesic effects.
Indications:	Pulseless ventricular tachycardia, ventricular fibrillation, ventricular tachycardia (w/pulse).
Contraindications:	Hypersensitivity to amide-type local anesthetics, supraventricular dysrhythmias, Stokes-Adams syndrome, 2nd- and 3rd-degree heart blocks, and bradycardias.
Precautions:	Hepatic or renal impairment, CHF, hypoxia, respiratory depression, hypovolemia, myasthenia gravis, shock, debilitated patients, elderly, family history of malignant hypothermia.
Dosage/Route:	Cardiac arrest: 1 to 1.5 mg/kg IV repeated every 3 to 5 min up to 3 mg/kg, follow conversion with a drip of 2 to 4 mg/min. Ped.: 1 mg/kg IV, repeat/3 to 5 min up to 3 mg/kg, follow conversion with a drip of 20 to 50 μg/kg/min. Ventricular tachycardia (w/pulse): 1 to 1.5 mg/kg slow IV. May repeat at one-half dose every 5–10 min until conversion up to 3 mg/kg. Follow conversion with an infusion of 2 to 4 mg/min. Ped.: 1 mg/kg, followed by a drip at 20 to 50 mg/kg/min.

Name/Class:	**LORAZEPAM (Ativan)/Sedative**
Description:	Lorazepam is the most potent benzodiazepine available. It has strong antianxiety, sedative, hypnotic, and skeletal muscle relaxant properties, and a relatively short half-life.
Indications:	Sedation for cardioversion and status epilepticus.
Contraindications:	Sensitivity to benzodiazepines.
Precautions:	Narrow-angle glaucoma, depression or psychosis, coma, shock, acute alcohol intoxication, renal or hepatic impairment, organic brain syndrome, myasthenia gravis, GI disorders, elderly, debilitated, limited pulmonary reserve.
Dosage/Route:	Sedation: 2 to 4 mg IM, 0.5 to 2 mg IV. Ped.: 0.03 to 0.5 mg/kg IV/IM/PR up to 4 mg. Status epilepticus: 2 mg slow IV/PR (2 mg/min). Ped.: 0.1 mg/kg slow IV/PR (2 to 5 min).

Name/Class:	**MAGNESIUM SULPHATE (Magnesium)/Electrolyte**
Description:	Magnesium sulphate is an electrolyte that acts as a calcium channel blocker, acting as a CNS depressant and anticonvulsant. It also depresses the function of smooth, skeletal, and cardiac muscles.
Indications:	Refractory ventricular fibrillation and pulseless ventricular tachycardia (especially *torsade de pointes*), AMI, eclamptic seizures.
Contraindications:	Heart block, myocardial damage, shock, persistent hypertension, and hypocalcemia.
Precautions:	Renal impairment, digitalized patients, other CNS depressants, or neuromuscular blocking agents.
Dosage/Route:	Ventricular fibrillation or tachycardia: 1 to 2 g IV over 2 min. Torsade de pointes: 1–2 g IV followed by infusion of 0.5 to 1.0 g/h IV. AMI: 1 to 2 g IV over 5 to 30 min. Eclampsia: 2 to 4 g IV/IM.

Name/Class: **MANNITOL (Osmitrol)/Osmotic Diuretic**

Description: Mannitol is an osmotic diuretic that draws water into the intravascular space through its hypertonic effects, then causes diuresis.

Indications: Cerebral edema.

Contraindications: Hypersensitivity, pulmonary edema, CHF, organic CNS disease, intracranial bleeding, shock, or severe dehydration.

Precautions: None.

Dosage/Route: 1.5 to 2 g/kg slow IV. Ped.: 0.25 to 0.5 g/kg over 60 min.

Name/Class: **MEPERIDINE (Demerol)/Narcotic Analgesic**

Description: Meperidine is a synthetic narcotic with sedative and analgesic properties comparable with morphine but without hemodynamic side effects.

Indications: Moderate to severe pain.

Contraindications: Hypersensitivity, seizure disorders, or acute abdomen before diagnosis.

Precautions: Increased intracranial pressure, asthma or other respiratory conditions, supraventricular tachycardias, prostatic hypertrophy, urethral stricture, glaucoma, elderly or debilitated patients, renal or hepatic impairment, hypothyroidism, or Addison's disease.

Dosage/Route: 25 to 50 mg IV, 50 to 100 mg IM. Ped.: 1 mg/kg IV/IM.

Name/Class: **METAPROTERENOL (Alupent)/Sympathomimetic Bronchodilator**

Description: Metaproterenol is a synthetic sympathomimetic amine, similar to isoproterenol that causes smooth muscle relaxation of the bronchial tree, decreasing airway resistance, facilitating mucus drainage, and increasing vital capacity.

Indications: Bronchospasm, as in asthma and COPD.

Contraindications: Hypersensitivity to sympathomimetic agents, tachydysrhythmias, and hyperthyroidism.

Precautions: Elderly, hypertension, coronary artery disease, and diabetes.

Dosage/Route: 0.65 mg via metered dose inhaler (2 sprays); 0.2 to 0.3 mL in 2.5 to 3 mL NS via nebulizer. Ped.: 0.1 to 0.2 mL/kg (5% solution) in 2.5 to 3 mL NS via nebulizer.

Name/Class:	**METARAMINOL (Aramine)/Sympathomimetic**
Description:	Metaraminol is a sympathomimetic similar to norepinephrine but less potent, with gradual onset and longer duration. It causes systemic vasoconstriction and increased cardiac contraction strength, increasing blood pressure and reducing flow to the kidneys.
Indications:	Hypotension in a normovolemic patient.
Contraindications:	Hypovolemia; MAO inhibitor therapy; peripheral or mesenteric thrombosis; pulmonary cdcma; cardiac arrest; untreated hypoxia, hypercapnia, and acidosis.
Precautions:	Digitalized patients, hypertension, thyroid disease, diabetes, hepatic impairment, malaria.
Dosage/Route:	100 mg/500 mL D_5W or NS, titrated to blood pressure: 5 to 10 mg IM.

Name/Class:	**METHYLPREDNISOLONE (Solu-Medrol)/Corticosteroid, Anti-inflammatory**
Description:	Methylprednisolone is a synthetic adrenal corticosteroid, effective as an anti-inflammatory and used in the management of allergic reactions and in some cases of shock. It is sometimes used in the treatment of spinal cord injury.
Indications:	Spinal cord injury, asthma, severe anaphylaxis, COPD.
Contraindications:	No major contraindications in the emergency setting.
Precautions:	Only a single dose should be given in the prehospital setting.
Dosage/Route:	Asthma/COPD/anaphylaxis: 125 to 250 mg IV/IM. Ped.: 1 to 2 mg/kg/dose IV/IM. Spinal cord injury: 30 mg/kg IV over 15 min, after 45 min an infusion of 5.4 mg/kg/h.

Name/Class:	**METOCLOPRAMIDE (Maxeran)/Antiemetic**
Description:	Metoclopramide is a dopamine antagonist similar to procainamide but with few antidysrhythmic or anesthetic properties. Its antiemetic properties stem from rapid gastric emptying and desensitization of the vomiting reflex.
Indications:	Nausea and vomiting.
Contraindications:	Hypersensitivity, allergy to sulphite agents, seizure disorders, pheochromocytoma, mechanical GI obstruction or perforation, and breast cancer.
Precautions:	CHF, hypokalemia, renal impairment, GI hemorrhage, intermittent porphyria.
Dosage/Route:	10 to 20 mg IM; 10 mg slow IV (over 1 to 2 min). Ped.: 1 to 2 mg/kg/dose.

Name/Class:	**METOPROLOL (Lopressor)/Beta-Blocker**
Description:	Metroprolol is a beta-adrenergic blocking agent that reduces heart rate, cardiac output, and blood pressure.
Indications:	AMI.
Contraindications:	Cardiogenic shock, sinus bradycardia < 45, 2nd- or 3rd-degree heart block, PR interval > 0.24, cor pulmonale, asthma, or COPD.
Precautions:	Hypersensitivity, hepatic or renal impairment, cardiomegaly, CHF controlled by digitalis and diuretics, AV conduction defects, thyrotoxicosis, diabetes, or peripheral vascular disease.
Dosage/Route:	5 mg slow IV/5 min up to 3 times.

Name/Class:	**MIDAZOLAM (Versed)/Sedative**
Description:	Midazolam is a short-acting benzodiazepine with CNS depressant, muscle relaxant, anticonvulsant, and anterograde amnestic effects.
Indications:	To induce sedation before cardioversion or intubation.
Contraindications:	Hypersensitivity to benzodiazepines, narrow angle glaucoma, shock, coma, or acute alcohol intoxication.
Precautions:	COPD, renal impairment, CHF, elderly.
Dosage/Route:	1 to 2.5 mg slow IV; 0.07 to 0.08 mg/kg IM (usually 5 mg). Ped.: 0.05 to 0.2 mg/kg IV; 0.1 to 0.15 mg/kg IM; 3 mg intranasal.

Name/Class:	**MILRINONE (Primacor)/Cardiac Inotrope, Vasodilator**
Description:	Milrinone is related to amrinone and increases the strength of cardiac contraction without increasing rate, increasing cardiac output without increasing oxygen demand.
Indications:	CHF or pediatric septic shock.
Contraindications:	Hypersensitivity.
Precautions:	Elderly, pregnancy, and nursing mothers.
Dosage/Route:	CHF: 50 µg/kg IV over 10 min, then a drip of 0.375 to 0.75 µg/kg/min IV. Ped.: (septic shock) 50 to 75 µg/kg IV, then a drip of 0.5 to 0.75 µg/kg/min.

Name/Class: **MORPHINE SULPHATE (Morphine)/Narcotic Analgesic**

Description: Morphine sulphate is a potent analgesic and sedative that causes some vasodilation, reducing venous return, and reduced myocardial oxygen demand.

Indications: Moderate to severe pain and in MI and to reduce venous return in pulmonary edema.

Contraindications: Hypersensitivity to opiates, undiagnosed head or abdominal injury, hypotension, or volume depletion, acute bronchial asthma, COPD, severe respiratory depression, or pulmonary edema due to chemical inhalation.

Precautions: Elderly, children, or debilitated patients. Naloxone should be readily available to counteract the effects of morphine.

Dosage/Route: Pain: 2.5 to 15 mg IV; 5 to 20 mg IM/SC. Ped.: 0.05 to 0.1 mg/kg IV; 0.1 to 0.2 mg/kg IM/SC.
AMI or PE: 1 to 2 mg/6 to 10 min to response.

Name/Class: **NALBUPHINE (Nubain)/Narcotic Analgesic**

Description: Nalbuphine is a synthetic narcotic analgesic equivalent to morphine, though its respiratory depression does not increase with higher doses.

Indications: Moderate to severe pain.

Contraindications: Hypersensitivity, undiagnosed head or abdominal injury.

Precautions: Impaired respirations, narcotic dependency.

Dosage/Route: 5 mg IV/IM/SC, repeat as 2 mg doses as needed up to 20 mg. Ped.: 0.1 to 0.15 mg/kg IV/IM/SC (rarely used).

Name/Class: **NALOXONE (Narcan)/Narcotic Antagonist**

Description: Naloxone is a pure narcotic antagonist that blocks the effects of both natural and synthetic narcotics and may reverse respiratory depression.

Indications: Narcotic and synthetic narcotic overdose, coma of unknown origin.

Contraindications: Hypersensitivity to the drug, non-narcotic-induced respiratory depression.

Precautions: Possible dependency (including newborns). It also has a half-life that is shorter than most narcotics; hence, the patient may return to the overdose state.

Dosage/Route: 0.4 to 2 mg IV/IM (2 to 2.5 times the dose ET), repeated/2 to 3 min as needed up to 10 mg. Ped.: 0.01 mg IV/IM (2 to 2.5 times the dose ET) repeated/2 to 3 min as needed up to 10 mg.

Name/Class:	**NIFEDIPINE (Procardia, Adalat)/Calcium Channel Blocker**
Description:	Nifedipine is a calcium channel blocker that reduces coronary artery spasm in angina. It also decreases peripheral vascular resistance, blood pressure, and cardiac workload.
Indications:	Severe hypertension and angina.
Contraindications:	Hypersensitivity or hypotension.
Precautions:	Monitor blood pressure carefully, since it can drop significantly with nifedipine use.
Dosage/Route:	One 10- to 20-mg capsule SL/PO.

Name/Class:	**NITROGLYCERINE (Nitrostat)/Nitrate**
Description:	Nitroglycerine is a rapid smooth muscle relaxant that reduces peripheral vascular resistance, blood pressure, venous return, and cardiac workload.
Indications:	Chest pain associated with angina and acute myocardial infarction, and acute pulmonary edema.
Contraindications:	Hypersensitivity, tolerance to nitrates, severe anemia, head trauma, hypotension, increased ICP, patients taking sildenafil, glaucoma, and shock.
Precautions:	May induce headache that is sometimes severe. Nitroglycerine is light sensitive and will lose potency when exposed to the air.
Dosage/Route:	1 tablet (0.4 mg) SL. May be repeated/3 to 5 min up to 3 tablets, or 1 to 2.5 cm of topical ointment, or 0.4 mg (one spray) SL up to 3 sprays/25 min.

Name/Class:	**NITROUS OXIDE (Nitronox)/Analgesic (gas)**
Description:	Nitrous oxide is a self-administered analgesic gas composing of 50% oxygen and 50% nitrous oxide. Its effects last only 2 to 5 minutes after administration ceases.
Indications:	Musculoskeletal, burn, and ischemic chest pain and severe anxiety (including hyperventilation).
Contraindications:	Possible bowel obstruction, pneumothorax or tension pneumothorax, COPD, head injury, impaired mental status, or drug intoxication.
Precautions:	Use in well-ventilated area. It may cause nausea and vomiting.
Dosage/Route:	Self-administered inhalation until the pain is relieved or the patient drops the mask.

Name/Class:	**NOREPINEPHRINE (Levophed)/Sympathomimetic Agent**
Description:	Norepinephrine is a naturally occurring catecholamine and causes vasoconstriction, cardiac stimulation, and increased blood pressure, myocardial oxygen demand, and coronary blood flow.
Indications:	Refractory hypotension and neurogenic shock.
Contraindications:	Hypotension due to hypovolemia.
Precautions:	Hypertension, hyperthyroidism, severe heart disease, elderly, MAO inhibitor therapy, patients receiving tricyclic antidepressants. Monitor blood pressure frequently and infuse the drug through the largest vein available as it may cause tissue necrosis.
Dosage/Route:	0.5 to 30 µg/min IV, titrated to BP. Ped.: 0.01 µg/kg/min (rarely used).

Name/Class:	**OXYGEN/Oxidizing Agent (gas)**
Description:	Oxygen is an odourless, colourless, tasteless gas, essential for life. It is one of the most important emergency drugs.
Indications:	Hypoxia or anticipated hypoxia, or in any medical or trauma patient to improve respiratory efficiency.
Contraindications:	There are no contraindications to oxygen therapy.
Precautions:	Chronic obstructive pulmonary disease and very prolonged administration of high concentrations in the newborn.
Dosage/Route:	Hypoxia: 100% by inhalation or IPPV.

Name/Class:	**OXYTOCIN (Pitocin)/Hormone**
Description:	Oxytocin is a naturally occurring hormone that causes the uterus to contract, thereby inducing labour, encouraging delivery of the placenta, and controlling postpartum hemorrhage.
Indications:	Severe postpartum hemorrhage.
Contraindications:	Hypersensitivity, prehospital administration before delivery of the infant or infants.
Precautions:	Before delivery may induce uterine rupture and fetal dysrhythmias, hypertension, intracranial bleeding, or asphyxia. Uterine tone, ECG, and vital signs should be monitored during administration.
Dosage/Route:	3 to 10 units IM after delivery of the placenta. 10 to 20 units in 1000 mL of D_5W or NS IV titrated to effect.

Name/Class: **PANCURONIUM (Pavulon)/Nondepolarizing Neuromuscular Blocker**

Description: Pancuronium is a nondepolarizing neuromuscular blocker that causes paralysis without bronchospasm or hypotension, nor does it cause the fasciculations associated with polarizing agents.

Indications: To facilitate endotracheal intubation.

Contraindications: Hypersensitivity to pancuronium or bromides, or tachycardia.

Precautions: Debilitated patients, myasthenia gravis, pulmonary, hepatic, or renal disease, or fluid or electrolyte imbalance.

Dosage/Route: 0.04 to 0.1 mg/kg IV. Ped.: same as adult.

Name/Class: **PHENOBARBITAL (Luminal)/Anticonvulsant**

Description: Phenobarbital is a long-acting barbiturate anticonvulsant with sedative and hypnotic effects that limits the spread of seizure activity.

Indications: Seizures, status epilepticus, and acute anxiety.

Contraindications: Hypersensitivity to barbiturates.

Precautions: Hepatic, renal, cardiac, or respiratory impairment, allergies, elderly, debilitated patients, fever, hyperthyroidism, diabetes, severe anemia, hypoadrenal function, and during labour, delivery, and lactation.

Dosage/Route: 100 to 300 mg slow IV/IM. Ped.: 6 to 10 mg/kg slow IV/IM.

Name/Class: **PHENYTOIN (Dilantin)/Anticonvulsant**

Description: Phenytoin is a derivative related to phenobarbital that reduces the spread of electrical discharges in the motor cortex and inhibits seizures. It also has antidysrhythmic properties that counteract the effects of digitalis.

Indications: Seizures, status epilepticus, or cardiac dysrhythmias secondary to digitalis toxicity.

Contraindications: Hypersensitivity to hydantoin products, seizures due to heart block, hypoglycemia, sinus bradycardia, and Adams-Stokes syndrome.

Precautions: Hepatic or renal impairment, alcoholism, cardiogenic shock, elderly, debilitated patients, diabetes, hyperglycemia, bradycardia, heart block, or respiratory depression.

Dosage/Route: Seizures, status epilepticus: 10 to 15 mg/kg slow IV. Ped.: 8 to 10 mg/kg slow IV. Dysrhythmias: 100 mg slow IV (over 5 min) to a maximum 1000 mg. Ped.: 3 to 5 mg/kg slow IV.

Name/Class:	**PHYSOSTIGMINE (Antilirium)/Parasympathomimetic**
Description:	Physostigmine inhibits the breakdown of acetylcholine, resulting in prolonged parasympathetic effects. It is sometimes used as an antidote for anticholinergic (atropine et al.) and tricyclic antidepressant overdoses.
Indications:	Tricyclic antidepressant (CNS and cardiac effects) and anticholinergic overdose.
Contraindications:	Asthma, diabetes, gangrene, cardiovascular disease, or narrow-angle glaucoma.
Precautions:	Reduce dose (or administer atropine) if increased salivation, emesis, or bradycardia develop.
Dosage/Route:	0.5 to 3 mg IV (not faster than 1 mg/min), repeat as needed. Ped.: 0.01 to 0.03 mg/kg/15 to 20 min to max 2 mg.

Name/Class:	**PRALIDOXIME (2-PAM)/Cholinesterase Reactivator**
Description:	Pralidoxime reactivates cholinesterase and reinstitutes the degrading of acetylcholine and restores normal neuromuscular transmission. It is used to reverse severe organophosphate poisoning.
Indications:	Organophosphate poisoning.
Contraindications:	Carbamate insecticides (Sevin), inorganic phosphates, and organophosphates having no anticholinesterase activity, asthma, peptic ulcer disease, severe cardiac disease, or patients receiving aminophylline, theophylline, morphine, succinylcholine, reserpine, or phenothiazines.
Precautions:	Rapid administration may result in tachycardia, laryngospasm, and muscle rigidity. Excited or manic behaviour may be noted after regaining consciousness.
Dosage/Route:	1 to 2 g in 250 to 500 mL NS infused over 15 to 30 min; or 1–2 g IM/SC if IV not feasible. Ped.: 20 to 40 mg/kg IV/IM/SC.

Name/Class:	**PROCAINAMIDE (Pronestyl)/Antiarrhythmic**
Description:	Procainamide prolongs ventricular repolarization, slows conduction, and decreases myocardial excitability.
Indications:	Ventricular fibrillation and pulseless ventricular tachycardia refractory to lidocaine.
Contraindications:	Hypersensitivity to procainamide or procaine, myasthenia gravis, and 2nd- or 3rd-degree heart block.
Precautions:	Hypotension, cardiac enlargement, CHF, AMI, ventricular dysrhythmias from digitalis, hepatic or renal impairment, electrolyte imbalance, or bronchial asthma.
Dosage/Route:	20 to 30 mg/min IV drip up to 17 mg/kg to effect, then 1 to 4 mg/min. Ped.: 15 mg/kg/IV/IO over 30 to 60 min.

Name/Class:	**PROCHLORPERAZINE (Compazine)/Antiemetic**
Description:	Prochlorperazine is a phenothiazine derivative similar to chlorpromazine with potent antiemetic properties and fewer sedative, hypotensive, and anticholinergic effects.
Indications:	Severe nausea and vomiting or acute psychosis.
Contraindications:	Hypersensitivity to phenothiazines, coma, or depression.
Precautions:	Breast cancer, children with acute illness or dehydration.
Dosage/Route:	5 to 10 mg IV/IM. Ped.: 0.13 mg/kg IV/IM/PR if > 10 kg or > 2 Y.O.

Name/Class:	**PROMETHAZINE (Phenergan)/Antiemetic**
Description:	Promethazine is an anticholinergic agent that enhances the effects of analgesics and is a potent antiemetic.
Indications:	Nausea and vomiting, motion sickness, to enhance the effects of analgesics, and to induce sedation.
Contraindications:	Hypersensitivity to phenothiazines.
Precautions:	Hepatic, respiratory, or cardiac impairment, asthma, hypertension, elderly, or debilitated patients.
Dosage/Route:	12.5 to 25 mg IV/IM/PR. Ped.: 0.5 mg/kg IV/IM/PR.

Name/Class:	**PROPAFANONE (Rythmol)/Antidysrhythmic**
Description:	Propafanone is an antidysrhythmic that stabilizes the myocardial membranes, reduces automaticity and the rate of single and multiple PVCs, and suppresses ventricular tachycardia.
Indications:	Ventricular and supraventricular dysrhythmias.
Contraindications:	Hypersensitivity, uncontrolled CHF, cardiogenic shock, sick sinus syndrome, AV block, bradycardia, hypotension, bronchospastic disorders, electrolyte imbalances, non-life-threatening dysrhythmias, COPD, or nursing mothers.
Precautions:	CHF, AV block, hepatic or renal impairment, elderly, or pregnancy.
Dosage/Route:	150 to 300 mg PO/8 h or 1 to 2 mg/kg IV at 10 mg/min.

Name/Class:	**PROPRANOLOL (Inderal)/Beta-Blocker**
Description:	Propranolol is a nonselective beta-blocker affecting both bronchial and cardiac sites. It reduces heart rate, myocardial irritability, contraction force, cardiac output, and blood pressure.
Indications:	Ventricular fibrillation and pulseless ventricular tachycardia refractory to lidocaine and bretylium and selected SVTs.
Contraindications:	2nd- and 3rd-degree heart blocks, CHF, cor pulmonale, sinus bradycardia, cardiac impairment, cardiogenic shock, bronchospasm, or bronchial asthma, COPD, adrenergic-augmenting psychotropic or MAO inhibitors.
Precautions:	Peripheral vascular disease, bee sting allergy, mild COPD, renal or hepatic impairment, diabetes, hypoglycemia, myasthenia gravis, Wolff-Parkinson-White syndrome, or major surgery.
Dosage/Route:	1 to 3 mg slow IV (over 2 to 5 min), not to exceed 1 mg/min, may repeat/2 min to 0.1 mg/kg. Ped.: 0.01 mg/kg slow IV.

Name/Class:	**PROSTAGLANDIN E$_1$ (Prostin VR Pediatric)/Vasodilator**
Description:	Prostaglandin E$_1$ is derived from fatty acids and causes vasodilation, inhibits platelet aggregation, and stimulates intestinal and uterine smooth muscles. It also helps maintain ductus arteriosus patency in newborn infants.
Indications:	Infant cyanotic heart disease.
Contraindications:	None.
Precautions:	Constant respiratory monitoring is required.
Dosage/Route:	Infant: 0.05 to 0.1 µg/kg/min IV/IO.

Name/Class:	**RACEMIC EPINEPHRINE (microNefrin, Vaponefrin)/Sympathomimetic Agonist**
Description:	Racemic epinephrine is a variation of epinephrine used only for inhalation to induce bronchodilation and to reduce laryngeal edema and mucus secretion.
Indications:	Croup (laryngotracheobronchitis).
Contraindications:	Hypersensitivity, hypertension, or epiglottitis.
Precautions:	May result in tachycardia and other dysrhythmias. Patient vital signs and ECG should be monitored.
Dosage/Route:	0.25 to 0.75 mL of a 2.25% solution in 2 mL NS once by nebulizer. Ped.: same as adult.

Name/Class:	**ROCURONIUM (Zemuron)/Nondepolarizing Neuromuscular Blocking Agent**
Description:	Prevents neuromuscular transmission by blocking the effect of acetylcholine. Paralyzes skeletal muscles including respiratory muscles.
Indications:	To maintain paralysis following intubation.
Contraindications:	Hypersensitivity.
Precautions:	Oxygen and resuscitative drugs available.
Dosage/Route:	0.6 mg/kg IV.

Name/Class:	**SALBUTAMOL (Ventolin)/Sympathomimetic Bronchodilator**
Description:	Salbutamol is a synthetic sympathomimetic that causes bronchodilation with less cardiac effect than epinephrine and reduces mucus secretion, pulmonary capillary leaking, and edema in the lungs during allergic reactions.
Indications:	Bronchospasm and asthma in COPD.
Contraindications:	Hypersensitivity to the drug.
Precautions:	The patient may experience tachycardia, anxiety, nausea, cough, wheezing, or dizziness. Vital signs and breath sounds must be monitored; use caution with elderly, cardiac, or hypertensive patients.
Dosage/Route:	Two inhalations (90 µg) via metered-dose inhaler (2 sprays) or 2.5 to 5.0 mg in 2.5 to 5.0 mL NS via nebulizer, repeat as needed. The duration of effect is 3 to 6 hours. Ped.: 0.15 mg/kg in 2.5 to 3 mL NS via nebulizer, repeat as needed.

Name/Class:	**SODIUM BICARBONATE (NaHCO$_3$)/Alkalizing Agent**
Description:	Sodium bicarbonate provides vascular bicarbonate to assist the buffer system in reducing the effects of metabolic acidosis and in the treatment of some overdoses.
Indications:	Tricyclic antidepressant and barbiturate overdose, refractory acidosis, or hyperkalemia.
Contraindications:	None when used in severe hypoxia or late cardiac arrest.
Precautions:	May cause alkalosis if given in too large a quantity. It may also deactivate vasopressors and may precipitate with calcium chloride.
Dosage/Route:	1 mEq/kg IV, then 0.5 mEq/kg/10 min. Ped.: same as adult (may be given IO).

Name/Class:	**SODIUM NITROPRUSSIDE (Nipride)/Nitrate**
Description:	Sodium nitroprusside is a rapid-acting hypotensive agent producing peripheral vasodilation and a mild increase in heart rate, a decrease in cardiac output, and a slight decrease in peripheral vascular resistance.
Indications:	Hypertensive crisis.
Contraindications:	Compensatory hypertension or impaired cerebral circulation (head injury, stroke).
Precautions:	Hepatic or renal impairment, hyponatremia, or hypothyroidism.
Dosage/Route:	0.5 to 0.1 µg/kg/min IV drip. Ped.: same as adult.

Name/Class:	**SOTALOL (Betapace)/Beta-Blocker, Antidysrhythmic**
Description:	Sotalol is a nonselective beta-blocker that slows heart rate and decreases AV conduction and irritability.
Indications:	Ventricular and supraventricular dysrhythmias.
Contraindications:	Hypersensitivity, bronchial asthma, sinus bradycardia, 2nd- and 3rd-degree heart block, long QT syndromes, cardiogenic shock, uncontrolled CHF, or COPD.
Precautions:	CHF, electrolyte disturbances, recent MI, diabetes, sick sinus rhythms, or renal impairment.
Dosage/Route:	1 to 1.5 mg/kg IV at 10 mg/min or 80 mg PO bid or 160 mg PO QD.

Name/Class:	**STREPTOKINASE (Streptase)/Thrombolytic**
Description:	Streptokinase is a thrombolytic that acts by activating the process that converts plasminogen to plasmin and results in the degradation of fibrin and fibrinogen and decreases erythrocyte aggregation.
Indications:	AMI, deep vein thrombosis (DVT), or pulmonary embolism.
Contraindications:	Active internal bleeding, aortic dissection, traumatic CPR, recent stroke, intracranial or intraspinal surgery or trauma (within 2 months), intracranial tumours, uncontrolled hypertension, pregnancy, hypersensitivity to anistreplase or streptokinase.
Precautions:	Recent major surgery (10 days), patients over 75 Y.O., cerebral vascular disease, GI or GU bleeding, recent trauma, hypertension, hemorrhagic conditions, ophthalmic conditions, or oral anticoagulant use.
Dosage/Route:	AMI: 1.5 million units IV over 1 hour. DVT and pulmonary emboli: 250 000 units IV over 30 min, then 100 000 units/h.

Name/Class:	**SUCCINYLCHOLINE (Anectine)/Depolarizing Neuromuscular Blocker**
Description:	Succinylcholine is an ultra-short-acting depolarizing neuromuscular blocker.
Indications:	Facilitated endotracheal intubation.
Contraindications:	Hypersensitivity, family history of malignant hyperthermia, penetrating eye injury, narrow-angle glaucoma.
Precautions:	Severe burn or crush injury; electrolyte imbalances; hepatic, renal, cardiac, or pulmonary impairment; fractures; spinal cord injury; dehydration; severe anemia; porphyria.
Dosage/Route:	1 to 1.5 mg/kg IV/IM. Ped.: 1 to 2 mg/kg IV/IM.

Name/Class:	**TERBUTALINE (Brethine, Bricanyl)/Sympathetic Agonist**
Description:	Terbutaline is a synthetic sympathomimetic that causes bronchodilation with less cardiac effect than epinephrine.
Indications:	Bronchial asthma and bronchospasm in COPD.
Contraindications:	Hypersensitivity to the drug.
Precautions:	The patient may experience palpitations, anxiety, nausea, or dizziness. Vital signs and breath sounds must be monitored; use caution with cardiac or hypertensive patients.
Dosage/Route:	Two inhalations with a metered-dose inhaler, repeated once a minute or 0.25 mg SQ repeated in 15 to 30 minutes.

Name/Class:	**THIAMINE/Vitamin**
Description:	Thiamine is vitamin B_1, which is required to convert glucose into energy. It is not manufactured by the body and must be constantly provided from ingested foods.
Indications:	Coma of unknown origin, chronic alcoholism with associated coma, and delirium tremens.
Contraindications:	None.
Precautions:	Known hypersensitivity to the drug.
Dosage/Route:	50 to 100 mg IV/IM. Ped.: 10 to 25 mg IV/IM.

Name/Class:	**VASOPRESSIN (Pitressin)/Hormone, Vasopressor**
Description:	Vasopressin is a hormone with strong vasopressive and antidiuretic properties but that may precipitate angina or AMI.
Indications:	To increase peripheral vascular resistance in arrest (CPR) or to control bleeding from esophageal varices.
Contraindications:	Chronic nephritis with nitrogen retention, ischemic heart disease, PVCs, advanced arteriosclerosis, or 1st stage of labour.
Precautions:	Epilepsy, migraine, heart failure, angina, vascular disease, hepatic impairment, elderly, and children.
Dosage/Route:	Arrest: 40 units IV. Esophageal varices: 0.2 to 0.4 units/min IV drip.

Name/Class:	**VECURONIUM (Norcuron)/Nondepolarizing Skeletal Muscle Relaxant**
Description:	Vecuronium is a nondepolarizing skeletal muscle relaxant similar to pancuronium with minimal cardiovascular effects.
Indications:	Facilitated endotracheal intubation.
Contraindications:	Hypersensitivity.
Precautions:	Hepatic or renal impairment, impaired fluid and electrolyte or acid/base balance, severe obesity, myasthenia gravis, elderly, debilitated patients, or malignant hyperthermia.
Dosage/Route:	0.08 to 0.1 mg/kg IV. Ped.: same as adult.

Name/Class:	**VERAPAMIL (Isoptin, Calan)/Calcium Channel Blocker**
Description:	Verapamil is a calcium channel blocker that slows AV conduction, suppresses reentry dysrhythmias, such as PSVT, and slows ventricular responses to atrial tachydysrhythmias. Verapamil also dilates coronary arteries and reduces myocardial oxygen demand.
Indications:	PSVT refractory to adenosine, atrial flutter, and atrial fibrillation with rapid ventricular response.
Contraindications:	Severe hypotension, cardiogenic shock, 2nd- or 3rd-degree heart block, CHF, sinus node disease, and accessory AV pathways, Wolff-Parkinson-White syndrome. It should not be administered to persons taking beta-blockers.
Precautions:	Hepatic and renal impairment, MI with coronary artery occlusion, or myocardial stenosis.
Dosage/Route:	2.5 to 5 mg IV bolus over 2 to 3 min, then 5 to 10 mg after 15 to 30 min to a max of 30 mg in 30 min. Ped.: newborn: 0.1 to 0.2 mg/kg (not to exceed 2 mg), age 1 to 15: 0.1 to 0.3 mg/kg (not to exceed 5 mg).

Glossary

10-code radio communications system using codes that begin with the word *ten*.

2,3-diphosphoglycerate (2,3-DPG) chemical in the red blood cells that affects hemoglobins' affinity for oxygen.

abandonment termination of the paramedic–patient relationship without assurance that an equal or greater level of care will continue.

abduction movement of a body part away from the midline.

ABO blood group two antigens known as A and B. A person may have either (type A or type B), both (type AB), or neither (type O). An immune response will be activated whenever a person receives blood containing A or B antigen if this antigen is not already present in his own blood.

acetylcholinesterase (AChE) enzyme that stops the action of acetylocholine, a neurotransmitter.

acidosis a high concentration of hydrogen ions; a pH below 7.35.

acquired immunity protection from infection or disease that is (a) developed by the body after exposure to an antigen, or (b) transferred to the person from an outside source.

action potential the stimulation of myocardial cells, as evidenced by a change in the membrane electrical charge, that subsequently spreads across the myocardium.

active listening the process of responding to your patient's statements with words or gestures that demonstrate your understanding.

active rescue zone area where special rescue teams operate; also known as the "hot zone" or "inner circle."

active transport movement of a substance through a cell membrane against the osmotic gradient; that is, from an area of lesser concentration to an area of greater concentration, opposite to the normal direction of diffusion; requires the use of energy to move a substance.

actual damages refers to compensatable physical, psychological, or financial harm.

acuity the severity or acuteness of your patient's condition.

acute effects signs and symptoms rapidly displayed on exposure to a toxic substance.

addendum addition or supplement to the original report.

adduction movement of a body part toward the midline.

adenosine triphosphate (ATP) a high-energy compound present in all cells, especially muscle cells; when split by enzyme action, it yields energy. Energy is stored in ATP.

adjunct medication agent that enhances the effects of other drugs.

administration tubing flexible, clear plastic tubing that connects the solution bag to the IV cannula.

administrative law a law that is enacted by governmental agencies at either the federal or the provincial and territorial level. Also called *regulatory law.*

adrenergic pertaining to the neurotransmitter norepinephrine.

advance directive a document created to ensure that certain treatment choices are honoured when a patient is unconscious or otherwise unable to express her choice of treatment.

advanced life support (ALS) refers to such advanced life-saving procedures as intravenous therapy, drug therapy, intubation, and defibrillation, cardioversion/pacing provided by advanced care paramedics (ACP) or critical care paramedics (CCP).

aerobic metabolism the second stage of metabolism, requiring the presence of oxygen, in which the breakdown of glucose (in a process called the Krebs or citric acid cycle) yields a high amount of energy. *Aerobic* means "with oxygen."

aeromedical evacuations transport by helicopter or fixed-wing aircraft.

affinity force of attraction between a drug and a receptor.

afterload the resistance against which the heart must pump.

against medical advice (AMA) your patient refuses care even though you feel he needs it.

agonist drug that binds to a receptor and causes it to initiate the expected response.

agonist-antagonist (partial agonist) drug that binds to a receptor and stimulates some of its effects but blocks others.

AIDS *acquired immunodeficiency syndrome*, a group of signs, symptoms, and disorders that often develop as a consequence of HIV infection.

air embolism air in the vein.

air-purifying respirator (APR) system of filtering a normal environment for a specific chemical substance using filter cartridges.

albumin a protein commonly present in plant and animal tissues. In the blood, albumin works to maintain blood volume and blood pressure and provides colloid osmotic pressure, which prevents plasma loss from the capillaries.

algorithm schematic flow chart that outlines appropriate care for specific signs and symptoms.

alkalosis a low concentration of hydrogen ions; a pH above 7.45.

allergy exaggerated immune response to an environmental antigen.

allied health professions ancillary health-care professions, apart from physicians and nurses.

alveoli microscopic air sacs where most oxygen and carbon dioxide gas exchanges take place.

amphiarthrosis joint that permits a limited amount of independent motion.

ampule breakable glass vessel containing liquid medication.

anabolism the constructive phase of metabolism in which cells convert nonliving substances into living cytoplasm.

anaerobic metabolism the first stage of metabolism, which does not require oxygen, in which the breakdown of glucose (in a process called glycolysis) produces pyruvic acid and yields very little energy. *Anaerobic* means "without oxygen."

analgesia the absence of the sensation of pain.

analgesic medication that relieves the sensation of pain.

anaphylaxis a life-threatening allergic reaction; also called *anaphylactic shock.*

anatomy the structure of an organism; body structure.

anchor time set of hours when a night-shift worker can reliably expect to rest without interruption.

anesthesia the absence of all sensation.

anesthetic medication that induces a loss of sensation to touch or pain.

anion an ion with a negative charge—so called because it will be attracted to an anode, or positive pole.

antacid alkalotic compound used to increase the gastric environment's pH.

antagonist drug that binds to a receptor but does not cause it to initiate the expected response.

anterior medial fissure deep crease along the ventral surface of the spinal cord that divides the cord into right and left halves.

antibiotics substances that destroy or inhibit microorganisms, tiny living bodies invisible to the naked eye. (*Antibiotic* means "destructive to life.")

antibody a substance produced by B lymphocytes in response to the presence of a foreign antigen that will combine with and control or destroy the antigen, thus preventing infection.

anticoagulant drug that interrupts the clotting cascade.

antidiuresis formation and passage of concentrated urine, preserving blood volume.

antidysrhythmic drug used to treat and prevent abnormal cardiac rhythms.

antiemetic medication used to prevent vomiting.

antigen a marker on the surface of a cell that identifies it as "self" or "not self."

antihyperlipidemic drug used to treat high blood cholesterol.

antihypertensive drug used to treat hypertension.

antineoplastic agent drug used to treat cancer.

antiplatelet drug that decreases the formation of platelet plugs.

antiseptic cleansing agent that is not toxic to living tissue.

antitussive medication that suppresses the stimulus to cough in the central nervous system.

apnea absence of breathing.

apoptosis response in which an injured cell releases enzymes that engulf and destroy itself; one way the body rids itself of damaged and dead cells.

appendicular skeleton bones of the extremities, shoulder girdle, and pelvis (excepting the sacrum).

aqueous humor clear fluid filling the anterior chamber of the eye.

arachnoid membrane middle layer of the meninges.

articular surface surface of a bone that moves against another bone.

ascending loop of Henle the part of the nephron tubule beyond the descending loop of Henle.

ascending tracts bundles of axons along the spinal cord that transmit signals from the body to the brain.

ascites bulges in the flanks and across the abdomen, indicating edema caused by congestive heart failure.

asepsis a condition free of pathogens.

aspiration inhaling foreign material, such as vomitus, into the lungs.

assault an act that unlawfully places a person in apprehension of immediate bodily harm without consent.

assay test that determines the amount and purity of a given chemical in a preparation in the laboratory.

atelectasis alveolar collapse.

atrophy a decrease in cell size resulting from a decreased workload.

auscultation listening with a stethoscope for sounds produced by the body.

autoimmune disease condition in which the body makes antibodies against its own tissues.

autoimmunity an immune response to self-antigens, which the body normally tolerates.

automaticity pacemaker cells' capability of self-depolarization.

autonomic dysfunction an abnormality of the involuntary aspect of the nervous system.

autonomic ganglia groups of autonomic nerve cells located outside the central nervous system.

autonomic nervous system part of the nervous system that controls involuntary actions.

autonomy a competent adult patient's right to determine what happens to his own body.

autoregulation process that controls blood flow to tissue by causing alterations in the tissue.

axial skeleton bones of the head, thorax, and spine.

B lymphocytes white blood cells that, in response to the presence of an antigen, produce antibodies that attack the antigen, develop a memory for the antigen, and confer long-term immunity to the antigen.

Babinski response big toe dorsiflexes and the other toes fan out when sole is stimulated.

bacteria (singular *bacterium*) single-cell organisms with a cell membrane and cytoplasm but no organized nucleus. They bind to the cells of a host organism to obtain food and support.

basic life support (BLS) refers to basic life-saving procedures such as artificial ventilation and cardiopulmonary resuscitation (CPR, automatic defibrillation) generally provided by EMS personnel at the primary care paramedic (PCP) level.

battery the unlawful touching of another individual without consent.

Battle's sign black and blue discoloration over the mastoid process.

beneficence the principle of doing good for the patient.

bioassay test to ascertain a drug's availability in a biological model.

bioavailability amount of a drug that is still active after it reaches its target tissue.

bioequivalence relative therapeutic effectiveness of chemically equivalent drugs.

bioethics ethics as applied to the human body.

biological half-life time the body takes to clear one-half of a drug.

biotransformation chemical alteration of a substance within the body; in the case of hazardous materials, the body tries to create less toxic materials.

blood pressure force of blood against arterial walls as the heart contracts and relaxes; the tension exerted by blood against the arterial walls.

blood spatter evidence the pattern that blood forms when it is spattered or dropped at the scene of a crime.

blood tube glass container with colour-coded, self-sealing rubber top.

blood tubing administration tubing that contains a filter to prevent clots or other debris from entering the patient.

blood-brain barrier tight junctions of the capillary endothelial cells in the central nervous system vasculature through which only non-protein-bound, highly lipid-soluble drugs can pass.

body armour vest made of tightly woven, strong fibres that offer protection against handgun bullets, most knives, and blunt trauma; also known as a "bullet-proof vest."

body substance isolation (BSI) a strict form of infection control that is based on the assumption that all blood and other body fluids are infectious.

Bohr effect phenomenon in which a decrease in pCO_2/acidity causes an increase in the quantity of oxygen that binds with the hemoglobin and, conversely, an increase in pCO_2/acidity causes the hemoglobin to give up a greater quantity of oxygen.

bolus concentrated mass of medication.

borborygmi loud, prolonged, gurgling bowel sounds indicating hyperperistalsis.

Bowman's capsule the hollow, cup-shaped first part of the nephron tubule.

bradycardia a pulse rate slower than 60.

bradypnea slow breathing.

brainstem the part of the brain connecting the cerebral hemispheres with the spinal cord. It comprises the mesencephalon, the pons, and the medulla oblongata.

branches functional levels within the IMS based upon primary roles and geographic locations.

breach of duty an action or inaction that violates the standard of care expected from a paramedic.

bronchi tubes from the trachea into the lungs.

bronchophony abnormal clarity of patient's transmitted voice sounds.

Broselow tape a measuring tape for infants that provides important information regarding airway equipment and medication doses based on your patient's length.

bruit sound of turbulent blood flow around a partial obstruction.

bubble sheet scanable call sheet on which you fill in boxes or "bubbles" to record assessment and care information.

buccal between the cheek and gums.

buffer a substance that tends to preserve or restore a normal acid-base balance by increasing or decreasing the concentration of hydrogen ions.

burette chamber calibrated chamber of Berutrol IV administration tubing that enables precise measurement and delivery of fluids and medicated solutions.

burnout occurs when coping mechanisms no longer buffer stressors, which can compromise personal health and well-being.

bursae sacs containing synovial fluid that cushion adjacent structures; singular *bursa*.

CAMEO® Computer-Aided Management of Emergency Operations; website developed by the EPA and NOAA as a source of information, skills, and links related to hazardous substances.

cancellous having a lattice-work structure, as in the spongy tissue of a bone.

cannula hollow needle used to puncture a vein.

cardiac contractile force force of the strength of a contraction of the heart.

cardiac cycle the period of time from the end of one cardiac contraction to the end of the next.

cardiac depolarization a reversal of charges at a cell membrane so that the inside of the cell becomes positive in relation to the outside; the opposite of the cell's resting state in which the inside of the cell is negative in relation to the outside.

cardiac monitor machine that displays and records the electrical activity of the heart.

cardiac output the amount of blood pumped by the heart in one minute.

cardiogenic shock shock caused by insufficient cardiac output; the inability of the heart to pump enough blood to perfuse all parts of the body.

carrier-mediated diffusion process in which carrier proteins transport large molecules across the cell membrane; also called *facilitated diffusion.*

cartilage connective tissue providing the articular surfaces of the skeletal system.

catabolism the destructive phase of metabolism in which cells break down complex substances into simpler substances with release of energy.

catheter inserted through the needle (intracatheter) Teflon catheter inserted through a large metal stylet.

cation an ion with a positive charge—so called because it will be attracted to a cathode, or negative pole.

cell membrane also *plasma membrane;* the outer covering of a cell.

cell the basic structural unit of all plants and animals. Cells are specialized to carry out all of the body's basic functions.

cell-mediated immunity the short-term immunity to an antigen provided by T lymphocytes, which directly attack the antigen but do not produce antibodies or memory for the antigen.

cellular swelling swelling of a cell caused by injury to or change in permeability of the cell membrane with resulting inability to maintain stable intra- and extracellular fluid and electrolyte levels.

cellular telephone system telephone system divided into regions, or cells, that are served by radio base stations.

central nervous system the brain and the spinal cord.

central venous access surgical puncture of the internal jugular, subclavian, or femoral vein.

cerebellum portion of the brain located dorsally to the pons and medulla oblongata. It plays an important role in the fine control of voluntary muscular movement.

cerebral perfusion pressure (CPP) the pressure moving blood through the brain.

cerebrospinal fluid fluid surrounding and bathing the brain and spinal cord (the elements of the central nervous system).

cerebrum largest part of the brain. It consists of two hemispheres separated by a deep longitudinal fissure. It is the seat of consciousness and the centre of the higher mental functions, such as memory, learning, reasoning, judgment, intelligence, and emotions.

certification the process by which an agency or association grants recognition and the ability to practise to an individual who has met its qualifications.

C-FLOP mnemonic for the main functional areas with the IMS—command, finance and administration, logistics, operations, and planning.

chemotactic factors chemicals that attract more white blood cells to an area of inflammation, a process called **chemotaxis.**

chemotaxis the movement of white blood cells in response to chemical signals.

CHEMTEL, Inc. Chemical Telephone, Incorporated; maintains a 24-hour, toll-free hotline at 800-255-3024; for collect calls and calls from other points of origin, dial 813-979-0626.

CHEMTREC Chemical Transportation Emergency Center; maintains a 24-hour, toll-free hotline at 800-424-9300; for collect calls and calls from other points of origin, dial 703-527-3887.

chief complaint the reason the ambulance was called; the pain, discomfort, or dysfunction that caused your patient to request help.

cholinergic pertaining to the neurotransmitter acetylcholine.

chronotropy pertaining to heart rate.

chyme semifluid mixture of ingested food and digestive secretions found in the stomach and small intestine.

circadian rhythms physiological phenomena that occur at approximately 24-hour intervals.

circulation assessment evaluating the pulse and skin and controlling hemorrhage.

circulatory overload an excess in intravascular fluid volume.

circumduction movement at a synovial joint where the distal end of a bone describes a circle but the shaft does not rotate; movement through an arc of a circle.

civil law the division of the legal system that deals with noncriminal issues and conflicts between two or more parties.

cleaning washing an object with cleaners such as soap and water.

clinical judgment the use of knowledge and experience to diagnose patients and plan their treatment.

clitoris highly innervated and vascular erectile tissue anterior to the labia minora.

closed incident an incident that is not likely to generate any further patients; also known as a contained incident or a stable incident.

closed questions questions that ask for specific information and require only very short or yes-or-no answers. Also called *direct questions.*

closed stance a posture or body position that is tense and suggests negativity, discomfort, fear, disgust, or anger.

cold zone location at a hazmat incident outside the warm zone; area where incident operations take place; also called the green zone or the safe zone.

collecting duct the larger structure beyond the distal nephron tubule into which urine drips.

colloids substances, such as proteins or starches, consisting of large molecules or molecule aggregates that disperse evenly within a liquid without forming a true solution; intravenous solutions containing large proteins that cannot pass through capillary membranes.

command post (CP) place where command officers from various agencies can meet with each other and select a management staff.

command the individual or group responsible for coordinating all activities and who makes final decisions on the emergency scene; often referred to as the incident commander (IC) or officer in charge (OIC).

common law law derived from society's acceptance over time of customs and norms. Also called *case law* or *judge-made law.*

communication the exchange of common symbols—written, spoken, or other kinds, such as signing and body language.

compensated shock early stage of shock during which the body's compensatory mechanisms are able to maintain normal perfusion.

competent able to make an informed decision about medical care.

competitive antagonism one drug binds to a receptor and causes the expected effect while also blocking another drug from triggering the same receptor.

concealment hiding the body behind objects that shield a person from view but that offer little or no protection against bullets or other ballistics.

concentration weight per volume.

conductivity ability of cells to propagate the electrical impulse from one cell to another.

confidentiality the principle of law that prohibits the release of medical or other personal information about a patient without the patient's consent.

conjuctiva mucous membrane that lines the eyelids.

connective tissue the most abundant body tissue; it provides support, connection, and insulation. Examples: bone, cartilage, fat, blood.

consent the patient's granting of permission for treatment.

constitutional law law based on the Canadian Constitution.

continuous quality improvement (CQI) a program designed to refine and improve an EMS system, emphasizing customer satisfaction.

CONTOMS Counter-Narcotics Tactical Operations; program that manages the training and certification of EMT-Ts and SWAT-Medics.

contractility ability of muscle cells to contract, or shorten.

convergent focusing on only the most important aspect of a critical situation.

cornea thin, delicate layer covering the pupil and the iris.

cortex the outer tissue of an organ, such as the kidney.

cortisol a steroid hormone released by the adrenal cortex that regulates the metabolism of fats, carbohydrates, sodium, potassium, and proteins and also has an anti-inflammatory effect.

cover hiding the body behind solid and impenetrable objects that protect a person from bullets.

crackles light crackling, popping, nonmusical sounds heard usually during inspiration.

cranial nerves 12 pairs of nerves that extend from the lower surface of the brain.

cranium vault-like portion of the skull encasing the brain.

creatinine a waste product caused by metabolism within muscle cells.

crepitation (or crepitus) crunching sounds of unlubricated parts in joints rubbing against each other.

cricothyroid membrane membrane between the cricoid and thyroid cartilages of the larynx.

criminal law division of the legal system that deals with wrongs committed against society or its members.

critical incident stress debriefing (CISD) a process used to help rescuers work through their responses to a critical incident within 24 to 72 hours after the event.

critical incident stress management (CISM) a system of related interventions usually performed by regional, nonpartisan, multidisciplinary teams composed of EMS peers and specifically trained mental health workers.

Critical Incident Stress Management (CISM) team monitors the emotional status of all on-scene personnel and provides the necessary support.

critical incident an event that has a powerful emotional impact on a rescuer that can cause an acute stress reaction.

critical thinking thought process used to analyze and evaluate.

crystalloids substances capable of crystallization. In solution, unlike colloids, they can diffuse through a membrane, such as a capillary wall; intravenous solutions that contain electrolytes but lack the larger proteins associated with colloids.

Cullen's sign discoloration around the umbilicus (occasionally the flanks) suggestive of intra-abdominal hemorrhage.

cultural imposition the imposition of your beliefs, values, and patterns of behaviour on people of another culture.

cytochrome oxidase enzyme complex, found in cellular mitochondria, that enables oxygen to create the adenosine triphosphate (ATP) required for all muscle energy.

cytoplasm the thick fluid, or *protoplasm,* that fills a cell.

decerebrate arms and legs extended.

decode to interpret a message.

decompensated shock advanced stages of shock when the body's compensatory mechanisms are no longer able to maintain normal perfusion; also called *progressive shock.*

decorticate arms flexed, legs extended.

defamation an intentional false communication that injures another person's reputation or good name.

defusing a short, informal type of debriefing held within hours of a critical incident.

degranulation the emptying of granules from the interior of a mast cell into the extracellular environment.

dehydration excessive loss of body fluid.

delayed effects signs, symptoms, and conditions developed hours, days, weeks, months, or even years after exposure to a toxic substance.

delayed hypersensitivity reaction a hypersensitivity reaction that takes place after the elapse of some time following reexposure to an antigen. Delayed hypersensitivity reactions are usually less severe than immediate reactions.

delirium an acute alteration in mental functioning that is often reversible.

dementia a deterioration of mental status that is usually associated with structural neurological disease.

demobilization establishment and staffing of a transition point with the object of providing crews time to regroup between a large-scale critical stress situation and going off duty or back to regular duty.

demobilized released resources—personnel, vehicles, and equipment—for use outside the incident when they are no longer needed at the scene.

demographic pertaining to population makeup or changes.

demylenation destruction or removal of the myelin sheath of nerve tissue; found in Guillain–Barré syndrome.

deployment strategy used by an EMS agency to manoeuvre its ambulances and crews in an effort to reduce response times.

depression a mood disorder characterized by hopelessness and malaise.

dermatome topographical region of the body surface innervated by one nerve root.

dermis true skin, also called the corium; it is the layer of tissue producing the epidermis and housing the structures, blood vessels, and nerves normally associated with the skin.

descending loop of Henle the part of the nephron tubule beyond the proximal tubule.

descending tracts bundles of axons along the spinal cord that transmit signals from the brain to the body.

desired dose specific quantity of medication needed.

detailed secondary assessment careful, thorough process of eliciting the history and conducting a physical exam.

devascularization loss of blood vessels from a body part.

diaphysis hollow shaft found in long bones.

diarthrosis a synovial joint.

diastole the period of time when the myocardium is relaxed and cardiac filling and coronary perfusion occur.

diastolic blood pressure force of blood against arteries when ventricles relax.

differential field diagnosis the list of possible causes for your patient's symptoms.

diffusion the movement of molecules through a membrane from an area of greater concentration to an area of lesser concentration.

digestive tract internal passageway that begins at the mouth and ends at the anus; also called the *alimentary canal*.

digital communications data or sounds are translated into a digital code for transmission.

dilation enlargement. In reference to the heart, an abnormal enlargement resulting from pathology.

disaster management management of incidents that generate large numbers of patients, often overwhelming resources and damaging parts of the infrastructure.

disentanglement process of freeing a patient from wreckage to allow for proper care, removal, and transfer.

disinfectant cleansing agent that is toxic to living tissue.

disinfecting cleaning with an agent that can kill some microorganisms on the surface of an object.

dissociate separate; break down. For example, sodium bicarbonate, when placed in water, dissociates into a sodium cation and a bicarbonate anion.

distal tubule the part of the tubule beyond the ascending loop of Henle.

diuresis formation and passage of dilute urine, decreasing blood volume.

diuretic a medication that stimulates the kidneys to excrete excess water; an agent that increases urine secretion and elimination of body water.

divergent taking into account all aspects of a complex situation.

Do Not Resuscitate (DNR) order a legal document, usually signed by the patient and her physician, that indicates to medical personnel which, if any, life-sustaining measures should be taken when the patient's heart and respiratory functions have ceased.

dosage on hand the amount of drug available in a solution.

dose packaging medication packages that contain a single dose for a single patient.

down-regulation binding of a drug or hormone to a target cell receptor that causes the number of receptors to decrease.

drip chamber clear plastic chamber that allows visualization of the intravenous drip rate.

drip rate pace at which the fluid moves from the intravenous bag into the patient.

dromotropy pertaining to the speed of impulse transmission.

drop former device that regulates the size of drops.

drug chemical used to diagnose, treat, or prevent disease.

drug-response relationship correlation of different amounts of a drug to clinical response.

due regard legal terminology found in the motor vehicle laws of most provinces and territories that sets a higher standard for the operators of emergency vehicles.

duplex communication system that allows simultaneous two-way communications by using two frequencies for each channel.

dura mater tough layer of the meninges firmly attached to the interior of the skull and the spinal column.

duration of action length of time the amount of drug remains above its minimum effective concentration.

duty to act a formal contractual or informal legal obligation to provide care.

dynamic steady state homeostasis; the tendency of the body to maintain a net constant composition, although the components of the body's internal environment are always changing.

dysmenorrhea menstrual difficulties.

dysplasia a change in cell size, shape, or appearance caused by an external stressor.

dyspnea the sensation of having difficulty in breathing.

echo procedure immediately repeating each transmission received during radio communications.

eddies water that flows around especially large objects and, for a time, flows upstream around the downside of an obstruction; provides an opportunity to escape dangerous currents.

edema excess fluid in the interstitial space.

efficacy a drug's ability to cause the expected response.

egophony abnormal change in tone of patient's transmitted voice sounds.

ejection fraction ratio of blood pumped from the ventricle to the amount remaining at the end of diastole.

electrolyte a substance that, in water, separates into electrically charged particles.

emancipated minor a person under 18 years of age who is married, pregnant, a parent, a member of the armed forces, or financially independent and living away from home.

embolus foreign particle in the blood.

emergency medical dispatcher (EMD) EMS person medically and technically trained to assign emergency medical resources to a medical emergency.

emergency medical responders (EMR) are responders who provide first-aid skills until more advanced personnel arrive.

emergency medical services (EMS) system a comprehensive network of personnel, equipment, and resources established for the purpose of delivering aid and emergency medical care to the community.

empathy identification with and understanding of another's situation, feelings, and motives.

EMS communications officer notifies hospitals of incoming patients from an MCI; reports to the transport officer and may also be called the EMS COM or MED COM.

EMT-Tacticals (EMT-Ts) EMS personnel trained to serve with a tactical Emergency Medical Services or a law enforcement agency.

encode to create a message.

endometrium the inner layer of the uterine wall where the fertilized egg implants.

endotoxins molecules in the walls of certain gram-negative bacteria that are released when the bacterium dies or is destroyed, causing toxic (poisonous) effects on the host body.

endotracheal intubation passing a tube into the trachea to protect and maintain the airway and to permit medication administration and deep suctioning.

enema a liquid bolus of medication that is injected into the rectum.

enteral drug administration the delivery of any medication that is absorbed through the gastrointestinal tract.

enteral route delivery of a medication through the gastrointestinal tract.

epidemiology the study of factors that influence the frequency, distribution, and causes of injury, disease, and other health-related events in a population.

epidermis outermost layer of the skin comprising dead or dying cells.

epididymis small sac in which sperm cells are stored.

epiphyseal plate area of the metaphysis where cartilage is generated during bone growth in childhood; *growth plate.*

epiphysis end of a long bone, including the epiphyseal, or growth plate and supporting structures underlying the joint.

epithelial tissue the protective tissue that lines internal and external body tissues. Examples: skin, mucous membranes, the lining of the intestinal tract.

erythrocyte red blood cell.

erythropoiesis the process of producing red blood cells.

erythropoietin a hormone produced by kidney cells that stimulates maturation of red blood cells.

ethics the rules or standards that govern the conduct of members of a particular group or profession.

ethnocentrism viewing your own life as the most desirable, acceptable, or best, and acting in a superior manner to another culture's way of life.

eustachian tube a tube that connects the ear with the nasal cavity.

excitability ability of the cells to respond to an electrical stimulus.

exotoxin a soluble poisonous substance secreted during growth of a bacterium.

expectorant medication intended to increase the productivity of a cough.

exposure any occurrence of blood or body fluids coming in contact with nonintact skin, mucous membranes, or parenteral contact (needle stick).

expressed consent verbal, nonverbal, or written communication by a patient that she wants to receive medical care.

extension tubing IV tubing used to extend a macrodrip or microdrip setup.

extension bending motion that increases the angle between articulating elements.

extracellular fluid (ECF) the fluid outside the body cells. Extracellular fluid comprises intravascular fluid and interstitial fluid.

extrapyramidal symptoms (EPS) common side effects of antipsychotic medications that include muscle tremors and parkinsonism-like effects.

extravasation leakage of fluid or medication from the blood vessel that is commonly found with infiltration.

extravascular outside the vein.

extrication group or branch responsible for removing patients from entanglements and transferring them to the treatment area; also known as rescue, or use of force to free a patient from entrapment.

facilitated diffusion diffusion of a substance, such as glucose, through a cell membrane that requires the assistance of a "helper," or carrier protein.

facilities unit selects and maintains areas used for rehabilitation and command.

facsimile machine device for electronically transmitting and receiving printed information.

fallopian tubes thin tubes that extend laterally from the uterus and conduct eggs from the ovaries into the uterine cavity.

false imprisonment intentional and unjustifiable detention of a person without consent or other legal authority.

fasciculus small bundle of muscle fibres.

fatty change a result of cellular injury and swelling in which lipids (fat vesicles) invade the area of injury; occurs most commonly in the liver.

feedback a response to a message.

fibrinolysis the process through which plasmin dismantles a blood clot.

fibroblasts cells that secrete collagen, a critical factor in wound healing.

field diagnosis prehospital evaluation of the patient's condition and its causes, based on your history and physical assessment.

filtrate the fluid produced in Bowman's capsule by filtration of blood.

filtration movement of water out of the plasma across the capillary membrane into the interstitial space; movement of molecules across a membrane from an area of higher pressure to an area of lower pressure.

finance and administration is responsible for maintaining records for personnel, time, and costs of resources or procurement; reports directly to the IC.

FiO₂ concentration of oxygen in inspired air.

first-pass effect the liver's partial or complete inactivation of a drug before it reaches the systemic circulation.

flanks the part of the back below the ribs and above the hip bones.

flexion bending motion that reduces the angle between articulating elements.

focused and problem-oriented secondary assessment process based on primary assessment and chief complaint.

free drug availability proportion of a drug available in the body to cause either desired or undesired effects.

gag reflex mechanism that stimulates retching, or striving to vomit, when the soft palate is touched.

galea aponeurotica connective tissue sheet covering the superior aspect of the cranium.

gauge the size of a needle's diameter.

general adaptation syndrome (GAS) a sequence of stress response stages: stage I, alarm; stage II, resistance or adaptation; stage III, exhaustion.

general impression your initial, intuitive evaluation of your patient.

glomerular filtration rate (GFR) the volume per day at which blood is filtered through capillaries of the glomerulus.

glomerular filtration the removal from blood of water and other elements, which enter the nephron tubule.

glomerulus a tuft of capillaries from which blood is filtered into a nephron.

glottis lip-like opening between the vocal cords.

glucagon substance that increases blood glucose level.

glucometer tool used to measure blood glucose level.

gluconeogenesis conversion of protein and fat to form glucose.

glycogenolysis the breakdown of glycogen to glucose, primarily by liver cells.

gold standard ultimate standard of excellence.

Good Samaritan laws laws that provide immunity to certain people who assist at the scene of a medical emergency.

granuloma a tumour or growth that forms when foreign bodies that cannot be destroyed by macrophages are surrounded and walled off.

great vessels the large arteries and veins located in the mediastinum that enter and exit the heart; the aorta, superior and inferior vena cava, pulmonary arteries, and pulmonary veins.

grey matter areas in the central nervous system dominated by nerve cell bodies; the central portion of the spinal cord.

Grey-Turner's sign discoloration over the flanks suggesting intra-abdominal bleeding.

gtts drops (Latin *guttae*, drops [*gutta*, drop]).

hate crimes crimes committed against a person wholly on the basis of the individual's actual or perceived race, colour, national origin, ethnicity, gender, disability, or sexual orientation.

haversian canals small perforations of the long bones through which the blood vessels and nerves travel into the bone itself.

hazardous material (hazmat) any substance that causes adverse health effects on exposure to humans.

health-care professional a properly trained and licensed or certified provider of health care.

heat escape lessening position (HELP) an in-water, head-up tuck or fetal position designed to reduce heat loss by as much as 60 percent.

HEENT head, eyes, ears, nose, and throat.

hematemesis vomiting blood.

hematocrit the percentage of the blood occupied by erythrocytes.

hematopoietic system body system having to do with the production and development of blood cells, consisting of the bone marrow, liver, spleen, kidneys, and the blood itself.

hematopoiesis the process through which pluripotent stem cells differentiate into various types of blood cells.

hematuria blood in the urine.

hemoconcentration elevated numbers of red and white blood cells.

hemoglobin oxygen-bearing molecule in the red blood cells. It is made up of iron-rich red pigment called *heme* and a protein called *globin*.

hemolysis destruction of red blood cells.

hemoptysis coughing up blood.

hemostasis the combined mechanisms that work to prevent or control blood loss.

hemothorax accumulation in the pleural cavity of blood or fluid containing blood.

heparin lock peripheral IV port that does not use a bag of fluid.

hepatic alteration change in a medication's chemical composition that occurs in the liver.

hilum the notched part of the kidney where the ureter and other structures join kidney tissue.

histamine a substance released during the degranulation of mast cells and also released by basophils that, through constriction and dilation of blood vessels, increases blood flow to the injury site due to vasodilation and also increases the permeability of capillary walls.

HIV *human immunodeficiency virus*, a virus that breaks down the immune defenses, making the body vulnerable to a variety of infections and disorders. *See also* AIDS.

hollow-needle catheter stylet that does not have a Teflon tube but is itself inserted into the vein and secured there.

homeostasis the natural tendency of the body to maintain a steady and normal internal environment.

hot zone location at a hazmat incident where the actual hazardous material and highest levels of contamination exist; also called the red zone or the exclusionary zone.

Huber needle needle that has an opening on the side of the shaft instead of the tip.

humoral immunity the long-term immunity to an antigen provided by antibodies produced by B lymphocytes.

hydrolysis the breakage of a chemical bond by adding water, or by incorporating a hydroxyl (OH^-) group into one fragment and a hydrogen ion (H^+) into the other.

hydrostatic pressure blood pressure or force against vessel walls created by the heart beat. Hydrostatic pressure tends to force water out of the capillaries into the interstitial space.

hypercarbia excess carbon dioxide in the blood.

hyperosmolar a solution that has a concentration of the substance greater than that of a second solution.

hyperplasia an increase in number of cells resulting from an increased workload.

hypersensitivity an exaggerated and harmful immune response; an umbrella term for allergy, autoimmunity, and isoimmunity.

hypertension blood pressure higher than normal.

hyperthermia increase in body's core temperature.

hypertonic having a greater concentration of solute molecules; one solution may be hypertonic to another.

hypertrophy an increase in cell size resulting from an increased workload.

hypnosis instigation of sleep.

hypodermic needle hollow metal tube used with syringe to administer medications.

hypo-osmolar a solution that has a concentration of the substance lower than that of a second solution.

hypoperfusion inadequate perfusion of the body tissues, resulting in an inadequate supply of oxygen and nutrients to the body tissues. Also called *shock*.

hypotension lower than normal systolic and diastolic blood pressure.

hypothalamus portion of the brain important for controlling certain metabolic activities, including the regulation of body temperature.

hypothermia decrease in body's core temperature.

hypotonic having a lesser concentration of solute molecules; one solution may be hypotonic to another.

hypoventilation reduction in breathing rate and depth.

hypovolemic shock shock caused by a loss of intravascular fluid volume.

hypoxemia decreased blood oxygen level.

hypoxia oxygen deficiency.

hypoxic drive mechanism that increases respiratory stimulation when blood oxygen falls and inhibits respiratory stimulation when blood oxygen climbs.

immediate hypersensitivity reaction a swiftly occurring hypersensitivity reaction (that occurs after reexposure to an antigen). Immediate hypersensitivity reactions are usually more severe than delayed reactions. The swiftest and most severe of such reactions is anaphylaxis.

immune response the body's reactions that inactivate or eliminate foreign antigens.

immunity (1) exemption from legal liability. (2) a long-term condition of protection from infection or disease; the body's ability to respond to the presence of a pathogen.

immunogens antigens that are able to trigger an immune response.

implied consent consent for treatment that is presumed for a patient who is mentally, physically, or emotionally unable to grant consent. Also called *emergency doctrine*.

impulsive acting instinctively without stopping to think.

incident management system (IMS) national system used for the management of multiple casualty incidents, involving assumption of responsibility for command and designation and coordination of such elements as triage, treatment, transport, and staging; sometimes called the incident command system.

incubation period the time between contact with a disease organism and the appearance of the first symptoms.

index of suspicion your anticipation of possible injuries based upon your analysis of the event.

infectious disease any disease caused by the growth of pathogenic microorganisms, which may be spread from person to person.

inflammation the body's response to cellular injury; also called the *inflammatory response*. In contrast to the immune response, inflammation develops swiftly, is nonspecific (attacks all unwanted substances in the same way), and is temporary, leading to healing.

inflammatory process a nonspecific defense mechanism that wards off damage from microorganisms or trauma.

informed consent consent for treatment that is given based on full disclosure of information.

infusion controller gravity-flow device that regulates fluid's passage through an electromechanical pump.

infusion pump device that delivers fluids and medications under positive pressure.

infusion rate speed at which a medication is delivered intravenously.

infusion liquid medication delivered through a vein.

inhalation drawing of medication into the lungs along with air during breathing.

injection placement of medication in or under the skin with a needle and synringe.

injury risk a situation that puts people in danger of sustaining injury.

injury intentional or unintentional damage to a person resulting from exposure to mechanical or any other form of energy or from absence of essentials such as heat and oxygen.

injury-surveillance program ongoing systematic collection, analysis, and interpretation of injury data important to public health practice.

inotropy pertaining to cardiac contractile force.

insertion attachment of a muscle to a bone that moves when the muscle contracts.

inspection the process of informed observation.

insulin substance that decreases blood glucose level.

intercalated discs specialized bands of tissue inserted between myocardial cells that increase the rate in which the action potential is spread from cell to cell.

intermittent claudication intermittent calf pain while walking that subsides with rest.

interstitial fluid the fluid in body tissues that is outside the cells and outside the vascular system.

intervener physician a licensed physician, professionally unrelated to patients on scene, who attempts to assist EMS providers with patient care.

intervertebral disc cartilaginous pad between vertebrae that serves as a shock absorber.

intracellular fluid (ICF) the fluid inside the body cells.

intracranial pressure (ICP) pressure exerted on the brain by the blood and cerebrospinal fluid.

intradermal within the dermal layer of the skin.

intramuscular within the muscle.

intraosseous within the bone.

intravascular fluid the fluid within the circulatory system; blood plasma.

intravenous access (cannulation) surgical puncture of a vein to deliver medication or withdraw blood.

intravenous fluid chemically prepared solution tailored to the body's specific needs.

involuntary consent consent to treatment granted by the authority of a court order.

ion a charged particle; an atom or group of atoms whose electrical charge has changed from neutral to positive or negative by losing or gaining one or more electrons. (In an atom's normal, nonionized state, its positively charged protons and negatively charged electrons balance each other so that the atom's charge is neutral.)

ionize to become electrically charged or polar.

iris pigmented portion of the eye. It is the muscular area that constricts or dilates to change the size of the pupil.

irreversible antagonism a competitive antagonist permanently binds with a receptor site.

irreversible shock shock that has progressed so far that no medical intervention can reverse the condition and death is inevitable.

ischemia a blockage in the delivery of oxygenated blood to the cells.

isoimmunity an immune response to antigens from another member of the same species, for example Rh reactions between a mother and her infant or transplant rejections; also called *alloimmunity*.

isometric exercise active exercise performed against stable resistance, in which muscles are exercised in a motionless manner.

isotonic exercise active exercise during which muscles are worked through their range of motion.

isotonic equal in concentration of solute molecules; solutions may be isotonic to each other.

jargon language used by a particular group or profession.

joint capsule the ligaments that surround a joint; *synovial capsule*.

joint area where adjacent bones articulate.

justice the obligation to treat all patients fairly.

kidney an organ that produces urine and performs other functions related to the urinary system.

Korotkoff sounds sounds of blood hitting arterial walls.

labia structures that protect the vagina and urethra, including the *labia majora* and the *labia minora*.

lacrimal fluid liquid that lubricates the eye.

laminae posterior bones of a vertebra that help make up the foramen, or opening, of the spinal canal.

larynx the complex structure that joins the pharynx with the trachea.

laxative medication used to decrease stool's firmness and increase its water content.

leading questions questions framed to guide the direction of a patient's answers.

legislative law law created by such law-making bodies as federal and provincial or territorial assemblies. Also called *statutory law.*

lesion any disruption in normal tissue.

leukocyte white blood cell.

leukopoiesis the process through which stem cells differentiate into the white blood cells' immature forms.

leukotrienes also called *slow-reacting substances of anaphylaxis (SRS-A);* substances synthesized by mast cells during inflammatory response that cause vasoconstriction, vascular permeability, and chemotaxis; mediators released from mast cells upon contact with allergens.

leur lock adapter with a rubber-covered needle used to puncture a blood tube's self-sealing top.

leur sampling needle long, exposed needle that screws into the vacutainer and is inserted directly into the vein.

liability legal responsibility.

liaison officer coordinates all incident operations that involve outside agencies.

libel the act of injuring a person's character, name, or reputation by false statements *made in writing* or through the mass media with malicious intent or reckless disregard for the falsity of those statements.

licensure the process by which a regulatory agency grants permission to engage in a given occupation to an applicant who has attained the degree of competency required to ensure the public's protection.

ligaments connective tissue that connects bone to bone and holds joints together.

ligamentum arteriosum cord-like remnant of a fetal vessel connecting the pulmonary artery to the aorta at the aortic isthmus.

living will a legal document that allows a person to specify the kinds of medical treatment she wishes to receive should the need arise.

local effects effects involving areas around the immediate site; should be evaluated based on the burn model.

local limited to one area of the body.

logistics supports incident operations, coordinating procurement and distribution of all medical resources.

lymphatic system a network of valveless vessels that drain fluid, called lymph, from the body tissues. Lymph nodes help filter impurities en route to the subclavian vein and thence to the heart.

lymphocyte a type of leukocyte, or white blood cell, that attacks foreign substances as part of the body's immune response.

macrodrip tubing administration tubing that delivers a relatively large amount of fluid.

major basic protein (MBP) a larvacidal peptide.

major trauma patient person who has suffered significant mechanism of injury.

malfeasance a breach of duty by performance of a wrongful or unlawful act.

management staff officers that handle public information, safety, outside liaisons, and critical stress debriefing; also known as the command staff.

mandible the jawbone.

manometer pressure gauge with a scale calibrated in millimeters of mercury (mmHg).

mast cells large cells, resembling bags of granules, that reside near blood vessels. When stimulated by injury, chemicals, or allergic responses, they activate the inflammatory response by degranulation (emptying their granules into the extracellular environment) and synthesis (construction of leukotrines and prostaglandins).

material safety data sheets (MSDS) easily accessible sheets of detailed information about chemicals found at fixed facilities.

maxilla bone of the upper jaw.

measured volume administration set IV setup that delivers specific volumes of fluid.

mechanism of injury combined strength, direction, and nature of forces that injured your patient.

medical direction medical policies, procedures, and practices that are available to providers either online or offline.

medical director a physician who is legally responsible for all of the clinical and patient-care aspects of an EMS system. Also referred to as *medical direction.*

medical supply unit coordinates procurement and distribution of equipment and supplies at an MCI.

medically clean careful handling to prevent contamination.

medicated solution parenteral medication packaged in an IV bag and administered as an IV infusion.

medication injection port a self-sealing membrane into which a hypodermic needle is inserted for drug administration.

medulla oblongata lower portion of the brainstem, containing the respiratory, cardiac, and vasomotor centres.

medulla the inner tissue of an organ, such as the kidney.

medullary canal cavity within a bone that contains the marrow.

menarche the onset of menses, usually occurring between ages 10 and 14.

meninges three membranes that surround and protect the brain and spinal cord. They are the dura mater, pia mater, and arachnoid membrane.

menopause the cessation of menses and ovarian function due to decreased secretion of estrogen.

menstruation sloughing of the uterine lining (endometrium) if a fertilized egg is not implanted. It is controlled by the cyclical release of hormones. Menstruation is also called a *period*.

mesentery double fold of peritoneum that supports the major portion of the small bowel, suspending it from the posterior abdominal wall.

metabolic acidosis acidity caused by an increase in acid, often because of increased production of acids during metabolism or from causes such as vomiting, diarrhea, diabetes, or medication.

metabolic alkalosis alkalinity caused by an increase in plasma bicarbonate resulting from causes including diuresis, vomiting, or ingestion of too much sodium bicarbonate.

metabolism the total changes that take place during physiological processes.

metaphysis growth zone of a bone, active during the development stages of youth. It is located between the epiphysis and the diaphysis.

metaplasia replacement of one type of cell by another type of cell that is not normal for that tissue.

metered dose inhaler handheld device that produces a medicated spray for inhalation.

microdrip tubing administration tubing that delivers a relatively small amount of fluid.

midbrain portion of the brain connecting the pons and cerebellum with the cerebral hemispheres.

minimum effective concentration minimum level of a drug needed to cause a given effect.

minimum standards lowest or least allowable standards.

minor depending on provincial or territorial law, this is usually a person under the age of 18.

misfeasance a breach of duty by performance of a legal act in a manner that is harmful or injurious.

mitosis cell division with division of the nucleus; each daughter cell contains the same number of chromosomes as the mother cell. Mitosis is the process by which the body grows.

mobile data terminal vehicle-mounted computer keyboard and display.

mons pubis fatty layer of tissue over the pubic symphysis.

morals social, religious, or personal standards of right and wrong.

morgue area where deceased victims of an incident are collected.

morgue officer person who supervises the morgue; may report to the triage officer or the treatment officer.

mucolytic medication intended to make mucus more watery.

mucous membrane tissues lining body cavities that communicate with the air; usually contain small, mucus-secreting cells.

mucus slippery secretion that lubricates and protects airway surfaces.

multiple-casualty incident (MCI) incident that generates large numbers of patients and that often makes traditional EMS response ineffective because of special circumstances surrounding the event; also known as a mass-casualty incident.

multiple organ dysfunction syndrome (MODS) progressive impairment of two or more organ systems resulting from an uncontrolled inflammatory response to a severe illness or injury.

multiplex duplex system that can transmit voice and data simultaneously.

muscle tissue tissue that is capable of contraction when stimulated. There are three types of muscle tissue: *cardiac* (myocardium, or heart muscle), *smooth* (within intestines, surrounding blood vessels), and *skeletal*, or *striated* (allows skeletal movement). Skeletal muscle is mostly under voluntary, or conscious, control; smooth muscle is under involuntary, or unconscious, control; cardiac muscle is capable of spontaneous, or self-excited, contraction.

mutual aid agreements or plans for sharing departmental resources.

myometrium the thick middle layer of the uterine wall made up of smooth muscle fibres.

myotome muscle and tissue of the body innervated by spinal nerve roots.

nares the openings of the nostrils.

nasal medication drug administered through the mucous membrans of the nose.

nasal septum cartilage that separates the right and left nasal cavities.

nasolacrimal duct narrow tube that carries into the nasal cavity tears and debris that have drained from the eye.

natural immunity inborn protection against infection or disease.

nebulizer inhalation aid that disperses liquid into aerosol spray or mist.

necrosis cell death; a pathological cell change; the sloughing off of dead tissue. Four types of necrotic cell change are *coagulative, liquefactive, caseous,* and *fatty. Gangrenous necrosis* refers to tissue death over a wide area.

needle adapter rigid plastic device specifically constructed to fit into the hub of an intravenous cannula.

negative feedback loop body mechanisms that work to reverse, or compensate for, a pathophysiological process, (or to reverse any physiological process, whether pathological or nonpathological).

negative feedback a mechanism of response that serves to maintain a state of internal constancy, or homeostasis. Changes in the internal environment trigger mechanisms that reverse or negate the change, hence the term "negative feedback."

negligence deviation from accepted standards of care recognized by law for the protection of others against the unreasonable risk of harm.

nephron a microscopic structure within kidney that produces urine.

nerve tissue tissue that transmits electrical impulses throughout the body.

net filtration the total loss of water from blood plasma across the capillary membrane into the interstitial space. Normally, hydrostatic pressure forcing water out of the capillary is balanced by oncotic force pulling water into the capillary for a net filtration of zero.

neuroeffector junction specialized synapse between a nerve cell and the organ or tissue it innervates.

neurogenic shock shock resulting from brain or spinal cord injury that causes an interruption of nerve impulses to the arteries with loss of arterial tone, dilation, and relative hypovolemia.

neuroleptanesthesia anesthesia that combines decreased sensation of pain with amnesia while the patient remains conscious.

neuroleptic antipsychotic (literally, *affecting the nerves*).

neuron nerve cell; the fundamental component of the nervous system.

neurotransmitter a substance that is released from the axon terminal of the presynaptic neuron on excitation and that travels across the synaptic cleft to either excite or inhibit the target cell. Examples include acetylcholine, norepinephrine, and dopamine.

neutropenia a low neutrophil count.

nocturia excessive urination at night.

noncompetitive antagonism the binding of an antagonist causes a deformity of the binding site that prevents an agonist from fitting and binding.

nonconstituted drug vial/Mix-o-Vial vial with two containers, one holding a powdered medication and the other holding a liquid mixing solution.

nonfeasance a breach of duty by failure to perform a required act or duty.

nonmalfeasance the obligation not to harm the patient.

nonverbal communication gestures, mannerisms, and postures by which a person communicates with others; also called *body language*.

nucleus the organelle within a cell that contains the DNA, or genetic material; in the cells of higher organisms, the nucleus is surrounded by a membrane.

ocular medication drug administered through the mucous membranes of the eye.

offline medical direction refers to medical policies, procedures, and practices that medical direction has set up in advance of a call.

oncotic force a form of osmotic pressure exerted by the large protein particles, or colloids, present in blood plasma. In the capillaries, the plasma colloids tend to pull water from the interstitial space across the capillary membrane into the capillary. Oncotic force is also called *colloid osmotic pressure*.

online medical direction occurs when a qualified physician gives direct orders to a prehospital care provider by either radio or telephone.

onset of action the time from administration until a medication reaches its minimum effective concentration.

open incident an incident that has the potential to generate additional patients; also known as an uncontained incident or an unstable incident.

open-ended questions questions that permit unguided, spontaneous answers.

open stance a posture or body position that is relaxed and suggests confidence, ease, warmth, and attentiveness.

operations carries out directions from command and does the actual work at an incident.

ophthalmoscope handheld device used to examine interior of eye.

opposition pairing of muscles that permits extension and flexion of limbs.

oral drug administration the delivery of any medication that is taken by mouth and swallowed into the lower gastrointestinal tract.

orbit the eye socket.

ordnance military weapons and munitions.

organ system a group of organs that work together. Examples: the cardiovascular system, formed of the heart, blood vessels, and blood; the gastrointestinal system, comprising the mouth, salivary glands, esophagus, stomach, intestines, liver, pancreas, gall bladder, rectum, and anus.

organ a group of tissue functioning together. Examples: heart, liver, brain, ovary, eye.

organelles structures that perform specific functions within a cell.

organism the sum of all the cells, tissues, organs, and organ systems of a living being. Examples: the human organism, a bacterial organism.

origin attachment of a muscle to a bone that does not move (or experiences the least movement) when the muscle contracts.

orthopnea difficulty in breathing while lying supine.

osmolality the concentration of solute per kilogram of water. *See also* osmolarity.

osmolarity the concentration of solute per litre of water (often used synonymously with *osmolality*).

osmosis the passage of a solvent, such as water, through a membrane; the diffusion pattern of water in which molecules move to equalize concentrations on both sides of a membrane; movement of solvent in a solution from an area of lower solute concentration to an area of higher solute concentration.

osmotic diuresis greatly increased urination and dehydration that results when high levels of glucose cannot be reabsorbed into the blood from the kidney tubules, and the osmotic pressure of the glucose in the tubules also prevents water reabsorption.

osmotic gradient the difference in concentration between solutions on opposite sides of a semipermeable membrane.

osmotic pressure the pressure exerted by the concentration of solutes on one side of a membrane that, if hypertonic, tends to "pull" water (cause osmosis) from the other side of the membrane.

osteoblast cell that helps in the creation of new bone during growth and bone repair.

osteoclast bone cell that absorbs and removes excess bone.

osteocyte bone-forming cell found in the bone matrix that helps maintain the bone.

otoscope handheld device used to examine interior of ears and nose.

ovaries the primary female sex glands, which secrete estrogen and progesterone and produce eggs for reproduction.

overhydration the presence or retention of an abnormally high amount of body fluid.

over-the-needle catheter/angiocatheter semi-flexible catheter enclosing a sharp metal stylet.

ovulation the release of an egg from the ovary.

oxidation the loss of hydrogen atoms or the acceptance of an oxygen atom. This increases the positive charge (or lessens the negative charge) on the molecule.

PA alveolar partial pressure.

Pa arterial partial pressure.

palpation using your sense of touch to gather information.

papilla the tip of a pyramid; it juts into the hollow space of the kidney.

parasympathetic nervous system division of the autonomic nervous system that is responsible for controlling vegetative functions. Parasympathetic nervous system actions include decreased heart rate and constriction of the bronchioles and pupils. Its actions are mediated by the neurotransmitter acetylcholine.

parasympatholytic drug or other substance that blocks or inhibits the actions of the parasympathetic nervous system. Also called *anticholinergic*.

parasympathomimetic drug or other substance that causes effects like those of the parasympathetic nervous system. Also called *cholinergic*.

parenchyma principle or essential parts of an organ.

parenteral drug administration outside the gastrointestinal tract.

parenteral route delivery of a medication outside of the gastrointestinal tract, typically using needles to inject medications into the circulatory system or tissues.

paroxysmal nocturnal dyspnea sudden onset of shortness of breath at night.

partial pressure the pressure exerted by each component of a gas mixture.

particulate evidence such evidence as hairs or fibres that cannot be readily seen with the human eye; also known as microscopic evidence or trace evidence.

passive transport movement of a substance without the use of energy.

pathogens microorganisms capable of producing infection or disease, such as bacteria and viruses.

pathology the study of disease and its causes.

pathophysiology the study of how disease affects normal body processes.

patient assessment problem-oriented evaluation of patient and establishment of priorities based on existing and potential threats to human life.

patient interview interaction with a patient for the purpose of obtaining in-depth information about the emergency and the patient's pertinent medical history.

pCO$_2$ partial pressure of carbon dioxide (*partial pressure* defined—see pO$_2$).

peak load the highest volume of calls at a given time.

pedicles thick, bony struts that connect the vertebral bodies with the spinous and transverse processes and help make up the opening for the spinal canal.

peer review an evaluation of the quality of emergency care administered by an individual, which is conducted by that individual's peers (others of equal rank). Also, an evaluation of articles submitted for publication.

pelvic space division of the abdominal cavity containing those organs located within the pelvis.

penis male organ of copulation.

percussion the production of sound waves by striking one object against another.

perforating canals structures through which blood vessels enter and exit the bone shaft.

perfusion the supplying of oxygen and nutrients to the body tissues as a result of the constant passage of blood through the capillaries.

perimetrium the serosal peritoneal membrane which forms the outermost layer of the uterine wall.

perineum muscular tissue that separates the vagina and the anus.

periorbital ecchymosis black and blue discoloration surrounding the eye sockets.

periosteum the tough exterior covering of a bone.

peripheral nervous system part of the nervous system that extends throughout the body and is composed of the cranial nerves arising from the brain and the peripheral nerves arising from the spinal cord. Its subdivisions are the somatic and the autonomic nervous systems.

peripheral vascular resistance the resistance of the vessels to the flow of blood: increased when the vessels constrict, decreased when the vessels relax.

peripheral venous access surgical puncture of a vein in the arm, leg, or neck.

peripherally inserted central catheter (PICC) line threaded into the central circulation via a peripheral site.

peristalsis wave-like muscular motion of the esophagus and bowel that moves food through the digestive system.

peritoneal space division of the abdominal cavity containing those organs or portions of organs covered by the peritoneum.

peritoneum fine fibrous tissue surrounding the interior of most of the abdominal cavity and covering most of the small bowel and some of the abdominal organs.

personal protective equipment (PPE) equipment used by EMS personnel to protect against injury and the spread of infectious disease.

pH abbreviation for *potential of hydrogen*. A measure of relative acidity or alkalinity. Since the pH scale is inverse to the concentration of acidic hydrogen ions, the lower the pH, the greater is the acidity; the higher the pH, the greater is the alkalinity. A normal pH range is 7.35 to 7.45.

phagocytosis process in which white blood cells engulf and destroy an invader.

pharmacodynamics how a drug interacts with the body to cause its effects.

pharmacokinetics how drugs are transported into and out of the body.

pharmacology the study of drugs and their interactions with the body.

pharynx a muscular tube that extends vertically from the back of the soft palate to the superior aspect of the esophagus.

physiological stress a chemical or physical disturbance in the cells or tissue fluid produced by a change in the external environment or within the body.

physiology the functions of an organism; the physical and chemical processes of a living thing.

pia mater inner and most delicate layer of the meninges. It covers the convolutions of the brain and spinal cord.

pinna outer, visible portion of the ear.

pitting depression that results from pressure against skin when pitting edema is present.

placental barrier biochemical barrier at the maternal/fetal interface that restricts certain molecules.

planning provides past, present, and future information about an incident.

plasma the liquid part of the blood.

plasma-level profile describes the lengths of onset, duration, and termination of action, as well as the drug's minimum effective concentration and toxic levels.

pleura membranous connective tissue covering the lungs.

pleural friction rub the squeaking or grating sound of the pleural linings rubbing together.

pluripotent stem cell a cell from which the various types of blood cells can form.

pneumothorax accumulation of air or gas in the pleural cavity.

Poiseuille's law a law of physiology stating that blood flow through a vessel is directly proportional to the radius of the vessel to the fourth power.

polyuria excessive urination.

pons process of tissue responsible for the communication interchange between the cerebellum, the cerebrum, midbrain, and the spinal cord.

posterior medial sulcus shallow longitudinal groove along the dorsal surface of the spinal cord.

postganglionic nerves nerve fibres that extend from the autonomic ganglia to the target tissues.

pO$_2$ partial pressure of oxygen; (*partial pressure* is the pressure exerted by a given component of a gas containing several components).

prearrival instructions dispatcher's instructions to caller for appropriate emergency measures.

prefilled/preloaded syringe syringe packaged in a tamper-proof container with the medication already in the barrel.

preganglionic nerves nerve fibres that extend from the central nervous system to the autonomic ganglia.

prehospital care report (PCR) the written record of an EMS response.

preload the pressure within the ventricles at the end of diastole, commonly called the *end-diastolic volume*.

premenstrual syndrome (PMS) a variety of signs and symptoms, such as weight gain, irritability, or specific food cravings associated with the changing hormonal levels that precede menstruation.

primary area of responsibility (PAR) stationing of ambulances at specific high-volume locations.

primary assessment prehospital process designed to identify and correct life-threatening airway, breathing, and circulation problems.

primary contamination direct exposure of a person or item to a hazardous substance.

primary prevention keeping an injury from ever occurring.

primary problem the underlying cause for your patient's symptoms.

primary triage triage that takes place early in the incident, usually on first arrival.

priority dispatching system using medically approved questions and predetermined guidelines to determine the appropriate level of response.

prodrug (parent drug) medication that is not active when administered, but whose biotransformation converts it into active metabolites.

profession refers to the existence of a specialized body of knowledge or skills.

professionalism refers to the conduct or qualities that characterize a practitioner in a particular field or occupation.

prostaglandins substances synthesized by mast cells during inflammatory response that cause vasoconstriction, vascular permeability, and chemotaxis and also cause pain. Prostaglandins also act to control inflammation by suppressing release of histamine and lysosomal enzymes.

prostate gland gland that surrounds the male urinary bladder neck and the first portion of urethra and is a major source of the fluid that combines with sperm cells to make semen.

protocols the policies and procedures for all components of an EMS system; principles for managing certain patient conditions.

prototype drug that best demonstrates the class's common properties and illustrates its particular characteristics.

proximal tubule the part of the nephron tubule beyond Bowman's capsule.

proximate cause action or inaction of the paramedic that immediately caused or worsened the damage suffered by the patient.

PSAP public safety answering point.

pseudo-instinctive learned actions that are practised until they can be done without thinking.

psychoneuroimmunological regulation the interactions of psychological, neurological, endocrinological, and immunological factors that contribute to alteration of the immune system as an outcome of a stress response that is not quickly resolved.

psychotherapeutic medication drug used to treat mental dysfunction.

public information officer (PIO) collects data about the incident and releases it to the press.

pulmonary embolism blood clot that travels to the pulmonary circulation and hinders oxygenation of the blood.

pulmonary hilum central medial region of the lung where the bronchi and pulmonary vasculature enter the lung.

pulse oximeter noninvasive device that measures the oxygen saturation of blood.

pulse pressure difference between the systolic and diastolic blood pressures.

pulse quality strength, which can be weak, thready, strong, or bounding.

pulse rate number of pulses felt in one minute.

pulse rhythm pattern and equality of intervals between beats.

pupil dark opening in the centre of the iris through which light enters the eye.

pus a liquid mixture of dead cells, bits of dead tissue, and tissue fluid that may accumulate in inflamed tissues.

pyramids the visible tissue structures within the medulla of the kidney.

pyrogen foreign protein capable of producing fever.

quality assurance (QA) a program designed to maintain continuous monitoring and measurement of the quality of clinical care delivered to patients.

quality improvement (QI) an evaluation program that emphasizes service and uses customer satisfaction as the ultimate indicator of system performance.

quality of respiration depth and pattern of breathing.

radio band a range of radio frequencies.

radio frequency the number of times per minute a radio wave oscillates.

rapid intervention team ambulance and crew dedicated to stand by in case a rescuer becomes ill or injured.

rapid trauma assessment quick check for signs of serious injury.

reabsorption the movement of a substance from a nephron tubule back into the blood.

reasonable force the minimal amount of force necessary to ensure that an unruly or violent person does not cause injury to herself or to others.

receptor specialized protein that combines with a drug resulting in a biochemical effect.

reciprocity the process by which an agency grants automatic certification or licensure to an individual who has comparable certification or licensure from another agency.

recirculating current movement of currents over a uniform obstruction; also known as a "drowning machine."

red bone marrow tissue within the internal cavity of a bone responsible for manufacture of erythrocytes and other blood cells.

referred pain pain that is felt at a location away from its source.

reflective acting thoughtfully, deliberately, and analytically.

renal pelvis the hollow space of the kidney that junctions with a ureter.

renin an enzyme produced by kidney cells that plays a key role in controlling arterial blood pressure.

repair healing of a wound with scar formation.

repolarization return of a muscle cell to its pre-excitation resting state.

reportable collisions collisions that involve more than $1000 in damage or a personal injury.

res ipsa loquitur a legal doctrine invoked by plaintiffs to support a claim of negligence, it is a Latin term that means "the thing speaks for itself."

reserve capacity the ability of an EMS agency to respond to calls beyond those handled by the on-duty crews.

resolution the complete healing of a wound and return of tissues to their normal structure and function; the ending of inflammation with no scar formation.

respiration the exchange of gases between a living organism and its environment; exchange of oxygen and carbon dioxide during inhalation and exhalation in the lungs and at the cellular level.

respiratory acidosis acidity caused by abnormal retention of carbon dioxide resulting from impaired ventilation.

respiratory alkalosis alkalinity caused by excessive elimination of carbon dioxide resulting from increased respirations.

respiratory effort how hard the patient works to breathe.

respiratory rate the number of times a person breathes in one minute.

response time time between when a unit is alerted until it arrives on the scene.

resting potential the normal electrical state of cardiac cells.

reticular activating system (RAS) a series of nervous tissues keeping the human system in a state of consciousness.

retina light- and colour-sensing tissue lining the posterior chamber of the eye.

retroperitoneal space division of the abdominal cavity containing those organs posterior to the peritoneal lining.

review of systems a list of questions categorized by body system.

Rh blood group a group of antigens discovered on the red blood cells of rhesus monkeys that is also present to some extent in humans.

Rh factor an antigen in the Rh blood group that is also known as antigen D. About 85 percent of North Americans have the Rh factor (are Rh positive) while about 15 do not have the Rh factor (are Rh negative). Rh positive and Rh negative blood are incompatible; that is, a person who is Rh negative can experience a severe immune response if Rh positive blood is introduced, as through a transfusion or during childbirth.

rhonchi continuous sounds with a lower pitch and a snoring quality.

rotation a turning along the axis of a bone or joint.

rules of evidence guidelines for permitting a new medication, process, or procedure to be used in EMS.

safety officer monitors all on-scene actions and ensures that they do not create any potentially harmful conditions.

scene safety doing everything possible to ensure a safe environment.

sclera the "white" of the eye.

scope of practice range of duties and skills paramedics are allowed and expected to perform.

scrambling climbing over rocks or downed trees on a steep trail without the aid of ropes. This can be especially dangerous when the surface is wet or icy.

scree loose pebbles or rock debris that can form on the slopes or bases of mountains; sometimes used to describe debris in sloping dry stream beds.

sebaceous glands glands within the dermis secreting sebum.

sebum fatty secretion of the sebaceous gland that helps keep the skin pliable and waterproof.

second messenger chemical that participates in complex cascading reactions that eventually cause a drug's desired effect.

secondary contamination transfer of a hazardous substance to a noncontaminated person or item via contact with someone or something already contaminated by the substance.

secondary prevention medical care after an injury or illness that helps prevent further problems from occurring.

secondary triage triage that takes place after patients are moved to a treatment area to determine any change in status.

secretion the movement of a substance from the blood into a nephron tubule.

section chief officer who supervises major functional areas of sections; reports to the incident commander.

sector interchangeable name for a branch, group, or division; does not, however, designate a functional or geographical area.

sedation state of decreased anxiety and inhibitions.

Sellick's maneuvre pressure applied in a posterior direction to the anterior cricoid cartilage that occludes the esophagus.

semantic related to the meaning of words.

semicircular canals the three rings of the inner ear. They sense the motion of the head and provide positional sense for the body.

semidecontaminated patient another term for field-decontaminated patient.

semi-Fowler's position sitting up at 45 degrees.

semipermeable able to allow some, but not all, substances to pass through. Cell membranes are semipermeable.

septic shock shock that develops as the result of infection carried by the bloodstream, eventually causing dysfunction of multiple organ systems.

septicemia the systemic spread of toxins through the bloodstream. Also called *sepsis*.

sequestration the trapping of red blood cells by an organ, such as the spleen.

serotonin a substance released by platelets that, through constriction and dilation of blood vessels, affects blood flow to an injured or affected site.

serum solution containing whole antibodies for a specific pathogen.

sesamoid bone bone that forms in a tendon.

sharps container rigid, puncture resistant container clearly marked as a biohazard.

shipping papers documents routinely carried aboard vehicles transporting hazardous materials; ideally should identify specific substances and quantities carried; also known as bills of lading.

short haul a helicopter extrication technique where a person is attached to a rope that is, in turn, attached to a helicopter. The aircraft lifts off with the person attached to it. Obviously, this means of evacuation requires highly specialized skills.

side effect unintended response to a drug.

simple diffusion the random motion of molecules from an area of high concentration to an area of lower concentration.

simplex communication system that transmits and receives on the same frequency.

singular command process in which a single individual is responsible for coordinating an incident; most useful in single-jurisdictional incidents.

sinus air cavity that conducts fluids from the eustachian tubes and tear ducts to and from the nasopharynx.

slander act of injuring a person's character, name, or reputation by false or malicious statements *spoken* with malicious intent or reckless disregard for the falsity of those statements.

solvent a substance that dissolves other substances, forming a solution.

somatic nervous system part of the nervous system controlling voluntary bodily functions.

span of control number of people or tasks that a single individual can monitor.

Special Weapons and Tactics (SWAT) Team a trained police unit equipped to handle hostage holders and other difficult law enforcement situations.

sphygmomanometer blood pressure measuring device comprising a bulb, a cuff, and a manometer.

spike sharp-pointed device inserted into the IV solution bag's administration set port.

spinal canal opening in the vertebrae that accomodates the spinal cord.

spinal cord central nervous system pathway responsible for transmitting sensory input from the body to the brain and for conducting motor impulses from the brain to the body muscles and organs.

spinal nerves 31 pairs of nerves that originate along the spinal cord from anterior and posterior nerve roots.

spinous process prominence at the posterior part of a vertebra.

spotter the person behind the left rear side of the ambulance who assists the operator in backing up the vehicle.

staff functions officers who perform supervisory roles in the IMS, rather than actually performing a task.

staging locations where ambulances, personnel, and equipment are kept in reserve for use at an incident.

staging officer supervises the staging area and guards against premature commitment of resources and freelancing by personnel; reports to the branch director.

standard of care the degree of care, skill, and judgment expected under like or similar circumstances by a similarly trained, reasonable paramedic in the same community.

standing orders preauthorized treatment procedures; a type of treatment protocol.

Starling's law of the heart law of physiology stating that the more the myocardium is stretched, up to a certain limit, the more forceful the subsequent contraction will be.

START acronym for the most widely used disaster triage system; stands for simple triage and rapid transport.

sterile free of all forms of life.

sterilizing use of a chemical or physical method, such as pressurized steam, to kill all microorganisms on an object.

stethoscope tool used to auscultate most sounds.

stock solution standard concentration of routinely used medications.

strainer a partial obstruction that filters, or strains, the water, such as downed trees or wire mesh, causing an unequal force on the two sides.

stress response changes within the body initiated by a stressor.

stress a hardship or strain; a physical or psychological arousal to stimulus.

stressor a stimulus that causes stress.

stridor predominantly inspiratory wheeze associated with laryngeal obstruction.

stroke volume the amount of blood ejected by the heart in one cardiac contraction.

subcutaneous emphysema crackling sensation caused by air just underneath the skin.

subcutaneous tissue body layer beneath the dermis; the layer of loose connective tissue between the skin and muscle.

sublingual beneath the tongue.

sudoriferous glands glands within the dermis that secrete sweat.

suppository medication packaged in a soft, pliable form, for insertion into the rectum.

surfactant substance that decreases surface tension.

sutures pseudo-joints that join the various bones of the skull to form the cranium.

sympathetic nervous system division of the autonomic nervous system that prepares the body for stressful situations. Sympathetic nervous system actions include increased heart rate and dilation of the bronchioles and pupils. Its actions are mediated by the neurotransmitters epinephrine and norepinephrine.

sympatholytic drug or other substance that blocks the actions of the sympathetic nervous system. Also called *antiadrenergic*.

sympathomimetic drug or other substance that causes effects like those of the sympathetic nervous system. Also called *adrenergic*.

synarthrosis joint that does not permit movement.

syncytium group of cardiac muscle cells that physiologically function as a unit.

synergism a standard pharmacological principle in which two substances or drugs work together to produce an effect that neither of them can produce on its own.

synovial fluid substance that lubricates synovial joints.

synovial joint type of joint that permits the greatest degree of independent motion.

syringe plastic tube with which liquid medications can be drawn up, stored, and injected.

system status management (SSM) a computerized personnel and ambulance deployment system

systemic effects effects that occur throughout the body after exposure to a toxic substance.

systemic throughout the body.

systole the period of the cardiac cycle when the myocardium is contracting.

systolic blood pressure force of blood against arteries when ventricles contract.

T lymphocytes white blood cells that do not produce antibodies but, instead, attacks antigens directly.

tachycardia a pulse rate faster than 100.

tachypnea rapid respiration.

tactical emergency medical services (TEMS) a specially trained unit that provides on-site medical support to law enforcement.

teachable moment the time shortly after an injury when patients and observers may be more receptive to teaching about how similar injuries may be prevented in the future.

tenderness pain that is elicited through palpation.

teratogenic drug medication that may deform or kill the fetus.

termination of action time from when the drug's level drops below its minimum effective concentration until it is eliminated from the body.

tertiary prevention rehabilitation after an injury or illness that helps prevent further problems from occurring.

testes primary male reproductive organs that produce hormones responsible for sexual maturation cells; singular *testis*.

thalamus switching station between the pons and the cerebrum in the brain.

therapeutic index ratio of a drug's lethal dose for 50 percent of the population to its effective dose for 50 percent of the population.

thrill vibration or humming felt when palpating the pulse.

thrombocyte blood platelet.

thrombocytosis an abnormal increase in the number of platelets.

thrombolytic drug that acts directly on thrombi to break them down.

thrombophlebitis inflammation of the vein.

thrombosis clot formation, which is extremely dangerous when it occurs in coronary arteries or cerebral vasculature.

thrombus blood clot.

tidal volume average volume of gas inhaled or exhaled in one respiratory cycle.

tiered response system system that allows multiple vehicles to arrive at an EMS call at different times, often providing different levels of care or transport.

tinnitus the sensation of ringing in the ears.

tissue a group of cells that perform a similar function.

tone state of slight contraction of muscles that gives them firmness and keeps them ready to contract.

tonicity solute concentration or osmotic pressure relative to the blood plasma or body cells.

topical medications material applied to and absorbed through the skin or mucous membranes.

tort a civil wrong committed by one individual against another.

total body water (TBW) the total amount of water in the body at a given time.

total lung capacity maximum lung capacity.

touch pad computer on which you enter data by touching areas of the display screen.

trachea 10- to 12-cm-long tube that connects the larynx to the mainstem bronchi.

transdermal absorbed through the skin.

transport supervisor coordinates operations with the staging officer and the transport supervisor; gets patients into the ambulances and routed to the hospitals.

transverse process bony outgrowth of the vertebral pedicle that serves as a site for muscle attachment and articulation with the ribs.

trauma a physical injury or wound caused by external force or violence.

trauma centre medical facility that has the capability of caring for the acutely injured patient. Trauma centres must meet strict criteria to use this designation.

trauma intervention programs (TIP) mental health workers and citizen volunteers specially trained to provide assistance to anyone emotionally traumatized by a crisis event.

treatment group supervisor controls all actions in the treatment group/sector.

treatment unit leaders EMS personnel who manage the various treatment units and who report to the treatment group supervisor.

triage tags tags containing vital information, affixed to your patient during a multi-patient incident.

triage a method of sorting patients by the severity of their injuries.

trocar a sharp, pointed instrument.

trunking communication system that pools all frequencies and routes transmissions to the next available frequency.

turgor normal tension in a cell; the resistance of the skin to deformation (in a normally hydrated person, the skin, when pinched, will quickly return to its normal formation. In a dehydrated person, the return to normal formation will be slower.)

turnover the continual synthesis and breakdown of body substances that results in the dynamic steady state.

ultrahigh frequency radio frequency band from 300 to 3000 megahertz.

UN number a four-digit number specific to a given chemical; some UN numbers are assigned to a group of related chemicals, but with different characteristics, such the UN 1203 designation for diesel fuel, gasohol, gasoline, motor fuels, motor spirits, and petrol. (The letters *UN* stand for "United Nations." Sometimes the letters *NA* for "North America" appear with or instead of the UN designation.)

unified command process in which managers from different jurisdictions—law enforcement, fire, EMS—coordinate their activities and share responsibility for command.

unit predetermined amount of medication or fluid.

up-regulation a drug causes the formation of more receptors than normal.

ureter a duct that carries urine from kidney to urinary bladder.

urethra the duct that carries urine from the urinary bladder out of the body; in men, it also carries reproductive fluid (semen) to the outside of the body.

urinary bladder the muscular organ that stores urine before its elimination from the body.

uterus hollow organ in the center of the abdomen that provides the site for fetal development.

vaccine solution containing a modified pathogen that does not actually cause disease but still stimulates the development of antibodies specific to it.

vacutainer device that holds blood tubes.

vagina canal that connects the external female genitalia to the uterus.

vallecula depression between the epiglottis and the base of the tongue.

vas deferens the duct that carries sperm cells to the urethra for ejaculation.

venous access device surgically implanted port that permits repeated access to central venous circulation.

venous constricting band flat rubber band used to impede venous return and make veins easier to see.

ventilation the mechanical process that moves air in and out of the lungs.

vertebre the 33 bones making up the vertebral column; singular *vertebra*.

vertebral body short column of bone that forms the weight-bearing portion of a vertebra.

very high frequency radio frequency band from 30 to 300 megahertz.

vial plastic or glass container with a self-sealing rubber top.

virus an organism much smaller than a bacterium, visible only under an electron microscope. Viruses invade and live outisde the cells of the organisms they infect.

visual acuity wall chart/card wall chart or handheld card with lines of letters used to test vision.

vital statistics height and weight.

vitreous humor clear watery fluid filling the posterior chamber of the eye. It is responsible for giving the eye its spherical shape.

volume on hand the available amount solution containing a medication.

warm zone location at a hazmat incident adjacent to the hot zone; area where a decontamination corridor is established; also called the yellow zone or the contamination reduction zone.

warning placard diamond-shaped graphic placed on vehicles to indicate hazard classification.

weapons of mass destruction (WMD) variety of chemical, biological, nuclear, or other devices used by terrorists to strike at government or high-profile targets; designed to create a maximum number of casualties.

wheezes continuous, high-pitched musical sounds similar to a whistle.

whispered pectoriloquy abnormal clarity of patient's transmitted whispers.

white matter material that surrounds grey matter in the spinal cord; made up largely of axons.

xiphisternal joint union between xiphoid process and body of the sternum.

years of productive life age at death subtracted from 65.

yellow bone marrow tissue that stores fat in semi-liquid form within the internal cavities of a bone.

zygoma the cheekbone.

Index

abandonment, 108–109, 203–204
abbreviations, 415, 417t
abdomen
    abdominal cavity, 613
    abdominal pain, 379
    abdominal vasculature, 611
    altered mental status, 377
    arteries, 612f
    ascites, 300, 301
    borborygmi, 300–301
    bruising, 370
    bruit, 300–301
    chest pain, 376–377
    children, 337
    Cullen's sign, 300, 370
    DCAP-BTLS, 369
    detailed secondary assessment, 387
    examination of, 300–301, 302f
    Grey-Turner's sign, 300, 370
    hollow organs, injury of, 370
    infants, 337
    intra-abdominal bleeding, 300, 370
    mesentery, 612
    muscles, 611f
    palpation, 301
    pelvic space, 610
    percussion, 301
    peritoneal space, 610
    peritoneum, 612–613, 613f
    rapid trauma assessment, 369–370
    respiratory distress, 376–377
    retroperitoneal space, 610
    retroperitoneal structures, 613
    subregions, division into, 610–611
abdominal aorta, 580
abdominal pain, 378–379
abdominal reflexes, 330
abdominal vasculature, 611
abducens nerve, 322, 533
abduction (joints), 503
ability to walk, 143
ABO blood group, 670
Aboriginal people, 92
absence seizures, 715
absorption
    as decontamination method, 196
    drugs, 699–700
    and hazmat exposure, 193
    metabolic absorption, 469
    reabsorption, 619
abuse
    of children, 15
    elder abuse, 15
    history of, 237
    sexual abuse, 15
Academic Emergency Medicine, 868
acarbose, 752
acceptance, 45
accessory nerves, 324
accident scenes, 113–114
"Accidental Death and Disability: The Neglected
    Disease of Modern Society" (NRC), 11
accidents, 241
accommodating conflict approach, 232
accountability, 6
    see also legal accountability
accuracy of documentation, 422
accurate information, 451–453
acebutolol, 730
acetaminophen, 712, 757, 869

acetylcholine, 549, 564, 566f, 584, 722
acetylcholinesterase (AChE), 194
acetylcysteine, 760
acetylsalicylic acid. *See* aspirin
Achilles reflexes, 330
Achilles tendon, 513
acid-base balance
    acid-base ratios relevant to pH, 485f
    acidosis, 483
    alkalosis, 483
    bicarbonate buffer system, 483–484
    bodily regulation of, 483–486
    buffer system, 483–484
    defined, 483
    hydrogen ions, 483
    kidneys, and pH, 486
    pH scale, 483
    respiratory component of, 485–486, 486f
acid-base derangements
    arterial blood gases, 645
    described, 644–645
    metabolic acidosis, 645
    metabolic alkalosis, 645
    respiratory acidosis, 644, 645
    respiratory alkalosis, 645
acidosis, 483, 644
acini, 573
acoustic nerve, 324
acquired immune deficiencies, 678–680
acquired immune deficiency syndrome. *See* AIDS
    (acquired immune deficiency syndrome)
acquired immunity, 668–669
acromioclavicular (AC) joint, 509
acromion process, 509
acronyms, 415, 443
action potential, 585
activated charcoal, 760, 870
active acquired immunity, 668–669
active listening, 236–237
active rescue zone, 160
active transport, 481, 620, 698
actual damages, 99
acuity, 438–439
acute abdomen, 378–379
acute effects, 193
acute inflammatory response, 672, 673f,
    674–675
acute phase reactants, 675
acute respiratory distress, 366
acyclovir, 756
addendum, 424
addictions, 38
Addison's disease, 750
additive effect, 708
adduction, 503
adenosine, 730, 870
adenosine triphosphate (ATP), 195, 469, 654
adjunct medications, 712, 713
administration of medications. *See* medication
    administration
administration staff, 140
administrative law, 93
adrenal cortex, 569t, 575, 750
adrenal glands, 472, 575–576
adrenal medulla, 561, 569t, 575
adrenalin, 575
adrenergic agonists, 727, 748
adrenergic antagonists, 727–728
adrenergic-inhibiting agents
    alpha$_1$ antagonists, 733–734

    beta adrenergic antagonists, 733
    centrally acting adrenergic inhibitors, 733
    combined alpha/beta antagonists, 734
    peripheral adrenergic neuron-blocking
      agents, 733
adrenergic receptor specificity, 727t
adrenergic receptors, 564, 683–684, 725, 725t
adrenergic synapse, 563f, 722
adrenocorticotropic hormone (ACTH), 572, 575,
    684
adult diseases, 241
adult-onset diabetes. *See* Type II diabetes
advance directives
    in Alberta, 112
    defined, 111
    do not resuscitate (DNR) orders, 15, 46,
      67–69, 111–113
    living will, 111
    in Ontario, 112
    potential organ donation, 113
advanced cardiac life support (ACLS), 380
advanced care paramedic (ACP), 9, 19
advanced care paramedic (ACP) competencies,
    844–850
advanced life support (ALS)
    defined, 9
    early programs, 11
    within eight minutes of onset, 17
    in hazardous terrain rescues, 180
    protocols, 452–453
adverse effects. *See* side effects
advice, 226
advocacy. *See* patient advocacy
aerobic metabolism, 654
aeromedical evaluations, 130
affinity, 705
afterload, 593
against medical advice (AMA), 431
age. *See* children; geriatric patients; infants
agent, 647
agents of infection. *See* infectious agents
aging of bones, 516–518
agonist, 706
agonist-antagonists, 706
AIDS (acquired immune deficiency syndrome),
    666, 679–680
air embolism, 814
air medical transport
    activation, 131
    advantages and disadvantages of, 130–131
    aeromedical evaluations, 130
    described, 130
    fixed-wing aircraft, 130
    helicopters, 130
    indications for use, 131–132
    landing zone, 133
    and mechanism of injury, 132
    patient preparation and transfer, 132–133
    rotocraft, 130
    scene safety, 133
    short haul, 178
air pressure, 133
air-purifying respirator (APR), 199
airbags, 171–172, 364
airway
    assessment, 355–357
    endotracheal intubation, 390
    facial fractures, and aggressive suctioning,
      383
    patency, 390

model verbal reports, 408–409
MODS. *See* multiple organ dysfunction syndrome (MODS)
molecule, 477
monoamine oxidase inhibitors (MAOIs), 719, 720–721
monoaxial joints, 503
monoblasts, 493
monocytes, 468, 490, 496
mons pubis, 624
mood, 320
moral issues, 91
morals, 63
morbidity, 647–648
morgue, 146
morgue officer, 146
moricizine, 729
morphine sulphate, 712, 893
mortality, 647
mortality rates, 15
mother-fetus ABO incompatibility, 670
motor activity, 267, 552
motor system, 325–328, 327f, 389
motor-vehicle accidents (MVAs). *See* motor-vehicle collisions (MVCs)
motor-vehicle collisions (MVCs)
    children, 59
    hazardous materials, potential for, 183–184
    injury prevention and, 60
    prevention of, 55
motor-vehicle laws, 96
mourning, 44–45
mouth, 286–289, 288f, 384, 533, 534f
movement, 469
moving patients. *See* lifting and moving patients
moving water rescues, 162–165
mucolytics, 744
mucous membranes, 597, 767–770
mucus, 597
multidisciplinary specialty teams, 8
multifactorial disorders, 646–647
multilumen airways, 357
multiple-casualty incident (MCI)
    see also incident management system (IMS)
    challenges of, 151–152
    command, 135–139
    common problems, 151
    defined, 133
    described, 133–134
    documentation, 433
    initiation of plan, 350
    location of all patients, 349–350
    and resource allocation, 71
multiple organ dysfunction syndrome (MODS)
    catecholamine release, 662
    clinical presentation, 663–664
    cumulative effects, 663–664
    defined, 662
    described, 662–663
    pathophysiology of, 662–663
    primary MODS, 662
    progression, 662
    secondary MODS, 662
    stages, 662
multiple responders, 455
multiple sclerosis, 652
multiple-service situations, 456
multiple symptoms, 247
multiplex communication system, 403
multivehicle responses
    ambulances, 128–129
    danger of, 54
murder, 205–206
murmurs, 300
muscarinic cholinergic antagonists, 723–724
muscarinic receptors, 564–565, 567t
muscle strength scale, 326t
muscle strength tests, 326t
muscle tissue, 470
muscle tone, 325, 325f

muscles
    see also muscular system
    abdomen, 611f
    ankle, 513
    arm muscles, 507f
    attachment to bone, 522f
    cardiac muscle, 518, 584, 585f
    elbows, 507–509
    eyes, 533
    hip and pelvis, 516
    intramuscular (IM) injection, 703, 792–796, 793f, 795f
    knees, 514
    neck, 536
    pairing of, 521
    of respiration, 544
    shoulder muscles, 512f
    shoulders, 510
    skeletal muscle, 518–521
    smooth muscle, 518
    tendons, 522
    thorax-associated musculature, 543–545
    tone, 522
    types of, 518, 521f
    wrists and hands, 506–507, 507
muscular system
    see also muscles; musculoskeletal system
    anterior view, 520f
    described, 471
    fasciculus, 521
    insertion, 521
    muscular tissue and structure, 518–522
    opposition, 521
    origin, 521
    posterior view, 519f
musculoskeletal system
    ankles, 308, 310f
    bone structure, 501–502
    children, 337–338
    crepitation, 305
    detailed secondary assessment, 389
    elbows, 305–308, 307f
    examination of, 304–314
    extremities, 305–311
    feet, 308, 310f
    hands, 305, 306f
    hips, 311, 313f
    infants, 337–338
    joint structure, 503–504
    joints, evaluation of, 304
    knees, 308–311, 312f
    muscle tissue, 470
    muscular tissue and structure, 518–522
    palpation, 304
    range of motion, 304–305
    shoulders, 308, 309f
    skeletal organization, 504–516
    skeleton, functions of, 500–504
    spine, 311–314, 315f
    swelling, 304
    wrists, 305, 306f
mutual aid, 23, 141
Mycobacterium tuberculosis, 665
mycoses, 666–667
mydriasis, 748
myeloblasts, 493
myocardial infarction, 636
myocardium, 577
myometrium, 626
myotome, 557

N-95 respirators, 41
nabilone, 747
NaCl (sodium chloride), 477
nails
    assessment of, 279
    described, 489, 489f
    yellowed or brittle, 314
nalbuphine, 893
naloxone, 712, 714, 893
names, remembering, 220

naproxen, 757
nares, 530
narrative writing
    assessment/management section, 427–428
    body systems approach, 427
    call incident format, 430–431
    CHART format, 429
    general formats, 428–431
    head-to-toe approach, 426–427
    narrative sections, 425–428
    objective narrative, 426–428
    patient management format, 429–430
    SOAP format, 428–429
    subjective narrative, 425–426
    vital signs, documentation of, 426
nasal bones, 529
nasal cavity, 384, 530, 597
nasal decongestants, 743
nasal medications, 769, 769f
nasal route, 703
nasal septum, 597
nasolacrimal duct, 597
nasopharyngeal airway, 357
nasopharynx, 533, 598
National Academy of Sciences, 11
National Association for Search and Rescue, 179
National Code of Ethics, 64
National Emergency Nurses Affiliation, 64
National Highway Traffic Safety Administration (NHTSA), 11, 23–24
National Occupational Competency Profile (NOCP), 7, 18, 20
National Oceanic and Atmospheric Administration (NOAA), 189
National Resource Council, 11
natural immunity, 668
nature of the illness, determination of, 352
nebulization facemasks, 771, 771f
nebulizer, 770–772, 770f, 771f, 773
neck
    airway structures, 535–536
    anatomy of, 535–536, 535f
    assessment of, 289–291, 290f
    chest pain, 376
    children, 335
    DCAP-BTLS, 366
    detailed secondary assessment, 384, 385f
    infants, 335
    jugular veins, 299, 366
    lymph nodes, 537f
    lymphatic system, 536
    muscles, 536
    other structures, 536
    rapid trauma assessment, 366, 367f
    respiratory distress, 376
    semi-Fowler's position, 366
    spinal column, 536
    subcutaneous emphysema, 366
    thyroid gland, 536
    vasculature, 535
necrosis, 639, 814
needle adapter, 802
needleless syringe, 779f
negative charges, 480
negative feedback loop, 473, 656
negligence
    actual damages, 99
    breach of duty, 98
    "chemical code only" treatment, 111
    comparative negligence, 101
    components of claim, 98–100
    contributory negligence, 101
    defences, 100–101
    defined, 98
    duty to act, 98
    malfeasance, 99
    misfeasance, 99
    nonfeasance, 99
    proximate cause, 100
    res ipsa loquitur, 99